Health care of women
A nursing perspective

Health care of women

A nursing perspective

CATHERINE INGRAM FOGEL, R.N., B.S.N., M.S.

Assistant Professor of Nursing,
University of North Carolina,
Chapel Hill, North Carolina

NANCY FUGATE WOODS, R.N., M.N., Ph.D.

Associate Professor, School of Nursing,
University of Washington,
Seattle, Washington

with 175 illustrations and 2 color plates

The C. V. Mosby Company

ST. LOUIS • TORONTO • LONDON   1981

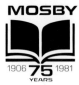

MOSBY

1906 **75** 1981
YEARS

A TRADITION OF PUBLISHING EXCELLENCE

The C. V. Mosby Company
11830 Westline Industrial Drive, St. Louis, Missouri 63141

Library of Congress Cataloging in Publication Data

Fogel, Catherine I   1941-
   Health care of women.

   Bibliography: p.
   Includes index.
   1. Gynecologic nursing. 2. Obstetrical nursing.
3. Women—Health and hygiene. 4. Women's health
services. I. Woods, Nancy Fugate, joint author.
II. Title. [DNLM: 1. Gynecology—Nursing texts.
2. Obstetrics—Nursing texts. WY156.7 F655h]
RG105.F63   610'.88042   80-17400
ISBN 0-8016-1605-0

GW/M/M 9 8 7 6 5 4 3 2   05/D/597

Contributors

NANCY B. ALEXANDER, R.N., M.S.N.

Assistant Professor, School of Nursing,
Duke University, Durham, North Carolina

PATRICIA HOLLERAN COTANCH, R.N., Ph.D.

Assistant Professor, School of Nursing,
Duke University, Durham, North Carolina

GRETCHEN KRAMER DERY, R.N., M.S.N.

Assistant Professor of Nursing,
Duke University, Durham, North Carolina

ANNE FISHEL, R.N., M.S.

Associate Professor of Nursing,
University of North Carolina,
School of Nursing,
Chapel Hill, North Carolina

CATHERINE INGRAM FOGEL, R.N., B.S.N., M.S.

Assistant Professor of Nursing,
University of North Carolina,
Chapel Hill, North Carolina

JANET LARSON GELEIN, R.N., M.S.N.

Associate Professor, Clinician II,
University of Rochester,
Rochester, New York

SALLY K. GRAHAM, R.N., M.S.

Formerly Instructor in Nursing,
University of North Carolina,
School of Nursing,
Chapel Hill, North Carolina

CONNIE HARRIS, R.N., M.S.N.

Coordinator, Decentralized Staff Development,
Psychiatric Nursing, University Hospitals of Cleveland;
Clinical Instructor in Psychiatric Nursing,
Case Western Reserve University,
Cleveland, Ohio

PAMELA HEIPLE, R.N., B.S.N.

Graduate Student, University of Rochester,
Rochester, New York

BARBARA HANSEN KALINOWSKI, R.N., B.S.N., M.S.N.

Practitioner/Teacher, Educational Consultant,
Coordinator of Surgical Nursing,
Rush-Presbyterian-St. Luke's Medical Center,
Chicago, Illinois

DEITRA LEONARD LOWDERMILK, R.N., M.N.

Clinical Assistant Professor,
University of North Carolina,
Chapel Hill, North Carolina

NANCY FUGATE WOODS, R.N., M.N., Ph.D.

Associate Professor, School of Nursing,
University of Washington, Seattle, Washington

JAMES S. WOODS, Ph.D., M.P.H.

Program Leader, Epidemiology and Environmental
Health Research Program, Health and Population
Study Center, Battelle Human Affairs Research
Centers, Seattle, Washington

Preface

During the 1960s and 1970s, two important forces converged to influence women's health: the women's movement and the women's health movement. Women entered the labor force in increasing numbers and more commonly sought employment in positions traditionally reserved for men. More women and men advocated self-actualization for women and egalitarianism in opportunities for self-development. At the same time women voiced their increasing dissatisfaction with health services and in many instances created alternative services that reflected new values concerning women, allowing them to reclaim control over their bodies and responsibility for their health. During this same period, the nursing profession, largely composed of women, began to recognize that many of the assumptions that limited the nature of nursing practice closely resembled many traditional assumptions about women. Nursing scholars began to address the similarities of the plight of the nursing profession to that of women in general. As a consequence of the women's health movement, the nursing profession began to recognize not only the ability women have to promote and maintain their own health but also the profession's responsibility to support women in their efforts.

Only recently has the nursing literature begun to focus on women's health problems, examining them from new perspectives. The purpose of this text is to provide practitioners of nursing with an overview of topics and issues that influence women's health in contemporary society. Women's health has been described, in large measure, only in relation to reproductive issues. We contend that to restrict our attention only to those topics usually addressed in obstetrics or gynecology textbooks would not only do a disservice to the complex health issues affecting women but would also deny the importance of nurses who are women as whole beings. Therefore, we have attempted to incorporate several aspects of health that infringe on the quality of women's lives, including the influence of the social context in which women live. We hope that this text will serve as a resource to students and practitioners in a wide range of clinical settings: community or hospital practice, health maintenance organizations, and acute care settings.

Unit one of the text, Women and the Health Care System, addresses the importance of the nursing practitioner's recognition of the most prevalent health problems affecting women, including mortality and morbidity patterns and the seemingly paradoxical relationships between these. It is equally important to recognize the special problems that impinge on women as providers of health care. An examination of the health care available to women includes an analysis of sexism in the delivery of health services and in the research on women's health, as well as a discussion of alternative models of health care and the consequences of the women's health movement.

Unit two addresses the importance of nursing practice with women (rather than *on* them). The sections on promotion and maintenance of health with women include a philosophy for nursing practice with women. The anatomy and physiology unique to women and issues that women must address throughout life provide a basis for assessment of women's health status.

Unit three addresses health problems that commonly affect women, including those involving violence, sexual dysfunctions, and pregnancy. Violence against women takes two forms: battering and sexual assaults. Sexual dysfunctions include a variety of problems with varied etiologies. Those problems that place the pregnant woman at risk are discussed with particular emphasis on the adolescent female and the client whose pregnancy is undesired. In addition Unit three includes discussions of a wide spectrum of women's health issues. The gynecologic triad consists of discharge, pain, and bleeding—the three most common symptoms bringing women to health services. Infertility requires a special awareness on the part of the clinician, not only in relation to the etiology but also to the problems women encounter living through and with the diagnosis. Surgery on the reproductive organs challenges women to cope with major changes in their bodies; discussions of the common reproductive surgeries and how nurses can help women cope with them are included. Malignancy of the reproductive system is one of the major causes of anxiety, mortality, and morbidity of women and as such merits special attention. Problems related to women's breasts elicit anxiety, as does the therapy for breast cancer; a discussion of prevention and management of breast problems is included.

Unit four of the text emphasizes women's health and its promotion and maintenance. Aging, exercise, work, nutrition, fertility control, and abortion merit special attention from health professionals who work with women. Alternative methods of childbirth are emerging from the women's health movement and involve issues related to childbirth, preparation, birthing, and early parenting. Lactation, a topic usually ignored, merits special attention here since many health professionals lack a knowledge base with which to help nursing women. The book concludes with an analysis of women's mental health and how women's mental health may be compromised.

We thank the special women in our lives who helped to bring this project (and us) to fruition, and we dedicate our work to them.

Catherine Ingram Fogel
Nancy Fugate Woods

Contents

Color plates

Women and the health care system

1

Women and their health

Nancy Fugate Woods

THE PARADOX

One of the most fascinating observations recorded by epidemiologists since their earliest investigations is the paradoxical relationship between morbidity and mortality for men and women: Although mortality rates for most causes of death are lower for women than for men, and women in the Western world live longer than men, women report more physical and mental morbidity and utilize health services at higher rates than their male counterparts.

The purpose of this chapter is to explore whether the assumptions about women being the "sicker" sex are justified; to examine the paradoxical relationship between sex differences in mortality and morbidity and use of health services. The chapter will conclude with a discussion of future trends in women's health states.

The discussion that follows will include comparisons of mortality rates for men and women and an analysis of the causes of mortality for both sexes. A comparison of sex-specific rates for morbidity and use of health services will be followed by an analysis of these differences and their possible meanings. Some explanations for the paradoxical relationships of mortality to morbidity and utilization of health services will also be offered.

MORTALITY—COMPARISON OF RATES FOR MEN AND WOMEN

Women in developed countries live longer than men. This can be verified statistically in a number of ways. Table 1-1 compares the death rates for men and women in nineteen Western countries. An easy way of calculating the excess male deaths is to calculate the ratio of male to female death rates (see column 3 of Table 1-1). When the ratios exceed 1.00, there is an excess of male deaths.

Death rates in the United States are compared in Fig. 1-1 and Table 1-3; data in Table 1-3 are used to compute the ratio of male to female deaths shown in Table 1-4. Table 1-5 is a comparison of male and female deaths

Table 1-1. Age-adjusted death rates per 1,000 in selected countries of low mortality, 1960*

Country	Death rates per 1,000 (all ages)		Ratio of male to female death rates
	Males	Females	
United States, white	10.5	6.4	1.6
England and Wales	10.5	6.6	1.6
Scotland	11.7	7.9	1.5
Australia[b]†	10.6	6.7	1.6
New Zealand‡	9.4	6.3	1.5
Canada	9.9	6.6	1.5
Union of South Africa§	12.3	7.8	1.6
Ireland	9.9	7.6	1.3
Netherlands	8.1	6.0	1.4
Belgium	11.2	7.3	1.5
France	10.6	6.4	1.7
Switzerland	9.7	6.7	1.4
Germany, Federal Republic	11.2	7.8	1.4
Denmark	8.6	6.7	1.3
Norway	8.0	5.8	1.4
Sweden	8.3	6.3	1.3
Finland	12.5	7.9	1.6
Portugal	12.8	9.5	1.3
Italy	10.5	7.5	1.4
Average			
1960	10.3	7.0	1.5
1950	11.1	8.5	1.3
About 1930	14.4	12.2	1.2
Standard deviation			
1960	1.4	0.9	0.12
1950	1.7	1.1	0.11
About 1930	2.4	1.7	0.07

*Adjusted on the basis of the age distribution of the total population of the United States, Census of April 1, 1950. Adapted from Spiegelman, M., and Erhardt, C. L.: International comparisons of mortality and longevity. In Erhardt, C. L., and Berlin, J. E.: Mortality and morbidity in the United States, Cambridge, 1974, Harvard University Press.
†Excludes full-blooded aboriginals.
‡Excludes Maoris.
§Europeans only.

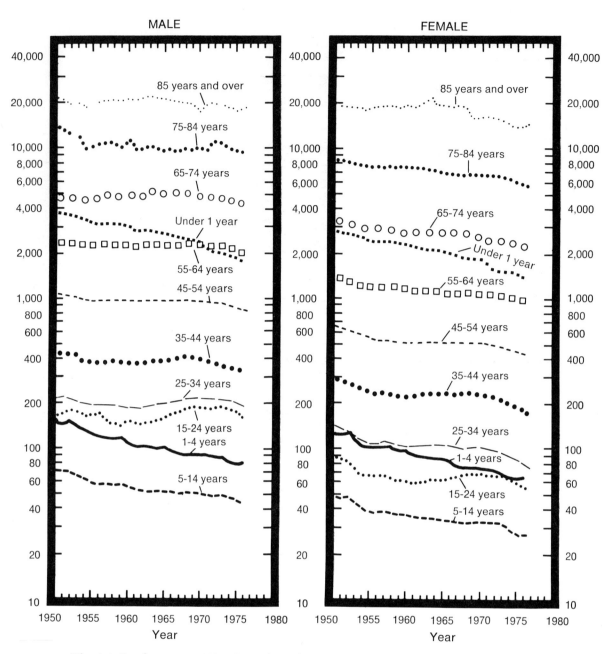

Fig. 1-1. Death rates per 100,000 population by age and sex: United States, 1950-1976. (For 1976, based on a 10% sample of deaths for all other years, based on final data.) (From Monthly Vital Statistics Report, Department of Health, Education, and Welfare.)

by specific causes. In all cases the rate for women is lower than that for men.

Not only has the advantage to women persisted worldwide, but also from 1930 to 1960 there has been a steady rise in the ratio of male to female mortality for each age group in the United States, indicating that the reduction of death rates during this period was more rapid for females than for males.

Relationships between the mortality rates for men and women in the United States population parallel the patterns seen in the other developed countries. Although more male than female infants are born alive (in a ratio of 106:100), death rates for males exceed those for females at all ages (Fig. 1-1). Death rates have become *more*, rather than less, divergent since the 1950s, although the increase in divergence of male vs female

Table 1-2. Life expectancy at birth for males and females*

Year	Females (yrs)	Males (yrs)
1900	48.3	46.3
1910	51.8	48.4
1920	54.6	53.6
1930	61.6	58.1
1940	65.2	60.8
1950	71.1	65.6
1960	73.1	66.6
1970	74.8	67.1
1971	75.0	67.4
1972	75.1	67.4
1973	75.3	67.6
1974	75.8	68.1
1975	76.5	68.7
1976	76.7	69.0
1977	77.1	69.3

*Data for 1900 to 1975 are from Statistical Abstracts of the United States, 1978, U.S. Department of Commerce; data for 1973 through 1976 are from Monthly Vital Statistics Report, Advance Report on Final Mortality Statistics, 1975 through 1978.

rates has slowed. The female advantage in life expectancy has increased dramatically since 1900. As illustrated in Table 1-2, males born in 1900 had an average life expectancy of 46.3 years and females born in the same year had a life expectancy of 48.3 years; thus males had a life expectancy 95.9% as long as that for females. Although males born in 1974 have an average life expectancy of 68.2 years, females born in the same year have a life expectancy of 75.9 years. This means that male life expectancy is now only 89.9% of that for females (Johnson, 1977). This relationship holds across racial groups (white vs nonwhite) although generally, nonwhites tend to have higher mortality rates than whites (Table 1-3).

Causes of disparity in death rates

The greater overall male death rate is attributable to a serious disadvantage for males reflected in most of the assigned causes of death.

International comparisons

An international comparison of causes of death is limited by the differences in the vital statistics systems of the countries as well as the social and economic habits of the populations. Sources of bias include the health habits of the population, the stage of illness at which health care was sought, the system of health care, training of health personnel, and the legal structure. To complicate matters, at any given time the countries may be using different versions of the International Classification of Disease. Finally, the use of crude death rates (rather than age-adjusted rates) may be misleading because of the aging of the population, increased medical care, and improved certification of death. With these limitations in mind, we can entertain some international comparisons of how the sexes fare.

The excessive increases in mortality rates among males 40 to 69 years of age from 16 Western countries* from the period 1930 to 1963 have been attributed to cardiovascular disease, cancer, and to a smaller extent, bronchitis. The deviations appear to have resulted from significant increases in adult male death rates from these diseases. National smoking propensities are highly correlated with changes in mortality from these three diseases. Slight increases in female mortality rates for the 40 to 69 year age group may reflect a decrease in maternal mortality for women during their earlier years (Preston, 1970).

United States

The age-adjusted death rates for selected causes of death in the United States for 1973 are given in Table 1-5. In every case except diabetes mellitus, male deaths outnumber female deaths. (Indeed, if only white males and white females are compared, fewer females than males die of diabetes.)

Although deaths from major cardiovascular-renal diseases have declined for men since 1940 and for women since 1920, the rate of decline has been greater for women. However, if one were to consider crude death rates rather than age-adjusted rates, one would find a dramatic increase in cardiovascular disease since 1915. Age-adjusted death rates for arteriosclerotic heart disease have also declined since 1950, although women retain their advantage (Johnson, 1977).

Before 1950 women had higher mortality rates from cancer than men, but death rates from cancer have since increased for men, with little change occurring for women since 1960. However, respiratory cancer rates demonstrate a totally different trend: age-adjusted death rates from lung cancer have risen for both men and women, and the sex ratios have narrowed considerably since 1960. This is attributable to a higher relative rate of increase among females. The sex mortality differential for other disorders of the respiratory system (bronchitis, emphysema, and asthma) has also been declining since 1965 (Johnson, 1977).

The sex differential for cirrhosis has been increasing

*Norway, Sweden, Belgium, United States, Scotland, England and Wales, Australia, New Zealand, Denmark, Netherlands, France, Austria, Germany, Portugal, Spain, and Italy.

Table 1-3. Deaths and death rates by age, color, and sex: United States, 1977*

Age	Total			White			All other		
	Both sexes	Male	Female	Both sexes	Male	Female	Both sexes	Male	Female
Number									
All ages	1,899,597	1,046,243	853,354	1,664,100	912,670	751,430	235,497	133,573	101,924
Under 1 year	46,975	26,875	20,100	33,199	19,229	13,970	13,776	7,646	6,130
1-4 years	8,307	4,720	3,587	6,198	3,541	2,657	2,109	1,179	930
5-9 years	5,834	3,556	2,278	4,579	2,798	1,781	1,255	758	497
10-14 years	6,745	4,344	2,401	5,449	3,487	1,962	1,296	857	439
15-19 years	21,443	15,573	5,870	18,056	13,209	4,847	3,387	2,364	1,023
20-24 years	26,543	20,047	6,496	21,273	16,255	5,018	5,270	3,792	1,478
25-29 years	23,292	16,937	6,355	17,488	12,804	4,684	5,804	4,133	1,671
30-34 years	21,641	15,641	7,000	16,283	11,005	5,278	5,358	3,636	1,722
35-39 years	24,036	15,531	8,505	17,883	11,583	6,300	6,153	3,948	2,205
40-44 years	34,073	21,421	12,652	25,814	16,314	9,500	8,259	5,107	3,152
45-49 years	55,483	35,094	20,389	44,086	28,093	15,993	11,397	7,001	4,396
50-54 years	89,640	57,038	32,602	73,608	47,325	26,283	16,032	9,713	6,319
55-59 years	125,574	80,315	45,259	106,153	68,530	37,623	19,421	11,785	7,636
60-64 years	167,098	106,505	60,593	144,509	93,031	51,478	22,589	13,474	9,115
65-69 years	209,496	129,873	79,623	183,434	114,844	68,590	26,062	15,029	11,033
70-74 years	236,099	138,157	97,942	209,645	123,782	85,863	26,454	14,375	12,079
75-79 years	247,048	129,552	117,496	223,046	117,355	105,691	24,002	12,197	11,805
80-84 years	243,550	112,387	131,163	226,422	104,030	122,392	17,128	8,357	8,771
85 years and over	306,151	113,309	192,842	286,576	105,183	181,393	19,575	8,126	11,449
Not stated	569	368	201	399	272	127	170	96	74
Rates per 100,000 population									
All ages	878.1	994.1	768.2	888.2	998.2	783.3	813.0	967.1	672.5
Under 1 year	1,485.6	1,659.0	1,303.5	1,266.2	1,429.7	1,094.8	2,546.4	2,780.4	2,304.5
1-4 years	68.8	76.5	60.8	62.5	69.7	55.0	97.6	108.1	87.1
5-9 years	34.0	40.6	27.1	32.1	38.4	25.6	43.0	51.6	34.3
10-14 years	35.1	44.4	25.5	34.0	42.5	25.0	41.0	53.9	28.0
15-19 years	101.6	145.7	56.4	101.2	145.8	55.2	103.9	145.0	62.8
20-24 years	133.5	201.9	65.3	125.0	190.0	59.3	184.1	276.6	99.1
25-29 years	132.1	193.9	71.4	114.4	167.3	61.4	246.9	382.0	131.7
30-34 years	140.9	193.2	90.0	121.2	164.2	78.3	279.6	415.1	165.6
35-39 years	195.5	259.5	134.8	166.6	219.3	115.6	393.2	560.8	256.1
40-44 years	304.7	393.3	220.6	264.5	339.7	191.7	580.0	793.0	404.1
45-49 years	482.3	625.8	345.8	434.9	565.1	309.7	832.5	1,100.8	599.7
50-54 years	754.7	998.7	528.7	695.1	925.4	480.1	1,244.7	1,624.2	914.5
55-59 years	1,138.1	1,524.3	785.1	1,068.0	1,440.0	726.2	1,775.2	2,310.8	1,307.5
60-64 years	1,784.9	2,431.1	1,216.5	1,704.3	2,338.0	1,144.0	2,561.1	3,360.1	1,895.0
65-69 years	2,480.4	3,473.5	1,691.2	2,431.8	3,436.4	1,632.7	2,886.2	3,795.2	2,176.1
70-74 years	3,847.1	5,319.9	2,766.7	3,727.7	5,233.9	2,634.6	5,156.7	6,196.1	4,298.6
75-79 years	6,073.0	8,153.1	4,739.7	5,957.4	8,104.6	4,603.3	7,408.0	8,650.4	6,450.8
80-84 years	8,814.7	11,363.7	7,393.6	8,949.5	11,597.5	7,494.9	7,351.1	8,986.0	6,265.0
85 years and over	14,725.9	17,299.1	13,542.3	15,292.2	18,041.7	14,039.7	9,595.6	11,286.1	8,673.5

*Refers only to resident deaths occurring within the United States. Rates per 100,000 estimated population in specified age group. Figures for age not stated included in "All ages" but not distributed among age groups. Calculated from the Current Mortality Sample is a 10% systematic sample of death certificates received each month in Vital Statistics Offices for each state. For mortality rates, 10% of the death certificates *received* in the office of Vital Statistics during a month period. The provisional underlying cause of death is likely to be biased with respect to the final cause of death reported to the National Center for Health Statistics so adjustments are made in the provisional data shown here. Data from Monthly Vital Statistics Report, December, 1979.

Table 1-4. Ratio of male to female crude death rates by age for whites and nonwhites: United States, 1977*

Age	Total	White	Nonwhite
All ages	1.29	1.27	1.44
Under 1 year	1.27	1.31	1.21
1-4 years	1.26	1.27	1.24
5-9 years	1.50	1.50	1.50
10-14 years	1.74	1.70	1.93
15-19 years	2.58	2.64	2.31
20-24 years	3.09	3.20	2.79
25-29 years	2.72	2.72	2.90
30-34 years	2.15	2.10	2.51
35-39 years	1.93	1.90	2.19
40-44 years	1.78	1.77	1.96
45-49 years	1.81	1.82	1.84
50-54 years	1.89	1.93	1.78
55-59 years	1.94	1.98	1.78
60-64 years	2.00	2.04	1.77
65-69 years	2.21	2.10	1.74
70-74 years	1.92	1.99	1.44
75-79 years	1.72	1.76	1.34
80-84 years	1.54	1.55	1.43
85+ years	1.28	1.29	1.30

*Computed from rates given in Table 1-3.

slowly, and the higher suicide rate for males has increased from 1970 to 1973 even though the overall rates have declined slightly for both sexes since 1960. Death rates from homicide have increased for both sexes since 1960, but the sex mortality ratio reveals no clear patterns: males continue to experience more deaths than females from motor vehicle and other accidents (Johnson, 1977).

Death rates from influenza and pneumonia have been fairly stable since 1950. However, the sex differential has continued to increase in recent years (Johnson, 1977).

The sex differential for diabetes mellitus is of interest because women have traditionally had higher rates than men. There is, however, a recent trend toward equality. Johnson (1977) points out that if this trend continues, one of the rare examples of a male mortality advantage will disappear.

Some explanations for sex differences in mortality
Biologic differences

One of the most obvious explanations for the sex differential in mortality—observed both in the United

Table 1-5. Age-adjusted death rates for selected causes, by color and sex: United States, 1974*

Cause of death	Total			White			All other		
	Both sexes	Male	Female	Both sexes	Male	Female	Both sexes	Male	Female
All causes	666.2	877.8	492.9	635.4	843.0	466.4	901.3	1,149.1	693.1
Major cardiovascular diseases, 390-448	310.8	413.7	228.1	302.9	409.1	217.8	374.8	449.1	313.5
Diseases of heart, 390-398, 402, 404, 410-420	232.7	323.6	159.2	228.8	322.8	152.9	262.8	325.8	210.8
Hypertension, 400, 401, 403	2.1	2.6	1.7	1.7	2.2	1.4	5.6	6.5	5.0
Cerebrovascular diseases, 430-438	59.9	66.5	54.9	56.4	63.0	51.4	90.9	98.3	84.7
Arteriosclerosis, 440	7.6	8.6	6.9	7.6	8.7	6.9	7.3	8.2	6.6
Malignant neoplasms, including neoplasms of lymphatic and hematopoietic tissues, 140-209	131.8	162.3	109.2	128.0	150.3	107.6	156.6	199.0	122.4
Accidents, E800-E949	46.0	69.4	23.8	44.3	66.6	22.9	58.5	92.3	29.0
Motor vehicle accidents, E810-E823	21.8	33.2	10.9	21.7	32.8	11.0	23.2	37.5	10.8
All other accidents, E800-E807, E825-E940	24.2	36.2	12.8	22.6	33.8	12.0	35.3	64.8	18.2
Influenza and pneumonia, 470-474, 480-486	16.9	22.6	12.8	15.7	21.0	12.0	25.4	35.1	17.5
Cirrhosis of liver, 571	14.8	20.7	9.7	13.4	19.0	8.6	25.0	34.0	17.4
Diabetes mellitus, 250	12.5	12.2	12.7	11.4	11.5	11.2	23.4	18.8	27.1
Suicide, E950-E959	12.2	18.2	6.7	12.8	19.0	7.1	7.2	21.7	3.3
Homicide, E960-E978	10.8	17.3	4.6	6.0	9.3	2.9	44.5	77.9	15.5
Bronchitis, emphysema, and asthma, 490-493	9.2	15.9	4.3	9.4	16.4	4.4	6.4	10.4	3.2
Tuberculosis, all forms, 010-019	1.3	2.1	0.7	0.9	1.5	0.5	4.6	7.2	2.5

*Based on age-specific death rates per 100,000 population in specified group. Computed by the direct method, using as the standard population the age distribution of the total population of the United States as enumerated in 1940; see Technical Appendix. Numbers after causes of death are category numbers of the Eighth Revision International Classification of Disease, Adapted, 1965. From Vital Statistics of the United States, Vol. II, Part A, Washington, D.C., 1978, U.S. Government Printing Office.

States and in other developed nations—is biologic. Because the inferior longevity of males is nearly universal throughout the animal kingdom and in humans, it would seem logical that differences in mortality rates are based on biologic differences between the sexes.

Although chromosomal and hormonal differences account for important biologic differences between males and females, genetically determined biologic differences appear responsible for only a small proportion of sex mortality differentials (Waldron, 1976).

Although there are some pathologic conditions caused by X-linked recessive mutations, which occur almost exclusively in males, Waldron (1976) estimates that deaths from these conditions account for less than 2% of the excess deaths experienced by males during the reproductive years. There is some evidence that genetic differences are responsible for sex differences in infant mortality (Naeye et al., 1971) and for the greater susceptibility of males to infectious disease during infancy and childhood (Michaels and Rogers, 1971). Two mechanisms are thought to be involved in females' greater resistance to infection. (1) The X chromosome carries quantitative genes for the production of immunoglobulin M, resulting in higher levels in the serum of females (Goble and Konapka, 1973). (2) The X chromosome is thought to permit greater options for variability in the female, since one of her X chromosomes may be active in some of cells and the other in occasional other cells; thus there can be more variation since different alleles may occupy a particular locus on each X chromosome (Naeye et al., 1971). Females have an additional advantage since estrogen and progesterone stimulate phagocytosis by macrophages (Vernon and Roberts, 1969). Although some investigators have hypothesized that estrogen is a factor in protecting premenopausal females from coronary heart disease, there is no evidence to support the theory that estrogen has a protective effect (Moriyama et al., 1971).

In the past, reproduction constituted a major cause of mortality for women of childbearing age. This is no longer the case in developed countries. Although there is still some risk of mortality associated with childbearing for females, it is not of sufficient magnitude to alter the sex mortality differential in favor of males.

Although an attempt has been made to account for the sex differences in mortality from coronary heart disease (CHD) by suggesting that men have a higher incidence because of higher levels of risk factors (higher serum cholesterol levels, higher systolic and diastolic blood pressure readings, higher incidence of left ventricular hypertrophy as evidenced by electrocardiogram, higher rates of cigarette smoking, and higher incidence of glucose intolerance) than women, this relationship held for those persons in the Framingham study ages 45 to 54 years old but not for those older than 54 years. For older persons, sex and CHD are related, and the primary factors and CHD are related, but sex is negatively related to the most important risk factors. Two explanations are suggested for these findings. First, the primary risk factors as measured at younger ages may be responsible for the sex mortality differentials at older ages. Next, the risk factors documented so far may not be the most important; the complex relationships between biologic factors and social life require further exploration (Johnson, 1977).

Although genetic and hormonal differences and reproductive experiences may be responsible for some differences in mortality between the sexes, their total contribution to mortality differentials is a minor one. In addition, the increases observed in mortality differentials for males and females over the past 50 years cannot be accounted for solely by biologic differences, since the genetic code varies too slowly for biologic differences to have made a significant contribution (Retherford, 1975). The great variability in mortality rates for males and females during the adult years suggests that other factors, such as changes in the environment, are most likely responsible. Because the effects of the environment on sex mortality differentials are mediated through the biologic differences between the sexes, both biologic differences and environmental influences must be taken into account.

Technologic improvements in health care

A number of changes in mortality have been attributed to technologic developments. As mentioned earlier, medical technology has aided in decreasing the maternal mortality rate. Improved detection and treatment of female reproductive cancers have also led to decreased mortality rates for women. Changes in proportionate mortality (that is, changes in the relative importance of various causes of death) represent an important way in which health technology has benefited females. As technology has assisted in limiting deaths from many acute illnesses, deaths from degenerative diseases, for which sex mortality differentials are especially large, are now weighted more heavily than in the past (Retherford, 1975). Thus technologic advances in health care have had profound positive effects on those acute illnesses that probably would have resulted in more similar mortality rates for men and women.

Stress

Stress produced by exposure of an individual to conflicting or ambiguous expectations regarding her or his behavior has been explored as an explanation for sex mortality differentials. However, as Nathanson (1977) points out, there has been little consensus among investigators about which sex experiences the most stress. Occupational or economic sources of stress have been suggested by some as determinants of male mortality (Retherford, 1975); others have implicated the traditional role of married women as a source of stress (Gove, 1973). Thus stress is not likely to adequately explain sex mortality differences.

Life-style

Several aspects of how men and women live their lives can influence how and when they die. Gove (1973) has listed three behavioral factors believed to create different life chances for men and women. First, norms regulating behavior for men and women may encourage higher mortality among men. For example, it is more appropriate for men than women to smoke and use alcoholic beverages. Second, life-style differences expose the sexes to different risks of death. Third, personality differences are probably involved; that is, the modal (usual or most common) male personality is more likely to be aggressive and take risks than the modal female personality. Waldron (1976) also cites risk-taking behavior as a factor in male mortality rates.

Differential exposure to smoking, a diet high in saturated fats, excess food, excessive use of alcohol, employment hazards, violence, and automobile accidents is probably responsible for excess male mortality from lung cancer and other lung disease (such as emphysema), cardiovascular disease, cirrhosis, fatalities from occupational accidents, and automobile fatalities.

Type A, coronary-prone behavior, also believed to be a risk factor for coronary heart disease, is typical of the societal expectations for males—aggressive competitiveness—whereas such behavior for females is not encouraged (Waldron, 1976).

Three elements of the life-styles of women have been cited by various investigators as having protective effects. The use of labor-saving devices in the home has been credited by some with improvement of women's mortality rates (Spiegelman and Erhardt, 1974). The trend toward limiting obesity may be another factor responsible for females' favorable mortality rates (Retherford, 1975). In addition, some investigators suggest that women's learned ability to adapt to role discontinuities during their lifespans may account for their relatively greater resilience during old age (Kline, 1975). Furthermore, Sinnott (1977) suggests that a person's ability to tolerate variations in sex roles is an indication of a kind of general flexibility associated with a longer lifespan and more successful aging.

When considering mortality from all causes, single, widowed, and divorced persons have higher rates than married persons. Men, however, seem to be afforded more protection from marriage than women. These differences are especially marked for causes of death for which the individual's psychologic state would be likely to affect her or his life chances (Gove, 1973).

A comparison of *suicide rates* for men and women across marital status categories shows that the disparity in completed suicide rates for married vs single, divorced, or widowed is greater for men than for women. Gove (1972) attributes this to the positive effects of marriage for men and the somewhat negative effects of marriage for women. Indeed, in some of the studies Gove cites, single women had lower suicide rates than married women, whereas the opposite pertained to men.

Predictions for the future

Sex differentials in mortality may be less striking in the future as women's roles in society change. For example, occupational hazards previously applicable to males will have more of an effect on the female population as more women enter the labor force. One group of 1717 female hourly employees in the rubber industry has already demonstrated an excess of lung cancer and myocardial infarction when compared with the United States population of women (Andjelkovic, 1976).

A reversal of the sex differences in mortality for male and female professionals has been seen for 1968–1972 in Wisconsin. More deaths from cancer, suicide, and motor vehicle accidents have been seen for professional women, and the male dominance in lung cancer rates has diminished. Ladbrook (1976) suggests three explanations for this unusual observance. First, women professionals are likely to be subjected to work overload when compared with men professionals. Second, women professionals are more likely than other women to adopt risk-rich behaviors, such as aggressive competitiveness, smoking, and drinking. Third, women professionals do not have the same kinds of socioemotional supports that are available to men from their spouses. Indeed, Ladbrook found that differential distribution of marital status across the sexes accounted for much of the reversal in previous mortality patterns.

A study of Type A coronary-prone behavior (Waldron et al., 1977) revealed that maximum values of Type A and "speed and impatience" scores were observed for employed women at ages 30 to 35, but the scores for employed men failed to show this peak. Furthermore, at younger ages (18 to 25) average Type A scores are significantly higher for employed men. Waldron suggests that women who are still employed at age 30 to 35 are Type A women, who are less likely to leave their jobs when they have children.

Table 1-6. Number of acute conditions per 100 persons per year, by condition group, according to sex: United States, 1978*

Condition group	Both sexes	Male	Female	Condition group	Both sexes	Male	Female
All acute conditions	218.2	207.1	228.5	Other digestive system conditions	4.2	4.3	4.1
Infective and parasitic diseases	24.7	22.8	26.5	Injuries	33.1	38.4	28.1
Common childhood diseases	1.8	1.8	1.7	Fractures, dislocations, sprains, and strains	11.2	13.3	9.3
Virus, N.O.S.	11.2	10.8	11.6	Fractures and dislocations	3.7	4.4	3.0
Other infective and parasitic diseases	11.7	10.3	13.1	Sprains and strains	7.6	8.9	6.3
Respiratory conditions	115.8	109.7	121.5	Open wounds and lacerations	8.1	10.8	5.7
Upper respiratory conditions	59.1	55.3	62.7	Contusions and superficial injuries	6.6	6.8	6.4
Common cold	45.6	42.4	48.6	Other current injuries	7.1	7.5	6.8
Other upper respiratory conditions	13.5	13.0	14.1	All other acute conditions	33.9	26.1	41.2
Influenza	50.3	48.3	52.2	Diseases of the ear	7.7	8.2	7.2
Influenza with digestive manifestations	2.6	2.2	3.0	Headaches	2.3	2.3	2.3
Other influenza	47.7	46.0	49.2	Genitourinary disorders	6.1	1.5	10.3
Other respiratory conditions	6.3	6.1	6.6	Deliveries and disorders of pregnancy and the puerperium	2.1	—	4.1
Pneumonia	1.6	1.3	1.9				
Bronchitis	2.7	2.6	2.8				
Other respiratory conditions	2.0	2.2	1.8	Diseases of the skin	1.7	1.8	1.6
Disgestive system conditions	10.7	10.1	11.3	Diseases of the musculoskeletal system	3.2	3.3	3.1
Dental conditions	2.8	2.6	3.1	All other acute conditions	10.9	9.0	12.7
Functional and symptomatic upper gastrointestinal disorders, N.E.C.	3.6	3.2	4.1				

*Data are based on household interviews of the civilian noninstitutionalized population. The survey design, general qualifications, and information on the reliability of the estimates are given in appendix I. Definitions of terms are given in appendix II.

NOTES: Excluded from these statistics are all conditions involving neither restricted activity nor medical attention.

N.O.S.—Not otherwise specified; *N.E.C.*—not elsewhere classified.

The appropriate relative standard errors of the estimates shown in this table are found in appendix I, figures I and VI.

Adapted from Givens, J.: Current estimates from the health interview survey: United States, 1978, Series 10, No. 130, Washington, D.C., Nov. 1979, U.S. Department of Health, Education and Welfare, National Center for Health Statistics.

MORBIDITY—COMPARISON OF RATES FOR MEN AND WOMEN

Although mortality data provide us with one index of ill health of a population, these data provide an incomplete picture. In developed countries, ill health frequently results from significant but nonfatal conditions such as mental illness or orthopedic and sensory impairments. The definition of morbidity used in conjunction with the National Health Interview Survey implies that *morbidity is a departure from physical or mental wellbeing that results from disease or injury and that has an impact on the individual's life inasmuch as she or he is aware both of the departure from health and the restrictions or disabilities resulting from the condition* (Cole, 1974).

Current estimates from the National Health Interview Survey data for 1978 show that in the United States women continue to report more illness than men and utilize health services at higher rates than men do. These estimates are based on data from a stratified random sample of households drawn from the civilian noninstitutionalized population of the United States. Several variables reflecting morbidity and health care utilization are measured.

Acute conditions

Acute conditions are those illnesses and injuries that have lasted less than 3 months and have involved one day or more of restricted activity or medical attention. The annual incidence of acute conditions is estimated by including only those conditions having their onset during the 2 weeks prior to the interview. Table 1-6 shows that the incidence of acute conditions for females exceeds that for males for nearly every condition, with the major exception of injuries. The higher rate of acute conditions for females appears less consistent during

Table 1-7. Number of acute conditions per 100 persons per year, by age, sex, and condition group: United States, 1978*

Sex and condition group	All ages	Under 6 years	6-16 years	17-44 years	45 years and over
Both sexes					
All acute conditions	218.2	387.6	272.9	224.5	129.1
Infective and parasitic diseases	24.7	64.5	36.9	22.3	9.4
Respiratory conditions	115.8	206.6	152.8	116.6	66.7
Upper respiratory conditions	59.1	133.9	80.2	55.9	29.8
Influenza	50.3	56.0	66.5	55.5	31.9
Other respiratory conditions	6.3	16.7	6.1	5.3	5.0
Digestive system conditions	10.7	14.0	13.3	11.2	7.4
Injuries	33.1	33.5	39.6	36.4	24.5
All other acute conditions	33.9	69.0	30.3	37.9	21.1
Male					
All acute conditions	207.1	403.5	261.6	202.7	114.4
Infective and parasitic diseases	22.8	72.1	34.0	17.2	7.7
Respiratory conditions	109.7	215.1	140.5	107.7	58.3
Upper respiratory conditions	55.3	134.5	70.1	51.0	26.6
Influenza	48.3	63.3	63.3	52.3	27.5
Other respiratory conditions	6.1	17.3	7.0	4.4	4.2
Digestive system conditions	10.1	10.7	14.0	10.6	6.5
Injuries	38.4	35.8	48.8	44.0	24.1
All other acute conditions	26.1	69.7	24.4	23.2	17.7
Female					
All acute conditions	228.5	370.8	284.6	244.9	141.4
Infective and parasitic diseases	26.5	56.6	40.0	27.1	10.7
Respiratory conditions	121.5	197.6	165.5	125.0	73.7
Upper respiratory conditions	62.7	133.2	90.7	60.5	32.5
Influenza	52.2	48.4	69.8	58.4	35.6
Other respiratory conditions	6.6	16.0	5.1	6.1	5.6
Digestive system conditions	11.3	17.5	12.7	11.9	8.2
Injuries	28.1	31.0	30.1	29.2	24.9
All other acute conditions	41.2	68.2	36.4	51.7	23.8

*Data are based on household interviews of the civilian noninstitutionalized population. The survey design, general qualifications, and information on the reliability of the estimates are given in appendix I. Definitions of terms are given in appendix II.
NOTES: Excluded from these statistics are all conditions involving neither restricted activity nor medical attention.

The appropriate relative standard errors of the estimates shown in this table are found in appendix I, figures I and VI.
Adapted from Givens, J.: Current estimates from the health interview survey: United States, 1978, Series 10, No. 130, Washington, D.C., Nov. 1979, U.S. Department of Health, Education and Welfare, National Center for Health Statistics.

the earlier part of the life cycle than at later ages (Table 1-7). For example, during the preschool years, males and females have similar rates. In all other age groups, females have higher rates than males in the majority of categories (Table 1-7). However, males (except those over age 45) consistently have higher rates for injuries (Howie and Drury, 1978).

Disability

Another variable measured by the Health Interview Survey is *disability*. "Days of disability" refers to a temporary or long-term reduction of an individual's activity

because of either acute or chronic conditions. Four types of disability days are reported in the Health Interview Survey: (1) restricted-activity days, (2) bed-disability days, (3) work-loss days, and (4) school-loss days. A restricted-activity day is one on which an individual reduces normal activity for the entire day because of an illness or injury. Bed-disability days are days during which the person spent all or most of the day in bed; these are also counted as days of restricted activity. Each day lost from work or school because of illness or injury is also counted as a day of restricted activity.

Females report proportionately more days of restricted activity than males (Table 1-8), with an average of 21.1 days of disability per year compared with 16.3 days for men. Women also report more bed-disability days per person per year than men and more work-loss days. In each case, the average number of restricted days is greater for women than for men. For both sexes, the trend appears to increase with age, although the pattern of more restricted activity for females would seem to be established before adulthood (female children have a greater number of school loss days than their male counterparts). Although the data given in Table 1-8 are for 1978, the patterns for the sexes have been the same in previous years (Howie and Drury, 1978).

Table 1-9 gives the number of restricted-activity days associated with acute conditions per 100 persons per year for 1978. One striking pattern observable from this table is the lower rate of disability from accidents and injuries experienced by females.

New York Telephone Co. study. Similar findings are borne out in a classic study of employees of the New York Telephone Company reported in 1960 (Hinkle, 1960). Ninety-six female telephone operators and 116 craftsmen from a single operating division who had been continuously employed for 20 or more years were included in the study. This involved approximately one third of all the female employees and one sixth of the males. Each person had a medical history and physical examination at the time of employment and at varying intervals throughout their careers, and none had shown evidence of a significant illness at the time they were hired. The employees were exposed to no significant occupational hazards, all lived in the same city, and all shared similar environmental exposure as well as socioeconomic characteristics. By reviewing their health records for the past 20 years, and by both reviewing records and making prospective observations over a 5-year period beginning with the end of the twentieth year of employment, the investigators found that both the number and nature of illness episodes differed greatly between males and females. On the average, women experienced 2.434 episodes of illness per year over the 20-year period, men 1.401. This amounted to 10.5 disability days per year for women as opposed to 4.30 for males.*

Hinkle and co-workers found that women had more of every type of syndrome but were much more likely to report upper respiratory infections, gastrointestinal disorders, myalgia, minor abrasions, headaches, and minor

---

*It should be noted that the disability days were reported as sickness absence days, and questions can be raised regarding the reason for employees using sickness days. It is certainly possible that employed women may have used days allocated to them for illness to care for sick children or other family members.

Table 1-8. Days of disability per person per year, by sex and age: United States, 1978*

Sex and age	Restricted activity days	Bed-disability days	Work-loss days
Both sexes			
All ages	18.8	7.1	5.2
Under 17 years	11.3	5.2	—
17-24 years	12.3	5.5	4.5
25-44 years	16.2	5.8	5.1
45-64 years	25.8	8.8	6.1
65 years and over	40.3	14.5	4.2
Male			
All ages	16.3	6.0	4.9
Under 17 years	10.7	4.9	—
17-24 years	10.5	4.1	4.2
25-44 years	13.9	4.5	4.4
45-64 years	23.2	7.3	6.2
65 years and over	35.1	14.2	2.9
Female			
All ages	21.1	8.2	5.7
Under 17 years	11.8	5.6	—
17-24 years	14.0	6.8	4.9
25-44 years	18.3	7.1	6.0
45-64 years	28.1	10.1	5.9
65 years and over	43.9	14.8	6.5

*Data are based on household interviews of the civilian noninstitutionalized population. The survey design, general qualifications, and information on the reliability of the estimates are given in appendix I. Definitions of terms are given in appendix II.

NOTES: Work loss reported for currently employed persons aged 17 years and over.

The appropriate relative standard errors of the estimates shown in this table are found in appendix I, figure II.

Adapted from Givens, J.: Current estimates from the health interview survey: United States, 1978, Series 10, No. 130, Washington, D.C., Nov. 1979, U.S. Department of Health, Education and Welfare, National Center for Health Statistics.

episodes of mood disturbances than men. Dysmenorrhea was a relatively common complaint among the women in the sample. After devising a "seriousness scale," which represented the probability that an untreated episode for any given illness would be fatal, the investigators classified each illness report according to its seriousness. Although the women employees incurred more illnesses than the men, there was a greater probability that men would die from their illnesses than women. Severity of illness, which was measured in terms of the amount of "prostration" it caused, was higher among women since they had significantly more episodes of disabling illness and thus more days of sickness absence than men.

Table 1-9. Restricted activity days associated with acute conditions per 100 persons per year by sex and condition group: United States, 1978*

Condition group	Days lost from school		Days lost from work		Days of bed disability		Days of restricted activity	
	Female	Male	Female	Male	Female	Male	Female	Male
All acute conditions	519.1	443.5	427.1	341.3	516.1	368.2	1120.7	849.1
Infective and parasitic diseases	85.5	65.4	26.4	23.8	56.5	42.1	103.9	83.5
Respiratory conditions	326.1	297.0	178.8	146.2	256.5	208.6	491.0	391.4
Upper respiratory conditions	143.6	114.1	57.2	47.5	82.7	67.4	189.7	151.4
Influenza	159.9	136.8	97.6	74.8	137.5	109.9	230.0	188.9
Other respiratory conditions	22.6	28.1	24.0	23.9	36.3	31.4	71.2	51.1
Digestive system conditions	23.0	19.1	23.6	22.2	23.6	23.7	54.7	42.5
Injuries	36.2	47.8	106.4	114.0	70.9	47.0	224.4	218.8
All other acute conditions	48.3	32.2	91.9	35.1	108.6	46.8	246.8	112.9

*Adapted from Givens, J.: Current estimates from the health interview survey: United States, 1978, Series 10, No. 130, Washington, D.C., Nov. 1979, U.S. Department of Health, Education and Welfare, National Center for Health Statistics.

Table 1-10. Percent distribution of persons with limitation of activity due to chronic conditions, by degree of limitation according to sex and age: United States, 1978*

Sex and age	Percent distribution			
	Total population	With activity limitation	With limitation in major activity	With no activity limitation
Both sexes				
All ages	100.0	14.2	10.6	85.8
Under 17 years	100.0	3.9	2.0	96.1
17-44 years	100.0	8.5	5.2	91.5
45-64 years	100.0	23.6	18.6	76.4
65 years and over	100.0	45.0	38.3	55.0
Male				
All ages	100.0	14.3	10.8	85.7
Under 17 years	100.0	4.2	2.2	95.8
17-44 years	100.0	9.1	5.5	90.9
45-64 years	100.0	24.3	19.7	75.7
65 years and over	100.0	48.2	43.2	51.8
Female				
All ages	100.0	14.1	10.3	85.9
Under 17 years	100.0	3.6	1.8	96.4
17-44 years	100.0	7.9	4.9	92.1
45-64 years	100.0	23.0	17.5	77.0
65 years and over	100.0	42.7	34.9	57.3

*Data are based on household interviews of the civilian noninstitutionalized population. The survey design, general qualifications, and information on the reliability of the estimates are given in appendix I. Definitions of terms are given in appendix II.

NOTES: Major activity refers to ability to work, keep house, or engage in school or preschool activities.

For official population estimates for more general use, see Bureau of the Census reports on the civilian population of the United States, in Current Population Reports: Series P-20, P-25, and P-60.

The appropriate relative standard errors of the estimates shown in this table are found in appendix I, figures IV and VII.

From Given, J.: Current estimates from the health interview survey: United States, 1978, Series 10, No. 130, Washington, D.C., Nov. 1979, U.S. Department of Health, Education and Welfare, National Survey for Health Statistics.

Table 1-11. Percent distribution of persons with limitation of activity by selected chronic conditions causing limitation, according to sex and age: United States, 1974*

Selected chronic condition	Percent distribution†											
	Both sexes				Male				Female			
	All ages	Under 45 years	45-64 years	65 years and over	All ages	Under 45 years	45-64 years	65 years and over	All ages	Under 45 years	45-64 years	65 years and over
Persons limited in activity	100.0	100.0	100.0	100.0	100.0	100.0	100.0	100.0	100.0	100.0	100.0	100.0
Tuberculosis, all forms	0.4	0.4	0.5	—	0.5	—	—	—	0.3	—	—	—
Malignant neoplasms	2.2	1.0	3.2	2.2	2.0	0.8	2.5	2.8	2.3	1.2	3.9	1.8
Benign and unspecified neoplasms	0.9	1.0	0.9	0.7	0.5	—	—	—	1.2	1.5	1.4	0.9
Diabetes	4.9	2.1	5.8	6.8	4.4	2.0	5.4	5.7	5.5	2.3	6.2	7.7
Mental and nervous conditions	5.1	6.2	5.8	3.4	4.8	5.9	5.2	3.0	5.5	6.5	6.3	3.8
Heart conditions	16.2	4.8	19.9	23.5	18.0	5.1	24.2	25.2	14.5	4.5	15.6	22.2
Cerebrovascular disease	2.7	0.4	2.8	4.9	3.0	—	3.2	5.8	2.5	—	2.4	4.3
Hypertension without heart involvement	6.7	2.5	8.8	8.7	4.5	1.6	5.9	6.0	8.9	3.4	11.8	10.9
Varicose veins	0.9	0.6	1.2	0.8	0.3	—	—	—	1.5	1.2	2.0	1.3
Hemorrhoids	0.3	—	—	0.4	0.4	—	—	—	0.3	—	—	—
Other conditions of circulatory system	3.9	1.8	4.0	5.9	3.3	1.0	3.7	5.5	4.5	2.7	4.4	6.3
Chronic bronchitis	1.0	1.1	1.0	0.9	1.1	0.9	1.1	1.2	0.9	1.3	0.9	—
Emphysema	2.8	0.5	3.5	4.4	4.5	—	5.1	7.9	1.2	—	1.8	1.6
Asthma, with or without hay fever	4.9	9.8	3.0	2.1	5.2	9.8	3.0	2.8	4.6	9.8	3.0	1.6
Hay fever, without asthma	0.7	1.7	0.3	—	0.8	2.1	—	—	0.7	1.3	—	—
Chronic sinusitis	0.7	0.6	0.7	0.6	0.6	—	0.7	—	0.7	—	0.8	—
Other conditions of respiratory system	2.1	1.8	2.3	2.1	2.9	2.0	3.4	3.3	1.3	1.5	1.2	1.1
Peptic ulcer	1.9	1.6	2.3	1.6	2.1	1.8	2.6	1.9	1.7	1.5	2.1	1.4
Hernia	2.4	1.4	2.9	2.8	2.6	1.6	1.2	3.2	2.1	1.0	2.6	2.4
Other conditions of digestive system	3.2	2.3	3.7	3.6	2.7	2.0	3.2	3.7	3.8	2.6	4.2	4.3
Diseases of kidney and ureter	1.2	1.3	1.3	1.0	0.9	0.8	1.0	1.0	1.5	1.8	1.7	1.1
Other conditions of genitourinary system	1.7	1.7	1.6	1.7	1.2	—	1.2	2.1	2.1	3.0	2.0	1.3
Arthritis and rheumatism	15.0	4.1	17.4	23.2	10.1	2.8	12.5	15.6	19.6	5.5	22.4	29.4
Other musculoskeletal disorders	5.9	6.3	7.9	3.2	6.0	6.7	7.8	3.0	5.7	6.0	7.9	3.4
Visual impairments	5.9	4.1	4.0	9.8	5.9	5.4	4.1	8.6	5.9	2.8	3.8	10.7
Hearing impairments	2.4	3.3	1.7	2.3	2.8	4.1	1.8	2.5	2.0	2.4	1.6	2.1
Paralysis, complete or partial	3.3	3.0	3.4	3.6	3.7	2.8	4.1	4.2	3.0	3.2	2.6	3.2
Impairments (except paralysis) of back or spine	7.0	10.4	7.3	3.2	6.8	9.2	7.5	3.1	7.2	11.7	7.1	3.3
Impairments (except paralysis and absence) of upper extremities and shoulders	2.1	3.6	2.1	1.0	2.6	4.0	2.7	1.0	1.5	2.0	1.5	1.0
Impairments (except paralysis and absence) of lower extremities and hips	6.4	7.7	5.7	6.0	7.2	9.4	7.0	5.0	5.7	6.0	4.4	6.9

*Data are based on household interviews of the civilian noninstitutionalized population. The survey design, general qualifications, and information on the reliability of the estimates are given in appendix I. Definitions of terms are given in appendix II.

†Percentages may add to more than 100 because a person can report more than one condition as a cause of his limitation; on the other hand, they may add to less than 100 because only selected conditions are shown. From Wilder, C. S.: Limitation of activity due to chronic conditions; U.S.—1974. In Vital and health statistics, Series 10, No. 111, Washington, D.C., June 1977, U.S. Department of Health, Education and Welfare, National Center for Health Statistics.

Chronic conditions

Limitation of activity because of a chronic condition is another variable examined in the Health Interview Survey. This refers to long-term reduction in activity, such as being unable to carry on the usual activity for one's age and sex group or being restricted in one's amount and kind of activity. Table 1-10 shows the degree of limitation experienced by different age groups. Table 1-11 lists the percent distribution of persons who are limited by various conditions.

Mental health
Relationship to physical health

In addition to studies of sex differences in reporting physical illness, investigators have considered sex differences in the reporting of psychiatric symptoms. Phillips and Segal (1969) have estimated the psychiatric symptomatology of a sample of 153 women and 149 men between 21 and 50 years of age selected from the city directory of Lebanon, New Hampshire. Two hundred seventy-eight of these persons were reinterviewed 1 year after the initial interview. Using the twenty-two item Mental Health Inventory developed for the Midtown Manhattan Study, the investigators attempted to rate the respondents in terms of psychiatric, psychophysiologic, physiologic, and ambiguous symptom indices. Also, the state of the subjects' physical health was measured by the respondents' reports on whether or not they currently had a number of illnesses or physical disabilities listed on what was described as a standard medical checklist.

Of interest is the fact that neither the items pertaining to physical illness and disability nor an item pertaining to emotional difficulties revealed a significant sex difference. There did not seem to be any sex differences in the prevalence or number of physical illnesses when the investigators considered either respondents' reports or physicians' diagnoses. More than one third of the women respondents had scores of four or more (disturbed) on the mental health index, compared to only about one fifth of the men. Furthermore, the percentage of respondents classified as disturbed increased as the number of illnesses reported increased. Among those reporting either zero or one illness, 13% of the men and 14.3% of the women scored high on the mental health index; of those reporting six or more symptoms, 41.4% of the men and 68.4% of the women scored high on the mental health index. It thus appeared that the number of illnesses reported had a greater influence than sex on psychologic disturbance, but the effect of illness was more pronounced among women than men. At high levels of illness sex differences became more apparent. The investigators suggest that while men and women may be similar inasmuch as their psychologic complaints are associated with physical illnesses, women are more expressive with regard to their mental health problems, particularly when their level of physical symptomatology is marked.

Respondents' patterns of utilization were also studied, revealing that in fifteen of twenty comparisons made according to position on each of the symptom indices and illness categories, a higher percentage of women than men sought help. When sex and number of physical illnesses were held constant, there was no relation between *any* of the measures of psychiatric symptomatology and medical utilization.

Marital status and sex roles

Gove, and Gove in association with Tudor, examined sex roles, marital status, and mental illness and mortality in a series of papers. Gove (1972b) explored the results of the major community-based mental health studies. Comparing the rates of mental disorder among married men and women as determined in seventeen community and treatment facility surveys, he found ratios of female to male rates ranging from 1.02 to 2.55. In no instance did a study reveal higher rates for mental disorder among married men. In the studies that dealt with single men and single women, four of these revealed a higher rate for women and eleven a higher rate for single men. In most studies there were higher rates for single persons than for married persons. Gove also computed an index to compare single persons to married by dividing the rate of mental illness of the never married by the rate of mental illness of the married. These calculations reveal that in only one study was the never married male "better off" than the married male. The results are somewhat similar for females with one notable exception: the index comparing the never married to the married is always higher for males than for females, in some instances males approaching a figure two to three times that for women. This would suggest that marriage affords much more protection to males than to females.

Gove (1972b) also provides comparisons of rates of mental disorder among men and women who were once married but are presently single. For divorced persons, eight of the studies showed that men have higher rates than women, and only three revealed the opposite. Data regarding widowed persons reveal a similar trend: seven of the studies show a higher rate of mental disorder among widowed men, and only two for women. Two studies that present rates for divorced and widowed persons combined indicate a higher rate of mental disorder among men than among women. Comparing the rates of mental illness of the formerly married was achieved by dividing the rate of mental illness of the formerly married by the rate of mental illness of the married. As one would expect, this ratio indicated a preponderance of mental illness among the divorced when compared with the married; this ratio was greater for men than for women, and in most instances the ratio was nearly twice as large for men as for women.

Computing this same ratio for the widowed and the married, similar findings emerge. In only one study did the widowed appear to be more mentally healthy than the married. Again, the trend is for males to have higher ratios than females. These same results hold for studies in which data for the widowed and divorced are combined in the analysis.

When considering the rates of residency as documented by a 25% sample of residents of mental hospitals for the 1960 census, the results are fascinating: In every instance but one the ratio of male to female residents is greater than 1.00 across categories of marital status. The only instance in which there was a preponderance of females was among the married.

Subsequent analyses that controlled for sociodemographic factors have revealed that socioeconomic status probably explains much of the variance that other investigators have attributed to marital status (Warheit et al., 1976).

It has been suggested that the higher rates of institutionalization of psychotic males and their longer hospital stays could be attributed to the fact that the role expectations for males are less tolerant of the behavior associated with mental illness. Furthermore, mentally ill males experience a more prompt and severe social reaction than mentally ill females (Tudor et al., 1977).

Depression

The bulk of evidence not only from clinical observations of patients coming for treatment but also from surveys of persons not under treatment, studies of suicide and suicide attempters, and studies of grief and bereavement indicates that more women than men suffer from depression. Several explanations have been considered:

1. The differences do not represent an artifact in reporting stress and distress; rather, women and men have different help-seeking patterns, with women seeking treatment more often.
2. Men may use alcohol or get into the penal correction system whereas women get medical help.
3. Evidence for genetic and hormonal mechanisms that would produce depression in women but not men is inconsistent at best.
4. The psychosocial milieu contributes to women's excess of depression by virtue of the social discrimination against women and the "learned helplessness" pattern of behavior to which women are socialized.

Furthermore, the incidence of depression may increase among women if the expectations of women rise but the social reality does not change to accommodate these rising expectations (Weissman and Klerman, 1977).

Utilization of health services

Information was obtained during the Health Interview Survey regarding the hospitalization experiences in each household during the year preceding the interview. While there were 16.3 hospital discharges per 100 persons per year for females, there were 11.8 for males. Close inspection of the data shows that the excess of female hospitalizations occurred during the childbearing portion of the life cycle. Although females were hospi-

Table 1-12. Number of physician visits and number of physician visits per person per year, by age and sex: United States, 1978*

Sex	All ages	Under 17 years	17-24 years	25-44 years	45-64 years	65-74 years	75 years and over
Number of physician visits in thousands							
Both sexes	1,016,647	242,441	134,897	266,438	229,439	91,203	52,230
Male	417,278	125,626	45,866	94,604	96,538	35,057	19,587
Female	599,370	116,816	89,030	171,834	132,901	56,145	32,643
Number of physician visits per person per year							
Both sexes	4.8	4.1	4.3	4.7	5.3	6.2	6.4
Male	4.0	4.2	3.0	3.4	4.7	5.5	6.4
Female	5.4	4.0	5.5	5.8	5.9	6.8	6.4

*Data are based on household interviews of the civilian noninstitutionalized population. The survey design, general qualifications, and information on the reliability of the estimates are given in appendix I. Definitions of terms are given in appendix II.
The appropriate relative standard errors of the estimates shown in this table are found in appendix I, figure V.

From Givens, J.: Current estimates from the health interview survey: United States, 1978, Series 10, No. 130, Washington, D.C., Nov. 1979, U.S. Department of Health, Education and Welfare, National Center for Health Statistics.

Table 1-13. Number and percent distribution of office visits by sex, color, and age of patient, according to principal diagnosis: United States, May 1973-April 1974*

Principal diagnosis classified by ICDA category†		Number of visits in thousands	Percent distribution									
				Sex		Color		Age				
			Total	Male	Female	White	All other	Under 15 years	15-24 years	25-44 years	45-64 years	65 years and over
All diagnoses		644,893	100.0	39.3	60.7	89.3	10.7	19.3	15.4	24.7	24.9	15.5
Infective and parasitic diseases	000-136	25,233	100.0	43.6	56.4	88.6	11.4	34.5	20.9	22.3	15.6	6.7
Neoplasms	140-239	12,713	100.0	36.2	63.8	90.5	9.5	—	—	18.2	39.0	31.4
Endocrine, nutritional and metabolic diseases	240-279	26,099	100.0	26.8	73.2	87.1	12.9	—	9.4	30.5	37.7	18.9
Diabetes mellitus	250	8,904	100.0	42.3	57.7	82.9	17.1	—	—	11.8	40.8	43.8
Obesity	277	10,136	100.0	12.3	87.7	88.3	11.7	—	17.0	46.6	31.7	—
Mental disorders	290-315	29,064	100.0	35.8	64.2	91.5	8.5	5.2	12.4	45.0	29.7	7.7
Neuroses	300	16,570	100.0	28.0	72.0	90.9	9.1	2.7	11.4	45.7	32.5	7.7
Diseases of nervous system and sense organs	320-389	50,841	100.0	44.3	55.7	92.9	7.1	27.6	9.7	15.9	26.4	20.4
Diseases and conditions of the eye	360-379	15,248	100.0	39.9	60.1	90.5	9.5	17.7	7.6	9.3	29.5	36.0
Refractive errors	370	9,175	100.0	35.1	64.9	92.6	—	18.8	19.0	17.9	32.7	11.6
Otitis media	381	10,523	100.0	57.5	42.5	94.6	—	72.1	—	—	—	
Diseases of circulatory system	390-458	59,240	100.0	42.1	57.9	88.5	11.5	0.8	1.8	11.0	41.6	44.7
Essential benign hypertension	401	22,752	100.0	35.7	64.3	87.1	12.9	0.6	1.6	11.6	47.6	38.6
Chronic ischemic heart disease	412	15,487	100.0	49.1	50.9	85.8	14.2	—	—	—	40.2	54.9
Diseases of respiratory system	460-519	97,383	100.0	45.8	54.2	88.7	11.3	36.9	14.0	20.3	19.9	9.0
Acute respiratory infections (except influenza)	460-466	50,859	100.0	45.5	54.5	88.8	11.2	44.9	15.6	18.5	15.5	5.5
Influenza	470-474	5,199	100.0	45.8	54.2	76.6	23.4	31.7	19.7	—	—	—
Hay fever	507	12,166	100.0	47.1	52.9	93.0	—	29.7	15.7	29.1	20.6	—
Diseases of digestive system	520-577	23,826	100.0	46.5	53.5	88.7	11.3	7.7	9.9	26.4	34.9	21.2
Diseases of genitourinary system	580-629	37,744	100.0	18.0	82.0	88.6	11.4	3.5	17.9	37.4	28.8	12.5
Diseases of male genital organs	600-607	3,596	100.0	100.0		92.0	8.0	—	—	31.1	33.2	—
Diseases of female genital organs	610-629	21,895	100.0		100.0	86.7	13.3	—	21.2	43.4	29.4	—
Diseases of skin and subcutaneous tissue	680-709	34,099	100.0	43.3	56.7	89.7	10.3	23.4	27.3	21.9	17.0	10.3

*From De Lozier, J. E., and Gagnon, P. O.: National ambulatory medical care survey: 1973 summary—U.S., May 1973-April 1974. In Vital and health statistics, Series 13, No. 21, Washington, D.C., Oct. 1975, U.S. Department of Health, Education and Welfare, National Center for Health Statistics.
†International Classification of Diseases.

talized at greater rates than males, length of stay was shorter for females (7.3 vs 8.7 days for males). Females were also more likely to make dental visits than males (Black, 1977).

During 1976 young adult females also tended to make more physician visits than did their male counterparts; males tended to make more physician visits than females if they were under 17 years of age (Table 1-12).

Preventive care

Data from the Health Interview Survey for 1973 indicate that women tend to have some selected procedures associated with preventive care* performed more often than men. More women respondents than men reported having had eye examinations and glaucoma tests. There were no sex differences for chest X rays, but more men (64.6%) than women (56.8%) had had electrocardiograms.

Three-fourths of the females in the sample had had a Pap smear, with the frequency being greatest in the 25 to 44 year age group and for whites. Three fourths of the women had had breast examinations performed by a physician, with the frequency being highest in the 25 to 44 year age group. On the average, pregnant women had about eleven prenatal visits per pregnancy. Frequency of preventive services increased with socioeconomic status.

Ambulatory care

The National Center for Health Statistics initiated the National Ambulatory Medical Care Survey to provide basic statistics about the public's use of ambulatory medical services in the United States. This survey is based on a continuing national probability sample and is unique in its incorporation of the need for seeking care as expressed in the clients' own words.† In brief, primary care utilization patterns demonstrated that women made 3.7 visits per person, a rate 50% higher than that for males (de Lozier, 1975).

Some explanations for sex differences in morbidity and utilization of health services

From the preceding discussion one gets an image of women as more frequently reporting illness than their male counterparts, more likely to seek preventive as well as therapeutic services, and less likely to be limited in activities from a chronic condition or institutionalized

---

*The procedures studied were believed to be used for the early diagnosis and treatment of illness and disease at early and treatable stages.
†One limitation of the survey is its inclusion of only patient-physician in-office encounters, neglecting the encounters made with primary care professionals, such as nurse practitioners, and those made outside the physician's office.

for mental illness. That women are more fragile than men might be a compelling explanation were it not for the sex differentials observed for mortality. Some alternative explanations for the sex differences in morbidity will be explored in the following pages.

Several explanations have been offered for the differences between men and women in morbidity and health services utilization patterns. These explanations include actual differences between men and women believed to be responsible for differences in illness as well as illness behavior, and problems pertaining to the methods used to study morbidity and utilization.

Differences between women and men in illness and illness behavior

Several differences between men and women have been cited in an attempt to explain the sex differences in illness and illness behavior. These are summarized in the box on pp. 19-20.

Some sex differences may be *biologic* in origin. For example, some of the restrictions in activity that women experience are attributable to childbearing and problems associated with pregnancy. Others suggest that physiologic differences in genetic makeup and hormonal milieu mediate sex differences in illness. Based on differences observed in illness behavior for males and females, some investigators infer that women may experience milder forms of physical and mental illness than men.

Some of the *psychosocial* differences between women and men form the basis of more compelling (though confusing) arguments. Although differences in illness etiology are attributed to women's roles being more stressful than men's, argument to the contrary has been offered. It has also been argued that males are exposed to more health risks than females, yet females report more acute morbidity and higher rates of utilization. It has also been suggested that sex differences in how symptoms are perceived, evaluated, and acted upon (illness behavior) influence the differential reports of both illness and illness behavior. That males are more often limited in carrying on their major roles has been attributed not only to males' roles being more strenuous than those of females, but also to the fact that women more often get diagnosed and treated for acute illness, and consequently suffer less limitation from chronic conditions.

Differences attributable to methods of study

Several difficulties in research methodology may be responsible for the sex differences observed in morbidity and utilization statistics. These include reporting biases introduced by proxy respondents, who are most fre-

Explanations for differences between females and males
in reported morbidity and utilization of health services

I. Differences attributable to differences between females and males
  A. Biologic differences
    1. Differences in illness
      a. Women may have higher prevalence of milder disease, an inference based on the fact that activity limitation for females is less than that for males even though prevalence for some chronic diseases is higher for females (Cole, 1974).
      b. Women may be afflicted with milder forms of mental illness than men because women report more symptoms despite the fact that hospitalization and mortality experiences are more positive than those of men (Cole, 1974).
      c. Females may have greater resistance to degenerative processes because of estrogen (Verbrugge, 1976; Moriyama, Krueger, and Stamler, 1971).
      d. Females have greater resistance to infectious processes than males have (Nathanson, 1977).
    2. Differences in illness behavior
      a. Restrictions in activity for women are in part attributable to deliveries and diseases associated with pregnancy (Cole, 1974).
  B. Psychosocial differences
    1. Differences in etiology
      a. Women's roles are more stressful; therefore they have more illness (Nathanson, 1975). Furthermore, there are several reasons why roles of housewives may induce emotional problems:
        (1) Housewives have no alternative source of gratification as males have outside the family.
        (2) Housework has little prestige and is considered unskilled.
        (3) Housewives have time to brood over their troubles since their work is unstructured and invisible.
        (4) Wives who work probably have less satisfactory jobs than men; therefore, working places more strain on women than on men.
        (5) Role expectations confronting women are diffuse and unclear (Gove and Tudor, 1972).
      b. Females and males are exposed to different physical risks of disease and injury that may account for part of the sex differences in morbidity.
        (1) Females tend to smoke, drink, and drive less than males.
        (2) Females are exposed to fewer occupational hazards than males.
        (3) Social roles of males may be more stressful, causing them to convert stress to physical symptoms or high-risk life-styles (Verbrugge, 1976).
    2. Differences in perception
      a. Females may be more sensitive than males to symptoms of bodily discomforts and more willing to report them (Verbrugge, 1976).
    3. Differences in illness behavior
      a. Women's roles and their predispositions lead to sex differences in how they perceive symptoms, the assessment of their importance, and readiness to take health action (Verbrugge, 1977).
      b. Females are more willing to report less severe conditions than males are (Cole, 1974). Men are more inhibited in reporting some symptoms than women (Mechanic, 1976). Furthermore, it is more socially acceptable for females to report discomfort (Nathanson, 1977).
      c. Women may utilize health services for more minor conditions than men do since their hospital discharge rates are similar for those of men and morbidity rates are known to be higher than those for men at given ages (Cole, 1974).
      d. Females are socialized to take care of themselves when ill rather than continuing their usual activity (Verbrugge, 1975).
      e. Women have more disability from acute conditions but less limitation from chronic conditions than males because they are diagnosed and treated earlier and their roles are less strenuous (Verbrugge, 1976).
      f. Women have fewer role obligations and therefore have more time to be ill than men have; the sick role is more compatible with women's role obligations than with men's (Nathanson, 1975; Rivkin, 1972).
      g. Higher prevalence of males unable to carry on their major activity may be due to their work being heavier than the usual

Continued.

Explanations for differences between females and males in reported morbidity and utilization of health services—cont'd

work for females rather than to any real differences in the health of men and women (Cole, 1974).

II. Differences attributable to methods of study

    A. Most interviews are done with women as "proxy" respondents for their spouses (Cole, 1974).

    B. Females may be, in general, more cooperative during interviews about their health and have better recall of their symptoms and health activities; they may be able to verbalize their complaints better (Verbrugge, 1976). Response bias resulting from perceived trait desirability, need for social approval, and naysaying would increase rather than decrease the sex differences reported in symptoms of mental illness (Clancy and Gove, 1974).

    C. Illness is defined in various ways in surveys, usually as it is experienced rather than as it is diagnosed or observed (Verbrugge, 1976).

    D. Large sex differences in symptomatology are found for subjective distress and psychophysiologic reactions. The behaviors seen more commonly in men, e.g., aggressiveness and violence, are less frequently measured. Furthermore, aggregate measures may be biased if they contain a preponderance of the symptoms most likely to be reported by females. Measures of mental distress need to be broadened to include more of the expressions of distress common to males (Mechanic, 1976).

    E. Morbidity data depend on behavior of individuals affected, so data used to measure sex differences in disease are instead measuring sex differences in symptom-reporting, utilization, or change in activity (Nathanson, 1977).

    F. Disability, as currently measured in surveys, may be more of a social than a physical concept (Mechanic, 1976).

    G. Utilization rates are often examined in the aggregate, rather than examining sex differentials for a given type of morbidity (Mechanic, 1976).

    H. Differences in rates of utilization may reflect *variations* in the following; however, these variables are rarely considered (Mechanic, 1976):

        1. Actual prevalence of symptoms

        2. Willingness to seek help from particular service

        3. Attitudes toward service

        4. Expectations regarding use of services

        5. Social accessibility of service

        6. Alternative services available

        7. Whether use of service is client- or practitioner-initiated (e.g., referral)

        8. Attitudes of practitioners toward men and women

        9. Process of health care for men and women who report same complaints

quently women. Other bias may be introduced by women's greater cooperativeness in interview situations, the way illness is defined in surveys, the kinds of symptoms assessed, behaviors associated with reporting symptoms (such as getting oneself into the health care system), and the numerous uncontrolled variables that can influence utilization rates.

Sex differences in the sick role following critical illness

A comparison of the recovery of fifty male and fifty female open heart surgical patients revealed that men were discharged slightly earlier than women and achieved self-sufficiency in bathing slightly earlier than women did (Brown et al., 1978). The amount of time spent in the recovery room, the amount of time elapsed before ambulation, and the number of pain medications and tranquilizers received were not significantly different for men and women. The authors conclude that the salience of sex-role expectations differs according to the specific sick-role behavior considered. Furthermore, the significance of sex-role expectations in determining the sick-role behavior of a seriously ill group of patients was slight. The authors also point out that although in acute treatment settings the sick role is enacted vis-a-vis health professionals whose attitudes and expectations influence the patient's sick-role behavior, the professional caring for the acutely ill person is more likely than those professionals caring for less ill persons to treat all patients alike (Brown et al., 1978).

Following open heart surgery, men relinquished the sick role more readily than women. There was, however, not a statistically significant difference in the percentage of men and women who returned to performing their usual instrumental roles after surgery. For men, the prime predictors of work performance were the amount of time off work prior to surgery, reports of somatic symptoms, age, functional heart class, and current and preoperative rejection of the sick role. In contrast, the prime predictor for women was awareness of physical symptoms, such that women with somatic symptoms were less apt to resume their preoperative work roles; age, presence of other health problems, and preoperative and current rejection of the sick role were also important determinants. Furthermore, males reported a greater rejection of the sick role prior to surgery; although faced with extremely dangerous surgery, they tended not to admit to poor health and its accompanying dependency, lack of power, and so on. The preoperative tendency to reject the sick role tended to have a surprising relationship to postoperative behavior. Both men and women who accepted the sick role preoperatively were more likely to return to work postoperatively (Brown and Rawlinson, 1977).

THE PARADOX EXPLORED

Having considered the paradoxical relationship between sex differences in mortality versus morbidity and utilization of health services, let us consider some explanations for the paradox. Crucial *biologic differences* between males and females may influence mortality and morbidity at early parts of the life cycle. However, their influence becomes less clear for older age groups where other variables come into play. Hormonal influences may also have some protective effects for females, but investigators of sex mortality differentials concur that the sharp increase in sex differences in mortality during this century cannot be explained by biologic factors. Thus it does not seem plausible that biologic factors are causing men to die at earlier ages than women. Rather, differences in exposure to nonbiologic variables have been implicated. Even if there were marked differences in biologic processes capable of explaining the changes seen in sex mortality differentials in this century, consideration must be given to sociocultural processes to explain the contradictions between women's seeming biologic advantage and their apparently unfavorable morbidity experience. An explanation that simultaneously takes multiple variables into account seems the most appropriate.

Although *social stress* has been suggested as a possible explanation for both the greater male mortality rates and greater female morbidity, this explanation is troublesome on several counts. First, there is controversy about the stressors associated with women's and men's lives: Whose roles are most stressful? Second, there does not seem to be a well-refined theory to account for the mechanisms by which sex differentials influence health. Is there a mechanism that causes males to die from exposure to social stressors and females to report

symptoms and use health services? Are there combinations of types of exposure to stressors and mechanisms of response that are more prevalent among women than men?

Changing *health technologies* may have had some influence on sex differences in mortality, morbidity, and use of health services, though these have not been carefully documented. Reduction in maternal mortality rates would need to be counterbalanced with some consideration of iatrogenic morbidity for females. Thrombophlebitis from birth control pills might provide one example illustrating how a decrease in mortality has been accompanied by an increase in morbidity attributable to changing health technologies.

Differences in *life-styles* have constituted one of the most appealing explanations of the paradox. According to this explanation, the way men and women live their lives is prescribed by the society in which they live and responsible for differences in health experiences. First, the different *norms* regulating women's and men's lives cause them to be exposed to different kinds of risks. Environmental and occupational hazards may account for higher mortality rates for men as well as their greater incidence of accidents and injuries and injury-linked disability. Furthermore, men are socialized to engage in high-risk behavior to a greater extent than women. Some modal personality differences, such as aggressiveness among males, may also predispose men to high-risk behavior and mortality rates. At the same time that societies prescribe exposure to the high-risk of mortality and morbidity, they restrain men from acknowledging illness (translated as weakness), altering their activities to accommodate illness, and seeking health services. Women, on the other hand, are encouraged to be more responsive to perceived illness and to avoid exposure to risks. Women may report more illness than men, therefore, because it is culturally more acceptable for them to do so. Furthermore, it has been argued that women are more able than men to accommodate illness into their other role responsibilities because of the more flexible nature of their roles. Thus the attitudes and activities ascribed to women are more self-protective than those ascribed to men (Nathanson, 1977).

Finally, the paradox may be attributable to ways in which the behavior and attitudes of health practitioners vary with respect to women and men as patients. It is likely that the sex differentials in both morbidity and utilization are influenced by practitioner behavior, as well as that of patients. Thus sex-role expectations held by the practitioner are likely to affect the definition and treatment of complaints presented by women and men. The effects of sex-role expectations held by clinicians may also be augmented by researchers who are inclined to equate "male" with "normal." For example, female utilization is sometimes regarded as "excessive" rather than reflecting what may be "appropriate" use of health services. However appealing, this last explanation is not well documented (see Chapter 3).

In summary, the most credible explanation for the paradoxical relationship between higher mortality rates for males and higher morbidity and utilization rates for females lies in the life-styles characteristic of men and women. It is also important for researchers as well as clinicians to consider the effects on diagnosis and treatment of assumptions about appropriate sex-role behavior for women and men.

DIFFERENCES BETWEEN GROUPS OF WOMEN IN ILLNESS AND ILLNESS BEHAVIOR

Nathanson (1975) suggests that examination of sex differences in health might well be supplemented by an examination of differences in illness and illness behavior between groups of women, and that such research might constitute a test of the models to explain sex differences in illness and illness behavior. She suggests that the following hypotheses be tested: Assuming that sociocultural conditioning is an important determinant of sex differences in illness and illness behavior, women for whom it is most acceptable to report illness (those with traditional, feminine sex-role expectations or norms) should report more symptoms, consult their physicians more frequently, and display more illness behavior. As shown in Table 1-14, the evidence is somewhat, though not universally, supportive of this notion.

A second approach to ascertaining the validity of some explanations for illness behavior is to examine the effects of women's roles on their behavior when ill (Nathanson, 1975). It would be predicted that women whose roles are most compatible with being ill (e.g., least demanding) would be more likely to report symptoms, utilize health services, or assume the sick role than women with more role obligations. The effects of employment on health status and illness behavior are equivocal, as are the effects of proliferation of roles and role demands. Likewise, the effects of employment and role demands on utilization of services reveal no clear trends.

The third hypothesis to be tested would relate stresses and strains associated with women's roles to their health (Nathanson, 1975). While being employed or married does not seem to directly affect mental health, being a mother is associated with more health complaints and fewer episodes of illness.

THE FUTURE: HEALTH OF WOMEN

The health of women in the future is most likely dependent on multiple variables, including changing health technologies, the life-styles that women adopt

(including the influence of social norms, exposure to hazards of the environment, and changes in the modal personality), institutionalized sex-role expectations as they influence health services delivery, and genetic/biologic changes.

Two outcomes from changing health technology are possible. First, improved early detection and treatment methods for diseases of women such as breast cancer may contribute to a longer lifespan and even more favorable sex mortality differentials than exist now. Second, development of health technologies may cause women to experience more iatrogenic mortality and morbidity than they currently encounter. Examples in this century include the appearance of vaginal cancer in DES daughters, and thrombophlebitis and increased risk of death from vascular diseases among women treated with birth control pills. Thus one must carefully weigh the costs with the merits of each development.

Likewise, the life-styles that women will adopt have the potential to improve as well as harm their health. As social norms change to allow equal opportunity for women in the labor force and more emphasis is placed on self-actualization, women may be increasingly exposed to toxic substances and other hazards of the workplace that currently account for work-connected disability and mortality among men. If women adopt health behavior, illness behavior, and sick-role behavior patterns more like those of men, it is possible that the protection once afforded them by use of services or self-care will be a lost advantage. On the other hand, if women maintain their previous patterns of self-care as well as utilization of services, they may be affected to a lesser extent than men by the hazards of the workplace. Furthermore, if sex discrimination in employment is abolished and women have equal opportunity to actualize their ambitions in their place of employment, their mental as well as physical health states may improve. On the other hand, if more women adopt the modal personality patterns currently prevalent among men, such as aggressive competitiveness, the advantages accrued by improved opportunities in the workplace may be erased.

As the current institutionalized sex-role expectations among clinicians are eradicated, the reported female "excess" incidence of some mental illnesses may decrease. However, the symptoms of mental illness reported by women and men may become more similar as sex-role expectations converge. As women's roles more closely approximate those of men (and vice versa) assumptions about appropriate therapies may require revision. For example, prescription of psychotropic drugs might be weighed more carefully for women as their effect on work functions becomes more visible. The self-care movement may make certain contacts with formal health services unnecessary (e.g., women may

Table 1-14. Summary of the literature relating women's norms and roles to health status and illness behavior

Independent variables	Dependent variables	Findings
Norms	Health status	Women who were less traditional in their sex role orientation had higher ego strength scores than those with more traditional norms (Gump, 1972).
		Women with contemporary sex role orientations reported more symptoms related to their mental health than women who had less contemporary norms (Powell and Reznikoff, 1976).
		No clear association existed between sex role norms alone and psychosomatic symptoms. However, women with traditional norms and traditional roles reported high numbers of psychosomatic symptoms more frequently than others. Women with nontraditional norms but who occupied traditional roles expressed protest instead of getting sick. These two responses were mutually exclusive only when the woman was less dependent on the family members, such as the husband (Levy, 1976).
		When controlling for race, education, and role, women with the most traditional sex role orientations reported the most symptoms of mental ill health (Woods, 1978).
	Illness behavior	Women high in familism (concern for the family above all else) tend to more inclined to adopt the sick role than those lower in familism (Geertsen and Gray, 1970).
		Traditional sex role norms predicted a greater likelihood of use of health services for illness among married women (Woods, 1978).
Roles	Health status	Employed women report fewer symptoms than housewives (Feld, 1963; Sharp and Nye, 1963; Finseth, 1975).
		Employment status was not associated with symptom reporting (Pope and McCabe, 1975).
		Depression was severe in one third of women seeking employment (Weissman, 1973).
		Women with least demanding immediate family situation and the most demanding social arenas reported the most morbidity for a 2 week recall period (Rivkin, 1972).
		Wives in a period of transition from outside employment to homemaking or beginning full-time employment from homemaking are under more stress than other women as evidenced by alcohol and drug use, psychiatric impairment, being sick in bed, and number of diseases uncovered on physical examination (Welch and Booth, 1977).
		Women who defined themselves as inadequate wives and mothers were more likely to define their health as poor than those satisfied with their role performance (Cole and Le Jeune, 1972).
		Being a mother was associated with having more symptoms of mental ill health than women's employment or spouse roles (Woods, 1980). The number of roles that the woman performed (including spouse, employee, and mother) had no direct effect on mental ill health (Woods, 1978).
		A positive relationship was found between an index of demanding roles and the number of symptom complexes that women reported. Also poorer socioeconomic status, illness in other family members, and number of children were important in explaining the variance in symptom complex reporting (Woods and Hulka, 1979).
	Illness behavior	Employed women use health services less frequently than homemakers (Finseth, 1975; Pope and McCabe, 1975).
		Employed women tended to use health services more than others, especially employed women who were married, had children, had positive attitudes toward the health care system and used few non-prescription drugs. Employed women were less likely to use disability days (Rivkin, 1972).
		Role proliferation had no direct effect on use of health services for illness (Woods, 1978).
		Number of demanding roles and employment did not influence seeking health care, self-medications, or use of lay referral system when ill. Women who were employed or had an ill child were less likely than their counterparts to cut down on their activity when ill. Women with young children were most likely to consult the lay network (Woods and Hulka, 1979).

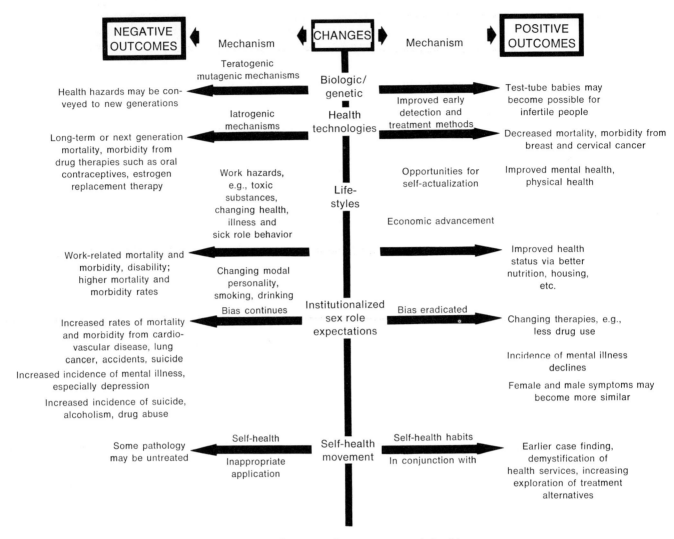

Fig. 1-2. Alternative futures in women's health.

choose to perform their own pelvic examinations and Pap smears rather than having a nurse practitioner or physician do so). This may have both positive and negative effects on women's health. Positive outcomes may accrue from women's improved knowledge of their bodies and accessibility of health services may no longer be a barrier to health maintenance.

Perhaps the single negative outcome of self–health care would be its inappropriate application to problems requiring consultation with those whose expertise is in pathology. As clinicians come to realize that women are knowledgeable about their health, however, social stratification between clinician and client is less likely to influence the process of health care. The de-

mystification of health that brought about the dissemination of health information to women is likely to result in consumers of services who are increasingly able to question decisions about treatment, explore alternative methods of healing, and carefully examine the ramifications of procedures such as surgery, drug therapy, and sterilization.

The change least likely to influence women's health in the future is changing biology. Given current knowledge of genetics, major changes in the human organism are not likely to occur rapidly. However, it is possible that health hazards will impinge on future generations as a consequence of contemporary environmental exposures.

REFERENCES

Aday, L. A.: The utilization of health services: indices and correlates, Springfield, Va., 1972, National Technical Information Service.

Andjelkovic, D., and Taulbee, J.: Mortality of female industrial workers, paper presented at the 104th Annual Meeting of the American Public Health Association, October 19, 1976.

Banks, M. H., and others: Factors influencing demand for primary care in women aged 20–44 years: a preliminary report, Int. J. Epidem. 4(3):189-195, 1975.

Beyond Tomorrow: Trends and Prospects in Medical Science, 75th Anniversary Conference, March 8, 1976, Rockefeller University, 1977.

Black, E.: Current estimates from the Health Interview Survey, United States, 1976, Vital and Health Statistics, Series 10, Number 119, Washington, D.C., Nov. 1977, U.S. Department of Health, Education and Welfare, National Center for Health Statistics.

Brown, J. S., Buchanan, D., and Hsu, L.: Sex differences in sick role behavior during hospitalization after open heart surgery, Res. Nurs. Health 1(1):37-48, 1978.

Brown, J. S., and Rawlinson, M.: Sex differences in sick role rejection and in work performance following cardiac surgery, J. Health Soc. Behav. 18(3):276-292, 1977.

Burbank, F.: U.S. lung cancer death rates begin to rise proportionately more rapidly for females than for males: a dose-response effect? J. Chron. Dis. 25:473-479, 1972.

Cherry, R.: The end of the medicine man. In Tripp, M., editor: Woman in the Year 2000, New York, 1974, Arbor House.

Clancy, K., and Gove, W.: Sex differences in mental illness: an analysis of response bias in self-reports, Am. J. Soc. 80(1):205-216, 1974.

Cole, P.: Morbidity in the United States. In Erhardt, C. L., and Berlin, J. E., editors: Mortality and morbidity in the United States, Cambridge, 1974, Harvard University Press, pp. 65-104.

Cole, S., and Le Jeune, R.: Illness and the legitimization of failure, Am. Soc. Rev. 37:347-356, 1972.

DeLozier, J. E., and Gagnon, R. O.: National Ambulatory Medical Care Survey: 1973 summary: U.S. May 1973-April 1974, Vital and Health Statistics, Series 13, No. 21, Washington, D.C., Oct. 1975, U.S. Department of Health, Education and Welfare, National Center for Health Statistics.

Doherty, E.: Are differential criteria used for men and women psychiatric patients? J. Health Soc. Behav. 19(1):107-116, 1978.

Ehrenreich, B., and English, D.: Complaints and disorders: the sexual politics of sickness, Glass Mountain Pamphlet No. 2, Old Westbury, N.Y., 1973, The Feminist Press.

Erhardt, C. L., and Berlin, J. E., editors: Mortality and morbidity in the United States, Cambridge, 1974, Harvard University Press.

Feld, S.: Feelings of adjustment. In Nye, F. I., and Hoffman, L. W.: The employed mother in America, Chicago, 1963, Rand McNally and Co., pp. 331-352.

Finseth, K., Dallal, G., Lynch, J. T., and Brynjes, S.: Health problems of employed women enrolled in an HMO, presented at American Public Health Association meeting, Nov. 1975.

Fisher, J.: Sex differences in smoking dynamics, J. Health Soc. Behav. 7(2):156-163, 1976.

Geertsen, H. R., and Gray, R. M.: Familistic orientation and inclination toward adopting the sick role, J. Marr. Fam. 32:638, 1970.

Goble, F. C., and Konapka, E. A.: Sex as a factor in infectious disease, Trans. N.Y. Acad. Sci. 2(35):325-346, 1973.

Gove, W.: Sex, marital status and suicide, J. Health Soc. Behav. 13:304-313, 1972a.

Gove, W. R.: The relationship between sex roles, mental illness and marital status, Soc. Forces 51:34-44, 1972b.

Gove, W. R.: Sex, marital status and mortality, Am. J. Soc. 79(1):45-67, 1973.

Gove, W. R., and Hughes, M.: Possible causes of the apparent sex differences in physical health: an empirical investigation, Am. Soc. Rev. 44:126-146, 1979.

Gove, W. R., and Tudor, J. E.: Adult sex roles and mental illness, Am. J. Soc. 78(4):812-835, 1973.

Greenberg, R. P., and Fisher, S.: The relationship between willingness to adopt the sick role and attitudes toward women, J. Chron. Dis. 30:29-37, 1977.

Gump, J. P.: Sex role attitudes and psychological well-being, J. Soc. Issues 28:79-92, 1972.

Hetherington, R., and Hopkins, C.: Symptom sensitivity: its social and cultural correlates, Health Serv. Res. pp. 63-75, Spring 1969.

Hinkle, L., Redmont, R., Plummer, N., and Wolff, H. G.: An examination of the relation between symptoms, disability, and serious illness in two homogeneous groups of men and women, Am. J. Public Health 50(9):1327-1336, 1960.

Howell, M. C.: Employed mothers and their families. I, Pediatrics 52(2):252-263, 1973a.

Howell, M. C.: Effects of maternal employment on the child, Pediatrics 52:327-343, 1973b.

Howie, L. J., and Drury, T. F.: Current estimates from the Health Interview Survey for 1977. Vital and Health Statistics, Series 10, Washington, D.C., Sept. 1978, U.S. Department of Health, Education and Welfare, National Center for Health Statistics.

Jarvis, G., and others: Sex and age patterns in self-injury, J. Health Soc. Behav. 17:146-155, 1976.

Johnson, A.: Recent trends in sex mortality differentials in the United States, J. Human Stress 3(1):22-32, 1977a.

Johnson, A.: Sex differentials in coronary heart disease: the explanatory role of primary risk factors, J. Health Soc. Behav. 19(1):46-54, 1977b.

Johnson, F., and Johnson, C.: Role strain in high-commitment career women, J. Am. Acad. Psych. 4(1):13-36, 1976.

Kitigawa, E. M., and Hauser, P. M.: Differential mortality in the United States: a study in socioeconomic epidemiology, Cambridge, 1973, Harvard University Press.

Kline, C.: The socialization process of women, Gerontologist 15:486-492, 1975.

Ladbrook, D.: Mortality of professional women, paper presented at the 104th Annual Meeting of the American Public Health Association, Women's Caucus, October 20, 1976.

Levy, R.: Psychosomatic symptoms and women's protest: two types of reaction to structural strain in the family, J. Health Soc. Behav. 17:122-134, 1976.

Lillienfeld, A. M., Levin, M. L., and Kessler, I. I.: Cancer in the United States, Cambridge, 1972, Harvard University Press.

Mason, K. O., and Bumpass, L. L.: Women's sex-role ideology, 1970, Am. J. Soc. 80(5):1212-1219, 1970.

McLaughlin, C., and Sheldon, A.: The future and medical care: a health manager's guide to forecasting, Cambridge, Mass., 1974, Ballinger Publishing Co.

Mechanic, D.: Sex, illness, illness behavior, and the use of health services, J. Human Stress 2:29-40, 1976.

Michaels, R. H., and Rogers, K. D.: A sex difference in immunologic responsiveness, Pediatrics 47(1):120-123, 1971.

Monteiro, L.: A comparison of male-female morbidity differentials. In Monteiro, L.: Monitoring health status and medical care, Cambridge, Mass., 1976, Ballinger Publishing Co.

Moriyama, I. M., Krueger, D. E., and Stamler, J.: Cardiovascular diseases in the United States, Cambridge, 1971, Harvard University Press.

Moss, A., and Wilder, M.: Use of selected medical procedures associated with preventive care, United States 1973, Vital and Health

Statistics, Series 10, No. 119, Washington, D.C., Mar. 1977, U.S. Department of Health, Education and Welfare, National Center for Health Statistics.

Naeye, R. L., and others: Neonatal mortality, the male disadvantage, Pediatrics 48(6):902-906, 1971.

Nathanson, C. A.: Illness and the feminine role: a theoretical review, Soc. Sci. Med. 9:57-62, 1975.

Nathanson, C. A.: Sex roles as variables in preventive health behavior, J. Commun. Health 3(2):142-155, Winter 1977a.

Nathanson, C. A.: Sex, illness and medical care: a review of data, theory, and method, Soc. Sci. Med. 2(1):13-25, 1977b.

National Center for Health Statistics: Vital statistics of the United States, Vols. I and II, Washington, D.C., U.S. Government Printing Office.

Phillips, D., and Segal, B.: Sexual status and psychiatric symptoms, Am. Soc. Rev. 34:158-172, 1969.

Pope, C., and McCabe, M.: The employment status of women and their health and well-being, presented at American Public Health Association meeting, Nov. 1975.

Powell, B., and Reznikoff, M.: Role conflict and symptoms of psychological stress in college-educated women, J. Consult. Clin. Psych. 44(3):473-479, 1976.

Poznanski, E. A., Maxey, A., and Marsden, G.: Clinical implication of maternal employment: a review of research, J. Am. Acad. Child Psych. 9:741, 1970.

Pratt, L.: Family structure and effective health behavior: the energized family, Boston, 1976, Houghton-Mifflin Co.

Preston, S. H.: An international comparison of excessive adult mortality, Popul. Studies 24:5-20, Mar. 20, 1970.

Retherford, R. D.: The changing sex differential in mortality, Westport, Conn., 1975, Greenwood Press.

Rivkin, M. O.: Contextual effects of families on female resources to illness, unpublished Ph.D. dissertation, Baltimore, 1972, Johns Hopkins University.

Selby, P.: Health in 1980-1990, a predictive study based on international inquiry, New York, 1974, S. Karger.

Sharp, L. J., and Nye, F. I.: Maternal mental health. In Nye, F. I., and Hoffman, L. W.: The employed mother in America, Chicago, 1963, Rand McNally & Co.

Shuvall, J., Antonovsky, A., and Davies, A. M.: Illness: a mechanism for coping with failure, Soc. Sci. Med. 7:259-265, 1973.

Sinnott, J.: Sex role inconsistency, biology, and successful aging: A dialectical model, Gerontologist 17(5):459-463, 1977.

Spiegelman, M., and Erhardt, C. L.: International comparisons of mortality and longevity. In Erhardt, C. L., and Berlin, J. E., editors: Mortality and morbidity in the United States, Cambridge, Mass., 1974a, Harvard University Press.

Spiegelman, M., and Erhardt, C. L.: Mortality and longevity in the United States. In Erhardt, C. L., and Berlin, J. E., editors: Mortality and morbidity in the United States, Cambridge, Mass., 1974b, Harvard University Press.

Spiegelman, M., and Erhardt, C. L.: Mortality in the United States by Cause. In Erhardt, C. L., and Berlin, J. E., editors: Mortality and morbidity in the United States, Cambridge, Mass., 1974c, Harvard University Press.

Tudor, N. W., Tudor, J., and Gove, W.: The effect of sex roles differences on the social control of mental illness, J. Health Soc. Behav. 18(2):98-112, 1977.

Verbrugge, L.: Females and illness: recent trends in sex differences in the United States, J. Health Soc. Behav. 17:387-403, 1976.

Vernon-Roberts, B.: The effects of steroid hormones on macrophage activity, Int. Rev. Cytol. 25:131-159, 1969.

Waldron, I.: Why do women live longer than men? Soc. Sci. Med. 10:349-362, 1976.

Waldron, I., and others: The coronary prone behavior pattern in employed men and women, J. Human Stress 3:2-18, 1977.

Warheit, G., and others: Sex, marital status, and mental health: a reappraisal, Soc. Forces 55(2):459-469, 1976.

Weissman, M., and others: The educated housewife: mild depression and the search for work, Am. J. Orthopsych. 43:563-573, 1973.

Weissman, M., and Klerman, G.: Sex differences and the epidemiology of depression, Arch. Gen. Psych. 34:98-111, 1977.

Welch, S., and Booth, A.: Employment and health among married with children, Sex Roles 3(4):385-397, 1977.

Wilder, C. S.: Health characteristics of persons with chronic activity limitations, U. S.—1974. In Vital and Health Statistics, Series 10, No. 112, Washington, D.C., Oct. 1976, U.S. Department of Health, Education and Welfare, National Center for Health Statistics.

Wilder, C. S.: Limitations of activity due to chronic conditions, U.S.—1974. In Vital and Health Statistics, Series 10, No. 111, Washington, D.C., June 1977, U.S. Department of Health, Education and Welfare, National Center for Health Statistics.

Wingspread Workshop: Women and development, presented at The Johnson Foundation, Racine, Wis., June 1976.

Woods, N. F.: Women's roles, mental ill health, and illness behavior, unpublished doctoral dissertation, Chapel Hill, 1978, The University of North Carolina.

Woods, N. F., and Hulka, B. S.: Symptom reporting and illness behaviors among married mothers: a comparison of employed women and homemakers, J. Commun. Health 5(1):36-45, 1979.

2

Women as health care providers

Nancy Fugate Woods

The number of women health care providers in the United States would suggest that they control a majority of the health services. Yet this overwhelming majority of the health labor force has little decision-making power. This chapter will examine the distribution of women in the health labor force in the United States, noting the stratification of this sector of the labor force by sex and economic class. Some explanations for stratification of the health labor force will be explored, with special emphasis given to the position of women in nursing. Nursing roots will be examined as a basis for explaining some of the problems nurses encounter today. The chapter will conclude with discussion of strategies for change on both a microsocial and macrosocial level.

WHERE WE ARE NOW
Distribution of women in the United States health labor force

The distribution of women in the United States health labor force for 1970 is illustrated in Fig. 2-1. Even a cursory examination suggests that health is women's work. Over 85% of all health service and hospital workers are women. Nursing is the largest health occupation and is populated almost entirely by female workers.

A more careful examination of the statistics shown in Fig. 2-1 reveals that although there is wide variation among the health occupations in the proportion of women workers, there is apparent segregation by sex. Women are underrepresented as health administrators, pharmacists, physicians, and dentists, but they comprise almost the entire complement of dental assistants, registered nurses, practical nurses, and dietitians. Thus it is not surprising that most of the health occupations could be stereotypically defined as female or male: the statistics reinforce the public image.

As Bullough and Bullough (1975) have noted, "The closer the health occupation is to the level at which decisions are made, the fewer are the women engaged in it and the more dominant the men." (p. 40) If one were

to rank the health occupations according to decision-making power and plot the percentage of women in each, the result would resemble Fig. 2-2. The data speak for themselves.

Disparity of income level is another clearly demonstrable phenomenon. Table 2-1 shows that the median income for the various health occupations varies widely, from high salaries for physicians and dentists to an income falling below the poverty level for some nonnursing health aids, dental assistants, nursing aides, and orderlies (Bullough and Bullough, 1975). Another phenomenon is the pervasive difference in salary for women vs men. When the health occupation is held constant, there is no instance in which the percent of men's salary paid to women reaches 100%; in most instances the salary is substantially less for women. Bullough and Bullough (1975) point out that educational discrepancies may account for the salary differential, yet these are apparent in only a few cases, most notably for health administrators. In most cases differential in median years of schooling does not exceed 1 year.

Stratification in nursing

A more careful look at the nursing sector of the health labor force reveals that not only is it predominantly female, but also it is highly stratified. Comparison of both median income and median number of years of education for registered nurses, practical nurses, nurse's aides, and orderlies confirms that these groups are stratified not only in the hospital hierarchy but also in the broader social milieu. If one also considers nursing administrators as part of the nursing labor force rather than as hospital administrators, the stratification only becomes more profound. Most nursing work is performed in institutional settings, with hospitals and nursing homes as the two primary employers of registered nurses, practical nurses, nurses aides, and orderlies (Fig. 2-3).

There is also sexual stratification within the nursing

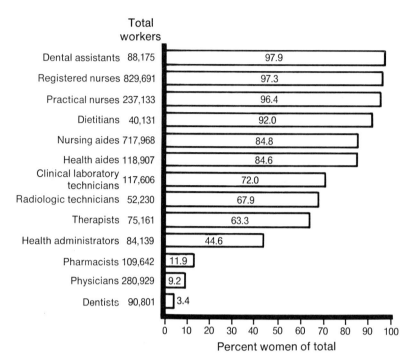

Fig. 2-1. Women workers in selected health occupations, 1970. (From American Public Health Association.)

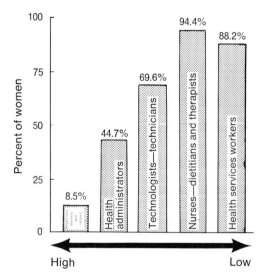

Fig. 2-2. Percentage of women in health work according to their input in decision-making. (Adapted from Bullough, B., and Bullough, V.: Sex discrimination in health care, Nurs. Outlook **23**[1]:40-45, 1975.)

Table 2-1. Income and educational distribution in the health occupations (1970)*

Occupation	Median income (dollars)		Percent of men's salary paid to women	Median school years completed	
	Men	Women		Men	Women
Physicians	25,000+	9,788	39	17+	17+
Dentists	21,687	6,351	29	17+	15.8
Optometrists	17,398	6,455	37	17+	16.8
Veterinarians	16,503	5,641	34	17+	17+
Pharmacists	12,065	5,565	46	16.6	16.4
Chiropractors	11,957	3,985	33	16.8	16.1
Health administrators	12,087	7,149	59	16.1	13.5
Laboratory technicians	7,242	5,560	77	14.7	14.6
Radiologic technicians	8,185	5,017	61	13.0	12.7
Dental hygienists	14,291	5,074	40	12.7	14.9
Health records technicians	5,852	5,687	97	14.5	14.0
Other technicians	6,976	4,473	64	14.6	12.8
Therapists	7,851	5,384	69	16.0	16.3
Registered nurses	7,013	5,603	80	13.5	13.3
Dieticians	6,037	4,462	61	12.7	12.9
Practical nurses	5,745	4,205	73	12.4	12.4
Nonnursing health aides	4,354	3,460	79	12.3	12.3
Dental assistants	4,094	3,405	83	12.6	12.5
Nurse's aides and orderlies	4,401	2,969	67	12.2	11.8

*From Bullough, B., and Bullough, V.: Sex discrimination in health care. Copyright 1975, American Journal of Nursing Co. Reproduced with permission from Nursing Outlook, **23**(1):42, 1975.

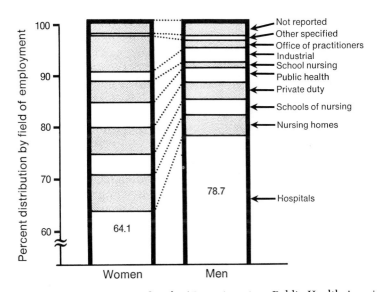

Fig. 2-3. Fields of employment of RN's. (From American Public Health Association.)

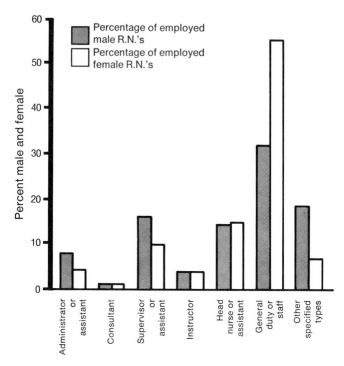

Fig. 2-4. Percent distribution of employed male registered nurses and female registered nurses by type of position, 1972. (From American Public Health Association.)

profession, with a larger proportion of men as administrators or supervisors and women as staff nurses (Fig. 2-4). Although more men appear to be entering nursing, their influence on the salary structure and the sex stratification within nursing remains to be seen.

Bullough and Bullough (1975) suggest that sexual segregation offers women in some of the health occupations little opportunity for mobility, and little incentive for study, research, or improvement of patient care. They observe that "those who are ambitious for advancement tend to leave the bedside and go into nursing education and administration." (p. 42) Because removing themselves from the clinical setting is a mechanism for gaining autonomy, nurses with the greatest career commitment tend to leave direct patient care.

In sum, stratification according to class and sex dictates the type of nursing functions individuals perform. Within the nursing labor force, men are often assigned the intellectual and managerial functions, women the manual labor. The educational preparation of the nursing labor force perpetuates a caste-like division of labor.

The distribution of women in the health labor force led Ehrenreich (1976) to comment:

I can summarize the status of women as health care providers in the U.S. very briefly: It is not good, and it does not look any better by comparison to the situation in other countries.

Whether we measure status in terms of income or in terms of more qualitative factors such as control over one's own work, input into institutional decisionmaking, or societal prestige, we find the same thing: Within the U.S. health industry, women occupy jobs characterized by lower income and less power and prestige than those occupied by males in the health industry, and even within the same job category, women receive lower incomes than men. The only exception to this generalization about sex stratification in the health industry occurs in the case of minority group males, who are concentrated at the very bottom of the occupational hierarchy. This pattern of race and sex stratification within the U.S. health industry has been documented again and again—in tones ranging from academic resignation to feminist outrage. (p. 7)

Some explanations for the status quo

Navarro (1975) comments that the occupational, class, and sex structure in the United States health labor force merely reflects that seen in the competitive sector of the economy. He compares the distribution of health workers by class and sex with the distribution of workers in other sectors of the labor force. Upper middle class men constitute the majority of physicians whereas lower middle and working class women comprise the remaining professionals, and service and clerical workers. Such a distribution of workers cannot be satisfactorily explained by simply examining problems of women;

rather, the distribution of political and economic power of men and women in the society must be examined. Navarro suggests that the social and economic systems controlled by men of defined class backgrounds control the status of working women.

According to Navarro, two socioeconomic factors explain the situation of women in the health labor force: (1) The main determinant of the division of labor in the U.S. economy is the social and economic roles men and women assume in the family. Women are cast in maintenance and reproducer roles, men as producers. Consequently, an employer who pays the producer for the work of one person actually gets the work of two people. (2) The economic utility of having a reserve army of workers probably is responsible for the distribution of women in the health labor force. Women are an exploitable pool of labor: when unemployment is high, they can be discouraged from entering the labor force; when there is a need for this reserve army of workers, (e.g., during World War II), they are available to the economic system.

Reinforcement of the division of labor in the family emanates from all the systems of communication and education in the country. The analogy between the roles of men and women in the family and in the health sector is apparent, with the predominantly female nurses and clerical and service workers being the dependents or appendages of the physician.

The same distribution of power can be seen in the political spheres of society and in health institutions. The boards of trustees of delivery institutions (hospitals) and reproductive institutions (foundations, private medical teaching institutions, and state medical teaching institutions) have a very low representation of women and lower-middle and working class individuals (Navarro, 1975).

Ehrenreich (1976) maintains that one must realize that medicine in the United States is above all a *private business,* loosely regulated and largely left to control itself as is other industry in a capitalist society. She contends that medicine in the United States has evolved over the last 70 years from a "preindustrial phase," characterized by the physician as an individual entrepreneur, to an "industrialized phase," characterized by the increasing centralization of resources in major medical institutions. Ehrenreich identifies several social forces that helped to reproduce sex stratification in the health professions. During the preindustrial phase these factors included:

1. Efforts to limit entry to the medical profession by limiting medical school admissions and lobbying against federal funding for medical school education.
2. Perpetuation of an ideology that the social division

of labor is determined by innate psychologic or physical differences between the sexes. This is not only perpetuated by limiting entrance of women to the professions but also several self-proclaimed experts have established women's presumed inferiority in their writings and public addresses. For example, Dr. Edgar Burman, a former advisor to Senator Hubert Humphrey, declared that women would not be fit for positions of responsibility because of their raging hormonal imbalances; see also Wilson's classic assertion that "the traits that compose the core of female personality are feminine narcissism, masochism and passivity." Ehrenreich points out that such comments were not only self-serving but also have been transformed into scientific fact merely because they were made by supposed men of science.

3. Failure of the government to socialize significant parts of women's work—child raising—has limited women's involvement in certain sectors of the health labor force. Absence of day care facilities has kept women out of occupations requiring lengthy or intensive training. Furthermore, medicine has been quick to point out the "pernicious effects" of day care, thus perpetuating the male dominance in the health labor force by advising against an institution that might undo the sexist division of labor.

Ehrenreich (1976) also identifies two features of the "industrialized phase" of medicine that determined women's status within the health labor force. First, an elaborate division of labor has evolved. *Much of the more costly labor of a multifunctional employee has been replaced with the less costly labor of semiskilled employees.* In the process of the proliferation of health workers, there has been a notable asymmetry in the sex distribution of employees. The cheap labor is female. Second, *planning and intellectual work is concentrated in a group representing a small proportion of the total labor force.* Physicians and administrators represent a decreasing proportion of the health labor force, yet they make major decisions affecting all other workers and the deployment of capital and other resources.

Ehrenreich (1976) contends that we are in the middle of a crisis in the legislation of authority. The rationalization of the work process in the health industry (such that full concentration of control rests in the hands of the hospital executives) cannot be complete for several reasons. First, hospital work is inherently unpredictable. People simply do not need services on a predictable schedule. Second, the material is human beings, which means that all the knowledge about the work process for the patient cannot be concentrated in any single individual. Instead all health workers are interdependent. Third, hospital workers tend to be highly motivated to provide good care. Thus, Ehrenreich concludes, it will never be possible to separate the intellectual from the manual effort, and workers who have little authority may make a greater contribution to the work process than do managerial level personnel. This leads to a crisis in the legitimization of authority. In the past, sex and race stratification of health workers made the authority structure appear natural. Yet, changes in the fabric of society seem to predict that the "natural" authority structure—white males at the top of the labor pyramid and females and minorities at the bottom—cannot persist.

Levitt (1977) agrees that the male domination in the health sector simply mirrors the division of political, economic, and social power in the American capitalist society. The differentiation of occupation by sex was reinforced as scientific medicine became the dominant mode of medical practice, with specialization, acute in-hospital therapy, high-level technology and drug therapy and surgery given first priority.

The Flexner report,* which legitimized the practice of scientific medicine, recommended closing several medical schools, among them those that trained women and blacks. The remaining programs required 4 years of expensive training, thus eliminating less wealthy students. Not only did the changing structure of medical education eliminate women and persons from the middle and lower classes, but it also fostered the production of fewer physicians. At the same time that highly specialized practices developed, women were stratified again—this time into areas such as pediatrics and psychiatry. The nature of scientific medicine seems to reproduce social stratification by sex, class, and race. Levitt asserts that while this is the case, changing the sex, class, and race differential is not the sole solution (or may be only a partial solution). We need an inquiry into the nature of medical practice to determine what is the best mode of health care and what will lead to better health.

Brown's analysis (1975) of the status of women in the health service industry suggests that "health service is women's work, but not women's power." Women are hired as health service workers because a labor force of women can be paid less than a similar labor force of men. Because it is also assumed that women are dedicated to service and will drop out of the labor force to raise children, the need for high salaries and promotions is precluded. Women are also readily available as a major

reservoir of unemployed persons. They are safe: it is believed that women are subordinates and will remain subordinates. Brown points out that many women acknowledge entering the health services because they want to help people and that caring for others is seen as women's work by society. Yet it could be argued that other higher paid health professionals help the sick, too.

Why, then, are women willing to accept low-paying subordinate positions? The answer, according to Brown, is that the economic opportunities available to women elsewhere are very limited compared to their occupational opportunities inside the health sector: women are actually paid much better in some of the health occupations. Furthermore, entry into the health labor force provides women with some skills that they can use now and in the future.

Brown contends that the current system is maintained by several mechanisms. Each health occupation (other than the unskilled) has a separate training program and entry criteria that lead to licensure or registration, and each has a professional society. The health professions, unlike the crafts, have rigid barriers between levels and rigid hierarchy. The top occupation—medicine—controls many other female occupations. Medicine has representation on the Joint Commission for Accreditation of Hospitals (JCAH), the American Hospital Association, and through the American Medical Association, the American Association of Medical Colleges, and the Commission on Medical Education medicine is able to control the creation of new health occupations and the division of labor. Support for physician control of the system is gained from universities, state legislatures, federal funding agencies, and government regulations. Only nursing seems to have escaped control of its own profession by physicians, yet the American Nurses Association and the National League for Nursing have no voice on the Joint Commission on Accreditation of Hospitals. Brown points out that the formal controls over the health workers are reinforced by the interpersonal relations at the work site, e.g., employer and employee, supervisor and supervised. Rank is maintained (as in the military) by uniforms and name tags listing the person's job. Professional training often reinforces the supremacy of the physician. Until recent times, nursing students were socialized to "know their place" in the hierarchy; the functions in which nurses are dependent on physician input (often called "orders") have been emphasized in nursing curricula to the exclusion of their independent functions.

In sum, several factors appear to maintain the current distribution of women in the health services occupations:

1. Distribution of roles in the family in this society, which creates the economic advantage of getting

---

*The Flexner Report (1910) (Medical Education in the United States and Canada) was an ostensible attempt to rate the existing medical schools according to their educational quality. Its consequences led to the closure of schools that did not meet their criteria.

an employee (producer) and wife (reproducer and maintainer) for one salary

2. Economic utility of having women as a reserve army of workers
3. Past efforts to limit the entry of women to some health professions
4. Failure of the government to socialize significant parts of women's work (e.g., child care)
5. Emphasis on practice of scientific medicine, which requires intensive and long-term training
6. Underrepresentation of women in policy-making groups, such as hospital boards of trustees

Women maintain their current positions in the health labor force for several reasons.

1. Their employment opportunities outside the health labor force are limited
2. They can acquire some skills for jobs that can be integrated with their other roles
3. They can make an important contribution to society
4. Their work is regarded as "women's work" by society

We have examined women's place in the health services and those factors that maintain the status quo. In the next section we will examine "nursing roots" in an effort to understand how modern nursing has been influenced by its history.

NURSING ROOTS: HOW WE GOT HERE

No other health profession has been shaped by the socialization of women to the same extent as the nursing profession. Although more men are attracted to the profession now than ever before, women constitute nearly 98% of the nursing labor force. As a result, the fate of women in society has been—and is—the fate of the nursing profession.

Education for women: effects on health

Examination of medical writings of the nineteenth century indicates that education for women was believed to be hazardous to their health. Hamilton (1885) wrote that "the best education for girls, then, is that which best prepares them for the legitimate duties of womanhood." He further asserted that attainment of high intellectual culture exacts too great a price and results in a "ruined or physically damaged constitution." Hamilton based his theory about education for women on a set of assumptions about physical and intellectual differences between the sexes. With respect to women, he asserted:

Extreme nervous impressibility; the strong reflex movements from the sexual system upon the intellectual nerve-centres, in health and disease; the notable lack of the logical faculty, as well as muscular power, show conclusively that the require-

ments in the education of the female are widely different from the opposite sex.

Hamilton proceeded to describe how "brain work" competes with the "vital forces of the body," and that such a diversion of "nerve power" to the mental labor involved in education could only lead to "greatly impaired or permanently ruined health, a life of sterility, general unhappiness, and uselessness." Hamilton went on to assert that the educational system is intrinsically faulty for it ignores the fact that girls cannot work effectively or safely during the menstrual period, and yet "co-education requires of them, during this period of disability, the same work exacted from the boys, who are not so disabled."

Such an explanation for women's supposed inability to survive educational experiences similar to those available to men and *still* be capable of reproducing is an example of how medical "science" has been used to justify exclusion of women from higher education. Of course, it would follow that the rigorous requirements of medical education would be hazardous to women's health! Such assumptions, then, were the basis for encouraging women to pursue work for which they were "naturally" suited and that required less rigorous education than that required for "male" professions.

Nineteenth century

During most of the nineteenth century there was not an organized nursing labor force in the United States. In the early part of the century most of the population was living in rural areas, and nursing care was performed on an informal basis by residents of the community. Indeed, Bellevue Hospital in New York City, the first institution solely dedicated to care of the sick, did not open until 1848. By the beginning of the Civil War, some efforts were being made to provide women with improved obstetric and gynecologic care. In 1860 the New England Female Medical College started a nursing school, and in 1861 the Women's Medical College of Philadelphia began their nursing program.

The Civil War demanded a large number of nurses, but they were largely untrained and most were male. Dorothea Dix enlisted the assistance of Elizabeth Blackwell, the first woman doctor to graduate from an American medical school, to help her train over 2,000 nurse volunteers. It has been suggested that the Civil War provided some women opportunities for leadership and gave them experience in educating nurses. Two types of efforts to increase the number of nurses were apparent following the Civil War. First, upper-class urban women interested in urban reform were instrumental in organizing Nightingale schools, such as Bellevue and Johns Hopkins. The image projected by nurses from these schools suggested that nursing could be a socially acceptable alternative to motherhood. As the need for nurses increased, a second source of nurses was tapped: working class women who had to work to earn a living.

The increase in the number of nursing schools for the 20 years from 1880 to 1900 is given below:

Year	Number of schools	Enrollment
1880	15	323
1890	35	1,552
1900	432	11,164

At the same time, the number of hospitals increased rapidly. Financial difficulties forced independent nursing schools to either close their doors or merge with hospitals. "The hospitals were willing to finance these schools, and also to establish new schools in return for their right to use the labor of the student nurses in their wards as well as the "private duty" services in the homes of the patrons of the hospitals." (Cannings and Lazonick, 1975; p. 193) As the Goldmark report* revealed, the integration of nursing schools with hospitals transferred a great degree of control from the nursing educators to the hospital and its superintendents.

In the late nineteenth century, the American Society of Superintendents of Training Schools of the United States and Canada was formed to oversee nursing education. In 1912 it became the National League of Nursing Education, now known as the National League for Nursing. In 1894, the professional organization for graduate nurses was formed: the Nurses Associated Alumnae of the United States and Canada. (This organization later was renamed the American Nurses Association.) The American Nurses Association began publishing the *American Journal of Nursing* in 1900 and encouraged registration of professional nurses. The nursing registration laws that were passed early in the twentieth century gave nursing some control over both education and practice.

One of the most important social structures to influence modern nursing was the hospital training school. A contractual agreement existed between the early nursing schools and the hospitals: The hospital ensured the use of its facilities for educational purposes. Learning by apprenticeship was the mode used in the Nightingale schools, along with instruction in scientific principles and practice of skills. Because the hospital schools in the United States did not have private endowments to ensure their financial backing, they agreed to give

---

*The Goldmark Report, officially entitled "Nursing and Nursing Education in the United States," was published in 1923. It revealed that there was a neglect of public health; that many schools had inadequately prepared faculty, deficient facilities, and unstandardized curricula; and that the chief nurse of the hospital was often also the head of the school of nursing (Deloughery, 1977).

nursing service to the hospitals that provided clinical experience for their students. Such an agreement encouraged the establishment of hospital schools of nursing. The situation that ensued is described by Ashley (1976): "The hospital was the master and the student was the apprentice, with the latter giving free labor to the former in return for informal training in the traditional manner." (p. 9) Ashley documents how the paternalistic system exploited the labor of students and led them to believe they were inferior and must remain subordinate to the medical profession. The educational system did not encourage students to question but rather to accept the status quo.

Thus the economic system of the hospital school mediated toward long hours of ward duty: the young nurses were not so much students as laborers. Students not only worked long hours but also were "allowed" to attend lectures only when it would not interfere with their duties. Often the medical profession expressed concern that nursing students were becoming overeducated. Thus control of information became an important tactic in reinforcing the sex stratification in the hospital family. Nurses were socialized to respond to "orders" from the physician and to stand when a physician entered the room, offer him her chair, or hold the door open for him (Ashley, 1976).

Early twentieth century

Nursing leaders, socialized in such schools, were not very radical. Lavinia Dock, a radical feminist, urged the profession to confront its predicament as early as 1903. She warned of the threat of male dominance of the nursing profession and urged nurses to recognize and use their powers. Instead, the profession identified with hospital development and sought the approval of hospital administrators and physicians rather than working toward their own liberation and establishing their own power base. Most members of the professional organization did not identify with the feminist movement or with the movement for women's suffrage. It is not surprising that the laws enacted to govern nursing practice merely gave public sanction to nurses' inequality and legitimized their subjection to the authority of the physician.

In the first three decades of the twentieth century the number of schools of nursing and the number of nurses expanded rapidly. Most nurses provided care for people in their homes and were referred patients by nursing registries or by physicians. During the 1920s and 1930s most nurses practiced in private duty. Only about 20% practiced in public health nursing and another 20% in institutions. Most hospitals found their labor supply in the numerous students enrolled in their nursing programs, and those without such programs hired cheap sources of labor—untrained workers.

While the Goldmark report recommended the definition and licensure of a subsidiary type of nursing service to work under the direction of a physician (practical nurses), the report also recommended that control over hospital education be given to educators affiliated with universities. This would have encouraged the transfer of power from the hospital hierarchy to the university.

Changing economic pressures reflecting the depression of the United States economy also influenced nursing. There were fewer demands for health services, and finally the ANA supported an 8-hour vs a 12-hour work day in order to share the work. During the Depression years, fewer private duty nurses were employed, and the number of nursing schools rapidly decreased.

In the 1930s, nursing practice shifted from the home of the patient to the hospital. Although childbirth experience was moved to the hospital from the home, this alone did not account for the shift in where nurses practiced. Cannings and Lazonick (1975) suggest that the change was partly attributable to the "development of capital-intensive medical techniques" that required centralization, but probably more important to the development of hospitals were insurance groups to bail out the hospitals that lacked paying patients. The number of graduate nurses employed in hospitals rose sharply, so that by the end of the 1930s, institutional nursing had replaced private duty nursing as the first employment category; public health nursing took third place.

As both registered nurses and practical nurses moved into the hospital setting, the hierarchy between them developed. The ANA rationalized the hierarchy, and licensing boards for practical nurses developed. During the 1940s there was a great expansion in the third group of hospital personnel—nursing aides. And so the groundwork for the Ginzberg principle: "Never use high-priced personnel for low-priced work." (Quoted in Cannings and Lazonick, 1975; p. 201.) Such a hierarchy within the nursing labor force seems to replicate the sex and race stratification seen in the rest of the health sector and has persisted to this day.

Nursing in the 1970s

Fitzpatrick (1977) contends that "of all the predominantly women's professions, nursing is perhaps the least understood and most ignored by those who champion the cause of equality for women." (p. 818) She continues to argue that because nursing epitomizes many of the characteristics and problems from which many women are attempting to dissociate, the women's movement has advanced entry of women into other professions and not supported their sisters in nursing.

Nursing education, whether in a hospital or a uni-

versity system, remains dominated by men: administrators of hospitals and universities, and their respective board of trustees, are predominantly male. In order to observe the allocation of resources in such systems, one has only to visit a campus or health (usually labeled medical) center and compare the physical facilities allocated to nursing and medicine (Grissom and Spengler, 1976).

Within many nursing programs, there are often few faculty role models to assist students; many nursing faculty conform to and perpetuate the feminine stereotype. Students are often not encouraged to be inquisitive or to challenge the status quo. For example, some nursing faculty do not believe that a discussion of the women's movement is an important part of their students' education.

Although most baccalaureate programs emphasize the autonomy of the profession, students experience a disparity between their expectations and the reality in most practice settings. Kramer's (1975) study emphasizes disenchantment that baccalaureate graduates experience as they discover the ways in which the health care system really works. Kramer recommends that nursing educators prepare students for the reality of the physician-dominated health care system, at the same time they are attempting to produce creative, independent agents of change.

As early as 1899 Teachers College, Columbia University, opened a program to prepare teachers of nursing and nursing service administrators; the first university-sponsored basic nursing program was opened in 1909 at the University of Minnesota. However, the American Nurses Association did not take a position with respect to levels of preparation of its professional practitioners until 1965. Following World War II, 2-year technical programs in nursing were introduced. However, the profession did not seem to be ready for this innovation. Baccalaureate, diploma, and associate degree prepared nurses all took the same licensure examinations and were hired for similar jobs in hospitals.

The 1965 Position Paper of the American Nurses Association advanced two levels of preparation for nurses: the associate degree for technical practice and the bachelor's degree for professional practice. At this writing three state nursing associations advocate legislation mandating a baccalaureate degree for entry into professional practice (Ohio, New York and Washington). Rather than fostering unity in the nursing labor force, these actions resulted in the competition among varying factions. Such competition has not only diluted the power inherent in the profession's numbers, but also limited the extent to which the profession can take a unified stand on many health issues.

During the 1970s several major changes occurred in the nursing profession:

1. Expanded roles offering increased autonomy became a reality as nurses pursued clinical specialization in hospital and community settings. The nurse practitioner movement legitimized roles for nurses in primary care.
2. Delivery of primary health care became increasingly valued. Nursing was described more often as health care rather than as illness care.
3. Doctoral education for nurses in the discipline of nursing became a reality.
4. Nursing became aware of its public image and began to make efforts to interpret nursing to the public.
5. Consumer input in planning nursing services was invited.
6. Nursing became a political force with a united political action body.

Nursing must confront several unresolved problems during the 1980s:

1. The struggle over professional domains will persist. Whether the practice of nursing can be truly interdependent with medicine remains to be seen.
2. The nursing labor force remains divided along educational and hierarchial lines, leaving it vulnerable to co-optation and diluting the strength of its numbers. The current debate over educational preparation for entry into nursing practice has the potential to unify the profession. If much energy is devoted to resisting change, however, there will be little energy remaining to exert political power in the sociopolitical arena.
3. The image of nursing held by the society as a whole still requires clarification if the public is to comprehend the range of health services nurses provide.
4. Society is slow in accepting the value of preventive health practices, and even slower to reimburse nurses for this type of care. The future of nursing will be closely tied to the policies for third party payment in both the private and the public sectors. Unless preventive and health maintenance services are provided for a national health plan, provision of nursing services may be limited to illness care.
5. Nursing as a discipline will continue to struggle for its place in academia. During the 1980s, nursing will have to contend with political and economic forces that threaten graduate education and the simultaneous challenge of providing doctoral education to the first generation of nursing Ph.D.'s.

STRATEGIES FOR CHANGE

Although the preceding discussion might suggest that the system of sex stratification among health care providers and the resultant stereotyping of nursing roles will persist, some have suggested strategies for change at both the micro- and macrosocial level. Change in the manner in which workers in the health labor force relate to one another will be explored as examples of strategies for microsocial change. Changes in the health care system and parts of the society as a whole will be discussed as examples of macrosocial change.

Microsocial strategies for change

A great deal of attention has been devoted to the study of ways in which members of the health labor force relate to one another. In particular, the interreactions between nurses and physicians have been shown to occur within a prescribed set of norms. One of the best known examples of these norms is the institution called "the doctor-nurse game" (Stein, 1967). The doctor-nurse game, which Stein classifies as a transactional neurosis, is based on the pretense that all decisions made about patient care are made by physicians. This, of course, cannot be true inasmuch as physicians are not present when most of patient care is given. Therefore, when nurses make a major decision they handle the situation by involving the physician and attempting to convince him that it was his idea.

Let us suppose that the physician has written a medication order that is inappropriate. The following statements might be made by the nurse in this situation:

Doctor, you have made an error.
Doctor, would you like to check this order?
Doctor, you always write such legible, appropriate orders, but
    if you have time, I wonder if you would clarify this order?
I'm so dense, I don't understand this order.

In 1974, a group of 103 hospital nurses and 40 physicians in California were given a questionnaire that included this item. None of the nurses sampled selected the first alternative, 56% chose the second, 41% the third, and 3% the last alternative. The same question was given to the physicians, and they were asked which of the responses they would prefer. Eleven percent chose the first, 86% the second, and 3% the third. No one chose the last option. When this as well as other items on the questionnaire were tabulated, it was found that nurses tended to choose indirect responses, suggestive of a certain amount of feminine gamesmanship; on the other hand, physicians preferred direct responses, especially those physicians who were younger (Bullough, 1975).

Such self-effacing communication as illustrated by nurses in the doctor-nurse game has been shown to reinforce the notion that the physician is the decision-maker, at the expense of nurses' ability to utilize their powers of assessment and decision-making. The physician also loses at this game inasmuch as he loses the opportunity to request direct feedback in a system where he is expected to be omnipotent. Moscato (1976) suggests that supervision, support, and self-exploration are mechanisms available to help nurses explore alternatives to the doctor-nurse game.

Supervision

Intradisciplinary supervision by a clinical specialist or other mentor can provide a role model for nurses by exposing them to new ways of relating to other professionals. The supervisory relationship can foster acquisition by nurses of new knowledge and skills with which to intervene, as well as facilitate their analytic skills, which they can then use to determine when and if the traditional caretaking roles are appropriate.

Support

Both *administrative* and *peer support* can be helpful in eliminating sex-role stereotyping from nursing practice (Moscato, 1976). The stance taken by nursing administration, including day-to-day practices as well as formal statements of philosophy, can reinforce or sabotage an atmosphere in which nurses can be exposed to intellectual and emotional resources. Measures to help nurses maintain their abilities and talents, such as workshops and training sessions, can foster professional development. Moscato (1976) points out that "too often the doctor-nurse game is played out between nursing administration and medical staff, while the new staff nurse is sacrificed and leaves the setting fatigued by 'playing it straight'!"

Rather than competing with one another, nurse colleagues can support one another (Moscato, 1976). Sharing of information and skills, as well as collaborating in the evolution of ideas, can create an atmosphere in which nurses can benefit from others' abilities and simultaneously obtain validation of their own abilities.

Self-exploration

Self-assessment, self-exploration, and growth can be fostered through individual activities such as reading, analyzing, and evaluating current sex-role issues. In addition, participation in a consciousness-raising group may foster a personal awareness of the causes and consequences of sex-role stereotyping, as well as alternative behaviors. Nursing education could provide "freeing educative experiences" that can help undo some of the traditional sex-role programming of its students (Moscato, 1976).

Education

Many schools of nursing are involved in consciousness-raising efforts on behalf of their students and are helping them become more assertive in their dealing with other health professionals. Nurses are also seeking advanced academic preparation, with many enrolled in masters and doctoral programs in an effort to improve the knowledge base of the profession. In some instances, nurses are pursuing advanced degrees in administration; subsequently they will influence the climate of the system by assuming positions as hospital administrators as well as top level nursing service administrators.

Continuing education programs are providing assertiveness training for graduates. Baccalaureate students in some schools are introduced to information on sex-role stereotyping and sexism in the health care system and the effects on nursing practice. Self-help and support groups for nursing students have become increasingly common. In some programs, faculty attempt to serve as role models for nonsexist behavior, modeling for students the ability to communicate directly, to be supportive, and to value other women.

Professional consciousness-raising

Wilma Scott Heide (1973), a past president of National Organization for Women (NOW) and a nurse, found it necessary to "leave nursing or suffocate psychologically." She sees many of the problems of nursing as symptoms of the oppression of women. For example, oppressed persons often find it safer to challenge others who are oppressed rather than those who are powerful. As a result, the struggles within and among oppressed groups lock them in internal power struggles when the real power lies elsewhere. Heide contends that nurses and nursing can be "leaders in bringing about a humanist society." Nursing, by engaging in a massive consciousness-raising effort, can affect not only the relations between two professions but also can assist in humanizing health care.

Macrosocial strategies for change

Several scholars of the United States health system have recommended strategies for change that involve not only efforts of a single profession, but also a reconceptualization of health and its relationship to the structure of society. Indeed, some hold out little hope for humanizing the system unless the basic assumptions of a capitalist health care system are challenged. Three strategies targeted at large institutions include: (1) changing the hierarchy within the health care system; (2) organizing workers to produce a change in the system of care itself; and (3) changing the economic structure of the system.

Changing the hierarchy: democracy in the health institutions

Ehrenreich (1975) attributes the increasing willingness of nurses to organize themselves as workers and to take job actions in order to win their demands to the rising feminist consciousness in the United States. She suggests that as the number of women in medicine grows, and as the women in health care become more militant, "sex differences will cease to be the automatic rationale for occupational stratification, and *sex defer-ence* [italics provided] will cease to be a palliative for class antagonism." (p. 12) Ehrenreich also predicts that we are probably entering a period during which the hierarchic divisions among women workers may consti-tute the greatest barrier to change. She cautions that such hierarchic divisions can lead to "a sterile profes-sionalism which uses the banner of feminism to advance the status of a particular occupational group." (p. 12) In sum, Ehrenreich recommends that we not devote so much effort to changing women's place in the hier-archy as to changing the hierarchy itself.

Navarro (1975) is somewhat less than optimistic about the possibility of changing the class and sex structure of the labor force in the health sector, observing that class loyalties appear to be far stronger than sex loyalties. For example, women elected to boards of trustees may behave similarly to their male colleagues and neglect the constituency of women they supposedly represent. Yet, it is apparent that for the status of women in the health occupations to improve, changes in the sex and class composition of those who govern the health sector and its institutions is essential. Navarro stipulates that one condition for liberating the majority of the women now in the labor force is the implementation of insti-tutional democracy in the health sector. The health institutions need to be controlled not only by those who work in them, but also by those who are served by them. The mere presence of women in positions of power would not be sufficient. Indeed, these wom-en must be representative of and accountable to all workers in the health sector, regardless of sex, race, or class.

Organizing workers

Brown's (1975) analysis would suggest that unionism as well as solidarity among the health occupations will be limited by the disinclination of different racial and sex groups to unite. Nursing, because of its strength of numbers and growing militancy, can risk such action; after all, in many instances there is not much to lose. The larger society, however, responds negatively to job ac-tions by hospital workers. Brown suggests that this is likely a response to the sex and race of the workers, rather than their sector of employment. Professionalism is often held out to health sector workers as the antith-esis to unionism. Yet many of the professional organi-zations (including ANA) are now engaged in collective bargaining and have economic and general welfare pro-grams for their workers.

Struggles against sexism and racism will require co-operation among various segments of the health labor force. Professionalism can be used as a mechanism for humanizing health care and relations between pro-viders of health care rather than as a mechanism for furthering racism and sexism in the hospital family.

Cannings and Lazonick (1975) suggest that restructur-ing the health care delivery system requires organization not only of consumer groups but also of worker groups. In the latter area, the nursing labor force is in a position of potential power. The divisions among the nursing labor force, however, must be overcome if a movement for better health services is to be successful. The authors point out that a movement for more worker control of the health industry is essential to the improvement of services. The increasing involvement of nursing in the direct delivery of services and their concentration in large institutions sets the stage for nursing workers to be instrumental in revolutionizing health services. The increasing commitment of nurses to remaining in the labor force and their strong commitment to changing the conditions for providing health care provide needed strength for a radical restructuring of the system of health care.

Changing the economic structure of the system

Cannings and Lazonick (1975) conclude that the status of women in health care and the revolutionary changes needed in the health care system cannot be considered without regard for the economic system in which it exists. Although the feminist movement may help unite health workers, it is not sufficient. "If any steps are to be of lasting significance, this consciousness itself must be developed into a socialist perspective on the delivery of health care and its relation to the rest of the capitalist system." (p. 214)

Levitt's (1977) analysis leads her to similar conclu-sions. She concludes that "we need to change both the sex differential in the provision of health care and the mode of practice of medicine to which it is tied." (p. 397) This would involve a greater emphasis on primary care and prevention of illness, less on the acute medical care and the medical-industrial complex.

REFERENCES

American Public Health Association: Women in health careers: chart book for International Conference on Women and Health, Wash-ington, D.C., June 16-18, 1975, Washington, D.C., Mar. 1976, The Association.

Ashely, J.: Hospitals, paternalism and the role of the nurse, New York, 1976, Teachers College Press.

Ashley, J.: Nurses in American history: nursing and early feminism, Am. J. Nurs. 75(9):1465-1467, 1975.

Ashley, J.: Nursing roots: impact on role change, paper presented at the Northwest Area Health Education Center Workshop, Winston-Salem, N.C., April 20, 1978.

Brown, C.: Women workers in the health service industry, Int. J. Health Serv. **5**(2):173-184, 1975.

Brown, C.: Roles for women health workers in the United States and China, Women Health **1**(2):11-13, Mar.-Apr. 1976.

Bullough, B.: Barriers to the nurse practitioner movement: problems of women in a woman's field, Int. J. Health Serv. **5**(2):225-233, 1975.

Bullough, B., and Bullough, V.: Sex discrimination in health care, Nurs. Outlook **23**(1):40-45, 1975.

Campbell, R.: California Nurse's Association, San Francisco, Minority Group Task Force, Minorities in Nursing, Jan., 1973.

Cannings, K., and Lazonick, W.: The development of the nursing labor forces in the United States: a basic analysis, Int. J. Health Serv. Res. **5**(2):185-216, 1975.

Clarke, E. H.: Sex in education; or a fair chance for girls, Boston, 1873, James R. Osgood and Co.

Cleland, V.: Sex discrimination: nursing's most pervasive problem, Am. J. Nurs. **71**(8):1542-1547, 1971.

Deloughery, G.: History and trends of professional nursing, St. Louis, 1977, The C. V. Mosby Co.

Edelstein, R. G.: Equal rights for women: perspectives, Am. J. Nurs. **71**(2):294-298, 1971.

Ehrenreich, B.: Health care industry: a theory of industrial medicine, Soc. Policy **6**(3):4-11, 1975.

Ehrenreich, B.: The status of women as health providers in the United States. In Proceedings of the International Conference on Women in Health, June 16-18, 1975, DHEW Pub. No. (HRA) 76-51, Washington, D.C., 1976, U.S. Department of Health, Education and Welfare, pp. 7-13.

Ehrenreich, B., and English, D.: Witches, midwives and nurses, Old Westbury, N.Y., 1973, The Feminist Press.

Epstein, C. F.: Woman's place: options and limits in professional careers, Berkeley, 1970, University of California Press.

Fitzpatrick, M. L.: Nursing, Signs **2**(4):818-834, Summer, 1977.

Grissom, M., and Spengler, C.: Woman power and health care, Boston, 1976, Little, Brown & Co.

Hamilton, S. H.: Female education from a medical standpoint, J.A.M.A., Sept. 19, 1885, pp. 318-320.

Heide, W. S.: Nursing and women's liberation: a parallel, Am. J. Nurs. **73**(5):824-827, 1973.

Howell, M. C.: A women's health school? Soc. Policy **6**(2):50-53, 1975.

Kramer, M.: Reality shock—why nurses leave nursing, St. Louis, 1975, The C. V. Mosby Co.

Levitt, J.: Men and women as providers of health care, Soc. Sci. Med. **11**:395-398, 1977.

Moscato, B.: The traditional nurse-physician relationship: a perpetuation of sexual stereotyping. In Kneisl, C., and Wilson, H. S., editors: Current perspectives in psychiatric nursing: issues and trends, St. Louis, 1976, The C. V. Mosby Co.

Navarro, V.: Women in health care, N. Engl. J. Med. **292**(8):398-402, 1975.

Piradova, M. D.: USSR—women health workers, Women Health **1**(2):24-29, May/June, 1976.

Proceedings of the International Conference on Women in Health, Washington, D.C., June 16-18, 1975, DHEW Pub. No. 76-51, HRA/OC-77-020, MacLean, Va., June 1975, Mitre Corp.

Reverby, S.: Health: women's work, Health/PAC Bull. **40**(15):20, 1972.

Stein, L.: The doctor-nurse game, Arch. Gen. Psych. **16**:699-703, 1967.

Women's work project of the union for radical political economics. USA—women health workers, Women Health **1**(3):14-23, 1976.

3

Women and health care

Nancy Fugate Woods

Increasingly, women are voicing dissatisfaction with health care. They not only have delineated the inadequacies of personal health services, research on women's health, public health services, and health policy, but they have also created alternative personal health services, begun their own research on women's health, and lobbied for health policy changes and for changes in public health practices. The 1980s promise to be years of continued activism as women increasingly shape the world of health care. Indeed, women have demanded a *redefinition* of health care.

Wilma Scott Heide (1978) points out that feminism has had a profound influence on definitions of health care. Health care is generally based on "relationships between people mediated and augmented by chemical and physical technologies." (p. 10) In the past the qualitative, expressive components of care have been overshadowed by the values assigned to instrumental technology. In other words, those qualities considered more "feminine," such as nurturance, have been undervalued in favor of the more "masculine" instrumental approaches. Because feminism has freed both sexes to express feminine *and* masculine behaviors, there has been increased attentiveness to and demand for the expressive qualities in those persons providing personal health services.

Woman have made it increasingly clear that medical care cannot be equated with health. Indeed, sometimes medical intervention has had the opposite effect: the Dalkon shield and estrogen replacement therapy are two examples. Feminist analysts of health care have concluded that at best there is an *illness care system* in the United States, and at worst it is not a system at all, but a loosely controlled medical-industrial complex designed for profit from illness (Corea, 1977; Daly, 1978; Ehrenreich and English, 1973).

The purpose of this chapter is to explore women's health care from the perspective of the woman herself. We will begin by exploring the problems women have faced in receiving personal health services, as well as the influence that education for health professionals and research on women's health has had on those professionals caring for women. Next we will consider women's health care worlds, including personal health services, public health services, research on women and health, and health policy impinging on women. We will consider the consequences of the woman's health movement, strategies for changing the quality of health care for women, and, finally, some predictions for women and their health.

HEALTH CARE: THE WOMAN'S PROBLEM

Health care has become *the* "woman's problem." Although there have been laudable changes in the nature of health services for women in the past decade, the health and social sciences literature is replete with accounts of sexism—in personal health services, in education of health professionals, and in research on women's health.

Sexism in personal health services

A number of investigators have addressed the problem of sexism in the delivery of personal health services. Most notably, there is evidence of sexist bias in diagnosis, treatment, prescription of medications, and admission to hospital for psychiatric problems. Sexist bias is less evident in the diagnosis and treatment of strictly medical conditions.

Diagnosis

Psychiatric. The now-classic study of Broverman and associates (1970) provides an early example of efforts to document sexist bias in diagnosis. Seventy-nine practicing psychologists, psychiatrists, and social workers were given a sex-role stereotype questionnaire. Each was asked to rate a healthy, mature, socially competent (1) adult (sex unspecified), (2) man, and (3) woman. These investigators found that a double standard of health exists for men and women, in which the general standard of health applies *only to men*. This double standard of health, which seems to stem from an "adjustment notion" of health, suggests that women should comply with the norms for female behavior, even though these behaviors are considered less socially desirable and less healthy for an adult person. Acceptance of this notion labels women who exhibit the positive characteristics of healthy adults, or men, as "unfeminine." Women who adjust to feminine norms must accept second-class adult status. The danger implied by these research findings is that clinicians who accept these stereotypes reinforce and perpetuate them not only with clients but also in their roles as experts who help form public opinion and health policy.

Aslin's (1977) study confirmed that the sex of the therapist can influence the expectations of mental health for women. Female community mental health center therapists and feminist therapists did not have separate perceptions of mental health for adults, females, wives, and mothers. However, male therapists differed significantly in their perceptions of mentally healthy adults, females, wives, and mothers. Furthermore, the male therapists' judgments of mentally healthy adults and mothers differed significantly from those judgments of female therapists. The male therapists responded to the adult instructional set in a significantly more male stereotypic way than they responded to the female, wife, or mother set. In this later study, however, perceptions of women reflected a more androgynous orientation than Broverman and associates (1970) had found in their earlier work. Perhaps this reflects changing ways of thinking about women, in that women can be allowed a wider range of behaviors than men. Another study of psychotherapists failed to confirm the effects of the therapist's own sex role attitudes and gender on judgments of the psychologic well-being of males and females (Gomes and Abramowitz, 1976). The only biases that were evident in this study favored the sex-role deviant female: she was judged as especially emotionally mature!

Medical. Although sexist bias has also been suggested in the assessment of women's physical complaints, McCranie and co-workers (1978) found that physicians viewed the patients' problems largely from an organic perspective regardless of the patient's gender. A clinical simulation was used to determine whether symptoms of females would be more likely to be diagnosed and treated as reflecting psychogenic illness than would the same symptoms reported by males. The investigators found there were no statistically significant differences in physicians' judgments of seriousness or of prognosis with and without treatment according to the sex of the patient. While there was a low incidence of prescription for psychotherapy or psychiatric testing for all patients, there was more frequent mention of use of psychotropic drugs, with no differences according to the gender of the patient.

Preliminary results of Verbrugge's (1978) analysis of the National Ambulatory Medical Care Survey data show that men and women are similar in the number of health complaints they present, the number of diagnoses they receive in ambulatory care settings, the specificity of their complaints, and the concordance between their complaints and medical diagnoses. The major sex differences appear to be that men seem to ignore symptoms or fail to perceive them; women rely more on physicians for emotional support than men do; women confuse reproductive and digestive symptoms more often than men (which is probably a function of the proximity of these systems in women). There was little evidence of sex bias in diagnosis. When men and women had the same complaint but were given a different diagnosis, it was because they had different underlying physical conditions. Women, however, seemed to have a more elaborate and broader vocabulary for describing their symptoms than men.

Lennane and Lennane (1973) caution that certain health problems that affect only women are likely to be labeled psychogenic in origin when, in fact, there is evidence of organic causation. They point out that dysmenorrhea, nausea of pregnancy, labor pain, and infantile behavioral disturbances are irrationally and ineffectively managed because of such assumptions.

Admission and referral for psychiatric treatment

Bart (1968) found that an element of selection operates in determining who is admitted to a neurology service vs who is admitted to a psychiatry service, and that this may be a function of the patient's vocabulary. She compared women who presented themselves as physically ill and who were admitted to a neurology service and subsequently discharged with a psychiatric diagnosis with those women who presented themselves as mentally ill and were admitted to a psychiatric service. Bart found that the former were more likely to be housewives who had not been employed since marriage, less educated, more rural by birthplace and current residence, of lower social economic status, and less likely to be Jewish than their counterparts. She suggests that the women who were admitted to the neurology service were less likely to have come from subcultures having "psychiatric vocabularies" than the women who were admitted to the psychiatric service.

Tudor and co-workers (1977) have attempted to explain sex differences in hospitalization for psychosis. They suggest that psychotic males are channeled into psychiatric treatment earlier (as young adults) and have a longer stay in mental hospitals than females because the role expectations for men are less tolerant of mental illness. Society reacts to psychotic males more promptly and severely than it does to females. Although neurotic males and females tend to seek treatment at about the same age, males tend to be hospitalized longer. These investigators suggest that because the boundaries of acceptable behavior are much more circumscribed for males than for females, the latter are treated earlier. They also point out that if health care is a scarce commodity, the greater access of males to treatment must be considered a "prerequisite of power."

There is evidence that bias is operative in psychiatric referral of children as well as adults. An examination of records from an outpatient child guidance clinic shows that more girls than boys are referred for psychiatric help for being defiant and verbally aggressive. More boys than girls are referred for being passive or emotional. In this study parents and graduate students in clinical and school psychology responded to hypothetical cases in which the same behavioral problems were attributed to a girl and a boy. The child who exhibited behavior divergent from that usually attributed to her or his sex was described as more severely disturbed, more likely to need psychiatric treatment, and as having a less positive future than were the children who exhibited sex stereotypic behavior (Feinblatt and Gold, 1976).

Psychiatric therapy

Once women seek help or are referred to helpers they may be subjected to sexist biases in the therapeutic process. Rice and Rice (1973) point out that freudian theory and practice, which constitutes a major body of psychotherapeutic knowledge, imbues therapists with an antifeminine orientation. Not only are there many disparaging references made to women in the literature, there are descriptions of women as the "abnormal" sex. To compound the problem, there is a predominance of male therapists, which undoubtedly has contributed to the delayed recognition of antifemale bias in the field.

Rice and Rice (1973) also point out that role unhappiness need not be assumed to be psychopathologic. Indeed, what is labeled pathologic from a psychoanalytic standpoint—not fitting into one's society—would be healthy behavior if viewed as an appropriate response to role conflict. Rice and Rice document that a number of forces perpetuate what therapists might regard as a "schizophrenia" of person for women: Women are encouraged to seek their identity through someone else. The traditional feminine housewife role seems futile, goalless, and repetitive, but it has been glorified by the media. The society rewards those in achievement roles; while motherhood is sanctified, it is not esteemed. The

consumer society encourages women to be objects rather than persons; consuming other objects becomes a substitute for identity and relationships.

Social programming of double-binds also affects women's self-image. They are encouraged to be virgins, but sexy; smart, but willing to hide it; achievers in school, but failures in work. Devaluing by the society of the personal characteristics one usually associates with femininity clearly perpetuates feelings of low self-esteem, depression, and lack of identity for women. Unless the *social* origins of these feelings are uppermost in the awareness of the therapist, the therapeutic process can only reinforce the status quo. Rice and Rice recommend that therapists help women probe the antecedents of feminine conflict, assist women to restructure their relationships with others, and assist them to explore new roles and models.

Recent research on counselor or therapist behavior suggests that the effect of the patient's sex on therapist's reactions is not pronounced, at least when therapists are required to respond to written case materials (Abramowitz et al. 1976). In addition, counselors seem to exhibit more behavioral biases with the "typical" clients than with those whose sex roles were atypical (Shapiro, 1977). It is interesting that in both of these studies female counselors or therapists demonstrated greater empathy for a patient (Abramowitz et al., 1976) and were more reinforcing and less punishing than male counselors (Shapiro, 1977). Shapiro points out that counselors have an inclination to shape clients into an image consistent with what they believe is appropriate, regardless of whether it is beneficial to the client. She warns that the growing acceptance of new roles for women may have created a climate in which the client who is most likely to be a victim of therapy is the more conventional woman rather than her liberated sister!

Drug therapy

Sexist bias has also influenced the prescription of medications. A higher incidence of prescription of mood-modifying drugs for women than for men has been documented. Cooperstock (1971) suggests that western women are permitted greater freedom in expressing feelings than are men. Because of this status women are more inclined to bring their emotional problems to the attention of a physician, who, influenced by the expectations that women will need such drugs more than men, prescribes a higher proportion of mood-altering drugs for women than men.

A number of explanations have been suggested for the differential rates of prescriptions for such drugs. How drugs are advertised and promoted may be one factor. Another is that "doing something" to decrease the patient's presenting symptom is easier than remedying the social conditions that promote the symptoms in the first place (Waldron, 1977).

Unnecessary surgery

Various studies indicate that hysterectomies rank from fourth to second of the most frequently performed types of surgery in the United States (Corea, 1977; Larned, 1977). It has been estimated that as many as one third of the hysterectomies and one half of the cesarean sections performed in the United States today are unnecessary (Seaman, 1972). In a review of a Teamsters audit done in the late 1950s and 1960s, it was estimated that twenty of the sixty hysterectomies reviewed were unjustified; in another 10% questions about justifiability could be raised (Morehead and Trussell, 1962).

More than twice as many hysterectomies are performed in the United States as in England and Wales. Bunker (1970) has identified several reasons for this higher surgical rate: a more aggressive approach to healing; less frequent use of consultation, which allows the physician to self-refer; maldistribution of physicians, resulting in many surgeons who do not have enough to do; and a fee-for-service payment method, which can provide an incentive for surgery. Additionally, the pervasive attitudes that the cause of all illness in women lies in the uterus and that the uterus is only good for having babies can create an approach to women that is cavalier at best.

Hysterectomy is becoming a routine procedure to be done for a variety of reasons—birth control, menstrual disorders, treatment of carcinoma, and cancer prevention. In some instances these may be valid reasons; however, a hysterectomy should not be done as an elective procedure or when more conservative treatment will suffice. The risks are too great.

Nature of health services

Marieskind (1975b) and others have noted that the nature of health services for women are different from those for men. In fact, several authors have commented that women get into the health care system via their reproductive organs. For many women, health care emphasizes the reproductive system, often to the exclusion of other aspects of their health.

Howell and Hiatt (1975), in a study of student health services in medical schools, found slightly different kinds of sex bias in the nature of health services. Usually there are few women physicians on the staff of these services, and women students did not have a choice regarding the gender of the physician they saw. In only 5% of the health services did respondents indicate that contemporary adult women often had needs that were different from those commonly addressed by traditional psychotherapists. In 50% of the student health services, women could not get a pelvic examination as part of a physical examination and/or primary care for an uncomplicated genital condition. The authors point out that many services may violate Title IX requirements for nondiscrimination.

Discharge from psychiatric institutions

A recent study of staff ratings of patients in an inpatient psychiatric therapeutic community demonstrated that although staff rated the illness severity of men and women similarly on admission, women were rated as having made significant improvement over time whereas men were not (Doherty, 1978). The staff ratings of pathology differentiated between men who were referred for further hospitalization vs discharged, but not between women who were referred or discharged. Instead, women who were single, unemployed, and young were more likely to be referred for further hospitalization than women who were married, employed, or older. Doherty suggests the women referred for further hospitalization are seen as more helpless, fragile, dependent, and in need of protection than their counterparts who are discharged.

SEXISM IN THE EDUCATION OF HEALTH PROFESSIONALS

Scully and Bart (1973) analyzed a number of commonly used gynecology textbooks to determine if the treatment of women might be based on inaccuracies or negative images of women in medical texts. Their research reveals that in many instances the information is inaccurate; for example, the findings of Masters and Johnson and Kinsey did not seem to influence content regarding the strength of women's sexual drives, the vaginal-clitoral orgasm misconception, and the prevalence of female sexual dysfunction. Not only did some textbooks advise physicians to counsel their women patients to simulate orgasms if they were not orgasmic with their husbands, one text likened the image of the gynecologist to God Almighty! Not only have women been portrayed as less adequate or less normal than men in these texts, but they have also been portrayed as inherently sick. One text actually states that the feminine "core" consists of masochism, narcissism, and passivity. With information such as this in textbooks written by authorities in gynecology, it is no surprise that women might be treated inappropriately by clinicians.

Widespread use of the masculine pronoun to denote physicians in texts may discourage those women interested in a certain specialty. Also, the language used to describe women in textbooks reinforces stereotypes about how women should behave (Roland, 1977). This remains the case even in most nursing books, where the masculine pronoun is used for physicians.

Advertising in medical journals. Another force influencing how women are treated is the advertising that appears in professional journals. Not only are women portrayed as mentally ill more often than are men, but also men are more often portrayed as physicians (Stockburger and Davis, 1978). In ads for mood-modifying drugs, women are shown significantly more often than men. In ads for other categories of drugs, pictures are used less often. All ads reviewed adhered to stereotypic gender roles in regard to patient as well as professionals (Mant and Darroch, 1975). Another review of advertisements for psychotropic drugs demonstrates that male patients are associated more frequently with rational appeals than were females (Smith and Griffin, 1977). While the illustration portions of the ads are usually associated with nonrational appeals, the headlines and texts are usually classified as rational appeals. Taken as a group, these studies reflect sexism in medical advertising. It is possible that such ads mirror medical practice, and also that the derogatory and demeaning images of women sell drugs (Smith and Griffin, 1977).

SEXISM AND RESEARCH ON WOMEN AND HEALTH

The effects of sexism have pervaded nearly every aspect of research, from the implicit assumptions guiding conceptual frameworks and selection of problems for study to the analysis of data and the conclusions inferred from study results.

Conceptual frameworks

The conceptual frameworks guiding research about women have been the products of the times in which the studies were conducted. Perhaps more important, they have been shaped by the prevailing academic orientations of the time. For example, social science research has been predicated upon certain domain assumptions about the social structure (Gouldner, 1970) and the family, such as the need for children to be raised in families in which men perform the "instrumental" roles and women the "expressive" roles* (Parsons and Bales, 1955). From here it is only a small leap to conceptual frameworks that confirm the rightness of such a social arrangement and predict negative consequences to children of women deviating from their "expressive" roles.

---

*According to Parsons and Bales, instrumental roles are those usually performed by men and involved negotiations outside the family. Expressive or feminine roles include intrafamily activities such as maintenance and nurturance.

Nowhere has the effect of a conceptual framework been more apparent than in the body of psychoanalytic research. Women who reject their "feminine" roles have been labeled sick, and so have those who accept them. Research directed by such a frame of reference can only confirm the inherent sickness in women.

Another example of the influence that conceptual frameworks play in research about women can be seen in medical textbooks and practice during the nineteenth century. Medicine defined women as sickly and in need of help, but simultaneously labeled them silly, self-indulgent, and superstitious. Such points of view led to experimentation with techniques such as the rest cure, in which there was nearly total sensory deprivation. It was superficially designed to help the frail, sickly, woman rest but, paradoxically, it had the function of making even the worst home life appear so much better than the treatment that women were miraculously "cured" (Ehrenreich and English, 1978). The "conservation of energy theory" was based on allegations that use of a woman's energy for any purpose but reproduction could only result in dysfunction of the uterus. Such a theory became a convenient justification for sex segregation in education as well as for experiments on curing the diversion of reproductive energy into sexual activities (Ehrenreich and English, 1979).

Unfortunately, contorted frameworks to guide research on women persist even now. The dominant frames of reference for women's health research remain illness-oriented, concerned with pathways to pathology, not wellness. Such normal events as lactation, childbirth, menstruation, menopause, and female sexual response have frequently been approached in the context of medical problems or pathologic events. Most notably menopause has been regarded as a deficiency disease to be treated with estrogens, thus justifying massive experiments with women. The "medicalization" of childbirth has led not to experimentation with self-help measures useful for women experiencing a natural event, but rather to experimentation with instruments such as fetal monitors designed to detect fetal or maternal pathology.

Another problem with women's health research is that frequently women's problems have been studied from a male perspective. Using males as a standard or norm has led to minimizing a woman's health concerns. For example, women are frequently labelled as "excessutilizers of health services" when males are used as the norm.

Choice of problems for study

The kinds of problems chosen for study could not help but reflect basic assumptions about women. The nature of the assumptions about women could easily provide the basis for differentiating research *for* women from research *against* women. As one example, the menstrual cycle literature contains a plethora of studies to detect the inherent "problems" women have because they menstruate: e.g., effects of the menstrual cycle on violent crimes, and accidents. Few studies of the positive effects of menstruation have been published to date.

In the past, the problems selected for study have focused on women's childbearing capacity, illnesses, or significant others, rather than on the women themselves. For example, studies have been largely directed at assessing the effects of exposures to toxic substances or effects of employment on the fetus or children rather than on the woman.

It is likely that each researcher chooses a problem for study that is interesting to her or him as an individual. Sechrest (1975) points out that killer diseases that primarily affect men, such as heart disease, receive a large share of researchers' attention, and comments, "Think how long it has taken to get around to doing a controlled clinical trial comparing the radical mastectomy to less mutilating operations." (p. 41)

It is also likely that the choice of problems for study is often a function of the research tools and traditions available at the moment. The biomedical orientation to research has emphasized specialization and superspecialization, an orientation that encourages thinking about molecular events. When this is the only avenue pursued in the selection of research problems, it is sometimes difficult for investigators to refer back to the object of the study: the total organism. Sophisticated instrumentation and superspecialization in substantive research areas are both likely to mediate toward research that regards a fragment of the woman rather than the woman as a whole person. The interdisciplinary research team might provide a mechanism fostering research directed at women as totalities, providing there are behavioral and social scientists who can explore new frames of reference.

Funding

One of the most compelling variables influencing research about women in this society is availability of funding. Large funding sources, such as the National Institutes of Health, define the nature of research about women, at least indirectly, inasmuch as they allocate scarce resources (money) for research programs. Institutes and foundations that fund research have the privilege of defining the nature of the programs to which they will allocate resources. This influence may be direct or indirect. Direct influences include Congressional mandates or the desire of a board of trustees. Indirect influence occurs via the peer review mechanism. For ex-

ample, the membership of the study section reviewing proposals for scientific merit and allocation of funding certainly influences the type of research funded. In the past, the largely male membership of these bodies had the opportunity to shape the nature of research about women. It is likely that the biomedical approach and the traditional orientations toward women's health would have prevailed unchallenged were it not for the increasing visibility of women on these bodies. Yet the medical research community is still dominated by males who staff funding agencies, study sections, research teams, and editorial boards of journals (Sechrest, 1975).

Sampling and informed consent

The samples chosen for medical experimentation have often been from populations of impoverished or relatively powerless women. Sechrest (1975) points out that the early research on oral contraceptives capitalized on the desire of poor and relatively uninformed Puerto Rican women to avoid pregnancy. In other instances, financial incentives, such as free drugs or free medical care for themselves or family members, may constitute not-so-subtle coercion. The fact that many women are socialized to docility and conformity would mediate against their confronting authority figures who recommend participation in an experiment. It is not difficult to imagine how the subtle but coercive differences between women subjects and male experimenters could interfere with obtaining informed consent. Not only would the woman who has been conditioned to be docile not be likely to ask for clarification, but also she might rightly assume that her medical care is contingent on her participating in the experiment. None of the ethical problems discussed above is unique only to women; they could apply equally well to minority groups. They do, however, necessitate certain precautions in the sampling of populations and assurance of informed consent. As Sechrest (1975) cautions, "Medical researchers who command resources which may be distributed to research subjects, or who can contribute in critical ways to the welfare of potential subjects who do not have access to ordinary support, or who can by force of personality, position, or authority produce compliance that would not otherwise be forthcoming are faced with an ethical problem." (p. 41)

Data analysis and interpretation

Bias can pervade the analysis of data and the interpretations of research findings. Benoliel (1975) points out that the "masculine agentic mode of scientific inquiry is insufficient for capturing the personal meanings of sensitive human experience." (p. 39) The tendency of researchers to only *quantify* findings rather than explore data via qualitative analytic approaches can contribute to a body of research that reduces human experience to numbers or rates. The development of high-speed computers has supported increasing sophistication in analytic strategies. Multivariate analysis allows investigators to look at the simultaneous effects of many factors on women's health. The temptation to use such high-powered analytic strategies may overshadow the need to deal with more "squishy" qualitative or categorical variables, such as human perceptions.

Another problem related to data analysis is that in some studies women are grouped with men, possibly masking sex differences in the dependent variable. In other instances, women are left out of the analysis altogether, as in some occupational health studies. Usually the investigator justifies this oversight by stating that the number of women was simply too small to warrant further analysis.

An important bias that exists in the interpretation of findings is the lack of attention given negative findings. One example is research dealing with the menstrual cycle. While numerous studies of effects of menstruation on everything from academic performance to incidence of homicide have appeared in the literature, Sommer (1978) points out that the bias against publishing research in which the null hypothesis was *not* rejected may explain our limited knowledge of menstrual cycle correlates.

Post hoc interpretation of findings is probably also a factor in our limited knowledge of women's health. When the findings do not fit a conceptual framework—or, more likely, domain assumptions—the inclination of some researchers might be to avoid publishing them altogether or to contort the logical underpinnings of the study to fit the data.

One final problem encountered in interpretation of findings is the use of data to indict the subjects. Sechrest (1975) points out examples of research in which minority racial groups and nurses who have participated in research projects find the data are used against them—to blame the victim or to confirm the researcher's domain assumptions.

In sum, what we know about women's health is a function of the prevailing conceptual frameworks about women, the problems chosen (and ignored) for study, the funding available to support research, the samples selected for study, and the approaches used for analysis and interpretation of data. What we don't know is simply astounding!

WOMEN'S HEALTH CARE WORLDS
Personal health services

The most striking change occurring in women's health care over the last decade has been movement from a nearly universal, traditional authoritarian approach in the delivery of personal health services to the pluralistic array of the late 1970s. While the evolution of some models for women's personal health services has been the result of humanistic movements within some of the professions, women themselves have had a profound influence on the structure of personal health services. In some instances, women created new kinds of services, such as self-help clinics, menstrual extraction groups, and home birth services provided by lay women. In other instances, the professionals co-opted some of women's efforts, creating modified forms of personal health services that remained under the thinly veiled control of the professionals (e.g., use of educational pelvic examinations). In still other instances, the economic threat from women who provided their own health care was sufficient to induce modifications in institutions. The home birth movement's competition for obstetric patients in an era of declining birth rates gave impetus to, if not precipitated, the trend for home-style delivery rooms in hospitals. As a consequence of both change from within the professions and pressures from women who were increasingly vocal about their dissatisfaction with their personal health services, there are now several models of services available to women. Although most women are still served by more traditional types of services, there are considerably more options available to some women than was the case in the late 1960s.

Types of health care worlds

Ruzek (1978), in an extensive study of the women's health movement, describes four ideal typical health care worlds: the traditional authoritarian, traditional egalitarian, traditional feminist, and radical feminist. Their differences in dominant role relationships, distribution of medical knowledge, division of labor, access to curatives, management of time and space, and assignment of risk are outlined in Table 3-1. In the traditional authoritarian health care world, as typified by public clinics and hospitals and some private physicians' practices, physicians believe that authority and decision-making remain in their hands. The doctor-patient relationship reflects an active-passive model. There is little sharing of medical information with the patient. There is a clear delineation of tasks in the setting with rigid distinctions maintained between categories of workers. Access to curatives is zealously guarded by professionals. Management of space and time reflects more concern for the professional's than the patients' convenience. Professionals attempt to provide risk-free care and usually do not encourage patients to make decisions about their own care, assuming that patients are unable to weigh the risks involved.

At the other end of the continuum is the radical feminist world of health care. In self-help clinics, menstrual extraction groups, and lay midwife–attended home births, women are encouraged and expected to be responsible for their own health care. Professionals are used as consultants. An attempt is made to widely disseminate knowledge about health, and all participants, including professionals, are expected to learn from one another. The division of labor is much less hierarchic, with each participant in a self-help group observing, advising, treating, and being treated. Women are encouraged to rely less on dangerous drugs, to utilize natural or low-risk curatives, and to question why access to some devices, such as diaphragms, is controlled by professionals. Indeed, some self-help groups assist women in fitting diaphragms and provide instructions for

Table 3-1. Characteristics of the ideal types of health care worlds*

Examples and characteristics	Ideal types of health care worlds			
	Traditional authoritarian	**Traditional egalitarian**	**Traditional feminist**	**Radical feminist**
Examples of settings	Public clinics, hospitals, some private practitioners' offices	Progressive clinics, some private practitioners' offices, "home-style" birthing rooms, private hospitals.	Feminist clinics, physician or nurse–midwife–attended home births.	Self-help clinics, lay midwife–attended home births, menstrual extraction groups.
Dominant role relationships	Authority and decision-making controlled by physician; patients expected to behave in passive mode; treated impersonally.	Professionals assume responsibility for and authority over care; patients expected to be somewhat informed and involved, but expected to follow doctor's orders; patients allowed some decision-making, but practitioners define parameters in which decisions can be made.	Care provided by female paraprofessionals; physicians do not see patients until after others have determined whether patient needs and is willing to see physician. Physicians act as consultants to clients. Women expected to be interested in and involved in own health care.	Patients encouraged to assume responsibility for own health care, with assistance of other lay women. Physicians relegated to technician status, usually hired to perform only those tasks restricted by law. "Women learn to perform basic health services for themselves" (p. 109).
Distribution of medical knowledge	Physicians believe they are only "reliable" source of information; monopoly on medical knowledge maintained.	Physicians believe that women with adequate information can make informed decisions about their care.	All participants, including physicians, are expected to increase their knowledge from contacts with multiple sources: lay health workers, family and friends, nurses, physicians, participation in health discussion groups and self-help clinics.	Same as traditional feminist.
Division of labor	Rigid distinctions maintained between worker categories; norms regulating division of labor are enforced; little interchange of responsibilities.	Same as traditional authoritarian.	Division of labor is less hierarchic. Lay women evaluate as well as observe physician's responsibilities and actions. Specialization, certification, hierarchic social relationships minimized. In self-help clinics, lay	Same as traditional feminist. Responsibility for routine care shifted from professional experts to women themselves. All participants encouraged to share in observing, advising, treating, and being treated.

*Adapted from Ruzek, S. B.: The women's health movement: feminist alternatives to medical control, New York, 1978, Praeger Publishers, pp. 103-142.

Continued.

Examples and characteristics	Ideal types of health care worlds			
	Traditional authoritarian	Traditional egalitarian	Traditional feminist	Radical feminist
			women rotate through a number of tasks. Division of labor similar to more traditional settings, inasmuch as less trained workers perform more simple or "boring" (to physicians) tasks.	
Access to curatives	Legal license to control access to drugs and perform procedures buttress physician authority.	Physicians less secretive about curatives, less possessive, e.g., women can choose nonprescription curatives.	Women's reliance on restricted drugs and technologies discouraged. Instead, dangers of certain curatives are discussed, unrestricted or natural alternative curatives are promoted, and certain devices, drugs, and procedures are defined as accessible to lay women, regardless of the law (e.g., menstrual extraction or diaphragm fitting).	
Management of space	Territories physician-controlled; women subject to rules and regulations of practitioners.	Women may have some control over some of the space and how it is used, e.g., home-style birthing rooms.	Space is less categorically defined, but still controlled by practitioners.	Spacial arrangements that reinforce status distinctions between patient and practitioner are minimized. Self-help territory is wherever women choose.
Management of time	Time managed to ensure steady flow of patients for practitioners, length of wait often greater for nonprivate patients; time spent with professional is minimal, often only a few minutes in some settings.		Waiting time to get an appointment is shorter, but clinic waits are still long, especially for "walk-in" or free clinics. Open scheduling or first-come, first-serve scheduling has been used to cope with "no-shows." Waiting time is used for educational purposes, history-taking. Usually 20 to 30 minutes allowed for each woman.	Self-help groups attribute equal value to time of each person participating. Time that would be used for waiting is spent observing procedures on other women in an effort to increase and share one's knowledge.
Assignment of risk	Efforts to promise risk-free care and preserve life at any cost are greatest here. Usually women are not encouraged to evaluate risks and make decisions about their own care.	In some settings women are given opportunity to weigh information about risks in making decisions about their own care.	Humanistic care combined with "safety and surety of modern medical science" may reduce risk as well as allow limited number of women to be treated humanely.	Participants are expected to be aware of risk and share information about risks.

their use. The turf of self-help groups is variable, and self-help clinic personnel minimize the distinction between patient and practitioner in the allocation of space. Time is of equal value to each member of the group, and all women are involved, so that "waiting" is not a function of the clinic's administration. Each woman is expected to be knowledgeable with respect to the risks of certain procedures, and information about risk is widely disseminated.

Between these two extremes are various permutations. The traditional egalitarian and traditional feminist are the middle categories Ruzek (1978) describes. There are, undoubtedly, several models that fall between the ideal types outlined in Table 3-1. The proliferation of new models for health care will probably continue, especially in the range between the traditional egalitarian and radical feminist portion of the continuum.

Development of women's health care worlds

Marieskind's (1975) chronicle of the women's health movement describes it as a grassroots organization dating from about 1970. She points out that the current women's health movement evolved from the women's liberation movement of the late 1960s and 1970s and parallels the popular health movement that accompanied the suffragism of the mid-nineteenth century. The women's health movement, like the popular health movement, seeks to provide alternatives to medical practice where they are needed and emphasizes preventive health concepts, self-awareness, and comprehension through a basic knowledge of bodily processes, and to demystify medicine. But the current women's health movement has strongly political interests and is a potential revolutionary force—feminist socialism. Recognizing the lack of control they have had over their reproductive potential (controlled as it was by men in government and in the top ranks of the health care industry), women have extended their concerns to gynecology and obstetrics. Not only has there been growing membership in women's groups providing diverse health services, but also there is identification of these groups as a social movement with a common goal for "improved health care for women and an end to sexism in the health system." The movement is also developing a growing literature on women's health and is receiving recognition by society.

The current status of the women's health movement has been described by Marieskind (1975) and more recently by Ruzek (1978). The movement's work focuses on changing consciousness, providing health services and trying to change established institutions. Although a number of approaches have been used, there are some pervasive commonalities among them. Most question the hierarchic structure of the system and promote the use of lay health workers, dissemination of information

and skills, and involvement of women in their own care. Challenging the existing division of health care labor and the profit motive, which influences the amount of surgery performed, is common among women in the movement. Collectivism allows women to experience mutual support and a nonhierarchic model. Self-realization is an important goal for women in this movement (Marieskind, 1975).

Feminists have also analyzed women's position in society and the health care system. Fee (1975) analyzes women and health care from the perspective of liberal feminism, radical feminism, and Marxist feminism. The data in Table 3-2 represent a summary of Fee's analysis. The three viewpoints range from proposals for changing the current system to those that would change the basic ideology and structure of American society.

Public health services

Although many women are directly affected by personal health services, it is important to note that public health services exist whose mission is the surveillance and promotion of the health of all people in the United States. The Bureau of Community Health Services (HEW) provides the majority of federally financed health services. In addition, the states and local governments provide funding for both personal and public health services.

Orientation of services

One example of the organization of services for women is seen in how funding is appropriated for various programs of Health and Human Resources' Bureau of Community Health Services. Funding is allocated specifically for Community Health Centers, Family Planning, and Maternal and Child Health Service Corps. The 1978 appropriation (in millions) is given below:

Community Health Centers	$262
Family Planning	135
Maternal and Child Health	333
National Health Services Corps	43

The separation of family planning centers from comprehensive community health centers is currently under scrutiny, with the government position reflecting the sentiment that separation of family planning from other primary health care services for women may be a detriment to women's health care. Yet traditional funding patterns are likely to prevail (Women and Health Roundtable, 1978).

In addition to separating family planning from primary care, the funding pattern also segregates maternal-child health. While the separate funding of each program area makes the health concerns of women *visible* in federal budgets, it also seemingly reinforces the segregation of "women's concerns" from the mainstream of primary care. No one has pointed out the obvious more clearly than Marieskind (1975): "We would think it very humorous to have men entering the health system through their penises, reproductive systems, and urologists; why do we not find it equally ludicrous that women's health care is principally organized around her uterus and reproductive potential?" (p. 48) Marieskind also points out that the organization of medical care mediates toward women receiving specialty care either from gynecologists or from a public maternal–child health program. Such an approach, recommended for young women from puberty onward, not only perpetuates women's identities as reproductive organs, but also leads to incomplete care for women. For example, physical examinations often consist of breast and pelvic examinations, excluding the other body systems, mental health, and social support systems. Marieskind (1975) proposes that the specialty be disbanded altogether; health care of women

would be returned to midwives and to internists trained in primary care, with surgeons and gynecologists used as consultants when necessary.

International concerns

The orientation of public health services for women in the United States reinforces the notion of women as a reproductive organism. As services are organized in developing countries, many aspects of the models used in the United States proliferate. The widespread use of devices, drugs, and surgery to limit population growth constitutes a major focus of health care for women. Products, such as infant formulas, are also introduced and advertised when the techniques they replace may be much safer (e.g., breast feeding). It is likely that in replicating the Western approach to biomedicine in developing countries, public health services will repli-

Table 3-2. A comparison of women's health worlds according to three feminist analyses*

Approach	Changes suggested by analysis of women's position in the society	Changes suggested by analysis of women's relation to health care system
Liberal feminism	Goals are to achieve equality with men, e.g., equal pay, equal opportunity, access to same choices available to men. Hierarchic structure of society is not challenged. Instead, attempt made to win rights and equality within established system.	Social subordination of women is reflected in sexual structure of medicine. Women are dealt with by physicians from position of power; authoritarian or parental manners are common. Women are accorded less respect whether well or ill. Emphasis placed on equalizing upper ranks of the health profession (medicine) by sex, offering feminist therapy, and changing the practice of gynecology and psychiatry.
Radical feminism	Goals are to entirely transform social institutions. Central struggle of history is between the sexes, not classes. Sexual oppression combated by special organizations of women's creation: consciousness-raising groups, rape crises centers, self-help groups. Attempts made to help women develop collective consciousness, to break down dominant ideology. Demystifying (e.g., the need for the patriarchal family) important component.	Medical profession is yet another system conforming to the patriarchal pattern of the family (doctor = father, nurse = mother, patient = child). Important to increase knowledge and ability of patients, so that they seek to inform and organize those receiving health care. Formation of feminist self-help groups has generated familiarity with health knowledge, awareness of one's body, skills in self-examination, and attitudes that confront the alienation that the culture imposes on females. Protest against medical management of childbirth and pressures for legalization of midwifery have characterized efforts. Women's health centers (alternatives to the present system) have been created, but confronted by the old order, lack of credentials, and shortage of funds. Much of the focus of women's programs for remaking health care was on reproductive problems, and funding has limited their focus on other aspects of health.

*Adapted from Fee, C.: Women and health care: a comparison of theories, Int. J. Health Serv. 5(3):397-415, 1975.

cate the problems inherent in the organization of services for women that we now experience. International programs for health services bear careful monitoring by women's health advocates. One area that deserves close attention is the use of fertility control drugs that would not be approved for use in the United States on women of third world nations. Another is the focus on women's reproductive capacities rather than on more basic problems such as malnutrition, that pose a serious threat to health.

HEALTH POLICY
Medicine as social control

Medical experts have influenced not only who can practice as healers, but also what is considered healthy. Ehrenreich and English (1978) illustrate the influence of medical "experts" on the roles that women were deemed healthy enough to perform in society and on housekeeping and childrearing. Daly's (1978) account examines how the practice of gynecology defines and reinforces the appropriate place for women, by reducing them to nothing, coercing them into ignoring their best interests, and participating in risky therapy. The "mind-menders," as Daly calls those practicing psychotherapy, have reinforced the control of women's power by labeling certain behaviors (e.g., those indicating rebellion against the status quo) as deviant and working to "correct" them.

Although feminist authors have addressed the problems women encounter in one-to-one relationships with healers, the enormous impact of such belief systems on the shaping of health policy has only begun to be explored. Some have suggested that despite the proliferation of academic publications about women's health

Table 3-2. A comparison of women's health worlds according to three feminist analyses—cont'd

Approach	Changes suggested by analysis of women's position in the society	Changes suggested by analysis of women's relation to health care system
Marxist feminism	Patriarchal assumptions regarding women's roles as wives and mothers support system in which women are paid lower wages. In turn this maintains low wages, increases profits, and divides the labor force along sex lines. Women can serve as reserve labor force, and for no pay perform domestic labor, and reproduce the labor force. Thus sexism is useful for capitalism. A necessary condition for liberation of women is rejection of capitalism with democratic socialism as a replacement.	American health system's deficiencies result from its commitment to profit rather than fulfillment of people's needs. Power rests in a handful of monopolistic institutions—a coalition of the AMA, commercial and insurance companies, research, teaching, community, and voluntary hospitals. Work force stratified by class, race, and sex, and labor is divided and specialized with "women's work" being given low value and divisions of the labor force being played off against one another. Health and illness are defined on the basis of ability to work, undoubtedly one reason why women's illnesses are seen as less serious than men's. Concentration is on objective causes of illness rather than on its social causes rooted in capitalism. Diseases that lack biomedical correlates are defined out of existence, or treated with placebos, such as tranquilizers. Other health conditions such as pregnancy are defined as medical problems and "controlled." System is not accountable to the American population it serves. Services reflect one's ability to pay, and specialization leads to fragmented care. While it is possible to provide excellent care to the entire population, the current control and organization of health care makes a complete reordering of priorities impossible within the current system. Democratic socialist system seems only way to liberate potential for improved care and prevention.

issues, academicians have relatively little input into public policy-making. Whether this is true because their research lacks relevance to policy decisions or because academicians have less influence than legislators and lobbyists should be explored. It is doubtful that the amount of energy currently invested in research on women and health is without merit for policy formulation. Yet most academic researchers have been socialized to objectivity, not activism. Perhaps women's health researchers need to be educated to be advocates as well as scholars! Perhaps the researcher advocate would then be able to deal more effectively with legislative bodies and regulatory agencies, and at least recognize the strong influence of economics on health policy.

NATIONAL HEALTH INSURANCE

A current health policy issue that embodies a number of women's concerns is national health insurance. At this writing, there is no national health plan, but several alternatives are being considered. Regardless of the plan adopted, there are a number of concerns about the impact of NHI on women's health. First, the scope of services included in an NHI plan may not be sufficiently attentive to the inequities that currently exist in our present payment system. Because women elect to use the system for "well-women" care (contraceptive services, pelvic examinations, screening, pregnancy and childbirth care), it is important that benefits from NHI *not* be limited to illness care. In addition, women may use more than one provider, for example, an internist and a nurse midwife. Some other important issues related to NHI are: eligibility structures that make NHI contingent upon employment status or husband's insurance policies; provider certification that is limited only to physicians and does not include free-standing clinics and other health care personnel such as nurse midwives; and incentives for reform of health delivery mechanisms

---

A woman's score card for National Health Insurance plans

	RESPONSE				RESPONSE	
	Yes	No			Yes	No
1. Will privacy and confidentiality be assured to women who participate?	☐	☐	d. Nutritionists?		☐	☐
2. Will the NHI plan provide for the following "well-woman" services:			e. Physical therapists?		☐	☐
			5. Is utilization of traditional physician services required?		☐	☐
a. Contraceptive or family planning services?	☐	☐	6. Will the woman who chooses to use more than one source of care (e.g., an internist and a nurse midwife) be penalized?		☐	☐
b. Screening for common gynecologic problems (e.g., Pap smears, breast examinations)?	☐	☐				
c. Care during pregnancy?	☐	☐	7. Does the plan allow for alternatives to the traditional medical care system?		☐	☐
d. Childbirth care?	☐	☐	a. Birthing centers		☐	☐
e. Treatment for common gynecologic problems (e.g., menstrual distress, vaginal infections, menopausal problems)?	☐	☐	b. Women's health care centers		☐	☐
			8. Will the plan provide coverage for women who work at home?		☐	☐
3. Will the plan cover a range of family planning services:			a. Will lower benefits be provided for women who work at home?		☐	☐
a. Basic family planning counseling?	☐	☐	b. More restrictive coverage?		☐	☐
b. Prescription devices or drugs?	☐	☐	9. Will coverage be contingent on marital status?		☐	☐
c. Female sterilization as well as vasectomy?	☐	☐	a. Will the plan cover single women to the same extent as married women?		☐	☐
d. Abortion?	☐	☐				
e. Infertility?	☐	☐	b. Will NHI coverage be protected in case the married woman becomes divorced or separated?		☐	☐
4. Does the plan allow for choices of health providers:						
a. Nurse midwives?	☐	☐	c. Must the woman remain in contact with her spouse in order to receive benefits?		☐	☐
b. Social workers?	☐	☐				
c. Nurse practitioners?	☐	☐				

that would limit women to a single provider (Lewis, 1976). It appears that NHI will be an outcome of the struggle between those whose greatest concern is the "economic costs of providing services" versus those whose concerns are with the "human costs of not providing the services" (Women and Health Roundtable, 1978).

CONSEQUENCES OF THE WOMEN'S HEALTH MOVEMENT

The women's health movement has had major consequences on both the established medical care system and the ways in which women view themselves and their health.

Ruzek (1978) lists five ways in which the women's health movement has attempted to deinstitutionalize medical authority. The first is by reducing the knowledge differential between client and practitioner. The informed client is able to challenge the authority of the professional, carefully analyze alternatives in treatment, and actively participate in planning her own care. Second, women have challenged the mandate or licensure of physicians to provide certain services. Access to devices such as diaphragms and to procedures such as pelvic examinations has changed dramatically as women have learned these skills and applied them in self-help groups. Third, women have reduced professional control and monopoly over related services and goods. The rise in numbers of home births has seriously challenged the professional control over this event and the services related to it. Fourth, the size of the profession relative to the clientele was once small; dissemination of health knowledge and skills has increased the numbers prepared to provide health services from an elite few to many. The pressure for nurses and non-physician professionals to provide primary health services has also changed the ratio. Finally, in some respects the clientele of health services has been transformed to a collectivity. Organized clients (as opposed to aggregates of clients) have seriously threatened institutionalized authority. Clients thus organized can lobby, educate, and shape the nature of health care delivery.

Ruzek (1978) describes a number of strategies for change. Some strategies to change health care within the medical professional model include education of clients, influencing legislation and public policy, judicial measures, selective utilization, and direct pressure. Some health activists have created alternate institutions. Whether these will provide stop-gap services or indeed will continue to compete in providing comprehensive care remains to be seen. Others have tried to redefine the boundaries of the traditional male medical authority.

Finally, women have attempted to alter the institutionalized medical authority in the society.

Seaman (1975) has outlined a set of four proposals for "pelvic autonomy." First, only women should be admitted to obstetrics and gynecology residencies. Second, all new research grants for study of the female reproductive system should be channeled toward training qualified women in reproductive biology. Third, the establishment and administration of laws related to female reproduction, abortion, and sterilization should be removed from the legal system and an agency modeled after the National Labor Relations Board or the Federal Communications Commission should handle these matters. Finally, Seaman recommends that neither the United Nations or the United States should sponsor or participate in international population activities or conferences unless women are represented in proportion to their numbers.

Howell (1975) proposes the establishment of a women's health school in which only women would be educated to provide health care for women. Rather than attempting to integrate care-giving into a traditionally male approach to practice, she suggests that it might be wise to acknowledge our differences and explore a model for an institution organized and served by women in which feminist values can be implemented.

As mentioned previously Marieskind (1975) has suggested that the specialty of obstetrics and gynecology might be disbanded altogether.

THE FUTURE

The future of the women's health movement will probably reflect an expansion in scope beyond primary gynecologic care to services addressing the well and ill, and youth through aged women. Mutual sharing of information may minimize distinctions in patient/provider relationships. The movement will continue to build its own body of knowledge, questioning that evolved by traditional medicine. The women's health movement is concerned not only with health but also with the potential for producing "social change in the fullest sense; a change in the consciousness of men and women freed from the binding roles of domination and submission." (Marieskind, 1975)

The women's health movement has increased social awareness of women's health issues; it has begun to determine health policy and to influence the institutionalization of some health reforms. The impact of the movement can be demonstrated by attitudinal changes in some patients and practitioners, alterations in modes of health care delivery, influences on sexism in medicine, and reassessment of use of hazardous drugs and devices. Government agencies have assumed sponsorship of some activities related to women's health, and some groups are learning how to influence public policy. Whether the net outcome of the women's health movement will be institutionalization of the values of the women's health movement, co-optation of their activities, or interdependence between traditional institutions and those born out of the women's health movement remains to be seen.

REFERENCES

Abramowitz, S. I., and others: Sex bias in psychotherapy: a failure to confirm, Am. J. Psych. **133**(6):706-709, 1976.

Aslin, A. L.: Feminist and community mental health center psychotherapists' expectations of mental health for women, Sex Roles **3**(6): 537-544, 1977.

Bart, P. B.: Does medicine care about women? Guthrie Bull. **47**:95-107, 1977.

Bart, P. B.: Social structure and vocabularies of discomfort: what happened to female hysteria? J. Health Soc. Behav. **9**(3):188-193, 1968.

Benoliel, J.: Self as a critical variable in sensitive research in women's health. In Olesen, V., editor: Women and their health: research implications for a new era, Washington, D.C., 1975, Department of Health, Education and Welfare DHEW (HRA 77-3138).

Broverman, I. K., and others: Sex-role stereotypes and clinical judgments of mental health, J. Consult. Clin. Psychol. **34**(1):1-7, 1970.

Cambell, M. A.: "Why would a girl go into medicine?" Old Westbury, N.Y., 1975, Feminist Press.

Chesler, P.: Women and madness, New York, 1972, Doubleday & Co.

Contraceptive insurance lacking, Nation's Health, May 1978, p. 9.

Cooperstock, R.: Sex differences in the use of mood-modifying drugs: an explanatory model, J. Health Soc. Behav. **12**:238-244, 1971.

Corea, G.: The hidden malpractice: how American medicine treats women as patients and professionals, New York, 1977, William Morrow and Co., Inc.

Doherty, E. G.: Are differential discharge criteria used for men and women psychiatric inpatients? J. Health Soc. Behav. **19**:107-119, 1978.

Ehrenreich, B., and English, D.: For her own good; 150 years of the experts advice to women, New York, 1978, Anchor Press.

Fee, E.: Women and health care: a comparison of theories, Int. J. Health Serv. **5**(3):397-415, 1975.

Feinblatt, J. A., and Gold, A. R.: Sex roles and the psychiatric referral process, Sex Roles **2**(2):109-121, 1976.

Feminist Counseling Collective: Feminist psychotherapy, Social Policy **6**(2):54-62, 1975.

Gomes, B., and Abramowitz, S. I.: Sex-related patient and therapist effects on clinical judgement, Sex Roles **2**(1):1-13, 1976.

Gouldner, A.: The coming crisis of western sociology, New York, 1970, Avon Books.

Heide, W. S.: Feminism: making a difference in our health. In Notman, M., and Nadelson, C., editors: The woman patient, New York, 1978, Plenum Press.

Howell, M. C.: What medical schools teach about women, N. Engl. J. Med. **291**:304, 1974.

Howell, M. C.: A women's health school? Social Policy **6**(2):50-53, 1975.

Howell, M. C., and Hiatt, D.: Do student health services discriminate against women: a survey of services in the U.S. medical schools, J.A.C.H.A. **23**:359-363, 1975.

Hutchinson, S. A.: Women's lib and psychotherapy, J. Psychiatr. Nurs., pp. 20-22, Nov.-Dec. 1975.

Jorgensen, V.: The gynecologist and the sexually liberated woman, Obstet. Gynecol. **42**(4):607-611, 1973.

Kahan, E., and Gaskill, E.: The difficult patient: observations on staff-patient interaction. In Notman, M., and Nadelson, C., editors: The woman patient, New York, 1978, Plenum Press.

Kaiser, B. L., and Kaiser, I. H.: The challenge of the women's movement to American gynecology, Am. J. Obstet. Gynecol. **120**(5):652-665, 1974.

Kjervik, D. K., and Palta, M.: Sex-role stereotyping in assessments of mental health, Nurs. Res. **27**(3):166-171, 1978.

Larned, D.: The epidemic in unnecessary surgery. In Dreifus, C., editor: Seizing our bodies: the politics of women's health, New York, 1977, Random House.

Lennane, K. J., and Lennane, R. J.: Alleged psychogenic disorders in women; a possible manifestation of sexual prejudice, N. Engl. J. Med. **288**(Part 1):288-292, 1973.

McCranie, E. W., and others: Alleged sex-role stereotyping in the assessment of women's physical complaints: a study of general practitioners, Soc. Sci. Med. **12**(2A):111-116, 1978.

Mant, A., and Darroch, D. B.: Media images and medical images, Soc. Sci. Med. **9**:613-618, 1975.

Marieskind, H. I.: Gynecological services and the women's movement: restructuring obstetrics and gynecology, paper presented at American Public Health Association 103rd Annual Meeting, Nov. 16-20, 1975a.

Marieskind, H. I.: Restructuring ob-gyn, Social Policy **6**(2): Sept-Oct. 1975b.

Marieskind, H. I.: The women's health movement, Int. J. Health Serv. **5**(2):217-223, 1975c.

Marieskind, H. I., and Ehrenreich, B.: Toward socialist medicine: the women's health movement, Social Policy **6**(2):34-42, 1975.

Morehead, M., and Trussell, R.: The quantity, quality and costs of medical care secured by a sample of Teamster families in the New York area, New York, 1962, Columbia University School of Public Health and Administrative Medicine.

Muller, C.: Methodological issues in health economics research relevant to women, Women Health **1**(1):3-9, 1976.

Muller, C.: Women and health statistics: areas of deficient data collection and integration, Women Health **4**(1):37-39, 1979.

Notman, M., and Nadelson, C., editors: The woman patient, New York, 1978, Plenum Press.

Oleson, V., editor: Women and their health: research implications for an era, Washington, D.C., 1975, Department of Health, Education and Welfare (DHEW HRA 77-3138).

Parsons, T., and Bales, R. F.: Family socialization and interaction process, Glencoe, Ill., 1955, The Free Press.

Prather, J., and Fidell, L.: Sex differences in the content and style of medical advertisements, Soc. Sci. Med. **9**:23, 1975.

Rice, J. K., and Rice, D. G.: Implications of the women's liberation movement for psychotherapy, Am. J. Psych. **130**(2):191-196, 1973.

Roland, C. G.: The insidious bias of medical language, Nurs. Digest **5**(1):53-55, 1977.

Ruzek, S. B.: The women's health movement: feminist alternatives to medical control, New York, 1978, Praeger Publishers.

Schwartz, A.: Women's issues in national health insurance, Nation's Health, p. 9, May 1978.

Scully, D., and Bart, P.: A funny thing happened on the way to the orifice: women in gynecology textbooks, Am. J. Soc. **78**:1045, 1973.

Seaman, B.: Free and female, Greenwich, Conn., 1972, Fawcett Publications, Inc.

Seaman, B.: Pelvic autonomy: four proposals, Social Policy, pp. 43-48. Sept.-Oct. 1975.

Sechrest, L.: Ethical problems in medical experimentation involving women. In Olesen, V., editor: Women and their health: research implications for an era, Washington, D.C., 1975, Department of Health, Education and Welfare (DHEW HRA 77-3138).

Shapiro, J.: Socialization of sex roles in the counseling setting: differential counselor behavioral and attitudinal responses to typical and atypical female sex roles, Sex Roles, 3(2):173-184, 1977.

Smith, M. C., and Griffin, L.: Rationality of appeals used in the promotion of psychotropic drugs: a comparison of male and female models, Soc. Sci. Med. 11:409-414, 1977.

Stockburger, D. W., and Davis, J. O.: Selling the female image as mental patient, Sex Roles 4(1):131-134, 1978.

Tudor, W., Tudor, J., and Gove, W.: The effect of sex role differences on the social control of mental illness, J. Health Soc. Behav. 18: 98-112, 1977.

Waldron, I.: Increased prescribing of valium, librium and other drugs: an example of the influence of economic and social factors on the practice of medicine, Int. J. Health Serv. 7(1):91-94, 1977.

Wildausky, A.: Doing better and feeling worse: The political pathology of health policy, Daedalus J. Am. Acad. Arts Sci. 106(1):105, 1977.

Withersty, D. J.: Sexual attitudes of hospital personnel: a model for continuing education, Am. J. Psych. 133(5):573-575, 1976.

Wolman, C. S.: Clinical applications of feminist theory, unpublished paper, 1978.

Nursing practice with women

4

Health promotion and maintenance for women: a nursing perspective

Nancy Fugate Woods

The nursing profession has traditionally sought new ways to meet human health requirements. The nature of nursing practice has changed frequently over the last century to respond to the needs of the populations served by the profession.* Such alterations in the nature of practice are currently exemplified by the increasing emphasis on delivering primary care services to populations not well served by traditional systems; for example, nurse practitioners have demonstrated an effective mechanism for providing primary care for rural populations as well as the urban poor. This tradition of providing services that reflect the health requirements of the population rather than the traditional structure and organization of the profession's practice enables the nursing profession to be responsive to the changing health requirements of special populations.

Nursing has traditionally been concerned with the well-being of the person as a whole. This view of humanity has been contrasted with the focus of other health professions. Medicine in this century has moved toward specialization around organ systems, diseases, and pathology, and toward increasingly microscopic levels of analysis. For example, biomedicine draws on the sciences of molecular biology and biochemistry. Other helping professions, such as social work, intervene with larger social systems such as the family, group, and community. A unique aspect of professional nursing practice is that its focus can be on the health of the client at the level of subsystems, as a total human being, or as part of a complex social network; all levels are considered simultaneously, along with the interaction among systems.

Nursing practitioners have attempted to foster active participation of clients in meeting their own health care requirements. Only in recent years have the general public and some health professionals come to the realization that health depends on the actions that individuals take to maintain and promote it. Yet the participation of clients in health activities was encouraged by even the earliest nursing scholars.

Virginia Henderson's definition of nursing, published in 1955, captures the essence of nursing and self-health: "Nursing is primarily assisting the individual (sick or well) in the performance of those activities contributing to health or its recovery (or to a peaceful death) that (s)he would perform unaided if (s)he had the necessary strength, will, or knowledge." (p. 4) Henderson further emphasizes that an important element of nursing's mission is to help the individual to become independent of nursing assistance as soon as possible. Other writers have reinforced the notion that an important dimension of nursing practice is promotion of the client's abilities to care for herself or himself (see Orem, 1971; Rogers, 1976; Roy, 1970; Weidenbach, 1964).

The nursing profession is almost entirely populated by women. Although the problems created by sex stratification in the health professions have serious consequences for health professionals and clients alike, the history of domination of the nursing profession by other, largely male, professions has heightened the sensitivity of some in nursing to problems women encounter in the society at large. While it is unfair to assume that female professionals will automatically be more sensitive to the needs of women than male professionals, some women have strong convictions about the necessity for women professionals to care for other women. For these women, the nursing profession may constitute a major resource for health care.

Because the nursing profession is able to alter its ap-

---

*Though some would suggest that the changes in nursing practice reflect the lack of direction of the profession rather than its concern with the health needs of populations, we will assume the latter to be the case in this chapter.

proach to practice to reflect the health needs of designated populations, because it is concerned with the well-being of the total person, because it is committed to fostering the active participation of clients in health promotion and maintenance, and because the profession is comprised almost entirely of women, it is likely that nursing will emerge as *the* profession most responsive to women's health needs. Furthermore, it is possible that the nursing profession will not only assume an advocacy position with respect to women and their emergent health requirements, but also will collaborate with (not co-opt) the self–health care movement for women. In view of the important contribution that nursing can make to women's health, the purposes of this chapter include the following: (1) to explicate a philosophy of nursing for a special population—women; (2) to describe processes by which nurses can assist women to promote and maintain their health; and (3) to delineate outcome criteria that can be used to evaluate the quality of nursing services for women.

HEALTH CARE FOR WOMEN: A PHILOSOPHY FOR NURSING PRACTICE

A philosophy for nursing practice requires that assumptions about nursing, health, health maintenance, and health promotion be made explicit. Assumptions about women and their health must also be delineated, inasmuch as they influence the nature of nursing practice with this special population.

Nursing

Hall (1977) defines nursing as "an abstract body of knowledge concerned with the life process in human systems as they interrelate in a complex hierarchy of individuals, families, groups, social organizations, communities, and societies." (p. 174) The practice of nursing includes application of this body of knowledge in clinical and teaching-learning as well as research situations. The goal of nursing practice is to promote and maintain the health of human systems.

In addition to being a body of knowledge, a profession, and an academic discipline, nursing can be characterized as *process*. The processes of assessment, intervention, and evaluation are sometimes alluded to collectively as *the* nursing process. As professionals, however, nurses incorporate many processes in their practice with clients. Hall (1977) has delineated several types of processes that are essential to nursing practice. Basic processes include perceiving, communicating, caring, knowing, problem-solving, creating, and valuing (see box). These processes are the most elemental of the human services skills. Hall also points out that these same processes might well describe the outcomes that nurses and clients seek in a nurse-client relationship.

These process-oriented skills are combined by the nurse in a special way to create the components of nursing practice. Hall identifies these components as assessing, intervening, and evaluating, which are combined to create the components of nursing practice. For example, perceiving and communicating are both important processes in assessing the health status of an individual or family. Problem-solving, creating, and caring might be combined in the intervention component of practice. Valuing, knowing, and perceiving might all be involved in the evaluation component.

In addition to the processes already mentioned, nurses employ several others to facilitate change in client systems. These include inquiring, helping, teaching, supervising, coordinating, collaborating, consulting, bargaining, confronting, and lobbying. These processes are not only employed by nurses to facilitate change in clients, but some can also be outcomes of the nurse-client relationship. For example, the client can be supported to confront others who impede her progress toward health; to inquire about her health state and how to promote it; to bargain and lobby for health care that is acceptable and accessible; and to teach others ways of healthful living. Hall asserts that nursing interven-

---

Basic process skills for nursing*

Perceiving is the process of differentiating the phenomenal field including the categorization of those internal and external stimuli which impinge upon the perceiver.

Communicating is the interpersonal process of sharing personal meaning in order to influence behavior.

Caring is the process of being responsive to the needs of others in relationships characterized by understanding, acceptance, and empathy.

Knowing is the on-going metamorphosis of ideas which provide for coherence and unity of feeling, thought, and action.

Problem-solving is the goal-directed process of seeking solutions to dilemmas through the utilization of a series of prescribed maneuvers including, in its simplest form, assessment, intervention, and evaluation.

Creating is the self-renewing process of total organismic involvement in self-selected activities in order to achieve significant, original, and imaginative outcomes.

Valuing is the organismic process of choosing, prizing, and acting in harmony with an internalized set of principles derived from experience which lend predictability in human behavior.

*From Hall, J.: Nursing as process. In Hall, J., and Weaver, B., editors: Distributive nursing practice: a systems approach to community health, Philadelphia, 1977, J. B. Lippincott Co., pp. 173-189.

tion is the "facilitation of process in clients" whether these processes are of a physiologic or interpersonal nature.

A process-oriented definition of nursing is consistent with the goal of facilitating health by fostering clients' abilities to make choices that promote and maintain their health. Individuals choose and follow courses of action judged to be beneficial to them. These choices are influenced by social norms, physiologic mechanisms, and the individual's response to the environment. Such choices create climates that are either favorable or unfavorable for human functioning. Self-care is "the practice of activities that individuals personally initiate and

---

Change process skills*

Inquiring is the cognitive process which questions assumptions and seeks knowledge in the pursuit of explanation, prediction and control.

Helping is a purposeful dynamic process within a time limited relationship directed toward enabling the client to achieve a more satisfactory level of functioning in a variety of life situations.

Teaching is the process of assisting clients to acquire the health-related knowledge, skills, and values which foster and maintain cognitive, interpersonal, and psychomotor functioning.

Supervising is the process of assisting people to function effectively by guiding their professional development and increasing their performance skills.

Coordinating is the process of bringing together diverse approaches to health care in such a way as to deliver quality health care to clients.

Collaborating is the process of working together in an egalitarian spirit to achieve mutually defined and desired goals.

Consulting is an interactional process between professionals in which the consultant shares specialized expertise to assist the consultee to solve work problems within the framework of the consultee's professional functioning.

Bargaining is the process of negotiating an agreement in which the persons involved settle the terms of the contract to their mutual satisfaction.

Confronting is the process of increasing awareness of different perceptions of reality through face-to-face communicative encounter.

Lobbying is the process of influencing the passage of legislation, the establishment of policy, and the implementation of administrative decision-making on the basis of special interests.

*From Hall, J.: Nursing as process. In Hall, J., and Weaver, B., editors: Distributive nursing practice: a systems approach to community health, Philadelphia, 1977, J. B. Lippincott Co., pp. 173-191.

---

perform on their own behalf in maintaining life, health and well being" (Orem, 1971; p. 13). Self-care is learned behavior and involves decisions about its performance. Some types of self-care are universally required, but some become necessary only in the event of illness, injury, or disease. According to Orem (1971), nursing systems are necessitated by the absence of the ability to maintain for oneself the amount and quality of self-care that is therapeutic in sustaining life and health, in recovering from disease or injury, and in coping with their effects. Nursing systems can be designed to help clients compensate entirely or in part for their inability to participate in self-care or to support and educate clients as they attempt to assume self-care responsibility.

Based on Orem's work, Kinlein (1977) has proposed a system of nursing in which the goal is to enhance the individual's self-care agency in maintaining or improving the health state. She outlines a process by which the nurse, in conjunction with the client, identifies the self-care practices in which the client currently engages. Nurse and client collaborate to delineate self-care assets and deficits. The therapeutic self-care demand is identified by the nurse (nursing diagnosis), and goal-setting with the client ensues. Finally, the nurse prescribes therapeutic measures to meet the client's self-care demand.

Consideration of a systems approach to nursing as described by Hall (1977) and the self-care concept as described by Orem (1971) and modified by Kinlein (1977) provides a model for nursing practice that reflects several assumptions about nursing:

1. Nursing is a body of knowledge concerned with life process in human systems as they relate to larger social systems and the environment.
2. Nursing can be regarded as process; assessment, intervention, and evaluation are important components.
3. Nurses intervene to facilitate the life process in clients.
4. Life processes (life, health, and well-being) are maintained by the self-care activities of individuals.
5. Nursing involves prescription of measures to enhance the client's self-care agency.

Implicit in the set of assumptions about nursing is a set of assumptions about clients. First, it is assumed that individuals have the *capability to make decisions* about their health and that they ultimately have *control of their own health* by virtue of the choices they make. It is also assumed that individuals have the *capability to provide their own self-care* with respect to their health. At times assistance may be necessary from a health professional, but the goal is always to restore the individual's self-care agency. These assumptions about clients, implicit in a systems approach to nursing and in use of the self-care concept, do not foster a provider-consumer dichotomy; rather they imply a collaborative kind of relationship in which information is freely exchanged with clients and informed decision-making is ideally the client's domain.*

Definitions of health

Defining health has been a problem for clinicians, researchers, and policy-makers in this century. Because of the difficulty associated in operationalizing concepts of health, clinicians, researchers, and policy-makers alike have often resorted to "the absence of disease" as an indicator of the concept. Of late, all groups have been somewhat more willing to commit to a definition. The familiar World Health Organization definition of health as "a complete state of physical, mental, and social well-being, not merely the absence of disease" expresses what health *ought* to be.

It should be pointed out, however, that the concept of health is socially determined, reflecting the structure of the society in which the individual lives. Kelman (1975) notes that there are two conflicting dimensions of health, which he refers to as "functional" and "experiential." The first might be regarded as the capacity to effectively perform the roles and tasks for which one has been socialized. The second, experiential health, reflects people's conceptions of what it is to be healthy. Experiential health would be perceived by the individual as a state of organismic integrity—not merely freedom from illness but also the "capacity for human development and self-discovery, and the transcendence of alienating social circumstances." (p. 629) Thus the experiential dimension of health is intrinsically defined, and although it is to some extent socially determined, as is functional health, it is the experiential dimension that is most congruent with the notion of nursing described here.

Health promotion and maintenance

The individual's and society's approach to health promotion and maintenance will, of necessity, reflect the values of the society, which are in turn determinants of the definition of health. If the functional definition of health is the criterion used to plan health policy and care, then health maintenance will consist of intervening between social stressors causing pathogenesis or treating the pathology once it exists. The goal of health maintenance will be the individual's ability to function in prescribed social roles. An example related to health

---

*This need not imply that nurses abdicate their responsibilities by refusing to make decisions when that is clearly what the client requests or perhaps even requires. There are instances in which clients may prefer to delegate the decision to the professional. What is crucial is that clients, even in these instances, have the right to decide—or to choose *not* to decide.

maintenance for women is presented to clarify the relationship between the definitions of health and health maintenance:

A homemaker with three children has become increasingly depressed over the past 2 years to the point that she is unable to take care of her home and her children. She is given a prescription for Valium based on the premise that she should be able to perform her normal tasks.

In this instance the health problem is attacked. Medication is interposed between the social stressor and the pathology to alter the individual's perception of the situation. Were the depression to continue despite medication, the pathology itself might be further attacked.

The same example might be used to illustrate how health can be promoted and maintained. Instead of treating the symptom of depression, the health professional ascribing to an experiential definition of health might involve the woman in describing her own assets and deficits and subsequently assisting her to discover her capacity for self-development and means of transcending or changing her situation. These goals might be fostered through membership in a support or consciousness-raising group.

Whereas the first approach to health maintenance is an attempt to help the client adjust to an alienating situation, the second is an attempt to help the client transcend the situation or in time to alter the environment to be more consistent with her own integrity. While the first situation describes therapeutic attempts to maintain the woman's health (e.g., the status quo with regard to her role performance), the second illustrates an attempt not only to help the woman to maintain her self-care agency but also to promote her health (that is, to grow).

Assumptions about women and their health

A philosophy for nursing of women must be based on explicit assumptions about women and their health. Rather than recounting assumptions about women that were relevant in the past, the purpose of this section is to make explicit a more recent view of women in society and their emergent health care requirements. In order to do so, it is necessary to consider demographic trends affecting women.

Women are living longer, marrying later and less often, remarrying less frequently after widowhood or divorce, having and expecting to have fewer children, and more often planning to have no children than their foremothers. Women are increasingly living alone as heads of households. Technology, legislation, and attitudinal and behavioral changes have joined to depress the birth rate in recent years. Women are showing some gains in educational level. They are also entering the labor force in increasing numbers and proportions, and remaining in it after marriage and during their early childbearing years. They initiate sexual activity at an earlier age and probably continue to be sexually active into their later years. Inflation and the energy crisis have conjoined to increase the economic squeeze experienced by families. At the same time, flexi-time arrangements for work and job sharing may become increasingly popular in the future. Television portrays alternative lifestyles for women much more openly than in the past, and the media's pervasive influence on women's lives has been used to disseminate health information as well. In addition, political consciousness has been raised regarding sex and racial discrimination (Lipman-Blumen, 1975).

Women's health and childbearing capacity

Popular concern about women's health has often been based on the assumption that a woman's health should be safeguarded because of her potential childbearing capacity. As a result, the clinical practices designed to care for a woman are often concerned with her reproductive health to the exclusion of other important aspects of her well-being. Women literally get into the medical care system via their reproductive organs. Such a limited concern for only reproductive function, of necessity, blinds health professionals to emergent physiologic as well as psychosocial interferences with health. For example, it is likely that the changing roles of women in western society will be associated with the kinds of stress-related health problems formerly more prevalent among males. Despite the fact that there is some evidence for this trend (e.g., with respect to alcoholism and cardiovascular problems), the thrust of occupational health research is often on elucidating sources of teratogenicity of causes of fetal anomalies rather than the effects of the work environment on the woman herself. Women's health is studied with federal dollars, but primarily those earmarked for maternal-child health. Therefore, an important assumption for nursing practice for woman is that *woman's health cannot be defined only on the basis of her childbearing functions.* A broader definition of health is needed to incorporate other aspects of physical and emotional well-being.

A somewhat related assumption is that women's mental health is not judged on the basis of her ability or willingness to perform certain sex-stereotypic roles and tasks. Rather *women's mental health should reflect her organismic integrity, the capacity for human development and self-discovery, as well as her capability to transcend socially alienating situations.* What is "normal" or "healthy" cannot be described as a discrete

point, but rather as a range of behaviors that subserve the woman's integrity. For many women, rejecting stereotypically "feminine" behavior—the normative or healthy behavior pattern according to some health sciences texts—is a sign of health.

Women's bodies

It should be noted that a woman's health is and can be uniquely influenced by several changes in her physiology: the onset of menstruation, pregnancy, interruption of pregnancy, childbirth, postpartum, nursing, and menopause. These events not only cause changes in the woman's body, but also may induce changes in the woman's relationship to her immediate social network and society at large. Female sexuality, childbearing, nursing, menstruation and menopause can be good, powerful, and pleasurable forces and should be regarded as healthy. Later chapters will discuss each of these forces in more detail.

By virtue of ownership, women have the right to control their own bodies. This implies that they have certain rights when they become clients in a helping relationship. These include rights to information regarding the advantages and disadvantages of various approaches to therapy, the right to end treatment when they choose, the right to be informed of the assessments of health professionals, and the right to knowledge about how their bodies function optimally and individually. This includes a right to shop for an appropriate practitioner.

When given adequate information and skills, the woman can be an expert in the care of her own body. The woman may gain expertise about her body either through regular self-examination or by sharing this experience with other women (Downer, 1975). Such expertise allows women to collaborate with the health professional in their self-care requirements. The intent here is not to co-opt the elements of the woman's health movement for use by the nursing profession in meeting self-serving objectives, but rather to foster self-care capabilities.

An assumption similar to that stated earlier is that given adequate information, a woman can exercise responsible reproductive control (Downer, 1975). Having an unplanned pregnancy may not be an indication of irresponsibility; rather it may indicate a lack of reliable, safe, and available contraceptive devices, or the lack of appropriate information with regard to their use.

Some feminists would insist that any specialized skills for assisting women with menstruation, orgasm, childbirth, and early abortion should be practiced by women only. While this might ensure the representation of a greater number of women in some of the currently male-dominated health fields (and might be a self-serving assumption for the nursing profession), one cannot assume that gender confers upon the health practitioner freedom from sexism and sex-role stereotyping. On the other hand, a woman should have access to a female health professional if that is her preference (Downer, 1974; Seaman, 1975).

NURSING PRACTICE FOR WOMEN

The philosophy of nursing presented earlier in this chapter outlines assumptions about nursing, health, health promotion and maintenance, and women and their health. These assumptions imply a special kind of relationship between nurse and client and an orientation to practice that reflects the emergent health requirements of women.

Structure and process of the relationship

Health promotion and maintenance can occur in the context of an egalitarian and collaborative relationship between the health practitioner and the client. The relationship can be one in which the professional power of the nurse is balanced with the power of the client; this is achieved by mutual recognition of one another's expertise, sharing of information, and defining goals in collaboration. The client is regarded as an expert about her own self-care and the nurse as an expert in the processes that can be used to facilitate health in the client. Information is shared freely between the two such that the client is availed of as much of the necessary data as

possible to make an informed choice about her health. This type of relationship fosters self-care rather than a kind of professional unionism designed to control information flow and enhance the status distinctions between client and professional. The client is an active participant in her own self–health care, not a passive recipient.

The focus of the relationship is on the woman as client, her "self," rather than her "role." This is not to say that the nurse does not consider the context in which the woman exists. Indeed, the nurse must be able to help the client analyze her immediate social networks and other social systems as they impinge on her as a woman and on her view of herself. The fact that a woman is a mother or a worker or a wife of the sole support of an aging parent—or any combination of these—will affect her health and her ability to cope with the stresses in her life.

A comparison of the structure and process of the relationship between nurse and client in traditional vs new systems of care is given in Table 4-1. There are important differences in power structure, information exchange, decision-making, integration of the client in the system, and the way in which women are viewed.

For example, a nurse practitioner who is employed in a family health center models the egalitarian and collaborative relationship described in Table 4-1 with her clients. Convinced that women have a fund of health

Table 4-1. Comparison of structure and process of the relationship between nurse and client in traditional vs. new systems

Dimension	Traditional system	New system
Power structure in relationship between nurse and client	Nurse seen as authority figure, more powerful than client.	Nurse and client have egalitarian, collaborative relationship. Power balanced between nurse and client.
Information exchange	Nurse maintains stratification in relationship by withholding some information from client; makes judgments about how much information client can "handle" or "needs to know." Minimal information obtained from client.	Information exchanged freely between nurse and client. Nurse recognizes client is expert in own self-care; nurse is expert in processes used to facilitate client's health.
Decision-making	Nurse may make some decisions which she judges client is unable to make. Usually this is subtle (e.g., only limited alternatives may be presented).	Client clearly the decider for own self-care. Nurse is consultant. Client chooses from all available alternatives.
Integration of client in system	Client clearly not a part of the "provider" system. Client passive recipient of prescriptions for health.	Client is component of system in which professionals and other clients strive for health. Client has an active role, and makes prescriptions for own health based on information about self-care.
View of women	Woman seen as a "role." Problems of population of women are defined on the basis of their reproductive roles in society.	Woman seen as individual, in social network; also viewed as part of population of women with emergent health care requirements.

information, she makes it a practice to ask her client's opinions ("What do you think about this?" "What do you think is causing the problem?") rather than merely sharing her own impressions. This nurse subsequently supplements the client's fund of information about the problem. She may recommend journal articles from nursing literature, or publications oriented to a nonprofessional audience, or she may use written materials she has produced for the clients in her practice. This nurse also attempts to expand the client's fund of information about treatment options, sharing their relative merits and disadvantages. The client is given responsibility for making an informed decision, and often prescribes regimens for promoting or maintaining her own health. This practitioner has a clear concept of the influence of the woman's social networks on her health and is alert to the emergent health needs of her clients. For example, her awareness of women's changing exposure to risk factors for cardiovascular disease and lung cancer prompts her to incorporate information about smoking and approaches to stopping smoking into the regular health assessments.

This type of nurse-client relationship gives rise to some subtle but important differences in the components of nursing process: assessment, intervention, and

evaluation. The content and process of each are altered as shown in Table 4-2.

Assessment

In the system advocated here, the data to be collected are relevant to the woman as an individual and as a whole person. They are not restricted to, nor do they emphasize, reproduction. The data are likely to relate to emergent health practices or problems characterizing the population of women from which the client comes. For example, in view of the increase in smoking and lung cancer among women, it would be important for the nurse to ask the woman about her smoking habits. Since many women use physical exercise to decrease stress, this is also a pertinent area to pursue in the history. Any additional data that the woman believes are relevant are also obtained. For example, women who have had recurrent vaginal or urinary tract infections are usually aware which medications are effective and which are not. Often they are able to diagnose their own problem and recommend the treatment that is most effective for them. Women who perform pelvic self-examinations can note very subtle changes in the cervix and often can describe the signs of ovulation.

The process of data collection involves an exchange

Table 4-2. Nursing process: a comparison of assessment, intervention, and evaluation in traditional vs. new systems

	Traditional system	New system
Assessment		
Data to be collected	Data relate largely to woman's reproductive structure and function. Other aspects of health may be minimized.	Data relate to woman's "self," individual problems, self-care assets. Data include potential or emergent health problems as defined by changing health patterns of populations of women.
Process of collecting data	Nurse decides what data are relevant, then collects them. Woman responds to questions initiated by nurse.	Woman provides nurse with own baseline data regarding health. Woman invited to share data she believes to be relevant. Nurse may point out other useful data to consider.
Data analysis	Nurse analyzes data to obtain nursing diagnosis, which is then shared with client. Woman is asked to validate nurses' inferences.	Woman is helped to analyze data. Nurse shares own impressions as nursing diagnosis. Woman's inferences regarded as valid.
Intervention		
Goal-setting	Goals are mutually derived.	Goals are woman's. Nurse delineates what she sees as possible for woman.
Process of intervening	Nurse performs intervention for client or teaches client to perform intervention. Intervention is to facilitate client's adaptation.	Nurse facilitates the woman's ability to perform processes important for self-care. Nurse collaborates with woman. Woman may be helped not to adapt to but to change environment.
Evaluation		
Criteria used for evaluation	Product-oriented; specify observable end-point in nurse-client relationship.	Process-oriented; specify processes woman has identified as important to fulfill self-care requirements.
Process for evaluating	Nurse compares mutually derived goals with product of the nurse-client relationship using product-oriented criteria.	Woman compares the goals she has set for herself with her self-care agency, using process-oriented criteria.

between nurse and client, and analysis is a shared responsibility. The woman is encouraged to provide as much baseline data and historical information as possible. Women who practice breast and pelvic self-examinations are encouraged to share this information and are reinforced to continue this self-care. The woman is encouraged to infer the nature of her problem from the data she has presented. The nurse contributes information relevant to the problem and facilitates the analysis. The nurse shares her own impressions with the client in the form of a nursing diagnosis.

Intervention

The goals to be pursued are those that the woman defines as important to her. The nurse, as consultant, may share what she sees as possible for the client. For example, if the woman is concerned about seeking employment but thinks she is too old at age 40 to enter the labor force, the nurse might share with her that many women in the same age group are seeking employment and are doing so successfully. The process of intervening in the new system of health care for women is a collaborative one in which the nurse facilitates the woman's abilities to perform those processes necessary for self-care. Rather than just facilitating the woman's adaptation to the environment, the nurse may facilitate the woman's ability to *change* the environment in which she lives. For example, the woman who is abused by a spouse is not encouraged to submit to further abuse or to learn to deny herself in order to avoid further abuse, but is often advised to remove herself from the dangerous environment and to learn to cope in another social situation. The woman who is unable to afford a nutritionally adequate diet is encouraged to obtain food stamps rather than become anemic. Women who have a diagnosis not covered by medical insurance, such as infertility, are helped and encouraged to lobby for better insurance coverage.

Evaluation

This component of the nursing process involves the woman's assessment of her self-care agency. She is invited to review the processes necessary for her self–health care and to compare her current status with her expectations for herself. The nurse validates the woman's observations and analysis and avails herself to the woman as a consultant. The evaluative component is guided by outcome criteria for health that the woman and nurse have established together.

Some general outcome criteria that nurses can use to evaluate their efficacy can be stipulated. First, it is important that the woman have an improved understanding of her health and self-care agency as a result of her

encounters with the health care practitioner. Second, the woman should have an improved ability to collect data about her health and make appropriate inferences from the data. Third, she should have expanded her ability to perform those processes important to self-care. Finally, she should have an improved capacity for making decisions about her health. If these criteria are met, then the nurse is effectively practicing the new system of care as delineated here.

Implicit in the foregoing discussion are two additional outcome criteria:

1. The woman will have her value system respected during her encounters with the health care system.
2. The woman's health problems or concerns will be managed in a way that is congruent with her biology, her view of herself, and her current role in society.

ORIENTATION TO NURSING PRACTICE FOR WOMEN

Nursing practice for women reflects a nurturing and empathic approach and an appreciation for the special problems of women. Its goals are not to make choices for clients about how to improve their health, but rather to allow them to make choices that expand their ability to perform self-care. It is based on an awareness of what it means to be a woman with respect to social systems as well as biology. It is based on the assumption that women and men should be regarded as equal. Women are not encouraged to be more feminine or more masculine; rather, an appreciation for the positive qualities commonly ascribed to both sexes (androgyny) is cultivated. Women are encouraged to pursue goals that are important to them, not only those that sex-stereotypic thinking would permit.

The nurse who practices with women needs an awareness of how the internalized consequences of sexism and sex-role stereotyping affect clients, as well as an appreciation of the accuracy of clients' descriptions of male oppression. The practice of nursing for women requires that the practitioner be aware of some of the problems that women encounter but that are rarely discussed openly: intimidation by men, rape, incest, battering, and sexual harrassment in employment. At times the nurse will find it essential to initiate discussion of these topics because of their painful and emotionally laden nature.

Nurses who provide health care for women also need to be proficient at social analysis. They must be able to empathize with women from different races, social classes, educational background, or political groups. Nurses need to be aware of the patriarchal influence on family dynamics and its effects; the "blame the mother" syndrome that has conveniently been used against women must be explored in an attempt to help women free themselves from unrealistic expectations and to help them appreciate their own mother's position. Nurses who work primarily with women clients can foster belief in the possibility of male-female equality in all settings.

Finally, nurses can foster woman-to-woman bonding and the development of female support systems for clients. Mother-daughter problems resulting from changing sex roles may require attention in some families. In others, role strain and similar existential conflicts affect women (Feminist Counseling Collective, 1975; Wolman, 1978).

The nurse practicing with women clients will find it essential to demystify the process of health care, help women reclaim responsibility for their own health, and reduce the alienating aspects of currently used health services. Above all, appreciation for the social as well as physiologic experiences affecting all women is essential.

This approach to nursing emphasizes health care as process, not product. It reflects the changing health desires of the population as well as the changing meaning of being a woman. Its proponents recognize the woman's health movement as an emergent alternative system for health promotion and maintenance. This philosophy of nursing practice for women welcomes alternatives to an illness care system that is currently ineffective with respect to promotion and maintenance of health. This philosophy implies that practitioners of nursing value the capability that women have for promoting and maintaining their own health. Those who ascribe to this philosophy do not wish to compete with or co-opt the women's self-health movement but recognize its contribution to the health and well-being of women and seek collaborative ties with these emergent systems.

REFERENCES

Bart, P.: Unalienating abortion, demystifying depression, and restoring rape victims, paper presented at the American Psychiatric Association, Anaheim, Calif., 1975.

Bart, P.: Taking our bodies back, paper presented to Division 35 of the American Psychological Association, San Francisco, 1977.

Benoliel, J. Q.: Self as critical variable in sensitive research in women's health. In Olesen, V., editor: Women and their health: research implications for a new era, Washington, D.C., 1975, Department of Health, Education and Welfare (DHEW HRA 77-3138).

Byrne, M., and Thompson, L. F.: Key concepts for the study and practice of nursing, St. Louis, 1978, The C. V. Mosby Co.

Donaldson, S. K. N., and Crowley, D. M.: The discipline of nursing, Nurs. Outlook **26**(2):113-120, 1978.

Downer, C.: Women professionals in the feminist health movement, Los Angeles, April 1974, Feminist Women's Health Center.

Feminist Counseling Collective: Feminist psychotherapy, Social Policy **6**(2):54-62, 1975.

Hall, J.: Nursing as process. In Hall, J., and Weaver, B., editors: Distributive nursing practice; a systems approach to community health, Philadelphia, 1977, J. B. Lippincott Co.

Hart, S. K., and Herriott, P.: Components of practice: a systems

approach. In Hall, J., and Weaver, B., editors: Distributive nursing practice: a systems approach to community health, Philadelphia, 1977, J. B. Lippincott Co.

Henderson, V.: The nature of nursing, New York, 1971, The Macmillan Co.

Howell, M. C.: A women's health school? Social Policy **6**(2):50-53, 1975.

Kelman, S.: The social nature of the definition problem in health, Int. J. Health Serv. **5**(4):625-642, 1975.

King, I.: Toward a theory for nursing, New York, 1971, John Wiley & Sons, Inc.

Kinlein, L.: Independent nursing practice with clients, Philadelphia, 1977, J. B. Lippincott Co.

Knowles, J., editor: Doing better and feeling worse: health in the United States, New York, 1972, W. W. Norton Co.

Lee, P.: Policy, women and health: same old system or something new? In Olesen, V., editor: Women and their health: research implications for a new era, Washington, D.C., 1975, Department of Health, Education and Welfare (DHEW HRA 77-3138).

Levin, L., and others: Self care: lay initiatives in health, New York, 1976, Neale Watson Academic Publications.

Lipman-Blumen, J.: Overview: demographic trends and issues in women's health. In Olesen, V., editor: Women and their health: research implications for a new era, Washington, D.C., 1975, Department of Health, Education and Welfare (DHEW HRA 77-3138).

Marieskind, H.: Restructuring ob-gyn, Social Policy **6**(2):48-49, 1975.

Marieskind, H., and Ehrenreich, B.: Toward socialist medicine: the women's health movement, Social Policy **6**(2):34-42, 1975.

Muller, C.: Methodological issues in health economics research relevant to women. In Olesen, V., editor: Women and their health: research implications for a new era, Washington, D.C., 1975, Department of Health, Education and Welfare (DHEW HRA 77-3138).

Nelson, C.: Reconceptualizing health care. In Olesen, V., editor: Women and their health: research implications for a new era, Washington, D.C., 1975, Department of Health, Education and Welfare (DHEW HRA 77-3138).

Norris, C.: Self care, Am. J. Nurs. **79**(3):486-489, 1979.

Olesen, V., ed.: Women and their health: research implications for a new era, Washington, D.C., 1975, Department of Health, Education and Welfare (DHEW HRA 77-3138).

Orem, D.: Nursing: concepts of practice, New York, 1971, McGraw-Hill Book Co.

Orlando, I. J.: The dynamic nurse-patient relationship, New York, 1961, G. P. Putnam's Sons.

Rogers, M.: An introduction to the theoretical basis of nursing, Philadelphia, 1970, F. A. Davis Co.

Roy, Sr. C.: Introduction to nursing: an adaptation model. Englewood Cliffs, N.J., 1976, Prentice Hall, Inc.

Ruzek, S.: Emergent modes of utilization: gynecological self-help. In Olesen, V., editor: Women and their health: research implications for a new era, Washington, D.C., 1975, Department of Health, Education and Welfare (DHEW HRA 77-3138).

Schlotfeldt, R.: The professional doctorate: rationale and characteristics, Nurs. Outlook **26L5**:302-311, 1978.

Seaman, B.: Pelvic autonomy: four proposals, Social Policy **6**(2):43-47, 1975.

Sechrest, L.: Ethical problems in medical experimentation involving women. In Olesen, V., editor: Women and their health: research implications for a new era, Washington, D.C., 1975, Department of Health, Education and Welfare (DHEW HRA 77-3138).

Weidenbach, E.: Clinical nursing: a helping art, New York, 1964, Springer Publishing Co.

Wolman, C.: Clinical applications of feminist theory, unpublished paper, 1978.

5

Woman's body

Nancy Fugate Woods

WOMEN AS INFORMED CONSUMERS

Women are becoming increasingly knowledgeable about their bodies and their health, as evidenced by their ability to participate more fully in their own self-care. Women have traditionally been more likely than men to use health maintenance and preventive services. With the advent of the women's health movement, women are assuming increasing responsibility for monitoring their own health states, and consequently may be well prepared to present their own accounts of past health problems, physical findings, and plans for health promotion and maintenance. In some instances they can recommend the therapy that has worked best for them in the past.

One mechanism of maintaining social control that has been characteristic of the medical care system in this society is control of information. Consumers are often not informed fully of normal and abnormal findings, a plan of care, alternative treatment options, and side effects. The assumption made by some providers is that consumers (especially women) lack the sophistication necessary to participate in a discussion of health problems or plans for health maintenance. This stance has been used to justify paternalistic patterns of care. As long as the practitioner can assume that the client is unable to comprehend health-related information, the logical conclusion is that the client cannot be expected to make appropriate judgments about issues such as the best of several alternative courses of therapy.

A second mechanism supportive of social control is stratification by social class. Usually the client and practitioner are not from the same social class. This is especially true in the case of women. (One has only to look at the distribution of women in the health professions to see that it mirrors the social and economic distribution of women in the society as a whole.) The women's health movement has attempted to eradicate the class/caste system in health care by equalizing the relationship between helper and helped. The key, at least for part of the population of women, seems to be self-health care; that is, women learning to meet their own self-care requirements and helping other women in an egalitarian relationship.

Control of information and social class differences have constituted important variables in health care for women in the past. The women's health movement has already made great strides in its attempt to inform women about their bodies. *Our Bodies, Ourselves* (Boston Women's Health Book Collective, 1976) is one example of a manual for women, designed to share the knowledge and power that comes with thinking about ourselves and our lives in an honest, humane, and powerful way. It is one example of a reference based not only on professional literature but also on valuable personal experience.

Women's changing attitudes about their bodies

Women who have come together to discuss their health often express a variety of feelings about their bodies. Women tend to make comparisons with one another and with an "ideal self." Often these comparisons have not been favorable. In fact, many women have negative feelings about their bodies, including a dislike for body hair or odors and discomfort with the genitals. There is often concern expressed about being inadequate—not measuring up to the "ideal" woman. Rather than valuing their uniqueness, women have often followed the injunctions of the advertising world to fulfill "the image."

Another difficulty women often experience is feeling that their bodies are not their own. The women from the Boston Women's Health Book Collective (1976) capture these feelings well:

Our "figure" is for a [potential] mate to admire. Our breasts are for "the man in our lives" to fondle during lovemaking, for our babies to suckle, for our doctors to examine. The same kind of "hands off" message is even stronger for our vaginas. We expect everyone else to be the final judge of how well we have displayed our "pluses" and minimized our "minuses," though we are somehow sure our "defects" will be noticed and remembered more than our "assets."

The women's health movement has encouraged women to feel ownership of their bodies, to appreciate their uniqueness as women, to increase their awareness of their physical bodies and the feelings associated with them, and to use their bodies in ways they choose to give them positive feelings. These goals are being fostered by women providing other women with information about their bodies and encouraging them to appreciate the connectedness of their bodies and minds.

Other consequences of the women's health movement are already reverberating throughout the traditional health services. Health care workers are recognizing the power of informed clients, and routinized regimens of care have given way to such innovations as birthing rooms. Women are being actively included in their care, for example, by being offered mirrors so that they can participate in the pelvic examination.

The power that women have attained through access to information has changed to some extent the status relationships that have characterized health services in the past.* It is no longer acceptable to many women to be excluded from establishing goals for their care or from planning "interventions." Women will increasingly collaborate with health professionals in establishing goals and creating a plan for how those goals will be attained. The change in power relationships mandates a shared responsibility for health.

The purpose of this chapter is to provide the nursing practitioner with knowledge about women's bodies that can be shared with women who are clients seeking nursing services or women seeking consultation and information. An overview of the structural and functional aspects of the female body will be presented first. Illustrations of many women's bodies will be presented to demonstrate the wide range of health and to dispel confusion between "healthy" and the mythical "ideal." A description of the visible features of women's bodies will be followed by a discussion of those features that are not directly visible. The procreative and recreative functions of anatomic structures will be compared and contrasted. Two important cyclic phenomena are the menstrual cycle and the female sexual response cycle; how the woman's body participates in each of these cycles will be described.

---

*This is not to say that individual approaches to demystifying one's body are sufficient to change the class structure in medicine that only mirrors that of the society as a whole. Rather, it is recognized that the self–health care movement has had limited success in reducing the harmful effects of status distinctions between some professionals and clients.

STRUCTURAL FEMALE ANATOMY
Breasts

Although in some western societies women are socialized to regard their breasts as symbols of their feminine attractiveness, and men are taught to regard the woman's breasts as sex objects, the female breasts are, in fact, organs that can subserve woman's procreative powers and recreative pleasures. Indeed, the mammary gland is the distinguishing feature of an entire zoologic class—mammals! These unique structures designed to serve woman's nurturance as well as her pleasure will be described from a health perspective in the following pages.

Visible structures

Location. The breasts are paired, highly specialized variants of sebaceous glands, located between the second and sixth ribs and between the sternal and midaxillary line. About two thirds of the breast lies superficial to the pectoralis major, the remainder to the serratus anterior.

Appearance. The breasts of healthy women are usually reasonably symmetrical in size and shape, although the breasts are often not absolutely equal. The skin covering the breasts is similar to that of the abdomen, and often hair follicles are noted around the pigmented area surrounding the nipple, called the areola. Women with fair complexions often can note a vascular pattern in a horizontal or vertical dimension. When present, this pattern is usually symmetrical.

The areolar pigment varies from pink to brown and the size is also highly variable from woman to woman. The nipple is located in the center of each breast, surrounded by the areola. Several sebaceous glands are seen on the areola as small elevations. The nipples are pigmented and protuberant; their size and shape are highly variable from woman to woman, and the same woman may notice a great deal of variation in the size and shape of her nipples depending on the extent to which they are contracted. Some women have inverted nipples, a condition in which the nipple is invaginated, or its central portion depressed. Some women have supernumerary nipples, nipples and breasts, or breast tissue. This supernumerary tissue develops along the longitudinal ridges extending from the axilla to the groin, which existed during early embryonic development (Fig. 5-1).

Visible changes in the woman's breast occur in conjunction with her development. Prior to age 10 there is little visible distinction between the male and female breast. At approximately age 10 the mammary buds appear in both breasts. The subareolar mammary tissue is most prominent at this point. The adult breast develops under the influence of estrogen and progesterone.

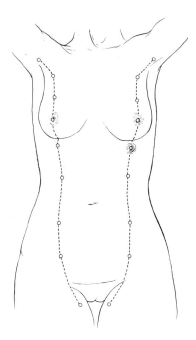

Fig. 5-1. Supernumerary nipples. Supernumerary tissue develops along the embryonic longitudinal ridges that extend from the axilla to the groin; these ridges are sometimes referred to as milk lines.

During the transition to adulthood, the prominent subareolar tissue of adolescence becomes receded into the contour of the remainder of the breast and the nipple protrudes.

Breast size seems to be influenced by nutrition, heredity, and the woman's individual sensitivity to hormones. Nodularity, tenderness, and size of the breasts may fluctuate with the menstrual cycle. Usually, the breast is smallest during days 4 to 7 of the menstrual cycle. An increase in breast volume, tenderness, heaviness, fullness, and general or nipple tenseness may be experienced 3 to 4 days premenstrually.

Short-lived changes of appearance are observed in many women during the human sexual response cycle, including protuberance of the nipple, increase in breast size, and so on. The breasts are highly erogenous organs for many women. They do not merely vary in shape and size with sexual excitement, there is also a great deal of variation from woman to woman in those parts of the breasts perceived as erotic. For example, some women perceive erotic sensations in the areolae, others from the nipple, and still others from the breast tissue near the axilla.

The breasts may double or triple in size during pregnancy. Striae, engorgement of veins, and increased prominence and pigmentation of nipple and areolae are common during pregnancy. The glandular tissue of the breast gradually involutes after menopause and fat is

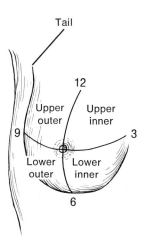

Fig. 5-2. Conventions for describing geography of the breast. The breast can be described in terms of quadrants or by analogy to the face of a clock.

deposited in the breasts. The breasts of postmenopausal women, therefore, take on a flattened contour and their appearance is less firm than it was prior to menopause.

A convention useful in describing the appearance of the breast is its division into four quadrants by vertical and horizontal lines that cross at the nipple. The axillary tail, a portion of breast tissue that extends into the axilla, is another important landmark. However, a more precise description of breast landmarks is one that incorporates an analogy to the face of a clock: thus a lump could be described at 2 o'clock, and the appropriate number of centimeters from the nipple.

Although some professionals encourage women to wear brassieres in order to prevent "Cooper's droop"—a drooping of Cooper's ligaments making the breasts appear pendulous—there is no compelling evidence that wearing a bra is an effective preventive strategy.

Components of breast tissue

There are three main components of tissue in the female breast: *glandular*, *fibrous*, and *fatty tissue*. The bulk of the breast is composed of subcutaneous and retromammary fat. Breast tissue is supported by fibrous tissue, including suspensory ligaments, extending from the subcutaneous connective tissue to the muscle fascia.

Glandular tissue. An important functional component of the breast is the glandular tissue, consisting of twelve to twenty-five lobes that terminate in ducts that open on the surface of the nipple. Each lobe is composed of twenty to forty lobules, each of which contains ten to one hundred alveoli (acini).

The alveolus is the basic component of the breast lobule. The hollow alveolus is lined by a single layer of milk-secreting epithelial cells, which are derived pre-

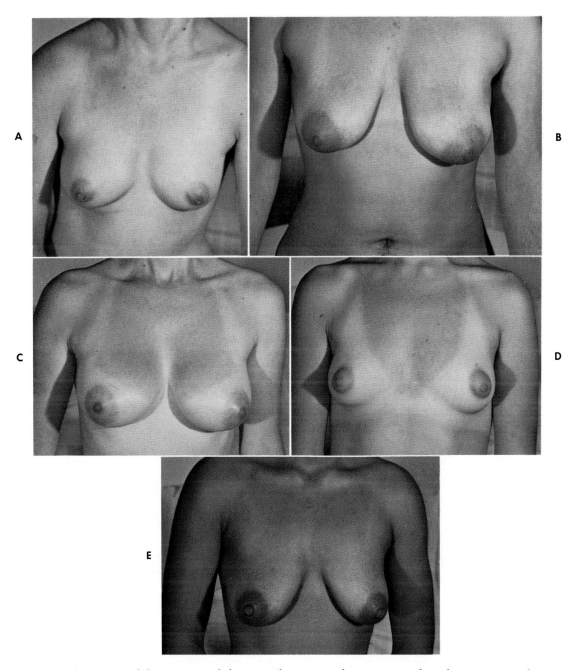

Plate 1. Variability in women's breasts. There is a wide variation in the color, contour, and size of women's breasts. The pigmentation and contour vary within and between racial groups as shown here.

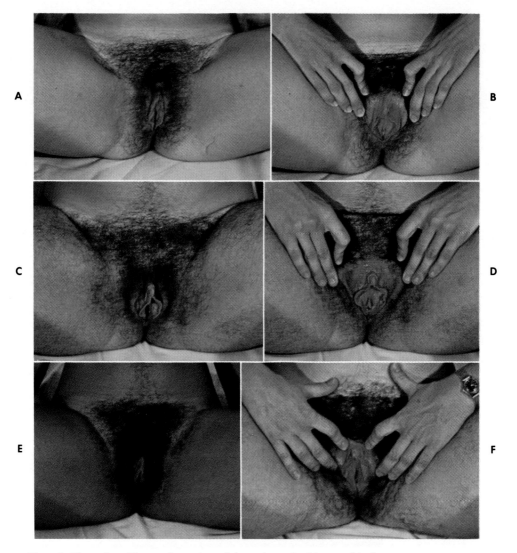

Plate 2. The vulva. The configuration of the vulva is highly variable from woman to woman. There is variation in skin color, texture of the pubic hair, and symmetry of the labia. The clitoris may vary in size and color. The appearance of the vulva may vary over the menstrual cycle. **A, C,** and **E,** The labia are shown in their usual position; **B, D,** and **F,** The labia are retracted to show the clitoris, vaginal opening, and other structures.

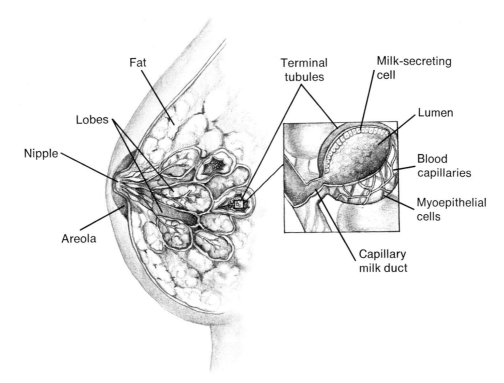

Fig. 5-3. Components of breast tissue. Breast tissue is comprised of glandular, fibrous, and fatty tissue. The alveolus is the basic component of the breast lobule and is lined with a single layer of milk-secreting epithelial cells.

natally from an ingrowth of epidermis into the mesenchyme between 10 and 12 weeks' gestation. These columnar cells enlarge greatly and discharge their contents during lactation. The individual alveolus is encased in a network of myoepithelial strands and is surrounded by a rich capillary network. The lumen of the alveolus opens into a collecting intralobar duct through a thin, nonmuscular duct. The intralobar ducts eventually end in the openings in the nipple, and these ducts are surrounded by muscle cells.

Supporting structures

Blood and nerve supply. The third and fourth branches of the cervical plexus provide the cutaneous nerve supply to the upper breast, and the thoracic intercostal nerves to the lower breast. The perforating branches of the internal mammary artery constitute the chief external blood supply, although additional arterial blood supply emanates from several branches of the axillary artery. Superficial veins of the breast drain into the internal mammary veins and the superficial veins of the lower portion of the neck, and from the latter into the jugular vein. Veins emptying into the internal mammary, axillary, and intercostal veins serve deep breast tissue.

Lymphatic drainage. The lymphatic drainage of the breast is of special interest and importance to women and health workers because of its role in dissemination of breast cancer as well as its ability to cope with infection. The lymphatic system of the breast is both abundant and complex. In general, the lymphatics drain both the axillary and internal mammary areas. Lymph from the skin of the breast, with the exception of areolar and nipple areas, flows into the axillary nodes on the same side of the body, whereas the lymph from the medial cutaneous breast area may flow to the opposite breast. The lymph from the inferior portion of the breast can reach the lymphatic plexus of the epigastric region. Drainage of lymph from the areolar and nipple areas flows into the anterior axillary (mammary) nodes. Lymph from deep within the mammary tissues flows into the anterior axillary nodes, but may also flow into the apical, subclavian, infraclavicular, and supraclavicular nodes. Lymph from areas behind the areolae and the medial and lower glandular areas of breast tissue communicates with the lymphatic systems draining into the thorax and abdomen.

Pelvic organs

Like her breasts, many of woman's pelvic structures serve her procreational powers and sexual pleasures. Despite the unique function served by their pelvic structures, many adult women are still unaware of the appearance of their external pelvic organs.

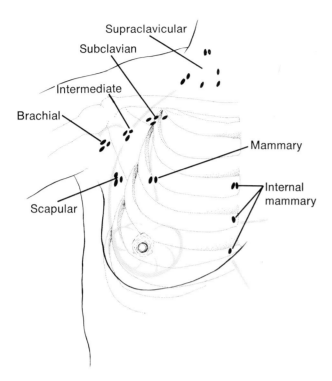

Fig. 5-4. Lymphatic drainage from the breast. Lymph from the skin of the breast flows to the axillary nodes on the same side of the body with lymph from the medial cutaneous area of the breast flowing to the opposite breast. Lymph from the inferior portion flows to the lymphatics of the epigastric region (not shown). Lymph from the areola and nipple flows into the mammary nodes.

Visible structures

Many of the structures of the woman's genitalia can be easily visualized with minor assistance from a mirror. The configuration of the genitals is strikingly unique to each woman and highly variable from woman to woman. For example, many paired structures, such as the labia, are not exactly symmetrical.

Vulva. The external female genitalia are commonly referred to as the vulva.* The most obvious feature on an adult woman is the *pubic hair*, which is rather coarse and curly and covers not only parts of the vulvar area (mons, labia majora), but also extends upward toward the abdomen. The flattened area of pubic hair over the abdomen forms the base of an inverted triangle sometimes referred to as the "female escutcheon." Although this is a somewhat typical pattern, it is not uncommon for healthy women to exhibit variation in this pattern. For example, hair growth may extend up toward the

*The vulva is sometimes referred to as the pudendum. The origin of this word, however, is from the Latin word meaning "to be ashamed." Therefore the term vulva will be used exclusively here.

umbilicus, to the anus, and inner portion of the thighs.

The *mons veneris* or mons pubis is composed of fat and lies over the symphysis pubis. The *labia majora* consist of two raised folds of adipose tissue. They are heavily pigmented, and in postpubertal women their outer surfaces are covered with hair while the inner surfaces are smooth and hairless. In postmenopausal women the hair on the labia becomes thinner and the labia and mons appear less full as a result of the loss of fatty tissue. The *labia minora* are two folds of skin heavily endowed with blood vessels that lie within the labia majora and extend from the clitoris to the fourchette (vaginal outlet). Each of the labia minora divides into a medial and lateral part. The medial parts join anteriorly to the clitoris to form the clitoral hood and the lateral parts join posterior to the clitoris. In some women the labia minora are completely hidden from view by the labia majora, but in other women the labia minora protrude between the labia majora. The color and texture of the labia minora are highly individual, varying from pink to brown. The clitoral hood covers the clitoris and is believed to protect this extremely sensitive organ from irritation. In some women the clitoral hood will adhere to the clitoris so that the hood cannot be pulled back very far to reveal the clitoris. For some women, clitoral adhesions or a tight clitoral hood can prevent stimulation during intercourse, and for women who perceive this as undesirable, lysis of clitoral adhesions is available.

The area between the labia minora is termed the *vestibule.* It contains both the urethral and vaginal orifices. The hymen, a membranous fold at the vaginal opening, may be intact, but more commonly is seen as small rounded fragments attached to the margins of the introitus. Skene's glands are multiple, tiny, paraurethral organs, the ducts of which open laterally and posteriorly to the urethral orifice. *Bartholin's glands*, located lateral and slightly posterior to the vaginal introitus, open into the groove between the labia minora and the hymen, at the 5 and 7 o'clock positions in relation to the vaginal orifice. Both Skene's and Bartholin's glands are usually not visible, although they are located in tissues that can be visualized, and their openings on the vulva can be seen in some women. The perineum consists of the tissues between the vaginal orifice and the anus.

Beneath the vestibule are two bundles of erectile tissue referred to as the bulbs of the vestibule. They are highly vascular and become congested during sexual response.

Clitoris. A woman's clitoris is an organ unique to all of human anatomy inasmuch as its sole purpose is to serve as a receptor and transformer of sensual stimuli. This unique structure is totally limited in its function to initiating or elevating levels of sexual tension (Masters and Johnson, 1966).

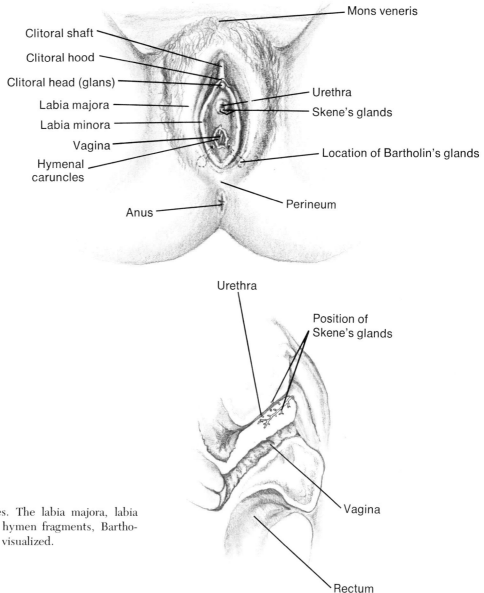

Fig. 5-5. Visible pelvic structures. The labia majora, labia minora, clitoris, vaginal opening, hymen fragments, Bartholin's glands, and perineum can be visualized.

The clitoris consists of two corpora cavernosa enclosed in a dense fibrous membrane that is made up of elastic fibers and smooth muscle bundles. Each corpus is connected by a crus to the pubic ramus and the ischium. The tip of the clitoris is referred to as the glans and is exquisitely sensitive. The clitoris is held in place by a suspensory ligament and two small ischiocavernosus muscles that insert into the crurae of the clitoris (Masters and Johnson, 1966).

Blood supply to the clitoris emanates from the deep and dorsal clitoral arteries that branch from the internal pudendal artery. The vasculature of the clitoris is impor-

tant in relation to changes in clitoral size during sexual response.

The length of the clitoral body (consisting of glans and shaft) varies markedly. The size of the clitoral glans may vary from 2 mm to 1 cm in healthy women, and is usually estimated at 4 to 5 mm both in the transverse and longitudinal planes. There is also variation in the position of the clitoris, a function of variation in the points of origin of the suspensory and crural ligaments. The glans is capable of increasing in size with sexual stimulation, and marked vasocongestive increases in the diameter of the clitoral shaft have also been noted.

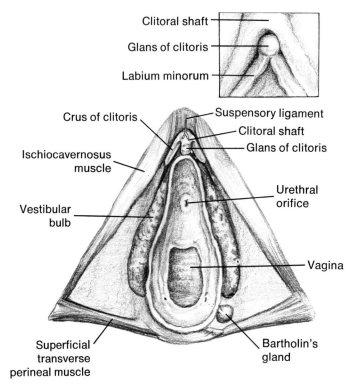

Fig. 5-6. The clitoris. The sole purpose of the clitoris is the reception and transformation of sexual stimuli. The glans and two corpora are held in place by a suspensory ligament and two ischiocavernosus muscles. The glans is exquisitely sensitive and increases in size with sexual stimulation as does the shaft of the clitoris.

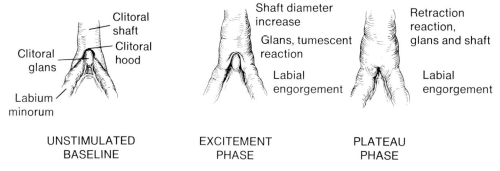

Fig. 5-7. The clitoris. The arrangement of the labia minora around the clitoris makes it possible for traction on the labia to indirectly stimulate the clitoris. (Adapted from Masters, W., and Johnson, V.: Human sexual response, Boston, 1968, Little, Brown & Co.)

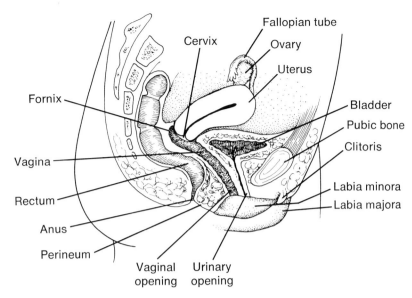

Fig. 5-8. The vagina. The vaginal canal is a potential rather than a real space and inclines posteriorly at about a 45 degree angle. The cervix pierces the anterior superior wall of the vagina. The recessed portion of the vagina adjacent to the cervix is the fornix.

The dorsal nerve of the clitoris is the deepest division of the pudendal nerve, and it terminates in the nerve endings of the glans and corpora cavernosa. Pacinian corpuscles are distributed in both the glans and the corpora but have a greater concentration in the glans. The pacinian corpuscles respond to deep pressure and probably play an important role in relaying afferent stimuli. Their distribution is highly variable from woman to woman, which probably accounts for the rich variation in women's self-pleasuring techniques. For example, some women prefer very light touch whereas others prefer deep pressure. In some women, the anatomic arrangement of the labia minora to form the clitoral hood makes it possible for mechanical traction on the labia to indirectly stimulate the clitoris. The clitoris is endowed with sensory nerve endings that respond to tactile stimuli as well as pressure. Although afferent stimuli can be received through afferent nerve endings in the clitoral glans and shaft, it is also thought that the clitoris may serve as the subjective end-point or transformer for the efferent stimuli from higher neurogenic pathways (Masters and Johnson, 1966). (See Chapter 9 concerning the relationship between neurogenic pathways and orgasm and sexual dysfunction.)

Vagina. Although it could be argued that the vagina is an internal structure, it can be easily visualized with the assistance of a speculum, light source, and a mirror. The vagina is a musculomembranous canal connecting the vulva with the uterus. It is lined with a reddish pink mucous membrane that is transversely rugated.

Under the stratified squamous epithelial lining is a muscular coat that has an inner circular layer and an outer fibrous layer.

The vagina is a potential rather than a real space. Although highly distensible, its collapsed length is approximately 6 to 7 cm anteriorly and about 9 cm posteriorly. The vaginal canal inclines posteriorly at about a 45 degree angle. The vagina is pierced by the uterine cervix anteriorly and superiorly. There is a recessed portion of the vagina adjacent to the cervix, which, together with the cervix, is called the vaginal fornix. The fornix has anterior, posterior, and lateral portions.

Unlike the clitoris, the vagina has procreative as well as recreative functions. One of the important physiologic functions of the vagina during sexual response is its ability to produce lubrication by means of transudation of mucoid material across its rugal folds. In addition, vaginal lubrication occurs in a rhythmic 90 minute cycle throughout the day and night. The venous plexus (including the bulbus vestibuli, plexus pudendalis, plexus uterovaginalis, and possibly the plexus vesicalis and plexus rectalis) encircling the vaginal barrel is believed to be responsible for this phenomenon. In addition to producing lubrication, the vagina demonstrates a fascinating distensive ability both during sexual response and childbirth. Both a lengthening of the vagina and a ballooning out of its inner portions have been observed during sexual response. The vascular changes occurring in conjunction with sexual response are profound. The reddish pink hue of the premenopausal vagina changes to a darker purplish vasocongested appearance. In postmenopausal women the color changes in the vagina and its expansion during sexual response are less pronounced. As the vagina distends, the rugae become flattened as a result of the thinning or stretching of the vaginal mucosa. The vagina, unlike the clitoris, is not well endowed with nerve endings; although there are deep pressure receptors in the innermost portion of the vagina, it is primarily in the outer third of the vagina that women report pleasurable sexual sensations (Masters and Johnson, 1966).

Cervix. Although the cervix might be regarded as an internal structure because it is a part of the uterus, it can be readily visualized with the aid of a speculum and a light source.

The cervix extends from the isthmus into the vagina and it is through the small cervical opening (os) that the uterus and vagina communicate. The cervical os may be enlarged or of an irregular shape in parous women. The cervix appears as an oval-shaped organ and is usually shiny and pink. In postmenopausal women it may be smaller and less colorful than in premenopausal women.

The stroma of the cervix consists of connective tissue with unstriated muscle fibers as well as elastic tissue.

The stratified squamous epithelium of the outer cervix (portio) is made up of several layers. The basal layer is a single row of cells resting on a thin basement membrane and is the layer where active mitosis is seen. The parabasal and intermediate layers are next. The intermediate layer is vacuolated because of the presence of glycogen. The superficial layer varies in thickness in response to estrogen stimulation. The desquamation of this surface layer occurs constantly. The superficial layer contains a large amount of glycogen as does the intermediate layer. It appears that glycogen plays an important role in maintaining the acid pH of the vagina. Glycogen released by cytolysis of the desquamated cells is acted on by the glycolytic bacterial flora of the vagina, forming lactic acid.

Just as the endometrium is influenced by the hormonal fluctuations of the menstrual cycle, so is the mucus produced by the secretory cells of the endocervical glands. This is especially noticeable in premenopausal women. The fluctuations of the cervical mucus over the menstrual cycle will be discussed later in this chapter. The endocervical canal shows an abrupt transition from the stratified squamous epithelium covering the vagina and the outer surface of the cervix to a tall, columnar epithelium rich in mucin.

Internal structures

The uterus, ovaries, and uterine tubes constitute the internal structures that are uniquely woman's.

Uterus. The uterus is a hollow, pear-shaped organ that

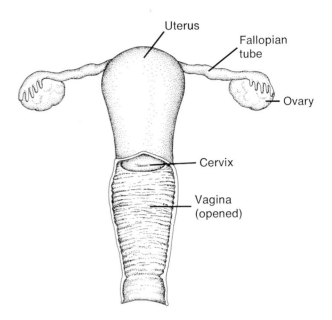

Fig. 5-9. The uterus, cervix, tubes, and ovaries.

is from 5.5 to 9 cm long, 3.5 to 6 cm wide, and 2 to 4 cm thick in nonparous women. The uterus of a parous woman may be 2 to 3 cm larger in any of these three dimensions. The uterus is usually inclined forward at a 45 degree angle from the longitudinal plane of the body. Usually, the uterus is anteverted and slightly anteflexed in position. However, it may also be retroflexed, retroverted, or in midposition.

The portion of the uterus above the cervix is referred to as the body and is constructed of a thick-walled musculature. It is covered with peritoneum on the exterior and lined with a mucous surface called the endometrium. The body of the uterus is divided into three portions: the fundus, the corpus, and the isthmus. The fundus is the prominence above the insertion of the fallopian tubes; the corpus is the main portion; and the isthmus is the constricted lower portion of the uterus adjacent to the cervix. The uterus is not a fixed organ, but can be moved about; for example, during the sexual response cycle the entire uterus elevates from the true pelvis into the false pelvis.

Tubes. Two uterine (fallopian) tubes function as oviducts for the transport of ova from the ovary to the uterus. They are inserted into the upper part of the uterus and run laterally to the ovaries. Each tube is approximately 10 to 12 cm long. The distal portions of the tube are fimbriated; the middle portion (ampulla) and the portion of the tube close to its insertion in the uterus (isthmus) are extremely narrow. The wider fimbriated end of the tube is not actually attached to the ovary but wraps part way around the ovary. The outer serous coat of the tubes covers a muscular portion con-

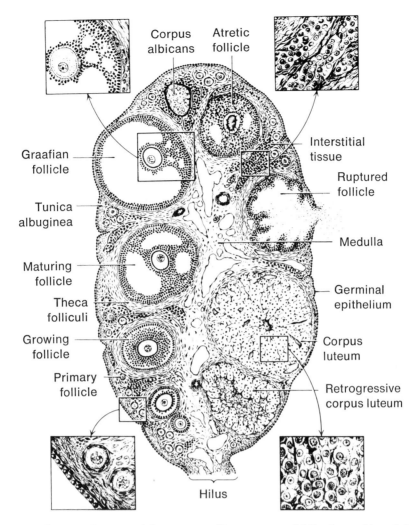

Corpus
albicans

Atretic
follicle

Graafian
follicle

Tunica
albuginea

Maturing
follicle

Theca
folliculi

Growing
follicle

Primary
follicle

Interstitial
tissue

Ruptured
follicle

Medulla

Germinal
epithelium

Corpus
luteum

Retrogressive
corpus luteum

Hilus

Fig. 5-10. Schematic diagram of the ovary. Different stages of follicular and luteal development are shown here. The events would occur sequentially, not simultaneously as shown. (From Mountcastle, V. B.: Medical physiology, ed. 13, St. Louis, 1974, The C. V. Mosby Co.)

sisting of an inner circular and outer longitudinal layer. The mucosal layer, composed of a number of rugae that become more numerous approaching the fimbriated portions, lines the tubes. The tubes are lined with cilia.

Ovaries. The ovaries are paired oval organs approximately 3 to 4 cm long, 2 cm wide, and 1 to 2 cm thick. They are located near the pelvic wall at the level of the anterior superior iliac spine. The ovaries float freely in the pelvis except for their attachment to the broad ligaments via the mesovaria. The external ovarian surface has a dull, whitish, opaque appearance. The ovary is composed of an outer cortex lined by a single layer of cuboidal epithelium. This layer contains a hilus through which blood vessels and nerves enter and leave. Beneath the outer layer is the stroma, which consists of spindle cells. The stroma of the ovary contains the primordial follicles. (The follicle and corpus luteum will be discussed later in conjunction with the menstrual cycle.)

Not only do the ovaries release gametes, but they also produce the steroid hormones estrogen and progesterone. The medullary portion of the ovary is composed of loose connective tissue, lymphatics, and blood vessels. The ovary has a rich lymphatic drainage, and an abundant supply of unmyelinated nerve fibers also enters the medulla.

At birth the human ovary contains about one million germ cells. The follicle is the functional unit of the ovary, the source both of the gametes and the ovarian hormones. Each follicle is surrounded by a theca folliculi. The theca contains an inner rim of secretory cells, the theca interna, and an outer rim of connective tissue, the theca externa. Within the theca, but separated from it by a layer of thin basement membrane, are the granulosa cells, which in turn surround the ovum. An acellular layer of protein and polysaccharide, the zona pellucida, separates the ovum from the granulosa cells. The theca

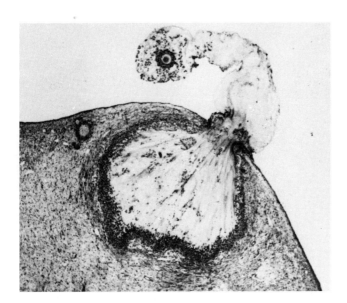

Fig. 5-11. Ovulation. At ovulation the ovum, surrounded by the corona radiata and floating in the follicular fluid, ruptures. The ovum and its corona of granulosa cells is extruded into the peritoneal cavity in a bolus of follicular fluid. (From Mountcastle, V. B.: Medical physiology, ed. 13, St. Louis, 1974, The C. V. Mosby Co.)

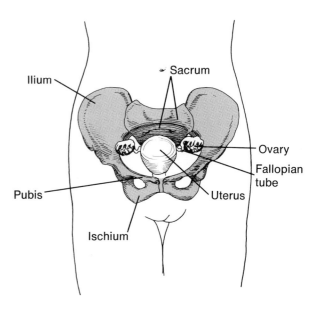

Fig. 5-12. The bony pelvis. The pelvis is composed of two innominate bones, the sacrum and the coccyx. The innominates are composed of the ilium, the ischium, and the pubis.

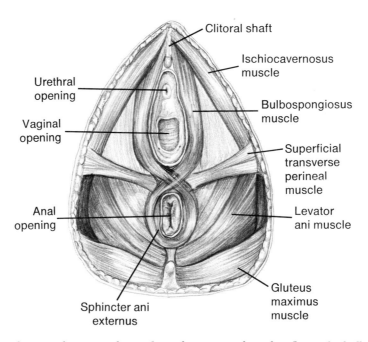

Fig. 5-13. Pelvic muscles. Several sets of muscles support the pelvic floor. The bulbocavernosus and the pubococcygeus have special significance for sexual sensory function.

interna is richly vascularized although neither the ovum nor the granulosa cells is in contact with any capillaries. Development and maturation of the follicle consist of proliferation of the granulosa cells and the gradual elaboration of fluid within the follicle. Accumulation of the fluid increases rapidly with follicular maturation and causes the follicle to bulge into the peritoneal cavity. As the follicle swells the ovum remains embedded in granulosa cells, the cumulus oophorus, which remains in contact with the theca. As fluid accumulates, the cumulus thins out until only a narrow thread of cells connects the ovum with the rim of the follicle. At ovulation the ovum, surrounded by the corona radiata and floating in the follicular fluid, ruptures. The ovum and its corona of granulosa cells become extruded into the peritoneal cavity in a bolus of follicular fluid. After ovulation, ingrowth and differentiation of the remaining granulosa cells fill the collapsed follicle to form a new endocrine structure called the corpus luteum. The corpus luteum regresses after about 2 weeks, leaving a remnant on the surface of the ovary called a corpus albicans. If a pregnancy ensues, the corpus luteum does not regress at this point.

Pelvic supporting structures

Bones, muscles, ligaments, blood vessels, and nerves form supporting structures of the pelvic organs.

Bony pelvis. The pelvis is composed of two innominate bones, the sacrum, and coccyx. The innominate bones, in turn, are made up of the ilium, ischium, and pubis.

The pubic bones join at the symphysis pubis. The pubic arch is formed by the inferior borders of the pubic bones and symphysis. The ilium joins with the sacrum posteriorly to form the sacroiliac joint. The female pelvis is wider and more shallow than the male's because of flaring of the female's iliac bones.

Muscle. Several sets of muscles attach to the bony pelvis to constitute the pelvic floor. These muscles actively and passively support the pelvis and are involved in the voluntary contraction of the vagina and the anus. The pubococcygeus muscle, part of the levator ani group, has particular significance in women, since it is important not only in sexual sensory function but also in bladder control and birthing for controlling relaxation of the perineum and expulsion of the infant. Also of importance for sexual pleasure is the bulb of the vestibule (bulbocavernosus).

Ligaments. Four pairs of ligaments support the uterus, ovaries, and tubes. These include the cardinal, uterosacral, round, and broad ligaments (Fig. 5-14). Stretching of these ligaments is sometimes associated with minor discomfort during strenuous exercise or during pregnancy.

Vasculature. The ovarian arteries arise from the abdominal aorta, supply the tube and ovary, and ultimately anastomose with the uterine artery. The uterine artery arises from the anterior branch of the hypogastric artery

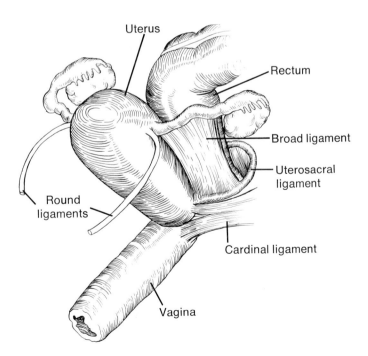

Fig. 5-14. Ligaments. Four pairs of ligaments support the uterus, ovaries, and tubes. These are the cardinal, uterosacral, round, and broad ligaments.

and supplies the cervix and uterus. The vaginal artery arises similarly from the anterior branch of the hypogastric artery. The uterine veins run along similar channels as the uterine artery. The ovarian veins from the vena cava pass through the broad ligament en route to the ovarian hilus. On the right, the ovarian vein empties into the inferior vena cava; on the left, into the renal vein.

Innervation. The internal genitalia are supplied by autonomic as well as spinal nerve pathways. The main autonomic supply to the uterus appears to consist of both sympathetic and parasympathetic fibers of the superior hypogastric plexus. The pudendal nerve is the main spinal nerve, providing the source of motor and sensory activation of the lower genital tract. Further discussion of the importance of the sympathetic and parasympathetic nervous system in the human sexual response cycle will be presented later in this chapter.

THE MENSTRUAL CYCLE
Neurohormonal control of menstruation

A discussion of the menstrual cycle assumes knowledge of hormone biosynthesis, metabolism, and the mechanism of action, as well as neuroendocrine control mechanisms. A brief overview of these topics as they relate to the menstrual cycle will be presented.

Hormones: biosynthesis, metabolism, and action

Biosynthesis. A hormone is a "substance that travels from a specialized tissue where it is released into the bloodstream to distant responsive cells where the hormone exerts its characteristic effect." (Speroff, 1978; p. 1) The hormones regulating the events of the menstrual cycle are derived from the same basic molecular structure as cholesterol. The sex steroids are commonly divided into three groups according to the number of carbon atoms. Corticoids and progestins comprise the C-21 series, all the androgens comprise the C-19 series, and the estrogens comprise the C-18 series. The normal human ovary is capable of producing all three classes of sex steroids: estrogens, progestins, and androgens. During steroidogenesis, the number of carbon atoms in the steroid molecule or cholesterol can be decreased, but not increased. The process of steroidogenesis can be accomplished by means of cleavage of a side chain from the cholesterol or steroid molecule, conversion of hydroxyl groups to ketones or ketones to hydroxyl groups, addition of hydroxyl groups (hydroxylation), or creation of double bonds by removal of hydrogen. Cholesterol is the basic building block in steroidogenesis, and all steroid-producing organs with the exception of the placenta are capable of synthesizing cholesterol from acetate. Thus the ovary can synthesize progestins, androgens, and estrogens in situ from a two-carbon molecule in ovarian tissue compartments using cholesterol as the common precursor. Blood cholesterol can enter the ovarian cells where it contributes to the biosynthetic pathways or can be esterified and stored as a precursor. The pathways for hormone synthesis are shown in Fig. 5-15 and appear to be governed by the cell type involved. For example, the follicular granulosa cells appear to produce progesterone whereas the thecal cells appear to be the principal source of estrogen and the stromal cells appear to produce androstenedione, DHA (dehydroepiandrosterone), and testosterone (Speroff et al., 1978).

About 80% of the principal sex steroids (estradiol and testosterone) are transported in the blood bound to a protein carrier called sex hormone–binding globulin, with about 19% loosely bound to albumin and only 1% unbound and free. Corticosteroid binding–globulin binds cortisol, progesterone, and other corticoid compounds. Although the precise purpose of the binding is unknown, it is believed that the biologic activity of a hormone can be limited by binding in the blood, thus preventing sudden shifts in hormone effects; or binding may prevent rapid metabolism of the hormone, allowing it to exist for a sufficient period of time to produce its biologic effect. It is known that the biologic effects of the sex steroids are produced by the free or unbound portion of the hormone (Speroff et al., 1978).

Metabolism. Androgens are common precursors of *estrogen.* Androstenedione is converted to testosterone, which is in turn converted to estradiol, the major estrogen secreted by the human ovary. Estradiol also arises from androstenedione by means of its conversion to estrone. Estriol is a peripheral metabolite of estradiol and estrone and, as such, a less active form. Such peripheral conversion of hormones is not always to an inactive form and is quite important. Indeed, the peripheral conversion of androstenedione to estrone accounts for 20% to 30% of the estrone produced each day. Therefore, the circulating estrogens in women include both the sum of direct ovarian secretion of estradiol and estrogen in addition to the products of peripheral conversion of C-19 precursors.

In nonpregnant women, peripheral conversion of steroids to *progesterone* is not observed. Progesterone production is from adrenal and ovarian secretion. Progesterone is excreted as pregnanediol glucuronide in the urine. Pregnanetriol is another excretion product of progesterone.

The ovary also produces *androgens,* primarily dehydroepiandrosterone (DHA) and androstenedione. Testosterone may become a significant secretory product when an androgen-producing tumor or excessive stromal tissue is present. The adrenal cortex also produces sex steroids as intermediate products in the synthesis of

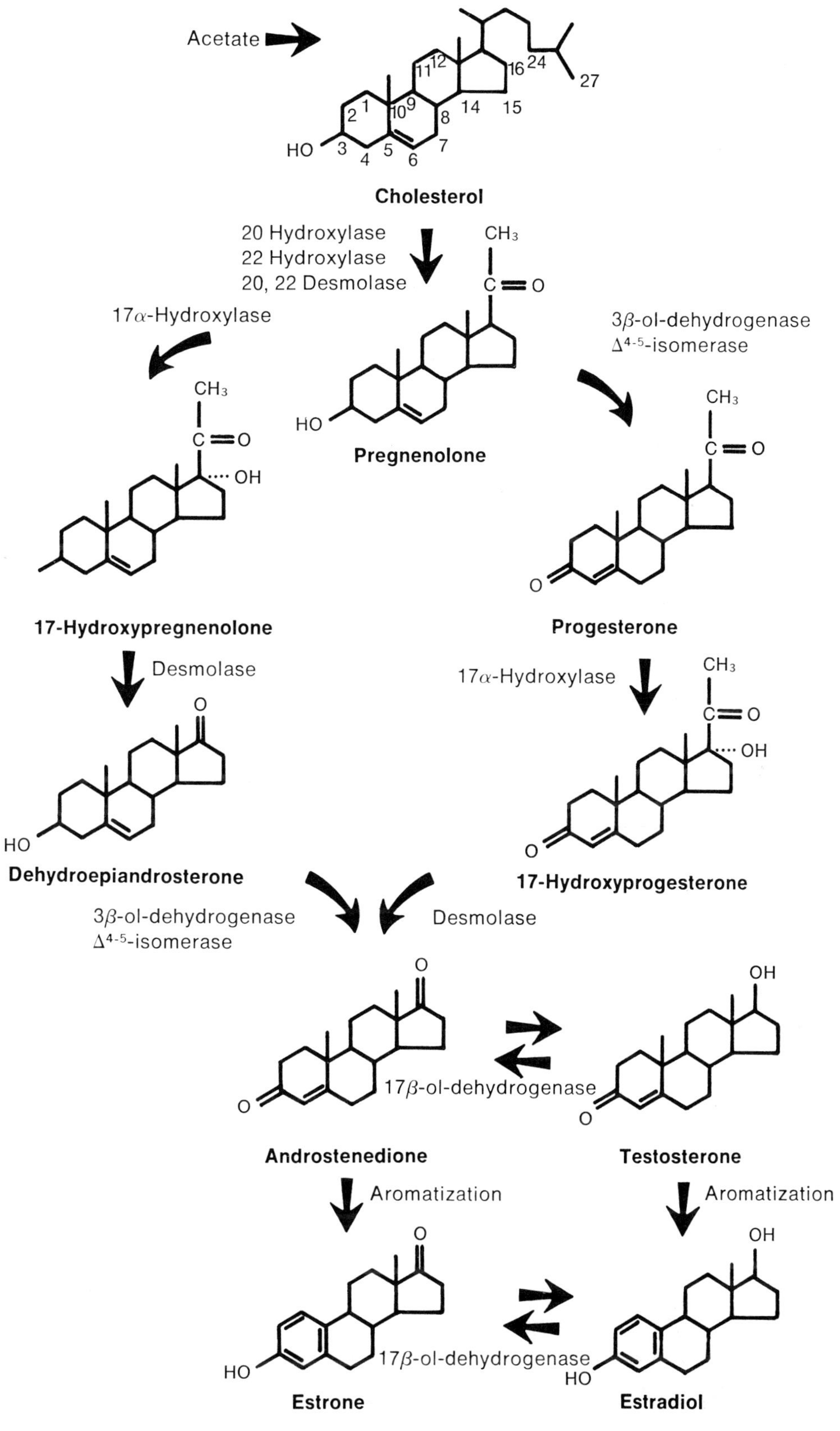

Fig. 5-15. Pathways for synthesis of estrogen and progesterone.

Table 5-1. Ranges of sex steroids in nonpregnant women*

Hormone	Follicular phase	Midcycle peak	Luteal phase
Estradiol (pg/ml)†	25-75	200-600	100-300
Progesterone (ng/ml)†	<1		5-20
Testosterone (ng/ml)	0.2-0.8	0.2-0.8	0.2-0.8

*Values from Speroff, L., and others: Clinical endocrinology and infertility, ed. 2, Baltimore, 1978, The Williams & Wilkins Co.
†pg = picograms; ng = nanograms

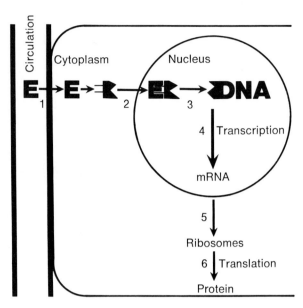

Fig. 5-16. Mechanism of action of steroid hormones. (Adapted from Speroff, L., and others: Clinical gynecologic endocrinology and infertility, ed. 2, Baltimore, 1978, The Williams & Wilkins Co.)

glucocorticoids and mineralocorticoids. Usually, the secretion of sex steroids by the adrenal is much less than that from the gonads. The binding capacity of testosterone appears to be decreased by the presence of androgens in both men and women, and therefore the binding capacity in women is higher than that in men. In women testosterone is produced by peripheral conversion of androstenedione as well as secretion by the ovary and adrenal gland.

Steroids and their metabolites are excreted in their conjugated sulfo-and glucuro- forms. Conjugation usually reduces or eliminates the activity of the steroids and is a step in deactivation prior to the hormone's excretion into urine or bile (Speroff et al., 1978). (See Table 5-1.)

Mechanism of action. In order to affect target cells, hormones require the presence of special mechanisms within the cells. Two types of hormone action can occur at the cellular level. The first involves specific cytoplasm receptor molecules in interaction with the smaller steroid hormones that are capable of readily entering the cells. The second mediates the action of tropic hormones at the cell membrane.

Steroid hormones owe their specificity of action to intracellular receptor proteins. The mechanism of action of the steroid hormones involves six steps. First, the hormone must diffuse across the cell membrane. Next it binds to cytoplasmic receptor protein, whose function it is to transport the hormone as a hormone-receptor complex across the nuclear membrane to the nucleus. Third, the hormone-receptor complex binds to nuclear DNA. Next, messenger RNA is synthesized (gene transcription). Fifth, messenger RNA is transported to the ribosomes, and finally messenger RNA–mediated protein synthesis occurs in the ribosomes.

The action of steroid hormones appears to be regulation of intracellular protein synthesis by means of the receptor mechanisms. Responsiveness to the hormone is determined by the presence of a specific receptor and the intracellular concentration of that receptor. For example, estrogen increases responsiveness to itself and

progesterone by increasing the concentration of its own receptors and intracellular progesterone receptors; progesterone, however, limits response to estrogen as it induces a decrease in estrogen receptors in the cytoplasm.

Only while the receptor is occupied with the hormone is its biologic activity maintained. As a result, the dissociation rate of the hormone from its receptor influences biologic response. Estrogen and its receptor complex have a long half-life, whereas progesterone-receptor complexes have short half-lives (Speroff et al., 1978).

The mechanism of action of the *tropic hormones* depends on the presence of a receptor in the cell plasma membrane of the target tissue. Thus tropic hormones do not enter the cells but only unite with a specific receptor on the surface of the cell. The union of the hormone with a receptor activates the adenyl cyclase enzyme in the membrane wall leading to the conversion of ATP to cyclic AMP. Cyclic AMP–receptor protein complex, in turn, activates a protein kinase. Cyclic AMP frees the catalytic subunit from the regulatory subunit of the kinase. Phosphorylation follows by means of the transfer of a phosphate from ATP to substrate proteins (Speroff et al., 1978).

Neuroendocrine control mechanisms

There are a number of complex interactions by which the brain controls the secretion of hormones by the pituitary. The hypothalamus appears to act as a transducer, functioning as a final common pathway by which internal and external environmental signals can be rec-

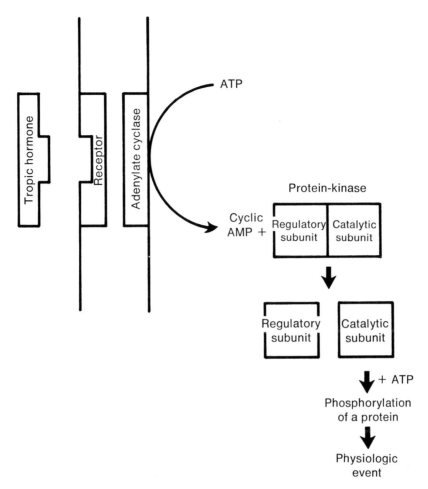

Fig. 5-17. Mechanism of action of tropic hormones. (Adapted from Speroff, L., and others: *Clinical gynecologic endocrinology and infertility,* ed. 2, Baltimore, 1978, The Williams & Wilkins Co.)

ognized, integrated, and reduced to neurohumoral directions to meet the body's physiologic needs.

A direct nervous connection does not exist between the brain and the anterior pituitary gland. Rather, the blood supply of the anterior pituitary originates in capillaries that lace the median eminence of the hypothalamus. It is possible that one's psychic experiences may influence hormonal events of the menstrual cycle by means of the effects of neurotransmitters on the hypothalamic releasing factors. For example, profound stress could produce amenorrhea by this mechanism. The hypophyseal portal system transports blood from the hypothalamus to the pituitary such that specific groups of hypothalamic cells appear to be linked with specific areas of the pituitary. There is much evidence that the control of the pituitary is achieved by means of neurotransmitters secreted by the hypothalamus into the pituitary portal system. The neurotransmitter controlling gonadotropins is called gonadotropin-releasing factor.

The control of prolactin is achieved by prolactin-inhibiting factor, which prevents prolactin release. It is not certain whether there are two separate releasing factors for luteinizing hormone (LH) and follicle-stimulating hormone (FSH) or if a single releasing factor is responsible for their control. The hypothalamic neural cells respond to signals in the blood and to neurotransmitters in the brain by the process of neurosecretion. By this process neurotransmitters are synthesized on the ribosomes in the cytoplasm of the neuron, put into a granule in the Golgi apparatus, and transported by active axonal flow to the neuronal terminal where it is secreted into the blood or across a synapse.

Tonic and cyclic centers of the hypothalamus control gonadotropic function, the tonic maintaining the basal level of gonadotropins by means of a negative feedback relationship with the steroids and the cyclic center responsible for the midcycle surge of gonadotropin in the female.

Tanycytes, ependymal cells that can transport ma-

Table 5-2. Average age at which rise in sex steroids is noted*

Hormones	Age
DHA	8 years
Androstenedione	8-10 years
Estrogens	10-12 years

*Data from Speroff, L., and others: Clinical endocrinology and infertility, ed. 2, Baltimore, 1978, The Williams & Wilkins Co.

terials from the ventricular cerebrospinal fluid to the portal system, and the secretions into the posterior pituitary pathway of vasopressin, oxytocin, and neurophysins also influence pituitary function. Gonadotropin production has been documented in fetal life; it surges during the middle of pregnancy, again during the first few months of life, then decreases markedly until puberty.

The ages at which the rise in sex steroids is noted are given in Table 5-2. It is believed that the hypothalamic-pituitary-gonadal feedback system operates prior to puberty but that it is suppressed. As the hypothalamic centers become less sensitive to the suppressive effects of sex steroids, the changes of puberty appear. In postmenopausal women, there are high levels of tropic hormones and low levels of ovarian hormones, but the rate at which these decline has not been carefully studied.

Phases of the menstrual cycle
Hormonal events and the ovarian cycle

The menstrual cycle is customarily divided into three phases to facilitate discussion: follicular phase, ovulation, and the luteal phase.

Follicular phase. During the follicular phase, hormonal influences lead the follicle through a period of initial growth. The initiation of follicular growth does not appear to be dependent on gonadotropin. In fact, follicular growth may have begun during the days of the previous luteal phase when the regressing corpus luteum secretes decreasing amounts of steroids. FSH is probably responsible for growth of the follicle whereas LH probably stimulates steroidogenesis. Initial follicular growth ends when a significant increase in estrogen becomes detectable, usually about 7 to 8 days before the LH surge preceding ovulation.

For continued growth, the follicle depends on gonadotropins. With the maturing of the follicle, the number of gonadotropin receptors increases, probably stimulated by estradiol, which has increased along with the gonadotropin. FSH and estradiol probably act synergistically to prepare the follicle to respond to LH. The following is thought to be the sequence of events:

Initial follicular growth
↓
FSH stimulation
↓
Estradiol production, increasing sensitivity to FSH by increasing the number of FSH receptors
↓
FSH induction of LH receptors that is enhanced by estradiol
↓
Differentiation of theca cells with increased estradiol production

During the latter part of the follicular phase, estrogens initially rise slowly, and reach a peak at ovulation. FSH declines as estrogen rises, but LH increases steadily, then surges at midcycle. High local estradiol concentration appears to increase the follicle's sensitivity to FSH.

From 24 to 36 hours before the LH peak, LH becomes detectable in follicular fluid. During follicular growth, LH binds to theca cells to promote steroidogenesis, thus becoming the principal source of estradiol until ovulation. At midcycle much of the estradiol is produced by the follicle that will ovulate. The remaining follicles become atretic, losing their receptors for estradiol, FSH, and LH. The increase in stromal tissue at this time is associated with increasing androgen levels in the plasma. Androgen is believed to have two effects: enhancing atresia within the ovary and stimulating libido.

Ovulation. It appears that the rise in estradiol sets off the gonadotropin surge in midcycle. It is thought that gonadotropin-releasing hormone (GnRH) causes the increase in both LH and FSH. LH brings about the processes of ovulation and luteinization whereas FSH may assist in the production of a normal corpus luteum by inducing LH receptors. There is a slight rise in progesterone at midcycle, which probably results from LH and luteinization; the small rise in progesterone probably enhances gonadotropin secretion by means of a central facilitative feedback. These high levels of gonadotropins exist for about 24 hours, decreasing during the luteal phase. The mechanism responsible for stopping the LH surge is unknown. Usually, the gonadotropin surge and the final maturation of the follicle coincide as the former is controlled by estradiol, which is, in turn, a function of growth of the follicle. The follicle usually ruptures within 24 hours after the LH peak. It is believed that the physical expulsion of the ovum results from an acute increase in prostaglandin triggered by LH (Speroff et al., 1978).

Luteal phase. After the follicle ruptures the granulosa cells increase in size and accumulate lutein to form the

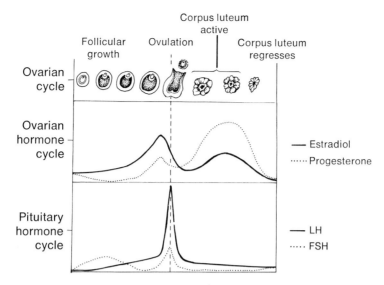

Fig. 5-18. The ovarian cycle. The pituitary hormone cycle and the ovarian hormone cycle can be plotted against the ovarian cycle. The follicle develops under the influence of estradiol, ruptures about the time of the LH surge; the corpus luteum develops under the influence of FSH, and 10 to 12 days after ovulation the corpus luteum begins to regress.

corpus luteum. By 8 or 9 days after ovulation the corpus luteum is highly vascularized, and this is associated with peak blood levels of progesterone and estradiol. The corpus luteum can synthesize androgens, estrogens, and progestins. From 10 to 12 days after ovulation, the corpus luteum begins to regress. The mechanism triggering regression is unknown, but is thought to be the production of estradiol. Pregnancy prolongs the corpus luteum by means of rapidly increasing levels of human chorionic gonadotropin (HCG), which maintains the steroidogenesis of the corpus luteum until placental steroidogenesis is established at about 9 to 10 weeks of gestation. During the luteal phase progesterone appears to interfere with aldosterone action at the renal tubule and estradiol stimulates an increased synthesis of angiotensinogen by the liver.

In sum, the key events of the menstrual cycle are influenced by estradiol. A decline in estradiol in the previous luteal phase leads to a rise in FSH. Estradiol induces FSH receptors, thus maintaining follicular sensitivity to FSH. Estradiol also works synergistically with FSH to induce LH receptors, thus enhancing follicular response to LH. The rapid rise in estradiol triggers ovulation (Speroff et al., 1978).

Uterine cycle

The uterine cycle consists of two phases, as does the ovarian cycle. Because the first portion of the menstrual cycle is dominated by follicular development and follicular secretion causes proliferation of the endometrium, it is called the follicular phase with respect to the ovary and the proliferative phase with respect to the endometrium. The second portion of the cycle is dominated by the corpus luteum and the increasing levels of progesterone evoke secretory changes in the endometrium. Therefore, this phase is referred to as the luteal phase with respect to the ovary and the secretory phase with respect to the endometrium.

Immediately following menstruation the endometrium is thin, only about 1 to 2 mm in thickness. The surface epithelium is made up of low cuboidal cells, the stroma is dense and compact, and the glands appear straight and tubular.

Proliferative phase. Under the influence of estrogen, the endometrium proliferates and increases in thickness. The endometrium becomes somewhat taller and the surface epithelium is now columnar. Although the stroma is still quite compact, the endometrial glands have become more tortuous. Mitotic activity is evident in both the surface epithelium and the basal nuclei of the epithelial cells lining the endometrial glands. Estrogenic effects are also seen in secretions of the cervical glands and in the vaginal lining. The variability in length of this phase of the menstrual cycle is greater than that for the luteal phase. Indeed, it is the varying number of proliferative or follicular phase days that accounts for the variation in total cycle length.

Secretory phase. As a consequence of the developing corpus luteum, progesterone evokes and increases the secretory changes in the endometrium. The surface epi-

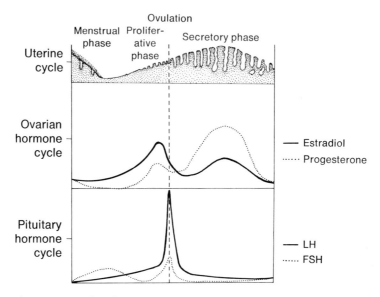

Fig. 5-19. The uterine cycle. The pituitary hormone cycle and the ovarian hormone cycle can be plotted against the uterine cycle. Under the influence of estrogen the endometrium proliferates and increases in thickness. As a consequence of the developing corpus luteum, progesterone evokes and increases the secretory changes in the endometrium. Menstruation is a vascular phenomenon, and it is believed to result from a stasis of blood flow to the coiled arteries of the endometrium. The stasis is thought to be the result of intense vasoconstriction produced by a prostaglandin.

thelium is now tall and columnar; the stroma is less compact than earlier in the cycle and somewhat edematous and vascular. The endometrial glands become increasingly tortuous and convoluted, while the nuclei of the epithelial lining cells have begun to migrate toward the luminal portion of the cell, thus producing a clear zone beneath referred to as a subnucleolar vacuole, presumptive of incipient ovulation. Glycogen is beginning to be secreted into the lumen of the glands, and mucin is also present.

Premenstrually, the surface epithelium is quite tall, about 8 to 9 mm. The stroma consists of large polyhedral cells mimicking decidua. The endometrial glands are very convoluted and serrated, resembling a corkscrew. The lining epithelium of the endometrial glands is less well demarcated and shrunken because of loss of glycogen into the gland lumen. A large number of lymphocytes and leukocytes are seen, probably as a result of the beginning necrosis of the endometrium brought about by impending menstruation.

Menstruation. Menstruation is a vascular phenomenon. The endometrium is supplied by two groups of blood vessels: the straight and the coiled arteries. The straight arteries, which supply the endometrium, do not change over the menstrual cycle. The coiled arteries supply blood to the upper and most of the middle third of the endometrium. As the endometrium grows over the menstrual cycle, the arteries become increasingly coiled as they increase in length more rapidly than the endometrium increases in thickness. Endometrial growth regresses a few days before the onset of menstruation; at the same time there is a stasis of blood flow to the coiled arteries, with intermittent vasoconstriction. Between 4 and 24 hours prior to the onset of menstrual bleeding, intense vasoconstriction occurs. The menstrual bleeding occurs from a coiled artery that has been constricted for a number of hours. It is thought that prostaglandins, synthesized in the endometrium as a result of progesterone stimulation, are released and produce even more vasconstriction. The dissolving of the endometrium liberates acid hydrolases from the cell lysosomes. The acid hydrolases further disrupt the endometrial cell membranes to complete the process of menstruation. Thus the fully developed endometrium is sloughed away, but not suddenly and completely; instead there is a gradual desquamation and petechial shedding of the upper two thirds of the endometrium. The lower layer (basalis) is retained and the stumps of the basal glands and stroma for the ensuing cycle grow from them. The surface epithelium regenerates rapidly and may begin even while other areas are in the process of being desquamated. The menstrual flow may last from 2 to 8 days. Menstrual fluid consists of cervical and vaginal mucus as well as degenerated endometrial par-

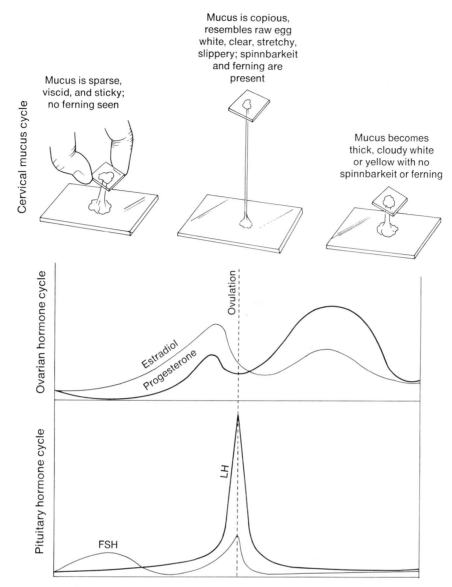

Mucus is copious, resembles raw egg white, clear, stretchy, slippery; spinnbarkeit and ferning are present

Mucus is sparse, viscid, and sticky; no ferning seen

Mucus becomes thick, cloudy white or yellow with no spinnbarkeit or ferning

Cervical mucus cycle

Ovarian hormone cycle

Ovulation

Estradiol

Progesterone

Pituitary hormone cycle

LH

FSH

Fig. 5-20. Cervical mucus. The cervical mucus undergoes predictable changes during the menstrual cycle. About midcycle the mucus demonstrates spinnbarkeit and ferning.

ticles and blood. Sometimes clots may appear in the menstrual fluid. Usually from 2 to 3 ounces of fluid is lost with the menses, but the amount of flow is highly individual.

Other target organs

Cervix. The cervical canal contains about one-hundred crypts referred to as glands; the secretory cells of these crypts secrete mucus into the endocervical canal. The mucus undergoes qualitative and quantitative changes during the menstrual cycle depending on the dominant hormones at the time. Immediately after menstruation the mucus is sparse, viscid, and sticky. If examined

under a microscope, an abundance of vaginal and cervical cells and lymphocytes can be seen. From about the eighth day of the cycle until ovulation, the quantity and viscosity of the mucus increase. Sometimes an obvious plug of yellow, white, or cloudy mucus of a tacky consistency is observed. At midcycle the mucus is a thin hydrogel containing only 2% solids and 98% water. The mucus resembles raw egg white, being clear, stretchy, and slippery. It will stretch without breaking or spin a thread (spinnbarkheit). Ability of the mucus to stretch at least 5 to 6 cm has been established as a guideline for determining adequacy of the cervical mucus to support sperm transport. When the midcycle mucus is allowed

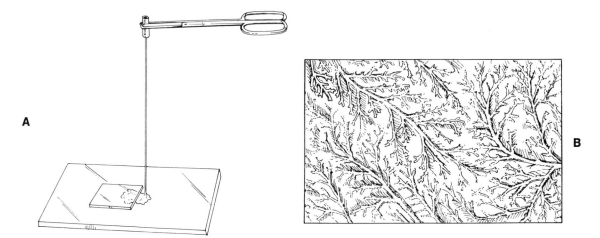

Fig. 5-21. A, Spinnbarkeit. At midcycle the mucus resembles raw eggwhite, being clear, stretchy, and slippery. It will stretch without breaking or spin a thread (spinnbarkeit). **B,** Ferning. When allowed to dry on a slide, the midcycle mucus gives a fern or palm-leaf pattern.

to dry on a slide it gives a fern or palm-leaf pattern. This pattern is absent after ovulation, during pregnancy, and after menopause. After ovulation the mucus may again become cloudy, white, or yellow and tacky and may disappear altogether. In sum, just prior to ovulation the cervical mucus should demonstrate the following:

1. A dribble to abundant cascade of mucus emanating from the cervical os
2. Moderate to pronounced uninterrupted mucus thread, which can be drawn half to all of the distance between the external os and the vulva
3. Partial to complete "ferning" of a sample viewed on a slide

Women can use the changes in cervical mucus as an indirect index of ovulation.

The cervix itself undergoes changes in anatomy during the menstrual cycle. During the proliferative phase the os progressively widens, reaching its maximum width just prior to or at ovulation. At the point of maximal widening, mucus can be seen extruding from the external os. After ovulation the os returns to a smaller diameter, with the profuse and watery mucus becoming scanty and viscid. These changes are believed to be estrogen induced and are not seen in prepubertal or postmenopausal women or in those whose ovaries have been removed. In sum, just prior to ovulation the cervix should be partially open to gaping; the mucosa should be pink to hyperemic and the cervical os open.

Fallopian tubes. The motility of the tubes is greatest during the estrogen-dominant portion of the menstrual cycle. They demonstrate a decreased motility during the progesterone-dominant phase.

Vagina. Estrogen stimulation leads to cornification of the vagina. Following progesterone stimulation the vaginal epithelium shows an increase in the number of precornified cells, mucus shreds, and aggregates of cells.

Breasts. Estrogen stimulates the growth of the ductal system of the breasts. Both nipple erectibility and areolar pigmentation are estrogen dependent. Progesterone in combination with estrogen stimulates the development of acinar buds of the milk ducts.

Menstrual cycle markers

The phases of the menstrual cycle have been marked by the basal body temperature, intermenstrual pain, and cervical mucorrhea. These three indicators seem to follow one another in time and to occur in a constant order. Following menstruation, the appearance of cervical mucorrhea (the discharge of physiologic cervical mucus into the vagina) precedes symptoms of intermenstrual pain by about 1.7 days. Intermenstrual pain (an acute peristaltic pain that occurs periodically in the left or right abdominal quadrant) precedes the rise in basal body temperature by about 2.5 days (Vollmann, 1977). In addition, invasive measures have been used to document events of the menstrual cycle, including radioimmunoassays of hormone levels in blood, cytologic changes in the endometrium and vaginal epithelium, and the direct visualization of the ovaries via laparoscopy used in conjunction with therapeutic goals. Because cycle length varies, even in the same woman, it is difficult to precisely document when menstrual cycle events will occur.

Basal body temperature (BBT). The most common

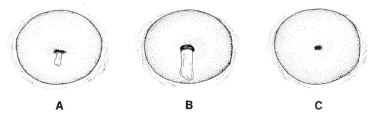

Fig. 5-22. Changes in the cervical os. The cervical os also changes over the menstrual cycle. **A,** During the proliferative phase mucus may be seen in the cervical os; **B,** at midcycle it appears open or even gapping. Prior to menstruation **(C)** the os becomes smaller and the mucus symptom may be absent.

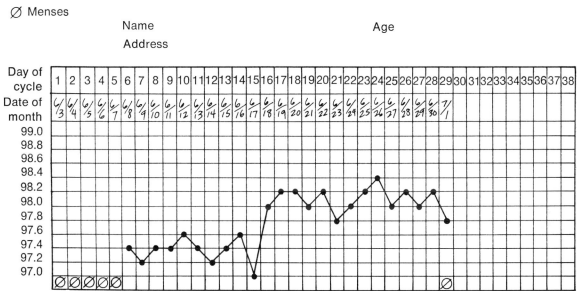

Fig. 5-23. Biphasic BBT chart. The basal body temperature is an important menstrual cycle marker. The temperature curve in healthy adult women should be biphasic between two episodes of menstruation with the lower temperature following the preceding menstruation and the elevated level preceding the next menstruation.

method used to mark phases of the menstrual cycle has been use of the basal body temperature. The basal body temperature, when taken immediately after awakening, shows less aberrant fluctuations than oral and axillary measurements. In healthy adult women there should be a biphasic curve between two episodes of menstruation, with a lower temperature recorded during the period of time following menstruation and an elevated level before the next menstruation. The temperature curve can be divided into a postmenstrual and a premenstrual phase by the intercept between the mean of all temperature measurements and the actual temperature curve. The length of the postmenstrual phase varies with the total cycle length whereas the premenstrual phase does not. The level of the mean BBT is highly individual and decreases with age. Monophasic temperature curves (showing no premenstrual rise) are common at menarche, may remain throughout maturity, and increase before menopause. Short premenstrual phases are also common in adolescent girls. The biphasic temperature curve is an integrated function of the ovarian activity as demonstrated by their absence in men, girls before menarche, women after menopause, and women after bilateral oophorectomy

(Vollmann, 1977). It is commonly assumed that a rise in the basal body temperature follows the LH surge, with ovulation presumably occurring at the low point prior to the continuous rise in temperature.

Intermenstrual pain. Intermenstrual pain (IP) consists of episodes of peristaltic pain localized in the right or left lower abdominal quadrant. Often the pain is initially localized in a small area approximately 2 inches medial to the anterosuperior iliac spine and 2 inches above the upper border of the symphysis. It may later radiate into the groin, labia, or vagina. IP episodes may follow one another in irregular intervals, sometimes ranging from 5 minutes to 1 hour and then fading over several hours. This pain is observed from menarche to menopause and is absent during pregnancy and amenorrhea. The length of the postmenstrual phase (time from onset of menstruation to IP follicular phase) varies with the length of the cycle. Monophasic BBT curves are found at a rate of 1.2% among menstrual cycles with IP (Vollman, 1977).

Cervical mucorrhea. Cervical mucorrhea has been described earlier. When the postmenstrual phase is determined by using the interval between onset of menstruation and the onset of the clear, watery mucorrhea, it varies with the length of the entire menstrual cycle. These markers can be useful to women who wish to avoid unplanned pregnancies, to monitor symptoms presumptive of ovulation, or to ascertain the onset of menstruation.

Correlates of menstrual cycle phase

Several correlates of the menstrual cycle have been identified. However, the behavioral changes associated with menstruation may be reflective of overestimates on the part of some researchers, as well as cultural folklore (Donnelson and Gullahorn, 1978).

Menstrual myths. Awareness of the menstrual myths is essential if one is to comprehend the origin of some belief systems regarding menstruation. Some myths are of the "protect her" genre. According to these, women

Table 5-3. Physiologic correlates of menstrual cycle phase

Investigators	Sample	Correlates	Findings
Janowsky, Berens, and Davis (1973)	11 female college-age volunteers studied for a total of 15 cycles	Daily weights, urinary K^+/Na^+ ratios, self-evaluation of negative affect	Potassium/sodium ratios and weight were elevated during the luteal premenstrual and early menstrual phases and decreased at other times.
Little and Zahn (1974)	5 students and 7 older married parous women studied for 10 and 3 cycles, respectively; monitored 6 days per week over 1 cycle	Skin temperature, skin resistance, heart rate, respiration, finger pulse volume, time interval estimation, mood adjective checklist, basal body temperature, reaction time	Significant rise in respiration and heart rate and fall in skin conduction level during the luteal phase. During ovulatory portion significant increases in autonomic responsivity with greater skin conductance responses and greater heart rate variability. These measures showing greater autonomic variability coincided with a peak in feelings of elation and vigor. BBT higher for older women, who also had less heart rate variability than younger women.
Patkai, Johannson, and Post (1974)	6 healthy women studied daily for 2 menstrual cycles	Urinary catecholamines and body temperature	No significant differences found in adrenaline and noradrenaline excretion between premenses, postmenses, ovulation, and postovulation periods.
Voda (in press)	20 menstruating, ovulating women 19 to 36 years old not using oral contraceptives	Basal body temperature; weight; finger and ankle girth; Moos MDQ; progesterone; aldosterone; sodium; potassium	Progesterone and aldosterone were correlated and increased toward the luteal phase, but not with any other variables; sodium and potassium were correlated; negative affect and concentration were correlated with a rise in the luteal phase; weight and finger and ankle girth were not correlated with one another or with any other variables.

are especially vulnerable to both physical and psychologic disturbances when menstruating. From this belief comes the injunction to protect oneself by avoiding cold, hard work, bathing, and washing one's hair.

More common are the menstrual myths concerning the danger associated with menstrual blood. Beliefs emanating from this myth are that menstruating women have the ability to harm growing crops, wither flowers, cause bread not to rise, and so on. Paramount of these myths is the belief that women are capable of contaminating their husbands and so sexual intercourse is contraindicated (see Leviticus, Chapter XV, and the Talmud). Many societies have such sexual taboos, and many isolate women from the rest of the society (e.g., in menstrual huts) (Delaney et al., 1977; Weideger, 1976).

Although menstruation has been viewed as dangerous or even dirty, menstrual blood has been attributed special healing powers and used in sorcery, as an aphrodisiac, and to ensure fertility (Delaney et al., 1977).

Although many of these myths have disappeared in the United States, there still is the tendency to regard the menstruating woman as vulnerable. It is probably this belief system that has most shaped the assumptions of researchers and health workers about correlates of the menstrual cycle.

Correlates of menstrual cycle phase. Physiologic correlates of menstrual cycle phase have not been extensively studied in recent years, but the few studies that have been reported recently reflect an attempt to elucidate autonomic nervous system correlates. One study demonstrates that urinary potassium/sodium ratios fluctuate throughout the cycle, as does weight, with both being elevated during the luteal premenstrual and early menstrual phases and decreased at other times (Janowsky et al., 1973), another shows that these changes are independent of one another and hormonal influences (Voda, in press). One study revealed that cyclic variation occurred in some autonomic nervous system responses (Little and Zahn, 1974) but another showed no significant differences in adrenaline and noradrenaline excretion (Patkai et al., 1974). Another demonstrated an increase in skin conductance level premenstrually, implying increased arousability at this time (Koeski, in press) (Table 5-3).

Behavioral correlates of menstrual cycle phase have generated much research interest, with mixed findings (see Table 5-4). It is of great interest that when men and women are compared, similar variability in both activity patterns (Dan, 1976) and symptoms (Wilcoxon et al., 1976) is seen. Women who have undergone hysterectomy but have functioning ovaries report differently with respect to mood and psychologic state from women who have not had a hysterectomy (Beumont et al., 1975).

This would suggest that expectations about symptoms may influence the association between cycle phase and symptom reports. This is borne out also by the fact that cyclic differences in symptoms are found only among women who believed they were premenstrual regardless of their actual cycle phase (Ruble, 1977).

There is evidence that sociocultural phenomena influence how women perceive and report cycle phase effects. For example, Japanese women report fewer breast symptoms during the perimenstrual period than other women, and Nigerians have a higher frequency of headaches (Janiger, 1972). Sex role norms also seem to influence how women describe their symptoms, with traditional women reporting more perimenstrual symptoms than others (Beck, 1970; Paige, 1973). Koeske and Koeske (1975) have shown that cultural expectations are responsible for the fact that while premenstrual symptoms are attributed to biology, good moods and rational behavior are not.

FEMALE SEXUAL RESPONSE CYCLES
Physiologic components of female sexual response cycles

Although female sexual anatomy had been studied early in this century by Dickinson, whose *Atlas of Human Sexual Anatomy* portrayed in detail changes in the human cervix and vagina resulting from sexual stimulation, and Kinsey (1953) had described the frequency and variety of sexual outlets available to women as well as their lack of marital sexual satisfaction, it was Masters and Johnson (1966) whose pioneering work in female sexuality and sexual physiology laid to rest an abundance of mythology and misconception about the events of the female sexual response cycle. Masters and Johnson attempted to determine what physical phenomena occur as humans respond to sexual stimulation as well as what psychosocial factors influence how people respond. They directly observed and measured the changes occurring during sexual response in 382 female volunteers whose age ranged from 18 to 78 years and 312 males ranging in age from 21 to 89. Their study population represented a wide range of educational levels and included nonwhites as well as whites.

Phases of the cycle*

To facilitate description of their observations, the investigators arbitrarily chose to divide the cycle into four phases: excitement, plateau, orgasm, and resolution. Excitement phase develops from any source of

---

*Adapted from Woods, N. F.: Human sexuality in health and illness, ed. 2, St. Louis, 1979, The C. V. Mosby Co.

Table 5-4. Behavioral correlates of menstrual cycle phase

Investigators	Sample	Correlates	Findings
Asso and Beach (1975)	20 women, ages 19 to 36 years who were not taking oral contraceptives; 8 female phobic patients on tranquilizers	Acquisition of a conditioned response	Both phobic and nonphobic women had significantly greater susceptibility to acquire response premenstrually vs intermenstrually.
Beck (1970)	37 women undergraduates	Headache, backache, pelvic discomfort, tension, depression, irritability	Headache, backache, and pelvic discomfort occurred more often in menstrual phase. Traditional sex-role attitudes were associated with premenstrual headache, tension, and irritability. During menstrual phase modern attitudes were associated with irritability and depression.
Beumont, Richards, and Gelder (1975)	25 menstruating women plus 7 women who had had hysterectomy	Three daily scores: mood, psychologic state, and physical state	Higher levels of symptoms were reported during premenstrual week and week of menstrual flow by menstruating women. Women who had had hysterectomies showed smaller cycle phase differences even though their hormonal assays were like those of menstruating women.
Dan (1976)	24 couples, ages 24 to 44 years; cycle phase studied with BBT and midluteal hormonal assays	Activity patterns	No significant differences found between husbands and wives in overall variability of activities.
Golub (1976)	50 normal adult women, 30 to 45 years of age	Depression adjective checklist; state-trait anxiety inventory	State anxiety and depression mean scores were higher during premenstrual phase, but lower than those of depressed female patients.
Morris and Udry (1970)	34 women	Activity based on pedometer readings	Activity peaked in midcycle, with two lesser peaks in the premenstrual and the menstrual phase.

bodily or psychic stimuli, and if adequate stimulation occurs, the intensity of excitement increases rapidly. This phase may be interrupted, prolonged, or ended by distracting stimuli.

The plateau phase is a consolidation period that follows excitement if adequate stimulation is maintained. Sexual tension becomes intensified to the level at which the person may experience orgasm. Like excitement, this phase may also be affected by distracting stimuli.

Orgasm, the involuntary climax of sexual tension increment, involves only a few seconds of the human sexual response cycle during which vasocongestion and myotonia are released. There appears to be greater variation of intensity and duration of orgasm among women than among men. Although the total body is involved, the sensual focus during orgasm is usually in the pelvic area.

During the resolution phase the person undergoes involutional changes that restore the preexcitement state. Women may, if adequately stimulated, begin another sexual response cycle immediately, before sexual excitement totally resolves. However, for the male a refractory period during which he cannot be restimulated is superimposed on the resolution period. Unless orgasm has been overwhelming, sexual tension is dissipated slowly. Usually the length of the resolution period parallels the length of the excitement phase.

Although Masters and Johnson state that the variety of patterns for females is almost infinite, they describe the three most prevalent patterns. In pattern A, the woman experiences multiple orgasms, with a fairly rapid resolution period. Pattern B depicts a nonorgasmic cycle in which several peaks are noted in the plateau phase and a longer resolution period occurs. Pattern C shows a

Table 5-4. Behavioral correlates of menstrual cycle phase—cont'd

Investigators	Sample	Correlates	Findings
Pallis and Holding (1977)	114 women admitted for suicide attempt (in Scotland)	Suicide attempt; severity of intent to die	Suicide attempts not related to cycle phase. Severity of intent to die was higher during premenstrual phase.
Parlee (1973)	44 college women	Volunteering behavior	Women more likely to volunteer at mid-cycle.
Ruble (1977)	44 women undergraduates who were not taking oral contraceptives and had not for 3 months prior to study; awareness of cycle phase manipulated experimentally	Moos menstrual distress questionnaire	Cyclic differences in symptoms were found for women who only *believed* they were premenstrual; learned associations may lead woman to overstate what she experiences or to perceive exaggeration of naturally fluctuating bodily states when she believes she is premenstrual.
Sommer (1972)	51 college women 33 oral contraceptive users	Critical thinking	No phase effects on critical thinking were found.
Surney et al. (1975)	82 undergraduate students	Application to counseling center	Initial contact for personal problems more likely to come during premenstrual and menstrual phases and least likely during ovulation; same results occurred with women taking oral contraceptive.
Udry and Morris (1968, 1970)	Working women	Sexual intercourse	Probability of intercourse highest at mid-cycle, with a decline in the luteal phase
Wilcoxon, Schrader, and Sherif (1976)	11 college women 11 college women using oral contraceptives 11 college men	Daily self-reports of pleasant events and activities, mood adjective check-list, personal stress inventory, and menstrual distress questionnaire	Only water retention and pain showed cyclic effects solely for females, but negative moods were associated with stressful events rather than cycle phase.

cycle in which the woman's excitement is first interrupted or distracted, an intense orgasm occurs, and resolution is very rapid.

Masters and Johnson describe only one sexual response pattern for males, although it is highly unlikely that it is invariant. In this pattern excitement proceeds rapidly, followed by a short plateau period, orgasm, and a resolution period.

There are two principal physiologic changes responsible for the events observed during the human sexual response cycle: vasocongestion and myotonia. Vasocongestion is defined as congestion of blood vessels, usually venous vessels, and is the primary physiologic response to sexual stimulation. Myotonia, increased muscular tension, is a secondary physiologic response to sexual stimulation. These two changes are responsible for the phenomena observed during the sexual response cycle.

A very important finding from the work of Masters and Johnson is that human sexual response is a total body response rather than merely a pelvic phenomenon. Changes in the cardiovascular and respiratory function as well as reactions involving skin, muscle, breasts, and the rectal sphincter are observed during the sexual response cycle.

Excitement phase

During the excitement phase of the human sexual response cycle, the clitoral glans becomes tumescent, or enlarged, and the clitoral shaft increases in diameter and elongates. The appearance of vaginal lubrication, caused by vasocongestion and likened to a sweating process, occurs within 10 to 30 seconds after initiation of sexual stimulation. The vaginal barrel expands about 3.75 to 4.25 cm in transcervical width and lengthens

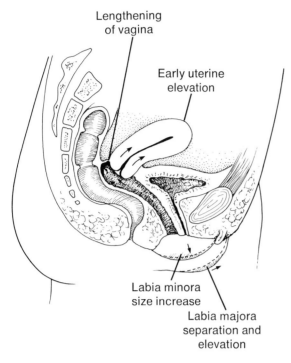
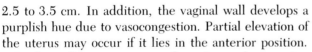

Fig. 5-24. Excitement phase.

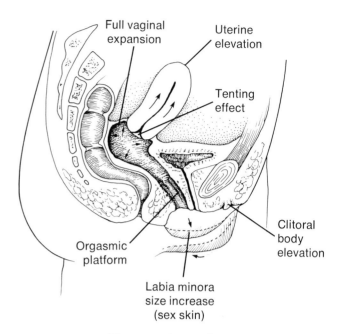

Fig. 5-25. Plateau phase.

2.5 to 3.5 cm. In addition, the vaginal wall develops a purplish hue due to vasocongestion. Partial elevation of the uterus may occur if it lies in the anterior position.

In the nulliparous woman, flattening and separating of the labia majora occur as in an apparent effort to open the entrance to the vagina. In the multiparous woman the labia majora move slightly away from the introitus due to a vasocongestive increase in their diameter. The vaginal barrel is lengthened approximately 1 cm as a result of the thickening of the labia minora. No changes have been observed in Bartholin's glands during this phase.

During excitement, vasocongestion causes vaginal lubrication. Elevation and flattening of the nulliparous labia majora, thickening of the multiparous labia majora, and extension of the labia minora are also vasocongestive reactions. Lengthening and broadening of the vagina also occur at this time.

During the excitement phase, changes also occur in the extragenital organs. In the female, nipples may become erect, breast size increases, the areolae become engorged, and the venous pattern on the breast becomes more obvious. The "sex flush," a maculopapular rash, may appear over the epigastric area, spreading quickly over the breasts. Some involuntary muscle tensing may be evident, as in the tensing of intercostal and abdominal muscles. The heart rate and blood pressure also increase as sexual tension increases.

Plateau phase

During the plateau phase, the clitoris retracts against the anterior body of the symphysis pubis, underneath the clitoral hood. Vasocongestion of the outer one third of the vagina and the labia minora causes an increase in size of this highly sensitive tissue, referred to as the orgasmic platform. Further increase in the depth and width of the vaginal barrel appears. The uterus becomes fully elevated, and as the cervix rises it produces a tenting effect in the inner part of the vagina. Irritability of the corpus uteri continues to intensify.

In both nulliparous and multiparous women, the labia majora continue to become engorged, with this phenomenon being more pronounced in the nullipara. The labia minora undergo a vivid color change from bright red to a deep wine-colored hue. This change in the "sex skin" is considered pathognomic of impending orgasm. During the plateau phase, a drop or two of mucoid material is secreted from Bartholin's glands; this secretion probably assists slightly in vaginal lubrication during prolonged coitus.

Several extragenital responses occur in the female during the plateau phase. Nipple erection and turgidity continue to develop along with an increase in breast size and marked engorgement of the areolae. The sex flush, which began during excitement, may spread over the body. Facial, abdominal, and intercostal muscles contract; muscle tension is increased both voluntarily and

that they have a nearly infinite capacity to be orgasmic. Consistent with Sherfey's analysis is the Hite data—several women reported that as the number of orgasms increases, the more stimulating, stronger, or more exquisite they became.

After orgasm, the women in Hite's study reported feeling tender and loving, strong and wide awake, energetic and alive, and wanting to be close. While some women preferred to have more than one orgasm, some said that they could not have multiple orgasms because the clitoris became too sensitive to touch.

Theories of orgasm

Freud hypothesized that women have two main erotogenic centers. During early stages of psychosexual development, the erotic activity centered in the clitoris. Freud reasoned that the clitoral orgasm, as often experienced during childhood masturbation, would be replaced by vaginal primacy in the adult woman. It was thus inferred from Freud's writings that the *vaginal* orgasm was the norm for adult women. The extension of Freud's theory led to the conclusion that women who required clitoral stimulation were neurotic and fixated at an earlier stage of development.

Masters and Johnson (1966) demonstrated the fallacy of the clitoral-vaginal transfer theory when they discovered that "an orgasm is an orgasm is an orgasm." Their work demonstrated that from a physiologic standpoint there is only one kind of orgasm regardless of which parts of the body are stimulated to produce it or who provides the stimulation. Furthermore, it is physically impossible to separate the clitoral from the vaginal stimulation in intercourse. Stimulation from thrusting of the penis (or any other kind of vaginal stimulation) affects the clitoris, labia, and lower vagina as one inseparable functional unit.

Kaplan (1974) suggests that no matter what kind of stimulation is provided, it is the clitoris that probably always evokes orgasm, but orgasm is always expressed by discharge of the circumvaginal muscles. The fact that there are touch fibers only within the entrance of the vaginal barrel and that proprioceptive and stretch sensory endings seem to be concentrated in the outer third of the vagina, while the clitoris is highly endowed with receptors, would substantiate the relative importance of the latter. Although stimulation of the 4 and 8 o'clock positions of the outer portion of the vagina have been found to be highly pleasurable, most women masturbate by pleasuring areas around the clitoris or the clitoris itself; few only insert objects into their vaginas.

The Singers (1972) have recently described three types of orgasmic experience: vulval, uterine, and blended orgasm. They suggest that the orgasm described by Masters and Johnson involving involuntary contractions of the orgasmic platform is a *vulval orgasm.* The *uterine orgasm* is one dependent on repeated deep stimulation of the cervix by the penis that displaces the uterus and ultimately causes stimulation of the peritoneum. The uterine orgasm is characterized by a gasping type of breathing that eventually culminates in an explosive exhalation. Like the vulval orgasm, the uterine orgasm is sexually gratifying. The *blended orgasm* is a combination of features of the vulval and uterine orgasms. The blended orgasm is perceived as "deeper than" the vulval orgasm. The Singers point out that none of the three patterns is preferable to the other. Rather, they seem to represent the variety of orgasmic experience available to women.

The theories of orgasm leave us confused regarding a single definition of the phenomenon. The subjective reports of women regarding their orgasmic experiences are richly variable and do not always directly correspond to physiologic correlates, such as vaginal contractions. Because there is no overt sign of orgasm corresponding to ejaculation (except perhaps vaginal contractions), it is difficult to document whether any two women are describing the same physiologic phenomena when they describe their orgasms. Also, some women describe sexually gratifying orgasms, but do not perceive vaginal contractions. The exact physiologic correlates underlying this experience are unknown (Williams, 1977).

Factors influencing the experience of orgasm

Many physiologic factors influence the woman's experience of orgasm. The first of these is stimulation. Not only can prolonged physical stimulation intensify the orgasmic experience but it also may result in multiple orgasmic experience. Age, parity, and menstrual cycle phase also seem to influence orgasmic experience. Women appear to reach their "sexual prime" at a later age than men do. With pregnancy, women develop a greater potential for vasocongestion of the pelvis (Sherfey, 1972). The elaboration of the pelvic vasculature is believed to be available to the woman after childbirth perhaps as a pleasurable legacy of her "labors." The luteal phase appears to be associated with an increase in sexual drive, probably a function of vasocongestion in the pelvis (Sherfey, 1972). Finally, both facilitating and inhibiting sensations and input can impinge on the reflex centers that supposedly govern orgasm. Thus inhibitory stimuli from the cortex can interfere with sexual response even in the presence of adequate physical stimulation; by the same token, facilitation of orgasmic experience from fantasy may make orgasm possible even in the absence of clitoral or vaginal stimulation (Kaplan, 1974). It is believed that androgen exerts important influences on the portions of the brain representing sexual experience, as well as the development and functioning of the genital organs. Androgen appears to enhance the erotic drives of both sexes. For example, women deprived of all sources of androgen by removal of the ovaries and adrenals appear to lose sexual desire and cannot be aroused by previously effective stimuli. Women given androgen replacement therapy show enhanced sexual arousal. Not much is known about the direct effects of estrogen and progesterone on sexual behavior, although women report individual differences in their libidinal responses to the cyclic fluctuations of these hormones (Kaplan, 1974). Studies of sexual behavior over the menstrual cycle indicate that intercourse and orgasm appear more likely to occur when estradiol levels are high, with rates of both dropping during the luteal phase (Udry and Morris, 1968).

INTERRELATIONSHIPS BETWEEN SEXUAL RESPONSIVENESS, BIRTHING, AND BREAST FEEDING

Niles Newton (1973) has delineated the similarities between three interpersonal acts unique to women: responding to sexual stimuli, giving birth, and breast feeding.

Women demonstrate similar behaviors whether responding to sexual stimulation or giving birth when unencumbered by drugs or iatrogenic disturbances. During the first stage of labor breathing becomes deeper with contractions, and the second stage of labor brings very deep breathing and breath-holding behaviors. Similar patterns of breathing can be seen during sexual response. During the first stages of sexual excitement breathing becomes more rapid and deeper; with impending orgasm, breathing may be interrupted or breath-holding may be observed. During the transition phase of labor the woman may experience a focusing on herself, decreasing attentiveness to external stimuli to the point of finding them noxious, heightened perception of pain or discomfort, and a yearning for expulsion that may parallel the introspection, response to external stimuli, heightened genital sensations, and a yearning for orgasm during sexual response.

During labor, particularly the second stage, women tend to make noises or to grunt. The same types of vocalization, gasping, or sucking noises may accompany approaching orgasm. Even facial expressions are similar. During the second stage of labor, the woman's face becomes intense, or stressed, leading an observer to believe that the woman is suffering. Similar facial expressions can be observed as orgasm approaches: the woman's mouth may be open, and her facial muscles tense. At both birth climax and with orgasm the woman's face

may resemble that of an athlete undergoing great physical strain.

With both birthing and orgasm, the upper portion of the uterus contracts rhythmically. Usually the mucous plug from the cervical os loosens during early labor and the same phenomenon may be experienced with sexual excitement, thus opening the cervical os for spermatozoa, rather than for the infant's birth. Just as the abdominal muscles contract periodically during the second stage of labor and a strong urge to bear down develops as delivery approaches, the abdominal muscles contract periodically during sexual excitement and the woman may relate sensations of bearing down with orgasm.* There are also similarities in central nervous system reactions during sexual excitement and childbirth. Just as women tend to become uninhibited during birth, especially as the baby's head descends the birth canal, inhibitions are often alleviated with impending orgasm. Sensory perception during birthing and sexual response are altered: during labor the vulva often becomes anesthetic as it is fully dilated with the baby's head, and there is a tendency for the woman to become less sensitive to the immediate surroundings as delivery of the infant approaches. However, following delivery, there is a sudden awareness. With coitus, there is a similar insensitivity to immediate surroundings, and with impending orgasm, there is sometimes a nearly complete loss of sensory perception. Following orgasm, there is a return of sensory acuity. Feelings of joy and well-being follow both childbirth and coital orgasm. Indeed, some women describe their childbirth experiences as sexually exciting and have characterized the birth climax as orgasmic.

Newton has also outlined similarities between lactation and coitus. First, it has been noted that uterine contractions occur with orgasm as well as suckling, as does erection of the nipples. Stroking of the breast and nipple stimulation occur both during breast feeding as well as during sexual play. Furthermore, the emotions aroused by sexual contact and by contact when nursing may produce similar changes in the vasculature of the breast and actually raise the skin temperature of the breast. It is known also that the milk-ejection reflex can be triggered by sexual excitement as well as by nursing. There is also a close resemblance between the

---

*Newton points out that the position for delivery resembles that commonly used for coitus in this culture. However, because of recent changes in birthing positions used by women in the United States and also because of the great variability of positions used for coitus by American women, this part of her analogy is less compelling than other portions.

emotions experienced during breast feeding and sexual arousal. Unfortunately, some women report feeling guilty about the sensual pleasures associated with breast feeding. It is thought that positive feelings about one's sexuality would be associated with positive feelings about breast feeding. Indeed Newton (1973) says that "the reason the sensuous nature of breastfeeding is so seldom recognized in our society may be the same reason birth orgasm is so seldom seen." (p. 84)

Social patterns have been quite effective in inhibiting breast feeding as well as female sexual response and natural, undisturbed childbirth. Perhaps as attitudes toward sexuality become more positive and childbirth practices become less encumbered by health professionals, society's attitudes toward breast feeding will become more positive.

Newton notes that there are important common characteristics shared among all three of these interpersonal acts. First, they are based at least in part on closely related neurohormonal reflexes. Next, they are sensitive to stimuli from the environment, and each can be inhibited during its earlier phases. (Fear and disturbance can have deleterious effects on labor, sexual functioning, and milk ejection.) Finally, all three appear to elicit caretaking behavior. Coitus, labor, and lactation all are interpersonal and psychophysiologic acts that are intertwined with affectionate partnership and caretaking behavior.

SUMMARY

From the foregoing discussion, it can be seen that there are several structures and functions unique to a woman's body. Both the menstrual cycle and the female sexual response cycle are important physiologic functions demonstrated only by the human female. Several of the structures of the woman's body serve both her procreative powers as well as her recreative pleasures, with the exception of the clitoris, an organ whose sole raison d'etre is to receive and transduce sexual pleasure. It has even been demonstrated that there are parallels between sexual responsiveness, giving birth, and breast feeding, thus suggesting that there are close interrelationships between the psychophysiologic processes that subserve these three reproductive and pleasurable interpersonal acts.

REFERENCES

Asso, D., and Beech, H. R.: Susceptibility to the acquisition of a conditioned response in relation to the menstrual cycle, J. Psychosom. Res. 19:337-344, 1975.

Bates, B.: A guide to the physical examination, Philadelphia, 1974, J. B. Lippincott Co.

Beck, A. C.: Chronological fluctuations of sex premenstrual tension variables. Doctoral thesis Purdue University, 1970.

Beumont, P. J., and others: A study of minor psychiatric and physical symptoms during the menstrual cycle, Br. J. Psych. 126:431-434, 1975.

Boston Women's Health Book Collective: Our bodies, ourselves, New York, 1976, Simon and Schuster, Inc.

Dan, A. J.: Behavioral variability and the menstrual cycle, presented at Annual Convention of the American Psychological Association, Washington, D.C., Sept. 1976.

Delaney, J., Lupton, M. J., and Toth, E.: The curse; a cultural history of menstruation, New York, 1976, New American Library.

Dickinson, R. L.: Atlas of human sex anatomy, ed. 2, Baltimore, 1949, The Williams & Wilkins Co.

Donelson, E., and Gullahorn, J.: Women: a psychological perspective, New York, 1977, John Wiley & Sons, Inc.

Fisher, S.: The female orgasm, New York, 1973, Basic Books, Inc.

Freud, S.: Some psychological consequences of the anatomical distinction between the sexes, Int. J. Psycho-Analysis, 8:133-142, 1927.

Golub, S.: The magnitude of premenstrual anxiety and depression, Psychosom. Med. 38:4-12, 1976.

Herschberger, R.: Adam's rib, New York, 1970, Harper & Bow, Publishers, Inc.

Hite, S.: The Hite report: a nationwide study of female sexuality, New York, 1976, Dell Publishing Co., Inc.

Janiger, O., and others: Cross cultural study of premenstrual symptoms, Psychosom. Med. 13:226-235, 1972.

Janowsky, D., Berens, S., and Davis, J.: Correlations between mood, weight, and electrolytes during the menstrual cycle: a renin-angiotensin-aldosterone hypothesis of premenstrual tension, Psychosom. Med. 35:143-154, 1973.

Kaplan, H. S.: The new sex therapy, New York, 1974, Brunner/Mazel.

Kinsey, A. C., Pomeroy, W., Martin, C., and Gebhard, P.: Sexual behavior in the human female, Philadelphia, 1953, W. B. Saunders Com.

Koeske, R., and Koeske, G.: An attributional approach to moods and the menstrual cycle, J. Pers. Soc. Psych. 31:473-478, 1975.

Little, B. C., and Zahn, T. P.: Changes in mood and autonomic functioning during the menstrual cycle, Psychophysiology 11:579-590, 1974.

Maddux, H. C.: Menstruation, New Canaan, Conn., 1975, Tobey Publishing Co., Inc.

Malasanos, L., and others: Health assessment, St. Louis, 1977, The C. V. Mosby Co.

Masters, W., and Johnson, V.: Human sexual response, Boston, 1966, Little, Brown and Co.

Morris, N. M., and Udry, J. R.: Variations in pedometer activity during the menstrual cycle, Obstet. Gynecol. 35:199-201, 1970.

Newton, N.: Interrelationships between sexual responsiveness, birth, and breast feeding. In Zubin, J., and Money, J., eds.: Contemporary sexual behavior: critical issues in the 1970's, Baltimore, 1973, Johns Hopkins University Press.

Paige, K.: Women learn to sing the menstrual blues, Psych. Today 7: 41-46, 1973.

Pallis, D. J., and Holding, T. A.: The menstrual cycle and suicidal intent, J. Biosoc. Sci. 8:27-33, 1977.

Parlee, M. B.: The premenstrual syndrome, Psych. Bull. 80:454-465, 1973.

Patkai, P., and others: Mood, alertness and sympathetic-adrenal medullary activity during the menstrual cycle, Psychosom. Med. 36:503-512, 1974.

Romney, S., and others: Gynecology and obstetrics: the health care of women, New York, 1975, McGraw-Hill Book Co.

Ruble, D.: Premenstrual symptoms: a reinterpretation, Science **197:** 291-292, 1977.

Ryan, C.: Our bodies, ourselves: the fallacy of seeking individual solutions for societal contradiction, Int. J. Health Serv. **5**(2):335-338, 1975.

Sherfey, M. J.: The nature and evolution of female sexuality, New York, 1972, Random House, Inc.

Shulman, A.: Organs and orgasms. In Gornick, V., and Morans, B., editors: Women in sexist society: studies in power and powerlessness, New York, 1971, Basic Books, Inc.

Singer, J., and Singer, I.: Types of female orgasm, J. Sex Res. **8**(4):255-267, 1972.

Sommer, B.: Menstrual cycle changes and intellectual performance, Psychosom. Med. **34**:263-269, 1972.

Speroff, L., Glass, R., and Kase, N.: Clinical gynecologic endocrinology and infertility, ed. 2, Baltimore, 1978, The Williams & Wilkins Co.

Surney, J. L., and others: Menstrual cycle and the decision to seek psychological services, Percept. Motor Skills **40**:886, 1975.

Udry, R., and Morris, N.: Distribution of coitus in the menstrual cycle, Nature **220**:593, 1968.

Vollman, R.: The menstrual cycle, Philadelphia, 1977, W. B. Saunders Co.

Waitzkin, H., and Waterman, B.: The exploitation of illness in a capitalist society, Indianapolis, 1974, The Bobbs-Merrill Co., Inc.

Weideger, P.: Menstruation and menopause, New York, 1976, Alfred A. Knopf.

Wilcoxon, L., and others: Daily self-reports on activities, life events, moods and somatic changes during the menstrual cycle, Psychosom. Med. **38**:399-417, 1976.

Williams, J.: Psychology of women: behavior in a biosocial context, New York, 1977, W. W. Norton and Co., Inc.

Woods, N. F.: Human sexuality in health and illness, ed. 2, St. Louis, 1979, The C. V. Mosby Co.

Yen, S. S. C., and Jaffee, R. B.: Reproductive endocrinology, physiology, pathophysiology, and clinical management, Philadelphia, 1978, W. B. Saunders Co.

6

Issues in the life cycle

Catherine Ingram Fogel

During her lifetime, a woman will have many experiences that are unique to her as a female. Events such as menarche and motherhood, the choices she makes about sexual preference, and the sexual options she exercises will all influence her development. Her self-concept and value system will be shaped by these choices and experiences.

From the moment of birth, a female receives messages about who she is and what it means to be a female in her particular culture. All too often these messages are negative and result in a self-concept that is less than positive.

Until recently it was assumed that all differences perceived between males and females were biologically based and therefore unchangeable—and this "anatomy is destiny" theory, first proposed by Freud, is still widely held. The resulting styles and practices of child-rearing and sex role socialization have had profound effects on the lives, mental health, and happiness of women. Sex role stereotyping of social and work roles, with the assignment of domestic, expressive, and nurturant roles to females, has allowed full development of only one aspect of the female being.

Many of the negative messages women receive about themselves and their bodies have their roots in folklore, stereotypes, and taboos that have a rather tenuous link with fact. As we discuss some of the stereotypes and taboos affecting women, we will cite recent studies dispelling some of these myths—and others that substantiate some of the behavioral differences between the sexes.

Nurses need to be aware of the issues in the life cycle of women that affect their health and health care. This means that nurses must also explore the ways in which these issues have affected them as well as their clients. Self-awareness and recognition of one's own value system will enable the nurse to separate her own from her client's interpretation of events. This measure of objectivity enhances the nurse's ability to assess, derive a

nursing diagnosis, and provide empathetic, client-centered care.

In this chapter we will discuss the biologic development of the female embryo, behavioral and other differences between the sexes, taboos associated with menstruation, female sexuality, and the roles of women in society. Issues specific to older women, childbearing, and infertility are presented in subsequent chapters.

GENDER IDENTITY

Individuals are assigned sex or determined to be sexual beings on three different levels: biologic sex, gender identity, and gender role. *Biologic sex* refers to chromosomal make-up, external and internal genitalia, hormonal status, and secondary sex characteristics. *Gender identity* is the belief that one is a male or female. This identity is the first stage in gender development and is firmly entrenched by age 3. Usually there is congruence between biologic sex and gender identity.

Gender role, or sex-typed behavior, is the second stage of gender development and refers to all that the individual says and does to indicate to herself and others that she is a female. It is the expression of those traits, roles, and responsibilities that are deemed appropriate to or expressive of femaleness. Gender role is the public expression of gender identity, while gender identity is the private experience of gender role (Money and Ehrhardt, 1972).

Money and Ehrhardt (1972) have developed a model for gender identity differentiation giving a developmental sequence of biologic and environmental events that interact to determine adult gender identity (Fig. 6-1).

Conception initiates the process of sexual differentiation that ends in a firmly established adult gender identity. Chromosomal sex is established at the moment of fertilization when the sperm contributor of an X or Y chromosome is paired with the X chromosome of the ovum. When the outcome is XX, female chromosomal sex is established. The XX chromosomal combination

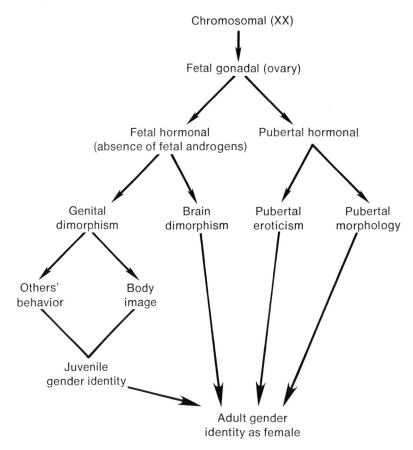

Fig. 6-1. Sequential and interactional components of gender identity differentiation in the female. (Adapted from Money, J., and Ehrhardt, A.: Man and woman, boy and girl, Baltimore, 1972, Johns Hopkins Press.)

determines that the undifferentiated fetal gonads will become ovaries at about 5 to 6 weeks' gestation.

Hormonal secretions from the fetal gonads influence further sexual differentiation between the seventh and twelfth week of fetal life. At this time fetal androgens must be added for a male to develop. If differentiation of the reproductive structures of a male is to occur, testicular hormones are imperative. Unless these are present in appropriate amounts at the critical times, male structures will not develop from the wolffian ducts. Additionally, it is thought that the müllerian-inhibiting substance prevents further development of the müllerian, or female, duct system. In the absence of fetal gonadal hormones, the fetus continues to develop the reproductive anatomy of a female. It does not appear that estrogen is essential at this stage for female development. Biologic sex is fairly well established by the twelfth week of gestation (Money and Ehrhardt, 1972).

While estrogens do not appear to be essential for the continued feminization of the fetal reproductive trait, they are released in the genetically female embryo. Even when the gonads are removed prior to the seventh

week of gestation, the fetus continues to develop as a female. Apparently, there is not an ovarian inductor substance necessary for female development. However, estrogens are necessary for complete development of the female genital trait. It is thought that the autonomous nature of female development occurred in response to the evolutionary dilemma of a need to bear live young without feminization of the male embryo with maternal estrogens (Money and Ehrhardt, 1972).

It is thought that there is a critical stage just prior to or right after birth when another set of sexual controls is introduced. In a process known as sex-typing of the brain, testosterone may influence the hypothalamus. The brain influenced by testosterone develops male, or acyclic, patterns for release of pituitary hormones, the gonadotropins. A cyclic pattern of gonadotropin release is established in the female-typed brain. Following this second crucial period, the individual is resistant or immune to the influence of either testosterone or estrogen depending upon his or her sexual differentiation (Money and Ehrhardt, 1972).

Animal research suggests that in a few critical days of

brain development, the prenatal hormonal environment exerts a determining influence on neural pathways that will subsequently affect differential sexual behavior. In humans the pathways have not been identified. The lower the animal is on the phylum scale the more likely its prenatally determined behavior is to be stereotyped and uninfluenced by later events. Human beings are more apt to be influenced by postnatal psychosocial factors (Money and Ehrhardt, 1972).

Once the infant is born, gender identity differentiation is most influenced by the response of others. As soon as the doctor or midwife says, "It's a girl!" a chain of responses and reactions is set in motion that will continue throughout life. Response on the basis of sex organs is one of the most universal and pervasive aspects of human interaction. From the time of delivery a female is held as a girl and in a way that is different from a boy. Scripting begins immediately. The differentiation of gender role and gender identity continues through identification with members of the same sex and complementary relationships with members of the opposite sex. Gender identity probably begins with an awareness that one belongs to one sex and not the other. Core gender identity—the earliest, probably unalterable form of gender identity—develops somewhere between 18 months and 3 years.

SEX DIFFERENCES

There are certainly differences between males and females, some of which are biologically determined. The question is, how many and which ones? It is important to distinguish between innate biologic differences and self-fulfilling prophesies.

Sex differences, at least in principle, could arise from at least five sources:

1. Intrinsic biologic differences present from birth
2. Cultural differences in assigned roles
3. Anticipatory socialization that is cultural but prepares the girl for actual biologic differences that become apparent later
4. Differential value, meaning, or reward assigned by the culture to gender-specific behaviors
5. Additional cultural elaboration of behaviors that develop as reactions to more basic responses

Among the basic undeniable sex differences, which are biologic and/or anatomic, are: Women can menstruate, conceive and bear children, and lactate; men cannot. The secondary sex characteristics of adulthood are reminders of the differences, as are the external sex organs. But are there any other differences between the sexes that are biologically determined?

Infants

Differences are apparent between male and female infants. Males tend to be larger, have more muscle mass, and be more active. Females tend to be more passive in motor responses and more sensitive to pain or tactile stimuli (Bardwick, 1971). As the infant and child develop, more and more sex differences develop. Bardwick hypothesizes that sex-typing of the brain causes an infant's personality to have qualities that are rewarded or punished by the parents in the light of their own perception of appropriate sex role behaviors.

Behavioral differences

According to widely held beliefs in our society, the average woman is passive, dependent, quiet, gentle, unintelligent, and generally inferior to the average male. Conversely, the average adult male is thought to be active, aggressive, independent, intelligent, rough, and superior in all respects to women. Traditional stereotypic adjectives often used to describe men and women are summarized in the following list:

Women	*Men*
Retiring	Aggressive
Dependent	Independent
Emotional	Hides emotions
Subjective	Objective
Easily influenced	Not easily influenced
Submissive	Dominant
Passive	Active
Noncompetitive	Competitive
Illogical	Logical
Home-oriented	Worldly
Nonadventurous	Adventurous
Feelings easily hurt	Feelings not easily hurt
Difficulty making decisions	Make decisions easily
Low self-confidence	High self-confidence
Not ambitious	Ambitious
Concerned with own appearance	Not concerned with own appearance
Talkative	Not talkative
Gentle	Rough
Sensitive to feelings of others	Not sensitive to feelings of others

Although these are commonly held beliefs, they have not all been substantiated by research data. Even though the data are incomplete and often inconsistent, it appears that actual differences between the sexes are not great. Table 6-1 summarizes many of the sex differences and similarities in men and women.

Aggression. The stereotype that men are more aggressive than women is supported by several studies. Research suggests that there may be a substantial biologic basis for sex differences in the areas of aggressive and dominant behaviors in males. The behavioral effects of exposure to testosterone have been documented in several animal studies. It appears that increased aggressiveness and male sexual responses are related to high testosterone levels. At present, however, the implication of such findings for masculine and feminine differentiation in humans are unclear (Parson and Ruble, 1978).

Males behave more aggressively than females at all ages. Females may not differ much from males in aggressive motivation or drive; however, their behavior differs significantly. It is thought that the differences in overt aggression may result in part from masculine sex typing of aggressive responses. Females are aware that aggressive behavior is defined culturally as unfeminine and therefore they become anxious when they respond aggressively, and will only exhibit such responses in private, permissible situations or indirectly. This is especially true in situations of overt physical aggression when sex differences are maximized (Ruble and Frieze, 1978).

Dependency. Females are believed to be more passive, dependent, and easily influenced than males. Whether or not this is really true is not clear. Differ-

Table 6-1. Sex differences and similarities*

Abilities	
General intelligence	No difference on most tests.
Verbal ability	Females excel after age 10 or 11.
Quantitative ability	Males excel from the start of adolescence.
Creativity	Females excel on verbal creativity tests; otherwise, no difference.
Cognitive style	No general difference.
Visual-spatial ability	Males excel from adolescence on.
Physical abilities	Males more muscular; males more vulnerable to illness, disease; females excel on manual dexterity tests when speed important, but findings ambiguous.
Personality characteristics	
Sociability and love	No overall difference; at some ages, boys play in larger groups; some evidence that young men fall in love more easily, out of love with more difficulty.
Empathy	Conflicting evidence.
Emotionality	Self-reports and observations conflict.
Dependence	Conflicting findings; dependence probably not a unitary concept.
Nurturance	Little evidence available on adult male reactions to infants; issue of maternal vs. paternal behavior remains open; no overall difference in altruism.
Aggressiveness	Males more aggressive from preschool age on.

*Reprinted by permission of Harcourt Brace Jovanovich, Inc. from *The Longest War: Sex Differences in Perspective* by Carol Tavris and Carole Offir, © 1977 by Harcourt Brace Jovanovich, Inc.

ences are particularly small in children. Studies of older children and adults have consistently found more women to rate themselves higher on dependence traits than men. This pattern may indicate learned conformity to sex-type expectations. Current research does not demonstrate consistent sex effects in dependency-related behaviors. Females are believed to be tactful, gentle, and considerate of others' feelings while males are not of these. Early research suggested that females are moderately more socially oriented and nurturant than males. In contrast, more recent studies have either found no differences or that differences were related to situational factors rather than innate sex differences. Overall, findings are inconclusive (Ruble, 1978).

Emotional stability. A very pervasive sex-role stereotype is that women are more emotional than men. The woman is unable to handle even minor crises. She is sensitive, moody, fearful, anxious, and cries easily. A review of relevant studies suggests that consistent sex differences in fearfulness and anxiety are found only with paper-and-pencil measures that are subject to stereotype bias. Whether or not females are actually more emotional than males has yet to be determined (Ruble, 1978).

Self-confidence. Males are stereotypically viewed as more self-confident than females. However, this has not been validated except in areas related to achievement. Even though stereotypic feminine attributes are devalued in comparison to male attributes, females do not consistently have a less positive self-concept than males (Ruble and Frieze, 1978). An exception in this was noted by Rosenberg and Simmons (1975) who, in a study of almost 2000 children and adolescents, found adolescent girls to be more self-conscious, more vulnerable to criticism, and more concerned with facilitating interpersonal harmony than boys. It was suggested that these differences reflect social definitions of sex roles.

Cognitive skills

Females have verbal skills that are superior to males. However, there appears to be substantial evidence that males have better spatial skills than females, and it is thought that the ability may have a biologic basis though the exact mechanisms mediating these biologic effects are not known (Parsons and Ruble, 1978). No differences in general intelligence have been documented (Tavris and Offir, 1977).

Summary of findings

Maccoby and Jacklin (1974) reviewed over 2000 works on psychologic similarities and differences between males and females. They conclude that many common assumptions about sex differences are unfounded, although there are some differences between males and females. Their findings are given here:

A. Unfounded beliefs about sexual differences:
1. Girls are more "social" than boys
2. Girls are more "suggestible" than boys
3. Girls have lower self-esteem
4. Girls are better at rote learning and simple repetitive tasks; boys are better at tasks requiring higher level cognitive processing and inhibition of previously learned responses
5. Boys are more analytic
6. Girls are more affected by heredity, boys by environment
7. Girls lack achievement motivation
8. Girls are auditory, boys visual

B. Sex differences that are fairly well established:
1. Girls have greater verbal abilities than boys
2. Boys excel in visual-spatial ability
3. Boys excel in mathematical abilities
4. Males are more aggressive

C. There is too little evidence or findings are ambiguous to state that girls and boys differ significantly in:
1. Tactile sensitivity
2. Fear, timidity, and anxiety
3. Activity level
4. Competitiveness
5. Dominance
6. Compliance
7. Nurturance and "maternal" behavior

There are differences between sexes: basic reproductive anatomy and physiology are different in the male and female, and there are some personality and cognitive differences. However, these differences are neither as great nor as numerous as common sexual stereotypes would have us believe. Some of the differences are founded in anatomy—namely, reproductive capabilities. With some few exceptions, however, anatomy is not destiny and it is not preordained that either women or men will think, act, and behave only in certain ways. It appears that gender identity rather than biologic sex determines many of the components of the sex role one learns. The evidence regarding early behavior sex differences and cross-cultural behaviors suggests that of all the behaviors commonly stereotyped as masculine or feminine, only aggression and spatial abilities differ regularly between the sexes. There is little if any evidence to support the theory of biologic or inborn personality or response differences between males and females. It appears that the differences seen in older children and adults are a result of socialization rather than biology. For the most part sex differences appear to be learned. Money and Ehrhardt (1972) believe that while the central nervous system, insofar as prenatal hormonal factors make it sexually dimorphic, is receptive to behavioral traits that are traditionally and culturally clas-

sified as predominantly male or female, these traits do not automatically determine gender identity but exert some influence on the ultimate pattern of gender identity. The predominant part of gender identity differentiation is accomplished by socialization in daily living.

MENSTRUATION

Menstruation is one of the three physiologic processes that belong exclusively to the female, the others being childbearing and lactation. Menstruation has been invested with enormous social significance, most of it negative. Throughout history menstruation has been viewed with a mixture of awe, pity, disgust, and fear. Myths about menstruation die hard and many people today feel uneasy about this basic physiologic process. Beliefs about this function are an important factor in discrimination against women and contribute to maintaining their second-class status.

Myths and taboos

Throughout history, menstruation has been regarded as undesirable by most and it is frequently the subject of superstition, restriction on behavior, and taboos. Men have been frightened and mystified by menstruation; it has been considered a source of dark power for women and a threat to men. The basis for many of the taboos is thought to involve the following (Martin, 1978):
1. Male castration fears were provoked by genital bleeding, which symbolized the vulnerability of the male's exposed genitals. Women were conceptualized as inferior; they were punished by deprivation of external or male genitals. In some way the monthly cyclic bleeding was a regular, threatening reminder of this.
2. Menses allowed the male to displace his deep-rooted guilt associated with his aggressive impulses.
3. Menses were seen as a prevention of incest. Women were believed to have increased sexuality during their menses and strict controls were needed to restrict their incestuous desires.
4. Taboos were a male projection upon women of the hatred and fear of the powerful father.

Most of these beliefs about menstruating women point to negative attributes. These beliefs fall into three basic categories which focus on weakness, evil power, or a capacity for doing good. Many menstrual myths center around protecting the woman and focusing on the woman's vulnerability to psychologic and physical damage. Other myths concern protecting others from the menstruating woman, implying the contaminating properties of menstruation. Menstruating women are viewed as dirty and dangerous. Many religious sanctions derive from the contamination fear, the most restrictive being the forbidding of sexual intercourse during menstruation and the need for ritual cleansing following menstruation.

A third set of beliefs sees "power in the blood." Although menstruation is considered dirty and dangerous, it is also thought to have healing powers and can ward off danger. While beliefs such as these are not common in the United States today, menstruation remains as something negative, which is embarrassing and to be ignored if possible.

Euphemisms commonly used to indicate the function of menstruation are another example of the prevailing negative view. The "curse" explicitly summarizes the traditional attitudes toward menstruation. Ernster (1975) finds that women tend to use such terms as a secret language when a straightforward statement about menstruation would be embarrassing. Men tend to use menstrual euphemisms that have sexual and derogatory connotations.

Belief systems such as these have resulted in negative feelings about cyclic physiology and have restricted women's power in the social order. Such obvious manifestations of femaleness are viewed with hostility or depression when the status of women is low and female roles are restricted. Menstruation is associated with pain, messiness, nuisance, uncleanliness, and indecency for many women.

Various socialization processes contribute to the negative feelings associated with menstruation. A study of the attitudes of white, middle-class, adolescent girls toward menstruation shows that the prevelant view of menstruation is "a sickness" (Whisnant and Zegans, 1976).

This same message conveyed through advertisements for feminine medication and hygiene products in which menarche is portrayed as hygienic rather than a maturational crisis. Commercial educational materials are important sources of information about menstruation for young adolescent girls. Whisnant and associates (1975) found that in these materials menstruation is presented as a source of embarrassment. Emphasis is placed on the mechanics of the process and ways in which to achieve hygienic control. Little acknowledgement or attention is put on the girl's emotional needs and anxieties. Attention is drawn away from the body, away from puberty and the resulting changes it brings, and is focused on how to conceal the evidence. Whisnant et al found that the old notions of menstruation as a disease or terrifying experience are not supported in educational materials, but neither is the development of a positive outlook concerning menstruation or menarche.

Hormonal influences on behavior

It is commonly believed that the menstrual cycle exerts a profound effect upon the lives and moods of most women, and the usual implication is that these effects are negative. However, research indicates that menstrual symptoms are not as debilitating as is frequently thought and that severe symptoms are not present in most women or in most cycles for a particular woman (Ruble and Frieze, 1978). Recent studies by Brooks and associates (1977) have shown that among 291 college women menstruation was accepted rather routinely and was not perceived as overly disruptive. In fact, Messent (1976) states that the "human female is exceptional with regard to hormones and sexual behavior since the effect exerted is at best very small."

However, other investigators have advanced various explanations for the apparent psychologic and behavioral fluctuations observed in association with the menstrual cycle (Ruble and Frieze, 1978). The most common view is that these are direct effects of the hormonal variations of the menstrual cycle. This particular school of thought attributes mood changes to the use and withdrawal of estrogen and progesterone in the organism. Another explanation centers on the effects of the enzyme monoamine oxidase (MAO). According to this theory, negative moods associated with the premenstrual and menstrual cycle are caused by changes in neural activity in the brain produced by MAO. Changes in the estrogen and progesterone levels during the second half of the cycle are associated with increased MAO activity.

The adrenal glands have also been suggested as a factor in mood changes (Ruble and Frieze, 1978). It is assumed that the balance of adrenal hormone levels is upset in some women during the premenstruation phase because of low levels of other hormones, specifically progesterone.

Most studies report correlations between phases of the menstrual cycle and psychologic status such as aggression, irritability, elation, and activation (Ruble and Frieze, 1978). To the extent that mood changes occur in the different phases of the menstrual cycle, the general pattern appears to be that negative symptoms are associated with the premenstrual or menstrual phase and positive feelings are reported at mid-cycle. Specific moods described in relation to phases of the cycle are a sense of well-being associated with the proliferative phase; heightened sexual desire at the time of ovulation; and feelings of passivity and depression as menstruation approaches, which linger on into actual menstruation (see Chapters 5 and 13 for additional discussions of behavioral changes associated with the menstrual cycle).

The main behavioral changes associated with the menstrual cycle are in sensory thresholds and emotional responses. The emotional changes that have been documented during the menstrual cycle are difficult to interpret. No hormonal involvement has been conclusively demonstrated, while the importance of psychologic and social factors in the development of emotional changes is given increasing credence. Much more research is needed to confirm the relationship between female hormones and human behavior (Messent, 1976).

Women react physiologically to menstruation and menarche in ways that are influenced by their culture. Brooks-Gunn and Ruble (1977) consider that attitudes about menstruation and associated symptoms are acquired at an early age. General cultural stereotypes, expectations about what will occur when menstruation begins, and specific information received from others all contribute to self-reported experiences of menstruation. Ruble and Frieze (1978) suggest that menstruation beliefs may affect women's and girls' actual experience as well as their perception of menstruation. Parlee's (1974) work supports this view; she has found that both men and women report virtually identical patterns of symptoms and symptom changes. Parlee suggests that stereotypic beliefs about the psychologic concomitants of menstruation may be the reason for this. Koeske and Koeske (1975) have found that when a woman acts negatively during the premenstrual phase of her cycle she is apt to label her behaviors as premenstrual tension. If the same behaviors occur at a different point in her cycle, they are not attributed to the effects of the menstrual cycle.

An additional cultural influence that has been associated with attitudes and reactions to the menstrual cycle is religion. Paige (1973) found that Catholics, Protestants, and Jews differ considerably in their attitudes toward menstruation and in level of anxiety experienced.

It may be that the cyclic changes in mood and behavior seen in many women are the result of the woman's emotional reactions to the physical symptoms associated with premenstruation or menstruation. Cramps may evoke hostility or irritability. Since menstruation is usually viewed as inconvenient, anticipation of the inconvenience or of dysmenorrhea could also cause irritability or anxiety. Not only can physical changes affect psychologic changes but psychologic reactions, such as stress or anxiety, may lead to change in hormonal levels, which may in turn create physical symptoms (Ruble and Frieze, 1978).

How a woman feels about menstruation depends on the interactions between her internalized values, her perceptions of society's and significant others' attitudes, her understanding of her reproductive processes, and the actual physiologic response of her body. Negative attitudes will predispose her to unpleasant experiences. Attitudes will in part determine whether she regards the normal variation of the menstrual cycle as abnormal or a natural physical response. Negative views of menstruation can decrease her sense of self as a woman—her self-worth and self-concept. The nursing practitioner can be instrumental in dissipating negative attitudes toward reproductive functions and thereby in enhancing a client's feelings of self-worth and value.

AGES AND STAGES OF THE ADULT WOMAN

Life is characterized by stages of development, nodal points in the life cycle, and developmental or maturational crises. The developmental cycles of adulthood last about 7 years. Adults move from one stage to the next as they begin to work on new developmental tasks and build new structures for their lives. By adulthood, it is assumed that a woman has achieved maturity. She views herself as independent, free to choose her intimates and to implement her own decisions. She recognizes her ability to love and influence others. Uncertainty can be tolerated and new experiences enjoyed. Each stage or passage of the adult female has definite characteristics. The following stages have been described by Gail Sheehy in *Passages* (1976b).

"Pulling up roots." Between 18 to 20, the individual removes herself from her family. She locates herself in a peer group role and in a sex role and anticipates a career. She has left the family home physically, and she begins leaving home emotionally. Rebounds back into the family structure are common. One part of the individual seeks to be separate while another wants to restore safety and comfort by merger with another. For a woman this often takes the form of marriage to one who she thinks will take care of her. Early marriage at this point can block growth. Usually a stormy passage through the stage aids normal progression of the adult life cycle.

"Trying twenties." During this stage the focus shifts from the inner self and the question "Who am I?" to the outer world and questions such as, "How can I put my goals into operation?" Tasks of this phase include shaping a vision of self, preparing for life work, finding a mentor, and developing a capacity for intimacy. Two impulses are always at work: to build a firm, safe structure for the future and to explore, experiment, and keep any structure tentative. The exhilaration of trying out the adult world is balanced by the fear that choices made are irrevocable.

"Catch-30." Between the ages of 28 and 32 feelings of being too restricted or too narrow are frequent. A common response is to tear up the life the twenties were spent putting together. Whatever course the woman has pursued, she now feels is too restricted and wrong. The woman previously content to be a wife and mother now wants a career, or vice versa. Almost everyone who is married, especially if for 7 years, feels discontent. Divorce or at least a serious review of the marriage and each partner's aspirations occurs. There is a lack of mutuality and an absolute need for more self-concern.

"Rooting and extending." During the early thirties, life becomes less provisional, more rational and orderly. Most individuals put down roots. Homes are bought and careers are pursued vigorously. Marital satisfaction declines.

"Deadline decade." Women begin to feel a sense of time squeeze about age 35. Whatever options she as a woman has already exercised she now feels an urge to review the options she set aside and those that aging and biology will close off in the foreseeable future. Several facts of female life combine to bring a sense of deadline to the fore:

1. Thirty-five is the age when the average mother sends her youngest child to school.
2. Thirty-five is the age when the average married woman reenters the working world.
3. Thirty-five is the age when infidelity becomes more probable.
4. Thirty-five is the most common age for runaway wives.
5. Thirty-five is the age when biologic reproductive boundaries are visible.
6. About age 35 is when the divorced woman is likely to remarry.

Questions such as "Why am I doing this?" and "What do I really believe in?" surface. Those parts of the personality that have previously been suppressed are now examined. The individual learns to be more accepting and tolerant of the less acceptable or attractive aspects of herself. Around the age of 40, the individual passes through a period of acute discomfort as she faces the discrepancy between youthful ambitions and actual achievements. The mid-life crisis is characterized by feelings of boredom, dissatisfaction with the way one's life has developed, and ambivalence and uncertainty about the future. The sense of time passing produces an urgency to accomplish goals—there is only one last chance. A woman may ask what she has given up to maintain her marriage or raise her children, or whether her career has deprived her of happiness. If she is childless she may wonder if there is still time. Women tend to reevaluate their lives as a whole.

Life patterns

Women choose one of several life patterns. The "caregiver" often marries in her early twenties or before and at that time does not wish to go beyond the traditional roles of wife and mother. The majority of women elect this role and a life of "cherishing, succoring, listening, and believing in other people." (Sheehy, 1976b, p. 206) Rather than pursue her own dreams the woman carries the dream of her husband and lives for her attachments. Her greatest fear may be abandonment by her significant others. In later years she may come to believe that this role is not sufficient and wish to add others. The "either-or woman" feels required to choose between love and children and work and accomplishments. She may be the nurturer who defers achievement and postpones a career in order to marry and start a family. She intends to pick up her career at a later

Table 6-2. Developmental model for sexual identity*

	Stage 1: Prenatal	Stage 2: Birth and childhood	Stage 3: Puberty	Stage 4: Sexual intimacy	Stage 5: Fertility/ parenthood	Stage 6: Loss of sexual powers
Biological events						
	Conception Fetal development	Birth Normal sexual morphology	Development of secondary sex characteristics Menarche	Sexual initiation Frigidity/impotence	Conception Pregnancy Parturition Lactation	Menopause Surgical loss Aging
Social events						
	None	Sex assignment Sex-role socialization Sex rearing Sexual exploration	Dating Popularity Sexual experimentation Sexual morality	Role conflict Assumption of marital role Resocialization regarding sexual behavior	Marital role Parental role	Freedom from fertility Wound to self-esteem Change in sex identity
Significant others						
	None	Parents Peers Physician	Peers	Partner(s) Peers	Spouse Parents Peers Community	Spouse

*From Laws, J.: Sexual scripts: the social construction of female sexuality, Hinsdale, Ill., 1977, Dryden Press.

time; however, the world does not wait and she often finds she can't catch up.

The "achiever" defers nurturing, postponing motherhood (and often marriage) in order to complete professional preparation and establish her career. At times this woman too forfeits her options by limiting her outlook so severely that she may not be able to reestablish a relationship.

The "integrators" attempt to combine career, marriage, and motherhood. Women in their twenties who attempt this rarely accomplish it successfully. It is quite possible at age 30 and decidedly possible at 35 when the personal integration necessary has developed. There are also some women who choose never to marry and other women who choose a transient impermanent life-style.

The nurse who is aware of the predictable stages of adult development in women and the possible life patterns they may choose will be able to provide her clients with anticipatory guidance that may facilitate successful passage from stage to stage.

FEMALE SEXUALITY

A woman's sexual identity is defined as her awareness of herself as a female and of those characteristics that make up her femaleness. These include knowledge of her body and its functions, images of femininity, sexual preferences, and sexual history. The earliest component of sexual identity is gender identity; other components of sexual identity build on the foundation of femaleness (Laws, 1977). Table 6-2 presents a model of the development of female sexual identity.

Effects of attitudes and values of society

Sexual behavior is based on the complex interactions of biologic, sociocultural, and emotional factors. Fig. 6-2 illustrates the determinants of sexual activity. Sexual identity and sexual behavior are strongly influenced by our values and attitudes, which define what is sexual and determine what we believe about the sexual nature of men and women.

Women presently live in a society that is sexually confused and repressed. Women's sexual roles reflect their roles in society. Historically, a woman's sexuality was bound up with her economic worth, childbearing functions, supposed inherent weakness, and second class status. Our most pervasive sexual attitudes are derived from Judeo-Christian teachings. The Hebreic view of women was that she is a possession, necessary for bearing children but essentially inferior. Women's bodies and functions were considered unclean and numerous purification rituals surrounded menstruation and pregnancy. The early Christians viewed woman as seductive

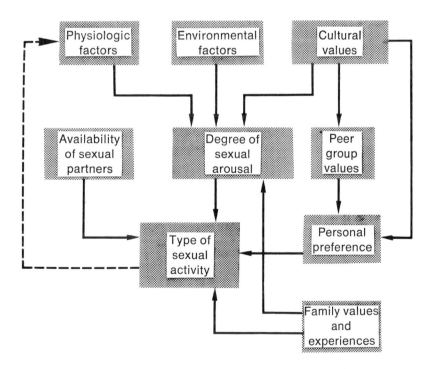

Fig. 6-2. Determinants of sexual activity. A number of factors interact to determine whether or not a person is sexually aroused and what type of sexual activity, if any, they engage in. People differ in the degree of importance attached to each factor. (From Frieze, I.: Sexual roles of women. In Frieze, I., and others, editors: Women and sex roles, New York, 1978, W. W. Norton & Co., p. 211.)

tempters of men. Women were not thought capable of considering the spiritual matters necessary for salvation; they were only concerned with earthly matters, specifically children. A woman's basic sexual nature was considered a constant threat to man's salvation because she was always distracting him from God with sex. "Good" women were not interested in sex and did all they could to avoid being aroused as sexual partners. The majority of women, however, were seductive, sexual, and morally inferior to men. Celibacy was considered the most holy state; however, marriage was acknowledged as a necessity for most men and women. The basic Christian beliefs that open sexual exposure is evil and that chastity is inherently good have been in evidence in our country since its Puritan origins (Frieze et al., 1978).

Many of the sexual attitudes held today can be traced to the Victorian era. The majority of middle-class Victorians believed sex to be dirty, dangerous, and disgusting. Premarital sex, sexual fantasies, and masturbation were wrong. Intercourse within the confines of marriage was acceptable, but only if it was performed infrequently, using acceptable positions, and did not involve "unnatural" practices. While the Judeo-Christian teachings discouraged sexual pleasure and advanced a narrow interpretation of normality on religious and moral grounds, the Victorians warned against sex for reasons of health and character. Women were divided into two groups: the good and the sexual. Good women did not enjoy sex, regarded it as a marital duty to be endured, submitted stoically, and were passive. Any woman who lustily enjoyed sex was automatically classified as bad or impure. However, despite the traditional message the Victorian women received, often there was a gap between actual behavior and beliefs, which resulted in guilt, anxiety, and remorse (Tavris and Offir, 1977).

Freud reflected much of the Victorian tradition in his basic belief system. He was, however, also a major influence for change in sexual attitudes. Although he expressed the belief that both sexes experience sexual desire, he thought women's sexual motivation was primarily the desire for a child while men's sexual desire was more direct. The sexual attitudes expressed in Freud's writing often provided a "scientific" foundation for or legitimized the already held Judeo-Christian beliefs. The basic inferiority of women and women's sexual orientation toward reproductive functions were upheld by Freud. He supported the historical belief in a greater sexual aggressiveness of males and the passivity of women. Freud also defined normal, mature, feminine sexuality as vaginal orgasm rather than clitoral. Moreover, Freud believed that postmenopausal women had no

sexual desires since they could no longer have children. Even though Freud's writing gave credence to many of the traditional erroneous beliefs about sex, at the same time he helped people accept that men and women have sexual feelings and that this is normal. He identified the negative effects of repressing sexual feelings and insisted that sexuality should be encouraged for all Frieze et al., 1978).

Although research on human sexuality by Alfred Kinsey and his collaborators in 1953 and by Masters and Johnson in 1966 and 1970 has had a tremendous impact in exposing myths about female sexuality, many still abound. At times it appears that one myth is dispelled only to be replaced by another. Some of the prevalent myths about female sexuality are summarized below:

1. *Women should satisfy men, since women's needs are secondary to men's.* This implies that a woman's sexuality is less than a man's, that his needs are greater and more important than hers.
2. *Each partner should be concerned with the sexual satisfaction of the other; sexual pleasure is the responsibility of the partner.* In this situation the person with the greater skills will be more successful. In general, women are taught to be concerned about others and men are socialized to be more self-oriented. A woman is often more apt to focus harder on pleasing her partner.
3. *Women arouse more slowly than men; it takes a great deal of stimulation to sexually arouse a woman.* The woman who is easily aroused may feel she is abnormal or unusual. In addition, there are enormous variations in women and men and within the same person at different times. It is impossible to generalize for an entire sex.
4. *Women who are raped ask for it; every woman wants to be raped.* Rape is a crime of violence, not a sexual crime. Most women do not want acts of violence committed against them nor do they knowingly and willingly provoke violence.
5. *Young girls should not be told about sex because it will put ideas in their heads.* Ignorance is dangerous and damaging. The myth reinforces stereotypes and the belief that sex is bad and must be ignored. When information is provided curiosity is satisfied and the possibility of experimentation lessened.
6. *Women are not sexually interested or generally responsive. They are incapable of multiple orgasms.* The classic research of Masters and Johnson has demonstrated that men and women experience sexual response in similar ways, that each is equally responsive.
7. *Women want sex only for procreation purposes.*

Total anorgasm	Climax only when alone, and with intense direct clitoral stimulation	Alone with erotic fantasy and direct stimulation	With lover and direct stimulation	Orgasm with coitus alone	Orgasm in response to nongenital stimulation and/or fantasy only
!	!	!	!	!	!

Women have the capability to enjoy sex on many levels as demonstrated by the research of Masters and Johnson and the writing of Sherfy.

8. *The man with a large penis is always a better sexual partner.* Within normal size ranges, the vagina expands to fit the erect penis. For most women, technique is a better indication of satisfaction than is size.

9. *Women are so sexually aggressive that they cannot be satisfied.* As the myth of women's passivity is dispelled, a new belief (or fear) of female insatiability has replaced it. There are not data to substantiate this myth.

10. *Female orgasms are life-changing experiences.* This is the reverse of the myth that orgasm for the woman is perverse or that women are asexual. Unrealistic expectations and concern over normality can result from this reverse standard.

Myths such as these about female sexuality have no foundation in fact. They do, however, serve the purpose of controlling anxiety about sexuality and hiding ignorance. To enjoy full sexual expression, myths must be questioned and ignorance replaced with fact.

Results of research

Until recently, very few meaningful statistics about female sexuality were available. The issue was further complicated by confusion about the relationship between female orgasm and coitus and what is normal and what is dysfunctional.

Much of the confusion is a residual of the old distinction developed by Freud between vaginal and clitoral orgasm. According to psychoanalytic theory, there are two kinds of orgasm—clitoral and vaginal; the clitoral is supposed to be neurotic, or less mature, while the vaginal orgasm is a healthy expression of adult sexuality.

Thanks to Masters and Johnson (1966) there is now considerable evidence to contradict the strict psychoanalytic position that there are two types of female orgasm—vaginal and clitoral—and that orgasm resulting from clitoral stimulation is pathologic. Masters and Johnson found that all orgasms, whether triggered by intercourse or direct clitoral stimulation, to be physiologically identical. Furthermore, female orgasms were not *either* vaginal *or* clitoral but had both components. Kaplan (1974) suggests that confusion could be reduced or eliminated if we could consider orgasm as a reflex having

both a motor and sensory component. There is no real controversy over the motor component, especially since the extensive research by Masters and Johnson. It is the sensory component that excites such controversy. For some reason, it is difficult to accept the notion that feelings in the vagina, pelvis, perineum, and uterus may result from stimulation of sensory nerve endings in the clitoris, which also has distinct, pleasurable, erotic sensations. Further, women differ in their orgasmic thresholds; there is a normal range to elicit response just as there is for any other type of reflex. It is not yet clear where normalcy ends and dysfunction begins. At one end of the spectrum are those women who have never experienced orgasm. Kaplan presumes that all physically normal women are capable of orgasm, and therefore the totally inorgasmic state represents dysfunction. But from then on the distinction between normal and pathologic becomes less and less clear. The spectrum might appear as above (Woods, 1979). Intercourse alone is a relatively mild stimulus (at least physically) and does not produce as intense a stimulation as does direct clitoral manipulation; therefore, women with relatively low orgasmic thresholds can climax on intercourse alone.

Kinsey (1953) found that 30% of the women in his sample did not have orgasm when first married, although only 10% were still nonorgasmic after 10 years of marriage. (It is believed that Kinsey meant orgasm by any means.) Fisher, in 1973, did a 5-year study of 200 middle-class women in New York City that failed to confirm many previously held beliefs. Fisher found no relationship between a woman's orgasmic responsiveness and the man's sexual technique, her source of sex education, her parents' attitudes toward sex, her religious beliefs, femininity, general mental health, traumatic sexual experiences or lack of them, sensitivity to stimulation, or premarital and marital experiences. Fisher's research did confirm other research that had shown that women who experience orgasm through vaginal penetration are no more emotionally mature than those who experience it through direct clitoral stimulation. In fact, a majority of his subjects (65%) expressed preference for clitoral stimulation. An additional finding was that highly orgasmic women are more likely than others to have been reared by dependable, caring, and demanding fathers who insisted upon meeting certain moral standards and expectations.

Two studies have added considerably to our knowledge of female sexuality and have documented the wide variability of sexual experiences and parameters of normalcy. Hite (1976) found that of the 82% of all females (3000) in her study who masturbated, 95% experienced orgasm. Further, the majority of these women reported that their physical sensations were more intense than those experienced with orgasm during intercourse; however, most women reported that overall pleasure and satisfaction were greater with intercourse than with masturbation. Hite also found that approximately 30% had orgasm with intercourse.

In marked contrast, a *Redbook* study found that 93% of married women were orgasmic during intercourse (15% all of the time, 48% most of the time, 19% sometimes, 11% once in a while) and 70% of women were coitally orgasmic premaritally. The *Redbook* research dealt very little with masturbation and did not measure orgasmic experience during masturbation.

Kaplan states that in our society 8% to 10% of the female population have never experienced an orgasm of any kind, while 90% of all women appear to achieve orgasm by some means or other. There are some clinicians who believe that a woman is sexually dysfunctional if she cannot achieve orgasm through intercourse, while others do not attach any particular importance to how orgasm is reached. A woman who is otherwise orgasmic but does not reach orgasm during coitus is neither frigid nor sick. In fact, this appears to be a normal variant of female sexuality.

Sexual life-styles

The adult woman faces basic role choices regarding her needs for intimacy, nurturance, and competency. During her adult years, the woman chooses the mode of sexual behavior that best suits her, decides whether to remain single or to marry, chooses between children or a childfree life-style, and makes decisions about her career. A woman today has more freedom than ever to choose her mode of sexual behavior. Increased permissiveness and improved contraceptive techniques mean that more options are possible. Autostimulation, heterosexual activities, and lesbianism are all available as alternatives for sexual fulfillment. More and more women are choosing premarital and extramarital sexual intercourse; more and more women are attempting to understand their sexual needs and meet those needs rather than accepting a stereotypic definition of them; and more and more women are defining their own personal creed of sexual behavior and morality rather than accepting society's stereotypic standards.

According to Kinsey (1953), while overt sexual activity in females is less at all ages than for males, the form of activity and frequency vary for different ages. Women peak in sexual activity in their thirties and remain at high levels until their late forties (Sheehy, 1976a). It is possible that the combined factors of increased experience, lessened fear of pregnancy, gradual loss of sexual inhibition, and potential for increased levels of vasocongestion from pregnancy result in the increased sexual capacity and activity in women in this age group. Although female activity is greatest at this point it is less, on the average, than the activity of men, perhaps because sexual activity is traditionally initiated on the basis of male rather than female desire.

More women than ever before are having premarital sex. In 1953 Kinsey found that 18% to 19% of his sample experienced premarital sex, while Zelnick and Kantner found in 1972 that almost 50% of their sample were no longer virgins by age 19. More recent studies indicate that premarital intercourse is becoming more common for all groups of women (Hunt, 1974). Tavris and Offir (1977) believe women experience premarital sex not for the sexual adventure itself but rather to maintain a relationship or prove love. Bardwick (1970) suggests that often young women comply because they fear they will lose their partner if they say no. Many of these women express insecurity, guilt, and fear associated with their sexual activities.

Kinsey found that women were less likely than men to experience extramarital sex. The incidence of extramarital sex in Kinsey's studies was approximately one in four or five. Hunt found in 1974 that the number of women under 25 years who had had extramarital sex had tripled since the 1950s. Although the number of women experiencing extramarital sexual activity may be increasing, differences between men and women still remain in terms of numbers of partners and motives. Twice as many men as women report sex with more than one extramarital partner. While men may explore the casual encounter for the sake of sex, women tend to correlate having extramarital sex with marital dissatisfaction (Tavris and Offir, 1977).

Sexual fantasy is now recognized as appropriate and normal for women; 60% of the women in Kinsey's studies reported having erotic fantasies about the opposite sex. He found, however, that women were less apt to be aroused by pornography and erotic material than were men. Recent studies, however, have found that men and women react similarly to erotic material and the majority of both sexes report physiologic signs of sexual arousal (Tavris and Offir, 1977).

Although both attitudes and behavior are becoming more open, and women are becoming more like men in their sexual activities, many people still cherish traditional attitudes and belief systems. Women's sexual behavior continues to be more strictly proscribed than that of men. The double standard—the belief that different sexual rules apply to men and women—still flourishes. These belief systems are manifest in the sexual behavior of men and women. Sexual dysfunctions often reflect sexual stereotypes and sexual proscriptions placed on women (see Chapter 9).

A woman in our society is expected to sexually arouse a man by her appearance. Men expect women to be attractive, and more emphasis is placed on a woman's physical appearance than a man's. If a woman's status is derived from the man she marries and she must be beautiful to attract a man, she is naturally going to be concerned about how she looks. Concerns over appearance and the need to attract a man through physical attributes are socialized into all young girls. Men use physical attractiveness as a criterion for dating; men are also judged by the attractiveness of "their" women. Because male status may be involved in a woman's attractiveness, its importance may be further emphasized (Frieze et al., 1978).

A sexual life-style is considered to be the pattern and expression of one's individual sexuality. Each sexual life-style has its own recognizable characteristics. The major choices for women are to be single or with someone, to be married or not married, to be monogamous or not, and to be heterosexual or homosexual.

Marriage

The expected, approved progression of relationships in the United States begins with dating, which evolves into serious courtship and then into monogamous marriage. In our culture if a woman does not marry she is considered defective. If she chooses a life-style other than marriage, she is thought to be bad because she experiences sex outside of marriage, or she is asexual and therefore an object to be pitied, or she is homosexual and therefore sexually deviant.

Monogamous marriage is the expected relationship for women. It is a status giving, prized institution. Marriage conveys an image of stability, maturity, and achievement. All adult female sexual conduct is expected to take place within marital bonds. The major advantages for women in monogamous marriage are: (1) sexual intimacy enhanced by emotional attachment and commitment to one partner, (2) the ability to be sexually active without negative stigma, (3) the establishment of trust, and (4) the assurance of a sexual and economic partner in old age. Monogamous marriage is disadvantageous in that it (1) routinizes sex, (2) restricts sexual options, and (3) brings the fear of infidelity.

Extramarital sexual relations are not an approved, accepted sexual life-style for a woman. Co-marital or extramarital sexual relations by both partners on a consensual basis is the life-style chosen by some. Reasons for opting for this life-style may be (1) escape from boredom, (2) increased experiences and thereby more pleasure, and (3) the wish to be "open" and honest about behavior already desired or practiced. Nonmonogamous sexual options may be difficult for many women to exercise. These require a high degree of self-confidence and security in the marital relationship. Sex and variety must be enjoyed, not just tolerated.

Single women

Some women may live alone for various periods in their lives or for a whole lifetime, by choice or necessity. Singleness has not been considered desirable in our society and has usually been viewed as a temporary period before the woman marries. However, a woman may choose to be single for economic reasons (the welfare mother or senior citizen on Social Security), because of divorce or death of a spouse, or because of emotional and sexual attractions to her own sex. Regardless of the reasons single women fall into two broad categories: those who view being single as a period in their lives and who do not want to remain single, and those who prefer to be single and independent.

The single woman has three sexual options: casual encounters, sex within a relationship, and abstinence. Two life-styles are also available—living alone and cohabitation. Two of society's most inviolate proscriptions for females—purity and value on female sexuality—are violated by casual sexual activity. A woman who has sex outside a relationship is considered loose and promiscuous. It is more difficult for the older female to find partners when casual sex is the objective. Casual sex conflicts with the socialization of women in regard to the proper context of sexuality. Most women link sex and love and it is difficult for them to think otherwise.

At times a single woman will choose to have sexual experiences within the context of a relationship without legal sanctions. The relationship may be with or without cohabitation. At present there is no research to indicate how satisfying or unsatisfying such relationships are.

Abstinence or voluntary rejection of an active sexual life is a possible life-style for a woman. It is often assumed that a woman who is not sexually active is either undesirable or "repressed." There are various situations and reasons why women who have previously been sexually active choose to abstain from sexual activity. At times a woman may refrain from sex because of health or hygienic reasons. Moral and religious conviction may cause a woman to refrain from sex until marriage or throughout her life. At times a woman may find herself in a stiuation that absorbs all of her energy and she does not perceive the lack of sexual activity as undesirable. Because we are conditioned to view sex as a need, abstinence is not considered a sexual option. The woman who chooses voluntarily to abstain from sex after her early twenties may receive negative responses from society. Abstinence as a temporary adjustment to a life situation appears to be relatively common and is not an automatic indication of repression or being undersexed or undesirable.

Homosexuality

Lesbianism—or homosexual activity and preference—is a difficult life-style for a woman. A lesbian is first of all a woman and therefore she experiences all of the socialization pressures common to women. She has many of the beliefs of women in general about sexuality. Often she experiences confusion, distress, and guilt when she first realizes her sexual preference. Lesbians are more similar to than different from heterosexual women. It is not well understood why certain women become lesbians. One of the primary determinants seems to be initial sexual experience. A very good initial sexual experience with a woman or a very traumatic one with a male may result in a woman becoming lesbian (Frieze et al., 1978). It is common for the first sexual contact to be with a friend with whom there has been a close nonsexual relationship. The benefits of lesbian relationships are: (1) they are more egalitarian, (2) they are less role-bound, (3) same-sex couples are more knowledgeable about each other's needs, and (4) women are more loyal and oriented to long-term relationships than men. Disadvantages of same-sex relationships are: (1) social stigma and the need to live a secret life, (2) fear of the partner's return to an easier straight life, (3) role stress because of lack of societally assigned roles, and (4) children—either the desire for them or the fear of losing them.

Socialization of women

Female sexuality involves far more than merely conceiving and bearing children. It is varied and rich with the potential for much enjoyment. The average woman also faces specific problems in her sex life. She must still face the prevailing view that sex is primarily for men. Women were raised to be sexually dependent on men, though sexual autonomy is a desired goal for women. Guilt is another problem for women, since they are socialized to believe sex is wrong. Lack of information hampers women in their sexual lives since they are socialized to believe that their concerns are unique and never experienced by other women. All of these factors decrease a woman's ability to be comfortable with her sexuality and herself as a sexual being.

Nurses can assist women to reach their full sexual potential by understanding the components of female sexuality and the wide variations of normality in expression and life-style. The nurse can identify potential problems and, through education and anticipatory guidance, eliminate or ameliorate them.

STEREOTYPES AND THE ROLES OF WOMEN
Effects of the stereotype

The effects of sex-role stereotypes on women vary; more often than not they are negative. It has been suggested that sex role stereotypes serve the function of controlling women—and specifically their sexuality. Stereotypes serve to reinforce and perpetuate the second-class status of women in our society. They are also used to justify an "inherent" female inferiority, as defined by men. Because sex-role stereotypes continue to be prevalent in Western culture, it is important to define them and examine their effects on women.

In every culture, normal female behavior has been defined by males, resulting in a concentration of power in men and the assignment of minor roles to women. The position of women has consistently been lower than that of men. Stereotypes of a woman designate her primary motivation to be a companion to a man and a mother. A woman has often been defined in terms of a man, rather than as an independent person. A woman is expected to be able to attract men; if she is successful, then she acquires a home and can fulfill her major goal in life—the nurturing role of wife and mother.

These stereotypes and the socialization process that results in this view of women appear to have differential effects on the personality development of male and females. For women the socialization process has fostered the nurturant, submissive, conservative aspects of the female role and has not facilitated the development of those attributes commonly defined as masculine—assertiveness, achievement-orientation, independence. In fact, these qualities have been explicitly discouraged in the socialization of females. Thus sex-role definitions of women are narrowed by the socialization process, which tends to inhibit their individuality, discourage their achievement, and restrict their autonomy.

Gump (1972) found that the view of femininity most acceptable to her research subjects recognized the importance and feasibility of assuming the roles of wife and mother while at the same time pursuing careers that would provide self-realization and achievement. However, the careers pursued were those traditionally associated with women, and most subjects wished for a husband and family. While these women were not traditional in viewing the roles of wife and mother as sufficient for fulfillment, they did not choose radical alternatives to the traditional stereotypic patterns. Gump also found that ego strength, a culturally estimated quality, was inversely related to the adoption of the female sex role (i.e., more purposeful, resourceful women were less traditional in their sex-role orientations).

The "fear of success" in women, as described by Horner (1971), is attributed to the fact that women anticipate negative reactions and challenges to their femininity as a result of high levels of achievement. When otherwise achievement-motivated young white women are faced with a conflict between their feminine image and their competence, they will adjust their behavior to be congruent with their internalized sex-role stereotypes. In order to feel or appear more feminine, women disguise their abilities or withdraw from nontraditional aspirations and achievements in our society (Horner, 1971). It is not known to what extent poor self-concept may be limiting; however, it seems reasonable to assume that internalized negative evaluations of female capabilities will promote withdrawal from competency.

Roles

One of the most important determinants of one's status in our society is the work that one does. Historically, women have worked either for free or in low-status, low-paying jobs. Today women usually are found in less powerful positions than men; they do not advance as quickly as men, and their jobs usually have a lower status. Most of the positions women hold do not satisfy their needs for achievement, recognition, or self-actualization.

Now, as in the past, the major roles for women are wife, homemaker, mother, and worker. Before the late nineteenth century, women, whether married or single, confined their activities to the home. Their work consisted of maintenance of the household, child care, food production and preparation, and the manufacturing of many of the necessary material goods. Only a few women worked outside the home as domestic servants or teachers. Early in the twentieth century, women began to work in clerical and sales positions, as factory workers and nurses, and teachers. During World War II, women made up the majority of the labor force and it was acceptable for a single woman to work. Upon marriage, however, she was to return to the home and devote the rest of her life to her family.

After World War II, shifts occurred in the relative emphasis placed on women's roles. Women married younger, were more likely to marry, and had more children sooner. Though a woman's life was still primarily focused on her children and home, for economic reasons, employment outside the home was common for both single and married women. By the end of the 1950s more women of all ages were entering the work force. Children were leaving home earlier. The woman's roles of mother and homemarker decreased. Changes in women's roles occurred even more rapidly in the 1970s.

Traditionally, the role of wife has been defined as taking precedence over all others. The role is assumed when a woman legally aligns herself with a male, and it implies the assumption of the related roles of mother and homemaker. Women are expected to perform household tasks out of duty and love, but generally, the status of homemaker is low. It is not always freely selected, it isolates the woman from other adults, and it heightens the woman's sense of powerlessness. The role of the homemaker does have some flexibility and autonomy, and in that sense it may compare favorably to other work available to a woman outside the home.

The role of mother is usually assumed through a biologic event; however, it is the *social* definition of motherhood that is crucial. A woman is expected to meet all the emotional and physical needs of her children.

Breaking out of the stereotype

Society's view of the roles appropriate to women have undergone rapid change recently. Factors altering the traditional belief that the only acceptable role for a woman is that of wife and mother include the following:

1. Women are marrying at a later age
2. Increasing numbers of marriages are ending in divorce
3. Contraceptive methods are greatly improved
4. Economic pressures have resulted in more women working
5. Birth rates have lowered
6. Societal views of working mothers are less negative than previously

Although society no longer holds that the only roles for women are those of wife, mother, and homemaker, these continue to be highly valued by both sexes. The result, in many cases, is that women try to fulfill more than one role by adding new ones onto their already existing roles. This can, of course, cause stress, and from two sources: First, the women who has assumed roles that violate the stereotypic view of women may well experience role conflict when she tries to fulfill too many sets of expectations. Second, role "overload" or discontinuity can occur simply from having too many commitments for too little time.

Role modification

Because it is impossible for any woman to comply with the expectations of the work role, motherhood role, wife role, and homemaker role all at the same time— and with equal success—modifications must be made in one or all of these roles.

Marriage. Although most women continue to choose marriage since it provides a stable context for the future, diverse marital patterns are emerging. For example, between 40% and 50% of married women with children now work outside the home, and this percentage is increasing. Modifications are also being made concerning who in the marriage has the most authority and decision-making power. Traditionally, the husband has enjoyed this power, but when marriages become more equal and less structured according to sex-role stereotypes, the balance of power becomes more equal.

Because divorce is more acceptable and available today, a marriage will likely continue only if the rewards are seen as equal to the effort put into it. As women discover they have desirable alternatives to remaining in an unhappy relationship, the likelihood of their remaining in an unsatisfactory marriage decreases. Each partner's ability to dominate the relationship may be tempered by the reality of the other's ability to leave the relationship (Frieze and Sales, 1978).

Motherhood. The role of motherhood is no longer simply assumed to be an automatic result of marriage. Because of effective methods of contraception and the availability of abortion, women can choose whether or not to have children.

Because the role of mother cannot be shed once it is assumed, the decision to have a child is being considered more seriously by more couples than has happened in the past. For many women the roles of career women and mother are not especially compatible, and a decision is made one way or the other.

Work role. When a woman works outside the home, role conflicts may quickly develop. Whether she works because of economic necessity, to expand her horizons, or to supplement the family income, conflicts may develop between family obligations and chances for advancement. When a married woman works, she faces decisions about who assumes responsibility for child care, who performs household maintenance, and whose career will dicate where the couple live. The emotional support of her husband is crucial for the working wife and mother. Even though men are generally more traditional in their view of sex roles, they are becoming increasingly supportive of women's efforts to change their roles.

Women often face discrimination from employment and expectations that they will behave in traditional female stereotypes. Their work may not be as objectively evaluated as a man's, and they may not receive promotion as rapidly as a man. Because of the very strong conflicts between career and marriage, most women currently tend to put family concerns first (Frieze et al., 1978). As a result, women are generally neither as productive nor as successful as men, thus reinforcing common stereotypes about women and work.

Women are currently experiencing rapid role change. It is an exciting time with the potential for both great personal growth and intense stress. The profession of nursing reflects many of the role conflicts and stressors confronting women. Nurses need to increase their awareness of the potentials and strains inherent in the multiplicity of women's roles. With this awareness nurses can be more supportive of themselves and their clients and enhance their own and their clients' positive growth.

REFERENCES

Bardwick, J. N.: Psychology of women: a study of bio-cultural conflicts, New York, 1971, Harper & Row, Publishers.

Block, J., Von De Lippe, A., and Block, J. H.: Sex role and socialization patterns: some personality concomitant and environmental antecedents, J. Consult. Clin. Psych. 41(3):321-341, 1973.

Brooks, J., Ruble, D., and Clark, A.: College women's attitudes and expectations concerning menstrual-related changes, Psychosom. Med. 39(5):288-298, 1977.

Brooks-Gunn, J., and Ruble, D.: Menarche: the interaction of physiological, cultural and social factors, presented at the Menstrual Cycle Conference, Chicago, Illinois, June 1977.

Ernster, V. L.: American menstrual expressions, Sex Roles, 1:3-13, 1975.

Fisher, S.: The female orgasm: psychology, physiology, fantasy, New York, 1978, W. W. Norton Co.

Frieze, I.: Sex roles of women. In Frieze, I., and others, editors: Women and sex roles, New York, 1978, W. W. Norton Co.

Frieze, I., and others, editors: Women and sex roles, New York, 1978, W. W. Norton Co.

Gagnon, J. H., and Greenblot, C.: Life designs: individuals, marriages and families, Glenview, Ill., 1978, Scott, Foresman & Co.

Gump, J. P.: Sex role attitudes and psychological well-being, J. Soc. Issues, 28(2):79-92, 1972.

Hite, S.: The Hite report, New York, 1976, The Macmillan Co.

Hunt, M. S.: Sexual behavior in the 1970's, Chicago, 1974, Playboy Press.

Kaplan, H. S.: The new sex therapy, New York, 1974, Brunner/Mazel Inc.

Kinsey, A. C., and others: Sexual behavior in the human female, Philadelphia, 1953, W. B. Saunders Co.

Koeske, R. K., and Koeske, G. F.: An attributional approach to moods and the menstrual cycle, J. Person. Soc. Psych. 31(3):473-78, 1975.

Laws, J. L.: Sexual Scripts: The social construction of female sexuality, Hinsdale, Ill., 1977, The Dryden Press.

Maccoby, E. E., and Jacklin, C. N.: The psychology of sex differences, Stanford, 1974, Stanford University Press.

Martin, L.: Health care of women, New York, 1970, J. B. Lippincott Co.

Messent, R. R.: Female hormones and behaviors. In Lloyd, B., and Archer, L.: Exploring sex differences, London, 1976, Academic Press, Inc.

Money, J., and Ehrhardt, A. A.: Man and woman, boy and girl, Baltimore, 1972, Johns Hopkins Press.

Paige, K. E.: Women learn to sing the menstrual blues, Psychol. Today, pp. 41-46, Sept. 1973.

Parson, J., and Ruble, D.: Is anatomy destiny? Biology and sex differences. In Frieze, I., and others, editors: Women and sex roles, New York, 1978, W. W. Norton Co.

Rosenberg, F., and Simmons, R.: Sex differences in the self-concept of adolescence, Sex Roles, 1(2):147-159, 1975.

Ruble, D.: Sex differences in personality and abilities. In Frieze, I., and others, editors: Women and sex roles, New York, 1978, W. W. Norton Co.

Ruble, D., and Frieze, I.: Biosocial aspects of reproduction. In Frieze, I., and others, editors: Women and sex roles, New York, 1978, W. W. Norton Co.

Sheehy, G.: Passages, New York, 1976b, E. P. Dutton & Co., Inc.

Tavris, C., and Offir, C.: Longest war, New York, 1977, Harcourt, Brace, Jovanovich, Inc.

Tavris, C., and Sadd, S.: The Redbook report on female sexuality, New York, 1971, Delacourte Press.

Whisnant, L., Brett, E., and Zegans, L.: Explicit messages concerning menstruation in commercial educational materials prepared for young adolescent girls, Am. J. Psych. 132(8):815-820, 1975.

Whisnant, L., and Zegans, L.: White middle-class adolescent girls' attitudes toward menarche, Nurs. Digest, pp. 52-54, Winter 1976.

Woods, N. F.: Human sexuality in health and illness, ed. 2, St. Louis, 1979, The C. V. Mosby Co.

Zelnick, M., and Kantner, J.: Some preliminary observations on pre-adult fertility and family formation, Stud. Fam. Plann. 3(4):59-65, 1972.

ADDITIONAL REFERENCES

Abernathy, V.: Cultural perspectives on the impact of women's changing roles in psychiatry, Am. J. Psych. 133(6):657-661, 1976.

Bernard, J. S.: The future of marriage, New York, 1972, World.

Broverman, I. K., Broverman, D., and Clarkson, F.: Sex role stereotypes and clinical judgments of mental health, J. Consult. Clin. Psych. 34(1):1-7, 1970.

Broverman, I. K., and others: Sex role stereotypes: a current appraisal, J. Soc. Issues, 28(2):59-78, 1972.

Heilbrunn, L., and Heit, P.: Menstruation and social health, Health Values 2(4):211-214, 1978.

Heurter, R.: Female sexuality. In Jervick, D. K., and Martinson, I. M.: Women in stress: a nursing perspective, New York, 1979, Appleton-Century-Crofts.

Hoffman, L. W., and Nye, F. L.: Working mothers: an evaluative review of the consequences for wife, husband and child, San Francisco, 1974, Jossey-Bass.

Hutchinson, J. B.: Biological determinants of sexual behavior, New York, 1978, John Wiley & Sons.

Kerr, C.: Sex for women, New York, 1977, Grove Press Inc.

Kleeman, J. A.: The establishment of core gender identity in normal girls, Arch. Sexual Behav. 1:101-116, 1971.

Loerisky, J.: Menstruation: alternatives to pharmacological therapy for menstrual distress, J. of Nurse-Midwif. 23:34-44, Fall 1978.

Maccoby, E.: Sex differences in intellectual functioning. In Bardwick, J. M.: Readings on the psychology of women, New York, 1972, Harper & Row Publishers.

Moscato, B.: Sex role stereotyping, Perspect. Roles, pp. 180-193.

Pleck, J. H.: Masculinity-femininity; current and alternative paradigms, Sex Roles, 1(2):161-178, 1975.

Parlee, M. B.: Stereotypic beliefs about menstruation: a methodological note in the Moos menstrual distress questionnaire and some new data, Psychosoc. Med. 36(3):229-240, 1974.

Rising, S. S.: Childbearing: its dilemmas. In Jernik, D. K., and Martinson, I. N.: Women in stress: a nursing perspective, New York, 1979, Appleton-Century-Crofts.

Roland, A., and Harris, B.: Career and motherhood, New York, 1979, Human Sciences Press.

Schriber, J. M.: Menstruation: culture and reproductive behavior," paper presented at Second Annual Interdisciplinary Research Conference on the Menstrual Cycle, St. Louis, 1978.

Schwartz, P.: Sexual life-styles. In Laws, J.: Sexual scripts: the social construction of female sexuality, Chicago, 1972, The Dryden Press.

Seaman, B.: Free and female, Greenwich, Conn., 1972, Fawcett Publication.

Spengler, C.: Conditioning of the female to her role in life. In Gressum, M., and Spengler, C., editors: Women and health care, Boston, 1976, Little, Brown and Co.

7

Assessment of health status

Catherine Ingram Fogel

Growing numbers of women are becoming dissatisfied with the health care currently available to them. From their perspective, the health care system is unresponsive, repressive, and often punitive. Nursing is frequently looked to to provide the type of health care women want and are beginning to demand. As defined by Kinlein (1977), nursing is "assisting the person in self-care practices in regard to [her or his] state of health." (p. 23) This definition is consistent with women's demands for health care that is based on their own assessment of what they need and that facilitates their involvement in their own health care.

If nurses are to meet these demands they must develop additional skills (and use those they already have more effectively) to provide primary health care to these women clients. Kinlein (1977) considers that a nurse may know as much as or more than a physician but the knowledge is used differently to achieve the goals of nursing care; this points to a need for nurses to become skilled in the assessment of health status. Nursing should facilitate the individual's self-care to maintain or improve her health state. Assessment skills and knowledge that the nurse possesses can enhance the collaboration between client and nurse to identify the client's self-care assets and limitations, and to determine what therapeutic measures are necessary to correct deficiencies.

This chapter provides the information needed to develop a data base for thorough assessment of a woman's individual health status. Implicit throughout is the assumption that a woman's primary worth is not just reproductive or sexual; rather, these are only two aspects of a multifaceted person. Therefore, a woman's health care is not focused solely on her reproductive capabilities, nor is her health defined solely in terms of her childbearing functions.

As stated elsewhere in this text women often enter the health system through their reproductive organs. This is the medical system's reflection of the wider social ideology, which views women as sex objects and reproductive organs. However, women are no longer dying from obstetric and gynecologic conditions, but rather from old age, chronic disease, and cancer. Women need health care that treats them as whole persons whose health care needs may be but are not necessarily obstetrically and gynecologically oriented.

Assessment must focus on the total being and include screening for those diseases for which women are specifically at risk. Emphasis should be placed on those life cycle events that are uniquely woman's and that alter physiologic functioning greatly: menarche, menstruation, pregnancy, abortion, childbirth, lactation, and menopause. Health care assessment must take into account the particular roles, societal influences, and cultural networks in which each woman exists.

The assessment process is a collaborative one between the client and nurse. The woman provides as much baseline data and historical information as she can; she is encouraged to contribute any information she believes relevant. The nurse contributes the information she has gathered through the use of all her assessment skills. The two sets of data are then jointly analyzed. The nurse has a responsibility to share the nursing diagnosis she has formulated with the client and to facilitate data analysis in any way possible. The cornerstone of the health assessment process is the development of a complete and accurate data base. The three components of the data base are client history, physical examination, and baseline laboratory data.

In order to assist the reader in developing a data base from which to formulate nursing diagnosis, various types of general and specific health histories, specific examination procedures, and various diagnostic tests are discussed in detail in this chapter. The assessment of general physical health is not presented here because the subject is discussed thoroughly in other basic textbooks.

HEALTH PROBLEMS DURING THE LIFE CYCLE
Adolescence

The most common health care problems for which adolescent girls seek treatment are dysmenorrhea, irregularities of the menstrual cycle, venereal disease, vaginitis, contraceptive problems, and pregnancy (Martin, 1978). The pelvic examination is essential to the diagnosis and treatment of all these problems. A woman's first pelvic examination, which often is done in adolescence, can have far-reaching significance. How a woman is treated during this examination—the messages she receives about herself and the impact on her body image, sexual identity, and sexuality—can influence her views about herself and her sexuality for many years. Establishment of a sexual identity is an essential developmental task during adolescence and can be enhanced or retarded by the attitudes and actions of the health care practitioner who performs the pelvic examination. It is essential that the procedure, which imposes physical vulnerability on a woman, be a self-appreciative experience rather than a destructive one.

Vaginitis is the most common gynecologic complaint in adolescent girls (Romney, 1976). At times the young girl is concerned about vaginal secretions that appear abnormal to her but are in reality a normal variation. For the adolescent, lack of knowledge and understanding of changes in her body and resulting differences in function can be frightening. It is crucial that the practitioner allay fears by providing support and appropriate information about pubertal changes. Much adolescent vaginitis becomes chronic because of the presence of unusual organisms and therapy-resistant bacteria; it is often associated with vulvitis, urethritis, and/or cervicitis. (Specifics of vaginitis are discussed in Chapter 13.)

Dysmenorrhea and menstrual irregularities are common problems in adolescence. There can be difficulties associated with the establishment of regular cyclic interaction between the ovary and pituitary. These irregularities can cause considerable anxiety since regular functioning is often equated with normal femininity. The girl may also worry about future fertility.

Zelnik and Kantner (1978) found that 40% of all adolescent girls were sexually active by age 19. (They also documented an increase in their use of contraception; why this has not resulted in a decline in pregnancy is not indicated.) Adolescent pregnancy has reached epidemic proportions in the United States today, and the practitioner who works with adolescent girls must be prepared to deal with these problems. Venereal disease is also a major health problem that is especially prominent among adolescents.

When one considers the number of health care problems associated with sexual or reproductive functioning, need for sex education and counseling becomes obvious. The adolescent girl needs help to anticipate body changes, understand sexual feelings, and demystify reproductive and sexual functioning. An understanding of menstruation can help to demystify it and possibly prevent negative attitudes. Sex education can prevent a great amount of sexually related morbidity. An understanding of conception, knowledge of one's value system, and ability to accept one's sexuality and sexual activity may help prevent unplanned pregnancy and venereal disease. Knowledge of contraceptives coupled with acceptance of one's own sexuality allows choice and control over one's body and life, thus helping to prevent unwanted pregnancy. The adolescent girl who is able to use effective decision-making and choice in determining her readiness for sexual activity has a greater opportunity to experience satisfaction in her sexual encounters and potentially less orgasmic dysfunction.

Adolescents are at risk for substance abuse—drug, tobacco, and alcohol. The health care practitioner needs to be aware of the signs and symptoms of substance abuse in order to accurately diagnose it. The adolescent needs to be made aware of the mortality and morbidity statistics from cirrhosis, lung disease, and arteriosclerotic heart disease, and understand how these can affect her future quality of life and functional capacity.

Nutritional problems affect adolescents in many ways. Obesity is often a problem. Nearly three million adolescents (more females than males) are obese in the United States, while many more are considered overweight (Murray and Zentner, 1975a). Adolescent females make up one of the most poorly fed groups in the United States. Anemia is common since their diets are often low in iron and calcium. Concern over appearance can lead to crash or fad dieting, which results in nutritionally poor intake. Further, teenagers are notorious consumers of junk foods. Adolescent pregnancy is another health problem related to nutritional needs; the relationship between poor nutrition and low birth weight infants is clearly documented.

Health assessment for adolescent girls should include an understanding of the leading causes of death among teenagers. Accidents, including motor vehicle accidents and poisoning, cause numerous deaths for both blacks and whites. Complications of pregnancy and abortions are also significant for both races, as are homicide and suicide. Pneumonia causes a significant number of deaths in both races while chronic rheumatic heart disease affects black teenagers (Martin, 1978; Robbins and Hall, 1970). Teenagers at risk can be identified and counseled in ways to reduce their risks; screening for all of these conditions should take place at every health care visit.

Reproductive years

The major health care problems of women during their reproductive years center around sexual and relationship difficulties, infective process of the reproductive and urinary tract systems, pregnancy and contraceptive difficulties, problems of menstruation, neoplasms of the reproductive organs and breasts, nutritional disorders, diabetes, and hypertension.

As women feel free to express concerns regarding their own sexuality and sexual dysfunction and to question the relationships they are involved in, these issues will more often become part of a thorough health assessment. More women are seeking help for a variety of sexual concerns and dysfunctional problems, as well as assistance in establishing, maintaining, and terminating relationships.

Finding a safe, reliable, acceptable contraceptive is a major concern for many women in the reproductive years. Contraceptive-related morbidity results largely from complications involving use of oral contraceptives or IUDs. Reassessment of contraceptive methods and updating of the client's information about her contraceptive choice are mandatory parts of health maintenance for women of reproductive age.

Problems relative to pregnancy are a major aspect of assessment of health status for this age group. Assessment of the pregnant woman, including determination of individuals at risk for complications, is essential, along with identification of each woman's specific needs for prenatal care. Determination of the need for problem pregnancy counseling should be included (see Chapter 12).

Menstrual problems make up a sizable portion of a woman's health care concerns during her reproductive years. Dysmenorrhea, variations in bleeding, and premenstrual tension syndrome are some of the difficulties encountered. Differentiation of normal from abnormal is necessary. Vaginal infections, urinary tract infections, pelvic inflammatory disease, and other infections of the reproductive system are also common among this age group (see Chapter 13).

Women today have a one-in-four risk of developing cancer and a one-in-ten risk that it will involve reproductive organs or the breast (Romney, 1976). History-taking should include data-gathering to identify the risk factors for cervical and breast cancer. Once the women at risk are identified, they can be made aware of potential danger signs. Pap smears and breast self-examination should be a part of every woman's assessment of health status. Lung cancer becomes a leading cause of death by age 35; it is becoming increasingly prevalent as more women smoke.

Nutritional disorders continue to plague women; obesity and anemia are the most common. Nutritional status becomes a crucial issue as women progress through their reproductive years. Good nutrition is essential for positive pregnancy outcomes; oral contraceptives also affect nutritional needs. Obesity is one of the factors that place women at risk for many of the diseases they are dying from in this age group. Arteriosclerotic heart disease is a leading cause of death by age 40. Development of adult-onset diabetes is greatly influenced by American habits of eating infrequent heavy meals and consuming large amounts of concentrated refined sugars. Alcoholism and cirrhosis become major problems between the ages of thirty and sixty; cirrhosis is one of the top ten causes of death in this age group.

Mental health issues are a major concern of women and frequently surface during the reproductive years. Depression is the most common psychiatric problem for women in any age group while anxiety is also present in many women. As the gap between traditional roles and new roles for women widens, it is expected that both problems will increase and intensify.

Late adulthood

Women in the late adult years often seek care for menopausal concerns; these may be related to irregularities of menses, abnormal bleeding, physical or emotional symptoms related to menopause, or possibly contraception. Menstrual irregularities become common and can be potentially very dangerous. Prompt diagnosis of abnormal bleeding in menopausal and postmenopausal women is essential. Cancer of the reproductive organs and breast continues to be a leading cause of death in this age group. Pap smears and breast self-examination are essential assessment tools. Other problems, such as pelvic relaxation, may also occur in this age group.

Many of the problems that arose in the late reproductive years continue. Obesity, hypertension, diabetes, anemia, and depression are health concerns of the older women also. Women age 65 and older often experience atrophic vaginitis, pelvic relaxation, osteoporosis, and various chronic diseases.

Women's self-care abilities and functional capacity differ greatly. Women often experience health problems that are not life threatening in and of themselves but that significantly affect the quality of life. For example, visual and hearing loss, limitations of activity because of arthritis, mental deterioration, and respiratory difficulties are common in the older age group. Pneumonia becomes a significant cause of death in the advanced years. This is the result of decreased resistance caused by poor nutrition, debilitation, and chronic illness. Cardiovascular disease continues as a major killer of elderly women. Cancer is also a significant mortality factor—not only cancer of the breast, cervix, and uterus but also of the stomach, rectum, and intestines. Finally, accidents contribute significantly to deaths among the elderly (Martin, 1978).

PERIODIC SCREENING

The importance of prevention and early disease detection is unarguable; however, there are practical questions about which tests to give, how often, and with what results. Frame and Carlson (1975) explored in detail the question of whether or not periodic health screening improves health or decreases mortality and morbidity significantly. They suggest that screening for a given disease should meet specific criteria before it is done. Screening is justified only when:

1. The disease significantly affects the quality or quantity of life.
2. There are acceptable treatment modalities currently available.
3. There is a long enough asymptomatic period of the disease involved so that diagnosis and treatment will significantly reduce morbidity and/or mortality.
4. Treatment begun in the asymptomatic period demonstrates results superior to results obtained when treatment is initiated in response to symptoms.
5. Diagnostic tests to detect the disease are available at a reasonable cost.
6. The incidence of the disease is high enough to justify the cost of screening.

Various diseases that are significant in the health care of women either in terms of mortality or morbidity are considered within these parameters, and recommendations as to health assessment and maintenance are proposed. The screening recommendations outlined below apply to asymptomatic adults. Women with symptoms or characteristics that place them at risk should be screened from an entirely different perspective. In addition, there are other conditions or health problems for which screening recommendations or procedures are not currently available. Screening is not a guarantee to good health; rather it is one factor in assessment of health status that optimally leads to high level wellness and maintenance of a state of good health.

Smoking

Although not a disease, smoking is a significant risk factor for many diseases. While the overall percentage of the adult population who smoke has decreased since the release of the first Surgeon General's report in 1964, this trend has not been as consistent for women. According to the American Cancer Society the percentage of overall decline in women is less than in men (34% to 29% for women as opposed to 52% to 39% for males in the years 1964 to 1975) and is not consistent across all age groups. The group ages 21 to 24 years had reversed the downward trend by 1975. Smoking rates for teenage girls, ages 13 to 19, have doubled since 1964 but have remained stable for teenage boys (McIntosh et al., 1978). The most recent Surgeon General's report, released in January 1978, indicates that women are starting to smoke earlier and continuing to smoke longer than previously, thus significantly increasing mortality and mor-

bidity risks. Generally, the more cigarettes smoked per day, the higher the risk of mortality. Mortality also increases with duration of the habit and the amount of smoke inhaled. Smokers have 1.7 times the mortality from coronary heart disease than nonsmokers have. Cerebrovascular disease is 38% to 114% higher in women smokers than in women nonsmokers. Smokers with chronic bronchopulmonary disease experience more symptoms and higher mortality rates. The most impressive statistics are those showing the relationship between lung cancer and smoking. Mortality rates are significantly higher for smokers than for nonsmokers. Mortality is also affected by the duration of smoking and degree of inhalation (Frame and Carlson, 1975).

There is no difficulty in diagnosing smoking by history; however it is a sociocultural phenomenon that is difficult to reverse. Risk factors contributing to the development of the habit are lower socioeconomic class, urban locale, religious belief, and parental smoking habits. It has been well documented that stopping smoking will substantially reduce the risk of morbidity and mortality from coronary heart disease, chronic bronchopulmonary disease, and lung cancer. For screening purposes it is recommended that a smoking history be taken initially and repeated at ages 30 and 40 (Frame and Carlson, 1978).

Lung cancer

Recently there has been an upward trend in the incidence of lung cancer, especially in males. There is a strong relationship between age and incidence of lung cancer. In addition there is a strong relationship between smoking—daily duration of habit, daily consumption, amount of smoke inhaled—and the risk of developing lung cancer (Frame and Carlson, 1978). Other risk factors include asbestosis and other lung conditions. Lung cancer is a fast-growing neoplasm with a short asymptomatic period and a rapidly fatal course. Early radiologic signs are subtle and easily missed; one third of the lesions are incurable before they are evident radiologically. The latency period between onset of symptoms and incurability is probably less than six months. Even with X-ray screening every 6 months, the five year survival rate increases only from zero to 5% to 8% (Frame and Carlson, 1978). Screening is not recommended at this time because, given present techniques, attempts at early diagnosis do not significantly decrease mortality.

Hypertension

It is estimated that fifteen percent of the adult population have hypertension, defined as a blood pressure of 140/90 or greater. It is more common in women than men and is race related; blacks are affected more often than whites. It is also related to age; the percentage affected increases with age (McIntosh, 1978). Hypertension also tends to be a familial problem. Hypertension significantly increases the risk of serious morbidity and mortality from coronary heart disease, cerebrovascular disease, and renal failure. Because adequate treatment will reduce the risk of these complications, diagnosis is crucial. There is a long asymptomatic phase to the disease. This is significant in light of the fact that complications increase in direct relation to both the degree and duration of hypertension. Further, medication is a reasonably effective treatment. Diagnosis is reliable, quick, and easy using a mercury sphygmomanometer and correct sized cuff. A single hypertensive reading should always be confirmed by subsequent readings. All adult women should have their blood pressure checked every 2 years (Frame and Carlson, 1978).

Arteriosclerotic heart disease

While men are affected more often than women, arteriosclerotic heart disease is the leading cause of death in women after age 40 (Robbins and Hall, 1970), and changes in the life-styles of women are narrowing the gap between the sexes in incidence and prevalence. It is believed that atherosclerotic processes may begin early in life, particularly if risk factors are present. Manifestations of the disease are myocardial infarction, angina, incidental diagnosis in the asymptomatic period, or death. Once the disease manifests itself, the risk of dying from it within 5 years increases five times. Risk factors for the development of arteriosclerotic heart disease include hypertension, hyperlipidemia, smoking, diabetes, obesity, sedentary life-style, family history and psychosocial tension.

Treatment in the earlier stages consists of identifying and eliminating risk factors so as to prevent and possibly reverse atherosclerotic changes. The standard diagnostic methods of physical examination, chest x-ray, or EKG are not reliable and often detect only the advanced cases (Frame and Carlson, 1978). The EKG is not recommended for general screening because detection of abnormality does not result in any unusual treatment regime and because the test is not very sensitive and can give false reassurance (Frame and Carlson, 1978). Recommended screening procedures are identification of risk factors by blood pressure checks every 2 years, blood cholesterol level determinations every 4 years, a smoking history every ten years, and determination of obesity every 4 years.

Stroke

Cerebrovascular disease is most common in people over age fifty-five. Risk factors include hypertension, elevated serum lipids, and diabetes. Stroke is often a sudden catastrophic event; however, about one third of the victims have had a prior transient ischemic attack with subsequent recovery. There is really no good way of predicting a stroke in advance. The only treatment in the asymptomatic stage is reduction of risk factors. All adult women should be screened for hypertension every 2 years and for hypercholesterolemia every 4 years (Frame and Carlson, 1978).

Diabetes

Maturity-onset diabetes usually develops insidiously over a period of years during which considerable mortality and morbidity related to vascular, infectious, ocular, and neurologic complications may develop. The major risk factors are heredity and obesity. Eighty percent of newly diagnosed adult-onset diabetics are obese. Diagnosis is easily made with a glucose tolerance test or 2 hour postprandial blood sugar test. Fasting blood sugars or urine sugar tests will detect overt diabetes.

The metabolic complications of diabetes, acidosis, and hypoglycemic shock can be controlled by treatment. There is considerable doubt and controversy about whether treatment can arrest or significantly alter vascular, ocular, neural, or renal complications. There is little evidence to date that treatment in the asymptomatic stage reduces long-term morbidity more effectively than waiting to treat until symptoms appear. Therefore, screening is not recommended for adults with no symptoms of diabetes. Screening is indicated as a part of an obesity work-up and in clients with a positive familial history.

Obesity

Thirty percent of American women are obese, defined as weighing at least 20% more than their ideal weight. The incidence of obesity rises with age. The most important risk factor is familial history. Obesity is characterized by gradual onset and progression. Weighing more than 20% to 30% above the ideal weight increases the morbidity risk from all causes by 50%; from cardiovascular and renal diseases by 50%; from diabetes by 283%; from cirrhosis by 150%, and from gallbladder and biliary tract disease by 52% (Frame and Carlson, 1978). Diagnosis presents no problem. The woman is weighed and her weight compared to ideal weight tables. Treatment is weight loss; success depends on motivation, and overall success rates are poor. Weight loss results in significantly lowered morbidity and mortality rates. Screening for obesity should be done for all adult women every 4 years.

Anemia

Approximately 10% of nonpregnant women are anemic and 85% to 90% of these cases are the result of iron deficiency. Often iron deficiency anemia is asymptomatic; there is no evidence that this anemia is harmful or that it is better to institute treatment before symptoms appear. Symptoms do not demonstrate any correlation with hemoglobin levels until values below 7 to 8 Gm per 100 ml are reached. The frequency of serious underlying disease is less than 10%. No routine screening for asymptomatic nonpregnant women is recommended (Martin, 1978).

Venereal disease

Most cases of syphilis occur in young and middle-aged adults. Syphilis is curable in the primary and secondary stages; but seventy-five percent of undetected cases will progress to irreversible complications with significant morbidity and mortality in the tertiary stage. There are several excellent, reliable, cheap serologic tests available. It is recommended that all persons between the ages of 20 and 50 be screened every 6 years and high-risk groups more often (Martin, 1978).

Although it is very common, readily diagnosed by culture, and easily treated by antibiotics, gonorrhea is not recommended for routine screening in asymptomatic women. It is asymptomatic in 75% of women and with such a low morbidity that screening is not justified in Frame and Carlson's (1975) opinion. If it were possible to eliminate the disease by systematic screening and treatment, the situation would be different; however, many experts consider it to be epidemiologically an uncontrollable disease (Fiumara, 1972). Therefore, given present technology and social values, it is believed that no routine screening is indicated. This is a controversial point of view and many will disagree. However, one population that should always be screened, asymptomatic or not, is pregnant women, because of potential risk to the fetus.

Cervical cancer

The Pap smear is an inexpensive, reliable test for cervical cancer. Further, it is well established that with early diagnosis and treatment, cervical cancer is a curable disease. The question is not really whether to screen for cervical cancer, but rather how often? Given the continuum of dysplasia to cancer in situ to invasive carcinoma of the cervix—with an average progression time of 44 months (Frame and Carlson, 1975)—it appears that the traditional recommendation of having a Pap smear every year may be not necessary. A reasonable compromise appears to be that all women over age twenty should have annual Pap smears for 2 years and then have a smear every other year indefinitely. High-risk groups, such as women from low socioeconomic populations or those with frequent and multiple sexual partners, should be screened more often.

Endometrial cancer

Endometrial cancer is a disease of menopausal and postmenopausal women primarily. The presenting symptom in almost eighty percent of cases is abnormal bleeding. Presently there is no good screening test to detect endometrial cancer prior to the appearance of symptoms. The best approach to screening seems to be client education to recognize and report any postmenopausal menorrhagia. Risk factors include diabetes, hypertension, and estrogen stimulation (Frame and Carlson, 1975).

Breast cancer

Breast cancer is the leading cause of cancer deaths in women. It is rare before age twenty-five, but becomes increasingly more common with age. The rate of growth and progression is exceedingly variable. Ninety percent of breast cancers are detected by self-examination; however, an average time lag of ten months occurs before treatment is sought. Screening recommendations are these: (1) thorough instruction regarding breast self-examination should be given to every woman at age twenty or on the first visit, with repeat instruction at ten-year intervals; (2) every woman should be encouraged to do monthly self-examinations; (3) breast examination by a health care provider should be made every two years until age fifty and then yearly; (4) women over fifty with large, fatty breasts should have annual or biannual routine mammography done.

GENERAL HEALTH ASSESSMENT
History

The collection of pertinent information—each woman's personal history—is essential to comprehensive assessment of health status. This history involves the collaborative effort of client and practitioner and should be kept in a form that is understandable to both. A format for gathering a general data base follows.

Personal information

Client's name, address, phone number, and date of birth or age are essential for identification purposes. Information relating to level of education, occupation, job satisfaction, religious affiliation, and ethnic group will assist in determining the client's sociocultural frame of reference. Marital status should be determined for its relevance and effect on reproductive and sexual behavior. Present means of support can give clues as to the client's ability to provide health care for herself.

Family history

Information is needed on the number of siblings and the health status of siblings and parents. It is often helpful to determine family history for the following:

hypertension, stroke, diabetes, tuberculosis, chronic respiratory problems, heart disease, cancer, thrombophlebitis, varicose veins, breast lumps or tumors, thyroid disease, kidney problems, and congenital defects (type). Which family members are affected should be noted for each condition. The client should be asked if there are any other conditions that she is aware of in her family that the practitioner has not asked about.

Medical history

The practitioner should explore with the client any previous medical problems the client may have experienced. Conditions to be explored include epilepsy, kidney or bladder disorders, migraine headaches, visual disturbances other than refractory error, cardiovascular disease, cancer, rheumatic fever, liver diseases, lung disorders, and nervous disorders. The client's drug reactions, allergies, and past immunizations should be recorded. Any hospitalization with date, type of illness, result, and follow-up should be noted also.

Surgical history

The type and date of surgery, diagnosis, what was done or removed, any complication that developed, and biopsy results (if applicable) should be ascertained.

Menstrual history

The client should be queried about the details of her last menstrual period: whether or not it was normal and if not, what the deviations were. Age at menarche, duration of period, amount of flow (described in terms of number of pads or tampons used), and irregularities in the cycle should be ascertained. Any difficulties such as dysmenorrhea should be explored. Episodes of amenorrhea should also be noted.

Contraceptive history

This includes current method being used (if any), duration of use, and any method-related problems or complaints. Information on previous methods used, including adverse effects and reasons for discontinuation, is helpful. Before asking about a woman's current contraceptive practices, the practitioner should determine whether she is "at risk" for pregnancy—of reproductive age and heterosexually active. Then she should be asked if she is currently planning a pregnancy or trying to avoid a pregnancy. Once this information is obtained, the interviewer can logically ask about current contraceptive practices and past experiences.

Obstetric history

Each of the client's previous pregnancies should be explored. Type of delivery, duration of pregnancy, birth weight and condition of infants at birth, and complica-

tions of pregnancy, labor, delivery, or postpartum should be described in detail. Spontaneous abortions with information as to duration of pregnancy, therapeutic measures, etc., should be recorded as well as any previous stillbirths and pertinent details. If the client has experienced therapeutic abortions, duration of pregnancy, method of abortion, and physical and psychologic complications should be noted.

Present health status

Thorough exploration of prior physical status, as described above, is helpful in assessing present health status. Maeck et al. (1978) suggest that a systems approach to the collection of past medical history in relationship to current, past, and potential illness has value. They propose the following model:

Gynecologic
  Current: Menstrual irregularities, dysmenorrhea, discharge, pruritus, sexual activity and orientation, dyspareunia, pelvic pain, breasts: pain, discharge, lumps
  Past: Menses: onset, duration, interval, last menstrual period and last regular menses (if LMP was different), contraception, venereal disease, abnormal Pap smears; breasts: lactation, previous breast diseases, or abnormalities
  Potential: Familial history of cancer; early and varied sexual activity as a risk factor in cancer of the cervix

Urinary
  Current: Dysuria, urgency, incontinence, hematuria
  Past: Renal disease, recurrent urinary tract infections, hematuria
  Potential: Familial history of polycystic disease

Endocrine
  Current: Changes in weight, abnormal hair growth, change in sexual activity, change in menses
  Past: Thyroid disorder, diabetes mellitus, menstrual disorders
  Potential: Exposure to radioactive material; familial history of diabetes mellitus, hirsutism

Gastrointestinal
  Current: Abdominal pain, melena, nausea, vomiting, diarrhea, changes in bowel habits, hemorrhoids
  Past: Ulcer, gallbladder disease, jaundice, other liver disease, diverticulosis, colitis
  Potential: Familial history of cancer, rectal polyps

Cardiovascular
  Current: Chest pain, dyspnea, edema of feet and ankles, varicosities, leg ulcers
  Past: Rheumatic fever, other heart disease, hypertension, phlebitis, embolitic disease
  Potential: Family history of hypertension, heart attack; limited physical activity, cigarette smoking, stress, obesity, high blood cholesterol levels

Respiratory
  Current: Chronic cough, hemoptysis, dyspnea, hoarseness
  Past: Tuberculosis, heavy smoker, asthma
  Potential: Smoking, familial history of cystic fibrosis

Neurologic

Current: Headaches, dizzy spells, drugs for seizures

Past: Seizures, paralysis, nervousness

Potential: Family history of Huntington's chorea

Psychiatric

Current: Anxiety, depression, difficulty sleeping, weeping, suicidal thoughts, overuse of alcohol or drugs

Past: Nervous breakdown, attempted suicide, psychiatric treatment

Potential: Drug abuse, family history of alcohol problems, suicide, mental problems before age 60

No matter what interview format is used for history-taking, an essential factor is establishment of a trust relationship between client and practitioner. This trust will facilitate the sharing of knowledge needed to arrive at a determination of health status. Throughout the process the client should be encouraged to share her perceptions of her health status and her presenting illness or health problem as well as broader concerns relating to her role and function. Assessment is best accomplished when there is a climate of openness between client and nurse, supported by mutual trust and respect.

In addition to general health status information, histories relating to specific problems can yield additional relevant information. History-taking related to specific health care problems of menstruation, vaginitis, abdominal pain, urinary tract infection, sexual dysfunction, and breast disorders will be covered in the relevant chapters in Unit Four.

HEALTH STATUS DURING PREGNANCY

Assessment of health status throughout pregnancy combines elements of the general health history and specific health care concerns. A comprehensive prenatal assessment includes a thorough history, physical examination, and specific laboratory tests. The prenatal history should include details about menstrual cycles, present pregnancy, previous pregnancies, past medical problems, family health history, sociocultural influences, and pregnancy plans.

Information about previous menstrual periods is important in determining the expected date of confinement (EDC). The client should be asked when her last period (LMP) was and what was it like. If the LMP was normal in onset, character, and duration then it can be used to determine the EDC by Nagele's rule: add 7 days to date, and subtract 3 months. If the LMP was different from usual—lighter, shorter, later than anticipated, or only spotting—conception may have occurred earlier. Some women will experience implantation bleeding about the time their period would have been due. A few women will experience slight bleeding for several cycles after pregnancy occurs. If the LMP was abnormal in any way, the woman should be asked if her prior men-

strual period was normal; if it was, the EDC is calculated from it. For the woman who has longer cycles, 35 days or more, the EDC may be 7 days later than that calculated by Nagele's rule.

The woman should be asked what makes her think she is pregnant. The common symptoms of early pregnancy, which include nausea, vomiting, breast tenderness or enlargement, urinary frequency, fatigue, constipation, and abdominal bloating, can help establish a diagnosis of pregnancy. The woman who presents later in pregnancy should be asked if and when she first felt fetal movement. Rule of thumb has it that quickening occurs at 20 weeks' gestation; therefore, identification of this point can assist in roughly calculating when to expect delivery. If the woman has not yet experienced quickening, she should be asked to note when it occurs and tell her practitioner.

Information about previous pregnancies can be predictive of potential high-risk status (see Chapter 10). The number of pregnancies is significant in that excessively high parity (over five pregnancies) is a high-risk factor. It is essential that the practitioner gather details about the exact outcome of each prior pregnancy. If there were premature deliveries, it is important to note how long each pregnancy lasted. If the woman has had a previous abortion, it is important to know if it was induced or spontaneous; when it occurred; and if spontaneous, whether it was complete or dilatation and curettage were performed. Repeated mid–second trimester abortions can indicate an incompetent cervix. Any indication of postmaturity, that is, pregnancies documented to have lasted more than 42 weeks, is important also. The birth weight and condition at birth of each infant can be predictive. Children of the same parents tend to be of similar birth weight, although weight increases slightly with each subsequent pregnancy. Excessively large infants (over 9 lbs) can suggest diabetes mellitus in the mother. Birth weight can give some clues as to length of gestation. The condition of the infant at birth and at present can provide information about congenital anomalies and complications of pregnancy and childbirth.

Information about previous labors and delivery can also be predictive. A history of very long or short labors can help the practitioner and client plan for the present experience. Prior indication of labor and the reasons for it can indicate problems that might affect the present pregnancy. Breech presentations tend to recur. Previous use of forceps should be noted since this can indicate a disproportion between maternal passageway and fetal passenger. A previous cesarean birth is always significant. The woman should be asked about any analgesia or anesthesia she has experienced and what her reactions were to them. Any complication of labor and delivery, such as preeclampsia, eclampsia, hemorrhage, or dystocia, should be explored in detail.

A family history of major illnesses can be predictive of problems during pregnancy. Diabetes, tuberculosis, heart disease, renal disease, hypertension, seizure disorders, or multiple births are particularly significant. The client should be asked about each; appropriate follow-up is indicated if positive answers are given. Information as to any prior or preexisting illnesses in the client should be gathered. Pregnancy may adversely affect preexisting cardiovascular disease, endocrine disorders, or problems of the gastrointestinal or musculoskeletal system. A history of depression can be significant postpartum. Any history of blood transfusions is significant since sensitization may have occurred. Prior gynecologic surgery may contraindicate vaginal delivery, particularly if uterine or pelvic floor repair was involved. It is important to know whether the client has had an appendectomy, particularly if the woman experiences abdominal pain during pregnancy.

The client should be asked about any present health problems and any medications she takes regularly. These can alert the practitioner to potential hazards or problems during pregnancy. Medications should be avoided whenever possible or at least minimized. Any history of allergies should be noted. This is necessary for safe treatment with medication and can give clues to possible allergies in the infant. Use of alcohol, drugs, or tobacco should be determined since substance abuse is associated with many factors affecting the well-being of the infant. Significant use of any of these places the pregnancy in a high-risk category. A thorough nutritional history should be taken that includes information about usual food practices, likes and dislikes, and diet modification currently being practiced, and food budget problems. The woman's knowledge about basic nutritional needs should be determined, as well as her interest and motivation.

It is important to know how the woman feels about her pregnancy in order to anticipate problems and explore alleviations. Asking her if the pregnancy was planned or not or if she was using contraception can lead to an exploration of concerns, stresses, or problems of the family. Information about a woman's social support system is important in identifying her needs for support, inclusion of others in care, her particular stresses and conflicts, and responses to treatment. Knowledge of financial needs and environmental risks is essential in planning comprehensive care. Each woman's social support system and cultural frame of reference are different and affect her ability to assume self-care practices and to be receptive to care from others.

The client should be encouraged to explore with her practitioner any requests, desires, or questions relating to childbirth. The client's ideas or decisions about natural childbirth, anesthesia, or analgesia for labor and delivery, partner involvement, method of feeding, or rooming-in provide valuable information about her attitudes, cultural frame of reference, and knowledge level. Some women are well informed and have already made many decisions about their childbirth experience; others have never considered such options and need much information.

Once the initial comprehensive prenatal history is taken and a data base established, it will need up-dating at each prenatal visit. The woman's general health and feelings are explored as well as any symptoms. Questions are asked so that the practitioner can differentiate between the so-called normal discomforts of pregnancy and those symptoms indicating a possible serious problem. Every pregnant woman experiences physical, physiologic, and emotional changes during pregnancy that are considered to be normal though uncomfortable. At times, however, the same symptoms can indicate potential danger. In order to differentiate between the normal and abnormal, a lengthy series of questions should be asked on each prenatal visit. A systematic approach is useful to avoid omitting any significant questions; it is often helpful to use a body systems approach. This is the format suggested here. The client is asked if she has experienced any of the following since her last visit:

1. *Headaches:* are relatively common in pregnancy, most probably caused by fluctuating hormone levels or possibly emotional tension. The following questions, which will differentiate between a single headache and a more serious problem, should be asked if the client indicates she is having headaches.

"Where does it hurt?" Pre-eclamptic headaches are described as throbbing and most severe on the top of the head. Sinus headaches are usually felt over the affected sinus. Tension headaches most often occur at the base of the neck while migraines are one sided.

"How often does it hurt and how long does it last?" Headache that occurs in pre-eclampsia is continuous, occurring after the twenty-eighth week gestation, and is often accompanied by vision problems. It does not go away. Headaches that last only a short time are usually not significant unless large doses of analgesics are taken.

"What relieves the pain?" Usually headaches that are relieved by simple pain relief medication are not significant unless they recur frequently. It is important to note what medication is being used, as some are contraindicated in pregnancy.

"Are they getting worse?" Any headache that is increasing in severity or intensity is cause for concern.

"Do you notice any other symptoms associated with the headache?" Blurred vision or changes in visual acuity can mean edema or vascular spasms. Vomiting or dizziness may be indicative of increased intracranial pressure.

If indicated by positive answers to the questions, the practitioner should screen for other signs of toxemia: visual problems, hypertension, sudden excessive weight gain, edema of hands and face, albuminuria, hyperreflexia.

2. *Visual problems:* Dizziness or spots before the eyes are not uncommon in pregnancy, again probably caused by hormonal changes. In rare cases anemia will cause dizziness. The main concern when a client describes visual disturbances is impending toxemia. Each client who describes these symptoms should be screened for the other signs of toxemia.

3. *Nausea and vomiting:* These are quite common in the first trimester of pregnancy and need to be differentiated from vomiting that results in more than a 5 lb weight loss or continues beyond the first trimester. Hyperemesis gravidarum, or excessive vomiting, occurs rarely, but when it does it jeopardizes fetal well-being through electrolyte imbalance and malnutrition, while also debilitating the woman.

The woman should be questioned as to the frequency and amount of vomiting and the relationship of symptoms to certain foods (such as fried), time of eating, and activity. The extent to which food and fluid intake has been restricted should also be ascertained. If nausea and vomiting are associated with abdominal pain or tenderness, with or without fever, it is essential that a differentiation between gastroenteritis and significant pathology such as appendicitis, pancreatitis, hepatitis, or intestinal obstruction be made. Vomiting can be a signal of flu, viral disease, or gastroenteritis. The effects of most viral diseases are not yet known; until sufficient data are available, flu-like symptoms should be noted in the prenatal chart. Finally, excessive or persistent vomiting beyond the first trimester can be a sign of hydatidiform mole and should be explored.

4. *Diarrhea:* This is not a common discomfort of pregnancy although some women experience it immediately prior to onset of labor. It is usually thought to be a symptom of flu or gastroenteritis.

5. *Constipation:* While not considered to be a danger signal, constipation can lead to straining and the development of hemorrhoids. It is often treated by over-the-counter preparations, which can be harsh. Constipation should be avoided in a woman with an incompetent cervix because straining is undesirable.

6. *Chest pains/shortness of breath:* Many women experience shortness of breath during strenuous activity or in the last trimester of pregnancy, when the enlarging abdomen encroaches upon the diaphragm. This needs to be differentiated from more serious problems. Cardiac problems may be exaggerated or become evident for the first time during pregnancy. The woman should be asked about the relationship between shortness of

breath and activity and the presence of dyspnea while lying down. Any woman who uses more than two pillows to sleep because of dyspnea or who experiences chest pain or shortness of breath with mild activity should be further evaluated for abnormality.

7. *Abdominal pain:* It is important to distinguish Braxton Hicks contractions and/or broad or round ligament pain, which are normal discomforts of pregnancy, from a serious medical problem. Braxton Hicks contractions can be perceived as early as the second month of pregnancy and may be intense and regular enough to prevent sleep. Most women who experience them learn to tolerate them. Ligament pain is caused by spasms that occur as the fundus rises and stretches the uterus. This type of pain usually lasts no longer than 20 minutes, does not require medication, and may be relieved by flexing the knees. If it is determined that the abdominal pain is not the result of Braxton Hicks contractions or ligament stretching, it is necessary to rule out such major difficulties as appendicitis, pancreatitis, hepatitis, cholecystitis, intestinal obstruction, or the possibility of labor. In determining the severity and character of the pain, the practitioner should ask what medication has been used whenever the pain interferes with sleep and usual activity, and whether the pain is continuous or intermittent.

8. *Fetal activity:* Changes in fetal activity can be significant and the pregnant woman should be asked on each visit if the baby is moving. After quickening has occurred, the client should be told to report any significant changes in fetal activity. No fetal movement for 24 hours is a danger sign.

9. *Vaginal bleeding or spotting:* In the first trimester bleeding can be indicative of a serious complication such as an ectopic pregnancy, spontaneous abortion, or hydatidiform mole; later in pregnancy it may indicate placenta previa or abruptio placentae. Minor conditions, such as vaginitis, cervicitis, or cervical polyps, may also cause episodes of vaginal spotting. Occasionally, the client will confuse bleeding caused by hemorrhoids or hematuria with vaginal bleeding. Every instance of vaginal bleeding or spotting should be explored with the client with questions such as the following:

"How much bleeding have you had?" The client should indicate this in amounts that are familiar to her—a teaspoon, a cupful. *"How many pads did you use?"* *"What size were they?"* *"Were they saturated?"* *"What color was the bleeding?"* *"When did it start?"* *"Were there any clots?"* If at all possible the practitioner should observe the bleeding or stained pad.

"When did you last have intercourse?" Spotting associated with intercourse is often a sign of cervicitis.

"Did you notice any pain?" Pain is often present with ectopic

pregnancy or abruptio placentae. Placenta previa is usually painless.

"Have you noticed any change in fetal movement or in how your uterus feels?"

10. *Vaginal discharge:* Most women experience increased vaginal discharge during pregnancy because of the hormonal changes that occur. Pregnancy increases a woman's susceptibility to monilia. Whenever a woman complains of increased vaginal discharge associated with pain, itching, foul odor, or burning upon urination, she should be screened for diagnosis. Some infections can be transmitted to the baby at time of delivery. These include monilia, which is thrush in the newborn; herpes, a virus that can be fatal; and gonorrhea, which can cause blindness in the newborn. Specific procedures for diagnosing types of vaginitis are found in Chapter 13.

11. *Back pain:* Back pain is common in pregnancy and can be caused by strain on the musculoskeletal system of the lower back as the uterus enlarges and the woman's center of gravity shifts. If a pregnant woman complains of back pain, it is important to determine the area of the pain. Pregnant women are predisposed to infections of the urinary tract, which can result in a complaint of low back pain. Pain or tenderness in the costovertebral angle (CVA) usually indicates a kidney infection. At times the pain is exquisite, or there may be only minimal discomfort associated with low-grade fever, urgency, dysuria, and/or burning upon urination. Occasionally, suprapubic tenderness, a sign of bladder infection, may also be present. Any pregnant women who complains of back pain should be asked about other relevant symptoms and checked for CVA tenderness. It is essential that any urinary tract infection be detected early, since kidney infections may predispose a pregnant woman to early labor and delivery of a low birth weight infant.

12. *Leg cramps:* Leg cramps can indicate the serious problem of thrombophlebitis or the less serious one of calcium or phosphorus imbalance. The incidence of thrombophlebitis increases during pregnancy as a result of alterations in clotting factors and increased dilation of vein walls due to increased fetal weight on pelvic veins. To distinguish thrombophlebitis from any other condition, the practitioner should check for tenderness, warmth, redness, and/or swelling over the affected extremity. A positive Homan's sign (pain upon forced dorsiflexion of the foot) may be present. If all signs of thrombophlebitis are negative, the pregnant woman should be asked about the amount of milk she drinks. Excessive milk intake can result in excess phosphorus while too low a consumption of milk can cause calcium depletion.

13. *Edema:* Lower extremity edema is a normal discomfort of pregnancy and is caused by retardation of venous return from the legs and subsequent fluid shift from capillaries to extravascular tissue. Edema is a serious problem when it occurs in the hands and face since this may be indicative of toxemia. When either hand or facial edema is present, it is essential to screen the pregnant woman for the other indicators of toxemia—hypertension, hyperreflexia, proteinuria, sudden excessive weight gain, and headaches or visual symptoms.

14. *Infectious process:* On every visit, the pregnant woman should be asked if she has experienced a cold, cough, or sore throat to determine the presence of upper respiratory infection. Any experience with chills and fever should be noted because any time a pregnant woman experiences an infection there exists the increased possibility of fetal infection. The pregnant woman should also be asked if she has been exposed to any infectious diseases; if she has, this should be noted in the chart. It is thought that many infectious diseases, particularly viral, can cause fetal damage.

15. *Medications:* At each visit the nurse should ask about any over-the-counter medicines or prescription drugs the client may have taken since the last visit. She should be asked about the kind and amount of each medication taken. No drug has been conclusively identified as safe for pregnant women. While medication should be avoided or kept at a minimum throughout pregnancy, this is particularly important in the first trimester when the fetus is extremely vulnerable.

16. *Emotional status:* Emotional changes are a part of normal pregnancy. Mood swings; changes in body image; fears of labor and delivery, pain, the unknown, of having an abnormal fetus, of loss of control, or death; changes in life-style and role all affect the emotional status of the pregnant woman. It is important to identify each woman's support system and to determine her emotional status on each of these issues. Follow-up concerning emotional status on each visit is mandatory for comprehensive care. Each practitioner has to decide how she will determine this and use an approach that she will be comfortable with.

Closely connected to emotional status is sexuality. Pregnant women frequently are hesitant to ask questions about sexual activity. The client should be given the opportunity to express any concerns or to ask any questions she may have about sexual activity, including safety of intercourse, positions to use, and alternatives to intercourse.

Quality prenatal care, which is founded on a thorough health assessment, is the right of every pregnant woman and the responsibility of her health care practitioner. Assessment and screening as described here will help ensure her rights and will assist the practitioner in carrying out these responsibilities.

GYNECOLOGIC EXAMINATION

Once the basic history has been collected, the woman usually has a physical examination. A complete gynecologic examination involves evaluation of the total woman. Basic data to be gathered prior to the actual examination include urinalysis, blood pressure, height, weight, and hematocrit; other tests should be performed as indicated. Screening using these laboratory tests is an essential part of determining health status.

Examination begins with the breasts. The breast examination has at least three purposes: detection of irregularities of the breasts, assessment of external appearance of the upper thorax, and instruction in breast self-examination. Breast examination must include palpation and inspection. The specifics of breast examination and a method of teaching self-examination are covered in Chapter 17.

Other assessment procedures done prior to the actual gynecologic examination include palpation of the neck for thyroid abnormalities and auscultation of the heart, lungs, chest, and thorax. The gynecologic assessment begins with the abdomen followed by an examination of the lower extremities. The abdomen is inspected for abnormalities, masses, and pregnancy contours; pubic hair distribution is noted. All four quadrants should be palpated covering the regions of the liver, spleen, and descending colon. Palpation and percussion of the liver should be a part of every examination because of the risk of benign liver tumors among birth control users. Any abdominal guarding and/or rebound tenderness should be noted and explored. The lower extremities should be examined for varicosities, edema, and other abnormalities.

The pelvic examination is generally perceived by women as being different from examination of other parts of their body. It is often viewed as uncomfortable, embarrassing, and unpleasant.

Fear prevents many women from obtaining regular gynecologic care. Some women are afraid of what the examiner may discover—some disease processes or dysfunction that they wish to keep secret or do not want to acknowledge themselves. A woman may have had discomfort during previous examinations, which causes her to dread another one. For others, it is fear of the unknown. Many are not knowledgeable about their anatomy and physiology and do not understand exactly what the examiner is doing and why.

An increasing number of women have become dissatisfied with traditional gynecologic care. Their complaints fall into four major areas: (1) patronizing, dictatorial attitudes, (2) lack of sensitivity, (3) sexist attitudes and biases, and (4) demeaning, humiliating pelvic examinations (Jorgenson, 1976). The first complaint is largely a power issue. The prevalent medical model today is still the parent (doctor)-child (patient) relationship. The physician has the power and authority while the patient is passive and dependent. Costanza (1972) describes the health care system as implying a relationship of "parent to child: of strong to weak, of giver to receiver, of active to passive." (p. xvii) Women are no longer comfortable with a patronizing approach but are demanding to be informed about their bodies and their medical care, and to be involved in the decision-making process. The physicians' lack of sensitivity, sexist attitudes, and sexual biases are often related to the fact that most gynecologists are men sharing with other men (and some women) the traditional views of women as both sex objects and inferior. Women may feel that male gynecologists are insensitive to them as women and as sexual beings. Often the male gynecologist is judgmental of his client's sexual activities and believes he has the "right to be the moral guardian of his woman patients" (Jorgenson, 1976). He may have society's sanction to be an advisor on sexual matters, but his education does not prepare him for this role. Women are beginning to demand that male gynecologists treat them as adult sexual beings, abandoning stereotypical views of women so as to treat their clients with dignity and respect.

Many women find the traditional pelvic examination to be demeaning and humiliating. Women often describe feeling embarrassed, powerless, helpless, and humiliated. Examinations are put off because of strong desires to procrastinate and feelings of resistance and discomfort (Debrovner and Stubin-Stein, 1975). The pelvic examination is a dreaded, unpleasant procedure involving an undignified position (supine in the lithotomy position), nakedness (covered only by a paper sheet or towel), and surrounded by an aura of mystery and lack of communication. Kaiser and Kaiser (1974) have described it thus: "The patient is literally helpless in that (gynecologist's) hands and feels that way: naked, supine, being manipulated with fingers and tools in her bodily orifices by someone hidden behind a sheet."

Medicine's basically authoritarian and dominant position where women are concerned has resulted in an emphasis on the technical and mechanical aspects of the pelvic examination. The emotional and psychologic components have been virtually ignored. Recently, perhaps because of growing dissatisfaction expressed by both the women's movement and the general health care consumers' movement, the importance of communication and of attention to the emotional and psychologic components of the pelvic examination and the woman's comfort are receiving attention.

A new format, which is called either the educational or the mirror pelvic examination, emphasizes the importance of communication with the woman before, during, and after the examination. A mirror is used to show the woman parts of her anatomy, thus providing an opportunity for learning. The woman is an active participant, voicing her concerns and sharing in the decisions about her health care. Dignity and self-respect are restored to women during the procedure and the integral role of sexuality in human beings is reaffirmed by dealing sensitively and openly about issues of sexual expression and reproduction. The educational pelvic examination seems to be gradually making the pelvic examination a less dreaded experience for those women who have experienced this new format (see Kaiser and Kaiser, 1974; Liston, 1978; Miller, 1974; Sarrel, 1978; Wells, 1977).

The practitioner can do several things to ensure that the experience of a pelvic examination is positive. Communication is essential from start to finish. It is important that the initial contact between practitioner and client take place on equal footing, while the client is dressed and before she is lying down on the examining table. Most women welcome the chance to talk to the practitioner before the examination, to establish rapport and discuss the examination and what to expect. It is essential that during the examination, the practitioner tell the client what she is going to do before doing it. A reminder to the woman that she will be touched can prevent tensing up and unnecessary discomfort. If the practitioner wishes the client to do something, directions should be specific. She should not say "relax" but rather ask the client to relax her abdomen or her perineum or whatever is needed. Small talk and jokes are inappropriate in this context, as is complete silence. What is needed is a sharing of information about the examination. A running dialogue about what is being done and what is being found is an excellent way of sharing information, encouraging questions, and getting the client involved in her health care.

Most women are afraid of the speculum, it looks and feels hard, unyielding, and cold. It must be warmed with warm water before insertion. For many women, the practitioner's casual handling of a speculum is viewed as an indication of disregard for her as a person. Demonstration of the speculum, allowing the client to see and feel it, will help to decrease the fears of having a speculum inserted. Insertion should always proceed slowly with steady pressure at an oblique angle.

Draping has become an issue for many women, who feel its use indicates there is something shameful about the procedure. Some think that drapes are used as a shield for the practitioner to hide behind, while for others it increases their apprehension because they cannot see what is happening. For other women, however, the drape provides a cover that they would be uncomfortable without, though they are wearing a patient gown.

The best solution is to have a drape readily available and let the client decide to use or refuse it. In either case the room should be warm, and maximum privacy for the woman should be ensured.

The pelvic examination provides a unique teaching opportunity. All of the excellent aids currently available for teaching a woman about her body are not substitutes for the real thing, her own body. Charts or models are based on anatomic norms and cannot illustrate individual variations. The practitioner, as she talks easily and points out various parts of the body, communicates acceptance of the female genitalia, an area that for most women still remains taboo. Without drapes and using a mirror, the practitioner can show the person being examined her external and internal reproductive organs. Without drapes, the examiner can see the client and maintain eye contact, thereby assessing facial expressions as to the amount and duration of discomfort, while also preventing an impersonal approach. With the client in a semi-sitting position and using a small mirror, the practitioner can point out structures of the external genitalia, including the outer and inner labia, anus, urethra, clitoris, and the vaginal orifice with its hymenal ring. By focusing on the proximity of the anus, vagina, and urethra, the practitioner can point out how easily bacteria can be spread from anus to vagina or urethra. Visualizing the clitoris and discussing its function can lead to voicing of sexual concerns or problems. After insertion of the speculum, the cervix and vaginal walls can be seen. If there are any abnormalities they can be shown to the client, who can then have some idea of what the problem is. She can take some responsibility for monitoring problems and reporting changes in subsequent examinations. Contrary to existing opinion, this does not appear to alarm clients but rather has the positive effect of increasing willingness to accept treatment when women can see the condition making it necessary. Women who experience this type of pelvic examination seem less fearful and resistant on follow-up visits. They are intelligent consumers of health care who are capable of understanding their bodies and who appreciate the need for periodic check-ups (Wells, 1977).

There are basically two parts to the pelvic examination: inspection and palpation. At the same time, various smears and cultures, notably the Papanicolaou smear and often gonorrhea culture, are obtained. The complete pelvic examination should include the following:

1. Inspection of the cervix and vaginal mucosa by speculum
2. Pap smear and gonorrheal culture
3. Palpation of the external genitalia
4. Palpation of uterus, including the cervix
5. Palpation of adnexa

6. Evaluation of perineal muscles and pelvic floor
7. Rectal examination

During inspection and palpation, the practitioner must be alert for the presence of an abnormal mass. An abnormal mass can be recognized as any unexpected mass, given the normal shape and composition of a pelvic organ or structure. When found, a mass should be evaluated in terms of consistency, mobility, shape, size, tenderness, texture, and color. Another abnormal finding is abnormal exudate—any fluid that differs from that normally secreted or excreted. It should be evaluated in terms of color, odor, viscosity, and amount.

Inspection of the external genitalia includes examination of the escutcheon (or mons pubis), clitoris, labia majora and minora, urethra, including Skene's glands, vaginal introitus, including the Bartholin's glands and hymen, and the perineum.

The *escutcheon*, or *mons pubis*, is examined for presence and distribution of pubic hair. Pubic hair usually appears about 1 year prior to menarche. The amount varies from woman to woman. Absence of hair in the woman over sixteen is considered abnormal. Excessive hair in itself is not abnormal unless it is associated with excessive hair growth elsewhere.

The *clitoris* is usually about 2.5 cm in length and 0.5 cm in diameter. Enlargement or atrophy is considered abnormal. The clitoris is a common site for syphilitic chancres in the young client and cancerous lesions in the older woman.

The *labia majora and minora* vary in size from woman to woman; before menarche the labia majora are poorly defined, and they atrophy following menopause. During the reproductive years they are prominent. The labia majora in the nulliparous woman are in close approximation; after a vaginal delivery the labia can be slightly gaping and shriveled. The labia minora are less prominent and often obscured by the labia majora. The labia are basically symmetrical. All surfaces are covered by epithelium that is uniformly pink. Abnormal findings include asymmetry or unusual enlargement, atrophy before menopause, or lack of prominence after age 16. Abnormal exudates, parasites, focal hyperpigmentation, depigmentation, varicosities, erythema, excoriations, ulcerations, and leukoplakia are considered common abnormalities. Leukoplakia may indicate precancerous growth. Upon palpation the labia should feel soft.

The *urethra* is normally pink and without exudate. It is abnormal to find erythema, exudate, or a mass. The Skene's, or paraurethral, glands are not normally visible. Visibility is considered abnormal, as are erythema, exudate, or a mass at or on the orifice.

Bartholin's glands, located just inside the vaginal introitus, are not normally visible or palpable. Swelling, erythema, duct enlargement, or discharge are abnormal.

There should be no protrusion, and no part of the vaginal walls should be visible at the *vaginal orifice*. Abnormalities include cystocele, rectocele, or uterine prolapse. The *perineum* is normally a firm, muscular body between the introitus and anus. If an episiotomy has been done during a vaginal delivery, there will be a scar, and the perineum will feel thinner and more rigid. Extreme narrowing of the perineal body or presence of a fistula or mass is abnormal.

Following examination of the external genitalia, the cervix is visualized with a speculum. The cervix should be observed for color, position, size, shape, surface characteristics, and discharge. The color of the cervix varies from woman to woman. It is usually pink; however, it is normally pale after menopause and cyanotic during pregnancy. Cyanosis can also occur with any condition that causes venous congestion or hypoxia. Inflammation can be a cause of hyperemia while anemia may cause pallor.

The cervix usually protrudes from 1 to 3 cm into the vaginal vault; any deeper projection can indicate uterine prolapse. The cervix is approximately 2 to 3 cm diameter in the nulliparous woman and 3 to 5 cm following vaginal delivery. It is usually round and symmetrical, though this may vary after childbirth. Prior to childbirth, the cervical os is small and appears either round or oval; after childbirth the os may appear slit-like or irregular, showing the effects of the stretching and/or lacerations of delivery (Fig. 7-1). Quite often lesions are seen on the cervix. Nabothian cysts, a relatively benign condition, are smooth, round, small, yellowish cysts. They are caused by obstruction of cervical gland ducts and accompany chronic cervicitis.

The portion of the cervix that projects into the vagina and can be seen on pelvic examination is called the ectocervix and is covered with smooth, pink, stratified squamous epithelium identical to vaginal epithelium. The endocervical canal is lined with columnar epithelium, which appears red and bumpy. The point at which the squamous and columnar epithelium meet is known as the squamocolumnar junction and has significance in the detection of cervical cancer (Fig. 7-2). Occasionally, the squamocolumnar junction may appear on the ectocervix causing the cervix to have the appearance of a red, relatively symmetrical circle around the os. This can be either a normal variation in the placement of the squamocolumnar junction or the result of childbirth laceration known as eversion or ectropion.

Ulcerations and excavations appear as irregular, rough, and friable tissue around the external cervical os. Erosion, a manifestation of chronic cervicitis, may also be seen, presenting as reddish areas around the cervical os, which bleed easily. Erosion is different from ulcerations in that no portion of the epithelium is miss-

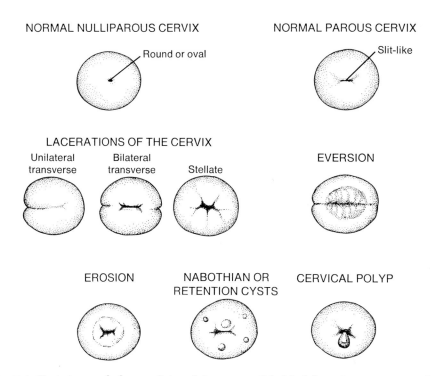

Fig. 7-1. Variations and abnormalities of the cervix. (Modified from Bates, B.: A guide to physical examination, Philadelphia, 1974, J. B. Lippincott Co.)

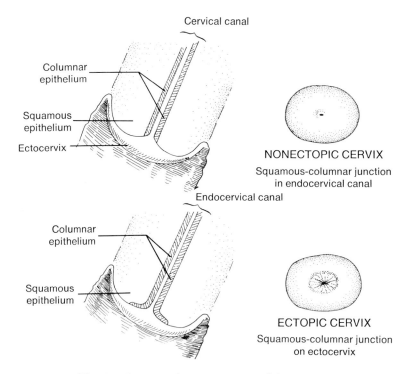

Fig. 7-2. Squamocolumnar junction of the cervix.

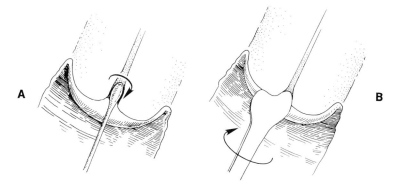

Fig. 7-3. Obtaining a Pap smear. **A,** Endocervical smear; **B,** cervical smear. (Adapted from Malasanos, L., and others: Health assessment, St. Louis, 1977, The C. V. Mosby Co.)

ing; rather, epithelium from the cervical canal has extended onto the cervical surface. Erosions should always be investigated further to distinguish early carcinoma.

Cervical polyps usually develop in the endocervical canal, only becoming visible when they protrude through the cervical os. They look light red, soft, and fragile. Normal cervical discharge varies with the menstrual cycle. It is always odorless and nonirritating; color and consistency vary from clear to white and from thick to thin to stringy. Discharge that is colored or purulent is abnormal.

The vagina is also examined during speculum insertion and withdrawal. Vaginal mucosa is normally unbroken, continuous, and covered with a clear, colorless, odorless secretion. During menstruation, the presence of bloody discharge is normal. Prior to menopause, mucosa is pink; after menopause it is pallid. During pregnancy, the vaginal mucosa appears cyanotic. Rugae, or wrinkles, are usually present in the nulliparous woman, becoming less prominent after delivery. Ulcerations, blood or blood clots of unknown origin, erythema, fistula, hemorrhagic lesions, leukoplakia, pallor prior to menopause, abnormal discharge, and cyanosis in the nongravid woman are all considered to be abnormal. One of the pathologic conditions most commonly found during vaginal examination is vaginitis. (See Chapter 13 for descriptions of specific types of vaginitis.)

The Pap smear and gonorrheal culture, when done, are taken during the speculum examination. The best time to collect a *Pap smear* is five to six days after the end of the menstrual period; however, Pap smears can be collected at any time, though presence of menstrual flow can make interpretation more difficult and obscure the presence of atypical cells. The woman should not have douched for 24 hours prior to collection, and no lubricating jellies should be used. Once the cervix is well exposed, it should be cleansed with a dry cotton ball to remove excess mucus. A cotton-tipped applicator is in-

Table 7-1. Classifications of Papanicolaou smears

Classification	Description
Class I	Normal
Class II	Atypical cells, not suspicious of tumor
Class III	Atypical cells, suspicious of tumor
Class IV	Probable malignancy
Class V	Definite malignancy

serted into the endocervical canal (Fig. 7-3) to the level of the internal os, rotated several times, withdrawn, and rolled onto a slide. The cervix is then examined to locate the squamocolumnar junction. A spatula is used to lightly scrape the squamocolumnar junction and cervical surface (Fig. 7-3, *B*). This is then smeared on a slide. Each slide should be immediately fixed to prevent the specimen from drying out and distorting the cells. Often, an additional specimen is taken from the vaginal pool in the area of the posterior fornix.

The Pap smear is a screening measure and further diagnostic tests are needed if results are abnormal. Pap smears indicate whether cervical cells are within normal limits or are suggestive of a malignancy. Originally, Dr. Papanicolaou developed numerical classifications to report findings (Table 7-1). These are not used very often any more because they are too broad. Descriptive reports are preferred because they are more useful in clinical decision-making. These reports describe more fully the cellular changes seen. In addition to notations regarding malignancy, specific infections often can be identified or hormonal evaluations provided. False negative reports of cervical lesions should not exceed 10% in a reliable laboratory. The most common reason for a false negative report is an inadequate sample taken improperly or improperly fixed. It is generally agreed that there is approximately a 5% false positive rate (Martin, 1978). The overall accuracy of the

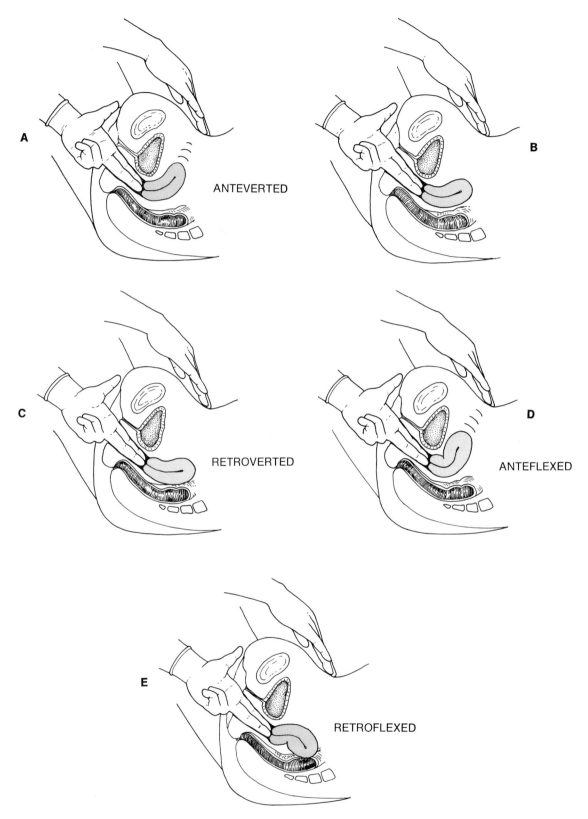

Fig. 7-4. Positions of the uterus. (Modified from Malasanos, L., and others: Health assessment, St. Louis, 1977, The C. V. Mosby Co.)

Pap smear for detecting cervical cancer is from 90% to 95%, making it one of the most reliable screening tests available.

For a *gonorrheal culture*, a specimen is obtained from the endocervical canal with a sterile cotton-tipped applicator. The swab is rolled on a specific culture medium plate (Thayer-Martin) and incubated. Culture for gonorrhea is necessary for diagnosis in women.

Neither a Pap smear nor a gonorrheal culture is done with every pelvic examination. They should be performed periodically. As noted earlier, all women over 20 (or before, if sexually active) should have a Pap smear every 2 years. Gonorrheal cultures should be done in the presence of symptoms, prior to IUD insertion, with a history of exposure, or at first prenatal visit.

Following the speculum examination, a bimanual examination is performed to palpate internal reproductive organs and assess pelvic support. Uterine size will vary according to the client's age and obstetric history. The nulliparous uterus is smaller than the uterus after pregnancy. Normally, the uterus is found in the midline and is symmetrical, freely mobile, nontender, and firm, although consistency varies with the life cycle and menstrual cycle of a woman. The uterus is more resilient near the end of the secretory phase of the menstrual cycle, softer during pregnancy, and firmer after menopause. The uterus is in one of three basic positions: anteversion, midposition, or retroversion; the uterus can also be anteflexed or retroflexed (Fig. 7-4). Abnormal findings include lack of symmetry, lateral displacement, limited mobility, abnormal masses, and tenderness.

The adnexa are palpated following uterine palpation. The primary structures examined are the ovaries and fallopian tubes. Differentiation of normal from abnormal is often difficult in adnexal areas because normal structures are often not palpable and abnormalities are mistaken for normal structures. In general, any mass that cannot be positively identified as a normal adnexal structure should be considered abnormal. Usually, the adnexa are mobile while abnormalities are fixed or have limited movement. The fallopian tubes have an extremely small diameter and are rarely palpable; ability to palpate suggests abnormal enlargement. Any abnormal mass should be noted; during the reproductive years this could signal an ectopic pregnancy. The ovaries are oval masses that feel smooth or slightly nodular. Normally, they are slightly tender upon palpation. Size varies with age and life events. The prepuberal and postmenopausal ovary is about 4 cm in length, while during the reproductive years one or the other may enlarge to 6 cm. This cyclic enlargement is normal only when it is unilateral and does not occur if the woman is taking ovulation-suppressant hormones. Abnormal findings of the ovaries include unusual nodularity, tenderness, unusual enlargement of one ovary or bilateral enlargement, fixation, and any abnormal mass on or within either ovary.

At some time during the pelvic examination, the integrity of the pelvic floor muscles and perineal muscles should be assessed. The pelvic floor muscles support the contents of the pelvic cavity. The tone is normally firm although childbirth trauma may weaken them. If the muscle tone becomes too weak, cystocele, rectocele, or stress incontinence may occur. Like the pelvic floor musculature, the perineal muscles are normally firm, although trauma during vaginal delivery can weaken them. The perineal body is often severed by an episiotomy. The perineal body is the common point of attachment for all the perineal muscles, and if it is damaged by poor surgical repair or weakened by numerous vaginal deliveries, it may not be able to fully contract. If too weak, the muscles contribute to stress incontinence as well as decreased sexual satisfaction.

Following palpation of the internal genitalia, a rectal examination is done to confirm uterine position, check for tumors of the posterior aspect of the uterus, and determine rectal sphincter tone.

Once the physical examination is completed and the medical history has been collected, the practitioner and client should discuss their findings and the meanings. Particular areas of concern should be identified and goals for improvement discussed. Finally, nursing care interventions and client self-care activities to improve the woman's health are decided upon and implemented. If appropriate, referral to the physician can be made.

Self-examination

Many women have elected to do pelvic self-examination in an effort to regain control of their bodies and avoid uncomfortable gynecologic examinations and dehumanizing, demeaning experiences. Initially, the woman often learns how to do pelvic self-examinations through a self-help group experience. She is taught to inspect her external genitalia, visualize and inspect her cervix, and examine her vagina. She learns what is normal for her throughout her menstrual cycle. With this knowledge of her body, the woman is then able to determine when an abnormality occurs and to seek appropriate treatment. She is able to make informed judgments about her need for care and to consult health professionals when their expertise is appropriate to the situation. This type of collaborative approach will facilitate preventive and maintenance self-care practices. One note of caution should be sounded, however. Self-assessment was developed as a health promotion technique and does not preclude the use of illness care services for the treatment of pathology.

Pregnancy tests

Recently "do-it-yourself" pregnancy determination kits have become available. While sensitivity and specificity of these tests await further clinical trials, they offer several advantages. In areas where pregnancy testing is not easily accessible or in those instances when privacy is essential, the opportunity for the woman to find out herself if she is pregnant is important. Many of these tests allow pregnancy to be determined earlier than the standard laboratory tests currently being used or by practitioner examination. For the client whose access to prenatal care is limited or delayed, the self-determination of pregnancy may allow her to begin healthful practices earlier. Early validation of her pregnancy may encourage a woman to seek prenatal care earlier than she would otherwise. However the availability of do-it-yourself pregnancy tests should not replace early entry to prenatal care or abortion counseling.

REFERENCES

Costanza, M.: Introduction. In Frankfort, E.: Vaginal politics, New York, 1972, Bantam Books, Inc.

Debrovner, C. H., and Stubin-Stein, R.: Psychological aspects of vaginal examination, Med. Aspects Hum. Sex. 9:163-164, Mar., 1975.

Fiumara, N. J.: The diagnosis and treatment of gonorrhea, Med. Clin. North Am. 56:1105-1113, 1972.

Frame, P. S., and Carlson, S. J.: A critical review of periodic health screening using specific screening culture, J. Fam. Pract. 2(1):29-36; 2(2):123-129; 2(3):189-194; 2(4):283-289, 1978.

Jorgenson, V.: Women's view of the gynecologist. In Glass, R. H., editor: Office technology, Baltimore, 1976, The Williams & Wilkins Co.

Kaiser, B. L., and Kaiser, I. H.: The challenge of the women's movement to American gynecology, Am. J. Obstet. Gynecol. 120:652-661, 1974.

Kinlein, M. L.: Independent nursing practice with clients, Philadelphia, 1977, J. B. Lippincott. Co.

Maeck, J. V., Braun, T. E., and Mead, P. B.: Patient evaluation. In Romney, S. L., and others, editors: Obstetrics and gynecology: the health care of women, New York, 1978, McGraw-Hill Book Co.

Malasanos, L., and others: Health assessment, St. Louis, 1977, The C. V. Mosby Co.

Martin, L. L.: Health care of women, Philadelphia, 1978, J. B. Lippincott Co.

McIntosh, H. D.: Hypertension—a potent risk factor, Heart Lung, 7(1):137-140, 1978.

McIntosh, H. D., and others: Introduction to risk factors in coronary artery disease, Heart Lung, 7(1):126-131, 1978.

Miller, G. D.: The gynecological examination as a learning experience, J. Am. Coll. Health Assoc. 23:162-164, 1974.

Murray, R., and Zentner, J.: Nursing assessment and health promotion through the life span, New York, 1975a, Prentice-Hall Inc.

Murray, R., and Zentner, J.: Nursing concepts for health promotion, New York, 1975b, Prentice-Hall Inc.

Robbins, L. C., and Hall, J. H.: How to practice prospective medicine, 1970, Methodist Hospital of Indiana.

Romney, S. L., and others: Obstetrics and gynecology: the health care of women, New York, 1978, McGraw-Hill Book Co.

Sarrel, P.: Adolescence. In Romney and others: Gynecology and Obstetrics, New York, 1978, McGraw-Hill Book Co.

Wells, G.: Reducing the threat of a first pelvic exam, Am. J. Mat. Child Nurs. pp. 304-306, Sept./Oct. 1977.

Wheeler, L.: Maternal assessment: Antepartal screening questions. Self-instructional package produced by Department of Maternal Child Health, School of Public Health, University of North Carolina, Chapel Hill, Dec. 1976.

Zelnik, M., and Kantner, J. F.: First pregnancies to women aged 15-19, 1976 and 1971, Fam. Plan. Persp. 10(1):11-20, 1978.

1975 Morbidity Statistics, U.S. Department of Health, Education and Welfare, National Center for Health Statistics, Washington, D.C., pp. 7-134 to 7-151.

ADDITIONAL READINGS

Bates, B.: A guide to the physical examination, Philadelphia, 1974, J. B. Lippincott Co.

Cohen, S., Buber, J. E., and Duperret, M.: Patient assessment: examination of the female pelvic exam. Part I. Am. J. Nurs. 78:1711-1744, Oct. 1978; Part II, 78:1913-1942, Nov. 1978.

Collen, M.: Periodic health examinations, Primary Care 3(2):197-203, 1976.

Delbanco, T. L.: The periodic health examination for the adult, Primary Care 3(2):205-214, 1976.

Dorsey, M., Lanterman, G., and Pack, J.: A research proposal: women's attitude toward the pelvic exam, Unpublished paper, Dec. 1978.

Hall, J. W., and Weaver, B. R.: A systems approach to community health, Philadelphia, 1977, J. B. Lippincott Co.

Jafari, K.: False negative Pap smear in uterine malignancy, Gynecol. Oncol. 6:76-82, 1978.

Lipman-Blumen, J.: Demographic trends and issues in women's health, Women's Health, DHEW Pub. No. 77-3138, 1972.

Liston, J., and Liston, E.: The mirror pelvic examination: assessment in a clinic setting, Obstet. Gynecol. Nurs. 7(2):47-49, 1978.

Little, D., and Carnevali, D. L.: Nursing care planning, Philadelphia, 1976, J. B. Lippincott Co.

Magee, J.: The pelvic examination—view from the other end of the table, Minn. Med. 59:99-100, 1976.

Marieskind, H. I.: Restructuring OB/GYN, Social Policy, pp. 48-49, Sept.-Oct. 1975.

Russo, N. G.: Protocol: women's health assessment, Nurse Pract., pp. 23-26, July-Aug. 1978.

Yura, H., and Walsh, M. B.: The nursing process, New York, 1973, Appleton-Century-Crofts.

Women and health problems

8

Women and violence

Connie Harris

In the late 1960s and early 1970s, the women's health movement emerged as an active force in the women's liberation struggle. Women were interested not only in their physical health but in their psychologic needs as well. Women's health clinics, consciousness-raising groups, and the feminist psychotherapy movement increasingly came into focus. Women were no longer content to just sit back and accept their fate. Rather they began to explore some of the problems and limitations imposed by the notions about women's roles. As a consequence, certain uncomfortable issues could no longer avoid public scrutiny. One such issue was violence against women. Tomkins (1972) suggests that violence plays a critical role in society: "Violence and suffering are critical in a democratic society, in heightening antipathy for violations of democratic values and in heightening sympathy for the victims of such violations." (p. 181)

American society is structured around family life. The idealization of the American family includes a successful marital relationship. Scott (1974) suggests that "a successful marital partnership is probably the most difficult of life's social requirements." (p. 433) Because many spouses have difficulty meeting each others' psychologic needs, violence may result. In addition, some people are socialized to believe that domestic violence is an acceptable way of dealing with the stresses of family life (Martin, 1976).

Women have typically played a dependent role in the family, while men have taken on the role of leader. In any system, a leader copes with many stressors, and the family, as a system, is no exception. Thus when people are socialized to use violence to cope with problems, the victim may not attempt to escape the violence; the aggressor may not cease using violence. Also, many women do not have the financial resources to flee the violent scene. As a result, wife abuse has become a significant issue in contemporary American life.

Rape is another form of violence against women currently plaguing communities. The incidence of reported forcible rape has increased nationally from 3 per 100,000 in 1933 to 11.6 per 100,000 in 1965 (Sutherland and Scherl, 1970). Others report increases ranging from 60% to 121% between 1960 and 1976 (Shaw, 1972; Horoshak, 1976; Klingbeil et al., 1976). Many rapes, however, remain unreported. If all rapes were reported, the number would easily be triple the above figures.

Many rapes are not reported because of the tendency of society to blame the victim. However, we have begun to examine the concept of victimization and the effect of violence on the victim and family. Communities are developing health care and counseling programs to assist women who are victims of rape or battering. Nursing contact with victims is increasing, especially in emergency care settings. In addition, nurses working in any setting can help identify these women, who may have concealed their violent experiences.

This chapter will discuss the etiology of violent behavior, the relationship of violence to wife battering and rape, the concept of victimization, and the implications for nursing practice.

ETIOLOGY OF VIOLENT BEHAVIOR

Rollo May (1972) suggests that violence is the logical result of a repressive culture. When people are denied what they are due, when they are made to feel impotent and stagnant, violence is the predictable outcome. "Violence is an explosion of the drive to destroy that which is interpreted as the barrier to one's self-esteem, movement and growth." (p. 182) Violence, unlike aggression, is not object related; the violent person swings out at whomever is in the way.

May describes five types of violence. *Simple violence* is a general protest against feelings of continuous impotence. *Calculated violence* involves exploitation by the leadership of the frustration and energy of people fighting for a cause. *Fomented violence* involves stimulation of "impotence and frustration felt by the people at large for the purposes of the speaker." (p. 186) *Absentee violence* is the support of violence occurring elsewhere, such as supporting a war with tax money. Finally, *"violence from above"* results when the person in power feels threatened that he or she will lose power.

May suggests that through violence people attempt to boost their integrity, self-esteem, and awareness of their own power. How people interpret the world around them is directly related to violence. Violent persons perceive the world as hostile and condescending. They will risk all, commit all, and assert all, while omitting rationality, in an effort to prove power and to establish a sense of self-worth (May, 1972).

Madden (1976) suggests that violent acts do not come from one cause alone but may be symbolic of various defects in the personality. Violent behavior may be related to unmet dependency needs in childhood; when these needs are not met, maturity may be stifled and personality development impaired, resulting in apathy, irresponsibility, and decreased sense of self. Madden summarizes several studies that point to the need for adequate parental-child relationships if dependency needs are to be met. Parental-child relationships have a direct bearing on dependency needs, which in turn are directly related to violence-prone behavior. Lack of success and feelings of powerlessness may also predispose people to violence.

Pinderhughes (1972) perceives projective identification and paranoia as significant mechanisms operating in violent interactions. "Paranoid dynamics with false belief systems based on projection can be observed in the midst of all intended violent human interactions." (p. 113) To commit violence, one must project evil onto the object of violence. The victim of violence "represents a renounced and projected part of the self, which, in the moment of violence, was perceived as totally evil." (p. 112)

Pinderhughes further suggests that people who perceive themselves as oppressed usually have little access to money, education, resources, etc. The oppressed experience few feelings of self-esteem or self-worth. When they attempt to free themselves from these feelings, confrontation occurs.

Menninger and Modlin (1971) point out that people prone to violent behavior may exhibit specific characteristics. These include (1) difficulty tolerating anxiety and stress; (2) a tendency to act rather than to delay; (3) limited, ambivalent relationships with significant others, characterized by relationships of paranoia; and (4) expressed feelings of weakness, inadequacy, and inferiority. Exploration of childhood history may reveal a tendency toward violence. Inadequate parent-child relationships, parental seductions, exposure to extreme violence, or behavior such as setting fires or cruelty to animals may indicate a predisposition to violent behavior (Menninger and Modlin, 1971).

Toch (1969) suggests that the cause of violence may be related to how people approach interpersonal situations. By studying "violence-prone" persons, such as inmates and parolees, Toch and colleagues have developed a catalogue of interpersonal relationships that might produce violent behavior. They suggest that persons who feel the need to defend or promote their self-image may utilize violent methods. Some persons, such as gang leaders, feel they must defend their public reputation and are allocated by the public a role that encompasses violence. These people may use violence to stay in the public spotlight. People may use violence to maintain norms they perceive as universal rules of conduct, to alleviate the threat of physical danger, or to cope with the pressure of difficult situations. Violence may also be used to bully or exploit others or for the purpose of self-indulgence. Finally, violence may be used as a method of catharsis or discharging internal pressure or uncomfortable feelings and moods (Toch, 1969).

RELATIONSHIP OF VIOLENCE TO WIFE ABUSE AND RAPE
Wife abuse

Studies by several investigators on wife abuse and rape provide supportive evidence for the above conceptualizations of violence. Pinderhughes (1972) notes that marital violence is commonly based on projective and paranoid relationships. When couples perceive their marital situation to be out of control, one spouse may use projection and paranoia to manipulate, control, or exploit the other. In Gayford's (1976) study, projective identification and paranoia were reported by 66% of the battering husbands portrayed as morbidly jealous. Scott's 1974 study also showed a relationship between unfavorable projective identification in the marital relationship and jealousy, usually on the husband's part.

In addition to jealousy, inadequate impulse control and inability to tolerate frustration were common characteristics of these battering men (Gayford, 1975b). In one of Gayford's studies (1976), 68% of the battered wives report that marital feelings revolve around indifference or hate.

Early exposure to violence and inadequate parent-child relationships also seem to be causative. In studies by Gayford (1976), 51% of husbands who had beaten their wives had witnessed violence between their own parents. As Geracimos (1976) notes, children who observe parental violence get mixed messages, including that it is all right to use domestic violence to cope with stress. Hilberman and Munson, in a study of battered women in rural North Carolina, found that battering husbands experienced emotional deprivation early in life and experienced early exposure to alcoholism, violence, and inadequate parental protection. In Gayford's study (1975a) 76% of battering husbands reported having poor interpersonal relationships with their parents.

Failure to acquire adequate social learning coupled with problems such as poverty, alcoholism, inadequate social supports etc., is also thought to be related to wife battering (Scott, 1974).

This is confirmed by Gayford (1975a), who reported that battering husbands tended to have poor school records, were often in trouble with the law, and were commonly heavy drinkers. Also, 33% of these men were unemployed resulting in family financial difficulties at the time.

Geracimos (1976), in an interview with a self-confessed "woman beater," was told that some men may use violence against women as a means of asserting manhood and position in an effort to maintain a public reputation of dominance and strength.

Rape

Metzger (1976) points out that the rapist asserts his "perceived socially, culturally, politically, and God-given rights." The woman "does not belong to herself. She is there for his use." (p. 406) In many cases, the attack is against *any* woman who happens to be around rather than against a specific woman. Metzger states that rape is an attempt by a marginally integrated member of society to affiliate himself with the community.

Burgess and Lazare (1976) describe rape as a way to control a woman over time. The rapist may perceive himself as having full sexual rights over the woman. Horoshak (1976) states that the rapist may be driven by a need for revenge against a female he hates. Thus, the rapist exploits his victim as a method of catharsis or discharge of uncomfortable feelings.

In summary, it must be emphasized that there is no single explanation for violent behavior. The above examples are presented as illustrations of the kinds of behavioral dynamics that may result in acts of violence against women. It is only with some understanding of the concept of violence that nurses can begin to appreciate the impact of victimization on women.

VICTIMIZATION: THE RESULT OF RAPE AND WIFE ABUSE

Battered wives commonly present complaints of vague somatic symptoms as well as signs of anxiety and depression. Many women feel drained and numb, and perceive themselves as incompetent, powerless, and deserving of the abuse. These women are high suicide risks because suicide is one way they can control their destiny (Gayford, 1975b). Insomnia and suicidal behavior are not uncommon. Psychologically, the women are immobilized by terror. They experience intense anxiety attacks at any unexpected event or at any event remotely connected with violence. Gayford (1975b) states that many of these women must be maintained on psychotropic drugs to cope with anxiety bordering on panic resulting from ever-present threat of violence. Unable to relax or sleep, many battered women experience conversion reactions and psychophysiologic responses, such as acute asthmatic attacks. It was also found that the beatings perpetuate problems related to already existing chronic diseases, such as uncontrolled diabetes.

Gayford points out that many women must tolerate battering because they fear further violence if they report the situation to the police. In addition, penalties for battering, such as fines and prison sentences, may only worsen the family situation. Both Pfouts (1977) and Lystad (1975) note that the battered wife may react to violence by taking her rage out on others, frequently her children.

Like wife abuse, rape has an intense emotional impact as well as physiologic implications for the victim and family.

Burgess and Holmstrom (1974) describe a cluster of symptoms that victims experience as a result of rape. This "rape trauma syndrome" is broken down into two phases, the acute phase and the adjustment or the reorganization phase. During the *acute phase*, victims may complain of disorganized sleep patterns, including insomnia and screaming out in their sleep. They may also experience a decrease in appetite, nausea when thinking about the incident, stomach pains, and various other physical complaints. They may present somatic complaints related to the area of the body that was the focus of the attack. Emotionally, in the acute phase, victims may experience feelings of overwhelming fear of physical injury, mutilation, or death. They may describe feelings of degradation, shame, guilt, humiliation, blame, anger, embarrassment, and revenge. Mood swings are not uncommon due to this wide range of emotional responses to the incident. Victims may overreact emotionally to interactions with other people, e.g., angry outbursts, crying for no apparent reason.

Burgess and Johansen (1976) describe a number of affective responses that may result from the rape. These include crying, inappropriate smiling, shaking, quivering, diaphoresis, or a quiet, guarded, and overcontrolled demeanor. Hilberman (1976) describes the overwhelming sense of powerlessness and helplessness connected with rape. Shaw (1972) suggests that the physical and emotional trauma of rape may result in fear of crowds and extreme guilt feelings of the victim that she may have caused the attack.

The victim may fear that the rapist is everywhere. She may respond quite differently to being touched by her partner after being raped.

It is not uncommon for the thoughts of the rape to continually haunt the victim. She is likely to have thoughts about how she might have been able to undo what has happened or how she might have been able to prevent what has happened, even though that is often unlikely.

Burgess and Holmstrom (1974) also emphasize that the disruption in life-style extends far beyond the acute phase into the long-term *reorganization* phase. Disruptions in life-style may include refusing to go out, moving away, changing phone numbers, etc. Dreams and nightmares may also be present on a long-term basis. Many victims develop fears and phobias specific to the rape situation. People with a past history of physical or emotional problems tend to regress. Also, some women experience a "silent" rape reaction in which the victim does not share the experience with anyone but rather bears the burden alone.

Sutherland and Scherl (1970) have found that the acute phase, lasting from a few days to a few weeks, was followed by a period characterized by outward adjustment. During this phase, the woman often returned to her work or school activities or assumed her role as homemaker. At this point she became outwardly composed and often indicated to health professionals that she needed no further assistance. It was thought by these investigators that among their sample this adjustment period contained much denial or suppression. They asserted that there was a real need for the woman to temporarily ignore the personal impact of the rape in order to cope with it.

However, after this phase of integration and resolution women experienced a sort of rebound need to talk and related feelings of depression. These investigators believed that it was during this final phase that the woman would integrate a new concept of herself.

Although it is essential for nurses to be cognizant of the emotional responses to victimization, they must not overlook the physical effects of violence. Often women are overtly injured, sometimes severely. Many women who have been raped have been stabbed or beaten as well, and they may have life-threatening injuries, such as subdural hematomas or ruptured internal organs. It is not surprising that immediately after the rape or beating women are likely to experience some physical reactions including bodily soreness, and pain from lacerations, as well as disturbance of sleep, upset eating patterns, and symptoms that are very specific to the force point of the attack.

These are just a few examples of victimization as it relates to wife abuse and rape. Clearly, both the physical and psychologic responses to violent acts are overwhelming and may have a profound effect on the victim and her significant others on a long-term basis.

NURSING PRACTICE

How do clients envision their need for help? How do they present themselves following rape? Burgess and Holmstrom (1976) found that the majority of clients in their sample were seeking *medical intervention*. They felt that they had been harmed or injured in some way and were looking for health professionals to help them. The second most common need was for *police intervention*. Next was the need for *psychologic intervention* or *emotional support*. A small percentage of women in this sample was uncertain about what they needed, if anything, and a very small percentage simply expressed a need for being controlled, because they felt out of control. The need for help as expressed by women who have been abused is not so well documented, but may parallel the same kinds of requests that are made by rape victims.

Many specific suggestions have been made for assisting the victim of violence, particularly in an emergency care setting.* All emphasize the importance of treating the patient with dignity and respect and providing adequate emotional support. There is need for an organized medical protocol for treatment, adequate follow-up care, and referral to community agencies as appropriate. Because nurses are key professional support people immediately following the attack, they must be adequately prepared to provide effective crisis counseling as well as physical care. The box on p. 143 presents a nursing protocol for assisting victims of violence in the acute care setting. This protocol is based on both the theoretic dynamics of violent behavior and the clinical literature on rape and wife abuse presented in this chapter.

Short-term intervention

Although not much research has been done to explore short-term interventions for women who have been abused, a number of investigators have described interventions for the woman who has been raped. In the context of rape crisis counseling, it is important that the counselor keep in mind considerations relative to the person's developmental level (Burgess and Holmstrom, 1975). For the *adolescent*, an issue may be maintaining independence rather than being brought back home from college; the adolescent woman who has been raped may, therefore, withhold this information until an occa-

---

*See Burgess and Holmstrom (1975); Burgess and Lazare (1976); Klingbeil et al. (1976); and Bellack and Woodard (1977).

**Protocol for nursing intervention
with victims of violence**

Examine and work through own attitudes concerning
rape and wife abuse.

See the client immediately. Avoid leaving a woman in
the waiting room where the environment will serve as
an added stressor. Avoid unnecessary stimuli, such as
numerous staff attempting to question her.

Explicitly define the nursing role for the client, and
clarify the roles of other health team members.

Explain necessary procedures and their rationale.

Prepare the client for required police procedures and
allow her to ventilate her concerns about them.

Provide for optimal client comfort. Secure medical
orders for somatic responses to violence such as nausea, intense anxiety, etc.

Allow the client to ventilate her concerns about the impact of violence on herself and her family. Help her
to identify adequate network supports to help facilitate crisis resolution.

Assist the client to explore conflicts in self-concept that
may be related to the violent experience, such as
guilt, self-blame, etc.

Explore the client's cultural beliefs about violence.

Discuss with the client which community agencies are
available for referral.

---

sion requires that she divulge it, such as diagnosis of
pregnancy or venereal disease. The *young adult* is at a
point in her life where development of intimacy is particularly important. For her, telling people, for example,
her parents, her boyfriend, or spouse, about the attack
may be particularly troublesome. The *adult* who is experiencing feelings of generativity is likely to be more
concerned about how the rape will affect others (spouse,
family, friends), whereas the older adult woman may be
primarily fearful of dying or being physically injured
rather than being sexually assaulted per se. Often elderly persons have a great deal of physical trauma along
with the psychologic residuals of the rape, particularly
if they are in fragile physical condition.

The model that Burgess and Holmstrom (1975) employ is a short-term approach that leads to improvement
in the woman's physical, emotional, social, and sexual
health. They employ a crisis intervention model that is
unique in one aspect: it is counselor initiated; that is,
the rape counselor takes the first step by initiating a
phone call to the victim. For victims whose rape is compounded by previous physical or mental health problems, Burgess and Holmstrom recommend maintaining
continuity with a primary therapist.

Other models for rape crisis counseling which have
developed over the last few years required that the *victim initiate contact.* While their services are certainly
valuable, crisis counseling centers using this approach
place an additional demand upon the client who must
not only initiate contact with the law enforcement authorities and a health service agency for validation of the
rape, but must also contact the crisis center.

Nurses employed in emergency care settings have an
obligation to interpret the available services for rape
crisis counseling to clients whom they see. Even more
desirable would be provision of such services as an ongoing part of the emergency care program. Such a program exists at Beth Israel Hospital in Boston.

Long-term intervention

It is essential that nurses and crisis counselors provide services beyond the point of immediate impact. It
is during the reconstitution phase that the woman may
actually need the most support. Her social network of
friends and relatives may not be adequate to sustain
her through the long arduous process of a trial should
she decide to press charges against the rapist or batterer.
For this reason the approach described by Burgess and
Holmstrom (1975) of providing follow-up counseling to
victims for several weeks after the rape seems particularly important. Certainly, these empathic kinds of services for victims may serve as a deterrent to the potential rapist or abuser by facilitating the victim's reporting
the crime. In addition, shelter services are available in
some communities so that women who have been
abused do not have to expose themselves or their children to the violence that may occur when they go home.
In some areas, the shelter personnel can actively assist
women in overcoming the economic obstacles that keep
them from leaving the situation in which they are
abused. A more difficult task is helping these abused
women overcome the low self-esteem that allows them
to believe they *deserved* the abuse.

Identification of victims

In addition to providing immediate and long-term
care for victims of violence, nursing responsibility for
identifying victims extends into most practice areas.
Pediatric nurses need to be aware of family dynamics
between children and other family members. For example, when a child is hospitalized, the nurse can observe
interrelationships in an effort to determine whether the
child's illness could be related to unhealthy family interactions characterized by violence. Hilberman and Munson point out that children of battered women may present a number of somatic, behavioral, and emotional
problems, such as stomach pains, headaches, attention-
seeking, and bedwetting. Child and adolescent rape victims may also experience these symptoms. The box on p.
144 describes other maladaptive behaviors that may

Maladaptive childhood behaviors: possible violence indicators

IF THE CHILD IS:
Aggressive
Passive aggressive
Defiant of authority
Quarrelsome
Hyperactive
School phobic
Unable to get along with other children
Fearful
Suspicious
Hypersensitive to criticism
Prone to temper tantrums
VIOLENCE MAY BE THE CAUSE

---

indicate that some form of violence is part of a child's life experience.

Children who present problems for which no medical reason can be found need an assessment of their family and social support systems. Nurses are in a good position to initiate this, since they work with patients and their significant others on a 24-hour basis.

Medical-surgical and maternity nurses are in an excellent position to help identify victims of violence because of the large number of women served in these fields. Nurses working with these patients need to be aware of signs of victimization, such as vague somatic complaints, lack of appetite, and inability to sleep. These women may be "silent" victims of violence.

Psychiatric nurses are also able to help identify rape and abuse victims. Many women who are experiencing victimization are referred to psychiatric units. Because many women conceal such acts of violence, they may be treated with drugs and/or psychotherapies without the source of the problem, the violent incident, being uncovered.

Finally, public health nurses play a vital role in helping to identify "silent" victims of violence. By visiting clients in the home they can observe firsthand the setting where many violent acts occur. They may actually observe some degree of violent interaction among family members and may need to assist families to deal with stress in a less destructive way.

If a nurse suspects a client is a victim of hidden violence, she should not attempt to "milk" the intimate details out of her. This may serve only to threaten or frighten the woman and cause her to withdraw even further. Instead the nurse should communicate to the client an attitude of interest and willingness to listen to her problems and to provide emotional support.

Meanwhile, the nurse can share with other members of the health team her concerns about the client's possible victimization. In this way, appropriate referrals can be initiated, and efforts can be made to determine whether victimization is truly a source of the client's problems.

In concluding, nursing staff play an important role in the care of victims of violence. As communities have begun to develop health care and counseling programs for rape and wife abuse victims, nurses are being called upon to provide physical care and crisis intervention for known victims, especially in emergency care settings. In addition, all nurses are in an excellent position to help identify possible victims of violence. They have the resources to initiate appropriate referrals both to assist the known victim and to confirm victimization.

ULTIMATE SOLUTIONS

Eliminating battering and rape altogether demands something more than the one-to-one types of interventions that have been discussed to this point; it demands more than courses in self-defense to assist victims to ward off attackers. Indeed, eliminating violence against women will involve a rather massive social change. Hilberman (1976), in an editorial from a recent issue of the *American Journal of Psychiatry*, summarizes this position when she states that "only when the sex roles of both men and women are defined by individual needs and talents rather than by stereotypic expectations based on sex and power motives will there be an end to rape." (p. 437)

Brownmiller, in *Against Our Will*, encourages society to place rape where it truly belongs: in the context of criminal violence and not within the purview of ancient masculine codes. We must regard rape as a crime against a person and not against property. A similar case can be made for wife abuse.

It is heartening to see that some change on the macrosocial level is already under way. Primarily spearheaded by the women's movement, changes are occurring in legislation that would protect the victim from becoming prosecuted: A New York State rape law, effective March 21, 1974, abolished all requirements for corroboration of the victim's testimony. Previously, the New York State laws had required that the testimony of a rape victim be corroborated by physical evidence of the victim's lack of consent. Other states are also recognizing that skepticism of women has been built into their laws. One New York district attorney commented that building skepticism of women into rape laws was not really necessary since it already existed in the police, the jury, the judges, and so on.

Further evidence of the impact of the women's movement is reflected by the recent funding of and establishment of a National Center for the Prevention and Control of Rape within the National Institute of Mental Health. This center will support research studies of the legal, medical, and social aspects of dealing with rape, the treatment of victims, and the effectiveness of existing programs to prevent and control rape. Demonstration projects to plan, develop, implement, and evaluate treatment and counseling programs for rape victims and their families, as well as to rehabilitate offenders will be included under the auspices of this agency.

The National Organization of Women (NOW) reports that there are currently over 300 chapters that have helped to form rape crisis centers, train and reform their local institutions, educate the public, establish governmental investigative bodies, and reform the rape laws in over half of the United States. NOW also actively supports efforts to create shelters for battered women. It has also worked to prevent any dangerous or sexist frauds from being perpetrated on the public. For example, it currently is pursuing charges of consumer fraud against self-proclaimed authorities on rape, hoping to prevent the spread of information on rape and self-defense that the organization considers potentially dangerous as well as degrading to women.

Ultimately, however, we will need to go beyond these efforts to draft legislation that views women as persons and not as property. We must move beyond consciousness-raising efforts at the National Institute of Mental Health. We need to move beyond the levels of intervention for individuals *after* they have been raped or beaten. Ultimately, what is necessary is intervention by women on a macrosocial and preventive level, rather than on the individual, or microsocial, level. Only when a woman is truly regarded as a person by the society will rape and battering come to be regarded as crimes against her person and not merely against her body.

REFERENCES

Bellack, J., and Woodard, P.: Improving emergency care for rape victims, J. Emerg. Nurs. 3:32-35, 1977.

Brownmiller, S.: Against our will: men, women, and rape, New York, 1975, Simon and Schuster.

Burgess, A., and Holmstrom, L.: Accountability: a right of the rape victim, J. Psych. Nurs. Mental Health Serv. 13:11-16, 1975.

Burgess, A. W., and Holmstrom, L. L.: Coping behavior of the rape victim, Am. J. Psych. 133(4):413-417, 1976.

Burgess, A. W., and Holmstrom, L. L.: Crisis and counseling requests of rape victims, Nurs. Res. 23:196-202, 1974.

Burgess, A. W., and Holmstrom, L.: Rape: victims of crisis, Bowie, Md., 1974, Robert J. Brady Co.

Burgess, A. W., and Holmstrom, L. L.: The rape victim in the emergency ward, Am. J. Nurs. 73:1741-1745, 1973.

Burgess, A., and Johansen, P.: Assault: patterns of emergency visits, J. Psych. Nurs. Mental Health Serv. 14:32, 1976.

Burgess, A., and Lazare, A.: Community mental health: target population, Englewood Cliffs, N.J., 1976, Prentice-Hall.

Fawcett, J., ed.: Dynamics of violence, Chicago, 1971, American Medical Association.

Gayford, J.: Battered wives, Med. Sci. Law 15:237-245, 1975a.

Gayford, J.: Battered wives—1, Nurs. Mirr. Midw. J. 143:62-65, July 15, 1976.

Gayford, J.: Wife battering: a preliminary survey of 100 cases, Brit. Med. J. 1:194-197, Jan. 25, 1975b.

Geracimos, A.: How I stopped beating my wife, MS, p. 53, Aug. 1976.

Hilberman, E.: Rape: the ultimate violation of the self, Am. J. Psych. 133:436-437, 1976.

Hilberman, E.: The rape victim, New York, 1976, Basic Books, Inc.

Horoshak, I.: Learn to fight rape—without hang-ups, RN 39:52-56, 1976.

Klingbeil, K., and others: Multidisciplinary care for sexual assault victims, Nurse Pract. 1:21, 1976.

Lystad, M. H.: Violence at home: a review of the literature, Am. J. Orthopsych. 45:328-345, 1975.

Madden, D., and Lion, J., editors: Rage, hate, assault, and other forms of violence, New York, Spectrum Publications, 1976.

Martin, D.: Battered wives, San Francisco, 1976, Glide Publications.

May, R.: Power and innocence: a search for the sources of violence, New York, 1972, W. W. Norton & Co., Inc.

McCombie, S., Bassuk, E., Savitz, R., and Pell, S.: Development of a medical center rape crisis intervention program, Am. J. Psych. 133(4):418-421, 1976.

Menninger, R., and Modlin, H.: Individual violence: prevention in the violence threatening patient. In Fawcett, J., editor: Dynamics of violence, Chicago, 1971, American Medical Association.

Metzger, D.: It is always the woman who is raped, Am. J. Psych. 133:405-408, 1976.

Notman, M., and Nadelson, C. C.: The rape victim: psychodynamic considerations, Am. J. Psych. 133(4):408-412, 1976.

Pfouts, J.: Coping patterns of abused wives, presented at the National Conference on Social Welfare, Chicago, 1977.

Pinderhughes, C.: Projective identification and paranoia in violent interactions. In Usdin, G., editor: Perspectives on violence, New York, 1972, Brunner/Mazel.

Scott, P. D.: Battered wives, Brit. J. Psych., pp. 433-441, 1974.

Shaw, B.: When the problem is rape . . ., RN 35:27, 1972.

Sutherland, S., and Scherl, D.: Patterns of response among victims of rape, Am. J. Orthopsych. 40:503-511, 1970.

Toch, H.: Violent men, Chicago, 1969, Aldine Publishing Co.

Usdin, G., editor: Perspectives on violence, New York, 1972, Brunner/Mazel.

9

Sexual dysfunction*

Catherine Ingram Fogel

Until recently, the sexuality of women was not acknowledged by society. Women were not expected to have sexual feelings nor were they allowed to respond sexually. With the advent of Masters and Johnson's (1966) revolutionary research into sexual response, society has begun to accept the idea of women as sexual beings who may experience disruptions in sexual functioning for a variety of reasons. With the new permission to acknowledge sexuality and a new awareness of dysfunctional patterns, women have begun to ask for help from nursing practitioners. In order to meet these increased expectations by clients, the nurse will need additional knowledge and skills. This chapter will examine the general causative factors of sexual dysfunction, identify general therapeutic approaches, discuss the causes and treatment of common psychogenic sexual dysfunctions in women, and explore the nurse's role in caring for clients with sexual dysfunction.

Physical factors as an etiologic basis for sexual dysfunction are limited (Gagnon, 1977). Only 10% to 20% of clients seeking treatment for sexual dysfunction are found to have a solely organic or physical basis for their difficulty (Haber, 1978). In addition, organic difficulties tend to play a lesser role in women than in men; female sexual physiology is less vulnerable to organic pathology than is the male (Kaplan, 1974a). For these reasons the focus of the chapter will be on psychogenic or nonorganic causes of sexual dysfunction.

Because very little is currently known about sexual dysfunction in lesbians, primary consideration is given to heterosexual dysfunction. It is thought, however, that similar principles may apply to both hetero- and homosexual female sexual dysfunction.

Haber (1978) defines sexual dysfunction as a "primarily psychosomatic disorder which makes it difficult or impossible for individuals to have and/or enjoy sexual experience." (p. 192) Pathology can force sexual expression to take a variety of distorted, inhibited, sublimated, and alienated forms in order to accommodate conflict. At times, actual physical impairments to the sexual response cycle may occur in response to the operant psychogenic factors (Kaplan, 1974a). Sexual dysfunction in women includes general sexual dysfunction, orgasmic difficulties, and vaginismus. Dyspareunia, which often has a physiologic basis, is discussed in Chapter 13.

OVERVIEW OF CAUSATIVE FACTORS

In many instances, sexual dysfunction arises from a lack of knowledge about sexuality, ignorance of sexual techniques, or general misinformation. For example, inadequate lovemaking can result solely from the couple's lack of information about sexual anatomy. Neither partner may know what the clitoris is or recognize the role it plays in sexual arousal. This is hardly surprising in a society such as ours, which places strong prohibitions on sexual behavior. Open, frank discussion about sex between couples or individuals has not been encouraged and is often strongly and actively discouraged. Also operating is the erroneous belief that the ability to adequately perform sexually is inherent in becoming an adult—that sexual prowess is instinctual and bestowed upon us when we come of age. If one has no knowledge of sex and sexual techniques and it is assumed that one does not need to be taught, the result is ignorance compounded by silence.

Another outcome of such a lack of knowledge coupled with an *expectation* of knowledge is the development of myths and misinformation. If one is expected to be knowledgeable, is not, but feels compelled to appear knowledgeable, human nature often responds with a myth or confused misstatement. We have only to consider the peer group discussions in adolescence that many of us participated in to realize how this phenomenon occurs. Several authors have documented the plethora of sexual myths and fallacies prevalent in the United States today (Masters and Johnson, 1978; McCary, 1975, 1978). The result of this can be a situation

---

*Portions of this chapter were taken from Woods, N.: Human sexuality in health and illness, St. Louis, 1979, The C. V. Mosby Co.

in which individuals have a set of expectations about sex, sexuality, and sexual performance based on a foundation of ignorance and misinformation. The couple who has no understanding of sexual anatomy may have intercourse as soon as erection occurs; ejaculation may happen without consideration as to whether the woman is sufficiently aroused. The couple may wonder why the woman is not orgasmic, and both partners contribute to sexual ineffectiveness. The woman cannot ask for the kind of stimulation she wants because she does not know what her needs are; the man is not aware that he is not a very effective lover. So in silence and ignorance they continue their unsatisfactory sexual habits (Kaplan, 1978).

It is important to understand how this ignorance and avoidance have developed in our society, and to move one step further to consider the second general basis of sexual dysfunction: guilt and anxiety. To comprehend society's negative attitudes toward sexuality, we must explore how sexual value systems develop and examine their impact on the individual's sexuality.

Value is defined here as an individual's view of the "good life." It determines what we want to do, the decisions we make, and the ways in which we behave. Sexuality is a powerful force that can be frightening to many. In order to handle the basic fear of sexual feelings and to provide guidelines for behavior, a whole variety of prescriptions or standards have been developed. These demands and expectations of society determine attitudes toward sexual matters. All cultures place specific restrictions on the expression of sexuality. These demands, expectations, and restrictions are internalized by individuals as they are socialized, and become a part of their value system. One of the strongest proscriptions in American society is avoidance of the topic of sex; with this lack of discussion many women have no opportunity to obtain accurate information. Discussions of sex in the home, school, or church, places where one ought reasonably expect to obtain accurate information, are frequently based on misinformation or biased information gathered from sources such as mass media and peers.

Much of the sex education received by children is negative—for example, labeling sexual organs as "private" or "dirty." Most 3-year-olds have pleasurable sexual sensations and positive attitudes toward sex. By the time of puberty, the child's normal reactions have typically been distorted by society's prevalent view of sex as evil and dirty. Added to this negative belief system are the common fears, ignorance, and misinformation about sex. Children are taught to suppress their sexual feelings and behaviors in order to be accepted by others. They often perceive that to have sexual feelings is wrong or bad and to act upon these feelings (in any way other than in a few limited, rigidly prescribed actions) is even worse. In a society presumably based on freedom of choice, sexuality represents an exception to the rule. Sex roles and acceptable sexual behaviors and rules are not to be transgressed. (For a discussion of women's sex roles and acceptable sexual behavior, see Chapter 6.)

The major restraining forces preventing the breaking of the rules are guilt and anxiety (Wilson, 1974). Sexual guilt seems to be the most influential factor in developing sexual attitudes and behavior. According to McCary (1978), sexual freedom is inhibited more by guilt than by any other cause. Even so, it does not appear that guilt in itself is necessarily an inhibitor of all sexual behavior; if it were, the human race in the United States would rapidly disappear! What appears to happen is that the guilt is minimized with repeated sexual behavior and gradually increased sexual involvement.

Many people grow up with unrealistic romantic ideals and expectations and are unprepared to deal with the probability that there are many persons whom they could love and perhaps marry. They may also be unaware that sexual fantasies of an infinite variety are normal. When the individual is confronted with feelings of attraction to more than one person at a time or with unacceptable fantasies, guilty feelings often occur, with resulting anxiety (McCary, 1978). It is important for sexual enjoyment that sex-oriented guilt be reduced to the minimum. Many studies document that the more guilt about sex one experiences, the less desire there is for sex, the fewer orgasms the person experiences, and the less one is able to respond sexually.

One of the major causative factors in the development of guilt is rigid religious conformity. According to Lehrman (1970), "unequivocally, absolutely, religious orthodoxy is responsible for a significant degree of sexual dysfunction, and it does not matter which of the three major religions is involved." (p. 17)

Almost invariably those experiencing sexual dysfunction have experienced negative conditioning in their formative years. As a consequence many couples are prevented from enjoying sex because of guilt and/or anxiety about erotic feelings. The partner may be actively discouraged from effective stimulation. What appears to happen is that the individual responds to sexual excitement by instantly stopping the activity that produces it. For example, the woman who begins to feel arousal does not encourage or savor these feelings but immediately encourages completion of the sexual act or pulls away from the contact (Kaplan, 1974b).

Like guilt, sexual anxiety is a potent etiologic factor in sexual dysfunction. Sources of sexual anxiety, which can be an obstacle to satisfactory sexual functioning, are fear of sexual failure, the demand for sexual performance, and fear of rejection.

Anticipation of not being able to perform is probably the most common cause of impotence and, to some extent, of orgasmic dysfunction. Once an episode of failure has been experienced, the fear of recurrence is great; unfortunately, a single sexual failure can set the stage for future failure. Anticipatory anxiety related to sexual performance can start a vicious cycle of fear of failure, consequent failure, increased fear of failure, which can escalate a single, transient failure into a state of serious, chronic dysfunction (Kaplan, 1974b).

It is difficult to determine why some individuals experience performance anxiety to a marked degree while others do not. Kaplan (1974b) suggests that generally insecure individuals and those whose behavior is excessively motivated by a need to compete and excel may be particularly vulnerable to fear of sexual failure. In addition, paranoid individuals tend to have a "pathologic" response to sexual failure. A further predisposing factor may be an insecure relationship with the spouse. However, Kaplan also points out that many persons whose sexual functioning is hampered by performance anxiety do not appear to be particularly neurotic or to have character disorders or a poor relationship with their spouse. According to Kaplan, regardless of other etiologic factors, an individual's fear that she may not perform adequately almost invariably plays a role in the general orgasmic dysfunctions of women.

A phenomenon that many people who are anxious about sexuality frequently experience is "spectatoring." If autonomic functions are to respond naturally, they must remain free of conscious control; therefore, for good sex, the individual must be able to suspend all distractions and lose herself in the experience. Those who are experiencing sexual anxiety frequently are unable to do this; they remain outside themselves, keeping a tight control over their emotions, and observing their sexual responses. In most cases the individual's expectations of herself are unrealistically high, and this perfectionism is usually coupled with lack of trust and insecurity. Thus we have the cast of the individual who is always "spectatoring" herself with resulting poor performance, which only serves to confirm her performance anxieties and fear of failure (Kaplan, 1974b; Masters and Johnson, 1970).

Closely related to the anxiety and subsequent sexual dysfunction resulting from fear of failure are the dysfunctions that follow demand for performance. General sexual dysfunction may result from a command or request to perform sexually. Vaginal lubrication is an automatic reflex that cannot be consciously produced. A request that is guilt-provoking or difficult to refuse can create enough fear and anger in the individual to make sexual responsiveness impossible in that situation. Performance demands are damaging and anxiety producing for both men and women; however, a woman can comply. To be sure, a woman cannot order up arousal upon command but she can allow a man to "use" her body. The man, however, must produce something visible—an erection. Demands for sexual performance can result in episodes of impotence in the man or nonresponsive patterns in the woman, which can then progress from fear of failure to chronic dysfunction. It should be noted that while the demand for performance more frequently comes from the partner, it may also come from the symptomatic client (Kaplan, 1974b).

Fear of rejection by the partner or an excessive need to please may also generate anxiety. To wish to give enjoyment and share pleasure with the partner is desirable and healthy. However, when this gets out of hand—becomes a compulsive need "to please, to perform, to serve, to not disappoint"—the emotion becomes dysfunctional (Kaplan, 1974b). Women are particularly vulnerable to rejection anxiety.

Poor communication or lack of communication has been implicated as a causative factor in sexual dysfunction. Couples may experience sexual dysfunction although they are generally satisfied with their nonsexual relationship and value it. These problems seem to be linked to a remarkable inability to talk about sex, limited knowledge of sex, and restrictive standards of acceptable sexual behavior. A vicious circle is once again set up—inability to talk about sex between partners perpetuates ignorance, lack of understanding, and misinformation; and these may be further complicated by the guilt engendered by a very restrictive sexual code. If couples have problems communicating in nonsexual areas, then their communications about sex will also be poor.

To communicate effectively about sex, both individuals need to be able to give and receive information about their needs, desires, and wishes. To convey information, an individual must be able to recognize a need or desire and then feel free to communicate it. To receive information, the individual needs to be aware of both overt and covert messages, and also be willing to receive and respond. Given all these variables, sexual communications can easily be ineffective. Poor communication can result not only from cultural factors but also from a variety of interpersonal/intrapsychic states, such as fear of emotional or physical abandonment, fear of loss of control, power struggles, low self-concept, fears about one's sexuality, and fear of intimacy.

It may be that lack of communication is not the cause of dysfunction, but rather this perpetuates a destructive sexual system and intensifies existing problems. For example, the woman who has some difficulty being orgasmic is fearful that if she asks her partner for more foreplay he will reject her. So she says nothing, does not validate her fears, and "fakes" orgasms, becoming more and more unresponsive. Since she has said nothing, her partner thinks everything is fine, is unaware of her lack of response, and assumes his satisfaction is hers. And with the assumption that everything is all right, he continues in his usual ineffective manner. Open communication would have prevented this pattern from developing (Levine, 1976).

Intrapsychic causes of sexual dysfunction, particularly psychologic conflict, have received considerable attention in the last few decades. Freud was the first to recognize and publicize the importance of sexual conflict in human behavior and to call attention to the power of sexuality in human behavior. A detailed description of the highly complex model of Freudian theories of sexual conflict and the etiology of sexual symptoms is beyond the scope of this chapter. However, a brief review of freudian theory as it relates to sexual dysfunction is useful here.

According to psychoanalytic theory, old fears of punishment for sexual expression learned as a child are reevoked by current adult sexual expression. The adult is victimized by these fears and attempts to make compromise solutions without being aware of the fears. In addition, there is material in the unconscious consisting of dangerous sexual memories and wishes that cannot be tolerated by the ego and therefore have been repressed. These sexual desires do not just disappear, however, but continue to seek alternative means of expression. When sex is subjected to conflict, sexual wishes are denied and then delayed, diverted, and expressed in distorted and neurotic ways.

A final concept important for understanding sexual disorders, according to Freud, is guilt—guilt about sexual pleasure, which is imposed by the conscious or superego and which also impairs sexual functioning without the person being aware of it. Freud thought that the common mechanism of dealing with unacceptable thoughts and feelings was to shove them into the unconscious to get rid of them. Anxiety warns the individual of the imminent return of these thoughts and mobilizes the individual's defenses to repress them. Thus, for Freud, repressed sexual wishes exert an enormous, though largely unrecognized, influence on our lives and are a common source of neurotic anxiety.

Freud also focused our attention on the importance of childhood experiences in shaping adult behavior. It is widely accepted today that sexuality is present at birth and plays a significant role in personality development. During childhood the most significant sexual material is repressed; the child learns to get rid of unpleasant feelings caused by dangerous and frustrating incestuous wishes by repression, by removing sexuality from the rest of the personality. However, these sexual impulses remain active in the unconscious to plague the individual later in life.

Elaborating upon his original premise, Freud developed a theory of three stages of psychosexual development—oral, anal, and genital. In the third stage, the child experiences the Oedipal period during which many of the sexual conflicts that may later surface are believed to be developed. The crucial feature of the Oedipal phase is that the child chooses the parent of the opposite sex as the object of his or her erotic aims. This "romance" arouses frustration, guilt, anxiety, and conflict in the child's relationship with the parent of the same sex. The little girl experiences intense sexual longing for her father and hates her rival, her mother, whom she also loves. The urge for incestuous sex and the hostile wishes evoke conflict. Loss of love and, to some extent, fear of genital injury are the controlling mechanisms that prevent the child from actively operating on her wishes. Resolution occurs when the conflict is suppressed, identification with her mother is achieved, sexual wishes toward her father are renounced, and later she marries an appropriate young man who has some of her father's desirable characteristics. According to Freud, unresolved Oedipal problems are the sole cause of sexual pathology. Sexual symptoms develop in the adult when current experiences activate those unresolved, dormant, and unconscious Oedipal conflicts of childhood.

Oedipal conflicts and the return of repressed conflicts can explain some types of sexual dysfunction; however, many individuals with unresolved Oedipal material do not experience sexual symptoms. Furthermore, sexual dysfunctions often occur in individuals who show no evidence of Oedipal problems. The ideas that early incestuous experiences are the only cause of sexual conflict and that sexual dysfunction is always caused by unconscious conflict have recently come under criticism. The newer treatment of sexual problems does not embrace this theory wholeheartedly, although the freudian concepts of unconscious motivation and the importance of childhood experiences in molding adult experiences have been retained. The concepts of repression and resistance are also useful. The "new" sex therapy does not reject the importance of the unconscious or the Oedipal conflict; however, the latter is considered only one of many factors that can play a role in development of sexual dysfunction.

An additional intrapsychic causative factor that warrants mention here is trauma. One reason why sexual dysfunction is so prevalent is that sexuality is an intensely pleasurable and powerful drive that cannot be repressed; at the same time it is a response that is readily associated with pain, and is easily traumatized, impaired, or distorted. Trauma may be physical or emotional, and the degree of sexual dysfunction may depend on the degree and extent of the trauma. After extreme trauma, an individual may never respond sexually again. However, so radical a consequence usually does not occur. Most persons adapt to the negative contingencies connected with sexual expression during childhood by varying degrees of denial of sexuality. Erotic impulses are not acknowledged or are dehumanized; or they may be considered dirty and shameful. Sexuality is not eliminated, however, since it is so powerful and pleasurable; what does occur is some form of sexual dysfunction. Few in our culture are so traumatized as to never function sexually at all; at the same time, few of us escape some contamination of our pleasure-imbuing erotic drive with sexual conflict.

Irrational fears may be another source of sexual anxiety. These may be considered causative factors since recognizing their existence, understanding their implications, and expressing the feelings attached to them can lead to improvement in sexual functioning. Several recurrent categories of irrational fear have been identified:

Conscience — "Sex is dirty, evil, wrong and will be punished."

Loss of control — "I will be swept away to an unknown terrible fate or I will get sick and die or I will be overwhelmed, engulfed, lost."

Aggression — "I might hurt myself or my partner."

Inadequacy — "My true nonworth will be discovered; I am unlovable; I will be abandoned; I'm nothing without my sexual organs."

Secret revelations — "My hidden fantasies or past will be revealed or discovered."

These are powerful, persistent, and sometimes unconscious ideas. They may exist in nondysfunctional persons, although with lesser impact; and, in fact, some of these fears are temporarily present during normal psychosocial development (Levine, 1976).

Two other intrapsychic explanations of sexual anxiety are more speculative and less specific. The theory of developmental influences has been advanced in an effort to understand the factors that account for the persistence of such things as irrational ideas, poor judgment about sexual behavior and partner choice, and prevention of Oedipal conflict resolution. It has been considered that these factors may not be sexual at all, but rather may depend upon the adequacy with which the person threaded the maze of psychosocial development during childhood. If the individual experienced events that made the resolution of psychosocial developmental tasks more difficult, then this may explain the tenacity of some sexual anxiety. Examples of possible causes for sexual anxiety in this framework are premature separation, excessive intimacy, parental rejection, sexual

trauma, and misrepresentation of reality supported by ignorance or religious orthodoxy. Levine (1976) makes the point that this conceptualization of causative factors is based on common sense and experimental data, not on fundamental research; therefore, it may be suspect.

An even more diffuse conception of intrapsychic causation is the view that sexual function and dysfunction are expressions of character. Because sexual life is the product of past conflicts, adaptations, and capacities, it is the potential reflection of the entire inner person. Dysfunction is thought to be affected by such things as capacity to form relationships, maturational accomplishments, self-concept, character style, energy level, tolerance for pleasure, and whatever current psychologic issues the individual is facing. This conceptualization is attractive in that it takes into account the interrelatedness of all psychologic forces; however, its very generality limits its usefulness (Levine, 1976).

A final general causative factor, which has been alluded to in the discussion of many of the other factors, is culture. The negative effects of our culture on sexual functioning are great. Many childrearing techniques are sexually restrictive, and sex-role stereotypes reinforce negative sexual self-concepts. The Victorian influence of sex roles is with us still and affects how we express our sexuality and what we expect of ourselves sexually. Specific cultural influences will be discussed under specific sexual dysfunctions (see also Chapter 6).

GENERAL THERAPEUTIC APPROACHES

Because sexual dysfunctions vary from person to person, a wide variety of treatment approaches and methods is used. The complexity of the cause is directly related to the ease or difficulty of treatment and its long-term success. In many cases the root of the difficulty is ignorance about sexual techniques or general misinformation about sex that can easily be corrected with sexual counseling. In other instances, in which the causes are more complex and dysfunction develops from fear of failure, of loss of control, of rejection, or performance anxiety, brief sex therapy focuses on improving communication skills between the couple and adding to their repertoire of sexual skills.

There are other clients whose performance anxiety and fear of rejection are more deeply rooted in marked conflict and severe insecurity. In this case therapy must include alleviating the conflict issues, whether intrapsychic or interpersonal; and the disturbed relationship of the couple and the poor self-esteem and guilt following sex must be considered. In these cases the therapist must be able to recognize the psychodynamics of unconscious conflict, know when to use sex therapy or psychotherapy, and be able to either provide appropriate therapy or refer the couple to another therapist. There is a final group of clients who are not appropriate candidates for sex therapy; their psychopathology is so profound and the defense systems they use are so rigid that extensive psychotherapy is needed before sex therapy can be beneficial (Kaplan, 1974a).

A variety of therapeutic approaches is being used today. In this chapter we will discuss the more commonly used and the more effective therapy modalities: psychoanalytic, behavioral, Masters and Johnson, Kaplan, and group approaches.

Psychoanalytic treatment

Traditionally, symptoms of sexual dysfunction have been considered to be almost invariably manifestations of deep-seated psychologic problems resolvable only with long-term individual psychotherapy. This approach assumes that dysfunction is caused by intrapsychic conflicts that occurred in early psychosexual development and that dysfunction comes from the same substrate as personality and neurotic disorders. In fact, Freud believed that anyone who was in any way abnormal was *invariably* abnormal sexually.

Other psychoanalysts have conceptualized psychopathology as collections of irrational beliefs and belief systems associated with expectation of injury or adverse effects, leading to maladaptive reactions and behaviors developed to prevent, minimize, or avoid the anticipated injury. At the same time behaviors are directed at repairing injuries already sustained or thought to be sustained. The basic goal of psychoanalytic therapy is extinction of the irrational belief systems, which are often unconscious. The conscious identification of the irrational belief system is considered crucial in psychoanalysis—it is the gaining of insight.

Despite increasing use of other therapeutic techniques psychoanalysts as a whole still rely heavily on insight. They believe that conscious awareness of the irrational beliefs underlying fears and maladaptive behavior offers the best chance for resolution of "neurotic" problems. If changes occur because the therapist gives permission, for example, the new behavior is dependent upon the relationship with the therapist and not on change within the individual (Bieber, 1974).

Psychoanalytic therapy is not thought to require special adaptation for use with a client experiencing sexual dysfunction (Wright, 1977). However, there do appear to be some problems specific to the treatment of sexual dysfunction. For example, although the nature of transference is thought to be the same in treatment of sexual and nonsexual dysfunction, when the content is overtly sexual, interpretation of the transference is more crucial in terms of the timing, tact, and comfort of the therapist.

The distinction must be made between a transference reaction and a client's sexual response to the therapist. To always consider a sexual response as a transferance reaction is to deny that there may be real responses by one individual who is attracted to another. Bieber (1974) states that the real problem is not the client's sexual response, but any anxiety, guilt, or shame the client feels. The analytic process assists the client to work through the *reaction*, not the sexual response. The analyst may also experience sexual feelings toward patients and these also may be biologic responses and not countertransference phenomena. Hopefully, the analyst is conscious of these feelings, comfortable with them, and can allow them to remain a sexual response on the part of one person to another. Recognition of these feelings is one thing; acting on them is another entirely. It is totally inappropriate for an analyst to act out sexual feelings in any way or to be seductive (Bieber, 1974).

If there is any area in which it is crucial that the therapist resolve his or her own irrational beliefs and biases, it is sex. A therapist who communicates doubts, uncertainty, residual guilt feelings, or questions about the normalcy of certain sexual behaviors will certainly hamper the client's chances to resolve sexual fears. Masturbation, incest, and promiscuity are particularly sensitive areas. However, an indiscriminate, all-permissive attitude about sexual behavior is also irresponsible.

The psychoanalytic model assumes that the conflict generating sexual dysfunction is not available to conscious thought. According to this school of thought, therapies that deal only with the present may succeed in modifying overt sexual behavior for a time, but since the underlying cause has not been dealt with, the "cure" will not last; relapse or symptom substitution will occur. Advocates of this method point out that clients who have gone through brief sex therapy often seek individual psychotherapy. These requests usually have three components: recognition of personal problems once the sexual difficulty is gone, operation of a transference left unresolved by previous sex therapy, and trouble with separation.

According to Wright (1977), no firm conclusions can be drawn as to the efficacy of psychoanalytic treatment of sexual dysfunction because the research studies reported are inconclusive, poorly done, and without controls. In selected cases the psychoanalytic approach alone might be most beneficial, particularly when the psychopathology is extensive and the defenses very rigid. This type of client is probably the exception rather than the rule, however; in the majority of cases of sexual dysfunction one of the other therapy modalities would be more helpful. It should be further noted that psychoanalysis is very expensive, time-consuming over an extended period of time, and generally used for individuals only.

Behavioral treatment

The behavioral method of treatment of sexual dysfunction is based on the assumption that human sexual behaviors are primarily the result of learning and conditioning, and that a specific learned behavior (the sexual dysfunction) must be unlearned before the dysfunction will disappear. In the absence of any physical pathology, sexual dysfunction is viewed as a learned phenomenon, maintained by performance anxiety internally and a reinforcing environment externally.

Learning theorists have identified precise conditions under which sexual symptoms may be acquired or developed. Behavioral therapists apply this knowledge to modify the dysfunctional behavior and replace it with more desirable responses. To do this, techniques based on learning principles are used. One such technique is systematic desensitization or "flooding" to relieve phobias. This has been particularly useful in treating vaginismus. The client is asked to imagine a situation that causes anxiety or tension; as soon as tension is felt, she is instructed to relax. Increasingly more intense situations are formalized until no anxiety or tension is produced.

Another important behavioral therapy technique involves the concept of sexual tasks. Specific therapeutic sexual tasks are designed, structured, and used to extinguish fears and inhibitions by gradually exposing the client to the feared situation. In addition, new and appropriate responses are learned by doing the tasks. Tasks are generally designed to reinforce more effective sexual responses and to gradually shape sexual behavior toward the goal of sexual competence. Modification of the couple's sexual system is also achieved so as to remove the rewards for sexually destructive behavior.

This therapy modality may be used for individuals, couples, and groups. The desensitization may be done in the office with the therapist or at home as a "homework" assignment. Masters and Johnson's concept of sexual tasks is based on a behavior modification approach, although they have added innovations of their own.

Behavior modification therapy is short term, less costly than psychoanalytic therapy, and may be particularly useful in dealing with phobic elements as in vaginismus. It does not consider underlying conflicts or multicausational factors of sexual dysfunction and, therefore, appears to be an incomplete method for some clients. Research data (Barbach, 1974; Labowitz and LoPiccolo, 1972) on its use in groups suggest that it can be very successful; however, other techniques and therapy modalities, such as conflict resolution and group support, are generally used in addition to desensitization and specific tasks.

The "new" sex therapy

Perhaps the greatest contribution to the treatment of human sexuality and to the ending of the "dark ages" of sex therapy was made by Masters and Johnson. The importance of their monumental pioneer research regarding the physiology of human sexual response cannot be overestimated. Their studies finally gave us an accurate picture of the basic physiology of human sexual functioning. This information opened the door to the development of rational and effective treatment of sexual disorders. Two such approaches will be described in detail.

Masters and Johnson

Before therapy is begun any organic factor causing sexual problems must be ruled out by a thorough physical examination. A basic premise of this therapy modality is that sexual response is a natural function. Human sexual behavior is a complex set of learned and instinctive phenomena that interact with cultural influences, personality dynamics, and hormonal factors. The reflex pathways of sexual functioning (penile erection and vaginal lubrication, for example) are not learned; however, psychosocial input can affect functioning, and anxiety, depression, or physical stress can disrupt it. A major misconception that operated among health care professionals for a long time is that sexually dysfunctional people can be taught to respond effectively; that is like saying we can teach someone to sweat or to breathe. Masters and Johnson emphasize that we can learn sexual behavior, but the potential to respond to sexual stimuli is instinctive. Therefore, we can learn to enhance biologic potential and can also learn ways of disrupting the natural physiologic responses. This opens the possibility of identifying obstacles to sexual functioning and suggesting ways to alleviate or circumvent them. In a similar way, negative attitudes can be unlearned and replaced with positive ones, and behavior and environmental coordinates to healthy responses can be identified and encouraged. According to Masters and Johnson, when this happens natural functioning will take over easily.

The second basic tenet is emphasis on the couple—the belief that the couple is the client and that there is no such thing as an uninvolved partner in a relationship in which there is sexual dysfunction. Masters and Johnson feel it imperative to educate both partners together rather than focusing only on the sexually dysfunctional individual. They recognize that the dysfunction may have preceded the relationship; that is, when sexual problems arise for the first time in a relationship where previously there had been no difficulty, the dysfunction may be caused by factors totally unrelated to the partner. However, at the lowest level, the functional partner is involved to the extent that sexual frustration is experienced, the relationship is disrupted, and other life areas are affected.

The third basic tenet is that a male-female therapy

team is necessary. This is rooted in the belief that men cannot fully understand female sexuality and vice versa. Neither sex can easily evaluate for the other the relationship between sexual identity and effective sexual functioning. The therapy team also serves as a role model for effective communication between a man and a woman. Moreover, it can counterbalance the possible tendency of a single therapist to inadvertently express his or her sexual value system to sexually vulnerable clients.

Masters and Johnson assume that imparting factual sexual information will relieve a significant amount of sexual dysfunction. Additionally, the couple study the dynamics of their own relationship, with a mutual educational model that allows the cotherapists to educate by modeling healthy interaction, interpreting material from both male and female perspectives, and reinforcing therapeutic content in different teaching styles.

Education is only one component of the therapy and is considered more valuable when combined with insights. Techniques of directly confronting fears about sexual performance and giving specific suggestions to overcome these fears are an integral part of the Masters and Johnson approach. Structured exercises that provide opportunity for sexual feelings to be experienced without any demands help to decrease performance anxiety and spectatoring. Verbalization of fears is encouraged as a method of reducing anxiety and also decreasing the need for spectatoring. The technique of reversing sexual dysfunction by concentrating on neutralizing performance fears and minimizing spectator roles is based on the knowledge that sexual response is a natural function and dysfunction is reversed by removing a psychologic barrier, not by teaching the individual how to function sexually.

With this conceptual framework, Masters and Johnson believe sexual dysfunction must be viewed in the context of the interpersonal relationship. While it is recognized that sexual dysfunction can be an isolated facet of a healthy relationship, their major contribution is the view that sexual distress usually arises from hostility, poor communication, double standards, unrealistic expectations, deception, etc. Therefore, therapy must focus on the relationship as a whole or important dynamics may be overlooked.

Specific therapy techniques are aimed at reestablishing positive, pleasurable sensations and attitudes toward sex and sexuality, and improving communication within the couple. Masters and Johnson believe that satisfactory sexual activity is always a way of enhancing communication between a man and woman. Sexual interaction has vast potential as a means of communication; it is a medium for exchanging trust and vulnerability.

With their belief in sex as a form of communication,

Masters and Johnson have developed techniques to improve communication skills. The focus first was on nonverbal aspects of communication and particularly the sense of touch, as the sense most identified with nonverbal communication. From this came their revolutionary concept of *sensate focus*. Sensate focus is defined as a "therapeutic technique which emphasizes the sense of touch in which body surfaces are gently, manually explored by self or partner to reestablish the sexual reactions of childhood." (McCary, 1978) For optimal effect, sensate focus is used to bring physical awareness in the partner who is touching and not specifically or solely for the sexual pleasure of the partner being touched.

In the early stages of therapy, anxiety related to performance is relieved. The emphasis is on touching as a personal sensual experience and only secondarily (if at all) as a sexual opportunity. The sensual experience consists of exploring the textures, contours, temperature, and contrasts of the partner's body in a manner and at a pace chosen by the one doing the touching. The sensate focus is usually carried out in a three-step program. In phase 1, purposeful erotic arousal (genital stimulation) is avoided. Tender gentle stroking is used to reestablish sensory reactions, remove fear of failure, and increase intimacy and mutual involvement. Intercourse is forbidden at this point. In phase 2, the couple is instructed in genital pleasuring, which involves gentle, teasing stimulation. The intent is to produce sexual arousal but not orgasm. Phase 3 is intended to produce orgasm by noncoital or coital means.

Masters and Johnson feel that for many people, verbal communication is more familiar and more comfortable, even when emotionally charged, than nonverbal communication. Therefore, a significant focus of therapy is on education in more effective communication techniques. The majority of time in therapy is devoted to this. Very often improved verbal communication skills release a couple's sexual feelings toward each other, thereby enhancing their sexual relationship.

Masters and Johnson require that a period of uninterrupted time be given to the relationship; they believe that this is essential to integrate the new techniques into existing life-style patterns. Social isolation is thought to enhance the quality of time. The couples leave their home, children, and familiar environment to participate in the therapy. The time frame is limited— daily sessions over a 2 week period. It is thought that there is significant cumulative return for clients who are exposed to sexual material on a day-to-day basis. It is easier to enhance communication skills when experiences are fresh in the mind. It is more clinically effective to evaluate sexual problems and questions as this happens, rather than after the fact. Daily exposure allows for immediate treatment of crisis (Belliveau and Richter, 1970; Masters and Johnson, 1970; 1976; 1978; McCary, 1978).

Masters and Johnson believe that traditional psychotherapeutic techniques have not been disregarded in their approach; rather, the focus of therapy has been changed. They see rapid treatment as emphasizing the interpersonal relationship and the couple rather than the individual's sexual needs or inadequacies. They do not believe that sexual dysfunction is always a symptom of underlying pathology. They do not deny that sexual dysfunction may be a symptom of underlying pathology, but they believe, emphatically, that sexual inadequacy is separate from psychopathology as often as it is a symptom of it. Also, they believe that when sexual inadequacy is a symptom, real psychotherapeutic gain might result from direct removal of the symptom. Their therapy program does not ignore individual psychodynamics and recognizes that identifying factors such as stress reactions, problems of self-esteem, psychopathology, and maladaptive defense mechanisms is essential to the efficiency and efficacy of therapy.

Masters and Johnson believe that classical patterns of transference distract from focusing therapy on the marital relationship, and move the focus to the relationship between the individual and one or both therapists. The therapy team minimizes the importance of transference. Aspects of transference are used, however, in that the authority and trust placed in the therapist can be particularly beneficial in the treatment of specific sexual dysfunctions (for example, vaginismus) (Masters and Johnson, 1976). Countertransference is also less apt to occur with a dual sex therapy team, according to Masters and Johnson. They take a strong position against any overt sexual activity between therapist and client.

The Masters and Johnson sexual therapy modality is very successful; their success rates for specific dysfunctions are high. It should be recognized, however, that their selection process is stringent and may be one reason for their high success rates. Their type of therapy is expensive because of large amounts of therapist time and the need for the couple to move from home into a motel. One additional disadvantage is that this approach is not applicable to a large part of the population (e.g., individuals, the poor, etc.). As done by Masters and Johnson, it is a highly selective therapy modality, although very successful for those who qualify and can afford it.

Kaplan

Kaplan's approach to sex therapy uses a dynamic interaction of specific sexual techniques and psychotherapy to relieve sexual dysfunction. She identifies two ways in which her sex therapy differs from other treatment mo-

dalities: (1) its goals are limited to relief of the client's symptoms, and (2) it departs from traditional techniques through the use of a combination of prescribed sexual experiences and psychotherapy. There are some commonalities with Masters and Johnson's approach, but there are essential differences as well.

The initial interventions are aimed at modifying the immediate causes and defenses against sexuality. The remote issues are dealt with only to the extent necessary to relieve the sexual symptom and to ensure the disability will not recur. Psychodynamic issues are interpreted and neurotic behavior is modified, but only if it is directly interfering with the client's sexual functioning or presenting obstacles to treatment. Treatment is considered successful when the difficulty is relieved; treatment is ended when the dysfunction is relieved and the factors directly responsible for the problem have been identified and resolved enough to assume the client's sexual functioning will remain stable.

Kaplan states that 80% of sexually dysfunctional clients can become symptom-free using sex therapy that limits itself to interventions that modify immediate blocks without making concurrent changes in basic personality structure or fundamental dynamics of the marital relationship. Kaplan's approach is first directed at immediate causation, with the understanding that deeper conflicts will be dealt with as necessary and that in the majority of cases this does not become necessary.

This approach depends upon synergy between the specific sexual task and the psychotherapeutic process. Dynamically oriented sex therapy does not use prescribed sexual interactions exclusively but an integrated combination of sexual experience and psychotherapy. Judiciously prescribed sexual interactions between the partners that are structured to relieve sexual difficulties are coupled with psychotherapeutic sessions that modify the intrapsychic and interpersonal blocks to sexual functioning and create a free, secure sexual system between the partners. This is the most effective treatment, in Kaplan's assessment. The sessions and experiences reinforce each other to reveal and remove blocks to sexual expression and also to identify and resolve personal and marital conflicts. On the basis of the initial evaluation, which includes a psychiatric examination, medical history, and physical examination if indicated, the sexual problem and possible underlying causes are provisionally diagnosed. This allows prescription of the initial sexual tasks. The couple's response to these tasks further clarifies the dynamics of the dysfunction.

Kaplan's therapy was modeled after Masters and Johnson; however, individual therapists of either gender are used. The rigid time schedule and specific sequences of sexual tasks have also been modified. No time limit is placed on treatment. The requirement of being away from home is not enforced. The most crucial difference appears to be in the conceptualization of the therapeutic process.

Kaplan's framework is more strongly rooted in the psychodynamic model and more committed to the resolution of underlying conflicts. Further, Kaplan employs a multicausal etiologic approach to sexual dysfunction that appears more eclectic than Masters and Johnson's approach. For Kaplan, the immediate causes seem more specific and similar for each of the sexual dysfunctions. When the deeper causes are considered more individual variation is taken into account.

Essentially, Kaplan views sex therapy as a task-centered form of crisis intervention, which presents an opportunity for rapid conflict resolution. To achieve this, various sexual tasks are used as well as insight therapy, supportive therapy, marital therapy, and any other psychiatric techniques that are indicated. Since a crucial ingredient of the therapy is participation in sexual exercises, only couples are treated; however, there is flexibility in the extent to which both must participate in the psychotherapeutic sessions.

Kaplan's therapeutic approach is flexible in that the various sexual and interactional tasks are used only as specifically indicated. None, including sensate focus, are routinely prescribed. The experiences are structured to achieve specific psychotherapeutic objectives, to deal with resistance to treatment, and to achieve sexual functioning. The prescribed sexual experiences appear to be effective because:

1. They alter the previously destructive sexual system and create a secure sexual environment in which the couple learns to make love in a freer, more enjoyable way.
2. The resolution of conflict is facilitated when previously avoided sexual acts are carried out.
3. The tasks stir up previously unconscious intrapsychic and interpersonal conflicts, which are thus available for psychotherapeutic intervention and resolution.

The therapeutic value of sexual tasks has been discussed before. For example, they assist the couple to unlearn destructive behavior, to get into touch with sensuous feelings, to learn new positive behavior, to resolve fear, to enhance their sexual pleasure, etc. In addition, experiential techniques have another value; they assist in the confirmation of the couple's problems. The couple's reaction to the task provides additional data to assess and confirm the problem and suggest future treatment strategies.

The sexual tasks are essential ingredients of sex therapy. Kaplan feels they are of limited value unless used with psychotherapy. The primary level of intervention or therapy is to modify immediate obstacles; these yield in part to education and clarification of sexual misinformation and to sexual experiential assignments. However, defenses and resistances are constantly mobilized by these experiences and must be handled by psychotherapeutic techniques. The unconscious conflicts or defense mechanisms must be understood and dealt with. The psychotherapeutic strategies used aim at modification of behavior by fostering insight into the unconscious forces that govern behavior. The conduct of the psychotherapeutic component of sex therapy is influenced by the limited objectives of relieving the sexual problem; therefore, interpretation is usually limited to those aspects of client behavior that directly influence sexual functioning—defenses against sexuality and/or resistance to the treatment process. The therapist first uses the simplest type of insight-producing tactics and proceeds to deeper levels only if necessary. Techniques to handle resistance may range from simple confrontation of self-destructive behavior patterns to analytic work with highly threatening unconscious material.

Kaplan's approach appears to be more flexible and more adaptable to individual couples than does the Masters and Johnson technique. It does not require the cotherapy approach or removal from the home environment, so the expense is somewhat less. The cure rates for various dysfunctions appear similar. The psychodynamic approach to sexual dysfunction appears to deal best with both the immediate and deeper causes of dysfunction (1974b).

Group therapy

Recently, group approaches to sex therapy have been used with good results. Barbach (1974), Labowitz and LoPiccolo (1972), and Baker and Nagata (1977) have all reported group approaches to treating sexual dysfunction. The group therapy modalities have generally used time-limited, behavior modification approaches. The groups have been composed of either all women, all men, or heterosexual couples. Focus has been on such problems as preorgasmic difficulties or dissatisfaction with sexual functioning. This type of therapy has promise in that the reported success rates are high, the cost is relatively low, and it offers therapy to an otherwise neglected population group—the individual with a sexual dysfunction who either does not have or cannot involve a partner.

The most common approaches to treating sexual dysfunction are summarized in Table 9-1. It can be seen that the approaches vary with respect to therapeutic focus, the body of theory guiding the approach, definition of the client, concepts forming the basis of therapy, the therapeutic process, and assumptions guiding the method.

Table 9-1. A comparison of approaches to treating sexual dysfunction*

	Intrapsychic	Dyadic	Behavioral-learning
Therapeutic focus	Intrapersonal conflicts	Relationship	Problem or symptom, specific and modifiable mechanisms of behavior
Theoretical base	Psychoanalytic theory	Systems theory	Social learning theory Behavior theory
Who is client?	Individual	The couple, the relationship	Individual or couple
Must both partners be involved in therapy (if there is a partner)?	No	Yes	No

What concepts form basis for therapy?	1. Concept of unconscious motivation, repression, resistance to treatment
	2. Influence of childhood experiences in shaping adult destiny
	3. Role of Oedipal conflict in production of sexual conflict
		1. Partner rejection, acceptance
		2. Communication problems
		3. Causes of marital discord including:
		  a. Transfer of feelings to partner from parents
		  b. Lack of trust
		  c. Power struggles
		  d. Contractual disappointments
		  e. Sexual sabotage such as:
		    (1) Using pressure and censure
		    (2) Using sabotaging timing
		    (3) Making oneself repulsive
		    (4) Frustrating partner's sexual desires and preferences
			1. Behaviors are conditioned
			2. When certain contingencies are present, certain behaviors occur; behaviors that are reinforced persist
			3. Behaviors, thoughts, and feelings become associated with negative labels
			4. Part of therapy is changing labels from negative to neutral or positive ones, or interrupting the connections between thoughts, feelings, behaviors, and negative labels

What points would be emphasized in sexual history?	Sources of conflicts, for example, experiences as child Developmental history emphasized	Developmental aspects important for each partner, but more important is how they *together* come to have sexual problem	1. Description of current problem 2. Onset and course, contingencies 3. Client's concept of cause and maintenance of problem 4. Past treatments and outcomes 5. Current goals and expectations
What role does therapist play?	Analyst of behavior	Counselor for relationship	Analyst of problem and its contingencies; teacher of new behaviors; can include: 1. Giving permission 2. Providing limited information 3. Giving specific suggestions 4. Providing intensive therapy

*From Woods, N. F.: Human sexuality in health and illness, ed. 2, St. Louis, 1979, The C. V. Mosby Co.

Table 9-1. A comparison of approaches to treating sexual dysfunction—cont'd

	Intrapsychic	Dyadic	Behavioral-learning
How does therapy proceed?	1. Superficial conflict is dealt with via use of techniques to attain symptom relief. Conflict is not necessarily eliminated by experientially oriented techniques, but these approaches may be more efficient than exclusive reliance on cognitive insight methods. Conflict is not ignored, but focus is on modifying immediately operating results of the conflict. *If necessary*, therapist may interpret and work with the patients' unconscious Oedipal material. 2. Many clients respond well to intervention in level of specific conflict alone. Others need additional conflict resolution. 3. Experiential techniques (structured sexual tasks) are used to foster conflict resolution by exposing client to feelings and aspects of self that have been avoided. 4. Attempt is made to help partners understand their problems intellectually, emotionally, and experientially. 5. Combination of experiential and psychoanalytic techniques (free association) is used.	1. Although primary emphasis is on sexual difficulties, this approach also focuses on pathogenic transactional dynamics. 2. Intervention focuses on modifying specific sexual interactions and communications. 3. Sometimes treatment of sexual problem can bypass marital obstacles. In other cases, basic resolution of the interactional problem must be effected first. 4. Changing sexual ambience to one of nondemand and low pressure is often essential first step.	1. Assessment of each sexual symptom and its contingencies 2. Plan for reinforcement or extinction contingencies 3. Use strategies to remove rewards from sexual symptom, to punish undesired sexual reaction, or to extinguish fear
What assumptions are basic to method?	Client's sexual symptoms are expressions of deeper conflicts that derive from childhood; sexual pleasure becomes associated with guilt as a result of child-rearing practices and constrictive upbringing.	Sexual difficulties spring directly from destructive sexual system.	Sexual symptoms occur because of reinforcing or negative contingencies. Sexual symptoms are learned inhibitions.

ETIOLOGY OF FEMALE SEXUAL DYSFUNCTION

Many of the causes or factors contributing to female sexual dysfunction are similar regardless of the dysfunction; what appears to differ are the coping abilities or defenses that evoke certain dysfunctional patterns and the immediate causes that trigger a dysfunctional response. To avoid repetition, an overview of common causes that contribute to all female sexual dysfunction will be given; the causative factors specific to each dysfunction will be considered later. Only etiologic factors having particular relevance to women will be considered; a basic review of causative factors in sexual dysfunction has already been presented.

Organic illness and drugs

Only a small percentage of female sexual dysfunction results from physical factors, according to Masters and Johnson (1970). Also, the female response cycle seems relatively less vulnerable to physical illness than the male. Chronic disease and age do not seem to affect sexual response as early or as severely as in the male. Very few diseases specifically affect sexual functioning in women, except as they cause general debilitation. Drug use and abuse can contribute to female sexual disorders; drugs that depress the central nervous system (narcotics, opiates, etc.), minor tranquilizers, and birth control pills have all been implicated. Again, men seem more vulnerable than women. Stress, fatigue, drugs, and illness can all have a detrimental effect on full sexual expression. Another physical factor that has not been clearly studied is obesity, which can interfere with sexual functioning on both an organic and psychogenic level (see Chapter 21).

Psychologic causes: situational

Female sexual dysfunction can be best understood in terms of the essential prerequisites of sexual response. First, adequate stimulation is essential for response to take place. Second, the woman must be sufficiently relaxed to be able to respond to the stimuli and to abandon herself to the sexual experience. Finally, if a specific learned inhibition of the orgasmic response is present, sexual functioning will be impaired.

Many women do not receive adequate stimulation during lovemaking and therefore the sexual response cycle does not begin. The arousal patterns of women are more variable than those of men: they are slower to respond, need more extensive gentle tactile stimulations, and need more reassurance. What stimulates also varies more. Frequently, the woman fails to assume responsibility for her own sexual pleasure, due in large part to cultural conditioning. There may also be deep-seated intrapsychic or interpersonal dynamics on the part of both or either partner that prevent effective stimulation.

Poor communication is often a chief offender. One reason why a man may not stimulate his partner adequately is that she does not tell him what she needs. Cultural conditioning plays a large part in many women's inability to communicate their needs. It should be noted that a woman's reluctance to express her needs is not always based on cultural stereotypes. Some men are repelled by assertive sexual behavior by women; if her partner is such a man, a woman may run a real risk of rejection if she behaves in a sexually assertive manner (Kaplan, 1974b).

It is common in our culture to assume that sex is the man's responsibility and that it is unfeminine to be sexually assertive. Another myth often perpetuated in our culture is that sexual compliance and self-sacrifice are equated with the perfect female lover. These beliefs are tied to the Victorian belief that sexual pleasure is sinful and shameful for women. To seek sexual pleasure evokes strong guilt feelings and anxiety on the part of many women. In our society sexual passivity has been the rule for women; actively seeking out sexual pleasure is considered to be aggressive, unfeminine, and selfish. A consideration of the Victorian views of sex helps explain where these myths and belief systems arose.

The Victorian era had a profound effect (primarily repressive) on female sexuality. The prevailing message was chastity and continence even in marriage; self-control was all important even though this meant denial of sexual desires and avoidance of all temptations, especially for the female. Sexual intercourse was permissible only for the purpose of procreation within the marital relationship. A female was to avoid all sources of possible sexual stimuli—everything from romantic novels to dancing to genital touching; the worst was masturbation, which brought the threat of disease, mental derangement, and future childbirth complications. Women were to be passive at all times in their interactions with men; boldness and immodesty were wrong because of their effect on the man, who might lose control. Remnants of this belief system can still be seen in the prevalent notion that it is up to the adolescent girl to say "no" and set the boundaries beyond which no sexual activity will take place.

Most women in the Victorian era, and even more recently, entered marriage ignorant of sex; emphasis was on avoidance and restraint. Women were expected to submit but experience no pleasure; orgasm was avoided since it supposedly interfered with conception. It should be noted that this derogation of sex was a residual of the ascetic doctrine of early Christianity. The effect of all of these views—as widely disseminated by physicians and the clergy—was to generate a climate of attitudes that have had a profound effect on our ideas about female sexuality and have influenced psychoanalytic views of female sexuality (Williams, 1977).

In dealing with a woman whose sexual dysfunction is based on inability to express or assume responsibility for her sexual needs, it is necessary to alter the couple's sexual system, rather than to teach new erotic techniques. The woman must learn to assume a share of the responsibility for her sexual pleasure, to develop a measure of sexual autonomy. Further, she must learn to feel comfortable with such autonomy. To achieve this, she must be able to communicate her sexual desires openly without demand or defensiveness; the partner also will need to learn this. In essence, the couple learns to negotiate and compromise realistically about sex (Kaplan, 1974b).

It was noted above that in order to have good, satisfying sex, the woman must be able to abandon herself to her erotic feelings and allow herself loss of control. Regardless of its source, anxiety about sex can give rise to defenses that prevent abandonment. Often the woman's ability to relax and give way to the sexual experience is blocked by fear of rejection. The inability of some women to become sexually aroused even with adequate stimulation probably indicates some underlying sexual conflict. If conflict is present, then erotic feelings awaken anxiety. When this happens, the woman prevents herself from feeling anxious by not only avoiding sexual stimulation but also by not allowing herself to feel sexually aroused through the use of defense mechanisms. A commonly used defense mechanism is obsessive intellectualization, which exerts conscious control over the sexual experience. The woman becomes a spectator of herself; she becomes judge and jury of her performance, always watching to see if she is performing "satisfactorily" or, more often, pleasing her partner. It should not surprise anyone that these mental exercises make it impossible for her to relax and to abandon herself to the erotic experience in a way that is essential to adequate sexual functioning.

Intrapsychic causes

Until recently, explanations of sexual dysfunction focused primarily on unconscious intrapsychic and transactional causes; situational, dyadic, and cultural factors were largely ignored. With the advent of brief treatment methods, which focus more on modifying immediate antecedents to dysfunction, often with dramatic success, the usefulness of the traditional approaches has been questioned. However, it is important to understand both, for while brief therapy will often remove immediate obstacles to adequate sexual functioning and restore it for the time being, there may be more deep-seated problems that need to be recognized and perhaps treated with longer-term therapy. The unconscious factors operating in female sexual dysfunction have their roots in early psychosexual development; they evoke negative emotional feelings during lovemaking, and defenses come into play to prevent the woman from experiencing these feelings. Kaplan identifies three factors most frequently implicated in the development of female sexual problems:

1. A woman's unconscious, unresolved conflicts about sexuality
2. A disturbed relationship with her partner
3. Unconscious guilt resulting from repressive culture in regard to expression of sexuality in general and impulses toward assertiveness and independence

Psychoanalytic theories identify two specific causes of dysfunction: Oedipal conflict and penis envy. If Oedipal conflict is not resolved, subsequent sexual behavior may be pathologic. For example, sexual response may be inhibited because a woman's partner reminds her of her father and reactivates her sexual feelings toward the forbidden love object. Or incestuous wishes and hostile feelings may make her feel too guilty to enjoy sex. Or there may be, on an unconscious level, a fear that if she abandons herself totally to sexual feelings, she will be either destroyed or abandoned by a jealous mother.

Penis envy supposedly occurs in girls ages 3 to 5 years; if it continues, then sexual dysfunction will occur later. Healthy adult psychosexual adjustment depends on the girl's reaction to her realization that she is deprived of a penis and on her ability to cope with the feelings of envy, rage, inferiority, guilt, etc., that supposedly occur with the realization. According to psychoanalytic theory, two types of outcomes are possible:

1. Healthy girls resolve their anger at being "short-changed" and are able to accept the feminine role with a minimum of conflict. (Feminine role here means being passive-receptive, having a sexual preference for "vaginal" orgasm, and repudiating clitoral eroticism.)
2. There are two neurotic outcomes. One is a flight from womanhood into being competitive, driving, and aggressive. The woman's aim is allegedly to deny that she does not have a penis by adopting stereotypic male sex-role behavior. Other women appear to be feminine on the surface, but harbor hatred toward men and behave in "castrating" or destructive ways toward them.

According to psychoanalytic theory, women who do not resolve their penis envy develop sexual dysfunction later—specifically vaginismus (which expresses the unconscious wish to castrate a man) and orgasmic difficulties because the transition from clitoral to vaginal orgasms is never made. Kaplan (1974b) states that what is frequently seen clinically is the sexually dysfunctional woman with evidence of unresolved Oedipal conflicts, which are expressed by the client's avoidance of sexual stimulation as a result of her unconscious tendency to equate marital sex with sexual pleasure with her father.

There have been numerous books and articles written to refute the hypothesis of penis envy. (The reader is referred to any of the current feminist literature.) An alternative, more rational hypothesis to explain the anger and envy that some women feel toward men can be found in the female sex-role stereotypes in our society in which women are repressed, insecure, and exploited. From early on, little girls are confronted with the differences between men and women and told that to be a man in our society is better—not anatomically, but from the standpoint of privilege and opportunities. Women are taught to be helpless and dependent upon men and often are taught that the price to be paid for security is submission to the needs of a man. The woman's worth as a person is seen only in terms of her mate. This can create conflict, particularly if the woman is bright and gifted. As women attempt to develop careers and to become persons in their own right, these conflicts may become increasingly apparent, with subsequent increase in sexual dysfunction.

Relationship issues often play a large part in female sexual dysfunction. The female's ability to respond is influenced by the quality of the relationship with her partner to a far greater extent than is true for the male. It is not clear to what extent this is culturally determined and related to learned dependency needs. And it may not be necessary to determine how much is biologic and how much is otherwise. What is important is that for a woman, the relationship must be good before sex can be good. She must be able to view her partner in a positive and loving way. Power struggles and hidden hostilities within the relationship are important sources of sexual dysfunction in women.

Fear of pregnancy may be another psychologic factor in sexual dysfunction. It is impossible to relax or let go if one is always unconsciously or consciously fearful of pregnancy. For some women, pregnancy fears haunt their reproductive years and they report becoming orgasmic for the first time when they are in fact pregnant or after menopause. Pregnancy fears may be linked with dependency fears and fears of rejection. Associated with this is lack of trust in birth control methods (Flowers, 1977).

Unconscious conflicts about sexuality, fear, shame, and guilt; conflicts about the female role, about independence/dependence, and activity/passivity; fear of men, of losing control, of rejection and abandonment, of pregnancy; poor self-concept, a negative marital relationship, and severe psychopathology can all be factors in causing any or all of the female sexual dysfunctions. They can exist, however, without causing any dysfunction.

Whether or not these factors cause dysfunction, depends more on how the woman handles them than on the causes themselves. Different defenses against the same conflicts will produce different sexual dysfunctions.

CLASSIFICATION OF SEXUAL DYSFUNCTION

Women's concerns about sexual functioning tend to cluster around three themes; orgasmic difficulties; pain associated with coitus, and lack of interest or feeling. In this section we will consider (1) general sexual dysfunction, (2) orgasmic dysfunction, and (3) vaginismus.

General sexual dysfunction

General sexual dysfunction is the most severe of the female inhibitions. The woman suffering from this type of dysfunction is basically devoid of erotic feeling and responses; she feels no sexual pleasure from sexual stimulation. On a physiologic level, there is no significant lubrication or sign of genital vasocongestion. Interestingly, sexually unresponsive women may vary considerably in their view of the sexual experience; many consider it an ordeal to be avoided if at all possible; they may find coitus disgusting or frightening. Others, while they do not find sexual contact particularly stimulating, may endure it to preserve the marital relationship. A third group of women, while not experiencing erotic pleasure in sexual contact, do enjoy the closeness, the cuddling and body contact, and derive distinct satisfaction from the emotional and physical closeness of intercourse. Some of these women, although they have no erotic feelings in foreplay and show no signs of sexual arousal, will experience orgasm rather easily once intercourse is begun.

Primary general sexual dysfunction occurs among those women who have never experienced erotic pleasure; secondary dysfunction occurs in those women who have responded at one time to sexual stimulation but no longer do so. Typically, these clients were aroused by petting but when intercourse became the exclusive object of sexual encounters, they lost the ability to respond. The more inhibited woman is the most difficult to treat. The prognosis is much better if the woman has some degree of responsiveness, or if she has been responsive in the past but is not now because of situational factors.

In contrast to men, women display far more variation in their reactions to their inability to respond sexually. For a man, erectile dysfunction is almost always a disaster; women's reactions to sexual inhibition range from intense distress to casual acceptance.

Some women endure the situation and use their bodies mechanically to bring intercourse to an end as soon as possible. Usually, these women eventually come to resent this situation. Always seeing another's intense sexual pleasure and satisfaction while feeling little or nothing eventually becomes frustrating and disappointing for these women. Some women appear to accept this while others develop antagonism toward sex and hostility toward their partner; still others become depressed, turning their anger inward. These women are often afraid to openly refuse to have sex and resort to subterfuge to avoid intercourse—the "not tonight, dear, I have a headache" syndrome. Illness, fatigue, and arguments are often used as excuses. Partners also vary greatly in their response to the woman's inability to respond sexually. Some accept it as a matter of course. Others attribute the woman's problem to their own inadequacies and may view it as a rejection. In order to deal with their own feelings of inadequacy, they may pressure the woman to perform, which only inhibits her further. Still other men are genuinely concerned about their partner's inability to respond and wish to assist in a positive way.

The differences between the psychologic responses of men and women to sexual dysfunction are in part cultural. In all cultures, the man is expected to perform sexually; therefore, inability to perform is pathologic. Women, at least until the present, have not been subject to the same pressure to be sexually responsive. In our culture today, two dichotomous view points are beginning to be seen: (1) woman's role in sexuality is to give pleasure and bear children, and (2) it is the woman's right (and perhaps responsibility) to respond sexually and to enjoy sex. When the former view is taken, we find physicians and clergy (especially male) assuring sexually unresponsive women that their lack of response is perfectly normal and advising them to adjust to their inorgasmic state. For those who hold the second view point, lack of sexual responsiveness in a woman is seen as a problem or a sign of pathology.

The point should be made that what produces emotional problems is not lack of sexual responsiveness or sexual abstinence per se, but rather the individual's negative attitude toward sexual deprivation. Kaplan (1974b) states that if an individual consciously gives up erotic gratification, accepts a nonsexual life and is not angered, frustrated, and disappointed by the deprivation, it is possible to sublimate and suppress sexual desire without visible psychologic damage. However, Kaplan emphasizes that the sequelae of general sexual unresponsiveness are not always benign; to the contrary. This may have severe adverse effects on a woman's mental health and on the quality of her marriage.

Treatment

Ellis (1961) recommends treatment through self-therapy combined with any other medical or psychologic treatment that seems indicated. Some of Ellis' suggestions are:

1. Selection of an appropriate time for sexual activity, when the woman feels rested and trouble free.
2. Discord between partners should be at a minimum when sex is attempted.
3. Most effective are expressions of kindness, love, and consideration.
4. The partner should be aware of those areas of the woman's body that are most responsive to sexual stimulation. These should be caressed.
5. Rest for a brief time between arousal efforts is often effective.
6. Genital, particularly clitoral, stimulation should precede intromission.
7. The use of sexual fantasy by the woman is helpful. Sexually arousing conversation may be beneficial.
8. The partner's emphasis on interest in the woman is helpful.
9. If arousal occurs but the woman is to some extent sexually insensitive, then one or more of the following procedures are recommended: steady and rhythmic pressure, intermittent or forceful stroking, and verbal encouragements. A woman's stimulating herself is often a valuable aid to her partner's attempts at arousing her.

Briefly, the objectives of treatment of general female sexual inhibition are to first make the sexual environment relaxed and nonthreatening so that anxiety and subsequent defenses against sex are not evoked. Second, the woman must be sensitized and helped to "get in touch" with her own sexual sensations; her conscious awareness of erotic feelings must be raised. Finally, the guilt and fear of rejection that many women experience and which blocks their ability to communicate with their partner—and their ability to ask for and receive effective stimulation—must be removed. To achieve these, Kaplan recommends a combination of systematically structured erotic experiences for the couple, with psychotherapy. The former (brief sex therapy) facilitates the achievement of all three objectives while the latter deals with the intrapsychic and transactional roots of the woman's difficulties as they crop up in the course of treatment. On an experiential level, the therapist prescribes sexual tasks that attempt to implement the goals of creating a nondemanding, sensous ambience, open communication, and heightening of the women's sexual awareness. These tasks are sensate focus exercises, genital stimulation, and nondemand coitus.

Each couple's prescribed experiences vary with their specific needs. Usually, however, the first week or two is a period of orgasmic and coital absence for both. Masters and Johnson's technique of sensate focus (described earlier) is an invaluable tool. The woman is taught to know what parts of her body are most sensitive to stimulation and what movements are most pleasurable. At first genital areas are omitted; later, as she begins to feel sensous pleasure, nondemanding genital play is introduced. By telling the woman to act first, guilt about receiving and fear of rejection are decreased. The woman is encouraged to be "selfish" by not being concerned about her partner at this point. The woman is freed of the pressure to perform or to "service" her partner. Freed of these pressures, often erotic, sensuous sensations are experienced for the first time. She begins to assume more responsibility for her own sexual fulfillment. She learns to be less passive and more active on her own behalf. She learns that her partner will not reject her if she asks for caressing and stimulation. The pleasure felt helps overcome shame and guilt. At the same time, therapy sessions are used to deal with resistance to sexual enjoyment and obstacles to treatment that are evoked by the experience.

Later, intercourse is introduced when a high level of erotic feeling is experienced during genital stimulation exercises. Often these women have little awareness of vaginal sensations; the initial object of coitus is to raise the woman's vaginal consciousness. The woman-superior position is considered to be most favorable; it allows the woman to direct coitus to her advantage. Women also find that Kegel exercises during thrusting produce new erotic sensations. If the partner's urge to ejaculate becomes too intense, the couple separates and the man stimulates the woman until intercourse can be resumed. The cycle is repeated until the woman feels that she can reach orgasm; if she does not want to try, the couple proceeds with intercourse until the partner climaxes. Nondemand, pleasure-oriented sexual experiences have several advantages. They are not as likely to mobilize anxiety and defenses that block erotic responses. The acts are designed specifically for erotic pleasure. Both the woman and her partner become more perceptive of the other's needs and responses.

Another essential ingredient is the stressing of basic tools of open communication; learning to talk to each other about such a sensitive topic without fear of recrimination or rejection is crucial. The new experiences may evoke intense feelings in both partners. Sexual activity is now governed by the woman; role reversal has occurred in many cases. This can be extremely threatening to both. Kaplan stresses that these experiences are integrated with psychotherapeutic sessions. This combination of experiential and psychodynamic treatment seems to be the most effective.

According to Munjock and Kanno's (1976) review of the literature on the effectiveness of various treatment methods for female sexual dysfunction, psychologic therapy is of some value, with the most successful outcomes reported for the short-term behavioral methods. Kinsey's (1953) research supports the conclusion that psychologic interventions effect change; he found that after 1 year, spontaneously remission of lack of or-

gasmic response occurred very slowly: 25% of females married 1 year were nonorgasmic during intercourse and it took 15 years for this figure to drop to 10%.

In a later study on the prognosis of treatment of female sexual inhibition, Munjock and Kanno (1977) concluded that a fair amount of evidence supports the following:

1. A good prognosis can be expected if the dysfunction results from misinformation or acute situational stress, particularly in women with previous satisfying sexual experiences.
2. No matter what the therapeutic approach, milder symptoms, short duration, and young age are associated with better results.
3. A good marital relationship is helpful for favorable progress.
4. If female sexual dysfunction exists in conjunction with marital discord, pervasive psychologic disturbance, or severe anxiety, these factors will interfere with psychotherapeutic efforts.
5. Extensive nonsexual psychopathology makes therapy more difficult and decreases the chance of success.
6. There is little research to support the notion that a cooperative, nonsymptomatic male sexual partner will facilitate therapy even though this appears to be common sense.
7. Research does not clearly support the superiority of unit treatment over individual.
8. The husband's presence is less crucial where there is a high level of sexual guilt and/or anxiety coupled with a good marital adjustment and treatment is by desensitization.
9. Dual sex therapy has not yet been proved to produce results significantly superior to the one therapist approach.

There is considerable research to support the following conclusions regarding the treatment of female sexual inhibition.

1. High levels of sexual anxiety (including performance anxiety), fear of failure, and severe traumatic sexual phobias indicate poor prognosis using methods other than desensitization. When there are specific, clear-cut fears inhibiting sexual pleasures, systematic desensitization can improve the prognosis substantially.
2. For clients without pervasive psychologic disturbances behavioral approaches using education, retraining techniques, and other learning strategies substantially improve treatment results while shortening therapy time.

Orgasmic dysfunction

Orgasmic difficulties are probably the most common sexual complaint of women and yet, as noted above, this is the most confused, muddled topic in sex therapy. In contrast to general sexual dysfunction, the woman with orgasmic dysfunction is sexually responsive, perhaps intensely so. She may seek out sexual contact, respond to sexual stimuli with erotic feelings, vaginal lubrication, and genital vasocongestion, and often enjoys intercourse and penetration, but she cannot get beyond the plateau stage. The orgasmic component of the sexual response cycle is inhibited. This type of dysfunction may be primary, in which the woman has never experienced an orgasm, or secondary if the disorder develops after a period of being able to reach orgasm. It may also be absolute or situational. If absolute, the woman is unable to achieve orgasm, either coital or clitoral induced, under any circumstances. If it is situational, she can climax but only under specific circumstances.

Some women adapt to the fact that they do not climax or have great difficulty in achieving orgasm without negative psychologic consequences. These women tend to deny the importance of orgasm and are able to enjoy the nonorgasmic aspects of sexuality. Some women simulate coital orgasm; after repeated "disappointments" over time, these women become progressively disinterested in sex. In other cases the woman's distress and her anticipation of failure may be intense enough to cause a secondary general lack of responsiveness that cannot be dealt with until the inhibited orgasmic reflex is restored. This is analogous to secondary impotence, which may occur in some cases of premature or retarded ejaculation. Finally, there are those women who are very upset and angry at their chronic inability to have an orgasm.

General causes of orgasmic dysfunction have already been discussed. Briefly, orgasm may be inhibited because it has acquired some symbolic meaning to the woman or because the intensity of the experience is frightening. Other factors involved may be ambivalence about the relationship, fears of abandonment or rejection, guilt, and hostility toward males. All combine to establish an involuntary "overcontrol" of the orgasm reflex. In nonorgasmic women, fear of losing control over feelings and behavior is very prevalent. The defense for this fear is "holding back" and overcontrol. The essential pathology—that is, the immediate one—is the involuntary inhibitor of the orgasmic reflex. It is easy to condition the female orgasm and it is highly susceptible to inhibition. Usually the woman is not conscious of the conditioning response.

Treatment. The primary objective is to decrease or obliterate involuntary overcontrol of the orgasmic reflex. Various forms of psychotherapy and counseling are excellent; again, an approach that combines both specific prescribed sexual experiences or tasks and psychotherapy appears to be most beneficial and successful.

The essential problem is to establish an environment that enables the woman to learn how to release the in-

voluntary control of her orgasmic response. Basically, she is taught to focus attention on sensations associated with increasing sexual excitement, particularly maximizing clitoral stimulation. At the same time, the woman learns to allow the sensations to flow freely to natural conclusion—orgasm—rather than inhibiting them. Through psychotherapy the woman becomes aware of her sexual conflicts and attempts to resolve them. Behavior modification is used to learn how to cease interfering with the natural progression of the sexual response cycle. Different specific techniques are used for the two types of orgasmic dysfunction and will be discussed separately.

The initial objective in treating a woman who has never had an orgasm is to help her have her first climax. This is usually most easily done by self-stimulation in a situation where stimulation is maximized and inhibition is minimized, usually by masturbation to orgasm while alone. Often guilt and fear about masturbation must be dealt with and worked through first. Therapy also often reveals that the woman does not know what to expect in orgasms; fears of dying or of liking it so much that she will become promiscuous are expressed. Early in the treatment, the nonorgasmic woman should be told what an orgasm is like and what to expect. Then instructions in clitoral stimulation are given. Stimulation may be manual or with a vibrator. Manual stimulation is preferable because it encourages the woman to become comfortable touching her body. Contraction of the pubococcygeus muscles and coital thrusting are also taught. Sometimes this is enough to produce orgasm. Usually, however, the inhibitions against sexuality and letting go are so strong that distraction through fantasy is necessary. Many women are guilty and anxious about their fantasies so that the content of the fantasies must be explored. The woman may need reassurance that fantasy of all sorts is normal and does not mean she is "sick," or "abnormal" or that she is going to act on the fantasy. Fantasy while stimulating herself is used to deactivate the usual intellectual processes. These tactics are usually highly successful and in a brief time period the woman is orgasmic with masturbation. This is a crucial transitional step in treatment, which then proceeds to attempt to have the woman experience orgasm with a partner.

Only about 8% of all woman are totally anorgasmic. Far more common is the situationally nonorgasmic woman. The woman can achieve orgasm under some circumstances—with masturbation alone but not with a partner; or with clitoral stimulation but not with coitus—or she has achieved it at some previous time. Treatment is aimed at removing the blocks to total orgasmic freedom. Some situationally nonorgasmic women have specific unconscious fears of letting go in the presence of men or a specific man. Fears of rejection and obsessive concern with another's pleasure also block release. There may be unconscious conflicts about coitus and penetration. These types of fears and conflicts must be dealt with through psychotherapy before orgasm can occur with coitus. Whatever the situational block is it must be discovered and dealt with.

Perhaps the most common complaint is that of the woman who is orgasmic with clitoral stimulation but not intercourse. As stated before it is questionable whether or not this is dysfunctional, but if it is a problem for the woman, then it is worthy of treatment. Several methods are used to increase clitoral stimulation during intercourse and to heighten vaginal sensations such as leisurely foreplay, female superior position, contraction of vaginal muscles during intercourse, etc.

Once the woman achieves orgasm alone, the second stage of conditioning is begun, which includes her partner. The approach is often gradual—orgasm while he is in the room, to while he is holding her, to his masturbating her to orgasm. The third step, following sensate focus and nondemand coitus, is a crucial technique called the bridge maneuver. The couple make love until the woman is aroused; then vaginal penetration using the female-astride or side-by-side position occurs. The man then stimulates the woman's clitoris with the penis in the vagina. When she is near orgasm, clitoral stimulation stops at her signal and active thrusting is begun to bring about orgasm. The shift in stimulation sometimes causes arousal to decrease, especially at first; if it does, the couple returns to the combined coitus—direct clitoral stimulation until the point just before orgasm is reached. Once again clitoral stimulation is stopped and quick coital thrusts are used to stimulate the clitorus between the two pubic bones. Orgasm almost always occurs! At times the woman is worried that the partner may find this tedious, and this needs to be discussed. Also, any psychologic material evoked by these experiences needs to be discussed (Kaplan, 1975a, 1978; McCary, 1978).

Masters and Johnson (1970) report an 83.4% success rate on their treatments of primary orgasmic dysfunction and 72.2% in situational dysfunction—80.7% overall. Kaplan (1974a) estimates that 90% of all American women are able to achieve orgasm through one way or another, although perhaps less than 50% reach orgasm regularly through intercourse.

Vaginismus

Vaginismus is a relatively rare female sexual dysfunction. Anatomically, the genitalia of a woman suffering from vaginismus are normal; but, whenever penile penetration is attempted, the vaginal muscles snap shut so tightly that intercourse is impossible. Vaginismus is a common cause of unconsummated marriage. The condition is caused by an involuntary spasm of the muscles surrounding the vaginal orifice, which occurs whenever an attempt is made to place any object in the vagina. Attempts to introduce the penis will cause agonizing pain.

In addition to the primary spasm of the vaginal inlet, women with vaginismus are usually afraid of vaginal penetration and intercourse. Vaginismus can be associated with other forms of female sexual dysfunction but this is not always the case. Many women who seek treatment for vaginismus are sexually responsive and orgasmic. It is necessary to treat vaginismus as a separate syndrome and to rule out any physical conditions that may be causing it. A pelvic examination must always be done.

Vaginismus cannot be treated lightly or ignored since it makes intercourse impossible. It can be devastating for both partners. Apart from the physical pain caused by repeated attempts to penetrate, the woman may feel frightened, frustrated, humiliated, and inadequate; fears of abandonment may also develop. It should surprise no one that with time, the woman attempts to avoid all sexual activities. This helps relieve the anxiety, which then reinforces the avoidance pattern and the maintenance of vaginismus. The man's reaction will vary depending upon his own psychologic and sexual vulnerability. He may be merely frustrated or experience her dysfunction as rejection. His sexual functioning may remain intact or he may develop secondary impotence.

Masters and Johnson (1970) believe that vaginismus is most often caused by the woman's reaction to an erectilely dysfunctional male whose repeated attempts at intercourse followed by failure so frustrate the female that she protects herself on a subconscious level by closing the vagina itself. Other important causes are fear or guilt about intercourse, including anticipated pain of first intercourse; prior sexual trauma such as rape; strict religious orthodoxy; and attempted heterosexual activity by woman with prior homosexual identification.

Kaplan (1974a) believes that any adverse stimuli associated with intercourse or vaginal entry can cause the conditioned response that results from association of pain or fear with attempts at or even fantasies of vaginal penetration. The original stimulus could be either psychologic or physical. Therefore, there can be a wide variety of factors causing the condition. Fear of men and ignorance about sex and childbirth can lead to anticipation of injury. Rigid restrictive attitudes that evoke guilt and anxiety can also cause vaginismus. Hostility toward or fear of her partner can be a contributing factor.

To summarize, the immediate cause of the vaginismic response seems to be specific. Vaginismus occurs when something negative becomes associated with the act or fantasy of vaginal penetration. The remote causes are not so clear-cut; they are multiple and may be any that produce pain or fear in association with intercourse.

Treatment

Treatment is aimed at modifying the immediate cause of the conditioned response. Deeper causes are dealt with only as this becomes necessary. The two most widely used approaches are those of Masters and Johnson and Kaplan; these will be considered in detail.

Masters and Johnson feel the most important step in treatment is physically demonstrating the existence of the involuntary vaginal spasm to both partners; anatomic diagnoses are also used. Once the couple is convinced of the vaginismus, treatment is done in privacy with the partner inserting graduated dilators under the woman's control. Intravaginal retention for several hours is encouraged. Usually the couple is ready to attempt coitus in 3 to 5 days. Once the physical symptom is relieved, Masters and Johnson feel the psychologic aspect is more easily dealt with. This includes explanation of the origin of the symptom and information to overcome the ignorance of sexual responsiveness usually found in these clients. The sensate focus exercises are used.

Kaplan (1974a) feels the unconscious meanings of vaginismus, while interesting, are of limited relevance to treatment. In addition, the insight-oriented approach is not uniformly effective. Her approach is aimed at modifying the immediate causative agent. Deeper causes are dealt with only as they interfere with the "in vivo desensitization/conjoint therapy approach" she advocates. The technique is quite simple, assuming pain-producing conditions have been corrected. Vaginal dilators or fingers are used as a method of deconditioning the muscle spasms that prevent entry.

Prior to this the woman's phobic avoidance of vaginal penetration must be ended since it will block the deconditioning therapy. Methods to treat the phobic element are psychoanalysis, hypnosis, and behavior therapy. In the latter two, systematic desensitization is used in which repeated imagery of feared situations occurs while the client stays relaxed. Most often the client fantasizes the feared sexual situation in a step-by-step manner until she can imagine penetration and remain relaxed. She then proceeds to vaginal dilation exercises using her finger, her husband's finger, or dilators.

Kaplan has seldom found it necessary to use the above-mentioned techniques to reduce the phobic element. Reassurance, support, rapid interpretation of the unconscious components of the client's fears, and confrontation of the client with the fact that she cannot be cured until she inserts something into her vagina appear to work for her. The client is taught to "stay with the unpleasant feeling." It is understood that inserting objects into her vagina is uncomfortable but she cannot be cured until she is prepared to do so. Avoidance of unpleasant affects and of the situations that evoke them is an important pathologic mechanism. It is essential that the patient achieve mastery over this. The unpleasant feelings are usually fear, tension, and anticipation of injury; most women are able to overcome these and find coitus to be a highly pleasurable experience. The period of greatest anxiety occurs just prior to the actual decision to give up the symptom, when the woman realizes she can be cured and it is now her responsibility. Anxiety usually decreases as soon as entry is successful.

Once the phobic element is dealt with, insertion of objects into the vagina progresses from one finger or small dilator to three fingers or a larger dilator. At this point, the woman usually realizes that if she can introduce three fingers without discomfort, she can probably accommodate a penis without discomfort. The sexual partner is now included by inserting his fingers in the progressive manner described above. When no muscle spasms occur, the couple is ready for penile penetration. The first intromission is crucial. The penis must be well lubricated and slowly inserted with the woman guiding it. Penile containment lasts for a few minutes and then is slowly withdrawn. The couple continues to remain close together and talk about the experience, discussing what will make the next experience easier.

Masters and Johnson (1970) report 100% cure of their 29 cases. Kaplan (1974a) states that 100% of clients can be cured by combined desensitization and progressive dilation, along with psychotherapeutic interventions as needed. However, Kaplan cautions that the cure of vaginismus may uncover other sexual dysfunctions that must then be dealt with.

NURSING ROLES AND RESPONSIBILITY

The nursing practitioner who works with women must be able to recognize a client's sexual problems and concerns, gather data, assess the client's situation, and arrive at an appropriate nursing diagnosis regarding a client's sexual dysfunction. Based on her determination of the problem, the nurse then decides whether she can intervene herself or must refer her clients to another resource for treatment. A framework for identifying clients at risk for sexual concerns and problems, and models for decision-making about the level of nursing intervention needed will be presented.

Many clients will spontaneously identify their sexual concerns or problems; however, other clients will not. A conceptual framework for identifying potential sexual problems can assist the nurse in recognizing and identifying specific sexual dysfunctions. Additionally, such a framework can alert her to potential problem areas,

Table 9-2. Framework for identification of client's sexual problems

Factor	Reason dysfunction occurs	Example
Behavior	Behavior seen as problematic by client because of excess or deficiency in frequency or duration; behavior not in appropriate form; does not occur under socially acceptable or expected conditions	Vaginismus; orgasmic difficulties
Anatomic disruptions	Changes in structural integrity (most often interruption of neural pathway)	Spinal cord injury; surgery; incompetent cervix
Physiologic alterations	Process of vasocongestion or sensory-motor conduction altered, extent of derangement and chronicity important influencing factors	Diabetes; cardiac disease
Pharmacologic agents	Drugs interfering with neurologic and circulatory mechanisms	Oral contraceptives; tranquilizers
Alteration in body image	Perception of self as unappealing with subsequent withdrawal and isolation; fear of sexual relations	Obesity; mastectomy; rape
Environmental influences	Influences inhibit or prevent ability to respond sexually	Hospitalization; institutionalization; lack of privacy in home; overcrowding
Life cycle	Certain events can influence, threaten, or disrupt sexual integrity	Menarche, pregnancy; menopause
Emotional alterations	Negative emotional states adversely affect libido and interfere with ability to form relationships	Anxiety; depression

thus facilitating case finding and anticipatory guidance. Table 9-2 presents a framework for identification of sexual problems.

Promotion of sexual health and interventions directed at eradicating sexual dysfunction are appropriate nursing roles today. Prior to assisting her clients with these concerns, the nurse must have accurate, in-depth information about human sexuality and sexual dysfunction. She must be aware of her own value system and be accepting of her own and others' sexual values, attitudes, and behaviors. The nurse should also have sufficient communication and interpersonal skills to relate easily to clients and to develop helping relationships.

The theoretical construct developed by Jack Annon (1974)—the PLISSIT model—has been used here as a framework for determining various levels of client need, nursing competence, and the need for referral. Annon believes that his model is applicable to many helping professions including nursing; it is a treatment model that does not require the extensive educational training necessary for other therapy modalities, such as the psychoanalytic or the "new" sex therapy.

The Annon model adapted for nursing is shown in Fig. 9-1. In this model, the vertical lines represent different sexual concerns or problems that clients have. The horizontal lines represent descending levels in complexity of interventions, which require increasing depth of knowledge, training, and skills on the part of the profession. With this model, the nurse can readily identify her particular level of competence, the types of skills necessary to intervene, and then decide when referral is needed.

Permission-giving means just that—often all an individual wants is sanction from someone he or she views as professional and knowledgeable. Many people want a sounding board to check out their concerns; to be reassured that they are not "bad" or "wrong" for having done, thought, or fantasized something sexual. Permission may also mean sanction *not* to do something. The nurse may give permission to think, read, talk, or fantasize about sex; to masturbate, to experiment sexually, to explore oneself or partner, to express one's sexual likes or dislikes. She may also give permission to not be sexually active or to refrain from harmful practices.

This level of intervention can usually be done in a brief time span. It can be done in a variety of settings where there is some privacy, and it does not require a great deal of special technique on the part of the nurse. The interpersonal and teaching skills that are an integral part of nursing education will usually suffice.

Permission-giving often helps decrease the client's anxiety about sex and to break the behavior → negative labeling → anxiety cycle that often occurs. The limitation to permission-giving is that no one can give blanket permission; there may be situations or acts that would have adverse consequences. It is the nurse's responsibility to be sure that clients are aware of all aspects and consequences of their actions; they must be able to make an informed choice. The extent to which the nurse will be comfortable giving permission will depend upon her knowledge of sexuality and her value system, which should allow for tolerance for a wide range of sexual behaviors, thoughts, and feelings.

Limited information, the second level of intervention,

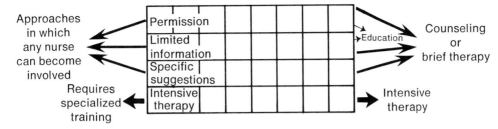

Fig. 9-1. Model for nursing intervention with clients experiencing sexual concerns.

may resolve concerns that cannot be resolved by permission-giving alone. Both of these levels are means of providing sex education for the client. Limited information provides the client with specific factual information that is directly relevant to her particular sexual concern. It is different from permission-giving, which is basically telling the client it is all right to continue doing what she has been doing. The second level gives the client factual knowledge, dispels myths about sexuality, and gives accurate information about sex and sexuality. This type of intervention can be both therapeutic and preventive; it can correct misinformation and prevent future problems by alleviating guilt and anxiety. It is essential that limited information be just that; the client is given factual information directly related to the *expressed, specific* concern. This is not a discourse on a broad range of sexual matters. Again, as in the first level, use of the intervention will depend on the individual nurse's comfort with sexual issues, her depth of knowledge, and her value system.

The third level, *specific suggestions,* is used when the first two levels do not seem appropriate or sufficient to resolve the client's sexual concern. It is assumed that before making any specific suggestions, the nurse would do a thorough nursing assessment including a sexual history. She should not just accept the client's labeling of the problem. The third level differs from the first two types of interventions in that it requires more action on the part of the client. The nurse has switched from a predominantly teaching role to one that employs more counseling techniques. Specific suggestions are direct attempts to help the client change behavior in order to reach the stated goal of improved sexual functioning.

It is important for the nurse to know that whatever suggestions are made are not contraindicated by any physical problem and that they do not transgress the client's value system. This level requires a great deal more knowledge and comfort than the previous ones. Specific suggestions may be used with clients who are experiencing organic as well as psychogenic sexual dysfunctions. As with the other levels, this one is preventive as well as therapeutic. The types of specific suggestions

range from the simple ones, such as suggesting the use of lubricating jelly to prevent dyspareunia to more complex ones such as masturbatory techniques for the preorgasmic female. Examples of specific suggestions include ways of enhancing orgasmic response for the female, techniques to improve marital communication, and different ways to give and receive sexual pleasure. Annon (1974) emphasizes that two sayings are frequently helpful to clients when using this level of intervention. First, "It is what you do with what you have, rather than what you have that counts." This can be particularly helpful for the client who has a negative self-concept. Second, "There is always another time or another day." This helps to decrease performance anxiety and spectatoring. At this level of intervention the nurse provides the client with specific suggestions that are designed to help her reach her identified goals.

The fourth level is required for those individuals or couples for whom the first three levels are inadequate and who are experiencing deeper or more prolonged intrapsychic or relationship problems. At this level the therapy modalities of Kaplan and Masters and Johnson are appropriate. It is unusual and probably inadvisable for the nurse to intervene at this level without extensive preparation beyond that offered in the basic nursing education program.

A sexual history may be a portion of a comprehensive nursing assessment or it may be the totality of an assessment. Its scope encompasses biologic, psychologic, sociocultural, and spiritual perspectives. This type of assessment will allow the nurse to decide if the concern is one in which she can become involved or one that needs to be referred elsewhere for treatment. Nurses may hesitate to elicit a sexual history, most likely because of their cultural conditioning, which dictates that sexual matters are not discussed. However, clients' sexual problems are a legitimate concern of the health care professional, and exploration of these problems through a sexual history is an indicated nursing responsibility. A sexual history provides a data base from which diagnoses can be made and a nursing care plan developed for education, counseling, or referral.

There is no one approach to obtaining a sexual history, or one specific form that must be used. There are, however, some general principles, which, if observed, will facilitate obtaining a sexual history. Privacy is essential. Not only is physical privacy mandatory, but also trust and confidentiality are necessary. History-taking itself can be therapeutic in that it allows the individual to discuss sexual matters in a nonjudgmental manner. The nurse has the opportunity (1) to give permission to the client to discuss concerns, (2) to validate that the client's concerns or behaviors are normal and acceptable, and (3) to provide limited information or suggestions to the client. It is important to use language that the client understands; without this an adequate picture of her concerns may not be obtained. Terms may need to be defined.

In gathering a sexual history, it is useful to move from less sensitive to more sensitive issues. The life-cycle approach provides a logical progression of events. It also often moves from less to more threatening topics. Asking questions that imply that a wide variation of sexual behavior is acceptable is less anxiety producing than a direct query about behavior. The nurse may also phrase questions in terms of "how" or "when" certain sexual practices were begun; this is less threatening than a "did you ever . . .?" approach. Inquiries may also be prefaced by statements that imply that the specific practice in question is not too unusual. It is best not to ask questions that require statistical answers; the client may give the answer she thinks the practitioner wants rather than the actual facts. No one wishes to appear abnormal. While it is usually best to approach questions regarding sexual practices in this manner, the nursing practitioner must be careful not to make unwarranted assumptions about her client's sexual behaviors.

While obtaining the sexual history, the nurse often has an opportunity to provide sex education. Misconceptions and misinformation can be corrected; terminology may be clarified. Additional attitudes may be communicated. Reassurances that normalcy is defined within the social and cultural unit may decrease anxiety and guilt about sexual behavior.

Various approaches for obtaining a sexual history are used by nurses. A brief sexual history can be integrated into a general health history. With this type only a few questions are asked. Areas addressed should include the person's sex roles, the way the person views herself as a sexual being, and sexual functioning. Even a brief history such as this will encourage clients to explore sexual concerns. Many clients will then state their problems without further questioning (Woods, 1979).

Annon (1974) suggests obtaining a sexual problem history, which can be used to supplement a brief history. The first component of such a history is a description of the current problem of concern in the client's own words. The onset and course of the problem are next explored. The age of the client at the time of onset as well as whether it occurred suddenly or developed over time is relevant. The course of the sexual problem, its functional relationship to organic phenomena such as drugs, alcohol, and changes over time should be discussed. The client's concept of the cause and maintenance of the problem is crucial. Prior treatments and their outcomes are explored next. This should include self-help activities as well as contact with any other health practitioner. Last, the client's current expectations and goals for treatment are examined. It is essential that the practitioner explore the client's expectations carefully since the client may wish to achieve goals that the nurse is unable to facilitate or that would be better achieved with another practitioner. If expectations are not made clearly, inappropriate treatment or referral may occur.

The following sexual history format represents a synthesis of approaches including those by Annon (1974) Masters and Johnson (1978), and Schiller (1973). Included are the following points:

1. Client's description of presenting problem, including onset, duration, and frequency; client's concept of cause and maintenance should be included
2. Determination of client's expectations of treatment and how realistic these are
3. Descriptions of the present relationship
4. Client's body image and self-concept
5. Special life cycle events, such as menarche, childbirth, midlife crisis, etc.
6. Environmental influences affecting sexual functioning
7. Client's sociocultural perspective or value system

Once the sexual history is obtained, the nurse can determine what the client's needs or problems are, what strategies will best meet these needs or solve the problems, and who best can implement the appropriate interventions. The nurse and client together can then discuss and decide what will be the best course of action for the client to pursue.

For the nurse involved in sexual counseling, there are several basic principles that should be observed. It is important that sexual counseling not transgress the client's religious values. If this does occur severe depression, anxiety, and guilt may result. All of us have strong convictions about what is right and wrong sexually; the nurse should not impose her values on the client. The timing of sexual discussion is important; the client should never be forced to talk about sex. The client will introduce subjects as she feels it is important to do so. Sex has many different meanings; it is not an all-or-none experience and this should be conveyed to the client. There are many ways to convey sexual information and different methodologies should be tried with different clients and at different times with the same client. Sexuality is a topic that should be continually open for discussion. Sexually dysfunctional persons experience changes in their psychosocial situation, which may produce new crises requiring resolution.

The roles of sex educator or counselor are legitimate ones for the nurse practitioner to assume. In order to do so, she must have an in-depth knowledge of the facts of human sexuality, be comfortable with her own sexual value system, develop a tolerance for the sexual values and behaviors of others, and have the ability to develop helping relationships that include mutual trust with her clients. With these skills and knowledge she will be able to successfully fill the role and meet the responsibilities of a sex educator and counselor.

REFERENCES

Annon, J. S.: The behavioral treatment of sexual problems, vol. 1. Brief therapy, Honolulu, 1974, Enabling Systems, Inc.

Apfelbaum, B.: On the etiology of sexual dysfunction, J. Sex Marital Ther. 3(1):50-62, 1977.

Baker, L., and Nagata, F.: A group approach to the treatment of heterosexual couples with sexual dissatisfactions, J. Sex Educ. Ther. 3(2):15-17, 1977.

Barbach, L. G.: Group treatment of preorgasmic women, J. Sex Marital Ther. 1(2):139-145, 1974.

Belliveau, F., and Richter, L.: Understanding human sexual inadequacy, Boston, 1970, Bantam Books, Inc.

Berman, E., and Lief, H.: Marital therapy from a psychiatric perspective, Am. J. Psych. 132(6):583-592, 1975.

Bieber, I.: The psychoanalytic treatment of sexual disorders, J. Sex Marital Ther. 1(1):5-15, 1974.

Bogen, I.: Orgasms are orgasms: whose responsibility? J. Sex Educ. Ther. 3(2): 1977.

Brady, J. P.: Behavior therapy and sex therapy, Am. J. Psychiatry 138(8):896-899, 1976.

Ellis, A.: The art and science of love, New York, 1960, Lyle Stuart, Inc.

Ellis, A.: Frigidity. In Ellis, A., and Abarabanel, A., editors: The encyclopedia of sexual behavior, vol. 1, New York, 1961, Hawthorne Books, Inc.

Fertel, N. S.: Vaginismus: a review, J. Sex Marital Ther. 3(2):113-121, 1977.

Fisher, S.: The female orgasm: psychology, physiology, fantasy, New York, 1973, Basic Books, Inc.

Flowers, G.: Female sexual dysfunction, J. Obstet. Gynecol. Nurs. Nov./Dec. 1977, pp. 12-16.

Franks, V., and Burtle, V.: Women in therapy, New York, 1974, Brunner/Mazel Inc.

Gagnon, J. H.: Human sexualities, Chicago, 1977, Scott, Foresman & Co.

Gornick, V., and Moran, B., editors: Woman in sexist society, New York, 1971, Basic Books, Inc.

Haber, J., and others: Comprehensive psychiatric nursing, New York, 1978, McGraw-Hill Book Co., pp. 192-194.

Hammer, S., editor: Women: body and culture, New York, 1975, Harper & Row, Publishers.

Hartman, W. E., and Fifthias, M. A.: Treatment of sexual dysfunction, New York, 1974, Jason Aronson, Inc.

Hite, S.: The Hite report, New York, 1976, The Macmillan Co.

Janeway, E.: Mans world, womans place, New York, 1971, Dell Publishing Co., Inc.

Kaplan, H. S.: The new sex therapy, New York, 1974a, Brunner/Mazel, Inc.

Kaplan, H. S.: The classifications of the female sexual dysfunctions, J. Sex Marital Ther. 1(2):124-138, 1974b.

Kaplan, H. S.: No nonsense therapy for six sexual malfunctions. Annual Editions. In Barbour, J. R., editor: Focus: human sexuality 77/78, Guilford, Conn., 1978, Dushkin Publishing Group, Inc., pp. 132-138.

Kegel, A. H.: Sexual functions of the pubococcygeus muscle, West. J. Obstet. Gynecol. 60:521-524, 1952.

Kerr, C.: Sex for women, New York, 1977, Grove Press, Inc.

Kinsey, A. C., and others: Sexual behavior in the human female, Philadelphia, 1953, W. B. Saunders Co.

Kutner, S. J.: Sex guilt and the sexual behavior sequence, J. Sex Res. 7(2):107-115, 1971.

Labowitz, W. C., and LoPiccolo, J.: New methods in the behavioral treatment of sexual dysfunction, J. Behav. Ther. Exp. Psychiatry 3:265-271, 1972.

Lehrman, N.: Masters and Johnson explained, New York, 1970, Playboy Press.

Levay, A. N.: Concurrent sex therapy and psychoanalytic psychotherapy: effectiveness and implications, J. Sex. Educ. Ther., pp. 25-33, 1976.

Levine, S. B.: Marital sexual dysfunction: introductory concepts, Ann. Int. Med. 84:448-453, 1976.

Maddox, J.: Sexual health and health care, Postgrad. Med. 58(1):54, 1975.

Masters, W., and Johnson, V.: Human sexual response, Boston, 1966, Little, Brown & Co.

Masters, W., and Johnson, V.: Human sexual inadequacy, Boston, 1970, Little, Brown & Co.

Masters, W., and Johnson, V.: Principles of the new sex therapy, Am. J. Psych. 133(5):548-584, 1976.

Masters, W., and Johnson, V.: Ten sexual myths explored. Annual Editions. In Barbour, J. R., editor: Focus: human sexuality 77/78, Guilford, Conn.; 1978, Dushkin Publishing Group, Inc.

McCary, J. L.: Sexual myths and fallacies, New York, 1975, Schocken Books, Inc.

McCary, J. L.: McCary's human sexuality, ed. 3, New York, 1978, D. Van Nostrand Co.

Miller, J. B.: Toward a new psychology of women, Boston, 1976, Beacon Press.

Munjock, D., and Kanno, P.: An overview of outcome in frigidity: treatment effect and effectiveness, Comp. Psych. 17(3):401-413, 1976.

Munjock, D., and Kanno, P.: Prognosis in the treatment of female sexual inhibition, Comp. Psych. 18(5):481-488, 1977.

Romney, S., and others: Gynecology and obstetrics: the health care of women, New York, 1975, McGraw-Hill Book Co.

Sadock, B., Kaplan, H., and Freedman, A.: The sexual experience, Baltimore, 1976, The Williams & Wilkins Co.

Schiller, P.: Creative approach to sex education and counseling, New York, 1973, Association Press.

Seagraves, R. T.: Primary orgasmic dysfunction: essential treatment components, J. Sex Marital Ther. 2(2):115-123, 1976.

Seamans, B.: Free and female, New York, 1972, Fawcett World Library.

Sharpe, L., and others: A preliminary classification of human functional sexual disorders, J. Sex Marital Ther. 3(2):106-114, 1976.

Sherfey, M. J.: The nature of evolution of female sexuality, New York, 1972, Random House, Inc.

Spengler, C.: Conditioning of the female to her role in life. In Gussum, M., and Spengler, C., editors: Woman power and health care, Boston, 1976, Little, Brown & Co., pp. 1-16.

Stahmann, R., and Hiliert, W.: Counseling in marital and sexual problems, ed. 2, Baltimore, 1977, The Williams & Wilkins Co.

Suitzer, E.: Female sexuality. In Focus: human sexuality 77/78, Annual Editions, Guilford, Conn., 1977, Dushkin Publishing Group, Inc., pp. 101-103.

Tavris, C., and Offir, C.: The longest war, New York, 1977, Harcourt Brace Jovanovich, Inc.

Tavris, C., and Sadd, S.: The Redbook report on female sexuality, New York, 1977, Delacorte Press.

Vincent, C. E.: Sexual and marital health, New York, 1973, McGraw-Hill Book Co.

Walbrek, A. J., and Walbrek, C.: Dyspareunia, J. Sex Marital Therapy 1(3):234-246, 1975.

Walbrek, A. J., and Walbrek, C.: Vaginismus, J. Sex Educ. Ther. Spring/Summer, 1976, pp. 21-24.

Weizberg, M.: Unwanted virginity, Female Patient, Apr. 1976, pp. 45-48.

Williams, J. H.: Psychology of women, New York, 1977, W. W. Norton & Co., Inc.

Wilson, R.: Introduction to sexual counseling, Chapel Hill, N.C., 1974, Carolina Population Center.

Witkin, M. H.: Ethical issues and sex therapy, J. Sex Educ. Ther. Spring 1978, pp. 8-10.

Woods, N. F.: Human sexuality in health and illness, ed. 2, St. Louis, 1979, The C. V. Mosby Co.

Wright, J.: The treatment of sexual dysfunction, Arch. Gen. Psych. 34:881-890, 1977.

ADDITIONAL READINGS

Adams, G.: The sexual history as an integral part of the patient history, MCN Ann. Mat. Child Nurs. 77:170-175, May/June, 1976.

Elder, M. S.: The unmet challenge: nurse counseling on sexuality, Nurs. Outlook 27:29-32, 1972.

LoPiccolo, L., and Neiman, J. R.: Sexual assessment and history interview. In LoPiccolo, J., and LoPiccolo, L., editors: Handbook of sex therapy, New York, 1978, Plenum Press.

Mims, F. H.: A model to promote sexual health care, Nurs. Outlook 26(2):121-125, 1971.

Mims, F. H.: Sexual health education and counseling, Nurs. Clin. North Am. 10(3):519-528, 1973.

Psznoy, M. S.: Taking a sexual history, Am. J. Nurs. 76(8):1279-1282, 1976.

Whitley, N.: The first coital experiences of one hundred women, J. Obstet. Gynecol. Nurs., pp. 41-45, July/Aug., 1978.

Zalar, M.: Human sexuality: a component of total patient care, Imprint 21(4):22, 1974.

Zeiss, A., Rosen, G. M., and Zeiss, R. A.: Orgasm during intercourse: a treatment strategy for women, J. Consult. Clin. Psych. 45(5):891-895, 1977.

10

High-risk pregnancy

Catherine Ingram Fogel

The majority of pregnancies have favorable outcomes—a healthy mother and infant and a happy family unit. This is not the case however for 10% to 20% of childbearing women, those women usually labeled as high risk for one reason or another.

By most predictions, 80% to 90% of all expectant mothers will have an uneventful pregnancy with a favorable outcome. According to Aubrey and Pennington (1973), 20% to 30% of the obstetric population give rise to 70% to 80% of perinatal mortality and morbidity. Pregnancy itself is not an illness but a normal life cycle event. There is, however, growing concern in the United States for the mothers and infants for whom something does go wrong. When a high-risk pregnancy occurs the challenge to nursing is tremendous. Extensive knowledge is essential for the nurse providing care to the client experiencing the biologic, emotional, and social crises of pregnancy at risk. This chapter will provide requisite knowledge by defining the concept of high-risk pregnancy, exploring the scope of the problem, presenting information about specific risk factors, providing assessment tools to identify the high-risk client, discussing diagnostic procedures for determining the client at risk, and analyzing appropriate nursing interventions.

DEFINITION AND SCOPE OF THE PROBLEM

Traditionally, a high-risk pregnancy has been defined as one in which the infant (or fetus) has a significantly increased chance of mortality or morbidity, either before, during, or after birth. Another traditional definition identifies the high-risk mother as one for whom childbearing entails special problems, usually defined in terms of medical/obstetric complications. The first definition is too confining for our purposes since it considers only the fetus; the second because it considers only medical problems. A broader definition is needed to allow for consideration of morbidity, accident, or mortality resulting from a variety of causative agents—physical, psychologic, or sociocultural—that place the ma-

ternal-fetal dyad at risk at any time during the childbearing cycle. This concept can easily be expanded to include the risk of a woman's being pregnant against her wishes, the risk of not being able to care for a child, and the risk of having too many children or deprived or neglected children. Thus the definition of "high risk" should include the risk of conceiving as well as the risks attendant upon pregnancy, labor and delivery, and postpartum.

The maternal mortality rate has shown a sharp drop in the United States over the past 35 years from 376.0 in 1940 to 12.8 in 1975 (expressed in deaths/100,000 live births). This represents a decrease of over 95%. Over the years the majority of maternal deaths have been caused by hemorrhage, toxemia, and infection; this triad still accounts for most of them. However, medical management for these complications has improved tremendously, which accounts for the vast improvement in mortality figures.

It could be argued that childbirth is much safer today if only maternal mortality rates are considered; however, maternal morbidity rates must also be considered and these are not available. Occasionally, statistics surface indicating, for example, that 6% to 7% of all pregnant women in the United States experience toxemia (Pritchard, 1976). However, since there is no uniform system of reporting maternal morbidity, there is no way of knowing what the incidence of maternal morbidity is or what the scope of high-risk pregnancy is. Further, our definition of high risk is not limited to, or measured in, medical complications or deaths alone. There are many other social, psychologic, and economic factors to be considered. In fact, even maternal morbidity rates alter dramatically when various risk factors such as age, race, and parity are considered. These will be discussed below in the section on specific risk factors.

In considering the scope of problems of high-risk pregnancy, two other rates need to be considered: infant mortality rates and perinatal mortality rates (the sum of fetal and neonatal death rates). Compared with other countries having comparable populations and technologies, the United States ranks fourteenth (Maniello and Farrell, 1977). Infant deaths rank fourth among all causes of death in the United States and equals all other deaths in the next four decades of life (Romney et al., 1975). Obviously, intrauterine life and birth are hazardous times.

The perinatal mortality rate has shown some gradual improvements over the years, decreasing from 29.3/1,000 live births in 1970 to 22.2/1,000 live births in 1975, yet the overall decrease is not as great as that of infant deaths. Statistics are not readily available for the incidence of birth defects and mental retardation, both of which can result from high-risk pregnancy. The incidence of low birth weight (less than 2,500 gm [5 lb 8 oz]) also has relevance to the magnitude of the problem, since these infants are more apt to be the product of a high-risk pregnancy and to have more problems in life.

Eight percent of all live births in the United States are infants who weigh less than 2,500 gm. There are really two types of low birth weight infants: preterm infants and those who are born at term but are too small for their gestational age. The risks of preterm and growth-retarded infants are so well documented that low birth weight in itself is considered a poor outcome of pregnancy. Deaths for low birth weight infants in the neonatal period are thirty times more frequent than for infants of average or normal birth weight. Bergner and Susser (1970) found perinatal mortality correlated to a far greater extent with birth weight than with length of gestation. It is now widely believed that if birth weight could be improved, mortality would be substantially reduced. Singer found low birth weight related to increased incidence of stillbirths, neonatal death, and poor infant development. Low birth weight is also associated with cerebral palsy, epilepsy, and various forms of mental retardation. Low birth weight children have more frequent hospitalizations for illness, more visual and hearing disabilities, and more learning problems in school (Worthington et al, 1977).

In 1950, 7.6% of all live births were considered to be low birth weight; by 1975 this figure had dropped only to 7.4% *(Vital Statistics).* The incidence is even more significant when considered by race: 7.1% for whites and 13.4% for blacks (Singer, 1977). The National Collaborative Perinatal Study has associated approximately 70% of each component of perinatal mortality (stillbirths and neonatal deaths) with low birth weight (Osofsky and Kendall, 1973). Advanced medical technology now enables the health care profession to save many of those infants who might otherwise have died, but these infants are at risk throughout life. They may grow up to become handicapped persons who are unable to compete in our increasingly complex society. The permanent damage,

measured in terms of man years of loss of life and productive living, exceeds that of other major catastrophes such as cancer, accidents, or cardiovascular disease (Romney et al., 1975). Ironically, society's greatest cost is not from the infants who die but from those who survive, sustain injuries, or emotional trauma and often face a lifetime of disability (Schwartz and Schwartz, 1972).

It is extremely difficult to identify the scope of the problem of high-risk pregnancy, since the statistics are not available; however the following offers a rough illustration (Babson et al., 1975). Of the 5 to 10 million conceptions occurring yearly in the United States:

- 2 to 3 million result in early, spontaneous abortion
- Nearly 1 million are legally or illegally terminated
- Of the more than 3.2 million pregnancies that reach 20 weeks' gestation, 40,000 fetuses die in utero; another 40,000 have severe congenital malformations; 90,000 will be mentally retarded (IQ below 70); another 150,000 will be poor learners

Another way of looking at the problem is to consider a group of 1,000 pregnancies, out of which we could expect the following:

Live births	900
Fetal deaths	100
Infant deaths	25
Premature births	66
Congenital anomalies	50
Obstetric complications	50
Nonmarital births	77

It should be noted that the numbers exceed 1,000 since one mother could account for more than one complication. And, unfortunately, this breakdown does not include other significant conditions for which statistics are not readily available, such as medical or emotional illness, socioeconomic problems, or unwanted pregnancies.

Reports of the statistics for high-risk and at-risk populations may vary somewhat from year to year, and the magnitude of the problem may not be altogether clear; however, this does not alter the fact that the high number of parents who are at risk is a challenge to nursing. Although medical expertise is necessary to diagnose and manage high-risk mothers, nursing expertise is essential in the screening, identification, and care of these clients.

RISK FACTORS

Traditionally, risk factors have been viewed only in the medical model framework; that is, only medical, obstetric, or physiologic risk factors were considered. Recently, it has been recognized that a more eclectic approach to high-risk pregnancy is needed. It is becoming increasingly apparent that the pregnant woman does not

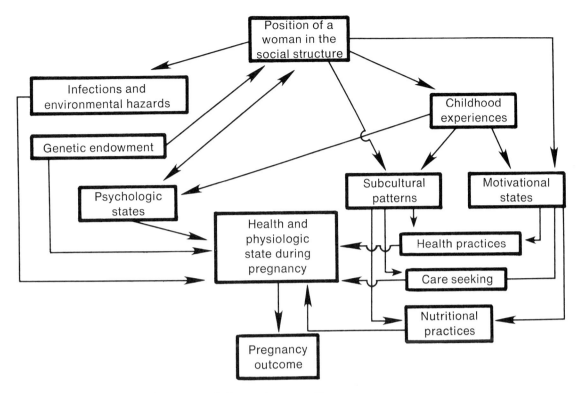

Fig. 10-1. Risk factors that may affect pregnancy outcome.

exist in a vacuum and that factors such as age, parity, emotional distress, poverty, and other environmental influences are as important to consider as specific disease entities such as toxemia or diabetes. Fig. 10-1 illustrates the way in which various risk factors may operate to affect pregnancy outcome.

It might be helpful to describe the "typical" mother at high risk. She is from a low socioeconomic class and more often than not nonwhite. She is at either extreme of the age continuum, and is pregnant for the first time or has had four or more previous pregnancies. She is probably unmarried and poorly nourished, often with a history of alcohol, drug, or tobacco abuse, chronic physical illness, or previous obstetric complications. Poor support systems and emotional disturbances may add further problems. Among the many factors that contribute to this picture, poverty underlies many of the other factors.

Poverty

For over half a century, it has been noted that the population most at risk is among the most underprivileged socioeconomically. Poverty seems to underlie many if not all of the other risk factors. Socioeconomic factors are highly correlated with low birth weight infants. Where adverse social conditions exist, infant death

rates are from two to four times the national figures. Much of the data is reported in terms of race; black children constitute only about 15% of the nation's children but nearly 40% of the nation's poor children (Schwartz and Schwartz, 1977). Other nonwhite races also are found in proportionately higher numbers in the lower socioeconomic groups. In 1975, 7.6% of all infants born were low birth weight; however, only 6.3% of all white infants were low birth weight. Manniello and Farrell (1977) found that from 1968 to 1974 black infants represented 94% of all premature births (measured in low birth weights). The infant mortality rate for nonwhite infants is almost twice as high as that of whites. As Schwartz and Schwartz (1977) point out, the fact that nonwhite infants die or are handicapped more frequently is not the result of race but of socioeconomic status. Socioeconomic level rather than race has been recognized as the significant variable since the study by Eastman (1947) in which he found prematurity rates were much higher for ward clients than for private clients. Although the highest rates were found in black clients, white clients living at or near the poverty level had very similar prematurity rates. Therefore, socioeconomic status may be considered the most significant variable although race cannot be ignored, since it is often an indicator of social class.

Two sets of issues emerge when one attempts to analyze the factors that predispose low-income women to high-risk pregnancy: general reproductive patterns and specific pathology. The phrase "too young, too old, and too often" succinctly summarizes the reproductive patterns of many poor women. The fetus and mother are at highest risk when the mother is at either extreme of age and parity. Both international and national data substantiate this (Osofsky and Kendall, 1973). Poor pregnancy outcomes are highest among the very young (below age 15) and the relatively old (over age 40). The number of pregnancies a woman has had is also closely related to perinatal mortality; mortality is high among first pregnancies, drops with the second, and begins to rise from then on, being highest after five or more pregnancies. Spacing of pregnancies also affects prognosis, with greater risk occurring when pregnancies are close together.

Low-income women tend to begin having children at an earlier age and to cease childbearing at an older age than do women in the population at large. In addition, the prevalence of high parity increases with the lowering of social class. Here education and racial background interact with economic level.

The poor enter pregnancy at risk because of poor general health and poor or nonexistent prenatal care. Low-income mothers often do not seek prenatal care at all or they do so late in pregnancy. When this is added to the already existing medical, emotional, and social conditions likely to have deleterious influences on pregnancy outcome, the problem is compounded seriously. These women are more likely to have low birth weight infants and are more likely to have medical complications of pregnancy, which predispose them either to perinatal mortality or to prenatal morbidity with increased risk of mortality. Low-income women are more apt to have a history of prior prenatal loss, which puts them at risk for fetal loss with a current pregnancy. Also, they are considerably more predisposed to intercurrent illnesses and obstetric complications during pregnancy.

Poverty also has an indirect effect on high-risk pregnancy in that other significant risk factors, such as nutritional status, emotional disturbances, and environmental influences, are affected by socioeconomic status. There soon becomes operant a cycle that is difficult to break and that has a spiraling negative effect on the high-risk mother and infant (Fig. 10-2).

Lack of prenatal care

Lack of prenatal care is a major factor in placing the pregnant woman at risk since the opportunity is lost for early diagnosis and treatment of obstetric complications. Dott and Fort (1975) found that even when race, pov-

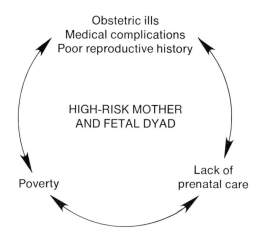

Fig. 10-2. Poverty influences on pregnancy outcomes.

erty, and birth weight were considered, infant mortality rates were four- to tenfold greater for women who had no prenatal care than for women who had more than nine prenatal visits. Some of the deterrents to obtaining and continuing prenatal care are: (1) ignorance of need for care, (2) negative attitudes toward prenatal care, (3) difficulties in arranging care, and (4) impersonal care.

Many women do not understand the need for early and continued prenatal care. Their orientation to medical care is one of treatment, not prevention and maintenance. The pregnant woman, regardless of income, may not know what kind of care is available, how to make an appointment, when she should go for the first time, or how to get this information. Weeks or months may elapse between the time the woman first suspects pregnancy and she first sees a physician. Others may be so frightened of physicians and the health care system that they delay or avoid seeking prenatal care.

Finances may also be a factor. The cost of care and transportation and the loss of work hours may create financial burdens that the client cannot assume. Financial arrangements for prenatal care are often difficult to make.

For some women, denial of pregnancy is a strong factor in delaying or not obtaining care. If the pregnancy is unwanted, the woman may attempt to deny it as long as possible. Obviously, regular prenatal care makes it impossible to deny the fact of pregnancy.

Many women complain about the depersonalization of care, and there is little incentive to return for care or initiate it in subsequent pregnancies. In too many cases, the visit is brief and routinized with little or no time for asking questions, discussing the client's concerns, or for client education. The waiting time is often measured in hours for a visit of minutes in which it appears nothing is done. If the preventive and maintenance measures are not explained to the client, the whole experience may be seen as valueless, time consuming, expensive, and irrelevant. The poor are frequently provided care by the least trained of the medical profession.

Age

Age has long been considered a crucial variable in determining high-risk pregnancy. It is obvious that there are basic physiologic differences existing at various stages in the childbearing period as well as important psychosocial variables in different age groups. As noted above, perinatal mortality is highest for women at either end of the age continuum in childbearing. The very young and very old mothers have the highest incidence of low gestational age and/or low birth weight infants even when socioeconomic status is not a consideration.

In regard to congenital defects, the influence exerted by age of the mother differs with the specific malformation. Anencephaly and hydrocephaly are seen more frequently in the infants of very young primigravidas; the incidence then decreases with age and parity until age 25, after which it rises until at age 40 the incidence is almost double that seen at age 25 (Aladjem, 1975). Trisomy 21, or Down's syndrome, is seen more frequently in infants of older women (1 case in 1,000 to 2,000 under age 25 years; 1 in 300 at age 35 to 40 years, and 1 case in 30 to 35 births over age 45 years). This is thought to occur because age may progressively affect the attachment of chromosomes to the spindle and therefore nondisjunction may occur more frequently (Clausen, 1977).

At one time it was believed that congenital heart defects were associated with maternal age; however, these are now believed to be more directly associated with higher birth order and only secondarily with increased age of the mother. The evidence of association with maternal age alone is greatly reduced when birth order is controlled.

Being surrounded by an aging mother is inimical to the fetus in many ways: Perinatal mortality and morbidity resulting from fetal abnormalities, intrauterine growth retardation, and maternal degenerative diseases (especially cardiorenal and diabetes) are greater. Poor implantation is more common in the older, multiparous woman, as is disturbed fetal nutrition in phases of organogenesis. The older woman also experiences an increased incidence of placenta previa, abruptio placentae, and antepartal hemorrhage.

According to Selvin and Cappinkel (1976) maternal age, paternal age, and parity all have separate and approximately equal and significant relationships with risk of fetal death. Resseguie (1976) however, rejects the premise that women who choose careers in their twenties, thus delaying pregnancy, will automatically incur elevated risk of stillbirth in their postponed pregnancies. He believes that the association of elevated rates of stillbirth with increased maternal age is an artifact of analysis; when other variables such as parity and socioeconomic levels are considered, age is no longer significant.

It has long been believed that toxemia was more common in the very young and those over age 35. Some research by Christianson (1974) suggests that not only is age significant but parity is also, and the multiparous woman is at greatest risk no matter what her age. Kajanoja and Widholm (1978) found that cesarean section rates were higher in women over age 40, while perinatal mortality was slightly elevated. Though maternal morbidity was relatively high, neither severe deterioration in maternal health nor maternal deaths occurred. They conclude that in today's society the "elderly woman has a good chance of giving birth to a healthy child after a safe pregnancy."

It has been assumed that the adolescent mother is at greater health risk than the mother who is between 20 and 34 years. However, recent medical studies do not always document this clearly (adolescent pregnancy is discussed more fully in Chapter 11).

There are also psychosocial effects associated with childbearing on both extremes of the continuum. Women having children late in the childbearing years may find caring for the child exhausts their physical capabilities; if social and economic conditions are also adverse, child neglect or abuse can result. The very young mother may find it difficult to assume the responsibilities of a child because of the repetitive and time-consuming nature of child care.

Parity

The number of previous pregnancies a woman has had may, of course, be related to her age, but there is also evidence that birth order itself can be a high-risk factor. First pregnancies are often high risk no matter what the age of the mother. The incidence of toxemia and difficult labor and delivery is higher in first births; and firstborns have higher rates of morbidity and mortality, although it is not clear whether this results from physiologic or sociologic factors. Infants born to unmarried mothers are known to have higher mortality rates and they are usually disproportionately represented in first pregnancies. High parity, especially more than five, closely spaced pregnancies, also brings greater risk.

Marital status

Marital status can be considered a high-risk factor since mortality and morbidity rates are higher for nonmarital than marital births. Further, unmarried women are less likely to obtain prenatal care than are married women. Even if prenatal care is obtained, the woman is less likely to follow the advice given her. An attempt to deny the pregnancy may be operating here. A higher number of nonmarital births occurs in the lower socioeconomic classes, which are at greater risk. Nonmarital pregnancies more often occur in the younger age group, age 15 and under, which is at extremely high risk for medical problems. Finally, there is some research to indicate that emotional stress (which may be found more often and at a higher level among unmarried mothers) may interfere with or have an adverse effect on fetal development. One theory suggests that emotional stress can predispose the woman to toxemia.

Medical complications

Medical complications of previous and current pregnancies, obstetric illnesses, and reproductive failures are numerous and well documented in every standard obstetric textbook. They will not be discussed in detail in this book; only the major ones will be summarized here. The more common causes of maternal mortality are hemorrhage, toxemia, and infection, which together account for nearly 60% of all reported maternal deaths. The major physiologic causes of maternal morbidity are:

1. Complications of a prior pregnancy, labor and delivery, or postpartum, which recur (for example, spontaneous abortion, toxemia, dystocia, hemorrhage, mastitis, previous unexplained stillbirth, premature rupture of membranes)
2. Medical complications/obstetric illnesses
   a. Anemia, particularly sickle cell disease or persistent anemia
   b. Diabetes
   c. Epilepsy
   d. Heart disease
   e. Hypertensive conditions (for example, toxemia or chronic hypertension)
   f. Infections, especially those that are sexually transmitted (i.e., gonorrhea and herpes)
   g. Kidney disease including urinary tract infections
   h. Pelvic surgery
   i. Thrombophlebitis
   j. Dysplasia and/or cancer of the cervix
   k. Cancer
   l. Rh factor

All of the above have the potential for placing the woman and fetus at high risk.

It has been recognized for many years that obstetric complications tend to recur in subsequent pregnancies. Further, it has been clearly documented that a woman with a history of a prior pregnancy loss is at increased risk for future losses. The etiology of this risk factor varies depending on when in the pregnancy it occurs. In early pregnancy the major risk factors are genetic abnormalities and structural anomalies of the reproductive tract. As pregnancy progresses, obstetric complications and chronic medical diseases of the mother become the major risk factors. Usually, the specific cause of pregnancy loss cannot be identified; however, there is a clear association between socioeconomic deprivation and increased fetal vulnerability. The various aspects of poverty discussed earlier seem to increase the risk of death in utero. Further, the poor are more likely to have chronic diseases, and when this is the cause of fetal loss, it is unlikely to change from one pregnancy to the next. Whatever the risks to the fetus from social deprivation, they change little from pregnancy to pregnancy (Schneider, 1973).

Nutrition

It is impossible to precisely identify nutritional influences in pregnancy because of the many complex, interrelated factors involved. Nevertheless, it is generally held that nutritional status is an important determinant of pregnancy outcome. There is a genetic design for growth and development of the fetus that cannot be fulfilled without adequate nutrition.

Studies indicate that height of the mother and her weight during pregnancy can affect fetal growth and subsequent birth weight and that these effects are independent and cumulative (Green et al., 1975). Thompson (1968) found that the babies of taller and heavier mothers weighed 500 gm more than the babies of shorter and lighter mothers. It is thought that maternal size may be a factor affecting the ultimate size of the placenta. There is also an interrelationship between infant birth weight and the amount of weight gained during pregnancy. Studies done during times of national deprivation, such as wartime or famine, indicate that acute, severe nutritional deprivation among pregnant women is associated with a significant lowering of birth weight and possibly of reproductive capabilities (Bergner and Susser, 1970; Pitkins, 1977; Worthington et al., 1977). This is supported by animal studies that suggest possible effects of malnutrition at different stages of gestation.

In the first trimester, severe limitation of the supply or transport of nutrients may cause restriction of the materials and energy needed for cell synthesis and cell differentiation, and thus produce malformations or death of the embryo. After the first trimester, malnutrition would not have teratogenic effects but could limit fetal growth. Nutrient requirements are greatest in the last trimester of pregnancy, when the cells are increasing in size and number. Even small nutritional restrictions could be serious at this time (Worthington et al., 1977).

The amount of weight gain desirable in pregnancy has been the subject of much controversy and numerous studies. Current thinking no longer places great emphasis on a specific number of pounds to be gained (20 to 30 lb is the usual recommendation today) nor on weight gain limitation. Higgins (1974) among others stresses the need for adequate protein and calorie intake throughout pregnancy and particularly in the last trimester, when the greatest amount of fetal growth takes place. The pregnant woman appears to need from 2,000 to 2,400 calories per day and her protein ingestion should be in the range of 80 gm per day. A minimal level of nutrients and calories must be available in order to obtain adequate birth weight. However, above this level, pregnant women can adapt themselves to a wide variety of food intake, both in quality and in quantity, without affecting birth weight. Other factors such as physical activity, prevalence of disease, age, and prepregnant maternal nutritional stores all affect an individual woman's needs.

The risks for the underweight pregnant patient (one who enters pregnancy 10% or more below standard weight for height) are significant. The probability of a low birth weight infant is appreciably higher and the risks of toxemia, antepartal hemorrhage, and anemia are also increased. The woman with inadequate weight gain (defined as a gain of 2.2 lb or less per month) is also at risk for having a low birth weight baby and for the effects of other nutritional deficiencies.

Obesity, the most common of all nutritional diseases, brings an increased risk of a number of complications including diabetes mellitus, chronic hypertension, and thromboembolic disease. Both maternal and perinatal outcome are compromised. It should be emphasized, however, that pregnancy is not the time to attempt to correct obesity. There is no evidence that weight loss or restriction has any effect on the complications of pregnancy of an obese woman. In fact, there is reason to believe it may be detrimental. Restriction of calories may result in restriction of other nutrients, particularly protein. Optimal protein utilization requires a certain energy intake to prevent amino acid metabolism to meet energy needs. Moreover, caloric restriction induces fat catabolism, which results in ketonemia; and the pregnant woman appears to be particularly susceptible to acidosis with starvation. It has been well documented that ketosis is poorly tolerated by the fetus and may actually cause mental retardation. Though excessive weight gain has long been thought to predispose to obstetric complications, in particular preeclampsia, this is not supported by recent research. It now appears that the only complication of excessive weight gain during pregnancy is the contribution it will make toward future obesity if the weight is not lost after delivery. Dietary restriction of nutrients in general, and of energy (calories and protein) and sodium in particular, has the potential

for impairing maternal capacity to make the needed physiologic adjustments to pregnancy and for interfering with fetal development (Pitkins, 1977).

As noted at the beginning of this section, the effects of nutrition are difficult to pinpoint conclusively, and they are in turn affected by multiple factors. Maternal nutrition can influence reproductive performance, especially of those women who are already at a high risk of delivering a low birth weight baby. Birth weight, which is a reflection of intrauterine growth, is a determinant of the infant's potential for survival and future health. The factors that place a pregnant woman at risk operate over her lifetime and continue to affect the nutritional status, growth, and development of her child. These include poverty, poor education, a deprived environment, and general poor health.

Environmental effects

There are specific environmental agents that have been reliably shown to affect fetal well-being and that therefore can be considered high-risk factors. These are alcohol, tobacco, certain drugs, radiation, specific maternal diseases such as diabetes, and certain infections.

Smoking. There is a strong, consistent relationship between maternal smoking during pregnancy and reduced birth weight. On the average, smokers' babies weigh from 150 to 250 gm less than nonsmokers' babies, and twice as many weigh less than 2,500 gm. It is generally accepted that the relationship between maternal smoking and reduced birth weight is direct and causal. Studies have also documented a direct increase in mortality risk as smoking level increases. The increased mortality results from premature delivery. These deaths are also associated with increases in the incidence of bleeding during pregnancy, abruptio placentae, placenta previa, and premature and prolonged rupture of the membranes. There may also be an increased risk for women who are anemic, of low socioeconomic status, or have prior poor obstetric histories, and who aggravate poor nutritional status by smoking (Meyer et al., 1976).

Hardy and Mellits (1972) attempted to determine the long-term effects of maternal smoking on infants, and they found that while these infants were lighter and shorter at birth and still shorter at 1 year than those of nonsmokers, this difference did not last. At 4 and 7 years there was no significant difference in either physical or intellectual development. Thus no long-term harmful effects were found among the children of pregnant smokers who survived the perinatal period.

Silverman (1977) attempted to determine whether smoking itself causes reduced birth weight or whether smokers are a self-selected group with different characteristics from nonsmokers that would account for production of lower birth weight babies. However, her study did not confirm the hypothesis that birth weight is dependent on innate characteristics of the mother rather than on the effects of the cigarette smoking.

It is essential to remember that the one consistent fact that has been substantiated is that smoking is associated with low mean birth weights and increased perinatal mortality. To summarize, the following facts are known:

1. Infants of mothers who smoke weigh less than infants of nonsmokers at all gestational ages. There is a two-fold increase in prematurity, and the weight difference is in direct proportion to the number of cigarettes smoked (Clark and Affonzo, 1976).
2. Neonatal mortality rates for single live births of low birth weight infants are significantly higher for infants of smoking mothers.
3. There is an increase in abortion rates but no significant increase in stillbirth or major fetal anomalies among women who smoke. There is some suggestion that there is an increased incidence of premature rupture of the membranes in smokers.

Alcohol. It has not been demonstrated clearly that the use of alcohol in ordinary social situations or for therapeutic reasons (such as inhibiting premature labor) is detrimental or has any acute effects on the fetus, increasing the risk for pre- and postnatal growth and developmental failures. Alcoholism often results in poor nutrition in terms of calories and necessary nutrients. Prenatal growth, particularly length is retarded, although birth weight is also decreased. The most commonly recognized sequelae in the offspring of alcoholic women is mental retardation, possibly the result of ethanol toxicity. Many are born with malformations of the heart, head, face, and extremities. Because of the magnitude and risk of mental deficiency in infants of alcoholic women, it is recommended that chronic alcoholics be on effective birth control measures. If the alcoholic becomes pregnant, she should be informed of the risks to the fetus and given the option of abortion. Apparently, these risks only apply while the woman is an active alcoholic (Streissguth, 1977).

Drugs. Drugs taken during pregnancy may adversely affect the developing fetus; these drugs may include those prescribed by a physician, those bought over the counter, or those commonly abused. Drugs can be teratogenic (cause congenital malformations), cause metabolic disturbances, produce chemical effects, or cause depression and/or alteration of the central nervous system function. When any medication is administered during pregnancy, the benefits must be weighed against the risks inherent in its use. Tables 10-1 and 10-2 summarize the potential effects on the fetus of many drugs and other environmental agents.

Drug abuse or narcotic addiction during pregnancy is a growing problem in the United States. In one study by Stone and co-workers (1971), over 90% of addicted women has inadequate or no prenatal care and the incidence of maternal complications markedly higher, especially prematurity, toxemia, breech births, and precipitate labor. In addition, the incidence of venereal disease and hepatitis is increased in drug addicts. All addictive drugs affect the infant, and the infant will demonstrate withdrawal shortly after delivery. There is a direct correlation between the length of addiction and the severity of the withdrawal symptoms in the infant. The symptoms suggest hyperactivity of the autonomic nervous system, with excessive weight loss and irritability. When the addicted pregnant woman receives treatment, the outlook is considerably brighter. There are two approaches available, detoxification and methadone-maintenance. In the detoxification program, com-

Table 10-1. Environmental agents that may cause birth defects*

Environmental agents not yet cleared of causing birth defects	Environmental agents for which there is no firm evidence for causation of birth defects
Chemical	**Chemical**
1. Blighted potatoes	1. Antibiotics (except streptomycin, tetracycline)
2. Corticosteroids	2. Antidepressants
3. Haloperidol	3. Anesthetics (general or local)
4. Oral contraceptives	4. Antiemetics
5. Streptomycin	5. Aspirin
6. Tolbutamide	6. Amphetamines
7. Tridione	7. Diuretics
8. LSD	8. Hypnotics (except thalidomide)
Infectious	9. Hypoglycemic agents (except tolbutamide)
1. Hepatitis virus	10. Marijuana
2. Influenza virus	11. Opiates
3. Mumps virus	12. Tranquilizers (except haloperidol)
	13. Vitamins
	Physical
	1. Heat
	2. Cold
	3. Light
	4. Vibration
	Maternal metabolism
	1. Fad diets
	2. Salt-restricted diets
	Infectious
	1. Bacterial infections

*From Aase, J. M.: Environmental causes of birth defects, Cont. Educ. Fam. Phys. 3(9):39-46, Sept. 1975.

Table 10-2. Environmental agents reliably known to cause specific congenital defects*

Agent	Effect	Comments
Chemical		
Alcohol	Prenatal and postnatal growth deficit, psycho-motor retardation, small eye fissures, joint abnormalities	According to recent estimates, this may be the third most common syndrome in which mental deficiency is a feature
Cigarette smoking	Low birth weight	Within limits, the diminution in average birth weight is dose-related
Coumadin	Dysplastic nose, stippled epiphyses, growth retardation, optic atrophy	May also be associated with other vitamin K antagonists
Cytotoxic drugs (aminopterin, methotrexate)	Prenatal growth deficit, hydrocephalus, limb abnormalities, frequent neonatal death	
Diphenylhydantoin	Broad face, low nasal bridge, dysplastic or absent nails, mild mental deficit, growth retardation	May occur in about 12 percent of pregnancies in women taking usual doses of diphenylhydantoin
Mercury (organic salts)	Mental deficit, hypertonicity, seizures	Cerebral palsy-like features as seen in Minimata disease in Japan
Tostosterone analogs, progestogens	Masculinization of the female fetus	
Tetracycline	Staining of primary and, rarely, secondary teeth	
Thalidomide	Phocomelia, abnormalities of external ear, facial hemangiomata, esophageal atresia, renal agenesis	
Physical		
Ionizing radiation	Microcephaly; leukemia	These effects seen with large doses (>150 rad), far in excess of usual diagnostic exposure. From a strict genetic point of view, however, no avoidable increase in radiation exposure can be considered "safe."
Radioiodine (^{131})	Destruction of fetal thyroid gland	
Maternal metabolism†		
Diabetes mellitus	Large fetal size, sacral agenesis (rare)	
Hyperphenylalaninemia	Faulty formation and function of central nervous system	
Infectious‡		
Cytomegalovirus	Mental deficit, hydrocephalus, chorioretinitis, microphthalmos	
Herpes simplex	Damage to central nervous system; skin lesions	
Rubella	Deafness, cataract, mental deficit, pre- and postnatal growth retardation, congenital heart disease	
Syphilis	Low nasal bridge, skeletal dysplasia, rhinorrhea	

*From Aase, J. M.: Environmental causes of birth defects, Cont. Educ. Fam. Phys. 3(9):39-46, Sept. 1975.
†These conditions, listed for completeness, are intrinsic to the mother, but may be considered "environmental agents" for the fetus, inasmuch as their effects must be mediated through the placental barrier.
‡Neonatal serologic testing is available for confirmation of these conditions.

plications for the mother and child are low birth weight, meconium-stained amniotic fluid (indicating fetal distress), and increased likelihood of breech presentation. The methadone program appears to have better results in that pregnancy complications are similar to the average obstetric population; however, low birth weight at term is frequent. The risks involved in multiple drug abuse are more complicated and not yet clearly understood; further, the long-term effects of intrauterine drug exposure, withdrawal syndrome, and treatment are not known (Aase, 1976).

Emotional factors

Under optimal circumstances, even a normal pregnancy brings profound physiologic and psychologic changes. There are numerous normal physiologic adaptations triggered by the extensive hormonal changes and the demands of the growing fetus. Psychologic adaptations are also great; even a normal pregnancy is a period of transient ego vulnerability. At another level, there are the anticipated changes in the family unit. McDonald (1968) has reviewed a wide range of studies that attempt to assess the role of emotional factors in complications of pregnancy. The literature does not provide conclusive evidence of any causal relationship between emotional factors and pregnancy complications. The most common finding is that women who subsequently have a complication of pregnancy have higher anxiety levels and fewer repressive type defenses than do women who experience normal pregnancy and delivery. McDonald suggests that anxiety can be a causative factor in the development of psychogenic obstetric complications.

A more recent study by Nuckolls and associates (1972) documents the necessity of jointly considering the woman's social or life stress and psychosocial assets. Singly, neither was related significantly to pregnancy complications but together they were predictive of obstetric complications of women who experienced highly stressful life situations. Those with psychosocial assets had only one third as many complications as those without assets. Without socially stressful situations, however, the presence or absence of assets was not related to the rate of complications. Gorsuch and Kay (1974) state that various psychosocial factors, especially anxiety, correlate with medical "abnormalities" in pregnancy. However, anxiety was often measured late in pregnancy and was not always examined in connection with life stress. In their study, anxiety during the first trimester was related to abnormalities of the childbearing cycle for mother and infant. Life stress that occurred in the second and third trimester was significantly associated with abnormalities. Anxiety and life stress were found to contribute to abnormalities of pregnancy independently of each other. Moreover, anxiety and stress were critical influences at different times in the pregnancy. Gorsuch and Kay found no evidence to suggest that either anxiety or stress before conception influenced the course or outcome of pregnancy.

These studies point to possible relationships between emotional factors and pregnancy complications. Among the most common complications cited are spontaneous abortion (especially habitual), prematurity, and toxemia. It remains difficult to delineate the specific effects that emotions and life changes have on pregnancy. More studies, correctly designed, are needed to answer these questions. On a final note, folklore and popular literature have long taken it for granted that acute anxiety, sorrow, or worry disturb the fetus and cause physical harm. It remains for someone to validate this (Schwartz and Schwartz, 1977).

Table 10-3 summarizes many of the psychosocial factors that may place the mother and/or infant at risk.

Table 10-3. Psychosocial factors that place the mother-infant dyad at risk

Risk factors	Examples
Maternal, paternal, or familial history of vulnerability (e.g., child abuse)	Inability to successfully have or raise a child
Preexisting major health problem (e.g., mental illness, alcoholism, mental retardation)	Low birth weight and other long-term sequelae
Poverty (e.g., noncompliance with health care); lack of prenatal care	
Insufficient support system (e.g., inadequate family support systems, systems prone to crisis, systems unable to fulfill family functions)	
Family disruption or dissolution (e.g., divorce, death, military service, abandonment)	
Role changes/conflicts (e.g., change in life-style, career, self, responsibilities, relationship; conflict about role expectations)	
Maturational crisis (e.g., difficulty in or inability to accomplish maturational tasks)	
Situational crisis (e.g., adolescent pregnancy)	
Noncompliance with cultural norms (e.g., nonmarital pregnancy)	
Dysfunctional behavior (e.g., anxiety, neurosis, depression psychosis)	
Poor coping skills	

IDENTIFICATION OF THE HIGH-RISK CLIENT

In order to decrease the hazards of childbearing it is essential to identify the client who is at risk. Identification of the high-risk pregnancy and specific risk factors possible is prerequisite to developing nursing strategies to reduce the risks. The sooner the client is identified, the greater are the chances for a favorable outcome for the mother and baby. Ideally, the potentially high-risk client should be identified at routine physicals, premarital examinations, or preconceptual evaluations so that diagnosis, specific treatment, and appropriate family planning can begin before pregnancy occurs. Unfortunately, this does not usually happen. Therefore, screening should begin with the initial prenatal visit. A study in North Carolina has shown that asking six crucial questions can greatly facilitate identification of high-risk groups (Scurletis, 1973). These questions are:

1. What is your age? (age factor)
2. How many pregnancies have you had? (parity factor)
3. How many years of education have you completed? (socioeconomic factor)
4. Have you had a previous fetal death? (reproductive loss)
5. Have you had a previous child born alive who is now dead? (possible low birth weight child)
6. What is your marital status? (nonmarital)

As can be seen, these questions touch on several of the risk factors discussed previously. With these questions the nurse can do a rough screening of clients to

Table 10-4. Categories of high-risk pregnancy

1. Age and parity factors
   a. Age 16 or under
   b. Primipara 35 or over
   c. Multipara 40 or over
   d. Interval of 8 years or more since last pregnancy
   e. High parity (5 or more)
2. Nonmarital pregnancy
3. Toxemia, hypertension, kidney disease
   a. Hyperemesis gravidarum
   b. Preeclampsia with hospitalization prior to labor
   c. Eclampsia
   d. Kidney disease—pyelonephritis, nephritis, nephrosis, etc.
   e. Chronic hypertension, severe (160/100 or over)
   f. Blood pressure 140/90 or above on two readings 30 minutes apart
4. Anemia and hemorrhage
   a. Hematocrit 30 or below in pregnancy
   b. Hemorrhage (previous pregnancy)—severe, requiring transfusion
   c. Hemorrhage (present pregnancy)
   d. Anemia for which treatment other than oral iron preparations is required (hemolytic, macrocytic, etc.)
   e. Sickle-cell trait or disease
   f. History of bleeding or clotting disorder at any time
5. Fetal factors
   a. Two or more previous premature deliveries (twins = 1 delivery)
   b. Two or more consecutive spontaneous abortions (miscarriages)
   c. One or more stillbirths at term
   d. One or more gross anomalies
   e. Rh incompatibility or ABO immunization problems
   f. History of previous birth defects—cerebral palsy, brain damage, mental retardation, metabolic disorders such as PKU
   g. History of large infants (over 9 lbs)
6. Dystocia (history of or anticipated)
   a. Contracted pelvis or cephalopelvic disproportion
   b. Multiple pregnancy in current pregnancy
   c. Two or more breech deliveries
   d. Previous cesarean section
   e. History of prolonged labor (more than 18 hours primipara; 12 hours multipara)
   f. Uterine anomaly
7. History of or concurrent medical conditions
   a. Diabetic or prediabetic
   b. Thyroid disease (hypo- or hyperthyroidism)
   c. Malnutrition or extreme obesity (20% over ideal weight for height; 10% under ideal weight for height)
   d. Organic heart disease
   e. Syphilis
   f. Rubella in first 10 weeks of *this* pregnancy
   g. Tuberculosis or other serious pulmonary pathology (e.g., emphysema, asthma)
   h. Malignant or premalignant tumors (including hydatidiform mole)
   i. Alcoholism, drug addiction
   j. Psychiatric disease or epilepsy (documented)
   k. Mental retardation
   l. Solitary ovary or tube (ectopic)
8. Those with previous history of
   a. Late registration
   b. Poor clinic attendance
   c. Home situation making clinic attendance and hospitalization difficult
   d. Mothers, including minors, without family resources (includes desertions, adoptions, injuries, separations, family withdrawals, sole support)

alert the health care team to a potential high-risk mother. Ironically, these questions are usually asked routinely on the pregnant woman's first visit to an obstetric clinic and yet few nurses ever put the answers into the perspective of high risk.

Screening tools may be used by nurse practitioners as guidelines for identifying high-risk clients. Screening tools serve two purposes: (1) they help the nurse easily identify problems or events that constitute threats to health during the childbearing cycle, and (2) they may serve as research tools in prospective surveys to identify high-risk clients among the childbearing population. Nesbitt and Aubrey (1967) have developed one screening tool, the Maternal Child Health Index (MCHC) (see

box) which has been repeatedly used to reliably identify the client at risk.

Aubrey and Pennington (1973) have developed another screening tool, the Labor Index (see Table 10-5), which allows them to identify additional clients at risk. They found that for clients who "failed" the total index (the MCHC Index and Labor Index combined) the relative risk was even higher, suggesting an additive effect in the two scores in terms of risk prediction. Table 10-6 gives a compilation of high-risk factors developed by the nurses in the Obstetrical Clinic at North Carolina Memorial Hospital, which can be used as a screening tool while interviewing. The list does not require scoring but helps the nurse remember special concerns.

Maternal-child health care index

Name: _____ Date: _____ EDC: _____ Hospital: _____

& Number: _____

The scoring system below is an attempt to categorize the degree of maternal and fetal risk based on the information available at the initial history and physical upon registration in our obstetric clinics. Please circle the numbers under each of the 8 categories which you feel apply and, at the bottom of this sheet, add up these numbers and subtract from a perfect score of 100.

I. Maternal age

Under 15	20
15-19	10
20-29	0
30-34	5
35-39	10
Over 40	20

II. Race and marital status

White	0
Nonwhite	5
Single	5
Married	0

III. Parity

0	10
1-3	0
4-7	5
Over 8	10

IV. Past obstetric history:

Abortions		Prematures		Fetal death		Neonatal death		Congenital anomaly		Damaged infants	
1	5	1	10	1	10	1	10	1	10	Physical	10
2	15	2+	20	2+	30	2+	30	2+	20	Neurological	20
3+	30										

V. Medical-obstetric disorders and nutrition:

Systemic illnesses		Specific infections		Diabetes		Chronic hypertension	
Acute, mild	5	Urinary:		Pre	20	Mild	15
Acute, serious	15	Acute	5	Overt	30	Severe	30
Chronic, nondebilitating	5	Chronic	25			Nephritis	30
Chronic, debilitating	20	Syphilis:		*Heart disease*			
		Treated	0	Class I or II	10		
		Untreated	20	Class III or IV	30		
		At term	30	History prior failure	30		

From Nesbitt, R. E. L., and Aubrey, R. H.: High risk obstetrics: value of semiobjective grading system in identifying the vulnerable group, Am. J. Obstet. Gynecol., April, 1969.

Maternal-child health care index—cont'd

Endocrine disorders		*Anemia*	
Definite adrenal, pituitary, or thyroid problem	30	Hgb, 10-11 gm	5
Recurrent menstrual dysfunction	10	Hgb, 9-10 gm	10
Involuntary sterility: Less than 2 years	10	Hgb, less than 9 gm	20
More than 2 years	20		

Rh problem		*Nutrition*	
Sensitized	30	Malnourished	20
Prior infant affected	30	Very close	30
Prior ABO incompatibility	20	Inadequate diet but not malnourished	10

VI. Generative tract disorders

Prior fetal malpresentations	10
Prior cesarean section	30
Known anomaly or incompetent cervix	20
Myomas: Over 5 cm	20
Submucous	30
Contracted pelvis: Borderline	10
Any contracted plane	30
Ovarian masses: Over 6 cm	20
Endometriosis	5

VII. Emotional survey (Grade 0-20 based on): Fears, attitudes, biases, hostilities, motivations, and behavioral patterns; prior pregnancies without supervision; time of registration; standard of child care and responsibilities; family unit, marital relationship; history of psychiatric illness in family

VIII. Social and economic survey (Grade 0-10 based on):
Employment—husband, patient; annual income adequacy, public assistance; education—husband, patient; housing—location, quality, facilities, and neighborhood environment

Total score of all 8 categories _____

100 less above score equals MCH Care Index _____

Table 10-5. Labor index*

Factors	Penalty points	Factors	Penalty points
Maternal factors		**Fetal factors**	
1. Prenatal care		1. Gestational age	
<3 prenatal visits	−10	<34 weeks	−30
No prenatal visits	−20	34-37 weeks	−20
2. Toxemia		>42 weeks	−20
Mild	−20	2. Multiple pregnancy	−20
Severe	−30	3. Previously undetected Rh sensitization	−20
3. Undetected diabetes	−20	4. Meconium staining	−30
4. Anemia–Hgb. < 10 grams	−10	5. Fetal heart rate abnormality (<115,	−30
5. Fever	−20	>165)	
Placental factors		Labor Index score = 100 − above penalties	
1. Bleeding before 20 weeks	−10		
2. Bleeding 20 weeks–term	−20	Total Index = 200 − (penalties from	
3. Bleeding with pain and/or hypotension	−30	MCHC Index and penalties from	
4. Ruptured membranes > 24 hours	−20	Labor Index)	

*From Aubrey, R. H., and Pennington, J. C.: Identification and evaluation of high risk pregnancy: the perinatal concept, Clin. Obstet. Gynec. **16**(1):3-29, Mar. 1973.

Table 10-6. Summary of high-risk factors influencing maternal-fetal dyad

Factor	Risk	Factor	Risk
First trimester			
Anatomic	Maternal	**Second trimester**	
	Ectopic pregnancy	Anatomic	Maternal
	Uterine abnormality		Uterine abnormality
	Retroversion		Incompetent os
Physiologic	Fetal		Fetal
	Gross chromosomal defect		Gross abnormality
	Hydatidiform mole		Acute hydramnios
	Multiple pregnancy		Multiple pregnancy
	Poor trophoblast invasiveness		Poor implantation
	Folate deficiency	Maternal complications	Rh incompatibility
	Endocrine deficiency		Cyanotic heart disease
	Hyperemesis gravidarum		Hypertension
	Defective sperm		Renal disease
Psychologic	Psychologic shock		Urinary tract infections
	Drugs		Accidents
Therapeutic	Social abortion (aspiration, saline, prostaglandin)		Anoxia of eclampsia
			Anoxia of epilepsy
	Drug therapy	Infections	Viral
	X-ray therapy		Polio
Infections	Viral		Hepatitis
Genetic	Sporadic mutation		Syphilis
	Inherited characteristics	Genetic	Amniocentesis
	Sex-linked disease	Idiopathic	Genetic death
Environmental	Poverty	Environmental	Poverty
	Drugs		Drugs
	Tobacco		Tobacco
	Alcohol		Alcohol
	Nutrition		Nutrition

*Associated with intrauterine growth retardation.

DIAGNOSTIC MANAGEMENT OF THE HIGH-RISK PREGNANCY

Closely allied with identification of the high-risk mother is management of the high-risk pregnancy once it is recognized. It is particularly important to determine the optimal time for delivery so that the fetus can achieve maximal benefit and maturity from the intrauterine environment on the one hand and avoid intrauterine death on the other. To this end several diagnostic tools have been developed that allow the health practitioner to more accurately determine fetal well-being and predict the optimal time for delivery.

Urinary estriol

There are times when it is essential to monitor fetal well-being over time, for example, when the pregnant woman is diabetic or has toxemia. One of the most use-

ful laboratory tests for this is the study of the woman's 24-hour urinary estriol excretion. Estriol is produced in a complex interrelationship between the fetus and the placenta, whereby maternal estrogen undergoes conversion in the placenta and fetal adrenals. Estriol is then conjugated in the mother's liver and excreted in her urine. Estriol excretion tends to increase progressively throughout pregnancy as long as the fetal-maternal-placental complex is healthy. By measuring the 24-hour urinary excretions of maternal estriol, one can estimate fetal well-being and get an idea of how well the fetal-placental unit is functioning. Estriol levels can be altered by abnormal functioning of the fetus, placenta, or maternal liver and kidneys. The pattern established is more important than any one absolute value. Any fall from previously normal values (12 to 15 mg/ml at term) is significant and must be confirmed by more than one

Table 10-6. Summary of high-risk factors influencing maternal-fetal dyad—cont'd

Factor	Risk	Factor	Risk
Third trimester		**Labor**	
Anatomic	Malpresentation Cord complications Placenta previa*	Anatomic	Head compression Malpresentation Cord prolapse Breech presentation Placenta previa Abruptio placentae Rigid soft tissues Multiple pregnancy Fetal hemorrhage Placental compression Excessive fetal size
Maternal complications	Hypertension* Rh incompatibilities Diabetes Thyrotoxicosis Autoimmune disease*		
Infections	Viral* Pneumonia		
Nutritional	Protein lack Iron deficiencies Abruptio placentae* Antibacterial drugs	Physiologic	Dehydration Ketosis Fetal acidosis Postural tachycardia
Therapeutic to mother	Tetracycline Antithyroid drugs Corticosteroids Anticonvulsants Anticoagulants	Maternal complications	Eclampsia
		Iatrogenic	Sedative depression Hypotension of anesthesia Anoxia of labor Prolonged labor Forceps Oxytocin
Conditions peculiar to pregnancy	Hypertensive disease* Postmaturity		
Fetal complications	Premature rupture of membranes Premature labor Hydramnios	Uterine and placental	Uterine hypotonicity, hypertonicity, inertia Placental insufficiency
Environmental	Poverty Drugs Tobacco Alcohol Nutrition	Environmental	Drugs Poverty

reading. In general, a drop of 25% from the baseline or average value indicates fetal distress and a drop of 50% indicates fetal death. Consistently low levels can indicate anencephaly, and an estriol reading of 4 to 8 mg/ml indicates impending death of the fetus.

Ultrasound or echo sounding

Ultrasonic echo sounding has recently added to the obstetrician's repertoire of diagnostic techniques to assess fetal growth and determine maternal problems. The technique consists of sending very short pulses of low-intensity, high-frequency soundwaves into the mother's uterus. The returning echo signals are transmitted onto a screen that builds up a two-dimensional picture of the intrauterine contents, which can then be photographed for a permanent record. Ultrasound gives five pieces of information:

1. *Gestational age:* The biparietal diameter of the fetal skull is measured; this measurement is then converted into a gestational age, which is accurate ±2 weeks. It should be noted that accuracy in determining fetal gestational age is decreased when the technique is used in the third trimester.
2. *Documentation of intrauterine growth retardation:* By doing a series of ultrasound readings over time (usually at 2-week intervals), it is possible to demonstrate growth or lack of growth in utero.
3. *Placental localization:* Locating the site of implantation is valuable in the diagnosis of placenta previa and when deciding where to do amniocentesis or cesarean section.
4. *Diagnosis of multiple pregnancy.*
5. *Diagnosis of congenital malformations:* Certain anomalies, such as hydrocephaly, anencephaly,

hydatidiform mole, or Siamese twins, can be diagnosed through ultrasound.

Ultrasound is a valuable tool for "dating" pregnancies and determining EDC in clients who are uncertain about when their last menstrual period occurred; this is especially critical when early delivery is anticipated, as with the client who is diabetic or Rh sensitized.

Prior to ultrasound, only the traditional and often very subjective methods were available. The woman's report of when her last menstrual period occurred or when she experienced quickening, the time when fetal heart tones were first heard, and fundal height measurements are examples of these less accurate methods of determining gestational age. Occasionally, radiographs of the fetal skeleton were taken to estimate fetal age as more or less than 36 weeks, since calcification of the distal epiphyses of the long bones occurs after 36 weeks' gestation. Radiographs were also used to diagnose multiple births and some congenital anomalies, such as anencephaly; it is still used to determine cephalopelvic disproportion.

Oxytocin challenge test

The adequacy of placental respiratory capabilities can be evaluated by the oxytocin challenge test (OCT) or stress test. This test is based on the premise that late decelerations of the fetal heart rate with uterine contractions indicate fetal hypoxia and distress. Uterine contractions decrease blood flow and therefore oxygen is not transferred to the placenta. If the placenta has adequate oxygen stores, then transient decreases will not cause changes in the fetal heart rate; however, if the fetus does not have adequate reserves and placental insufficiency is present, the fetal heart rate decreases at or slightly after the peak of the contraction. Late deceleration of the fetal heart indicates that the fetus cannot tolerate stress—that there is uteroplacental insufficiency and the fetus is in jeopardy.

In the stress test (OCT) (done in the last trimester if there is a question of fetal distress), oxytocin is administered intravenously continuously in increasing amounts until mild uterine contractions are produced. This constitutes a "stress situation" for the fetus. Oxytocin administration is continued until three or four contractions, lasting 30 seconds and of good quality, are observed in a 10-minute period. A test is considered positive if persistent late decelerations occur in association with normal uterine contractions when the patient is lying on her side. At this point delivery is considered advisable and fetal maturity studies (ultrasound, amniocentesis) are done. A suspicious test result is one in which occasional late decelerations occur. The test is then repeated in 2 to 3 days. In a negative result there are no late decelerations when adequate contractions are present. In this case OCT should be repeated in 1 week.

Recently, some health care teams managing high-risk pregnancies have begun to use a test known as the "passive" fetal activity test (FAT). In this test, fetal monitoring equipment is attached to the pregnant woman so that fetal activity (usually fetal heart tones) can be monitored with normal, unstimulated uterine activity. It is believed that this less complex, nonintrusive procedure can also give adequate data about fetal well-being.

Amniocentesis

The structural chemical components and activity of fetal cells in amniotic fluid can provide valuable information regarding fetal well-being and maturity.

Amniocentesis is the transabdominal aspiration of amniotic fluid from within the uterine cavity. It is a safe and accepted procedure that may be done in the outpatient clinic. While it is obviously not done routinely, the risks of infection, fetal injury, and fetal hemorrhage are very small (one complication in 1,000 procedures). The amniocentesis procedure is as follows:

1. After the surgical preparation with an antiseptic and sterile draping of the abdomen, the obstetrician determines the most suitable site for insertion of the needle. The three sites used are illustrated in Fig. 10-3.
   a. If the head is not fixed in the pelvis and can be displaced superiorly, the area used is that between the vertex and the symphysis pubis. In this area, one goes through the thinnest part of the uterine wall in a region where the placenta is seldom found.
   b. The second site of choice is that area between the vertex and the shoulder where there is almost always a pocket of amniotic fluid.
   c. The third site of choice is that region where the small parts are palpable. This site is most often chosen when the head is not palpable or fixed in the pelvis.
2. After selection of the proper site, local anesthesia is infiltrated into the skin and anterior abdominal wall.
3. The needle, usually a 20-gauge spinal needle, is inserted through the abdominal wall, peritoneum, myometrium, and into the amniotic sac.
4. This is then followed by withdrawal of the amniotic fluid, usually 10 to 15 ml.

The studies most commonly done on amniotic fluid to determine fetal maturity and well-being are the following:

Color. This is obviously the easiest and most readily apparent sign. As the fluid is drawn into the syringe, one can easily see whether it is clear or stained. The presence of meconium (a brown to blackish appearance) indicates fetal distress and possible fetal death. At times the amniotic fluid will appear whitish or opaque. This is not necessarily a cause for alarm.

Bilirubinoid pigments. Bilirubin is produced from the breakdown of red blood cells, and is thus present at certain levels in normal amniotic fluid. Peak levels are

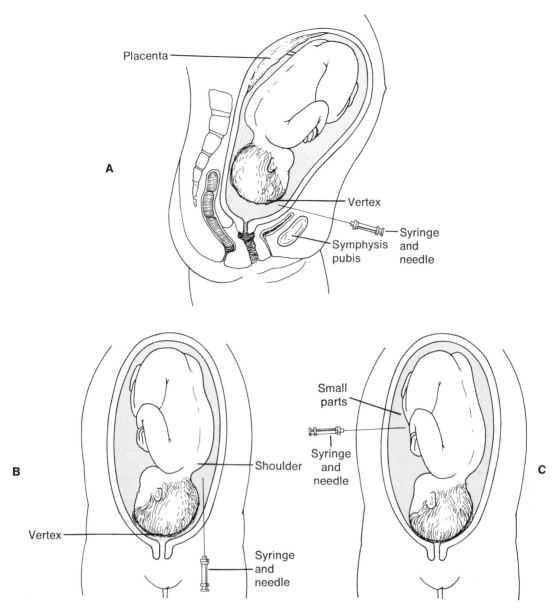

Fig. 10-3. Sites for amniocentesis.

obtained between 16 and 30 weeks' gestation, and a steady decline occurs thereafter with disappearance occurring by 36 weeks. Excessively high levels of bilirubin usually occur with erythroblastosis and may be an indication of fetal distress.

Creatinine concentration. Levels of creatinine in the amniotic fluid increase with gestational age and therefore are useful in determining fetal maturity. When the creatinine level is less than 1.5 mg/100 ml, the fetus is immature; 1.2 to 2.0 mg creatinine is borderline, and greater than 2.0 mg indicates probable fetal maturity. However, it should be noted that lower values are reported in diabetic mothers, and thus the creatinine concentration test alone is not enough to establish maturity.

L/S ratio. This ratio has proved to be of considerable value in determining fetal pulmonary maturity, indicating surface active phospholipids. The concentration of sphingomyelin (S) slightly exceeds lecithin (L) until the twenty-sixth week at which time there is an abrupt increase of lecithin until after the thirty-fifth week of gestation. At 35 weeks, there is a marked increase in the lecithin and none in sphingomyelin. This has led to the conclusion that once the surge of lecithin has occurred (at 35 to 36 weeks), pulmonary maturity is sufficient to avoid respiratory distress syndrome if delivery occurs at this time. The ratio looked for is 2:1 and when this occurs, there is a 97% chance that the fetal lungs are mature.

Table 10-7. Summary of diagnostic tools for fetal maturity*

Test or tool	Fetal maturity
Last menstrual period (LMP)	Determine EDC (subjective, often inaccurate)
Fetal heart	If present at 20 weeks by fetoscope (subjective)
Quickening	Begins 14-16 weeks but often not recognized by mother until 20 weeks (subjective to objective depending on who recognizes and documents)
Fetal distal femoral epiphysis	36 weeks (by X-ray often difficult to determine)
Fetal proximal tibial epiphysis	38 weeks (by X-ray often difficult to determine)
Fetal biparietal diameter	8.5-36 weeks ± 2 weeks gestation objective—more accurate than LMP test
Amniotic fluid assessments	
L/S ratio	2.0 or more, usually after 34-36 weeks
Creatinine	2.0 mg% (objective; accurate)
Fat cells	18%

*Adapted from Romney, S., and others: Gynecology and obstetrics: the health care of women, New York, 1975, McGraw-Hill Book Co.

Cytology. Desquamation of the fetal skin occurs in the amniotic fluid and as the fetus approaches maturity there is an increasing number of fat-containing cells from the sebaceous glands of the more mature skin. These are readily demonstrated by the use of a special fat stain (Nile blue sulfate). After staining, a fat cell count is done. If more than 10% fat cells are present in the amniotic fluid, the pregnancy is probably 37 weeks' gestation or more. In addition, a maturation index is now beginning to be used. The squamous cells are rated on a scale of 1 to 4 (immature basal cells = 1; mature squamous cells = 4). The ratio of mature squamous cells to immature basal cells is determined. At term very few immature cells are found.

Bubble tests. This is a test to determine whether or not surfactant has been laid down in the fetal lung. Surfactant is essential for expansion of the lungs at birth and for normal respiration thereafter. If the lungs are mature, stable foam will be generated on the surface of amniotic fluid when ethanol is added. This test is probably the most rapid, simple, and inexpensive test we have to date that produces conclusive results.

NURSING CARE

It is well documented that pregnancy is a crisis both physiologically and psychologically. Usually the crisis is maturational; however, the crisis may also be situational when the pregnancy becomes high risk. The family experiencing a high-risk pregnancy has anxieties and complex problems that require individualized, in-depth nursing care. The obvious physical problems, coupled with the psychologic and emotional impact of a high-risk pregnancy, create a highly stressful situation. Because pregnancy and illness are uncommon experiences, the usual coping mechanisms will not work and new ways of behaving must be developed. The high-risk mother must accomplish three different sets of developmental tasks: (1) the task of pregnancy, (2) tasks resulting from illness, and (3) the tasks of the two together—a high-risk pregnancy. The developmental tasks of pregnancy, as conceived by Rubin (1970), are:

1. Seeking a safe passage for herself and her child through pregnancy, labor, and delivery
2. Ensuring acceptance of her child by her significant others
3. Bonding to her unknown child
4. Learning to give of herself

The behavioral tasks of illness have been thoroughly documented in nursing literature; as they relate to pregnancy they are: adaptation to the sick role, acceptance of an uncertain outcome, possible adaptation to a chronic disability/illness with successful grieving, and assumption of the appropriate role in the therapeutic regimen. The treatment of pregnancy as high risk is often a shock and causes anxiety about the outcome for both mother and child. The stages of the grief process must be worked through for healthy resolution and acceptance. During the shock and denial phase the woman may experience a period of self-doubt. Self-questioning often occurs. If the pregnancy was planned, the woman may wonder if she is doing the right thing in attempting a pregnancy; if the pregnancy was unplanned, the woman may feel she is being punished in some way. Often clients attribute the problem to something they did or did not do; an element of self-blame is present. For example, the diabetic may feel she ate too many sweets or the woman who has high blood pressure may think she worried too much. Many women move from blaming themselves to blaming others, moving from the shock and denial phase into the anger phase of the grief process. They may ask why the physician did not prevent the problem or discover it sooner. Often the nurse is the recipient of this anger and must learn to accept it, understand its implications for the client, and allow its expression without reacting defensively—a tall order. After these initial reactions have occurred, the client can begin to consider the implications of a diagnosis of high-risk pregnancy for herself and her family. It is crucial that the client arrive at this in order to ultimately accept her pregnancy, herself, and her illness or problem; without this acceptance, compliance with medical management cannot be achieved, and the potential for magnifying the complications of a high-risk pregnancy increases.

One of the essential tasks of high-risk pregnancy is acceptance of self as a high-risk mother. Everyone has a positive mental body image or concept of oneself as healthy. To accept oneself as high risk is difficult because it implies lack of perfection, a state of illness, or ill health. The risk factor may be newly diagnosed or a long-term illness, but in either case the woman must incorporate a new aspect of herself—pregnancy and illness—with new and threatening meanings. The woman needs to retain as positive a body image as possible throughout her pregnancy. An essential part of the nurse's role is to support all efforts of the client to view herself in a positive way.

Frequently, the high-risk mother wonders whether the "pregnancy will accept her"; that is, she fears losing the fetus and being childless forever. Whether the pregnancy was planned or not, or wanted or not, often does not affect the concern about the possibility of being childless. Many women value their ability to bear children and want to be able to choose whether to have children or not. Being a high-risk mother may be seen as a threat to self-concept as a woman and as a mate. The woman may fear rejection from her partner and family, depending upon her value systems and theirs.

The maturational task of accepting pregnancy is made more difficult in the high-risk situation. The normal fears a woman has for herself and the infant are intensified, and understandably so, since they are based in reality. All the fears about the infant being normal and about death of self or the infant are increased. Frequently, the pregnant woman considers the cost involved in energy, time, and money—for herself and her family—and wonders if all of this can be paid. It is difficult to accept the pregnancy as it truly is—a high-risk, stressful situation. Sometimes the woman does not feel or look sick and does not understand the necessity for all the clinic visits and tests. Acceptance of the sick role may be particularly difficult in the United States today with increased emphasis on the naturalness of pregnancy and childbirth.

Many adaptations are required of the high-risk mother in order to achieve the maternal tasks of pregnancy. In order to secure a safe passageway for herself and her child she may be asked to change her entire pattern of daily living. A woman may be willing to endure almost anything to "guarantee" safety for herself and her baby. This attitude may ensure client compliance with medical management, but this type of belief is not entirely based in reality. No one can promise a mother that her good behavior will ensure the birth of a healthy, normal infant. Often the nurse must deal with the client's need

to hope, the importance of following the physician's orders, and the necessity of not instilling false hope. It is impossible to promise any woman unconditionally that she and her infant will be healthy.

The high-risk mother frequently experiences many fears and fantasies about what her infant will be like and how she and the infant will be accepted. Questions such as, "Can I be a good mother," and "How will the father react" are common. It is often difficult for the high-risk mother to become emotionally bonded to the unborn child; the desire for the first positive signs of baby's wellness is crucial to her. Any preparations for the new baby may be delayed until after delivery. There may be no signs of nesting at all, even in the third trimester.

The high-risk pregnancy is a crisis situation for the client and family, calling for highly individualized nursing care. The high-risk mother frequently has depleted energy resources to give of herself. She has made so many sacrifices and changes and undergone so much stress that she may have difficulty summoning the resources to cope with new stressors. Crisis intervention can be used effectively to provide the high-risk mother the immediate help she needs. The goal is to work through the immediate crisis in the following steps: (1) initial assessment of the mother and her problem, (2) development of therapeutic interventions, (3) intervention, and (4) crisis resolution and anticipatory guidance directed toward future crisis. The actual interventions must be directed and flexible, in order to help the mother intellectually understand the crisis, consciously realize and identify her feelings, explore possible coping mechanisms, and anticipate future crises and make plans to prevent them.

The information about risk factors presented in this chapter, the various assessment tools described, and an understanding of the stressors of high-risk pregnancy can suggest areas to be explored with the mother. But while we can generalize about areas in which to anticipate problems, it is essential that the nurse listen to what the mother is saying about her needs, concerns, and stressors. The assessment should also include a careful evaluation of the family and social situation. The social support system, particularly the family and partner, is highly significant in assessing stressors, coping abilities, and planning nursing care. The family is very important in terms of support, role shifts, and security. By recognizing the influence the family has on the client, the nurse can assess the strengths of the family and use them as she works with the client. The cultural heritage of the client affects all aspects of her life and personality including attitudes toward pregnancy, health, and disease. Cultural attitudes that affect prenatal behavior are (1) responsibility for fetal growth as reflected in dietary habits, sexual practices, and guilt when complications occur, (2) concern for the pregnant woman, (3) pregnancy as proof of sexual prowess, (4) pregnancy as a time of increased vulnerability and debilitation, and (5) pregnancy as a time of shame and reticence (Lytle, 1977). Religion will influence attitudes toward abortion, women's role in life, pregnancy, and family planning. Cultural attitudes toward disease and illness vary considerably. Illness may evoke a major emotional response in one culture while it may be considered less important in another. In the United States, where independence, perfection, and achievement are valued positively, the need to be taken care of may create conflict. Examples to be explored by the nurse in the assessment follow:

1. Family: members; number and ages of children; is father of the baby present; are there pressing problems or illnesses in other family members
2. Support system: Is the family stable; how close is the extended family; are there close friends; who else lives in the house; who is the main support person; whom can woman turn to for help; whom can she talk to
3. Financial situation: who works; what is family's income; what are the expenses; is the wife's income essential; is there third-party insurance
4. Attitudes toward pregnancy: planned or not; wanted or not; what are worries or concerns; what does family worry about most; has childbirth preparation been planned
5. Stress factors: are there other pressures or stressors in nuclear or extended family that directly affect client
6. Strengths: how are mother or couple handling the pregnancy; marital relationship mature and reality based
7. Plans: what are long-term plans and expectations

After all data have been gathered and a nursing diagnosis of the problems has been developed, the plan of care is devised. Development of a helping relationship with the high-risk client is essential; trust and continuity of care greatly facilitate nursing care. The nursing role includes teaching and explanation since the client must have a thorough understanding of her condition. She should understand the probable course of her pregnancy, the procedures involved, her particular risk factor, and any hospitalizations anticipated; in addition, the parameters of normal pregnancy—what to expect, diet, exercise, emotional changes—should be explained to her. All of this will help her to intellectualize the crisis and anticipate future problems. The problem-solving method of teaching seems to be most successful. The nurse assists the client to think of alternative solutions given the necessary facts, rather than just telling client ready-made answers. When the client works out a solution for herself it seems to be more lasting and more effective, and she is more likely to follow through with it.

Being a high-risk mother is an enormous task. It is a physical, emotional, maturational, situational, and social crisis. Nursing care of the high-risk maternity client should be developed and carried out to assist the client to maximize strengths and minimize stressors.

REFERENCES

Aase, J. M.: Environmental causes of birth defects, Cont. Educ. Fam. Phys. 3(9):39-46, 1975.

Aladjem, S.: Risks in the practice of modern obstetrics, St. Louis, 1975, The C. V. Mosby Co.

Aubrey, R. H., and Pennington, J. C.: Identification and evaluation of high risk pregnancy: the perinatal concept, Clin. Obstet. Gynec. 16(1):3-29, 1973.

Babson, S. G., and others: Management of high risk pregnancy and intensive care of the neonate, St. Louis, 1975, The C. V. Mosby Co.

Bergner, L., and Susser, M.: Low birth weight and prenatal nutrition, Pediatrics, 46(6):946-966, 1970.

Blair, C. L., and Salerno, E. M.: The expanding family: childbearing, Boston, 1976, Little, Brown & Co.

Blinick, G., and others: Drug addiction in pregnancy and the neonate, Am. J. Ob/Gyn. 125(2):135-142, 1976.

Budd, K. W.: Behavioral tasks of the high risk maternity patient. In Lytle, N., editor: Nursing of women in the age of liberation, Dubuque, Iowa, 1977, William C. Brown, Publishers.

Christianson, R. E.: Studies on blood pressure during pregnancy. I. Influence of parity and age, Am. J. Obstet. Gynecol. 125:509-513, 1974.

Clark, A. L., and Affonso, D. D.: Childbearing; a nursing perspective, Philadelphia, 1976, F. A. Davis Co.

Clausen, I., and others: Maternity nursing today, New York, 1977, McGraw-Hill Book Co.

Contrasts in health status, Vol. 1: Infant death: an analysis by maternal risk and health care, Washington, D.C., 1973, Institute of Medicine, National Academy of Sciences.

Correy, J. F., and Campbell, S. N.: What is meant by the 'at risk' pregnancy? Austral. Phys. 6:205-212, 1977.

Crane, G. P.: A high-risk pregnancy management protocol, Am. J. Obstet. Gynecol. 125(2):227-235, 1976.

Davids, A., and DeVault, S.: Maternal anxiety during pregnancy and childbirth abnormality, Psychosom. Med. 24(5):464-469, 1962.

Dott, A. B., and Fort, A. T.: The effect of availability and utilization of prenatal care and hospital services on infant mortality rates, Am. J. Obstet. Gynecol. 123:854, 1975.

Eastman, N.: Prematurity from the viewpoint of the obstetrician, Am. Pract. 1:343-352, 1947.

Forfar, J.: Drugs that cause birth defects, Contemp. Obstet. Gynecol. 4:61-65, 1974.

Galloway, K.: The problem solving approach in high risk pregnancy, Am. J. Mat. Child Nurs., pp. 294-299, Sept./Oct. 1974.

Gorsuch, R. L., and Kay, M.: Abnormalities of pregnancy as a function of anxiety and life stress, Psychosom. Med. 36(4):332-362, 1974.

Green, M., and others: Prenatal exposure to narcotics, Ped. Ann., pp. 418-423, July 1975.

Halstead, L.: The use of crisis intervention in obstetrical nursing, Nurs. Clin. North Am. 9(1):69-76, 1974.

Hardy, J., and Mellits, E. D.: Does maternal smoking during pregnancy have a long-term effect on the child? Lancet, pp. 1332-1336, Dec. 23, 1972.

Higgins, A. C.: Nutritional status and the outcome of pregnancy, J. Canad. Diet. Assoc., pp. 17-35, 1974.

Jacobson, H.: Weight and weight gain in pregnancy, Clin. Perinatol. 2(2):233-242, 1973.

Jones, M. B.: Antepartum assessment in high risk pregnancy, J. Obstet. Gynecol. Nurs., pp. 23-27, Nov./Dec. 1975.

Kajanoja, P., and Widholm, O.: Pregnancy and delivery in women aged 40 and over, Obstet. Gynecol. 51(1):47-51, 1978.

Kennedy, J. C.: The high risk maternal infant acquaintance process, Nurs. Clin. North Am. 8(3):459-556, 1973.

Larson, V.: Stresses of the childbearing year, Am. J. Pub. Health 36(1):32-36, 1966.

Lechtig, A., and others: Influence of maternal nutrition on birth weight, Am. J. Clin. Nutr. 28:1223-1233, 1975.

Lechtig, A., and others: Effect of food supplementation during pregnancy on birthweight, Pediatrics 54(4):508-520, 1975.

Leon, J.: High risk pregnancy: graphic representation of the maternal and fetal risk, Am. J. Obstet. Gynecol., pp. 497-504, Oct. 1973.

Lucey, J. F.: Drugs and the intrauterine patient. Proceedings Symposium on the Placenta, Its Form and Functions, Birth Defects Original Article Series, Vol. 1, No. 1, Apr. 1965.

Luke, B.: Maternal alcoholism and fetal alcohol syndrome, Am. J. Nurs. 77(12):1924-1926, 1977.

Lytle, N. A.: Nursing of women in the age of liberation, Dubuque, 1977, Wm. C. Brown, Publishers.

Manniello, R., and Farrell, P.: Analysis of U.S. neonatal mortality statistics from 1968 to 1974 with specific reference to changing trends in major causalities, Am. J. Obstet. Gynecol., pp. 667-674, Nov. 15, 1977.

McDonald, R. L.: The role of emotional factors in obstetrical complications: a review, Psychosom. Med. 30(2):222-237, 1968.

Meyer, M., and others: Perinatal events associated with maternal smoking during pregnancy, Am. J. Epidemiol. 103(5):464-476, 1976.

Meyer, M. B., and Fonascia, J. A.: Maternal smoking, pregnancy complications and perinatal mortality, Am. J. Obstet. Gynecol. 128:494-502, 1977.

Moore, M. L.: Realities in childbirth, Philadelphia, 1978, W. B. Saunders Co.

Naylor, A. F., and Myrianthopolous, N. P.: The relation of ethnic and selected socioeconomic factors to human birthweight, Ann. Hum. Gen. 31:71-83, 1971.

Nesbith, R. E. L., and Aubrey, R. H.: High risk obstetrics: value of semiobjective grading system in identifying the vulnerable group, Am. J. Obstet. Gynecol., pp. 972-985, April 1, 1967.

Nuckolls, K., and others: Psychosocial assets, life crisis of the prognosis of pregnancy, Am. J. Epidemiol. 95(5):431-441, 1972.

Osofsky, H. J., and Kendall, N.: Poverty as a criterion of risk, Clin. Obstet. Gynec. 16:103-109, 1973.

Peckham, C., and Christianson, R.: The relationship between pregnancy weight and certain obstetric factors, Am. J. Obstet. Gynecol. 3(1):1-7, 1971.

Pernoll, M. L., and others: Review: prenatal diagnosis, Obstet. Gynec. 44(5):773-783, 1974.

Pitkins, R. M.: Nutritional influences during pregnancy, Med. Clin. North Am. 61(1):3-15, 1977.

Pritchard, J. A., and MacDougald, P. C.: Williams obstetrics, ed. 5, New York, 1976, Appleton-Century-Crofts.

Resseguie, L. J.: Comparison of longitudinal and cross-sectional analysis: maternal age and stillbirth ratio, Am. J. Epidemiol. 103(6):551-559, 1976.

Romney, S., and others: Gynecology and obstetrics: the health care of women, New York, 1975, McGraw-Hill Book Co.

Rose, P. A.: The high risk mother infant dyad, Nurs. Forum 6(1):94-102, 1967.

Rothman, I. J., and Fyler, D. O.: Sex, birth order, and maternal age characteristics of infants with congenital heart defects, Am. J. Epidemiol. 104(5):527-534, Nov. 1976.

Rubbelke, L., and Waller, M. V.: Maternal health index—a nursing aid to decision on priorities of services, ANA Clin. Sess., pp. 175-184, 1969.

Rubin, R.: Cognitive style in pregnancy, Am. J. Nurs. 70:502, 1970.

Schenkel, B., and Vocheu, H.: Nonprescription drugs during pregnancy, J. Reprod. Med. 12(1):27-34, 1974.

Schneider, J.: Repeated pregnancy loss, Clin. Obstet. Gynec. 16:120-133, 1973.

Schwartz, J. L., and Schwartz, L. H.: Vulnerable infants, New York, 1977, McGraw-Hill Book Co.

Scurletis, T., and others: High risk indicators of fetal, neonatal and postnatal mortalities, N. Carolina Med. J., p. 183-192, March 1973.

Seaman, B.: How late can you wait to have a baby? MS, Jan. 1976.

Selvin, S., and Cappinkel, J.: Maternal age, paternal age and birth order and the risk of fetal loss, Hum. Biol. 48(1):223-230, 1976.

Silverman, D. T.: Maternal smoking and birth weight, Am. J. Epidemiol. 105:513-521, 1977.

Sinclair, J. C.: Nutritional influences in industrial societies, Am. J. Des. Child. 129:549-553, 1975.

Spellancy, W. N.: Management of the high risk pregnancy, Baltimore, 1975, University Pub. Press.

Stone, M., and others: Narcotic addiction in pregnancy, Am. J. Obstet. Gynecol., pp. 716-723, Mar. 1972.

Streissguth, A. P.: Maternal drinking and the outcome of pregnancy, Am. J. Orthopsychiatry 47(3):422-430, 1977.

Thompson, A. M., and others: The assessment of fetal growth, J. Obstet. Gynecol. Br. Comm. 75:903, 1968.

U.S. National Center for Health Statistics: Vital statistics of the United States, 1977 Annual, Washington, D.C., 1977, U.S. Government Printing Office, p. 70.

Wallack, R.: Comparison of pregnancies and births during methadone detoxification and maintenance, Ped. Ann. 4:46-61, 1975.

Willis, W.: Perinatal loss, socioeconomic factors, J. Obstet. Gynecol. Nurs., pp. 44-47, Mar./Apr. 1977.

Worthington, B. S., Vermeersch, J., and Williams, S.: Nutrition in pregnancy, St. Louis, 1977, The C. V. Mosby Co.

11

Adolescent pregnancy

Catherine Ingram Fogel

Adolescence is a crisis period that must precede maturity; it is highlighted by inconsistency, uncertain feelings, and unpredictable reactions. The developmental tasks for the adolescent are experimentation, a struggle for independence, a search for self, a need to accept a changing body image, and acceptance by peers. The adolescent's two normative tasks are achieving independence (she must emancipate herself from her home and family of origin) and self-discovery (she searches for her identity as a woman). During adolescence, the female must integrate growth in physical, social, and psychologic areas into a meaningful whole; accept, develop, refine, and master a new identity; lay the groundwork for long-term mutual interpersonal relationships; and develop patterns of work behavior that are consistent and reasonable for an adult occupation or career. All of this must be accomplished in a relatively short period (less than 10 years) and at a time when the adolescent feels particularly vulnerable.

The tasks of adolescence are accompanied by emotional lability, ambivalence, heightened sensitivity, and a fluid, vulnerable ego state (Clark and Affonso, 1976; Shouse, 1975). A complicating factor is that in our culture physical maturation occurs much earlier than does the assumption of adult responsibilities. Readiness to assume a responsible position in life and to support a family comes much later than do sexual drives.

According to Erikson (1950) the developmental tasks of this period in life are: (1) establishment of one's own identity (crisis of adolescence), (2) development of intimacy in relationships (crisis of young adulthood), and (3) creation and nurturing of life (crisis of adulthood). The adolescent who becomes pregnant finds herself struggling to solve both the crisis of adolescence and of adulthood; often the tasks of young adulthood are never completed.

Childbearing at any age is a significant event for a woman. For the teenager it is often accompanied by more complex and more serious problems than the older woman experiences. Adolescent pregnancy is two, if not three, separate crises superimposed one upon the other: the teenager who becomes pregnant must resolve the developmental crises of adolescence and adulthood plus the developmental crisis of pregnancy; together these create a situational crisis—adolescent pregnancy. In addition, there are often medical and social complications that the adolescent must deal with. The teenager often is unmarried, which can cause additional psychosocial stress.

The challenge to nursing in assisting the pregnant teenager to successfully resolve these crises and to experience positive growth is enormous; and it is growing every year as adolescent pregnancy reaches epidemic proportions in the United States.

The purpose of this chapter is to provide the nurse with the knowledge and processes needed to meet this challenge. The epidemiology of adolescent pregnancy is reviewed, with consideration given to both its distribution and determinants. Health risks and emotional and sociocultural influences are also discussed. Finally, nursing strategies are considered.

SCOPE OF THE PROBLEM

Teenage pregnancy has now reached epidemic proportions in the United States. According to a zero population growth (ZPG) report (1977), 1 million teenagers become pregnant every year. Nearly 600,000 births in 1975 were to mothers under 20 years of age; they comprised 20% of the total births for the year. While birth rates for women 20 years of age and older have fallen sharply, the rate of childbearing for teenagers has not followed this pattern. This is particularly true for girls age 14 and younger and for 15- to 17-year-olds. (Those women who are 18 to 19 years old have actually experienced a fertility decrease similar to that of older women [ZPG, 1977; Vital Statistics, 1977].)

In 1975, three out of every ten women aged 20 had borne at least one child. One in ten teenagers from age 15 to 19 becomes pregnant each year, resulting in about 1 million pregnancies; and approximately 30,000 girls age 14 and under conceive. Nearly 40% of these pregnancies are the result of nonmarital conception and account for 52% of the total nonmarital births in the country. Of these pregnancies six in ten end in live births, almost three in ten are terminated by elective abortion, and one in ten ends in spontaneous abortion (ZPG, 1977). Teenagers account for one third of all legal abortions performed in the United States.

These statistics documenting a rise in both the actual number of teenage pregnancies and the rate at which pregnancy is occurring appear particularly alarming when we consider the unfortunate circumstances often surrounding birth to an adolescent girl. The infant is more likely to be of low birth weight, and to be born to a mother with less than a high school education and whose prenatal care and nutritional status are inadequate (Vital Statistics, 1977). That there are increased numbers of teenage pregnancies is particularly frustrating and puzzling considering the general decline in fertility of women, the increased availability of family planning services, and the legalization and resultant increased use of abortion.

The girl who becomes pregnant while still a teenager faces a multitude of problems. Potentially severe medical complications place both the mother and infant at risk for illness and death. And apart from the numerous biologic dangers she faces, the adolescent's life is disrupted. Prospects for completing her education are severely compromised. She faces motherhood prematurely, usually before her own maturation has been completed—and pregnancy in our society often is not a maturing experience for an adolescent. Furthermore, the very young lack the resources and experience to rear a child; the adolescent girl must first achieve her own developmental goals, since this is crucial to her performance as a mother. Among pregnant teenagers, incomplete education, low income level, psychologic and developmental problems, high parity, and potential social dependency are common. What results is a "syndrome of failure" for the pregnant adolescent when she fails to (So. Med. J., 1969):

1. Fulfill the developmental tasks of adolescence
2. Remain in school
3. Establish a stable family
4. Be self-supporting
5. Have healthy infants
6. Limit the size of her family

SOCIAL COST OF TEENAGE PREGNANCY
Education and income

There are three general reasons why adolescent mothers tend to have low incomes: (1) they are more likely to be single and dependent upon what they can earn or what government subsidies provide; (2) their education is interrupted and they lack the training and experience necessary to obtain well-paid, steady employment; and (3) if married, they are more likely to have married a young man who interrupted his education or who lacks the requisite experience to obtain and hold a job that pays well (Nye, 1977).

Pregnancy and motherhood are the major reasons why young women drop out of school. Eight out of ten women who become pregnant at 17 years of age or younger never finish high school. Among the very young (15 years and below) the statistics are even more alarming: nine out of ten never finish high school and four out of ten do not complete the eighth grade.

Moore and Waite (1977) have found that early childbearing is strongly associated with low levels of educational attainment, particularly for those girls attending school at the time of the birth of their first child. This association holds true even when other factors known to influence educational attainment, such as family background, race, and educational aspirations, are considered. The negative impact of early childbearing on educational attainment probably results from the difficulties of running a household, the costs of child care, the need to earn a living, and possible pressure from family and friends to be a full-time mother and caretaker. There is no evidence to suggest that the teenage mother is able to catch up with her peers who remain childless; in fact, the opposite all too often occurs. Teenage mothers fall further and further behind former classmates who postpone parenthood. While both black and white adolescent girls are handicapped by early childbearing in respect to their schooling, the effect appears to be greater for the white adolescent. Moore and Waite hypothesize that this is the result of more accepting social attitudes and the presence of more social mechanisms in the black community for dealing with the phenomenon of teenage pregnancy.

Given the association between education and such factors as occupation and income, it seems likely that early childbearing greatly diminishes the overall success of women. Inadequate schooling has potentially placed adolescent mothers at a permanent disadvantage. Because many do not complete high school and the vast majority have no work experience, they are doubly disadvantaged in job competition. Child care responsibilities often further restrict employment opportunities. Thus adolescent mothers are more apt to be unemployed, receiving welfare and/or existing incomes that are below poverty level.

Divorce

According to Nye (1977), many adolescent mothers marry the father of their baby. A large percentage of teenage marriages are unanticipated prior to conception and are the means to deal with an unplanned pregnancy. Teenage marriages are extremely vulnerable; they are two to three times as likely to end in divorce as marriages which begin with the couple in their twenties (ZPG, 1977). Bacon (1974) found that the divorce rate for women rises as age decreases; the rate for the youngest group is twice the average rate for all women. Given that the current national divorce rate is about one in two marriages, the teenage marriage appears to have almost no chance at all. Two thirds of marriages of school-age girls end in divorce in the first 5 years (Nye, 1977) and half of the marriages of girls pregnant in high school dissolve in four years (Furstenburg, 1976). In addition, many marriages end in desertion or other permanent separations. Those marriages that do survive tend to be disadvantaged in terms of occupation, income, and material assets.

High parity and high-risk pregnancy

Women who were teenage mothers are more likely to have a larger completed family and to have their children closer together than other women do. Women who have their first child at age 17 or younger will have thirty percent more children than women who begin childbearing at ages 20 to 24 (ZPG, 1977). More babies are now being born to very young mothers and these young mothers account for a larger proportion of all births. This increase has been observed in both whites and nonwhites (Vital Statistics, 1977). The health of babies born in rapid sequence is likely to be poorer than that of the first infant. In addition, the woman's health suffers when pregnancies occur more closely than 2 years apart.

Babies born to teenage mothers are more likely to be of low birth weight than are infants born to mothers in their twenties, and the incidence of low birth weight increases as age of the mother drops. This association between age and incidence of low birth weight occurs regardless of race and marital status. That is, although the proportion of low birth weight infants is higher among blacks than among whites and higher for nonmarital than for marital pregnancy, the incidence of low birth weight is *always* highest among infants born to the youngest mothers (Vital Statistics, 1977). (See Chapter 10 for a discussion of the significance of low birth weight and its effect on the well-being of the infant and child.)

Teenagers are less apt to receive adequate continuous prenatal care than are older mothers. Young teenage mothers are also more likely to obtain no prenatal care or to seek it relatively late in pregnancy. The proportion of 15-year-olds who first obtain prenatal care in the third trimester is almost twice that for 19-year-old mothers and five times that of mothers 25 to 29 years old. Simi-

larly, the younger the mother, the less likely she is to begin prenatal care in the critical first trimester of pregnancy. The relationship between age of the mother and onset of prenatal care holds regardless of race. However, on the average, white mothers of all ages begin care earlier than do black mothers, and the incidence of no prenatal care is somewhat lower for white than for black mothers except in the under-15 age group (Vital Statistics, 1977). As noted in Chapter 10, inadequate prenatal care is a significant risk factor in the childbearing cycle.

Nonmarital pregnancy

Because the overwhelming majority of teenage girls are not married—more than ninety-five percent of those 17 years old and under in 1970—the majority of pregnancies occurring to teenagers will be nonmarital. There has been a steady increase in the total number of nonmarital births. At first glance this appears to be very alarming—an "epidemic" of nonmarital pregnancies, so to speak; however, the figures are somewhat misleading and should be interpreted in light of other variables. For example, a significant proportion of teenagers are *not* sexually active and therefore are not at risk for pregnancy. When conventional nonmarital pregnancy rates are recomputed taking this into account, they show a decline in recent years in the proportion of sexually active teenagers who bear children out of wedlock (Zelnick and Kantner, 1972). It is important to be aware that while the actual number of adolescent females at risk is increasing as more teenagers become sexually active, and more babies are being born to single mothers each year because the population of potential teenage mothers is growing, the rate of this increase in single parent births is declining.

According to Zelnick and Kantner (1978) from 1971 to 1976 the proportion of white teenagers who had ever been pregnant increased at a rate roughly equal to the rate of increase in sexual activity. Thus among white sexually active females, there was no change in the incidence of pregnancy. Blacks showed approximately the same rate of increase in sexual activity; however, the number who became pregnant remained essentially unchanged; therefore, the incidence of single parent pregnancy actually declined. In 1976 more than seven in ten first pregnancies occurring to teens were premaritally conceived (nine in ten to blacks and more than six in ten to whites). Teenage pregnancy places at least two people at risk—the mother and the infant—and these risks are biologic, psychologic, and social. There appear to be synergistic effects from the factors of age, race, socioeconomic status, marital status, parity, and adequacy of prenatal care; acting together they produce a risk greater than any one produces alone. And the teen-ager is vulnerable in all these respects.

ETIOLOGY

Much has been written about why adolescent girls become pregnant—assuming that there exist causes over and above the biologic one of sperm fertilizing egg. In the past one single cause was usually identified to explain all aspects of the problem; more recently, there has been some acknowledgement of the possibility of multiple factors, and a belief that no one single factor explains everything. To date the research has not sufficiently identified the factors related to adolescent pregnancy nor sufficiently differentiated between motivation for sexual intercourse and desire for pregnancy. There are many theories of causality for adolescent pregnancy, motherhood, and nonmarital pregnancy. At present no one theory, be it psychologic or sociologic, can be satisfactorily modified or extended to explain adolescent pregnancy in general. However, it is helpful to know what the prevailing theories are in order to understand the many factors that can interact to produce an adolescent or nonmarital pregnancy.*

"Fallen women" model

In the early 1900s, the nonmarried mother was considered a "fallen woman" or "born bad." Then followed a brief period during which the nonmarried mother was classified as a mental defective. After World War I, she was seen as a product of "the wrong side of the tracks" or a bad environment. She was typically viewed as uneducated, ignorant, and poor. The "sinful daughters of Eve" theory has now fallen into ill repute; however, remnants of this belief still operate today. The view that sexual activity will increase if teenagers are provided sex education has its basis in the older belief, as does the idea that promiscuity (and, by extension, pregnancies) will increase as a population moves from a traditional to a modern, secular society. This latter view is rooted in the traditional religious belief that the threat of earthly or divine punishment results in low rates of nonmarital sexual activity. However, as Cutright (1971) clearly documents, no such phenomenon occurs; analysis of the nonmarital pregnancy rates in a variety of countries, including the United States, demonstrates that this is not so. For example, both church membership and attendance and nonmarital pregnancy rates rose

---

*The majority of past and present theories of causation do not clearly differentiate between nonmarital and adolescent pregnancy because most adolescent pregnancies are nonmarital and it is believed many of the same factors are operant. However, this belief has not yet been clearly substantiated by research data.

significantly between 1940 and 1965 in the United States.

Psychologic model

Psychologic theories of causality abound in the literature and are based on the assumption that some feature of the young girl's psyche causes her to risk sexual intercourse without contraceptive protection because pregnancy meets a psychologic need (see Pliones, 1975; Stewart, 1976; Young, 1954). From a psychoanalytic perspective, the girl is considered a victim of unconscious motivation resulting from a dysfunction in early parent-child interactions. Nonmarital pregnancy has been commonly viewed as an expression of the girl's ambivalent feelings toward her parents. The pregnancy is seen as systematic and purposeful—an attempt by the personality to ease an unresolved conflict. Leontine Young (1954) presents a classic example of this theory of causality. In her research Young found a consistent pattern of domination in the home by one parent, and the lack of happy, mature, loving parents.

Khlentzos and Pagliaro (1965) found four major emotional states to be characteristic of unwed mothers: ambivalence, rebelliousness, loneliness, and feelings of unworthiness. Although all characteristics might be present in the same girl, one usually dominated.

Much of the difficulty with these theories is that they were developed from small populations that are already screened (for example, girls under psychiatric treatment) and are only selectively applicable to white middle class population. Findings in these studies may be valid, but only for the teenagers in the particular study. No generalizations can be made from such studies to a general population of teenagers. The Pauker (1971) longitudinal study indicates that no one personality or motivational causality model can explain all nonmarital pregnancies.

For some girls a sexual relationship involves a search for the love that is not available from the parents. In such cases, pregnancy is an undesired outcome that was not intended or anticipated. A closely related case might be the woman who feels alone, abandoned, or depressed and who is seeking a relationship to overcome these feelings. She turns to someone who can give tenderness and intimacy without considering the consequences; in this case, neither pregnancy nor motherhood is desired. Similarly, when a significant loss has occurred, there is a need to fill the void. Some girls consciously seek to fill it by becoming pregnant and having a baby. They wish for something to love and to be loved by, something that belongs only to them; they fantasize that a baby will fill the void.

Other young girls become sexually active and subsequently pregnant in an effort to get attention, particularly from their mothers. For others, getting pregnant is an act of rebelliousness and a way to retaliate when they perceive they have been hurt. It is thought that in such cases the girl experiences conflicting feelings of love and hate toward her parents and expresses them through pregnancy, which is both an act of hostility and a cry for love. It should be noted that if this is the underlying causation, the act of having a baby will not relieve the need for treatment or get at the cause. In all of these situations involving psychologic causality several factors are operating:

1. The conscious or unconscious meaning of pregnancy to the girl and (usually) her parents
2. The girl's state of mind when the pregnancy occurs
3. Her current life situation
4. Her mode of expressing her wishes, particularly if she has a pattern of acting out unconscious wishes in an impulsive manner or has a tendency to overlook realities when under pressure

Sociologic model

Another major theoretical explanation of nonmarital motherhood is the sociologic model, which was particularly popular in the 1950s and early 1960s. Vincent (1961), for example, theorized that "illicit" sexual behavior is learned through interaction and identification with family, peers, and other significant cultural reference groups. He suggests that nonmarital motherhood is a function of the girl's socioeconomic position and affiliation with professional, religious, and political groups.

"Culture of poverty"

According to one sociologic theory, there is a "culture of poverty," particularly among black low-income groups, that promotes nonmarital pregnancy. Proponents of this explanation subscribe to the notion that cultural scripting dictates that no marriage is better than a poor marriage, and many women feel that a consensual union allows increased freedom and flexibility. Such stereotypes are rooted in the following specific cultural theses: (1) that high rates of nonmarital pregnancy stem from the matriarchal culture developed during slavery, (2) that no stigma is felt by a black nonmarried mother, and (3) that sexuality in the lower classes is spontaneous and uninhibited.

No longer is the "culture of poverty" theory given much credance, since research has not supported this belief system. Liben (1969) notes that there has been a tendency to assign intrapsychic causes for nonmarital pregnancies to middle-class white women, while social factors and laxity of norms continue to be stressed as causative for lower-class, nonwhite women. Only a few middle-class pregnancies are seen as genuine accidents,

while in the lower class, nonmarital pregnancy is said to be accidental and incidental to early sexual experiences.

A review of the literature (Pliones, 1975) indicates that the high incidence of pregnancy in this subculture is the result of ignorance about contraceptives and economic and social obstacles to difficulty obtaining abortions. Furstenburg (1969, 1970, 1976), who rejects the "culture of poverty" theory, has found that the majority of the pregnant black, urban teenagers and their mothers are unhappy about the pregnancy and negative toward it. Rainwater (1960) found that the poor are less sexually spontaneous and are more inhibited than other classes. Schlakman (1966) refutes the sociologic theory of premarital pregnancy by pointing out the inadequacies of the data. Although there is an association between poverty and early pregnancy the problem is the result of limited access to contraceptive services.

Johnson (1974) points out the two-way interaction between poverty and adolescent pregnancy: Not only does poverty increase the chances of adolescent pregnancy, but pregnancy also increases the chances of continuing poverty. Other authorities believe that the girl may be using pregnancy as an escape mechanism—a way out of school or a poor family situation. Still other researchers believe that nonmarital pregnancy is a result of a family pattern, the expectation that daughters will repeat their mothers' actions.

Cultural factors

In a second theory based on the sociologic conceptualization the scope of social factors implicated in early pregnancy is much broader. In this view, early pregnancy is promoted not only by the culture of poverty but also by the dominant American culture. According to Kleeman (1975), the factors contributing to the incidence of adolescent pregnancy are (1) the fact that teens are dependent and have no meaningful role in society, (2) the cultural stereotype of women's role, and (3) the ambiguity about what society says and does about sex.

Nonmarital pregnancy has also been considered a reflection of the different values held by society about sexuality (Vincent, 1961). The assumption is made that nonmarital pregnancy will increase as individuals come to have more favorable than unfavorable definitions of intercourse outside the marital relationship. American society, with its emphasis on sexual stimulation, particularly through the media, simultaneously encourages the cause and censures the results.

Rains (1971) has taken the concept of conflicting sexual norms and extended it to include the process of achieving sexual identity. She hypothesizes that causality lies in the adolescent's attempt to come to terms with sexuality and responsibility. She observes that many adoles-

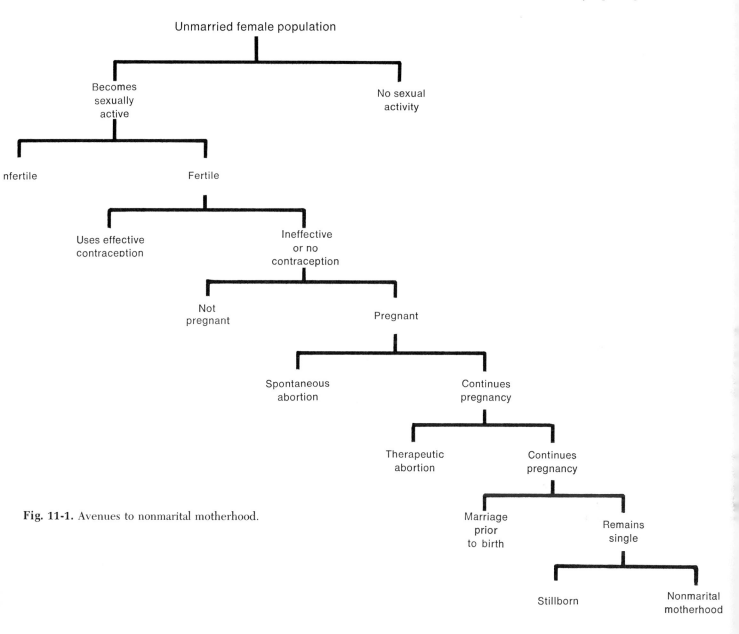

Fig. 11-1. Avenues to nonmarital motherhood.

cents are sexually active outside marriage and do not get pregnant, and those who do often do not end up as married mothers. As can be seen from Fig. 11-1 the steps toward nonmarital motherhood are many and varied.

Self-respect and reputation are crucial factors in a girl's premarital sexual behavior (Rains, 1971). Use of contraception is involved with a girl's self-concept as a sexually active being. For many girls in our culture, acceptance of sexual intention and of one's own sexuality is inherent in contraceptive usage. The implication is that a girl who uses contraception will be viewed as promiscuous, and her reputation will be damaged. To avoid this, adolescents develop techniques of denial and neutralization of the facts! "I didn't believe it could happen to me." Such denials imply that nice girls are

not sexually active. The value system that allows sex only if it is spontaneous and the result of overwhelming passion only reinforces this behavior. It appears there is a universal fantasy among adolescent girls that they will not get pregnant. It is a paradox that girls believe that nice girls do not prepare for intercourse but nice girls also do not get pregnant. Sex education and accessibility of contraception cannot effectively deal with this point of view because the issue is moral, not informational.

Another factor in causing adolescent or nonmarital pregnancy may be the role definitions of women that exist in the United States today and society's view of childbearing. Society, to a large extent, defines a woman's worth in terms of her childbearing capacities and childrearing abilities; a woman's sexuality is another aspect of her feelings of worthiness. Further, pregnancy is seen as a demarcation between childhood and adulthood. Once a female has borne a child she is no longer a child herself. Childbearing is also a creative endeavor; for some it may be their only expression of creativity. For many women childbearing has great positive value in their measurement of self-worth. It becomes a way of enhancing a positive self-concept because it has so many positive sanctions in our culture. And for some teenagers these positive values outweigh all of the negative sanctions against an adolescent or nonmarital pregnancy.

Lack of information

Lack of information and failure to use contraception are also causes of adolescent pregnancy. Coupled with this lack of information may be considerable peer pressure to become sexually active once dating has begun. Even though many adolescents have reservations about premarital sex, the peer group provides techniques to neutralize the norms (Furstenburg, 1976; Sorenson, 1973). Furstenburg's (1969, 1970, 1976) research refutes the view that premarital pregnancy is wanted or motivated; he has found pregnancy to be often unintended and unwelcome. His studies demonstrate that the majority of adolescents would use birth control if it were accessible and if they were assured it was safe and effective. The two significant factors in determining whether a teenager gets pregnant, says Furstenburg, are the number of years she has been sexually active and whether or not she uses contraceptives. Furstenburg, and Zelnick and Kantner (1978) have validated that pregnancy for those teens who keep their infants is not the result of promiscuous or casual sex. Most of the adolescents have a stable, long-term relationship with the father of the child.

The episodic and unanticipated (for whatever reason) nature of sex among adolescents is one of the greatest deterrents to contraception. Sorenson (1973) found that many teenagers admit carelessness and/or forgetfulness. Lack of information about contraception greatly contributes to the problem. Some teenagers do not believe they can become pregnant if intercourse is infrequent; this belief is reinforced when adolescents become sexually active in their early teens, often before ovulation has been established, and hence do not become pregnant even when sexually active. Zelnick and Kantner (1972, 1978) have found that some nonusers of birth control unrealistically discount the possibility of pregnancy; but over half who unintentionally became pregnant thought there was a good chance it might happen. An explanation for this seemingly irrational behavior lies in the low degree of confidence teenagers have in the most available (drugstore) methods. Many teenagers have little or no notion of the relative effectiveness of various birth control methods; many consider oral contraception the only effective method that is also easy to use. Other methods are considered to be too much trouble and not particularly safe. Some adolescents use only methods that do not require the assistance of a professional—withdrawal, douching, or the rhythm method—all highly ineffective. Many teenagers are not aware of the implication of sexual behavior and do not realize what they are doing or what the end results may be. Compounding this problem is the reluctance of parents to provide adequate, accurate sex education. Furstenburg (1976) found parents to be reluctant to discuss birth control, and quite willing to ignore the fact that their daughters were sexually active. Even when discussed, it was only in very vague terms and often with the implication that it was the partner's responsibility.

Not knowing where to go for information, assistance, or birth control devices is another problem. Even if the girl knows where to obtain birth control information, she may be put off by health care professionals and their attitudes. Many are afraid to seek contraceptive services because they fear the physician or nurse will tell their parents or will refuse services; they may be too self-conscious to discuss their needs, or they are afraid of the medical examination. For others, the cost of contraception is a problem; they cannot afford private medical care and are unaware of free services available.

The etiology of adolescent pregnancy is complex and no one theory of causality will stretch to fit all teenagers who become pregnant. It is probable that all the factors related to nonmarital and adolescent pregnancy have not yet been sufficiently identified. And none of the theories can be satisfactorily modified or extended to explain adolescent pregnancy in general. It is often difficult to pinpoint what the causative agents are in a specific instance and frequently more than one is apparent in the same person. The nurse needs to have an understanding of the multiple causality of the problem in order to accurately make assessments and determine nursing diagnoses. It is only then that nursing care can be individualized for each client, which is crucial in the care of the pregnant adolescent.

HEALTH RISKS
Physical health

It has been assumed that the pregnant adolescent has greater health risks than 20- to 34-year-old women. However, various studies attempting to document maternal health risks in adolescent pregnancy show confusing and often contradictory results. It has been difficult for researchers to demonstrate that risks result solely from age. However, one thing is apparent: not all pregnant teenagers are subject to the same risks. Age, race, socioeconomic status, marital status, parity, and adequacy of prenatal care act synergistically and the critical factor is the sum of these factors, not age alone. (See Menken, 1972; Stepto et al., 1975; Stickle, 1975; Kreutner et al., 1978.) Further, nutritional status appears to be highly significant in all pregnancies, but particularly in adolescents. Two extensive reviews of medical literature (Baizerman, 1971; Grant and Heard, 1972) have reached the same conclusion: the effects of race, socioeconomic status, parity, and prepregnancy obesity are more significant than age in determining the risks of pregnancy. Further, age alone is a risk factor but is not as significant as the other factors alone or in combination (Stepto et al., 1975).

The actual age of the adolescent appears to influence her potential for a high-risk pregnancy. The older the adolescent the closer her pregnancy risks are to those of the older woman. Girls 14 years and under appear to be at significantly greater medical risk when pregnant than 15- to 17-year-olds, while for teenagers ages 18 and 19, medical risks are essentially the same as the woman who is 20 to 24 years. There is a higher incidence of toxemia, uterine dysfunction, and contracted pelvis among mothers 14 years and younger (Coates, 1970).

Toxemia, which includes pre-eclampsia and eclampsia, appears to be the greatest health risk in adolescent pregnancy; the younger the adolescent the higher the rate (Stepto et al., 1975). However, it is difficult to compare studies because they lack a standard definition of toxemia and lack controls for age, race, and adequacy

Table 11-1. Studies of obstetrical risk in adolescent pregnancy*

	Researchers and date of study			
	Israel and Woutersz, 1963	Hassan and Falls, 1964	Mulka and Schaaf, 1968	Clark, Niles, and Wong, 1967
Subjects				
Age	Under 20 yrs	12-15 yrs	15 or younger	10-16 yrs
Race	52% b; 48% w	27.7% b; 72.3% w	85% b; 15% w	Largely black
Parity	71% primipara, 29% multipara	Primipara	Primipara	82% primipara, 16% segundipara, 1% tertigravida
Number	3,995	159	139	291
Controls				
Age	Over 20 yrs	22 yrs	19-21 yrs	10-16 yrs
Race	25% b; 75% w	12% b; 88% w	88% b; 12% w	Largely black
Parity	Unknown	Primipara	Primipara	Unknown
Number	40,709	78	119	400
Conditions†				
Anemia	+	N	0	N
Pre-eclampsia	+	+	N	N
Hypertension	0	N	−	N
Toxemia	0	+	N	+
Prolonged labor	0	+	0	N
Cephalopelvic disproportion	0	+‡	0	N
Comments	Pre-eclampsia, toxemia, and anemia rates higher for blacks than for same age whites. Control group not matched at early point in study. Prolonged labor risk might be due to parity difference in study and controls.	Greatest risks to 14-year-olds. Blacks had higher pre-eclampsia toxemia rates than whites.	Lack of contrast in risks to subjects and controls may indicate race is more important than age in incidence of anemia and hypertension, which had high rates in both groups.	Studies and controls differed only in adequacy of prenatal care, controls having adequate care. Comparisons made in study of adolescents and adult controls not reliable.

*Modified from Stewart, K. R.: Adolescent sexuality and teenage pregnancy: A selected annotated bibliography with summary forewords, Chapel Hill, 1977, State Service Office, Carolina Population Center, The University of North Carolina at Chapel Hill. Reprinted by permission of publisher.

†Notes: + indicates greater risk for subjects than controls; − indicates less risk for subjects than controls; 0 indicates no difference in risk; N indicates condition not included in study.
‡Only in 12- to 13-year-olds.

of prenatal care. For the very young teenager both age and race are important risk factors in toxemia (Hassan and Falls, 1964; Coates, 1970). Israel and Woutersz (1963) found that for the older teenager race was a more important factor than age. Nonwhites of all ages were found to have higher toxemia rates than whites of any age. (It should be noted that race is also associated with less access to prenatal care and lower socioeconomic levels.) A third variable—prenatal care—is also important. Those who receive little or no prenatal care have much higher rates of toxemia than do those adolescents who receive adequate prenatal care (Clark, 1967). Although research to date has not conclusively determined the effect of age alone in obstetric risks associated with adolescent pregnancy, there is strong evidence that toxemia in general, and pre-eclampsia specifically, are a greater risk for adolescent mothers than for mothers in their twenties.

Other risks often cited for teenagers are cephalopelvic disproportion, anemia, and prolonged labor. Again the supporting evidence is mixed. The pregnant adolescent over age 15 usually has an obstetric performance similar to older women in labor and delivery. In adolescents whose bone growth is not completed there appears to be a higher incidence of contracted pelvis and feto-pelvic disproportion. The dividing line between pelvic adequacy and disproportion usually occurs between ages 14 and 15; if pregnancy occurs after age 15 and the mother does not experience anemia, toxemia, or premature labor, she may have a benign obstetric course (Stepto et al., 1975). It appears that if fetopelvic disproportion does not exist, labor may be shorter for the adolescent than for older women.

There are other health risks for the pregnant teenager that deserve mention. Sexually transmitted diseases have become epidemic in the United States particularly among teenagers. According to Kreutner and associates (1978) all obstetric clinics in the United States are reporting increased frequency of sexually transmitted infections in pregnant adolescents. Gonorrhea, syphilis, and herpes simplex type II pose particularly grave risks for both the mother and infant. During pregnancy, infection increases the risk of fetal wastage, congenital defects, and prematurity. Adolescent girls may also be subject to infections common to childhood such as otitis media, streptococcal infection, and pertussis.

Drug abuse is a complex problem and may be more common in teenagers than in older women. Infectious hepatitis, malnutrition, syphilis, thromboembolic processes, repeated recurrent infections, anemia, and possible drug intoxication or withdrawal place additional grave stresses on an already high-risk pregnancy (Stepto et al., 1975).

Teenagers are notorious for their poor dietary habits; they are reported to have the least favorable diets of all age groups. Adolescent females often have poorer diets than males, even though the adolescent girl is experiencing the most pronounced physical growth spurt of her life. The adolescent whose nutritional reserves are depleted by inadequate diet and who has increased nutritional needs for growth and development will be ill-prepared for pregnancy. This problem may be further complicated if she is of a lower socioeconomic level with a lifetime of poor nutritional intake (King and Jacobson, 1975).

Both prepregnant obesity and underweight have been implicated as obstetric hazards. Also of concern is low weight gain (less than 11 lb) in pregnancy, which is associated with a high incidence of low-birth weight infants (Kreutner et al., 1978) (see Chapter 10). Poor nutrition in the early months of pregnancy affects development of the embryo and its capacity to survive, while poor nutrition in the later stages of pregnancy affects fetal growth.

Any discussion of the health risks of adolescent pregnancy must include the risks to the infant. The most frequently mentioned health risks to the infants of teenage mothers are prematurity, low birth weight, and increased neonatal and infant mortality. Babies born to teenagers are two to three times more likely to die in the first year than are those born to women in their twenties. Jakel and associates (1975) found that risks of prematurity and perinatal death are higher for teenage mothers, particularly those having subsequent pregnancies while still in their teens. In their study of Louisiana teenagers, Doth and Fort (1976) found that the offspring of teenage mothers were at greater risk for stillbirth, perinatal mortality, prematurity, and infant mortality. Zlatnik and Burmeister (1977) demonstrated that low "gynecologic age" (defined as chronologic age minus age at menarche) increases the risk of delivery of a low birth weight infant. Pregnant adolescents are disadvantaged biologically, culturally, and socioeconomically and those conceiving closest to menarche may be most disadvantaged of all.

Nutritional influences may also be involved. The growth spurt usually occurs prior to menarche and growth is not completed until 4 years after menarche. Therefore, a pregnant adolescent with a low gynecologic age must satisfy nutritional needs for her own growth as well as for those of the fetus. Failure to meet these nutritional needs may result in intrauterine growth retardation and perhaps premature labor. Race is also correlated with low birth weight infants and young age of the mother. The Niswander-Gordon (1972) study found that the occurrence of low birth weight infants was higher among blacks than among whites. (For an expanded discussion of the sequelae of low birth weight infants see Chapter 10.)

Mental health

The psychologic importance of pregnancy and childbirth depends on three variables: psychodynamic, situational, and cultural. The woman's feelings and perceptions of herself as a woman and as a potential mother are examples of psychodynamic implications of pregnancy. Determinants of the intrapsychic response to pregnancy and childbirth include the woman's psychic history, relationship to her mother, resolution of previous developmental stages and tasks, self-image, body image concept and how comfortable she feels about her body, and her motivations for being pregnant.

Situational variables are those inherent in the immediate environment. Her relationship (or lack thereof) with the father of the baby, her employment and educational status, life changes required by the birth of a child, and her emotional and financial resources will all influence her adaptation to this life cycle milestone.

Pregnancy is also a cultural event of major significance and there are many cultural meanings of childbearing. These include attitudes and beliefs about pregnancy, birth, and motherhood, values attached to female reproductive functions, and expectations of behavior for the pregnant woman and mother. Childbirth often defines a woman's relationship to society; it is a transition from childhood to adulthood and the (usually) irreversible state of parenthood.

All pregnant women experience mood swings, introversion, passivity, and fears, but these may be intensified in the already vulnerable adolescent. In addition, because it is the obvious outcome of sexual relations, pregnancy may enhance any conflict the adolescent may have about her own sexuality or sexual behavior. There is an increased need for stable relationships, and these may not be available. The pregnant woman's need for dependence may conflict with the adolescent's need to be independent. Intense conflict may occur between the rush to grow up and the need to be secure. Many adolescents report strong feelings of guilt and anxiety, particularly when the pregnancy is nonmarital. These feelings are increased when external supports—both cultural and interpersonal—are needed but not available. In our culture when the established codes of conduct—marriage before pregnancy—are transgressed, support is often withdrawn. The adolescent may experience rejection or abandonment by society, parents, peers, or her sexual partner.

Other conflicts may also develop in an adolescent pregnancy. Role conflicts for the young female are not uncommon; she is simultaneously daughter and mother. Achieving motherhood is a critical life event requiring the woman to take on many complex, demanding roles, while other roles are abandoned or modified. When motherhood occurs early in life, it is probable that the stress caused by acceleration of role transitions will be pathologic. Additionally, peer relationships are altered, and this complicates the girl's resolution of the task of solidifying her identity since she no longer has the advantage of peer support and feedback. Development of a positive self-concept is further complicated by all the body image issues inherent in pregnancy itself. With all of these conflicts of task resolution occurring within a short time period, it is no wonder that the pregnant adolescent may appear bewildered, overwhelmed, anxious (often to the point of panic), hostile, apathetic, withdrawn, or guilty—a fearsome burden for the teenager and a tremendous challenge for the nurse.

Other significant risks have been identified earlier in the chapter—the risks of marital instability, disruption of education, economic problems, and difficulty in regulating family size and childrearing. Early motherhood is closely associated with a high incidence of marital dissolution, poverty and shortened education. The following statement by Arthur Campbell (1968) eloquently summarizes these risks:

The girl who has . . . a child at the age of 16 suddenly has ninety percent of her life's script written for her. She will probably drop out of school; even if someone else in her family helps to take care of the baby, she will probably not be able to find a steady job that pays enough to provide for herself and her child; she may feel impelled to marry someone she might not otherwise have chosen. Her life choices are few, and most of them bad. Had she been able to delay the first child, her prospects might have been quite different assuming that she would have had opportunities to continue her education, improve her vocational skills, find a job, marry someone she wanted to marry and have a child when she and her husband were ready for it.

The adjustments of adolescence, marriage, and parenthood are three of the most difficult adjustments a woman will have to make in her lifetime. The thought of combining all three adjustments at once is overwhelming. This is the basis for the view that the psychologic, educational, economic, and marital risks of adolescent pregnancy are greater than the medical risks. It is easy to imagine the distress, fear, and desparation of the pregnant teenager, and these are seen repeatedly by nurses. However, Stewart (1976) makes the point that documentation of all these risks is not complete. There is a need for more research on those risks of nonmarital pregnancy and subsequent marriage that fall outside the category of medical risks. The educational, economic, psychologic, and marital risks are the result of both the sociocultural environment and pregnancy. The risk elements change as society changes.

NURSING STRATEGIES

Nursing care of the pregnant adolescent must be multidimensional to include preventive, restorative, and maintenance elements. Fig. 11-2 illustrates points in the process of adolescent pregnancy where the nurse could possibly intervene.

All nurses have opinions about the appropriateness of becoming pregnant, both why and when. These opinions are based on the individual's value system and may involve particularly strong feelings in the case of adolescent pregnancy. The opinions and feelings vary; each nurse will respond differently depending on who is pregnant and how she is coping with the pregnancy. It is essential for the nurse to be aware of her feelings and to identify the value system underlying them. Unless she is aware of these, she may limit her effectiveness by (1) overidentifying with the client, (2) stereotyping the individual, or (3) reacting punitively to the young girl.

Assessment

It is essential that the nurse approach each pregnant adolescent client without prior assumptions. Assumptions about how a specific client feels or perceives her pregnancy are of little use and may hinder assessment. The nurse needs to ascertain how stressful the situation is for the client, what her particular strengths and weaknesses are, and what her coping abilities are. Table 11-2 summarizes pertinent areas of assessment to be considered. When the nurse has this information she can assist the client in viewing her situation realistically, determining alternatives, and making responsible decisions.

Goals

Each adolescent who is pregnant has specific needs, however, it is helpful for the nurse to have in mind general goals toward which she and the client can move if the girl chooses to carry the pregnancy to term. These are three-fold:

1. The girl's emergence from pregnancy with as positive an image of herself as her personality and circumstances will permit
2. Use of the pregnancy by the girl as a point of departure for maturation and growth as an individual and a woman
3. A healthy mother and infant as an outcome of the pregnancy.

Management strategies

Crisis theory provides a useful framework for nurses who work with pregnant adolescents. The use of crisis intervention techniques facilitates problem-solving and increases the potential for self-understanding and ma-

turity. The nurse can be one of the balancing factors that help to restore equilibrium and thereby avoid the development of future crises through (1) establishing realistic perception of the event, (2) finding adequate support systems, (3) developing useful coping mechanisms, and (4) anticipating potential future crises. (See Chapter 12 for further discussion of crisis theory and intervention.) The assessment process will indicate to the nurse when tension, anxiety, depression, and inability to function make a diagnosis of crisis appropriate. During assessment the nurse should be able to determine what positive factors are present for the establishment of equilibrium and what are missing. Finally, the assessment process itself is a crisis intervention technique in that it raises feelings onto a conscious level and can be used to gain intellectual understanding. It can be anticipated that for the adolescent girl periods of disequilibrium with inadequate coping mechanisms can occur at the following times:

1. Discovery and acceptance of the pregnancy
2. Communication to significant others and their response
3. Decision to have an abortion or carry the pregnancy to term
4. Labor and delivery
5. The decision on adoption versus foster care vs keeping and rearing the child
6. Making future plans (marriage, education, occupation)

For the pregnant adolescent any or all of these have the potential of crisis. Anticipating these and intervening may be helpful in decreasing stress, thereby avoiding disequilibrium.

The nurse who works with pregnant adolescents must be able to develop satisfactory helping relationships with her clients. The nurse's ability to do so is influenced by her own psychologic functioning and value system, as well as her ability to evaluate her own behavior and perceive her own capacities and limitations accurately. She must be genuinely interested in and warmly accepting of her clients and be able to convey this. It is important to be honest for only then can trust be established and a helping relationship develop. The nurse must convey to the client her belief that she is worthy in order to reduce feelings of abandonment and guilt. In this climate increased confidence, an acceptance of self, and an enhanced self-esteem can come about; when this occurs denial is decreased and realistic perception of events is increased (Petrella, 1978).

The nurse must help the pregnant adolescent accept the reality of her situation. It is essential that the nurse not foster denial because psychologic equilibrium is achieved only when events are perceived accurately. Often the nurse may unconsciously prolong a client's

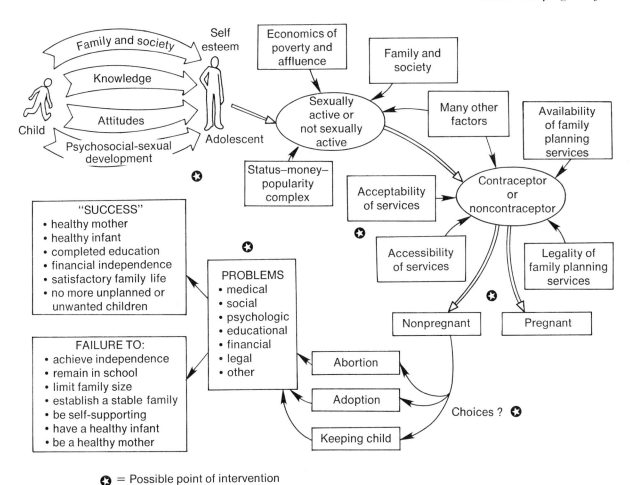

Fig. 11-2. Interjection points in the adolescent pregnancy process.

denial by trying to protect her from the hurt she will experience when reality is accepted. If the potential for growth inherent in crisis is to be realized, denial must be stripped away and loss or grief experienced. When abortion is chosen, the loss is early and obvious—perhaps more a loss of a fantasized baby than a real one. But loss of a fantasy can be painful too. The degree of difficulty in adjusting to the loss will depend on how much emotion was invested in the fantasy, how much the fantasy can be acknowledged and mourned, and how actively the client participates in the decision-making process. When adoption is chosen, there is a painful separation from a live being. The baby must first be acknowledged as a being separate from the mother, then the mother must separate from the infant and mourn as if the baby had died. Mothers who keep their babies also experience a loss—loss of a life-style and loss of a vision of self as the ideal mother providing the ideal life for her child. This type of partial loss and separation and the resultant pain may be even more difficult to deal

with because the situation is so unclear. Loss involves suffering and pain but there is more to it than that. Separation can lead to a heightened sense of self and of what is important. From this can come responsible decision-making and emotional maturity (Polsby, 1974).

The key to helping the adolescent mother realize her growth potential is to encourage her to assume responsibility for herself and to determine what she wants for herself and her offspring. A common obstacle to this occurs when the nurse becomes so caught up in the painful aspects of the girl's situation that she wants to take care of her. To some extent this is not bad; the adolescent needs physical care and loving concern and the nurse can provide this while also meeting her health care needs. But the key is knowing when to stop and how to avoid being trapped into doing too much. It is all too easy to make decisions for the client, although legally, biologically, and emotionally the client is responsible for the decisions about herself and the fetus.

Table 11-2. Assessment tool for adolescent pregnancy

Categories of assessment	Specific factors to ascertain	Significance
Sociocultural status	Racial background Ethnic heritage Socioeconomic level Educational attainment	Culture defines what stigma, if any, is attached to being an adolescent or single mother. There may be moral proscriptions or concern over economic hardships the girl faces. Cultural values give the nurse some idea of the impact the pregnancy will have on client. These will then need to be validated with client. An important part of assessment should be cultural position on abortion and adoption since these may be alternatives the client will be considering. It is important to know what resources and community services are available to the client. Socioeconomic status is a part of one's cultural background and may offer additional information regarding the significance pregnancy will have for the adolescent. In part, one's educational background and attainment will affect one's socioeconomic status.
Support system	Parents living, dead, separated or divorced With whom does client live? Client's place in family constellation Number, ages, and sex of siblings Who is most significant support person? Is there extended family available? Relationship of client with her mother Relationship with sexual partner Responses of family, significant others, partner to her pregnancy	The nurse needs to know who is significant to the pregnant adolescent and what her relationship is to them. Information on the family constellation and the client's place in it will help the nurse develop a plan of care with her client, using whatever supports are available.
Informational needs	What does client want to know? What are her specific concerns or fears? Knowledge level regarding prenatal care, nutrition, labor and delivery, contraception, childrearing, and parenting. What kinds of information has she been given by mother, female relatives, peers about pregnancy? What does she expect labor to be like?	Before the nurse can develop a plan of care with client, she must know what the adolescent knows and does not know about a variety of subjects. It is axiomatic that the nurse who wishes to be effective in client teaching must begin at the client's level of understanding and knowledge; the client will learn best what she is motivated to learn.
Sexuality and sex education	When did she become sexually active? Use of birth control (kind, how often?) How does she feel about her sexual activity? What type of sex education has she received and from whom? Was this pregnancy planned?	A female's way of relating sexuality, her use of contraceptives, and her general knowledge of sex are crucial to assess, since this information will provide the basis for counseling during and after pregnancy. It will also help the nurse in her presentation of available options to client in deciding the resolution of her pregnancy (for example, did she choose not to use birth control with the knowledge that abortion would be available if needed?).
Emotional status and coping abilities	How does she feel about being pregnant? What options has she considered for resolution of the pregnancy? What are her relationships with her family, peers, and father of the pregnancy now? Does she feel nervous, upset, anxious, depressed? What does she do when she feels upset? Whom does she confide in?	The nurse must be able to identify the stresses client is experiencing and how she is coping with them. Level of anxiety being experienced should be identified.

Table 11-2. Assessment tool for adolescent pregnancy—cont'd

Categories of assessment	Specific factors to ascertain	Significance
Emotional status and coping abilities—cont'd	Nonverbal observations: stuttering; excessive activity, repetitious or constant talking; selective inattention Does she appear to use disassociation, denial, or distortion of reality? Report of symptoms such as insomnia, excessive fatigue, diarrhea, nausea, palpitation, loss of appetite.	
Medical and obstetric status	See Chapters 7 and 10.	Because of potential risks of adolescent pregnancy, nurse should be alert for high-risk indicators; signs and symptoms of toxemia, anemia, and malnutrition are of particular significance.
Relationships with health professionals	Prior hospitalization Previous experience with nurses What has she been told by peers or relatives about hospitalization? Cultural definitions of health, illness, expectations of health care system.	The adolescent's response to nurse and her willingness and ability to form a helping relationship will be influenced in part by her prior experience with health care systems and her expectations of nursing.
Future plans	Pursuit of education Career goals Child care arrangements Means of support How does she plan to feed and care for infant? Has she chosen a name for infant? What preparations for the infant have been made?	

This is the key concept: the client is the person responsible and she must make the decisions. The most important thing for the counselor to do at first is *to listen.* Good listening means checking the impulse to rush in with advice, assurances, or truisms. It is important to hear the pain, frustration, and confusion. It is not the nurse's job to take away the pain—we do not have the answers. But we can hear the teen's pain and acknowledge the hurt. We can reflect her thoughts back so that she can hear her own thoughts, fears, and desires. By letting her know that we hear and that she matters, we have begun the helping process.

Next the nurse needs to objectively inform the client about all the resources and options available. In order to make a responsible decision, the client must know the choices. Considering all of the options can lead to better decision-making and an increased sense of individual competence and self-worth. (See Chapter 12 for a discussion of the options available.) The nurse can support the girl in smaller decision-making activities, such as when to make her next appointment for prenatal care, whether to see the baby before it is placed for adoption, what to name the baby, etc., for it is through making smaller decisions that the client learns to assume the responsibility for making the larger ones. Once a decision

is made, the nurse can continue to reinforce that decision, to reflect back the advantages and disadvantages of the choice as seen by the client, and support the girl in her ambivalence when needed.

Nonjudgmental counseling by the nurse is essential if the adolescent is to work through her feelings about the pregnancy and reach the best decision for herself. The nurse can enhance the client's abilities to cope with stress, guilt, and ambivalence if a nonthreatening relationship can be developed. The one most effective tool of the nurse is herself—to communicate effectively and project herself as a caring person.

Often the nurse will encounter indifference, anger, hostility, or apathy. This may be a reaction of the girl to the "system," to authority, or to a perceived threat to her self-esteem. The most effective approach in this instance may be to take the initiative in establishing trust, to communicate persistent interest, to listen attentively to the client, and to be consistent and constant about visits, promises, and information given to the client. It is imperative to communicate what the client can expect of the nurse and to let the client know that the nurse sees her as unique (Bomar, 1975).

A three-step nursing approach that establishes a helping relationship and trust, allows for the surfacing of dependency needs, and ultimately fosters independence is helpful. It is often difficult to establish a helping relationship and effective communication with these clients, because adolescents often appear withdrawn, passive, or even hostile. One way to demonstrate concern is to focus on the client's immediate needs or concerns, allowing her to discuss what she wishes. Once a trust relationship is established, dependency can surface as a normal phenomenon of maturation as a part of the relationship. Each adolescent and her dependency needs should be assessed individually as the nurse decides how much dependency to allow. The decision should be based on an assessment of the girl's personality, experience, coping abilities, and present life stresses. By accepting dependent behavior, the nurse assists the adolescent to move toward maturation and more independence. Independent functioning is the ultimate goal, but reaching this is a gradual process characterized by regressive dependent behavior and increasing self-reliance.

The pregnant adolescent's need for information is varied. These clients often seem to need information about their own bodies and about the internal and external changes that are occurring before they can utilize information about prenatal care, labor, and delivery. Teenagers seem to harbor more misconceptions than older women, and they are very often influenced by "old wives tales." It is mandatory that the nurse provide accurate information at the client's level of understanding.

Feelings of safety and comfort are enhanced by decreasing the scope of the unknown. By meeting the client's need for information the nurse can create an environment in which potentially threatening events can be explored realistically and the unknown becomes known. Body image issues are particularly crucial; there is often an intense preoccupation with self; perhaps this is the way the adolescent accepts her changing self. An invaluable nursing contribution is to build self-esteem and reinforce the adolescent's sense of positive self-value.

Information about nutrition is also essential to the well-being of the adolescent mother and her baby (see Chapter 21). Information about labor and delivery is also crucial to reduce the girl's fear of the unknown. Finally, the adolescent needs to be aware of the common danger signals of pregnancy as well as any specific to her own condition. This ensures that she will be able to act responsibly and knowledgeably in her own self-care.

For the nurse, working with pregnant teenagers can be both rewarding and frustrating; she may often wonder if she is accomplishing anything. It requires optimism and infinite patience. Success is measured in slow, small, often intangible changes. The nurse is most effective when she provides consistency and reality in her nursing care, allows the development of a trust relationship, and fosters the maturational process of the adolescent.

SERVICES

In the United States today there is a tremendous desire on the part of concerned professionals and the lay public to do something about pregnant teens. A great deal of energy is expended and programs are begun without a clear idea of what it is they wish to accomplish. A review of the literature (Stewart, 1976) reveals several goals of existing programs for teenagers: (1) reduction of complications of pregnancy and delivery, (2) delay of subsequent pregnancies, (3) continuation of the mother's education, (4) education of the woman for pregnancy, delivery, and parenthood, (5) development of a system of social supports to help the girl care for herself and her child, and (6) facilitation of satisfactory psychologic adjustment to the pregnancy so that responsible decision-making is possible. These goals may be met in part or whole by a variety of programs.

The multidisciplinary team approach has been found successful in providing high-quality health care to pregnant adolescents and has also been very satisfying for staff and clients (Packer and Cooke, 1976). The composition of the team will vary with each client; however, there should always be a core of workers who share a common approach to the client based on a knowledge of pregnancy, adolescent development, and group process. The team approach offers the client the advantages of shared knowledge and cooperative decision-making. The team approach also provides the adolescent with consistency and continuity of care. It has the additional benefit to the community of being potentially more economical.

Existing programs for pregnant teenagers are usually either hospital based or school based, and they reflect a different emphasis on goals depending upon their origin. Hospital-based programs have as their primary goal a lowering of health risks in pregnancy and delivery; the literature indicates that this is successfully accomplished (Stewart, 1976). However, these programs are not always effective in delaying subsequent pregnancies or ensuring continuation of the teenager's education. The school-based programs are more successful in assisting the adolescent to continue in education and delay future pregnancies. It is not clear how successful they are in reducing risk rates, however, a consistent problem for all programs is evaluation. The need for comprehensive, objective evaluation is tremendous, particularly given the current push to "do something."

PREVENTION

The sexually active teenager should be designated as a high priority target population for sex education and family planning services. Numerous studies have shown that adolescent girls are receiving inadequate sex education and contraceptive information.* Realistic sex education, which includes information about pregnancy risks, contraception, the alternative of abortion, pregnancy testing, early symptoms of pregnancy, and where services can be obtained should be available to all teens via schools, churches and mass media. There is a need for increased federal and state funding for preventive as well as maintenance services. Restrictive laws regarding contraception, sex education, and abortion need to be modified so that services are widely available. Research to determine why teenagers do not use available contraceptive measures needs to be instituted, and efforts to discover safe, effective contraception for both men and women need to be expanded.

For pregnant teens pregnancy counseling needs to be available that provides nonjudgmental information about all available options. Furthermore, there needs to be adequate obstetric and pediatric care for teenagers who choose to carry their pregnancy to term. Provisions should be made for education, employment, and social services for teenage parents as well as day care for their infants. The possibility of national health insurance coverage for all health services related to adolescent pregnancy and childbearing, with provisions to protect the privacy of minors should be explored.

Prevention of adolescent pregnancy and the subsequent development of high risk mothers and infants is certainly cost effective. But equally important are the savings in terms of the quality of life. Each individual has the right to some quality in her life, which is enhanced when a teenager does not get pregnant. This is certainly true for herself and her potential offspring, but also for her family, for her partner and more indirectly for society.

---

*See Malo-Greneva, 1970; Simmons, 1972; Connell and Jacobsen, 1971.

REFERENCES

Babikiar, H. N., and Goldman, A.: A study in teenage pregnancy, Am. J. Psychiatry **128:**755-760, 1971.

Bacon, L.: Early motherhood, accelerated role transition, and social pathologies, Social Forces, **52**(3):333-341, 1974.

Baizerman, M., and others: Pregnant adolescents: a review of the literature with abstracts, 1969-1970. Pittsburgh, 1971, Maternal Child Health Section, Graduate School of Public Health, University of Pittsburgh.

Bomar, P. J.: The nursing process in the care of a hostile, pregnant adolescent, Mat. Child Nurs. J. **4**(2):95-100, 1975.

Campbell, A.: The role of family planning in the reduction of poverty, J. Marriage Family **30**(2):236-245, 1968.

Clark, A.: The crisis of adolescent unwed motherhood, Am. J. Nurs. **67**(7):1465-1469, 1967.

Clark, A., and Affonso, D.: Childbearing—a nursing perspective, Philadelphia, 1976, F. A. Davis Co.

Clark, A., and others: The pregnant adolescent, Ann. N.Y. Acad. Sci. **142**(3):813-816, 1967.

Coates, J.: Obstetrics in the very young adolescent, Am. J. Obstet. Gynecol. **108**(1):68-72, 1970.

Cutright, P.: Illegitimacy: myths, causes and cures, Family Plan. Perspect. **3**(1):26-48, 1971.

Doth, A., and Fort, A.: Medical and social factors affecting early teenage pregnancy, Am. J. Ob Gynecol. **125**(4):532-536, 1976.

Erikson, E. H.: Childhood and society, New York, 1950, W. W. Norton Co.

Furstenburg, F., and others: Unplanned parenthood: the social consequences of teenage childbearing, New York, 1976, The Free Press.

Furstenburg, F.: Premarital pregnancy among black teenagers, Transaction **7**(7):52-55, 1970.

Furstenburg, F., and others: Birth control knowledge among pregnant adolescents, J. Marriage Family **31**(2):34-42, 1969.

Grant, J., and Heard, F.: Complications of adolescent pregnancy, Clin. Ped. **11**(12):567-570, 1972.

Hassan, H. M., and Falls, F.: The young primipara: a clinical study, Am. J. Obstet. Gynecol. **88**(2):256-269, 1964.

Jakel, J. F., and others: Comparison of the health of index and subsequent babies born to school age mothers, Am. J. Public Health **65**(4):370-374, 1975.

Johnson, C. L.: Adolescent pregnancy: intervention into the poverty cycle, Adolescence **9**(35):391-402, 1974.

King, J. C., and Jacobson, H. N. In Zackler, J., and Brandstadt, W., editors: Nutrition and pregnancy in adolescence. The teenage pregnant girl, Springfield, Ill., 1975, Charles C Thomas, Publisher.

Kleeman, L.: Adolescent pregnancy: the need for new policies and new programs, J. School Health **45**(5):263-267, 1975.

Kreutner, A., Kessler, K., and Hollingsworth, D. R.: Adolescent obstetrics and gynecology, Chicago, 1978, Year Book Medical Publishers, Inc.

LaBarre, M.: Pregnancy experiences among married adolescents, speech presented at 1967 annual meeting of American Orthopsychiatric Association, Washington, D.C.

Liben, F.: Minority group clinic patients pregnant out of wedlock, Am. J. Public Health **59**(10):1868-1881, 1969.

Malo-Greneva, D.: What pregnant teenagers know about sex, Nurs. Outlook **18**(11):32-35, 1970.

Menken, J.: The health and social consequences of teenage childbearing, Family Plan. Perspect. **4**(3):45-53, 1972.

Moore, K. A., and Waite, L. J.: Early childbearing and educational attainment, Family Plan. Perspect. **9**(5):220-225, 1977.

Niswander, K. R., and Gordon, M.: The women and their pregnancies, Philadelphia, 1972, W. B. Saunders Co.

Nye, F. I.: School age parenthood. Extension Bulletin 667, Washington State University, April 1976 (rev. Jan. 1977).

Osofsky, H. J.: The pregnant teenager, Springfield, Ill., 1968, Charles C Thomas, Publisher.

Packer, J., and Cooke, C.: The interdependent team approach in caring for the pregnant adolescent, J. Obstet. Gynecol. Nurs., pp. 18-25, July/Aug. 1976.

Pauker, J.: Girls pregnant out of wedlock, J. Oper. Psych. **1**(1):15-19, 1971.

Petrella, J. M.: The unwed pregnant adolescent, J. Obstet. Gynecol. Nurs., pp. 22-26, July/Aug. 1978.

Pliones, B. M.: Adolescent pregnancy: review of the literature, Soc. Work **20**(4):302-307, 1975.

Polsby, G.: Unmarried parenthood: potential for growth, Adolescence, 9(34):273-284, 1974.

Rains, P.: Becoming an unwed mother—a sociological account, Chicago, 1971, Aldine Publishing Co.

Rainwater, L.: And the poor get children, Chicago, 1960, Quadrangle Books.

Schlakman, V.: Unmarried parenthood: an approach to social policy, Social Casework 47(8):494-501, 1966.

Shouse, J. W.: Psychological and emotional problems of pregnancy in adolescence. In Zackler, J., and Brandstadt, W., editors: The teenage pregnant girl, Springfield, Ill., 1975, Charles C Thomas, Publishers.

Simmons, J. P.: Sex education of the adolescent female, Ped. Clin. North Am. 19(3):765-778, 1972.

Sorenson, R.: Adolescent sexuality in contemporary America, New York, 1973, World Publishers.

South. Med. J.: Pregnancy in young adolescents—a syndrome of failure. 62:655, 1969.

Steinman, M. E.: Reaching and helping the adolescent who becomes pregnant, Maternal Child Nursing, pp. 35-37, Jan./Feb. 1979.

Stepto, R. C., Keith, L., and Keith, D.: Obstetrical and medical problems of teenage pregnancy. In Zackler, J., and Brandstadt, W., editors: The teenage pregnant girl, Springfield, 1975, Charles C Thomas, Publishers.

Stewart, K. R.: Adolescent sexuality and teenage pregnancy, Chapel Hill, N.C., 1976, Carolina Population Center.

Teenage childbearing: United States, 1966-1975. Monthly Vital Statistics Report, 26(5), Suppl. Sept. 8, 1977.

Vincent, C.: Unmarried mothers, New York, 1961, Free Press.

Young, L.: Out of wedlock, New York, 1954, McGraw-Hill Book Co.

Zackler, J., and Brandstadt, W., editors: The teenage pregnant girl, Springfield, Ill., 1975, Charles C Thomas, Publisher.

Zelnick, M., and Kantner, J. F.: First pregnancies to women aged 15-19: 1976 and 1971, Family Plan. Perspect. 10(1):11-20, 1978.

Zelnick, M., and Kantner, J.: Some preliminary observations on pre-adult fertility and family formation, Stud. Family Plan. 3(4):59-65, 1972.

Zero Population Growth: Teenage pregnancy: a major problem for minors, ZPG Report, Aug. 1977.

Zlatnik, F. J., and Burmeister, L. F.: Low gynecologic age, Am. J. Obstet. Gynecol. 128:183-186, 1977.

ADDITIONAL READINGS

Adolescent fertility—risks of consequences, Population Reports, J-10, July 1975.

Anderson, C.: The lengthening shadows: a case study in adolescent, out-of-wedlock pregnancy, J. Obstet. Gynecol. Neonatal Nurs. pp. 19-22, July/Aug. 1976.

Babikiar, H. N., and Goldman, A.: A study in teenage pregnancy, Am. J. Psychiatry. 128:755-760, 1971.

Bonam, A. F.: Psychoanalytical implications in treating unmarried mothers with narcissistic character structures, Social Case. 44:323-329, 1963.

Connell, E., and Jacobsen, L.: Pregnancy, the teenager and sex education, Am. J. Public Health 61(9):1840-1845, 1971.

Deutsch, H.: The psychology of women, Vol. II, New York, 1945, Grune & Stratton, Inc.

Fischman, S. H.: The pregnancy resolution decisions of unwed adolescents, Nurs. Clin. North Am. 10(2):217-227, 1975.

Frye, B., and Barham, B.: Reaching out to pregnant adolescents, Am. J. Nurs. 75(7):1502-1504, 1975.

Gispert, M., and Falk, R.: Sexual experimentation and pregnancy in young black adolescents, Am. J. Obstet. Gynecol. 126(4):459-466, 1976.

Hertz, D. B.: Psychological implications of adolescent pregnancy: patterns of family interaction in adolescent mothers to be, Psychosomatics 15:13-16, 1977.

Howard, M.: Only human, New York, 1975, The Seaburg Press.

Khlentzos, M., and Pagliaro, M.: Observations from psychotherapy with unwed mothers, Am. J. of Orthopsych. 35(4):779-786, 1965.

Marinoff, S., and Schonbaly, D. H.: Adolescent pregnancy, Ped. Clin. North Am. 19(3):795-802, 1972.

Shainess, N.: Psychological problems associated with motherhood, Am. Handb. Psych. Vol. 3.

Stickle, G.: Pregnancy in adolescents: scope of the problem, Contemp. Ob/Gyn., June 1975, Reprint.

Tellack, W. S., and others: A study of premarital pregnancy, Am. J. Public Health 62(5):676-679, May 1972.

Trail, L., and Woutersay, T.: Teenage obstetrics, Am. J. Obstet. Gynecol 85(5):659-668, 1964.

Vadies, G., and Pomeroy, R.: Pregnancy among single American teenagers, Adv. Plan. Paren. 10(4):198-203, 1975.

Worthington, B. S., and others: Nutrition in pregnancy and lactation, St. Louis, 1977, The C. V. Mosby Co.

12

The unwanted pregnancy

Catherine Ingram Fogel

An unwanted pregnancy is one of the most stressful situations that a woman is likely to experience in her lifetime. It demands decision-making within a short time period if all options are to be considered. It is an agonizing dilemma fraught with pain, stress, and anxiety, caused not by the simple biologic fact or inconvenience of pregnancy but rather by the fact that human lives are affected by the way in which the woman deals with the unwanted pregnancy.

Any nurse who works with women for even a short time will come in contact with clients experiencing unwanted pregnancy. It is, therefore, essential that they have the requisite knowledge and skills to provide appropriate pregnancy counseling to clients. Assisting the woman who is experiencing an unwanted pregnancy (and her mate when possible) to arrive at a decision and counseling her about preventing any future unwanted pregnancies are important aspects of care. The role is one of accepting and supporting the woman's decision and facilitating a positive experience of personal growth.

To be an effective pregnancy counselor the nurse needs specific skills and knowledge. In this chapter we will:

1. Describe the magnitude of the problem
2. Discuss causative factors of unwanted pregnancy
3. Consider available options
4. Discuss prevention of unwanted pregnancies

Woven throughout are the appropriate nursing assessment and management strategies and the ethical issues relevant to women's health care.

PREVALENCE

It is difficult to estimate how widespread the problem of unwanted pregnancy is because this statistic is not usually collected by the Bureau of Vital Statistics. Also, many women may be reluctant to admit that a pregnancy is undesired or unplanned if the fetus is carried to term and the woman keeps the child. Of course, even those women who passionately desire children and have minutely planned conception and pregnancy will experience ambivalence as a normal phenomenon of pregnancy; there will be times when, if asked, they would describe their pregnancy as unwanted. Even with these reservations, however, it is possible to infer from some known statistics and parameters an estimate concerning the number of unwanted pregnancies.

It has been variously estimated that from 5% to 20% of all pregnancies (to both married and nonmarried women) carried to term are unwanted (Cates et al., 1977; Fussel and Hatcher, 1975). This, of course, does not include those pregnancies that are terminated by abortion. The number of abortions in 1977 was reported to be 1,000,000 (U.S. Department of Vital Statistics). Cates and associates (1977), using several data sources, put the total number of unwanted pregnancies in the United States in 1974 at a conservative 969,700; however, this figure does not include the number of unwanted pregnancies that were terminated by spontaneous abortion (which occurs at a rate of one in five of all pregnancies). In addition, according to Tanis (1977), only an estimated 20% of young couples using contraception succeed in having wanted pregnancies at spaced intervals.

It is obvious that unwanted pregnancy is of considerable magnitude—an estimated 15% of all pregnancies occurring in the United States today are unwanted and at least 1 million women suffer the agony of an unwanted pregnancy.

WHY DOES IT HAPPEN?

How does this happen in this day and age of enlightened sexuality and effective contraception? The reasons are many and varied, but appear to follow a few common themes: cultural norms, ignorance, professional barriers, difficulties with contraceptive methods, and psychologic issues.

Cultural norms

Over and over again research* confirms society's sanctions against planned sex for nonmarried women, and because of this many women use contraceptives erratically, if at all. Because our culture does not usually sanction any sexual behavior except that occurring within the marital relationship, unpremeditated sex, when involvement is controlled by emotion, is seen as less immoral than planned sexual experiences.

In the United States today there has been a shift of responsibility for contraception from the male to the female. At the same time, the nonmarried woman is made to feel that her use of contraception is not socially acceptable. She is twice damned if she has sex outside of marriage and also uses contraception. Using contraceptives, particularly a reliable method of birth control, suggests a commitment to sex—as if using the "pill," a diaphragm, or an IUD is a symbol of planned sex. This would be further validated by a visit to a physician, which certainly constitutes planning ahead.

The cultural belief that women are promiscuous or immoral if they use birth control may encourage women to leave themselves vulnerable to pregnancy. Also, the inconsistency between a value system that prohibits nonmarital sex and a woman's own sexual activity is often handled by rationalizing that sex occurred in the "heat of passion." "Spontaneous" sex, which is technically unplanned, has a measure of virtue, and failure to use a contraceptive is assumed to be evidence of one's relative innocence. (There may also be an element of absolution in the "2-week sweats" each month, a form of punishment for the "wrong" act of sexual intercourse.)

Less effective methods of birth control seem to be less stigmatizing and less threatening than safer methods. These methods allow the woman to demonstrate some concern for avoiding pregnancy and yet imply that nothing more is planned than the one encounter. The woman does not need to feel "always ready" and does not need to openly acknowledge sexual activity to herself or to anyone else. Our culture also programs the woman to see herself as vulnerable to the male and that she must be seduced; when this occurs she can be the "violated virgin," a variation on the "heat of passion" theme. In a culture that positively values virginity until marriage (while the peer group does not) many girls preserve a "technical" virginity; they are still virgins as long as the penis does not penetrate the vagina. Unfortunately, this method of preserving virginity does not preclude pregnancy.

There are basically three forms of *denial* that can

*See Barr, 1977; Buford and Peters, 1973; Tanis, 1977; and Zimmerman, 1977.

operate in the occurrence of unwanted pregnancy. First is the very prevalent belief, especially among teenagers, that "it can't happen to me"; this is most often linked to a feeling of invulnerability and the belief that "nice" girls do not get pregnant. Another form of denial is linked to abrogation of personal responsibility either by denying the responsibility and possible consequences for one's actions or by shifting responsibility to someone else (expecting the partner to use contraception). A third type of denial involves an inability to see oneself as a sexually active person, which may be tied to societal norms restricting nonmarital behavior for all women, not only teenagers or those just becoming sexually active.

Guilt is a powerful emotion that often operates in the etiology of unplanned pregnancies. The woman, married or not, who believes that sex is for procreation purposes only is going to experience guilt if the possibility of pregnancy is eliminated. Many women state that they would experience embarrassment and shame if others found out about their sexual activity and need for contraception. They do not want to be seen going to a physician, the only way of obtaining reliable methods of birth control.

The taboo for many women against handling or touching their genitalia may prevent some of them from using many forms of birth control, thus increasing their risk of an unwanted pregnancy.

Closely allied with the cultural belief system we have been considering is the inability to accept the fact that much of behavior is not the result of cautious forethought; rather it is the outgrowth of emotions or feelings. The power of emotion over the intellect is tremendous but seldom recognized or acknowledged. The woman who states she does not plan to be sexually active again (usually right after delivering an unwanted infant) is proof of this lack of acknowledgement. Most people grossly underestimate the power of sexual drive and desire. It is an accurate assumption that once a woman becomes sexually active she will remain so as long as health and opportunity allow. Both fear and sex are strong emotions; however, in the end they are not equal. Sex has a way of subduing fear and, given the right circumstances, time, and opportunity, sex will overcome fear—even the fear of pregnancy.

Ignorance

In a society in which sexual stimuli, conversation, and awareness abound, there is still an appalling amount of myth, misconception, and misinformation concerning sex. Some women do not understand their own reproductive anatomy or physiology. Some are afraid that without the possibility of pregnancy they will become overly aggressive sexually.

Anxiety or fear may arise from mistaken beliefs about the effects or side effects of various contraceptives (for example, that weight gain is inevitable with oral contraceptives, or that use of certain contraceptives will be detrimental to the sexual organs). Many women have mistaken ideas about how contraceptives work, their effectiveness, and when contraceptives are needed. It is not true, for example, that a woman cannot become pregnant during menstruation, while breastfeeding, or during menopause. Lack of understanding can also lead to incorrect or sporadic use of contraceptives, if they are used at all. Sometimes a lack of faith in one method is generalized to a belief that *no* type works. Unwanted pregnancy may also occur simply because the woman does not know where to obtain birth control.

Professional barriers

Unfortunately, some women become pregnant because of barriers imposed by health care professionals. Women may not seek help because they fear judgmental attitudes from health professionals. The physician or nurse who makes punitive statements to the nonmarried woman or who refuses to give contraceptives to the teenager makes these women vulnerable to unwanted pregnancy. Professionals must examine their own value systems since any negative feelings toward sex, birth control, and the clients they serve will affect the care they give.

Family planning may be viewed either as a way of controlling population (often implying the control of particular groups) or the opposite end of the spectrum—an undesirable interference with nature. Some nurses have negative attitudes toward the poor, believing, for example, that they are stupid, sexually irresponsible, or unable to use contraception effectively. These attitudes are quickly perceived by clients.

Some nurses do not feel comfortable with family planning education as a part of their nursing practice. They may feel inadequate to counsel and reluctant to gain requisite knowledge. Others feel it is an invasion of privacy to discuss sexual matters with clients. A nurse may also feel guilty about her own contraceptive practices, have conflicting moralistic views, a lack of commitment to contraception, or be unable to discuss sexuality comfortably. Cultural norms play a strong role here since the nurse may consciously or unconsciously believe that sex is sinful and pregnancy a just punishment. Tolerance for a wide variety of sexual standards and behaviors is necessary for nurses who offer contraceptive counseling.

Once a woman has decided upon a method of birth control, accepted the fact of her sexual activity and its attendant need for responsible behavior, it is not within the province of the health professional to try to change her behavior. The nurse's role is to counsel, reassure, provide information, and allow the woman to make her own decision. Instilling fear, guilt, shame, or loss of esteem in clients is inappropriate.

There have been cases in which mistakes by health care professionals have led to unwanted pregnancies (giving a woman the wrong information, taking a woman off one type of contraceptive without replacing it with another, or spending insufficient time with the client to ensure she completely understands how to use the contraceptive method she has chosen). Delay in confirming a pregnancy may also necessitate a woman carrying an unwanted pregnancy to term. All of these errors on the part of health care workers contribute to the problem of unwanted pregnancies.

Difficulties with contraceptive methods

Unfortunately, a sizable number of women who use a given contraceptive method correctly and faithfully still become pregnant; no contraceptive method yet devised is 100% foolproof. Still other women dislike any type of contraception that distracts from the spontaneity of sex. This may become more and more of an issue as many women who have used oral contraceptives and the IUD become disenchanted with these methods and switch to other methods that are viewed as medically safer but require planning and interruption of the sex act. Finally, severe crisis in a woman's life, such as family problems, job change, or death of a loved one, can cause her to cease functioning in a logical, consistent manner, and this often includes contraception.

Psychologic issues

There are many reasons of an emotional or psychologic nature that may cause a woman to risk an unwanted pregnancy. For example, a couple may become lax in contraceptive usage or alter their use because of changes in their sexual activity. This can happen when the future of the relationship is uncertain or needs clarification. The thought of a breakup is too threatening to deal with on a conscious level, so the couple avoid direct action but precipitate a confrontation with the advent of an unplanned pregnancy. Sexual intercourse, when it is used as a way to initiate, maintain, or prolong a relationship, is often associated with a feeling of desperation that allows the woman to accept the possibility of pregnancy. Intercourse can also be used as a weapon to gain control in a relationship. If a woman is using an effective method of contraception, she can no longer control the frequency of intercourse through reminders about the possibility of pregnancy. In a similar manner a male may fear that without threat of pregnancy the female sexual drive will be beyond his capabilities to fulfill. For these reasons either may resist contraceptive use.

One partner may force contraception on the other, who, resenting it, will abandon it as a way to be in control. Sexual identity conflicts can also result in lack of contraceptive usage and thus an unwanted pregnancy (for example, the woman who feels feminine only when she knows she can conceive or the man who has a strong need to impregnate repeatedly as proof of his virility and masculinity). Likewise, some women see pregnancy as proof of womanliness and may experience conflict between the need to feel sexually attractive and the need not to be pregnant again. Fertility is also equated with youth and creativity. Those whose self-esteem is low or whose sexual identity is closely tied to fertility will not do well with contraception and will often find themselves with unwanted or unplanned pregnancy.

A sense of personal worthlessness may cause the woman to allow herself to be used sexually. Pregnancy can enhance this self-punishment. Some women believe strongly that fate rules their lives. These women may feel too apathetic and helpless to make plans and follow them through, since they cannot deal with the normal fears and insecurities of life on a conscious level. Finally, ambivalence toward pregnancy, childbirth, parenthood, and sex often is present and may cause the woman to neglect or avoid using contraception effectively, thereby leaving the matter unresolved and possibilities open in both directions.

For too long, women have been blamed by society for becoming pregnant when they did not wish to. Unwanted pregnancy occurs for many different reasons. It is important that the nurse understand the many factors that may produce the phenomenon of an unwanted pregnancy.

COUNSELING IN UNWANTED PREGNANCY

An unwanted pregnancy has the potential for being one of the most intense life crises a woman encounters. Anxiety is almost always present, usually at a very high level, and can complicate the woman's decision-making abilities. In order to counsel effectively, the nurse should understand why the anxiety is produced. Most women will experience conflict, fear, guilt, and shame. For some, these feelings may arise from the knowledge that they have disappointed their parents and have not met parental expectations regarding sexual conduct and future plans. Others fear the partner's reaction. They may be afraid he will leave if he finds out about the pregnancy or that he will deny any responsibility for it. Anxiety may also spring from a wish to have nothing more to do with the sexual partner.

Some women grieve for lost dreams and hopes and are afraid that they may not be able to attain personal goals, such as higher education or a career. Anxiety can be generated by feeling trapped into marriage, or belief that marriage is a poor solution. Pregnancy and subsequent childrearing impose severe burdens, and many woman have limited resources available. A woman may feel that she simply does not have enough resources—financial, material, or emotional—to provide for another human being. Many women feel incapable of handling the physical or emotional strain of pregnancy, childbirth, and its attendant responsibilities. They may be aware of their own need to mature and may feel they have too little to give a child emotionally. For some women, anxiety is generated by a wish to prevent anyone from knowing about the pregnancy. They may be fearful of ostracism and criticism from friends, family, and church. Feelings of shame can create tremendous anxiety.

An unwanted pregnancy has a tremendous potential for trauma and possible disastrous consequences both to the woman and to her partner, family, and potential offspring. All women should have the right to control their own fertility and this includes choosing to continue or terminate the pregnancy.

Crisis intervention

Pregnancy counseling is a type of crisis intervention that takes place at a time when the woman may have decreased coping abilities, a weakened sense of self-esteem, and is experiencing considerable anxiety, fear, or panic. It takes place within a forced-choice situation; the decision will be made either through consideration of alternatives and subsequent choice or through default as the biologic process continues. The goals or objectives of the counseling experience should be (Wilson, 1973):

1. Exploring with the woman her feelings about the pregnancy and her understanding of options available to her
2. Structuring the counseling so that the woman is able to make an informed decision
3. Supporting the woman's decision
4. Facilitating the resolution of the decision with whatever information is needed
5. Helping the client gain a better understanding of herself through an understanding of what led to the unwanted conception
6. Preventing a subsequent unwanted pregnancy

Since problem pregnancy counseling is a form of crisis intervention, it is important that the nurse understand the concept of crisis and crisis intervention theory and methodology. Briefly, each individual strives to live in a state of emotional equilibrium; the goal in a crisis is always to return to or maintain that state. Each person has his or her own usual methods of problem-solving techniques with which to deal with problems. When these cannot be used to deal with a particular situation, the equilibrium is upset. The individual has to either solve the problem or adapt to nonsolution; in either case a new state of equilibrium will result. When there is a problem that cannot be solved, frustration increases and symptoms of anxiety appear with decreased ability to function. This is a transition period during which there is both the danger of increased psychologic vulnerability and the opportunity for personal growth. The outcome of the crisis is governed by the types of interactions that occur between the person in crisis and the key figures in her life.

Predictable potential crisis points occur when periods of greatest social, psychologic, and physical change are coupled with biologic and social role transitions (for example, menarche, marriage, and parenthood). Crises come in two forms: maturational and situational. Maturational crises are the normal processes of growth and development; they evolve over an extended period of time and often require many alterations in the individual's character. There may be some awareness of increased feelings of disequilibrium, but the individual usually does not intellectually correlate these feelings with a realization that developmental change is occurring. Situational crises are caused by external events that are stressful to the individual. The birth of a baby can be both a situational and a maturational crisis.

It is important to look at those factors that will determine whether a person will regain a state of equilibrium or enter a crisis state. Three factors have been identified that seem to make the difference: (1) perception of the event, (2) situational support, and (3) coping mechanisms. Fig. 12-1 illustrates the paradigm of the effects of a stressful event on the human organism. The first balancing factor, *perception of the event*, refers to the meaning the event has for the individual. Is the event perceived realistically or is perception distorted? If the event is perceived realistically, there is recognition of the relationship between the event and feelings of stress. In this case, problem-solving can be directed appropriately toward reduction of tension and successful resolution is more probable. When perception is distorted, the relationship between the event and stressful feelings will not be identified, problem-solving efforts will be ineffective, and tension will remain.

Social supports are those persons in the environment upon whom the woman depends for assistance and caring. To whom can she talk or turn? Who is available to depend on? Loss, threatened loss, or feelings of inadequacy in relationships can increase the vulnerability of the individual so that when a stressful situation happens, disequilibrium and crisis can occur.

The final balancing factors are *coping mechanisms*. These are those methods learned by the individual to cope with anxiety and reduce tension. Coping mecha-

nisms are what people usually do when faced with a problem. These tension-reducing mechanisms can be overt or covert and consciously or unconsciously activated. They are generally classified as the following behavioral responses: aggression, regression, withdrawal, and repression. The selection of the response is based on what has worked successfully in the past to relieve anxiety and reduce tension. Each response has been used at different times by the individual, found to be effective in maintaining stability, and has become a part of the person's method of meeting and dealing with the stresses of living (Aguilera and Messick, 1978).

The goal of crisis intervention is resolution of the immediate crisis with focus on return to a precrisis level of functioning. The role of the therapist is direct, supportive, active participation. Techniques are varied and flexible but there are specific steps involved in crisis intervention. Although it is not possible to place each step in a clearly defined category, typical intervention would pass through the following phases (Aguilera and Messick, 1978):

1. Assessment of the woman and her problem. This requires the therapist to be skilled in focusing techniques in order to gather all the data necessary to define the problem clearly so as to obtain an accurate assessment of the precipitating event and the woman's perception of it.
2. Development of a plan of intervention based on the individual's needs and situation.
3. Intervention techniques:
   a. Assisting the woman to gain an intellectual understanding of the crisis.
   b. Helping the woman express her feelings about the situation openly.
   c. Assisting the woman to explore alternative methods of coping and solutions available to her.
4. Resolution of the crisis and anticipatory planning to prevent future similar crisis.

Alternative counseling

Alternative counseling, a form of crisis intervention, is a model for problem pregnancy counseling that is particularly effective. This type of counseling has several defining features that differentiate it from more general types of counseling and other forms of crisis intervention. Generally, alternative counseling is characterized by: (1) limited counselor-client contact with high emotional intensity, (2) a variety of possible circumstances, (3) complexity of issues, (4) information exchange, and (5) necessity for a decision by the client.

Usually, a relatively brief time period is spent in counselor-client contact. If more than three sessions are necessary, it is important that the nurse recognize the additional time needed to deal with the issues involved and that more highly specialized therapy skills may be needed. In this instance, she should assess her own capabilities as a therapist to provide what is needed and consider referral if appropriate. Usually, the actual time spent with each woman in alternative counseling is limited by the urgent nature of the problem and sometimes by agency and personnel limitation. Alternative counseling is a response to a choice crisis which is usually resolved in a relatively short period of time.

The brief time period in no way implies that intense feelings are not present. Problem pregnancy counseling is marked by intense emotions and is often accompanied by a decreased ability to effectively cope with such intensity. The present crisis situation may cause past emotional conflicts to surface, which only intensifies the present situational stress. When feelings and emotions run high in counseling sessions, it may be very difficult for the client to consider alternatives and decide on a course of action.

Another characteristic of problem pregnancy counseling is the wide variety of situations and circumstances that may surround the pregnancy and the differences between individual women's abilities to cope with an un-

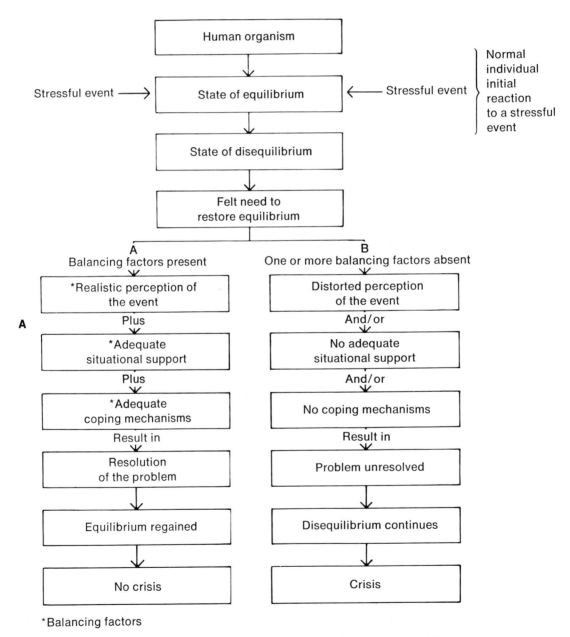

*Balancing factors

Fig. 12-1. A, Paradigm: effect of balancing factors in a stressful event.

wanted pregnancy. The nurse must be able to listen effectively and assess individuals of various backgrounds, ages, family situations, and personalities. The crisis of unwanted pregnancy and the need to make a decision are common to all these women, but it would be poor nursing judgment to assume that all women will react similarly; circumstances and individual coping resources vary tremendously. The nurse needs to be flexible enough to help each woman examine her own situation and to mobilize all of her available resources to solve her problem.

Resolution of the crisis of a problem pregnancy is made more difficult because of the number and complexity of external or environmental issues involved, including legal, economic, sociopolitical, religious, and cultural factors. These issues have to be considered by each woman and are the framework within which her decision is made. The issues relevant to each woman's personal world are different, and therefore the problems and pressures involved in resolution will vary. The counselor needs to understand on an objective level those issues that affect problem pregnancies in general but must also be able to ascertain which issues and pressures are preventing a particular woman from effectively making a decision.

The alternative counseling method involves a substantial amount of information exchange during counselor-client interactions. This is particularly important since the counseling contact is brief, often intense, and involves complex issues. The first phase of information

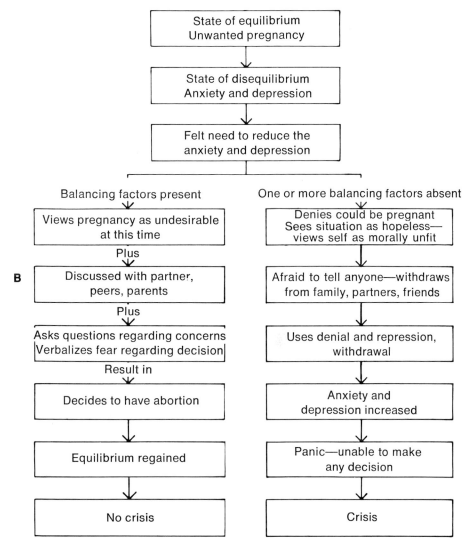

Fig. 12-1, cont'd. B, Paradigm applied to unwanted pregnancy. (**A,** From Aguilera, D., and Messick, J.: Crisis intervention, St. Louis, 1978, The C. V. Mosby Co.)

exchange in this type of helping relationship is *information-gathering by the counselor.* The interaction centers on gathering enough data from the client to adequately assess the problem and its various dimensions. The focus is on helping the client define and elaborate the problem rather than on offering suggestions or exploring alternatives. A special problem that often occurs in problem pregnancy counseling and clouds the picture is that the client has already made a decision. These pre-counseling decisions are usually the product of fear and panic, and the counselor needs to provide initial reassurance that the alternative chosen is possible and then move to explore the problem more fully. In data gathering, several areas of information are important. These include information about (1) relevant background experiences, (2) typical behavior and personality of the woman, and (3) the woman's life circumstances.

Information about past experiences is important in that these experiences help determine in large measure the present response of the woman to the unwanted pregnancy. Information about socioeconomic status, age, previous pregnancies, relationship with the man involved, and prior developmental life crises and experiences can all help the nurse make an assessment. Prior learning and experiences have implications that come to the surface in crisis and can be barriers to effective problem resolution. Knowledge about personality and behavior of the woman helps the nurse to understand what kind of person the client is. This is important because specific behaviors and personality attributes have their origins in significant past experiences, which influence the client's ability to cope and make decisions in the present.

It is crucial to know what the present life circumstances of the woman are if the nurse is to help her arrive at a realistic decision. The relationship with the male involved is especially important—an unwanted pregnancy arising from an assault is vastly different from that occurring within the context of a loving relationship that precludes children for financial reasons.

The second phase of information exchange centers on *processing the information received from the client.* Organizing the information enables the counselor to better understand the client and thus define the direction of the counseling process. Further information from the client is combined with information that the counselor has available and that can be shared later with the client. The gathering, processing, and organization of information occur simultaneously. At the verbal level, the counselor is attempting to discover enough information to adequately assess the problem. At a cognitive level the counselor is trying to eliminate irrelevant data and organize what remains into a meaningful whole to better understand the client.

The final stage of information exchange is called *information-sharing.* This happens only after enough data have been collected and assessed so that the counselor can make accurate nursing diagnoses regarding the problem. Many different directions can be taken. First, the nurse can aid the client by providing information relevant to her present problem, particularly by helping her perceive her present situation and the circumstances of her pregnancy more objectively. In addition, the client can be assisted to explore the positive and negative aspects of all available alternatives and their implications. Finally, information can be shared that will help the client to clarify and more clearly understand her feelings and emotional reactions to the unwanted pregnancy and to the decision process. It should be stressed that discovery, processing, and sharing of information are cyclical and several cycles may be required before adequate solution and closure are reached by the client. Further, the nurse needs to give the client all factual data about the various alternatives available to her but only after exploration and data-gathering are completed. If information is offered too soon it may block open consideration of all alternatives, free decision-making, and successful resolution.

The type of information given the client may range from specifics of reproductive anatomy and physiology to the legal aspects of abortion and adoption to available community resources and cost. This information is crucial to the decision-making process. What type of information is needed will vary from woman to woman. It is important that the nurse not assume that all women need certain types of information but rather respond to their individual needs. The decision-making process can only be hampered by too much information or information that is nonessential for a particular situation. However, relevant facts help the client weigh alternatives, look at the advantages and disadvantages of each, and clarify her feelings and more clearly understand them.

A final characteristic of alternative counseling is the necessity for the client to *make a decision.* Focus should remain on the decision-making process within the context of the circumstances of the unwanted pregnancy, the alternatives available, and the resources possessed by the client. The overall direction is exploration of alternatives and making a decision, although there may be subgoals in the counseling process. Focus is on the ultimate decision to be made and not on "therapy," which implies changing some aspect of behavior or reducing tension by some means other than crisis resolution. These may become part of the counseling process at some later date but are not inherent in alternative counseling for problem pregnancies. Methods used by the counselor include acceptance of the woman and her situation and helping her mobilize all available resources to aid in deciding. In essence, the counselor's role is to help each woman move from her present position to an acceptable decision regarding the problem pregnancy (Wilson, 1973).

Each woman facing the biologic fact of an unwanted pregnancy has a decision to make and time is her master. The decision-making process for each woman is similar and follows a similar sequence. Mace (1972) has outlined the following steps: (1) defining the problem fully, (2) exploring and understanding the implications of the present situation, (3) assessing and understanding feelings about the situation, (4) accumulating information about all relevant aspects of the situation, (5) examining the positive and negative aspects of all available options, and (6) making the decision and following it through.

Available alternatives

Basically, the alternatives or options available for the woman facing an unwanted pregnancy are (Fig. 12-2):
1. Marriage, if not already married; carrying the pregnancy to term and raising the child
2. Single parenthood
3. Releasing the child for adoption
4. Abortion
5. Suicide (This is certainly not a meaningful alterna-

tive but some women have seen this as the solution to their problem.)

Marriage. This has been the option most frequently chosen for the past 100 years. Women feared the condemnation of society and did not want their child to bear the stigma of "bastard." For many women the thought of adoption was also intolerable. More recently, however, marriage has become increasingly less popular as women realize the disadvantages of an unhappy marriage. Neither the prospect of a high probability of divorce nor a life of unhappiness and resentment is appealing. A "forced" marriage may be viewed as having little meaning, and little value is seen in raising a child in such an environment (Buford and Peters, 1973). Women considering marriage because of pregnancy must examine their motives realistically. Is guilt a factor? Are sympathy and pity factors in the decision? Will one or the other partner feel tricked or trapped in later years? These questions often become important in subsequent pregnancies when old feelings are resurrected (Moore, 1978). Vincent (1961) points out that the couple should realize that the question, "Would he have married me if . . .?" is unanswerable and part of a very universal problem. All couples, at some point in their marriage, will drag up the past into arguments, and premarital pregnancy is only one issue available to be resurrected. Premarital

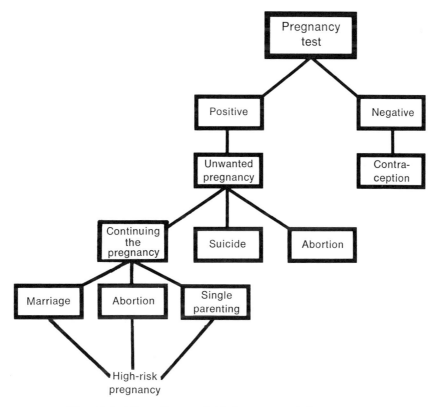

Fig. 12-2. Alternatives available in an unwanted pregnancy.

pregnancy is not itself an absolute contraindication to marriage, although waiting until after the child is born and then making the decision about marriage might be a reasonable alternative (Moore, 1978). If marriage is chosen, it is more desirable to have the type of wedding the couple would have had no matter what the circumstances. A hurried secretive affair may be long remembered and haunt them in years to come.

Single parenthood. The decision to enter into single parenthood is becoming more popular and more acceptable to women today. It is influenced by cultural norms and individual circumstances. Women in low socioeconomic groups are more likely to attempt single parenthood; many are the products of single parent families themselves. Another factor that increases the likelihood that a woman will choose to keep her baby is support from her parents for this choice. McCoy and Muth (1973) state that older women already maintaining their own homes, women who have a continuing relationship with the father, women who consider future marriage a possibility, and women who have had prior pregnancies not carried to term are more apt to keep their child.

The woman who chooses single parenthood faces real, pressing concerns about which she must decide in a short time period. She must decide where she will live: with her parents or other relatives? with the partner? with friends? alone? in a maternity home? in foster care? Another crucial issue is increased financial needs and how these will be met. Most single mothers who keep their infants will have financial problems regardless of their socioeconomic status. The median income for families headed by women in 1977 was $6,400 compared to a median income of $13,800 for husband-wife families (Moore, 1978). Each woman needs assistance in realistically assessing the expenses of pregnancy and child-rearing vs her available funds. The nurse can assume part of this role in conjunction with the social worker. A variety of resources are potentially available, such as employment; assistance from the father of the child, parents, or relatives; medicaid and other governmental programs; and community resources. The nurse can provide information, listen to feelings, and help the mother explore alternatives and eventually arrive at the decision best for her. The single mother needs to decide how she will obtain adequate medical care for herself and her infant, and how will she begin or continue a job or her education. There is the chance that a woman's choice to be a single parent is based on a notion about the joys of motherhood rather than an objective evaluation of the situation. It is essential that the woman consider all of the relevant issues and arrive at a realistic solution.

Adoption. Traditionally, adoption has been second to marriage as the most popular alternative. It is a particularly difficult choice to make and extracts a high cost both economically and emotionally. There are all the expenses of a pregnancy, labor, and delivery, plus the painful reality of giving the baby away. Support should be available to the mother as she struggles through the initial decision and then the weeks and months that follow. She will need reassurance as she questions whether or not she is doing the right thing. A review of how she arrived at the decision and of the advantages and disadvantages is the most helpful means of support from the nurse. These clients need a lot of empathy, particularly as delivery becomes imminent and when the baby is taken to the adoption agency. The mother should always know that the decision to place a baby for adoption is not irrevocable until after the baby is born and for some interval of time thereafter (e.g., 30 days from the signing of the papers). Long-term resolution of guilt and sorrow is difficult to achieve. Many women who have placed a child for adoption later state that they wish they had terminated the pregnancy by abortion (Buford and Peters, 1973). Butts and Sporakowski (1974), in a study to determine which type of woman chooses to bear a child in a maternity home rather than have an abortion, found the following characteristics: Maternity home clients are younger, less educated, go to church more regularly, are less aware of abortion, less sexually permissive, have a poorer relationship with the putative father, and are less likely to be satisfied with their pregnancy decision than those who chose abortion. This is important since it indicates areas of intervention for nursing: increased knowledge may affect what decision is made; and certain clients may need certain types of information. Finally, contrary to popular belief, girls choosing abortion were more satisfied than those who chose adoption. Perhaps the question of satisfaction with alternatives and potential guilt associated with alternatives needs to be more carefully examined by the practitioner.

Abortion. Abortion is and should be a realistic and available alternative for each woman. Legal abortion is not acceptable to everyone but for many women it is the solution to their problem (see Chapter 23). Nurses have a responsibility to support a legal abortion when the client makes this choice.

SUMMARY

In summary, it is essential that nurses remember that there is no one right answer or panacea for the resolution of an unwanted pregnancy. Who is to say what an individual woman should or should not do? Each has to make her own decision and then act on it. Solving the dilemma of an unwanted pregnancy may be the single most important decision a woman will ever have to make. Regardless of whether she chooses to continue the pregnancy or terminate by abortion, it is her decision alone.

It is the nurse's role to facilitate the decision-making processes by whatever interventions are available, to support the woman's decision with understanding, safety, and caring, and to help her live with the decision as well as possible.

REFERENCES

Aguilera, D. C., and Messick, J. M.: Crisis intervention, St. Louis, 1978, The C. V. Mosby Co.

Barr, S. J.: A woman's choice, New York, 1977, Ranna Association Publishers, Inc.

Buford, R., Jr., and Peters, R.: Unwanted pregnancy, New York, 1973, Harper & Row Publishers.

Butts, R. Y., and Sporakowski, M. J.: Unwed pregnancy decisions, J. Sex Res. 10(2):110-117, May 1974.

Cates, W., and others: Abortion as a treatment for unwanted pregnancy: the number two sexually transmitted condition, Adv. Planned Parent. 10(3):115-121, 1977.

Clark, A. L., and Affonso, D.: Childbearing: a nursing perspective, Philadelphia, 1976, F. A. Davis Co.

Fussel, J., and Hatcher, R.: Women in need, New York, 1975, The Macmillan Co.

Mace, D. R.: Abortion: the agonizing decisions, New York, 1972, Abington Press.

McCoy, G., and Muth, F.: The alternatives in continuing the pregnancy. In Wilson, R., editor: Problem pregnancy: a counseling and resources manual, Chapel Hill, N.C., 1973, Student Graphics, University of North Carolina—Chapel Hill.

Moore, M. L.: Realities in childbearing, Philadelphia, 1978, W. B. Saunders Co.

Tanis, J. L.: Recognizing the reasons for contraceptive non-use and abuse, Am. J. Mat. Child Nurs. Nov./Dec. 1977, pp. 364-369.

U. S. National Center for Health Statistics: Vital statistics of the United States, Washington, D.C., 1977, Annual.

Vincent, C.: Unmarried mothers, New York, 1961, The Free Press.

Wilson, R. C.: Problem pregnancy: a counseling and resources manual, Chapel Hill, N.C., 1973, Student Graphics, University of North Carolina—Chapel Hill, pp. 15-23.

Zimmerman, M. K.: Passage through abortion, New York, 1977, Proege Publishers.

ADDITIONAL READINGS

Abernathy, V.: Prevention of unwanted pregnancy among teenagers, Prim. Care 3(3):399-406, 1976.

Abernathy, V.: The abortion constellation, Arch. Gen. Psych. 29:346-350, 1973.

Abernathy, V., and others: Identification of women at risk for unwanted pregnancy, Am. J. Psych. 132(10):1027-1031, 1975.

Baldwin, B.: Problem pregnancy counseling: general principles, Chapel Hill, N.C., 1973, Student Graphics, University of North Carolina—Chapel Hill.

Bracken, M.: Abortion, adoption, or motherhood—an empirical study of decision making during pregnancy, Am. J. Obstet. Gynecol. 130(3):251-262, 1978.

Cutright, P.: Illegitimacy: myths, causes and cures, Family Plan. Perspect. 3(1):26-49, 1971.

Hartley, S. F.: Illegitimacy, Berkeley, 1975, University of California Press.

Keller, C., and Copeland, P.: Counseling the abortion patient is more than talk, Am. J. Nurs. 72(1):43-46, 1972.

Parad, H. J.: Crisis intervention: selected readings, New York, 1965, Family Services Association of America.

Romney, S. L., and others: Gynecology and obstetrics, New York, 1975, McGraw-Hill Book Co.

Shea, F. P.: Survey of health professionals regarding family planning, Nurs. Res. 22(1):17-24, 1973.

Westoof, C. F., and Ryder, N. B.: The contraceptive revolution, Princeton, N. J., 1977, Princeton University Press.

13

The gynecologic triad: discharge, pain, and bleeding

Catherine Ingram Fogel

Throughout her life, the average woman will experience bleeding, pain, or discharge associated with her reproductive organs or functions. Many women will seek out nurses as advisers, counselors, and caregivers for these concerns. To meet their clients' needs, nurses must have information. Any symptom may indicate pathology or disease, or it may be a normal variation of the menstrual cycle. Past experiences, cultural knowledge, and societal expectations may influence the client's or nurse's interpretation of symptoms. Feelings of fear, guilt, and anxiety are commonly experienced. The nursing practitioner must be able to distinguish the normal from the abnormal, identify pathology when it exists, and understand the meaning of the symptoms or illness for the client. This chapter provides the needed information to meet these objectives. Each symptom is discussed in terms of (1) its meaning, (2) common causes, including representative diseases, (3) normal characteristics and pathologic alterations, and (4) specific management strategies. Nursing interventions and client self-care activities are emphasized throughout.

DISCHARGE AND PRURITUS

Although not life-threatening, these symptoms unquestionably diminish the quality of life for the woman who suffers from them. Vaginal discharge and itching of the vulva and vagina are among the most frequent reasons a woman seeks help from a health care provider. More women complain of leukorrhea, or vaginal discharge, than any other gynecologic symptom (Parsons and Sommers, 1978). These symptoms are perceived differently by individual women; one woman may experience severe physical discomfort and another only minor distress. A client may be very anxious or only mildly concerned. The woman's reaction will depend on many factors including her previous experience, knowledge, cultural conditioning, and the number and severity of symptoms.

Normal vaginal discharge and odor are often considered to be offensive. Body odors in general are not acceptable in our society, and this is intensified when the odor is related to sexual organs. One has only to consider the host of products developed by the cosmetics industry to clean, deodorize, and perfume to realize how uncomfortable many women are with their normal body odors. The great concern women express over concealing menstruation exemplifies the unacceptability of their physiologic processes.

Increased vaginal discharge, malodor, or itching may be perceived as "dirty." Anxiety may result from the misconceptions that discharge or itching is indicative of cancer or venereal disease. Infection and itching are often closely associated in the client's mind. Because infections with a gynecologic origin may have a shameful connotation, clients may delay seeking help until the symptoms become unbearable. Fears of offending may be heightened; the women may be very concerned about the nurse's reaction to these symptoms. The nurse has a responsibility not only to assist in the resolution of the disease process causing the discharge or itching but also to help the client accept and understand her body.

Normal characteristics

Vaginal secretions are a normal, regularly occurring experience for women during their childbearing years. There are numerous variations in the amount and characteristics of vaginal secretions, which are determined by physiology, emotions, and pathology. Women who have adequate endogenous or exogenous estrogen will have vaginal secretions. The major source of vaginal secretion is the cervical mucosa. Small amounts are secreted by the Bartholin's, sebaceous, sweat, and apocrine glands of the vulva, and rarely by the uterus or oviduct. The vaginal mucosa, which contains no glands, is not truly secretory; however, copious vaginal lubrication known as "sweating" does occur during sexual excitement. Normal vaginal secretions are odorless, acidic, nonbloody, and colorless. An alkaline, glairy mucoid substance is secreted by the cervix. This is more abundant and less viscous at ovulation. Normal vaginal secretions are acidic, with a pH range of 3.8 to 4.2. The *Lactobacillus*, or Döderlein's bacillus, is the most common vaginal flora. Physiologic vaginal secretions usually are not malodorous. Increases in vaginal secretions occur at ovulation, several days before menstruation, and during sexual excitement (Romney, 1975).

Life cycle changes

The female newborn may have a mucous discharge for one to ten days following delivery as a result of in utero stimulation of the uterus and vagina by maternal estrogen. A similar mucoid discharge may be seen a few years before and after menarche as a result of increased estrogen production by the maturing ovary. Pregnancy often substantially increases mucus production with a resulting profuse discharge. A similar discharge may occur in the woman taking oral contraceptives (Romney, 1975).

Before menarche and following menopause, when estrogen levels are low, vaginal secretions are minimal. The vaginal epithelium is inactive and thin, the cells contain very little glycogen, Döderlein's bacilli are absent, and the vaginal pH is between 6 and 7. This inactive, unstimulated mucosa is particularly susceptible to infection while the estrogen-stimulated vaginal mucosa during the present reproductive years is less so.

Vaginal secretions normally vary throughout the menstrual cycle. During the immediate postmenstrual phase when the estrogen level is low, the mucosa is thin and relatively inactive and there is little cervical cell secretion. Vaginal cells proliferate and exfoliate rapidly as estrogen production increases; at the same time the cervical cells secrete more and more mucus. Maximal estrogen production occurs at ovulation and causes a profuse watery discharge, primarily from the cervix. Secretions then decrease until just prior to menstruation.

Concept of infection

Vaginal discharge is most often caused by infection or irritation. Occasionally, however, a serious disease is the underlying cause. It is important that the nurse understand the many influences that determine the development of vaginal infections.

Until recently it was thought that disease processes in the vagina involved introduction of pathogens into the vagina, combined with decreased resistance because of pH alteration or increased glycogen in the vaginal mucosal cells. However, it now appears that cyclic vaginal glycogen is not a major factor in altering vaginal flora.

Also, many organisms capable of producing disease are present in significant numbers in the genital tracts of asymptomatic women (Martin, 1978). Thus the traditional explanation for vaginal infections no longer seems valid. A more comprehensive view of the host-pathogen relationship is needed. Genetic, physiologic, emotional, social, and environmental factors may all be involved. For example, differences have been found in the number and types of bacteria present in the genital tracts of women in different social classes and with differing sexual activity (Romney, 1975). Nutritional status may influence infections since morbidity is higher when the individual is malnourished, and particularly with protein-caloric deprivation.

A number of systemic illnesses cause decreased resistance to infection. Intense or prolonged stress is also often associated with the onset of systemic illness or the precipitation of acute minor illness. Lower socioeconomic status has been linked with a higher incidence of disease probably in association with nutritional or stress factors. The health care practitioner should take a broad approach in caring for clients with vaginal infections. While central, it is not sufficient to simply identify the offending organism and prescribe the appropriate drug. The many other factors that may be contributing significantly to the client's problem need to be recognized and dealt with.

Common causes

The most common causes of vaginal discharge are (1) infectious processes such as *Hemophilus vaginalis, trichomonas vaginalis,* and *Candida albicans;* (2) parasites such as pinworms; (3) mechanical irritants; and (4) contact allergens. Many of the venereal diseases also cause vaginal discharge. (These will be discussed in the section on pain because pain is usually the primary symptom that brings the client to seek help.) Chronic cervicitis accounts for most discharges not associated with itching, pain, or sensitivity. Oral contraceptives and intrauterine devices have also been found to cause vaginal discharge. Each of these causes is associated with a fairly typical history and characteristic physical findings. Table 13-1 summarizes the causes, symptoms, characteristics, and recommended treatment. Effective treatment is based on accurate diagnosis, which includes identifying the causative agent and determining contributing variables.

Diagnosis

There are three components to making an accurate diagnosis: history, physical examination, and laboratory tests. Each component will provide significant data upon which to make an assessment; no step should be omitted.

Table 13-1. Common causes of vaginal discharge

Cause	Symptoms	Diagnostic measures	Treatment
Infections			
Candida albicans (<50% of all vaginitis)	White, curd-like, cheesey discharge; characteristic patches on vaginal walls and cervix; itching; inflamed vagina and cervix	KOH slide shows hyphae and/or spores; Nickerson culture	Monistat (miconozole) cream used daily for 14 days Nystatin suppositories daily or b.i.d. for 14 days
Trichomonas vaginalis	Yellowish to greenish, frothy, copious discharge; "strawberry spots" of cervix; foul odor; severe burning, itching, and dyspareunia	Saline wet smears show *Trichomonas*	Flagyl (metronidazole), 250 mg t.i.d. for 7 days *or* 2 Gm stat for both partners Symptomatic therapy
Hemophilus vaginalis	Grayish white, homogenous discharge; scant amount; fishy or foul odor	Saline wet smear demonstrates typical "clue" cells	Oral antibiotics for both partners: ampicillin, 500 mg q.i.d. for 5 days; Flagyl (metronidazole), 250 mg t.i.d. for 7 days
Foreign body	Blood tinged, serosanguineous or purulent discharge; usually foul odor; discharge may be thick or thin	Visualization of object	Removal of object; antibiotics specific to secondary infection
Allergens or irritants	Increase in usual type and amount of secretions, itching, burning, rash	By exclusion of other possible causes; identification of possible allergen or irritant	Removal of possible allergen or irritant; topical steroid ointment as needed
Cervicitis	Yellow, mucopurulent discharge erosion seen on cervix; cervix appears inflamed and irritated with varying amounts of ulceration; nabothian cysts; mucosa around os everted	Pap smear; visualization of cervical lesions; gonorrhea or other culture to identify infecting organism	Cauterization; antibiotics; conization of cervix For *Chlamydia* infection: tetracycline, 250 mg, q.i.d., for 14 days for both partners

History

Onset of symptoms. It is important to know when discharge began. Recent onset indicates an acute condition while a chronic condition such as cervicitis is typified by symptoms of long duration.

Characteristics of discharge. The *color* and *consistency* of the discharge can suggest specific causes. Discharge that is thick and purulent suggests gonorrhea or bacterial infection; a white, curd-like or watery discharge is characteristic of *Candida infection; Trichomonas* often causes a frothy, green or yellowish discharge; *Hemophilus* infection is characterized by grayish white, scant, cloudy discharge; any discharge that is serous or blood-tinged may be caused by a foreign body or malignancy. *Odor* is a third characteristic to inquire about. *Trichomonas, Hemophilus,* and foreign bodies often cause a foul-smelling odor.

The *amount* of discharge can be significant also. When asking about amount it is important to have the women quantify her answer, since amounts and perceptions of amount can vary greatly. Discharge is considered copious if it soaks through the woman's underpants onto her outer clothing, or stains her underpants sufficiently to require wearing a tampon or pad.

Associated symptoms. *Itching* is often associated with vaginal discharge. *Trichomonas* characteristically is associated with intense itching of the vulva although any infection that causes labial and vulvar irritation and erythema can result in itching. Uncontrollable nocturnal scratching is indicative of pinworms. Itching of the upper mons and vulva associated with pinprick spots of blood on the panties is often seen with pediculosis pubis.

Other symptoms often associated with vaginal discharge are dysuria resulting from local irritation of the urinary meatus, abdominal cramping, or a sense of pelvic fullness. Pelvic fullness may suggest endometritis, salpingitis, cystitis, or pelvic congestion.

Medications. Oral contraceptives can increase vaginal discharge. There also appears to be an increased susceptibility to gonorrheal infections in women taking oral contraceptives who are exposed to the disease. Both oral contraceptives and antibiotics have been implicated in the increased incidence of candidiasis (Meeker, 1978). Until recently it was believed that antibiotics caused more candidal vaginal infection through suppression of normal protective vaginal bacterial flora, resulting in an overgrowth in *Candida*. Current thinking suggests that the mechanism involved is direct stimulation of *Candida* by antibiotics. Meeker reports that the most recent studies show no difference in the incidence of candidiasis between oral contraceptive users and nonusers. Contraceptive agents such as foams, jellies, and creams may cause allergic reactions with vaginal discharge. IUD-caused endometritis or cervicitis may increase vaginal discharge.

Personal hygiene. Frequent douching, particularly with harsh or concentrated solutions, may irritate vaginal tissue. Douching more than once a week can alter the vaginal environment and predispose the woman to infection. Sprays, deodorants, powders, perfumes, and antiseptic soaps or ointments used in the perineal area can cause irritation and/or allergic reactions. Nylon panties or tight fitting pants that do not allow free air flow and absorption of moisture can cause chafing and irritation. Good perineal hygiene is essential to prevent vaginal infections and is important to inquire about.

Previous history. Recurrent vaginal infections can be caused by a number of factors. Diabetes predisposes the woman to recurrent *Candida* infections. Reinfection, or the "ping-pong" syndrome between the male and the female, is common with trichomoniasis. Any of the sexually transmitted diseases can be passed between partners. Inadequate therapy, whether through practitioner error or a lack of patient compliance, can result in recurrent infection. Emotional factors can also cause recurrent vaginitis (Martin, 1978). If prior treatment resolved the infection and the current symptoms are the same, it may be stress induced or psychogenic in nature. If previous treatment was unsuccessful, then the prior diagnosis was incorrect, the course of therapy was inadequate, or client compliance was poor.

Physical examination and laboratory tests

Once these basic areas have been discussed with the client, further data collection should proceed based on the nursing diagnosis. After the history is taken, a pelvic examination, including speculum and bimanual examination, and collection of specimens are indicated. It is important that the examination be done when symptoms are present and the client has not douched or used any medication so that adequate laboratory specimens can be obtained. The following points should be included in the pelvic examination.

External genitalia. The vulva, perineum, and labia should be examined for swelling, redness, and excoriation. These may be mild to severe and involve all or only a portion of the area. Bright red, inflamed labia are indicative of *Candida* infection. There may be lesions or eruptions on the external genitalia. Condylomata acuminata or venereal warts appear as pale, irregular clusters of wartlike lesions. Herpes vaginalis appears as vesicles filled with clear fluid and ulcerations (see section on pain). Any lesion that cannot be identified or appears suspicious should be biopsied to rule out carcinoma.

Speculum examination. The client should be asked to empty her bladder to decrease possible discomfort. The vagina is examined using a warm dry speculum. No lubricating material should be used because it may alter the results of specimens taken. During the speculum examination, vaginal discharge is observed and various smears and cultures are obtained. Each of the common vaginal infections causes a characteristic discharge. Confirming laboratory tests should also be done.

Candida albicans is characterized by a white, lumpy, cottage cheese–like discharge that is found in patches on the vaginal walls, cervix, and labia. Often the vagina and cervix look bright red and swollen (Figs. 13-1 and 13-2). Itching of the vulva is characteristic. Smears should be taken from the patches. Both saline wetprep and potassium hydroxide (KOH) slides should be done. The KOH slide is diagnostic for *Candida* as it lyses other vaginal cells and leaves the *Candida* intact. The characteristic spores or hyphae of *Candida* can be seen (Fig. 13-3).

Trichomonas vaginalis discharge is usually yellowish to greenish, frothy, mucopurulent, copious, and with a foul odor. Fleury (1978) notes that the discharge is often more gray then green and that bubbles are present in only 10% of patients. Typically, the discharge worsens during and after menstruation. Often the cervix and vaginal walls will demonstrate the characteristic "strawberry spots" or tiny petechiae, and the cervix may bleed on contact (Figs. 13-4 and 13-5). In severe infections, the vaginal walls, cervix, and occasionally the vulva may be acutely inflamed. The client may experience burning, dysuria, itching, and dyspareunia with severe infection. *Trichomonas* is readily detected by a wet smear in over 90% of cases (Fleury, 1978). If there is any question, a KOH smear can be done to rule out *Candida*. The typical one-celled flagellate trichomonads are easily distinguished (Fig. 13-6).

Hemophilus vaginalis causes a grayish white, homogenous, foul-smelling discharge. Usually the discharge is scant and no itching, burning, or soreness are present (Fig. 13-7). The odor has a characteristic "fishy" smell. Diagnosis is most easily done by wet smear in which the typical "clue" cells are seen. These are vaginal epithelial cells that are covered by the small gram negative bacillus (Fig. 13-8).

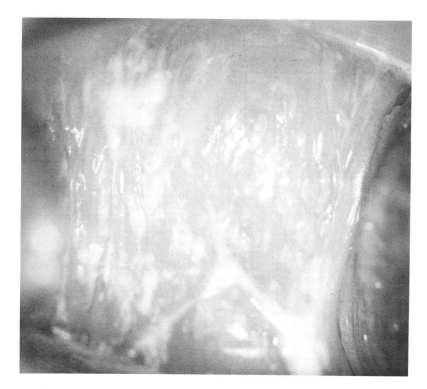

Fig. 13-1. Candidal vaginitis. (Courtesy Ortho Pharmaceutical Corp.)

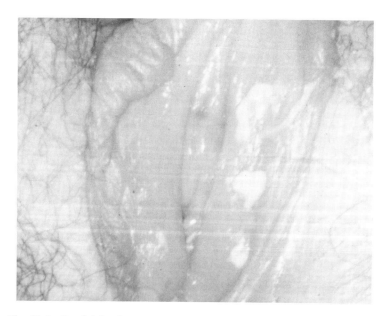

Fig. 13-2. Candidal vulvovaginitis. (Courtesy Ortho Pharmaceutical Corp.)

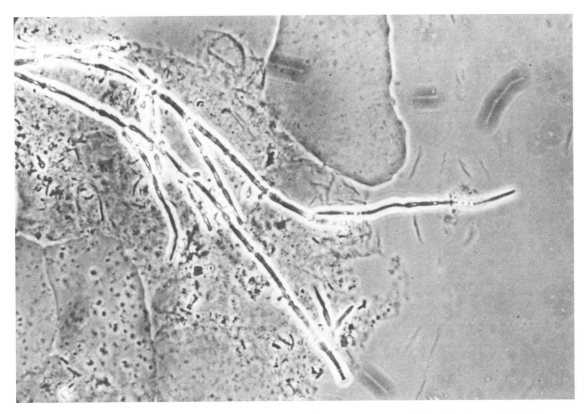

Fig. 13-3. Candidal organisms. (Courtesy Dr. Fred Fleury, University of Illinois, Springfield, Ill.)

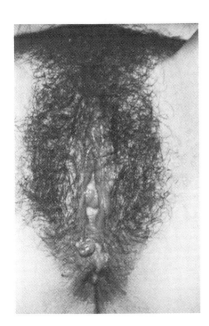

Fig. 13-4. Trichomonal vaginitis. (From Gardner, H. L., and Kaufman, R. H.: Benign diseases of the vulva and vagina, St. Louis, 1969, The C. V. Mosby Co.)

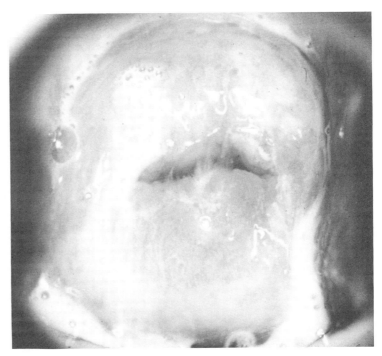

Fig. 13-5. *Trichomonas vaginalis* with cervical erosion. (Courtesy Ortho Pharmaceutical Corp.)

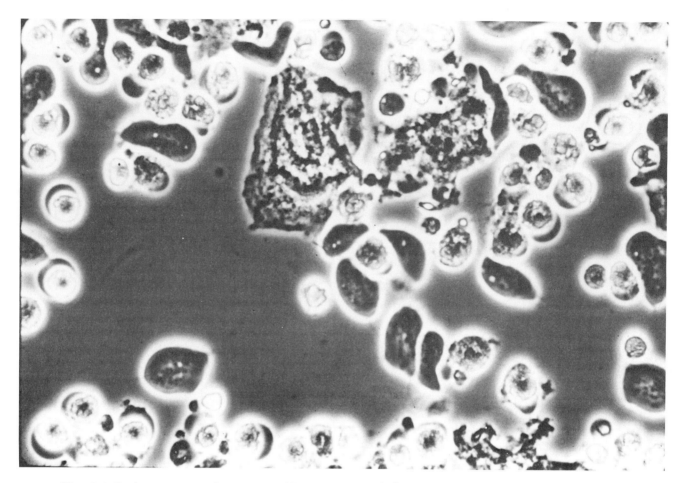

Fig. 13-6. *Trichomonas vaginalis* organisms. (Courtesy Dr. Fred Fleury, University of Illinois, Springfield, Ill.)

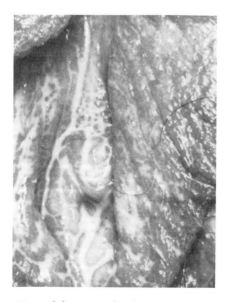

Fig. 13-7. *Hemophilus vaginalis* discharge. (From Gardner, H. L., and Kaufman, R. H.: Benign diseases of the vulva and vagina, St. Louis, 1969, The C. V. Mosby Co.)

Foreign bodies in the vagina result in a foul-smelling, blood-tinged, serosanguineous or purulent discharge, which may be either thick or thin. Upon speculum examination, the foreign body should be visible, frequently lodged in the posterior fornix. Foreign bodies commonly found include tampons, diaphragms, and condoms. If there is a secondary infection with inflammation and purulent discharge, it should be cultured.

No one specific discharge is characteristic of *allergic* vaginitis. There may be an increase in the usual type and amount of secretions as well as itching and burning. Rashes in the vulvar area are often present. There is little upper vaginal or cervical irritation. The diagnosis is often made by exclusion and confirmed by the alleviation of symptoms once the allergen is removed.

When discharge is present in *cervicitis*, it is usually yellow and mucopurulent caused by an infecting organism such as *E. coli.* Fleury (1978) estimates that over 50% of clients with purulent mucoid discharge have *Chlamydia* infections. There is often erosion of the

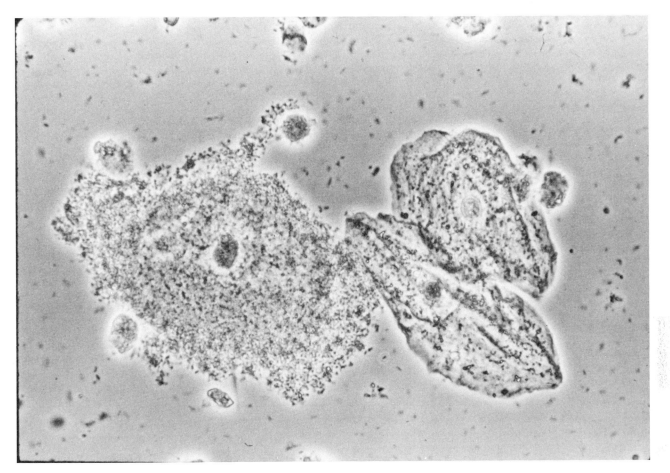

Fig. 13-8. *Hemophilus vaginalis* organisms. Clue cell is on left, normal cell on right. (Courtesy Dr. Fred Fleury, University of Illinois, Springfield, Ill.)

cervix, which appears as an area of granular, irritated, friable tissue with varying amounts of ulceration. There may be single or multiple retention or nabothian cysts. Diagnosis of the infecting organism is often by exclusion. Gonorrhea and herpes should always be ruled out.

Gonorrhea causes a yellow purulent discharge from the cervix. This disease and other sexually transmitted diseases will be discussed in the section on pain.

A characteristic symptom of *malignant neoplasms* of the lower genital tract is discharge. Any growth in this area may cause a continuous serous, mucoid, sanguineous, or purulent discharge. Bloody discharge should be a clue to the possibility of malignancy. If the neoplasm becomes infected or necrotic, the discharge will be purulent, malodorous, and offensive. Copious amounts of thin watery discharge, which collects in the vagina and drains from the cervix, may indicate fallopian tube carcinoma in the postmenopausal woman.

Age of the client can affect the type of vaginal discharge present. *Atrophic vaginitis* is characterized by watery discharge (although it may be mucopurulent), and by burning and itching of the vagina or vulva. This is a superficial, irritating, sometimes bacterial infection of the thin, poorly vasculated vaginal epithelium of the postmenopausal woman. Diagnosis is made by examination that reveals the typical estrogen-lacking epithelium and atrophy of vaginal structures. Vaginitis caused by lack of estrogen stimulation may also occur in children.

Parasites, particularly pinworms, can cause vaginitis in children. Diagnosis is usually made by microscopic examination of a piece of clear tape placed on the perineum of the child while asleep. The tape will show the typical ova of the pinworm, which are deposited outside the rectum at night.

Data gathered from the client's history, a description of symptoms, the practitioner's direct observations through examination, and the results of various laboratory tests are combined to make a nursing diagnosis. The key points of the common types of vaginal discharge are summarized in Table 13-1.

Treatment

The treatment for vaginal discharge or itching is often specific to the offending pathogen. The usual treatments for the common causes of vaginal discharge are as follows:

Candida albicans is treated with Monistat (miconazole) or Sporostacin (chlordantoin) cream applied twice daily for 14 days. Mycostatin (nystatin) vaginal suppositories, one or two daily for at least 2 weeks, are also used. Monistat has been found to be more effective than Mycostatin (Shuster and Giulian, 1976; Davis et al., 1974; Culbertson, 1974), although both are currently used. If there is extensive irritation, swelling, and discomfort of the labia and vulva, topical anti-inflammatory creams may help relieve the discomfort. Sitz baths may also decrease inflammation. The client must be made aware that completing the full course of treatment prescribed is essential to completely removing the pathogen. The client should be told to continue medication even during menstruation. If possible, intercourse should be avoided during treatment; if this is not feasible, the woman's partner should use a condom to prevent introduction of more organisms.

Trichomonas vaginalis has traditionally been treated with Flagyl (metronidazole), 250 mg t.i.d., for 10 days. A single dose of 2 Gm is currently being recommended. Although the male partner is usually asymptomatic, it is recommended that he receive treatment also since he often harbors the trichomonads in the urethra or prostate. When oral Flagyl is taken, the client must be advised not to drink alcoholic beverages, or she will experience side effects of nausea, vomiting, and headache. She may also notice a sharp, unpleasant metallic taste in her mouth. Gastrointestinal symptoms are common whether alcohol is consumed or not. Flagyl is contraindicated in pregnancy, because it crosses the placental barrier. It is also contraindicated in clients with blood dyscrasias or central nervous system disease because in rare cases Flagyl may affect the hematopoietic or central nervous system (Parsons and Sommers, 1978). Flagyl has become the object of concern since recent studies have indicated that it causes mutation in bacteria in controlled testings (Voogd et al., 1974). Drugs causing bacterial mutations are suspected of being carcinogenic (Martin, 1978). Voogd et al. have concluded that "metronidazole . . . should be used with caution, at least for the time necessary for a retrospective study of patients." (p. 490) At present it appears best to avoid the use of Flagyl unless other therapies are ineffective. Tricofuron (furazolidone and nifuroxime mixture) suppositories can be prescribed, 1 twice daily vaginally for one week and then one every day for 2 to 3 weeks. This medication also is effective against Candida and is safe during pregnancy. The woman should be instructed to continue therapy during menses and refrain from intercourse if possible.

Hemophilus vaginalis infection is treated by oral antibiotics for both partners. Traditionally, ampicillin, 500 mg q.i.d. for 5 days or Cephalosporin, 500 mg q.i.d. for 5 to 6 days have been used. Recently, Flagyl has proved superior to these; doses of 250 mg t.i.d. for 7 days have a 95% cure rate (Fleury, 1978). Only symptomatic clients should be treated. And Flagyl should be used only with resistant cases. Sulfa vaginal creams such as AVC are often used—one applicator-full a day for six to fourteen days. These provide symptomatic relief, though Fleury reports that their effectiveness has been seriously questioned recently (Fleury, 1978).

Removal of the allergen or irritant is the treatment for *allergic* or *irritative vaginitis*. The practitioner should explore any possible areas of irritation. Preventive health measures (p. 229) can be very effective with this type of vaginitis. When the client is experiencing considerable discomfort, local relief measures may help. Sitz baths several times a day can reduce inflammation. Hydrocortisone cream can be used to reduce the local inflammatory reaction. If vaginitis is caused by a foreign body, removal of it will alleviate symptoms in a few days. If infection is present specific antibiotic therapy should be started once the pathogen is identified.

Acute cervicitis usually can be treated with local antibiotics given orally or parenterally. Chronic cervicitis may require conization of the cervix (see Chapter 14). Cervical laceration or erosions are usually cauterized with silver nitrate sticks or electric cautery.

Recurrent vaginitis can be extremely discouraging and frustrating for both the client and the practitioner. It is important to identify the reason for the recurrence. Is it due to reinfection? poor compliance? incorrect treatment? If the client does not complete the entire course of treatment, the organisms have probably not been eradicated, and another complete course of treatment is needed. Sometimes medications are absorbed inadequately because heavy vaginal discharge has interfered or the woman has used tampons or douched shortly after inserting the medication. Douching should precede insertion of medication to clear away a heavy discharge. Tampons, which can absorb much of the medication, should not be used.

Possible pockets of organisms in sheltered sites should be explored. Skene's glands, Bartholin's glands, the urethra, bladder, or rectum can all act as sources of reinfection. The sexual partner should also be considered as a possible source of reinfection.

Recurrent *Candida* infection associated with oral contraceptive use is difficult to eradicate. It may be necessary to switch to another type of birth control to completely cure the infection. Women who have repeated

Candida infections should be checked for diabetes with a glucose tolerance test. Recurrent *Trichomonas* infection may be prevented by vinegar douches to maintain vaginal acidity (pH 4.5 to 5.0).

Vaginitis can recur when the client is under unusual stress. If other causative agents have been eliminated, the woman may come to see that emotional conflicts are being expressed in vaginal symptoms. She should also be helped to realize that this is not unusual. It has been estimated that 60% to 65% of all gynecologic problems have psychosomatic aspects (Beloff, 1974). If this diagnosis is established, treatment options include counseling, psychotherapy, and/or psychotropic medications.

At times the client or practitioner may wish to use alternative intervention to attempt to resolve vaginitis. Suggestions for these are summarized in Table 13-2.

Preventive measures

Preventive measures are important for all types of vaginal infection and particularly for women with recurrent vaginitis. Prevention begins with good personal hygiene. The perineal area needs to be washed frequently to remove perspiration and smegma accumulations. The client should be instructed to pat the area dry rather than rub it. Towels and washcloths should be clean and never shared. The proper technique of wiping after voiding and defecation should be taught. One should always wipe from front to back (never the reverse) to avoid introducing bacteria into the vagina or urethra. Sprays, soaps, powders, and deodorants that are perfumed or irritating in any way should not be used. Any chemicals that irritate the skin or vaginal mucosa or alter the vaginal environment should be avoided. Clothing that is too tight, does not allow free airflow to the perineum, or traps moisture should be avoided. Underpants and pantyhose should always have a cotton crotch. Douching should be avoided or kept to a minimum. Douching can strip the vagina of its normal flora, introduce bacteria, aggravate inflammation. Sexual partners should be clean. If there is doubt, condoms should always be used. If lubricant is needed during intercourse, a sterile, water-soluble type should be used. A final cautionary note might be: "Don't put anything in your vagina you wouldn't put in your mouth."

Vaginal discharge is a common problem for women of all ages. Although it is usually self-limiting and relatively minor, it is extremely uncomfortable both physically and emotionally. The nurse can do much to alleviate a client's discomfort by teaching preventive measures, instructing her in recognition of symptoms, and assisting her with self-care activities to prevent and treat vaginitis.

PAIN

The most common problem that women have is pain in the pelvic area. Twenty percent of gynecologic patients experience this type of pain as their primary concern (Guerriero, 1971). Parsons and Sommers (1978) state that "women tend to focus their attention on the uterus and adnexa and attribute the majority of their ills to this source—even though they are wrong fifty percent of the time." (p. 341) It is often difficult to determine the origin or cause of gynecologic pain; in fact, it is estimated that somewhere between 5% and 25% of all gynecologic clients experience functional pelvic pain without associated organic cause.

Table 13-2. Alternative therapy for vaginitis

Infection	Intervention	Dosage	Administration
Monilia	Gentian violet	Few drops/qt water 0.25% to 2% (over-the-counter drug)	Douche or local application
	Vinegar (white)	1 tbs/pint water	Douche every day for 5-7 days; twice daily for 2 days
	Acidophilus culture	2 tbs/pint water	Douche twice daily
	Acidophilus yogurt Plain yogurt	1 application hourly and as needed to labia for symptom relief	
Trichomonas	1 handful chapparel chamomile	Steep in 1 qt water for 20 minutes	Douche 2-3 times per week for 2 weeks
Nonspecific	1. Vinegar douche	5 tbs/2 qt water	Every other day for 1 week
	2. Salt (sea)	1 tbs/qt water	Every other day for 1 week
	3. 1 tsp. goldenseal 1 clove minced garlic	Steep in 1 qt boiling water	Douche every day for 7 days
	4. 1 tsp goldenseal	Steeped in 1 pt water; strain with cloth	Douche every day for 7 days
	5. Betadine gel		Twice daily for 7 days

Women have difficulty describing or localizing pelvic pain. A woman's description of the character of her pain can often be misleading because pain can originate from two primary sources: (1) cutaneous and muscle innervations involving so-called A nerve fibers, and (2) visceral innervations involving C fibers. The A fibers are responsible for acute pain, which is described as stinging, pinprick, or knife-like. Often this pain can be located with some accuracy by the client. Pain of this type may originate in the labia, vagina, and abdominal wall. C fibers are responsible for the burning and aching that are usually characteristic of chronic pain. These fibers are slow conductors of the pain impulse; often pain originating in these fibers is referred pain. Thus pain originating in the uterus, tubes, ovary, or bladder may be experienced directly but may also be referred to other sites. The site identified by the client may not be the source of the pain but its referred site. Pelvic pain is thus often confused or distorted by the client because of the way she experiences the pain. It is more difficult to describe the quality, site, or severity of pelvic pain than pain from other sources. The meaning the pain has for the individual also influences her ability to describe the pain.

Pain is a warning, a sign that there is something wrong. For many women pain associated with the reproductive organs may be particularly frightening because of its double significance. To have something wrong with her reproductive organs may be a direct threat to a woman's self-concept or body image. It may mean that she will be unable to fulfill reproductive or sexual functions. The early twinges of a spontaneous abortion may be perceived as excruciating pain because of its additional significance—the loss of a pregnancy. Pain can be a reminder of female bodily functions and therefore either welcomed or disliked. Dysmenorrhea may be more severe in the woman who dislikes her feminine role. Pain can also be an expression of emotional conflicts; it can be the expression of anger, fear, guilt, anxiety, or sexual distress. The woman who experiences vaginismus is often expressing emotional conflict through a physical response.

Cultural norms are important influences on an individual's reactions to and expectations of pain. Moral and religious meanings are also associated with pain. The traditional view that women must suffer in childbirth has both a religious foundation and a moralistic message that it is woman's lot to suffer. Anticipation of pain as unavoidable in a given situation, for example, childbirth, is a learned response. Acceptance of pain is characterized both by a willingness to experience pain and a belief that it is unavoidable; this usually reflects cultural beliefs. For example, labor pain is often expected as part of childbirth; in one cultural group it is not acceptable and various methods are used to alleviate it; in other cultures it is expected and accepted, and little or nothing is done to relieve it (Zabrowski, 1958). Ways of reacting to pain are prescribed by our culture. Positive and negative values are ascribed to particular pain experiences depending on whether the pain is viewed as having positive or negative effects on the welfare of the individual or group. Pain is culturally more acceptable in certain parts of the body and may elicit more sympathy than pain in other sites.

It is not possible to define pain. It is a subjective and personal experience and therefore not subject to a rigid definition. McGaffery (1972) states that "pain is whatever the experiencing person says it is and exists whenever he says it does" (p. 8). The nurse must listen to the client's assessment of pain and act on this rather than on her own estimation of what a client is or should be feeling. The pain experience includes all of a person's sensations, feelings, and behavioral responses and has three phases: anticipation, presence, and aftermath (Martin, 1978). Pain is both a sensory experience and the behavioral response to this stimulus. Pain behaviors are physiologic and psychosocial. Nursing interventions should be directed at both the sensory level and the pain behavior; nursing care is ineffectual otherwise. The woman as a whole experiences pain and the nurse must take this into account. In order to provide realistic care, the nurse must be aware of the common causes of gynecologic pain, the ways in which these are diagnosed, the treatments specific to alleviation of the cause, and appropriate nursing interventions.

Differential diagnosis

It is often very difficult to determine the source of gynecologic pain. At times the source is obvious, as in the client who presents with severe perineal pain associated with the ulcerations and excoriation of genital herpes; more frequently, however, the source is much less obvious. It is important to distinguish between pain from functional and benign causes and pain arising from pathologic processes. A thorough, meticulous assessment that includes a history, physical examination, and diagnostic tests is essential.

Pain resulting from pathologic processes is caused by (1) sudden distention, (2) vigorous contraction of hollow viscera, (3) rapid distortion of the capsule of a solid organ, (4) crushing or stretching of blood vessels, (5) chemical irritation of the peritoneum, (6) anoxia of functioning muscle tissue, and (7) nerve impingement by fibrosis or inflammation. It is thought that pathologic processes affecting the cervix and surrounding tissues, the lower uterine segment, the urethra, trigone of the bladder, and the rectum cause pain that is localized in the lower sacral area or buttocks and radiates down the

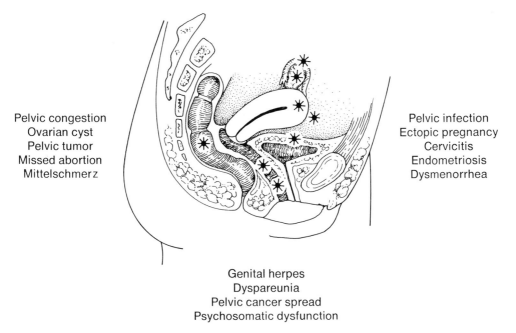

Pelvic congestion
Ovarian cyst
Pelvic tumor
Missed abortion
Mittelschmerz

Pelvic infection
Ectopic pregnancy
Cervicitis
Endometriosis
Dysmenorrhea

Genital herpes
Dyspareunia
Pelvic cancer spread
Psychosomatic dysfunction

Fig. 13-9. Causes of gynecologic pain.

leg. Painful stimuli from the uterine fundus and bladder are experienced in the lower abdomen from the umbilicus to groin (Parsons and Sommers, 1978) (Fig. 13-9). It should be noted that the client may also experience pain in these sites from other causes. This merely underscores the necessity for a meticulous assessment.

History

Frequently, it is difficult to collect an accurate history for pelvic pain because the woman is unable to describe her pain clearly. The traditional method of assessing (Martin, 1978; Romney, 1975; Parsons and Sommers, 1978) should be used with particular attention paid to those aspects that are unique to women.

Onset. The way the pain begins often suggests its cause. Pain that begins suddenly and reaches intensity rapidly suggests perforation, rupture, or ischemia (for example, rupture of an ectopic pregnancy or abruptio placentae). Pain that begins gradually and develops over several days or weeks, or pain for which an exact time of onset cannot be clearly determined, is more apt to be the result of obstruction, infection, inflammation, or congestion. Examples of this type of pain are cystitis, pelvic inflammatory disease, endometriosis, and dysmenorrhea.

Location. As indicated before, the site of the pain can indicate the location of the pathologic process. Unilateral lower quadrant pain may indicate an ectopic preg-

nancy, ovarian cyst, or mittelschmerz. Cystitis is experienced as a suprapubic pain. Pelvic congestion and uterine tumors may cause midabdominal or lower back discomfort. Infectious processes cause pain that is often bilateral and involves the entire abdomen.

Character. The client should be asked to describe the pain in her own words, as specifically as possible. Her choice of words will reflect her vocabulary and educational level, what she thinks is the cause of her pain, her level of medical knowledge and understanding, and her prior experience with pain. Some adjectives commonly used to describe gynecologic pain are:

1. Cramping—intermittent, short-term, poorly localized pain, indicating congestion, obstruction, irritation, or inflammation.
2. Sharp—intense, stabbing, wave-like pain that may be characterized by cycles of intense pain followed by pain-free or dull aching intervals. Location can often be pinpointed. Pain is often associated with neoplasms, thrombosis, and ureteral stones.
3. Burning—may be associated with a feeling of heat; often acute, and may be caused by mucosal irritation such as of the bladder or urethra. Pain may be present with many vaginal infections.
4. Aching—dull, continuous, steady pain that may be generalized and fluctuate in severity. Congestion, muscle spasm, and swelling may cause this type of pain.

5. Throbbing—a pulsing sensation, a regular waxing and waning of painful feeling. It is seen with infections, inflammation, and arterial spasms.
6. Fullness—a feeling of bloating or distention may be experienced with conditions such as pelvic congestion or premenstrual tension syndrome.

Intensity or severity of pain is not an accurate indicator of the seriousness of the condition, since people differ greatly in their perception and communication of pain. It is important to note how much interference with normal activities the pain causes. If the client can continue her usual daily routine, the pain is probably not too intense. Interference with sleep patterns can also give clues as to the severity of the pain. What pain relief measures are being used and how successful they are will also indicate severity of pain.

Associated factors. It is essential to explore with the client what precipitates pain, what makes it worse, and what relieves or diminishes it. These factors may assist in determining the cause. For example, pain that occurs following a meal is usually the result of a bowel condition; pain that occurs during or after urination results from urinary tract infection.

Attention should be paid to the client's gynecologic history, particularly her menstrual history. Acute abdominal pain following one or two missed periods suggests an ectopic pregnancy. Pain occurring about midcycle suggests mittelschmerz, and pain that occurs after the menstrual period may be related to salpingitis. Dysmenorrhea and pelvic congestion usually occur prior to the onset of the menstrual period. Menstruation may exacerbate chronic pelvic inflammatory disease. Pain associated with endometriosis often begins after ovulation.

Pain associated with intercourse should be explored. Pain that occurs with penetration may be related to infection or inflammation of the vulva or vagina. It may also be psychogenic, as in vaginismus. When deep penetration results in pain it is apt to be organic in nature. Endometriosis, tumors, and pelvic inflammatory disease (PID) can cause deep pelvic pain associated with intercourse.

The client's past medical and surgical history should be explored to ascertain whether prior illness or surgery could be responsible for current pain and to rule out any possible causes. For example, adhesions are common following abdominal surgery. A history of gonorrhea might suggest pelvic inflammatory disease. If a hysterectomy has been performed, obviously uterine pathology would not be a consideration.

Finally, the woman's current life-style and recent changes and stressors should be considered. Stressful situations can be translated into somatic complaints; for women this often appears to be associated with the reproductive organs. The nurse should assess the current stress level of the client in order to determine its relevance to the client's condition.

Physical examination

The physical examination provides additional data for determining the cause of gynecologic pain. Vital signs should always be taken: temperature elevations indicate infection or inflammation; rapid pulse and respiration are also associated with fever, although these may be present in extreme anxiety or with severe pain. An abdominal examination is always done. Auscultation should be performed to determine bowel sounds as well as any abnormal sounds. During this assessment any areas of tenderness, rigidity, or guarding are noted. The presence of any pelvic masses should be determined. A pelvic and rectal examination, as described in Chapter 7, is always performed. While inspection is always done to determine visible abnormalities, the bimanual examination is usually more helpful. Gentleness is essential. The nurse should use whatever techniques she can command to facilitate relaxation. Deep breathing often helps to prevent or decrease muscular tension, thereby decreasing discomfort. It should be remembered that the client is already in distress and the necessary examinations may exacerbate this. Careful identification of areas of tenderness, masses, thickening, and fullness is essential. Cervical tenderness upon movement associated with bilateral adnexal fullness or masses (Chandelier's sign) indicates pelvic inflammatory disease. Uterine tenderness is often associated with endometriosis. An ectopic pregnancy may be indicated by cervical congestion, minimal uterine enlargement, and a unilateral adnexal mass that is tender. Definite masses are described in terms of their size, shape, mobility, and tenderness.

Laboratory tests

Various laboratory tests may be performed to provide additional data. Complete blood counts are often ordered. An elevated white blood cell count may indicate infections such as pelvic inflammatory disease. The presence of anemia caused by blood loss, as documented by decreased hematocrit and hemoglobin, can suggest a ruptured ectopic pregnancy or abruptio placentae. An elevated erythrocyte sedimentation rate may suggest pelvic inflammatory disease. A clean catch urinalysis should always be obtained when there is any suggestion of urinary tract infection. The nurse may want to incorporate a clean catch urine collection as a part of the routine assessment of all clients who present with pain of a suspected gynecologic nature.

Common causes of gynecologic pain

Infectious processes account for much gynecologic pain. The most common are gonorrhea and resultant pelvic inflammatory disease, herpes genitalis, and urinary tract infections. Each of these is discussed below.

Gonorrhea

The most serious infectious disease in the United States is gonorrhea. Over 945,945 women were reported to have gonorrhea in 1974 (Center for Disease Control, 1975), and that figure probably represents a minority of the actual cases experienced by women. Often cases are not reported by the physician, or the disease may be asymptomatic and unrecognized. It is estimated that about 60% of women with gonorrhea are asymptomatic. While *Neisseria gonorrhoeae* infection is not usually life-threatening, it may result in upper genital tract infection, salpingo-oophoritis, tubal occlusion, and/or pelvic abscess formation with resultant infertility. Reported gonorrhea cases in females rose 8.8% from 1974 to 1975. Pelvic inflammatory disease (PID) occurs in 17% of all women known to have had gonorrhea and about 4.5% of women with PID are surgically sterilized as the only effective cure for their infection. About 5,750 girls miss school each day because of gonorrheal infection (Phipps, Long, and Woods, 1979).

Much attention has been given to reasons for the recent "gonorrhea epidemic." Although increased promiscuity (or sexual relations not restricted to one partner) has been suggested as a reason for the increase in gonorrhea cases, studies have shown that most clients diagnosed in clinics are not promiscuous. In one study 66.4% of the clients who had venereal disease had only one sexual contact (Darrow, 1975). Prostitution was implicated as a cause prior to World War II. Today, however, most persons who have gonorrhea are single and under age 25 while the majority of prostitution clients are married, older men (Phipps, Long, and Woods, 1979). The birth control pill has revolutionized contraceptive practices and has been blamed for the increased cases of gonorrhea on three counts: removal of the fear of pregnancy as a bar to sexual activity, decreased use of the condom, which acts as a mechanical barrier to the organisms, and alteration in the vaginal and cervical environment, which is believed to increase a woman's susceptibility significantly. Women with decreased levels of estrogen (for example, before menarche or after menopause) appear to be at greater risk for the development of gonorrheal vulvovaginitis. Fiumara (cited in Ledger, 1974) found an increased incidence of upper genital infections among women using oral contraceptives who had been exposed to the gonococcus. IUDs are associated with relatively high risks of PID, which is most frequently caused by gonorrhea; however, it cannot therefore be assumed that the IUD causes increased gonorrhea rates.

Prevention of gonorrhea and other venereal diseases is becoming increasingly important as the epidemic grows. Probably the only way to completely prevent the disease is to make sure that two virgins begin their sexual life together and lead a completely monogamous life thereafter. To eradicate gonorrhea completely we would need annual VD treatment days during which everyone received a penicillin shot (Martin, 1978). This is both impossible and ridiculous. Although efforts toward mass education and screening have not yet been effective, they need to be considered. Educational efforts should be directed toward enhancing public awareness of all sexually transmitted diseases, ways to control and treat them, and their serious consequences, as well as the broader issues of responsible sexuality and sexual behavior. (Screening measures are discussed in Chapter 7.) Methods of tracing sexual contacts need to be improved. Improved diagnostic methods and treatment measures are also needed but require additional research. The nurse's role is two-fold: she may focus on the individual woman and her need for information as well as on community education.

For most women, venereal disease is something to be afraid of, ashamed of, and hidden. Many have heard that venereal disease can cause blindness, insanity, sterility, and death. Venereal disease is equated with immorality, promiscuity, social stigma, and low social status. However, punitive, moralistic views are counterproductive for all involved. Such attitudes on the part of health care professionals do not deter clients from sexual behavior but do prevent them from seeking adequate diagnosis and treatment. Any individual who chooses multiple sexual partners or less traditional sexual behavior needs to understand that she increases her risk of contracting venereal disease. The risk factors increase with frequent changes in sexual partners and with casual sexual encounters. Regardless of these facts, anger is often felt when venereal disease is diagnosed; the woman is angry at the supposedly irresponsible sexual partner. Problems increase when a marital or committed relationship is involved. Sexual activity outside the relationship by one or both partners must be acknowledged. Anger, guilt, accusations, and recriminations are often experienced. The relationship may be threatened or in extreme cases dissolved. Physical abuse against the woman may occur. The way in which the relationship is defined will determine how a diagnosis of venereal disease will affect that relationship. The woman who holds to a traditional double standard sanctioning male extramarital sexual activity may have expected such acts and may accept them as a part of her life. The woman who expects fidelity may be crushed with evidence of her partner's infidelity. In the relationship that includes previously agreed-upon sexual freedom, venereal disease may be considered a potential but unfortunate risk. A further concern for women may be the implication of the disease for subsequent fertility.

Gonorrhea is caused by *Neisseria gonorrhoeae*, a gram negative bacteria that can invade any mucosal surface—most commonly the endocervix, urethra, Skene's glands, and Bartholin's glands in women. Rectal and nasopharyngeal gonorrhea is also seen. Direct physical contact, primarily sexual, is the method of disease spread. An endotoxin is produced three to twenty-one days after exposure, which results in redness and swelling. The disease process may be localized or spread by bloodstream invasion, direct tissue extension, or both. Most commonly, spread occurs through the endocervical canal to the endometrium to the fallopian tubes to the peritoneal cavity. Menstruation facilitates direct spread because the endocervical canal is dilated, the mucous plug gone, and necrotic tissue and serum from menstrual discharge are available for the organisms' nourishment. Infection of the endometrium is usually transient unless factors such as recent delivery, abortion, or surgical procedures have decreased resistance. The mucosa of the fallopian tubes, which are patent during menstruation, is invaded. Exudate is produced and often drains into the peritoneal cavity with resulting degrees of pelvic peritonitis. Progression of the disease causes thick, edematous, hyperemic tubes and resulting occlusion, inability to drain, and abscess formation.

Key factors in the progression of infection are organism virulence, innate or host tissue resistance, and availability and adequacy of treatment. Most women who have gonorrhea are asymptomatic or have minor symptoms that they overlook. Most gonorrhea is diagnosed by culture, history of contact, and/or presenting symptoms.

A diagnosis of gonorrhea is based on the client's history and substantiated by culture. Routine screening of asymptomatic clients is done when this is practical and economically feasible. Gonorrheal cultures should be obtained on every woman who is seen for contraception and prenatal care. The client's history is still the most accurate diagnostic tool initially. Areas of exploration should include the following:

Symptoms. Any symptoms the client mentions should be explored. She should be questioned about vaginal discharge, itching, burning, and pain. Although vaginal discharge is uncommon with gonorrhea, when it is present it is yellow and purulent. This is most commonly seen in women with poor estrogen support to vaginal mucosa. Pain upon urination, frequency, and involuntary loss of urine may be experienced within the first few days following contact. Pain may be experienced if the Skene's or Bartholin's glands become obstructed. If discharge from the cervix drains onto the vulva, edema, redness, excoriation, itching, burning, and pain may develop. Abdominal pain or cramping indicates upper reproductive tract involvement. The on-

set of pain during the first week of the menstrual cycle suggests gonorrheal salpingitis (Martin, 1978). Fever associated with abdominal pain and pelvic tenderness suggests pelvic inflammatory disease.

Menstrual history. Changes in menstruation can indicate gonorrheal infection. Usually there is increased flow and cramping. Irregularities may also be reported.

Sexual history. Any change in sexual partners increases the risk of exposure to venereal disease. Dyspareunia caused by deep pelvic thrusting can signal PID. It is important to explore the possibility of exposure with the client. If there is known exposure, it is mandatory that the nurse determine if the man was treated and at what point relative to exposure. The nurse should also ascertain whether the client has ever had gonorrhea and how it was treated.

Culture. Culture for gonorrhea is essential to confirm a diagnosis. When a single site is cultured it should be the endocervical canal since 85% of infected clients harbor organisms there (Martin, 1978). Both endocervical and anal cultures are recommended for diagnosis; and endocervical cultures are used for screening purposes (CDC, 1975; Bhattacharyra, 1974). Modified Thayer-Martin medium, which encourages the selective growth of gonococcus and inhibits growth of the usual vaginal and rectal contaminants, is used for culture. Menstruation is an excellent time for culturing because large numbers of organisms are shed at this time (Quirk and Huxall, 1975).

The treatment of choice in uncomplicated cases is aqueous procaine penicillin G, 4.8 million units in a single dose, injected half in each buttock. This dose is preceded by giving of 1 Gm probenecid orally 30 minutes prior to injection. Probenecid decreases the excretion time of penicillin in the urine, thereby elevating serum levels. Some strains of gonorrhea are resistant to penicillin, and large doses are needed for treatment. Spectinomycin, 4 Gm intramuscularly, has also been found effective. If the client is allergic to penicillin, tetracycline, 1 Gm initially followed by 0.5 Gm q.i.d. for 4 days, is recommended. Since some foods, especially dairy products, interfere with tetracycline absorption, oral forms should be given 1 hour before or 2 hours after meals. Pharyngeal gonorrheal infections are often more difficult to treat than anal or genital infections. If the standard penicillin regimen is not effective, tetracycline should be used. The client should return for follow-up cultures 7 to 14 days after treatment. She should know that cures following a single treatment are more difficult to obtain now than they once were, thus the need for follow-up.

Nursing responsibilities are multiple. Clients who have a sexually transmitted disease must be informed about their disease. When a woman seeks help for a problem, she wishes to get well. She is often highly motivated and receptive to information and advice. Once a diagnosis is made, the focus should be on treatment—effecting a cure and preventing complications and reinfection. Clients must be informed about drug action, effectiveness, side effects, chance of cure, and need for follow-up. The woman also needs information about self-care. In order to care for herself knowledgeably, she needs to know how the disease is transmitted and the possibility of reinfection and infection of her sexual partner or partners. She should be informed that her sexual partners need to be checked for signs of infection, to know what the symptoms are, and to obtain care if necessary. Clients should refrain from intercourse until cured or the partner should use a condom if abstinence is not possible. This may be an advantageous time to teach general hygiene and personal health practices to reduce the possibility of secondary infection, recurrence, or other genital infections. Specific instructions on care of any lesions on the body should be included. Often opportunities arise to provide information about diet, nutrition, exercise, contraception, and reproduction. Clarification of attitudes about sexual activity and sexuality may also be possible.

For the prevention and control of gonorrhea, contact investigation is essential. The client is asked about her sexual contacts, and those named are then examined and treated when necessary. Often the woman is reluctant to name her sexual contacts. She may fear that her or her partner's parents will find out. Reporting venereal disease may be seen as a threat and the woman may hesitate to get another person in trouble. She may fear recriminations or punishment from a spouse or other person named as a contact. The woman should be asked about contacts at the initial visit, preferably after she has been treated and her condition discussed with her. At this time concern with herself may be lessened and she may be more willing and able to identify her contacts.

Pelvic inflammatory disease (PID)

The most common complication of gonorrheal infection is pelvic inflammatory disease. It occurs in 10% to 17% of those women who have the disease and is directly or indirectly involved in almost 20% of all gynecologic problems (Martin, 1978). PID is an infectious process that may involve the fallopian tubes, ovaries, or pelvic peritoneum, veins, or pelvic connective tissue. Infection may be confined to one structure or involve the entire pelvis. Salpingitis refers to inflammation of the fallopian tube and is the most common site for PID. The infection can be either acute or subacute.

Pain is the universal symptom. It is usually present in both lower quadrants. The pain may be dull, cramp-ing, and intermittent; or it may be severe, persistent, and incapacitating. Adnexal tenderness is present upon examination and Chandelier's sign is present. In acute PID, a fever of 102° F with nausea and vomiting suggests abscess formation and peritoneal involvement. Pelvic examination reveals an adnexal mass and abdominal rigidity. Laboratory data showing an elevated white blood cell count and elevated sedimentation rate suggest acute infection. It should be pointed out that only 40% of clients with gonococcal PID are febrile; 60% have an elevated white count and 70% have an elevated sedimentation rate.* Relevant history includes use of an IUD, exposure to gonorrhea, recent abortion or dilatation and curettage, purulent vaginal discharge, irregular bleeding, and a longer, heavier menstrual period.

Subacute PID is far less dramatic; there is great variation in the severity and extent of symptoms. At times they are so mild that the woman ignores them. Symptoms that suggest subacute PID are chronic lower abdominal pain, dyspareunia, menstrual irregularity, urinary discomfort, low-grade fever, low back ache, and constipation. Diagnosis is made on the basis of a careful history and physical examination, including pelvic and laboratory data. Cervical and rectal cultures should be done to identify the causative organism and determine appropriate therapy.

The majority of clients with PID are hospitalized; occasionally, subacute PID is managed on an outpatient basis. If patient compliance or reliability concerning follow-up is questionable or if there is no response to treatment, hospitalization is mandatory. The most important treatment is intensive antibiotic therapy. Penicillin (or tetracycline in the penicillin-sensitive woman) is the drug of choice for gonorrheal PID. Intravenous fluids are important for hydration in the febrile client. Often the woman is given nothing by mouth, particularly if bowel sounds are absent. The client is placed on bed rest in a semi-Fowler's position to facilitate dependent drainage so that abscesses will not form high in the abdomen. Comfort measures include analgesics for pain, heat to the abdomen to improve circulation, and all other nursing measures applicable to a client confined to bed. Vital signs are taken every 4 hours until the client is afebrile; nursing observations include degree of pain and changes in the amount, color, odor, and consistency of vaginal discharge.

The most common reason today for major gynecologic surgery is acute and chronic salpingitis (Romney, 1975). Exacerbation and/or reinfection may require surgery to relieve chronic pelvic pain or menstrual abnormalities.

---

*Gonorrhea infection: discussing complications, Contemp. OB/GYN **5:**36-48, 1975.

Acute PID that does not respond to antibiotic therapy is a surgical emergency; often an emergency total abdominal hysterectomy and bilateral salpingo-oophorectomy are necessary to cure the disease.

Infertility secondary to PID is also possible. The incidence in the United States is unknown; however, Scandinavian studies reveal infertility rates of 15% to 40% following a single acute episode of PID. It is reasonable to assume that the incidence in the United States is equal or higher (Romney, 1975).

The residual effects of PID are difficult to predict; it is known that tubal scarring and adhesions can develop on an initial attack. There is no immunity against reinfection. Subsequent attacks increase the probability that tubal function will be impaired. There is some question as to whether PID is a chronic disease. It has been suggested that symptoms are caused by reinfection rather than exacerbation of an existing condition (Arnas et al., 1974). Adhesions and scarring in the lower abdominal cavity resulting from pelvic peritonitis are a potential cause of continued discomfort and lower abdominal pain.

The woman who suffers from PID may be acutely ill or experience long-term discomfort. Either or both take an emotional toll. Pain in itself is debilitating and this is compounded by the infectious process. The potential or actual loss of reproductive capabilities can be devastating to the woman's self-concept. Part of the nurse's role is to help the client adjust her self-concept to fit reality and accept these alterations in a way that promotes health.

Herpes genitalis

Herpes genitalis, caused by the herpes simplex type II virus (HSV-2), is an acute inflammatory disease of the genitalia. It is being seen with increased frequency. According to Gardner and associates (1974), "genital herpes is responsible for over ninety percent of all vesiculoulcerative disease of the female genitalia." The incidence of herpes genitalis in private clients exceeds the combined incidence of all other major venereal diseases. The infection, once contracted, is always present and may become active at any time. There is no satisfactory treatment, and there are no effective epidemiologic control methods.

Nearly all genital lesions are caused by HSV-2; only 5% are caused by HSV-1. HSV-2 is transmitted by sexual contact. The symptoms of HSV-2 infection in adult women vary; about 45% may be subclinical or asymptomatic. A primary infection usually appears within 3 to 7 days after exposure. This is usually more severe than recurrent infections and tends to be seen more often in teenagers and young adults. The characteristic lesions are vesicles; the basic pathology is localized tissue necrosis. Mild paresthesia and burning of the external genitalia may be experienced before the lesions become evident. Vesicles develop early and rupture quickly, resulting in shallow painful ulcers. Lesions often coalesce to form large ulcerations. The lesions are frequently extensive, involving the labia, perineum, vulva, vagina, and bladder.

The primary site of infection is thought to be the cervix. Most women experience extreme tenderness and severe pain. Primary infections are often accompanied by fever, headache, malaise, chills, anorexia, and generalized adenopathy from viremia (Edwards, 1978). Urination is extremely painful and urinary retention is not uncommon. Urethritis may occur with a watery purulent discharge. Secondary bacterial infection can develop as long as the lesions are open. Primary lesions last 3 to 6 weeks and then heal spontaneously unless secondary infection is present. Healing does not result in scarring unless bacterial infection occurs.

The disease can recur throughout the individual's lifetime. Recurrence can be spontaneous or be triggered by other infectious diseases, fever, menstruation, or emotional stress. It is thought that the virus is capable of lying dormant in sensory nerve ganglia, usually sacral. It is also thought that following primary infection, an equilibrium between host and virus develops. When this equilibrium is altered, the disease recurs. Although recurrent HSV-2 infection is not life-threatening it causes much anxiety and discomfort. The infections are disrupting and lead the woman to perceive herself as not well.

The frequency of HSV-2 infections in pregnant women is about three times that in nonpregnant women (Edwards, 1978). HSV-2 infections are apt to be more severe during pregnancy; the virus is active longer, cervical involvement is more severe, and recurrent infections are more difficult to diagnose. HSV-2 affects the fetus in three ways. First, there are increased abortion rates in infected mothers. There is a five-fold increase with a primary infection and a three-fold increase with recurrence. Second, premature births are increased in women with primary infections. And third, congenital malformations have been associated with the virus. Infants infected in utero have shown marked microencephaly, severe mental retardation, retinal dysplasia, patent ductus arteriosus, intracranial calcification, and vesicles filled with yellow purulent discharge (Nahmias, 1975). The majority of babies contract herpes during delivery through an infected birth canal. There is a 60% risk of neonatal herpes if the delivery is vaginal or occurs by cesarean section more than 4 hours after the membranes rupture. The disease may be either localized or disseminated. The disseminated disease, which occurs more often, is more serious, with a mortality rate of 82% (Edwards, 1978). Both disseminated and localized infections have central nervous system and ocular sequelae, and recurrences are common during the first 5 years of life. Because of the grave risks to the infant, current recommendations are cesarean section for the woman with lesions in the third trimester. If the membranes have been ruptured for more than 4 hours, the incidence of ascending infection increases markedly and a cesarean section is not done.

Although a direct causal relationship has not been established, a link is believed to exist between HSV-2 and cervical cancer. Women with HSV-2 have a greater incidence of cervical cancer and precancerous lesions than do women who have not been infected. Also, these women have a higher incidence of antibodies to HSV-2. HSV-2 has been detected in cervical tumor cells from carcinoma in situ. HSV causes chromosomal aberrations in tissue culture, a feature of neoplasms. HSV is the virus that most often affects the cervix and is known to have affected the area where malignancy appears later. There is the possibility that human cervical cancer may be a venereally transmitted disease and that HSV-2 plays a role in its etiology (Edwards, 1978). Other theories suggest that HSV-2 is carcinogenic, initiating a chain of events beginning in late adolescence and ending in middle age with invasive cervical cancer. The cells of the cervix are more vulnerable to carcinogens immediately before puberty and in early pregnancy because then they are undergoing transformation from columnar to squamous epithelium. The fact that incidence of HSV-2 infection is highest in adolescents and there is a higher incidence of cervical cancer in women who begin sexual activity in their early teens ends credence to this theory.

There is no known cure for herpes genitalis, nor is there any way to prevent primary infections or recurrences or to decrease the length of infection. Various therapies have been tried in adults, but all have proved ineffective and some are dangerous. One of the most recent therapies to be used is photodynamic inactivation of the virus with a tricyclic dye. However, this has been shown to be ineffective and potentially dangerous. It was at first thought that healing time of the lesions was shortened, length of time between recurrences increased, and the number of recurrences decreased. However, recent studies have demonstrated that healing time is unaffected in both primary and recurrent infections (Adams et al., 1976). It is recommended by some that this treatment no longer be used because of evidence that cells transformed as a result of photodynamic inactivation may have oncogenic properties (Nahmias, 1975).

Much of the treatment currently recommended is aimed at symptom relief. Topical steroid creams, antihistamines, alcohol, camphor, and dilute povidone-iodine (Betadine) solution have been used with varying results. Analgesics, sitz baths, boric acid solution, or Burow's solution compresses may afford some pain relief. Application of ethyl ether has been tried for immediate relief of discomfort and itching. The effectiveness and safety have yet to be proved; application of ether is initially very painful.

Nursing care should be supportive and directed toward assisting the client to find relief for the discomfort. Client education should include facts about recurrence, stressing the need for follow-up care. Pap smears should be done routinely because of the link with cervical carcinoma. Long-term follow-up of affected neonates is essential because of the possibility of long-term sequelae. The need for emotional support of the client is often great. The client's concern and distress are increased by the recurrent nature of the disease, the extreme discomfort, the lack of a cure, and the possibility of cancer.

Urinary tract infection

Most women experience dysuria, or painful urination, at some point in their life. About half of the time it is caused by urinary tract infection (UTI). These infections are the most frequent infectious problem of women and they are often seen in women of childbearing age. Several factors are involved in the high frequency of female urinary tract infections. Infectious organisms are introduced to the urinary tract through the urethra. Vaginal secretions, sexual intercourse, sexual stimulation, insertion of tampons, close fitting of clothing, and perineal pads all have potential for bringing pathologic organisms into contact with the meatus. Another source of contamination is the rectum; personal hygiene habits are closely associated with fecal soiling.

Some authorities believe that the relatively short female urethra may allow introduction of organisms to the bladder. Overdistention commonly occurs because of the infrequent voiding pattern of many adult women. Additionally, many women do not empty their bladder completely upon voiding, leaving a reservoir of urine. These two factors create an excellent culture medium for bacteria growth. Although many factors may predispose a woman to urinary tract infections, there are also a number of factors that contribute to a favorable prognosis for cure. Most clients are healthy with normal urinary tracts. The majority of infecting organisms are relatively sensitive to available antibiotics. In addition, most antibiotics are concentrated and excreted via the kidneys and urinary tract so that high levels of antibiotics are present at the infection site.

Few women can tolerate acute dysuria for any length of time. It is painful and can be frightening. A process that usually makes one more comfortable—that is, voiding—now causes burning, shooting pain. Frequency makes a woman void more often and urgency makes her feel she will lose control of urine at any minute. It is impossible to concentrate, focus on usual activities, or become comfortable. Relief is usually sought quickly. These symptoms, particularly if accompanied by hematuria, can be frightening. Most women are aware of the alarming consequences of kidney disease. Acute illness is frustrating, particularly if it occurs at times of stress. With recurrent infections, the client's self-concept may be lowered and feelings of helplessness may develop.

Some women develop dysuria following sexual intercourse. The syndrome known as trigonitis or "honeymoon cystitis" often occurs when the pattern of sexual activity alters from little or no activity to vigorous and frequent activity. Symptoms of dysuria, urgency, frequency, and bladder irritation not associated with infection are characteristic of this noninfectious inflammatory process. It is caused by trauma to the urethra during prolonged or very active intercourse. It is more common in nulliparas whose perineum is high with a tight introitus and undisturbed pelvic sling musculature. The penile shaft comes in close contact with the anterior vaginal wall; with frequent vigorous thrusts under the urethra and against the base of the bladder, trauma, capillary rupture, edema, and inflammation can occur.

Changes in sexual patterns or sexual partners can introduce new pathogens and thereby cause an infection. Women may associate urinary problems with their sexuality. For the woman susceptible to trigonitis, sexual intercourse becomes closely associated with dysuria. The resultant pain and discomfort are clearly apt to make her less eager for sexual activity. Sex causes pain rather than pleasure. Many women first experience urinary tract difficulties when they are pregnant. Postpartally many women have difficulty voiding, and urinary retention and infection are common problems. Inability to completely control urine flow may first occur following a traumatic delivery.

Urinary tract infections are diagnosed on the basis of the client's history, specific laboratory tests, and physical examination. When a woman says she is having dysuria, the nurse should gather the following data about her problem:

Symptoms. It is important that the client describe her symptoms. Dysuria, urgency, and frequency are common in infection and inflammation of the urinary tract. Fever and flank and back pain are associated with kidney involvement. A recent onset indicates an acute process while symptoms experienced over time imply chronicity.

The times when the pain occurs may be significant. Urethritis is characterized by pain at the onset of voiding; trigonitis is signaled by postvoiding pain. Constant dysuria and frequency accompany lower urinary tract infection and inflammation. Hematuria is significant and can indicate where the sources of inflammation or infection lie. Lower urinary tract infection is rarely accompanied by fever. A high fever (102° to 105° F), chills, nausea, vomiting, and flank pain are typical of pyelonephritis. Frequently, vaginitis can cause urethritis; increased vaginal discharge or itching can signal this. Flank or back pain is typical of renal disease, while mild lower abdominal pain may be present with cystitis. The amount voided can be significant; small frequent voidings indicate diminished bladder capacity. Dysuria with larger amounts voided indicates urethral or trigone involvement.

Associated factors. Any activities that might irritate the urethra should be identified. These include changes in sexual activity, long jolting auto rides, and riding narrow-seated bicycles. Some women experience a feeling of urinary irritation immediately prior to menstruation. Changes in soaps, creams applied to the vulva, or tampons can cause irritation.

History. Any previous urinary tract infections and the treatment should be noted. The presence of known renal disease should be documented. Recent childbirth or gynecologic procedures can cause inflammation, irritation, or the introduction of infecting organisms.

Physical examination. The client's temperature should be taken to determine the presence of fever. This can help determine whether there is upper or lower urinary tract involvement. Suprapubic tenderness is ascertained on abdominal examination and can indicate cystitis. Percussion of the costovertebral angle (CVA) is essential. Renal infection is signaled by sharp pain or exquisite tenderness upon light tapping of the CVA. Pelvic examination is done if it appears there may be a vaginal infection.

Urinalysis. A clean catch urine specimen is usually obtained for examination. Catheterization is to be avoided because of the potential for introducing infection into the bladder. Urine is examined for the following indications of infection:

1. Red blood cells—one or two cells visualized per microscopic examination is normal; a larger number indicates hematuria. Bleeding without other indications of kidney disease is usually from the lower urinary tract.
2. White blood cells—large numbers indicate infection; clumps of cells suggest urinary tract infection.
3. Bacteria—not a normal constituent of healthy urine.
4. Protein and glucose—urine should also be checked by dipstick for pH, protein and glucose; neither protein nor glucose is normally present in urine.

Culture. Whenever the client is symptomatic,

urine specimens should be cultured. In specimens obtained by the clean catch method, colony counts of greater than 100,000 bacteria per milligram of urine are considered diagnostic of infection. Following catheterization, colony counts of 10,000 or more indicate infection. Sensitivity studies should be done to determine which antibiotic will be effective against the infecting organism.

The most common urinary tract infections, their symptoms, and diagnostic points are summarized in Table 13-3.

Urinary tract infections in women with symptoms and positive urinalysis are treated with antibiotics. Often medication is begun before results of culture and sensitivity results are available. Most infections are caused by gram negative bacteria, and drugs that are effective against these organisms are generally used. Table 13-4 summarizes the most common drugs and appropriate dosages.

Initial infections are most often caused by *Escherichia coli*, and respond well to drugs effective against gram negative bacteria. Treatment should last 10 to 14 days;

Table 13-3. Common urinary tract infections

Disease	Symptoms	Physical examination	Laboratory data
Urethritis	Persistent dysuria; frequency and urgency; hematuria with initial voiding; no fever, malaise, nausea, or vomiting	No CVA tenderness or abdominal discomfort	Urinalysis of first voiding shows significant WBC and bacteria; midstream voiding is negative; culture is positive
Trigonitis	Persistent dysuria; frequency and urgency; often sexual intercourse 36 to 72 hours prior to onset of symptoms; no systemic symptoms or hematuria	No abdominal discomfort or CVA tenderness	Urine culture is negative
Cystitis	Acute: 24-hour dysuria; urgency and frequency; hematuria at end of voiding; no systemic symptoms	Suprapubic tenderness; no CVA tenderness	Midstream voiding has WBC and bacteria; culture is positive
	Chronic: mid (if any) bladder irritation	None	Urinalysis demonstrates WBC and bacteria; culture is positive
Pyelonephritis	Acute: fever, malaise, nausea and vomiting, back or flank pain; dysuria, urgency, frequency, and hematoma may or may not be present	Severe CVA tenderness; usually unilateral	Midstream voiding shows high concentrations of WBC, bacteria; pyuria may or may not be present; urine culture is positive
	Chronic: no dysuria or bladder irritation; no systemic symptoms	CVA tenderness may or may not be present	Proteinuria and WBC are often found; urine culture may or may not be positive

Table 13-4. Medications commonly used for urinary tract infections

Medication	Dosage	Precautions	Comments
Gantrisin	1 to 2 Gm every 4-6 hrs for 10-14 days	Avoid if allergic to sulfa	Safe, economical
Azo-Gantrisin (gantrisin and pyridium)	1-2 Gm every 4-6 hrs		Gives urine an orange red color
Ampicillin	250 to 500 mg every 6 hrs for 10-14 days	Avoid if allergic to penicillin	Used when client is allergic to sulfa
Tetracycline	250 to 500 mg q.i.d. for 10-14 days	Do not take with food, dairy products	Used when client is allergic to sulfa or penicillin
Furadantin or macrodantin	100 to 150 mg q.i.d. for 10-14 days		Urinary antiseptic
Mandelamine	1 Gm q.i.d.	To be used with an acidifying agent. Should not be given with a sulfonamide as insoluble precipitate forms in urine	Used for prophylaxis in recurrent infections
Pyridium	600 mg every 24 hrs in divided dosages	Turns urine orange red	Urinary tract analgesic

the client's urine should be rechecked in 2 to 3 days, at which time it should be sterile. A repeat urinalysis culture should be done in 14 days after treatment is completed. Three additional follow-up cultures at 3-month intervals, and two more at 6-month intervals are suggested. The client should be cautioned to take the full course of medication prescribed even though her symptoms disappear in 48 to 72 hours. She should drink large amounts of fluids and void often. If the medication should not be taken with food, dairy products, or antacids, the client should be informed of this.

Prevention. Preventive measures are extremely important for women who experience recurrent urinary tract infections. Proper technique in wiping after voiding or defecation is essential to prevent bacterial contamination of the urethra from the rectum. Women should always wipe from front to back. Good personal hygiene will also discourage bacterial growth. The woman who has experienced repeated urinary tract infections should be encouraged to shower rather than take tub baths. Good bladder habits can be taught. Many women tend to void infrequently; they should be encouraged to empty their bladder regularly so that urine does not stagnate. Increased fluid intake will flush the urine out of the bladder frequently. Emptying the bladder before and after sexual intercourse will help to wash bacteria away from the urinary meatus. Cleansing of the perineal area prior to intercourse will also reduce the number of bacteria available to be introduced into the urinary tract.

Dysmenorrhea

One of the most common gynecologic problems of women of all ages is dysmenorrhea, or painful menstruation. Eighty percent of women have some discomfort associated with menses, while about 10% are incapacitated to such an extent that they miss work or school (Romney, 1975). Green (1977) states that 35% of all older adolescent girls, 25% of female college students, and 60% to 70% of single women in their thirties and forties experience discomfort severe enough to interfere with normal activities for 1 to 2 days. Dysmenorrhea, occurring 1 day prior to or at the onset of menstruation, is characterized by pelvic pain that disappears or markedly improves by the end of menses. It can be either primary or secondary. Primary dysmenorrhea occurs in the absence of organic disease while secondary dysmenorrhea is associated with organic pelvic disease.

Almost all women have some indication or awareness that their period is about to start; this is not necessarily perceived as pain. There is some discomfort normally associated with ovulatory menstruation, often called the premenstrual syndrome; however, this is not dysmenor-rhea. Dysmenorrhea may be associated with these prodromal symptoms or it may occur with few or no symptoms. Characteristically, the pain of dysmenorrhea begins with the onset of menstruation, although some women will experience mild cramping or lower abdominal aching 24 to 48 hours prior to bleeding. Dysmenorrheal pain is usually colicky and cyclic, although it may also be a nagging, dull ache. It is usually localized in the lower midline or radiating down the back of the legs.

Primary dysmenorrhea usually develops 1 to 2 years after menarche when ovulatory function is established. For the most part, anovulatory bleeding, common in the first few months or years after menarche, is painless. The pattern is for the first cycles to be painless, followed by cramping, which begins when the ovary is fully developed, maturation of the ova occurs, and progestin is secreted. Primary dysmenorrhea appears to be self-limiting for it is primarily a problem of teenagers and young adults and often disappears or is markedly improved by age 25 or following pregnancy. The pain is either a sharp cramp-like pain, similar to colic or abortion, or a steady dull ache accompanied by bearing down sensations with referred pain to the legs and suprapubic area. Approximately 60% will experience cramps, while the rest experience pelvic ache and discomfort (Parsons and Sommers, 1978). Many women also experience abdominal distention, breast tenderness, nausea and vomiting, dizziness, headache, palpitations, and flushing.

Many theories have been advanced to explain the cause of dysmenorrhea. Endocrine imbalances were long believed to cause dysmenorrhea. It was postulated that the normal estrogen/progesterone ratio was disturbed during the luteal phase of menstruation. This idea was based on the fact that the normal stimulant of uterine contractions is estrogen, the normal inhibitor is progesterone, and the characteristic cramps are related to exaggerated uterine contractility. However, studies have not demonstrated imbalances, and the menses appears to be normal with ovulation and a normal hormonal milieu. Furthermore, anovulatory cycles are characteristically painless.

Various anatomic and obstructive factors were also once thought to be the cause of primary dysmenorrhea. Uterine hypoplasia was thought to be a factor, the rationale being that a uterus that was too small or poorly developed would not be able to cope with the secretory products of menstruation. There is no evidence to support this theory. Cervical stenosis or any condition, such as polyps, that would occlude the cervical canal could cause dysmenorrhea, probably through contraction of uterine musculature as it attempts to propel menstrual products through the cervical canal. However, the incidence of this is low and related to secondary, not primary, dysmenorrhea. Conditions that cause general debilitation, such as anemia, severe fatigue, diabetes, or other chronic illness, are associated with a higher incidence of dysmenorrhea; however, they probably act as exacerbating factors rather than causative agents.

Primary dysmenorrhea is commonly considered to be caused either partly or wholly by psychogenic factors. Many current medical textbooks emphasize the supposed psychologic basis of primary dysmenorrhea (see Green, 1976; Parsons and Sommers, 1978; Lennane and Lennane, 1973). Some of the postulated causes are: taboos and superstitions about the genitalia; fear of an adult sexual life; ambivalence and severe conflict about developing a sexual identity; self-punishment for masturbation; and attention-seeking. According to Romney and associates, there may be a strong psychologic factor in dysmenorrhea, particularly when it does not fit the typical pattern of occurring 2 years after menarche and lasting for the first day of flow. It is suggested that (1) pain is used to view menstruation as an illness and to deny its sexual and reproductive significance; (2) it is used as an isolation technique to avoid exhibiting increased sexual and aggressive feelings; (3) the pain has secondary gain in that the woman is taken care of; and (4) pain can be used to deny feelings.

While it may be that there are individual women whose dysmenorrhea is founded in emotional conflicts, there is no reason to ascribe these causes to all women. While some women may have manipulative motivations associated with their expression of menstrual pain, this should not be generalized to other women without a carefully documented history. The implication is that a client's faulty outlook causes the condition, not that a client's personality may affect the amount of suffering or complaining associated with an organic illness. If the pain were a result of emotional factors alone, one would expect it to start at the time of the initial psychologic shock—at menarche—not 2 years later. The pain is dependent upon the occurrence of ovulation and is frequently alleviated by ovulation suppression; this does not support a psychogenic etiology.

Present evidence suggests a relationship between prostaglandins and dysmenorrhea. Prostaglandin E_2 produces myometrial relaxation, while prostaglandin $F_{2\alpha}$ stimulates an increase in the amplitude and frequency of uterine contractions. Prostaglandin $F_{2\alpha}$ is the predominant prostaglandin found in the endometrium during the luteal phase and menses (Abraham, 1975). Excessive activity of the myometrium may occur in dysmenorrhea in response to prostaglandin $F_{2\alpha}$. Increased synthesis of prostaglandin $F_{2\alpha}$ is thought to occur during the luteal phase of painful menstrual cycles. The subsequent excessive release of prostaglandin during menstrual shedding of the decidua causes an increase in uterine smooth muscle contractibility. In addition, there is increased absorption of prostaglandin F_2 from the endometrium caused by poorly coordinated fundal contractions. There may also be increased sensitivity of the endometrium and myometrium to $F_{2\alpha}$ and decreased sensitivity to E_2. Severe contractions with resulting ischemia cause the cramp-like pain of dysmenorrhea. The systemic symptoms of dysmenorrhea, such as nausea and vomiting, diarrhea, and syncope, may result from systemic absorption of prostaglandin into the bloodstream (Meckler and Jordan, 1980; Halbert, 1976; Ylibarkala and Dawood, 1978).

Secondary dysmenorrhea is defined as painful menstruation that develops after a pattern of relatively comfortable periods has been established. It is associated with organic pelvic pathology. Most of the pain is produced by pelvic vascular congestion associated with pelvic lesions. The pathologic conditions most commonly causing secondary dysmenorrhea are pelvic inflammation, anatomic disruptions such as cervical stenosis or malpositioned uterus, and endometriosis. Careful history and diagnosis are essential to distinguish between primary and secondary dysmenorrhea and to identify the organic pathology operant in secondary dysmenorrhea. Only then can appropriate treatment be started.

History

A thorough menstrual history is essential to obtain an accurate diagnosis. Areas to explore include the following:

Menarche. The practitioner must know when the client's periods began since this is a critical factor in the diagnosis of primary dysmenorrhea. The nurse should explore with the client the type of preparation or education the woman received prior to onset. Determining both the client's and her parents' attitudes toward menstruation will help identify any emotional component.

Characteristics. Frequency and duration of menstruation are important to note in order to determine where the client falls within the range of normal. (See Table 13-5 for a summary of average composition of the menstrual cycle.) Changes in the character and amount of flow should be explored with the client. Any clotting should be noted. The time when cramps begin, their duration, and severity should be determined. The natural history of menstrual cramping will help to ascertain whether pathology is involved. The relationship between pain and bleeding is significant.

Reproductive factors. It is important to note what contraceptive is being used, since this may affect cramping. For example, the IUD is often associated with more severe cramps while oral contraceptives suppress ovulation and thereby alleviate dysmenorrhea associated with ovulation. The client's reproductive history is also sig-

Table 13-5. Characteristics of the menstrual cycle

Menarche	Occurs between 11 and 16 years of age; extremes are 9 to 18 years; average age is 12.
Duration	Average is 2 to 5 days; remains relatively constant for a given woman; wide variation between women.
Interval	Usually about 29.5 days; range is 18 to 40 days; considered normal as long as variation of interval does not exceed 5 days; variation from cycle to cycle in one woman or between woman may be considerable.
Amount	Average blood loss is 30 to 100 ml; some women lose up to 200 to 300 ml without anemia.
Character	Mixture of endometrium, blood, mucus, and vaginal cells; dark red; usually does not clot; less viscous than blood.

nificant; traumatic labor and delivery, cervical lacerations, infections, and gynecologic procedures can all predispose to secondary dysmenorrhea. Often primary dysmenorrhea is alleviated following pregnancy.

Emotional factors. It is important to assess the individual woman's response to dysmenorrhea. Exploration of attitudes to menstruation, including her family's attitude, may assist the practitioner to determine whether a psychologic overlay exists. The client's pain threshold and response to pain should also be ascertained.

Experience. It is important to determine the extent to which dysmenorrhea causes disruption of the client's life. Can she continue with her usual daily activities or must she be in bed? How long the pain lasts and what seems to relieve it (and for how long) should be determined. The nurse should inquire as to what other symptoms the woman experiences.

Treatment

The treatment of dysmenorrhea is multifaceted and depends upon the severity of the disability and the individual client's response; with secondary dysmenorrhea it must be directed at the cause. Many women are able to cope with mild menstrual cramps by using mild analgesics. Aspirin, which in sufficient doses is a prostaglandin antagonist, and heat are often all that is needed. For those clients experiencing severe pain and systemic symptoms, prostaglandin inhibitors may be effective in controlling the symptoms. Halbert (1976) recommends the use of Indocin (indomethacin), 25 to 50 mg initially with additional doses as needed. Indocin inhibits prostaglandin synthesis but does not affect prostaglandins already present. Halbert (1976) indicates that Indocin would be more effective if started on day 21 or 22 of the cycle. Currently, it has not been approved for use for dysmenorrhea and is contraindicated in individuals under 14 years of age. The effects of this drug, such as

nausea, dizziness, and pounding headache, are so annoying that client compliance is low. Schwartz (1974) found that flufenamic acid, another prostaglandin inhibitor, in doses of 125 mg q.i.d. provides relief from dysmenorrhea with a much lower incidence of side effects. This compound appears to not only neutralize preformed prostaglandins but also to inhibit prostaglandin synthesis; therefore, treatment is necessary only during menses.

Hormonal therapy has also been used with some success in the treatment of dysmenorrhea. Duphaston (dydrogesterone), a synthetic pure progesterone, has been used to control cramps without suppressing ovulation. This medication, taken in daily doses of 10 to 20 mg from day 5 to day 25 of the menstrual cycle, has successfully relieved dysmenorrhea (Aydar, 1965). However, the drug is expensive and is associated with breakthrough bleeding. Oral contraceptives have been used to suppress ovulation and therefore relieve or prevent dysmenorrhea. When ovulation is suppressed, the effect of estrogens on the endometrium is inhibited before much endometrial growth has occurred. The reservoir of prostaglandins is insufficient to cause the severe uterine contractions of dysmenorrhea (Carey, 1975). Oral contraceptives should only be used with clients who are sexually active. For treatment of dysmenorrhea they are contraindicated in young adolescents or in women with documented history of irregular menses.

Nonpharmacologic therapies are often effective in minimizing menstrual distress. While these are all valid alternatives to chemotherapy, the individual client will need to find out which ones work best for her. A woman has specific dietary needs during menstruation and many of the symptoms of menstrual distress may be caused by altered metabolic activity and resulting deficiencies. Therefore, it might be possible to alleviate discomfort by a diet that replaces deficits. Maintenance of good nutrition at all times constitutes primary prevention of menstrual distress. By decreasing sodium intake the week prior to menses, mild sodium retention can be reduced. Foods that are natural diuretics, such as asparagus and coffee, can also decrease fluid retention. Vitamin B has been suggested for relief of those symptoms associated with high estrogen levels premenstrually. The B vitamins improve hepatic inactivation of excess estrogen and also increase protein utilization. Fatigue, tension, and depression are symptoms of both vitamin B deficiencies and premenstrual tension syndrome. Diets high in vitamin B may help relieve these symptoms. Carbohydrate metabolism may be altered premenstrually with resulting increased sugar tolerance and hypoglycemia. A high protein diet with frequent feedings should help relieve hypoglycemia symptoms (Lovesky, 1978).

Regular exercise will help prevent menstrual discomfort; and specific exercises done daily can prevent or relieve pain. Muscle toning and breathing exercises are helpful in dysmenorrhea. This is explained by the theory that hypoxia of muscle tension and muscle tension itself exacerbate painful sensations. Maddox (1975) recommends swimming as the exercise most beneficial in building muscle tone and preventing menstrual problems. Specific exercises to relieve discomfort are the "pelvic rock" and "dry-land swimming."

Mild heat has distinct pain-relieving properties since heat decreases hypertonus of muscles. Additionally, vasodilation increases blood flow to the affected area, relieving ischemia. Heat also increases elimination of menstrual fluid. Many women find a heating pad, tub bath, or shower to be very effective.

The need for sleep is increased during menstruation and increased sleep time can be therapeutic in relieving tension. Massage has also been found to be a successful pain relief measure. The pain threshold increases when a second stimulus (such as massage) is applied at an intensity below the discomfort level. Effleurage, or a soft rhythmic rubbing of the abdomen in a circular manner, is often effective. This provides a distraction and alternate focal point. For some women, strong manual pressure on the abdomen is more successful. In many of these pain relief measures, the important factor is that the woman can decide for herself what works best and can thereby decrease her dependency.

Orgasm has been reported to relieve cramps in some women (Annon, 1974). It appears that the physiologic contractions of orgasm during the sexual response cycle facilitate menstrual flow and relieve pelvic congestion. Orgasm is effective if cramping is relieved by the heavier flow of the menses. In addition, orgasm can serve as a tension release as well as a pleasurable sexual release.

Cox (1978) has reported successful reduction of painful cramping of primary dysmenorrhea following systematic desensitization. Medication usage, invalid hours, negative attitudes, and symptom complaints were all decreased. Heczey (1978) successfully reduced dysmenorrhea and other menstrual discomfort through the use of individual and group autogenic relaxation training. Various other techniques such as Hatha Yoga, progressive relaxation and meditation may also offer pain relief for some women. Fleischauer (1973) has successfully used modified Lamaze breathing and exercise to assist clients to deal with menstrual cramps.

As stated by Lovesky (1978), "A long history of negative social attitudes toward menstruation has resulted in internalized negative feelings toward menstruation, the female body and female sexuality." (p. 43) These feelings influence the amount, quality, and intensity of perceived menstrual distress (see Chapter 6). An integral component in the alleviation of menstrual distress is education to facilitate positive attitudes. The nursing practitioner can do much to correct misinformation, provide facts about what is normal, and support the client's feelings of positive sexuality and self-worth. The nurse can be an important factor in helping a woman change her self-image and self-concept.

In addition to educational and supportive interventions, the nurse can offer several alternatives for alleviating menstrual discomfort. The client can thus explore alternatives and decide which ones work best for her. The best alternatives will be those that provide the client a sense of autonomy so that she achieves independence, ego strength, and increased self-respect. The most successful treatments for relief of dysmenorrhea are those that work on several levels—physiologic, psychologic, and sociologic.

Premenstrual syndrome

The menstruating woman experiences a monthly, hormonally determined, physiologic cycle. Often she experiences somatic symptoms and mood fluctuations associated with this cycle. Almost all women have some awareness of when their period is to start. For some women this is merely an awareness of normal alteration in her physical and emotional state, which causes little or no discomfort. For other women, the changes are more uncomfortable and cause more disruption. The incidence of premenstrual syndrome is estimated to vary from 5% to 95% of all women and includes a wide variety of symptoms. It is more common in women in their late twenties and older and often increases in severity as the woman nears menopause. The syndrome may vary from mild abdominal or pelvic fullness, slight breast tenderness, and mild irritability to severe, incapacitating symptoms such as nervousness, fatigue and exhaustion, crying spells, depression, decreased concentration, hypoglycemia and cravings for sweets, weakness and fainting, trembling, low abdominal pain and/or bloating, headache, generalized aching, nausea and vomiting, diarrhea, constipation, and severe breast tenderness. These symptoms are usually most severe just prior to onset of menstruation and begin to subside as flow begins. Some women report positive sensations such as feelings of increased creativity, ability to concentrate, and increased mental and physical activity.

Epidemiologic studies have correlated a wide variety of symptoms and behaviors with the premenstrual phase of the menstrual cycle. Crimes of violence, increased suicide attempts, schizophrenic episodes, admissions to psychiatric wards, and increased accident rates have all been attributed to the premenstrual phase of the menstrual cycle (Benedick, 1959; Bardwick, 1971; Dalton, 1964). Often these findings have been generalized to create a picture of women who are irrational, impulsive, intellectually impaired, and a pawn of their "raging hormones." Many of these studies have grave methodologic problems and are not scientifically accurate. Psychologic studies of the premenstrual syndrome have not established a class of behaviors and moods that fluctuate throughout the menstrual cycle or that are characteristic for any one phase of the cycle (Parlee, 1973). Studies of cyclic behavior in adult menstruating women need to be evaluated through comparison studies of possible cyclic changes in behavior in nonmenstruating persons. Conclusions regarding the physiologic basis of disruptive effects of premenstrual syndrome may be biased because of the source of the data—self-report questionnaires (Ruble, 1977). Cultural affective influences must be separated from physiologic influences. Dan (1976), in a study that compared behavior of husbands and wives, found that the menstrual cycle could not be said to add variability to women's behavior in comparison with men. Golub (1976) found that premenstrually anxiety and depression scores were significantly higher than at midcycle but were much lower than those of patients with psychiatric disorders. She concluded that the magnitude of premenstrual mood changes was small, with little effect on personality and no effect on cognitive function.

Although its exact effect on behavior is not known, a loosely defined complex of symptoms associated with the premenstrual phase of the menstrual cycle, known as the premenstrual syndrome, does appear to exist. No specific cause is known at present. Various hormonal explanations have been sought; however, there is no general agreement about which hormonal change, if any, causes premenstrual syndrome. It is known that phasic changes in gonadotropins, prolactin, progesterone, estrogen, androgens, and mineralocorticoid secretions occur; however, the effect these may have on the development of premenstrual syndrome is unclear. Estrogen-progesterone imbalances, vitamin B_6 deficiencies, activation of renin-angiotensin-aldosterone system, and changes in monoamine oxidase (MAO) activity have all been explored without success (Steiner and Carroll, 1977).

The lack of clarity regarding etiology is reflected in the long list of treatments recommended and used with varying success. Because weight gain and generalized edema are often associated with the premenstrual syndrome, it has been considered that measures that would counteract these symptoms would relieve distress. Estrogen, which is sodium sparing, was thought to be the cause of the many symptoms associated with sodium and fluid retention. Progesterone, which is thought to counter this effect of estrogen, was given to relieve symptoms. At times this worked, but at other times it appeared to have no effect or even to aggravate symp-

toms. Diuretics are often given to relieve generalized edema; they may provide good relief in some women. Tranquilizers have been prescribed to alleviate depression, nervousness, and irritability; likewise, psychotherapy has been recommended by those practitioners believing the syndrome to be primarily psychogenic in origin. Oral contraceptives, aldosterone antagonists, lithium, vitamins, physical therapy, and a high protein diet have all been suggested. At present no single treatment is universally accepted as effective. Treatment is mainly aimed at relief of the most uncomfortable symptoms. The client can probably assist the practitioner best in determining the therapeutic regimen. Again, educational and supportive measures to facilitate self-care and control seem to be helpful.

Mittelschmerz (intermenstrual pain)

Many women experience cyclic lower abdominal pain associated with ovulation. The source of discomfort is thought to be increased intrafollicular pressure prior to rupture or leakage of small amounts of follicular fluid or blood into the peritoneal cavity causing localized pelvic peritonitis. Usually the pain occurs suddenly, lasts a few hours or a day, is sharp initially, and then changes to a dull constant ache associated with fullness or pressure. Some women notice an associated pinkish discharge occurring at the same time. The discomfort is rarely incapacitating and resolves spontaneously.

Endometriosis

Endometriosis is a disease in which endometrial tissue, which responds to hormonal stimulation, is found outside the uterine cavity. It can cause severe discomfort and may be extremely debilitating. Although the exact incidence is difficult to determine because it can exist without causing symptoms, it is estimated that about 25% of women have endometriosis (Berger et al., 1978). At one time it was thought that endometriosis was more prevalent among white middle and upper class women; however, more recently racial differences have been found not to exist. It was once believed that the problems attributed to lower socioeconomic groups, such as pregnancy and tubal blockage caused by gonorrhea and other venereal diseases, prevented the disease. It is more likely, however, that the symptoms once attributed to pelvic inflammatory disease were actually symptoms of unrecognized endometriosis. Active endometriosis is most common in women between the ages of 30 and 40. It does not occur prior to menarche since it depends on hormonal stimulation for propagation. It is rarely found in clients under the age of 20 or in postmenopausal women. There appears to be an inherited tendency to develop endometriosis although the exact mechanism is not known (Romney et al., 1975).

An endometrial lesion with a good blood supply responds to estrogen and progesterone in the same way that uterine endometrium does. The monthly menstrual discharge is absorbed by the surrounding tissues, causing inflammation and constricting scar tissue. The scar tends to restrict subsequent blood supply, thus modifying subsequent hormonal stimulation and response. During menstruation, however, pressure from within may cause the lesion to burst at its weakest point, spilling pieces of endometrium and blood into the abdominal cavity onto new peritoneal surfaces, or extravasating into adjacent tissues. Pain results from inflammation, irritation, encroachment, and obstruction.

Two basic etiologic theories are widely held today: (1) retrograde transportation of the endometrium and (2) transformation of tissue. Transportation is thought to occur by spontaneous implantation of endometrium that is moved through the fallopian tubes via menstrual reflux into the peritoneal cavity where it implants. It has been suggested that some women develop endometriosis from retrograde menstruation because of a lack of immunologic resistance or because of prostaglandin involvement. In direct extension the endometrium invades the uterine muscle causing endometriosis or adenomyosis. Metastasis of endometrium may occur through the lymphatic or venous system resulting in endometriosis of the lungs, eyes, or brain. Endometriosis may also occur through inadvertent implantation of endometrium during a surgical procedure.

The transformation theory is based on the mutation capabilities of tissue. It is believed that any tissue that arises out of colonic fetal tissue can later differentiate into endometrium-like tissue. Transformation would

have to be stimulated by factors such as inflammation, infection, or endocrine imbalance. Familial tendencies may be operant here.

Nutrition has also been associated with the development of endometriosis (Berger, 1978). Intercourse during menstruation and use of tampons have also been suggested as causative factors. It had been thought that these might increase the incidence of reflux; however, that is unlikely.

Symptoms are often related to the location of endometrial lesions (Fig. 13-10). The classic symptoms are dysmenorrhea, deep dyspareunia, and sacral backache. Chronic pelvic pain is often present. Generally, symptomatology falls into three categories: (1) pain, such as dyspareunia, dysmenorrhea, or pain associated with bowel movements; (2) infertility; and (3) menstrual abnormalities. The pain is usually dull, aching, or cramping in the lower abdomen or back, most often associated with menstruation and decreasing as flow begins. However, pain is not always associated with menses; it may begin following ovulation and continue as a vaginal aching, cramping, or bearing down sensation. Pain may be constant or intermittent and show no variation with menses. It is caused by irritation of the peritoneum, tissue distention, and/or traction from adhesions. A history of pain that increases in intensity over time is suggestive of endometriosis; onset is often gradual. The amount and severity of pain offer no clue to the extent of the disease; pain is related to the site of endometriosis, not the extent.

The two major complications of endometriosis are infertility and progression of the disease with increasing pain and interruption of the woman's life and possible

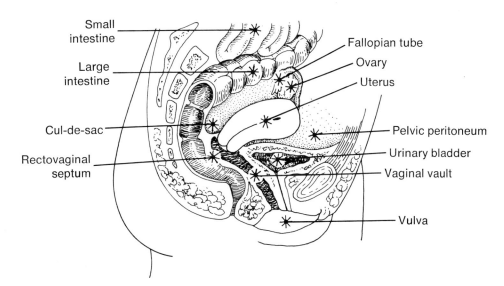

Fig. 13-10. Common sites for endometriosis.

rupture of a large endometrioma and abdominal catastrophe. The fertility rate for women with endometriosis is 66% compared with a rate of 88% for the general population.

Treatment is highly individualized, since endometriosis may cause no symptoms or be severe and disabling. Diagnosis is made by history, pelvic examination, and visualization of lesions. When the client experiences symptoms of discomfort enough to interfere with her life-style, treatment should be instituted. The decision about treatment must take into account the woman's age and desire for future children. When symptoms are mild, education about the disease and supportive concern may enable the client to cope with the discomfort. Mild analgesics may help with dysmenorrhea. Hormonal therapy is recommended for the woman whose discomfort is moderate, who wishes to have subsequent children, or who is not a surgical candidate by her own choice or because of other contraindications. Pregnancy is therapeutic to endometriosis in that it suppresses ovulation and menses; therefore, drugs that also cause amenorrhea are indicated. Agents formerly used include androgens and estrogens; however, these caused severe side effects. Currently, danazol, an antigonadotropin, is being used with good results. This drug leads to decreased pituitary-ovarian stimulation and thus causes decreased endometrium and endometriosis activity (Ranney, 1975). Recommended dosage is 600 to 800 mg/day in divided doses for 6 to 9 months. At present there is about a 60% cure rate (Berger et al., 1978). Danazol provides rapid relief of symptoms, is safe, and has few side effects. However, it is expensive, and some clients experience weight gain, edema, and breakthrough bleeding.

Surgery is often necessary for severe, acute, or incapacitating symptoms. Surgery is the definitive treatment. Decisions as to the extent of the surgery depend on age, desire for children, and extent and location of endometrial lesions. When the client is of reproductive age, desires children, and the disease does not preclude this, reproductive function should be retained by careful and thorough resection of endometriosis with retention of ovarian functioning. Where preservation of reproductive function is not required, total hysterectomy and excision of areas of endometriosis are usually curative; a success rate of 97% to 100% is achieved (Taylor, 1978). Some ovarian tissue should always be retained in the premenopausal female; castration is not necessary. Nursing care of the client who has surgery for endometriosis not only includes general postoperative measures (as outlined in Chapter 15), but also must take into account the emotional significance the client may attach to her disease and its reproductive and sexual implications.

Pregnancy

Pain may be associated with reproductive functions of women. The disruptions in reproductive processes that may cause the client to seek care are ectopic pregnancy, spontaneous abortion, and abruptio placentae.

When implantation of the ovum occurs outside the uterine cavity, pain often results. The most common site of an *ectopic pregnancy* is the fallopian tube. Pain is caused initially by distention as the tube can no longer accommodate the enlarging conceptus. Trophoblastic invasion of the tubal wall results in lower abdominal and pelvic pain, which is first experienced as a dull ache and changes to a sharp localized pain as the pregnancy progresses. Tubal rupture is then imminent. Following tubal rupture, the pain is temporarily relieved; however, generalized abdominal and pelvic pain of increasing severity develops as bleeding occurs into the peritoneum. Ectopic pregnancy is more common in the poor and blacks. The incidence is one out of every one hundred to two hundred pregnancies. It can be a life-threatening condition if bleeding becomes profuse.

Usually, the client describes a history of missed periods and suspected pregnancy. She may have experienced spotting or irregular bleeding and pain. The pain can be intermittent over several days or progress rapidly with increasing severity. Urinary frequency may be present as well as defecatory urges if there is blood in the cul-de-sac. Often the woman has abdominal tenderness and guarding, as well as pelvic and adnexal tenderness, which is more pronounced on the affected side. If bleeding is severe, signs of shock are present. When a woman of childbearing age complains of lower abdominal pain, the possibility of ectopic pregnancy should be considered. Once diagnosis is made, surgical removal of the pregnancy and the affected fallopian tube is performed. Treatment for shock and blood replacement are also indicated.

The woman who has an ectopic pregnancy requires much physiologic and emotional support. Often her physical condition is so serious that emergency surgery is done without the possibility of adequate psychologic preparation and adjustment prior to surgery. She is in pain before and after the operation, and she may need blood and fluid replacement therapy. She may or may not have known she was pregnant. The pregnancy may have been desired or unwanted. She may be afraid she will not be able to conceive again or carry a subsequent pregnancy to term. All these factors need to be assessed for each woman, with nursing actions based on the individual assessment. The nurse should remember that the client is in a crisis situation, that her coping skills will be impaired, and that her self-concept may be lessened. The client's cultural frame of reference in regard to childbearing may also influence her perception of what has happened to her and the significance it holds for her.

Up to 20% of all pregnancies are terminated in *spontaneous abortion* (Romney et al., 1975). Pain is often experienced when a woman is aborting; however, bleeding is a more universal symptom and therefore this process will be discussed later.

Acute, severe abdominal pain that occurs in late pregnancy may be caused by *abruptio placentae*. This is premature separation of the placenta with retroplacental hematoma formation and infiltration of the myometrium with blood. The degree of pain is correlated with the degree of separation. There may be no pain or only mild discomfort when separation is minimal, whereas total premature separation causes severe pain. The pain is constant and may be felt in the abdomen or referred to the back. The woman may experience only mild discomfort upon abdominal palpation or she may experience severe pain and have a boardlike rigidity of the abdomen. Mild and moderate abruptio placentae are characterized by mild to moderate abdominal pain and vaginal bleeding, which begins almost immediately. Severe abruptio is characterized by severe abdominal pain and little or no bleeding. Fetal well-being may not be compromised in less severe cases of abruptio, while total abruption almost always results in severe fetal distress or death.

Care of the woman experiencing abruptio placentae is aimed at prevention or treatment of hypovolemic shock, continuous monitoring of maternal and fetal states, and termination of the pregnancy in the most advantageous manner possible. The pregnant woman is always cared for in the labor and delivery area since this represents a critical care nursing situation. Nursing responsibilities include assessment of bleeding status; careful, accurate monitoring of vital signs and determination of shock; preparation for possible emergency delivery or cesarean section; monitoring of fetal state; and detection of uterine activity.

The woman who is pregnant and experiencing pain and bleeding is anxious and very frightened. She should never be left alone. Allowing her to express her concerns will provide the nurse with opportunities to correct misconceptions, offer information, and realistically reassure her. A sense of trust is essential for the client in such a stressful situation.

Sexual activity

Some women experience pain associated with sexual activity, most commonly dyspareunia, or pain upon intercourse. This problem and other associated conditions are discussed in Chapter 9.

Pelvic masses

Pelvic masses can cause pain or abdominal discomfort. The woman frequently experiences a vague ache and a sense of fullness or heaviness in the pelvis. At times the pain is associated with intercourse, menstruation, or defecation. Acute pain is experienced when the mass twists on its pedicle, when bleeding into a cyst occurs, or when a cyst ruptures.

Many ovarian cysts are functional and develop from the graafian follicle or corpus luteum. They are not neoplastic but pathologic variations of normal physiologic events. These are the most common cause of detectable ovarian enlargement. Follicular cysts can develop at any time during the reproductive years and usually do not cause symptoms. Some women notice menstrual irregularities, mild pelvic discomfort, low back pain, or deep dyspareunia. Corpus luteum cysts are found in ovulating women only and are apt to be symptomatic. Menstruation may be delayed and then prolonged or irregular. Unilateral pelvic discomfort is common. Acute abdominal pain occurs with ovarian cysts when torsion or loss of blood supply, hemorrhage into the cysts, or rupture with intraperitoneal spillage occurs.

Fibroids or leiomyomas are the most common benign tumors of women and are found more commonly in nullipara. Pregnancy appears to facilitate regression, although spontaneous abortion and infertility are more common in women with these tumors.

Discomfort associated with uterine fibroids is likely to be an aching or dragging fullness in the pelvis. Discomfort is most often caused by encroachment on the adjacent bladder or rectum. Excessive flow and/or irregular bleeding may also be experienced. Pelvic examination frequently establishes the diagnosis.

Pelvic pain may also be caused by malignant neoplasms. Usually this does not happen until increased size and/or metastasis have occurred. Pain as a component of gynecologic malignancy is discussed in Chapter 16.

Psychogenic pelvic pain

Lower abdominal or pelvic pain in the female may have a psychogenic rather than organic origin. For some individuals pain is a method of coping with intrapsychic or interpersonal conflict. The child learns that expression of pain can result in comforting, and she may come to associate pain with interpersonal relationships. Pain can also be linked with punishment in the individual's mind. Pain can be expiation for guilt or be equaled with power and attention getting.

Pain can be a symptom of conversion reaction, a psychic mechanism by which an idea, fantasy, or wish in regard to another person is expressed in somatic terms and is experienced by the individual as a physical rather than mental symptom. The idea, wish, or fantasy is unacceptable to the individual at a conscious level and is thus "converted" to a bodily symptom. Conversion symptoms often develop from intrapsychic conflict. The symptoms provide the client with primary gain, for she is protected from the anxiety, guilt, shame, or hopelessness that might result if she had no other way of dealing with the unacceptable, unconscious feelings. There is also secondary gain realized from the change that occurs in relationships because she is sick.

It has been suggested that lower abdominal and pelvic areas are frequently used to express emotionally engendered pain because of their association with sexual and reproductive function, which are highly significant emotionally (Engel, 1970). It may be that the minor functional pains frequently occurring in these anatomic areas provide the neural pathways for the activation or exaggeration of pain impulses. Psychogenic pelvic pain is characterized by inability of the client to specifically locate the site of pain or precisely describe it. It usually begins after awakening, does not awaken the client, and develops as stresses mount. It is often dull, vague, and continuous. Pain does not follow neural pathways but is generalized, variable, and shifting. It does not appear to improve or worsen over time. Interpersonal conflicts often precipitate its development. No organic cause can be identified.

The pain, although it has no organic basis, is real to the woman and must be accepted as such. In order for treatment to be effective, this fact must be accepted by the practitioner. A careful history is essential to rule out an organic cause and to detect psychogenic pain. McGuire (1978) identifies several behavioral patterns suggesting an important psychogenic component to the pain:

1. Either no relief or only sporadic, inconsistent relief is obtained from medications.
2. Symptoms are diffuse, widespread, and alter over time.
3. The impact that the client's illness or symptoms has on her life is out of proportion to the severity of the disease. Secondary gain can be inferred.
4. Physicians are changed often, pointing to the client's difficulty in forming interpersonal relationships and her need to never complete treatment or be cured.
5. Bizarre symptomatology, excessive detail, and morbid fascination with physical functions and symptoms may be seen.
6. The client often presents herself in a manner that alienates the person treating her and discourages further exploration. Clients may be verbal, hostile, obnoxious, and demanding.

Recognition of these behavioral patterns in clients with pelvic pain may facilitate identification of the client for whom pelvic pain is a dysfunctional response to environmental stress.

It may be helpful to discuss with the client as the diagnostic process evolves the possibility that her symptoms are a result of stress, tension, or conflict. Involvement in the decision-making process can facilitate insight into her particular problems. If she feels she is involved and contributes to determining her diagnosis, the woman is less apt to feel betrayed, rejected, or labeled. At times the assessment process itself will provide sufficient self-knowledge and insight for resolution of conflicts and symptoms. The client may be able to deal more directly with the conflicts or stressors and thereby end the need for conversion to physical symptoms. The process may also facilitate her acceptance of counseling or psychotherapy. Use of medication must be carefully thought out. It is possible to develop physical or emotional dependence; addiction is not uncommon in the woman with chronic pelvic discomfort. Use of any drugs should be short-term pending a definite diagnosis.

Unfortunately, some women are unable to accept the fact that their pain is psychogenic. They may refuse psychotherapy or counseling and demand that the practitioner *do* something. The secondary gain is too strong or the emotional conflict too deep to be resolved. Such women frequently have multiple needless surgeries and may indeed end up with physical causes for their pain.

The nurse's role in assessment and exploration of the client's pain is a significant one. The trust inherent in the helping relationship can be a therapeutic strategy to assist this client in self-exploration and development of insight into interpersonal and intrapersonal conflicts expressed as pain. Support as the learning process continues will be essential for a successful outcome.

BLEEDING

Gynecologic bleeding, or lack of it, is the most common symptom of disease seen by women's health care practitioners (Romney et al., 1975). A study done at the University of Minnesota Family Practice Unit found that at least one client with abnormal vaginal bleeding was seen every week (Beck et al., 1972). Bleeding that is perceived as abnormal or unusual produces fear and anxiety. Blood is seen as the life-giving and life-sustaining substance, and its loss is therefore viewed as life-threatening. Bleeding provides a sense of urgency and a need to *do* something.

Bleeding is a frequent gynecologic symptom. When menarche occurs, the presence of blood may elicit apprehension and fear of uncontrolled hemorrhage. While this apprehension does not usually continue in most women, any irregularity or change will quickly reawaken the fear and anxiety. Any abnormal bleeding can make a woman feel more vulnerable and threatened.

Differences in cyclic bleeding patterns or bleeding that is perceived as abnormal may evoke fears regarding sexual or reproductive abilities. Sexual identity and role are closely tied to menstrual functioning for many women; therefore, any occurrence that alters this function may be perceived as a threat to sexual identity. The female nurse will also need to be aware of her own feelings about gynecologic bleeding and its meaning in order to provide comprehensive nursing care for the client. She must examine her values and see how these may influence her ability to collect and assess data, derive a nursing diagnosis, and implement nursing strategies.

Many often confusing terms are used to describe the various types of gynecologic bleeding. The following terms will be used in this chapter:

Metrorrhagia: uterine bleeding at any time other than during the menstrual period
Menorrhagia (hypermonorrhea): excessive menstrual flow
Hypomenorrhea: deficient amount of menstrual flow
Oligomenorrhea: abnormally infrequent menstruation
Amenorrhea: absence of menstruation
Metrorrhea: any pathologic discharge from the uterus
Polymenorrhea: increased frequency of menstrual bleeding
Dysfunctional uterine bleeding: abnormal endometrial bleeding without demonstrable organic pathology

Spotting refers to "small amounts of bloody vaginal discharge, usually intermenstrual." (Romney, 1975, p. 179) The color varies from pink to dark brown. Pink spotting usually indicates minor bleeding mixed with other secretions; dark brown spotting is usually old blood; bright red spotting represents recent bleeding.

Bleeding is considered abnormal in a woman (1) who has never established a regular pattern, (2) whose pattern changes, or (3) who bleeds between periods. Abnormal bleeding may occur at any age and for a variety of reasons. (See Table 13-6 for a summary of the common causes of gynecologic bleeding throughout the life cycle.) Bleeding may last only a few hours or persist for several weeks. It can vary from spotting to hemorrhage and may be associated with passage of clots. Abnormal gynecologic bleeding is presumed to be uterine in origin until proved otherwise. It may be associated with a range of symptoms varying from severe pain and cramps to no discomfort at all. Bleeding associated with pregnancy is usually accompanied by some type of abdominal pain and often by nausea, breast fullness, abdominal bloating, and edema. Abnormal bleeding not associated with pregnancy is less often associated with pain or other symptoms (Romney et al., 1975).

Most women seek care for one of three reasons associated with bleeding: absence or amenorrhea; spotting; and changes in the menstrual cycle that are perceived to be abnormal.

Amenorrhea

Amenorrhea can cause much distress and concern. Defined as the absence of menstruation, it is classified as primary or secondary. In primary amenorrhea the female has never menstruated. Secondary amenorrhea occurs when a previously normally menstruating woman

Table 13-6. Causes of abnormal gynecologic bleeding through the life cycle*

Childhood	Childbearing years	Postmenopausal
Foreign bodies: cotton, paper, safety pins, sand, sticks	Pregnancy complications	Carcinoma
Self-inflicted lacerations	Anovulation	Estrogen therapy
Vaginitis: nonspecific, can be gonococcal	Oral contraceptives	Endometrial hyperplasia
Rectal and urethral bleeding may appear to be vaginal	Intrauterine contraceptive devices	Polyps
Pinworms: excoriation from scratching	Cervical erosion	Fibroids
Systemic disease: leukemia	Vaginal infections	Coital injuries due to atrophy
Medications: griseofulvin, oral contraceptives	Vaginal or cervical lacerations	Atrophic vaginitis
Consider precocious puberty; vaginal adenosis of DES daughters	Uterine fibroids (after age 25)	
	Cervical polyps (after age 25)	
	Medications: phenothiazines, hypothalamic depressants, anticoagulants, anticholinergics, thiazide diuretics	
	Systemic disease: hypothyroidism, blood dyscrasias	
	Psychogenic factors	
	Endometrial hyperplasia (after age 35)	
	Endometriosis and adenomyosis (after age 35)	

*Developed from information in Beck, W. W., and others: Abnormal gynecological bleeding: when a youngster bleeds vaginally, Patient Care, pp. 56-70, Nov. 1, 1973; Abnormal gynecological bleeding: diagnosis and treatment during childbearing years, Patient Care, pp. 20-60, Oct. 15, 1973; Vaginal bleeding, Nurs. Times, p. 998-1000, June 30, 1977.

ceases to do so. Any defect or interruption in the hypo-thalamic-pituitary-ovarian-uterine axis may cause failure of menstruation. An abnormality in one or more of the following areas can cause the interruption: anatomic, physiologic, biochemical, genetic, or emotional.

Primary

Primary amenorrhea is considered to exist if the adolescent girl reaches the age of 18 and has never menstruated. The average of menarche is 12 or 13 years with normal ranges of 10 to 16 years. The client or her parents will usually have sought health care prior to the age of 18; however, if the girl is 17 years of age or less and has normal growth and development, including secondary sex characteristics, definite diagnostic measures will be delayed until age 18. Discussion of ranges of normal pubertal development, reassurances about ranges of normal, and exploration of family history can be helpful. Girls tend to menstruate at about the same time as their mothers and grandmothers, and a family history of late menarche can be significant. If any signs of physical abnormality are present or the girl appears to have delayed growth and development or if she is 18, diagnostic measures are begun.

Primary amenorrhea may be caused by a variety of factors, such as failure of the müllerian ducts to fuse embryologically, chromosomal defects, hormonal imbalances, systemic disease, psychologic factors, nutritional status, and occasionally ovarian tumors. Table 13-7 summarizes the major causes of primary amenorrhea. Almost one half of the clients who have primary amenorrhea have chromosomal or developmental defects; one fourth to one third are chromosomally abnormal. Only 20% of girls with primary amenorrhea can be induced to menstruate. Fertility is often compromised; the later the age of menarche, the less the chances of bearing a child (Parsons and Sommers, 1978).

Primary amenorrhea is diagnosed by careful history, physical examination (including pelvic), buccal smear to detect chromosomal aberrations, and progesterone and estrogen-progesterone withdrawal tests. Progesterone, 50 mg intramuscular, is given. Withdrawal bleeding indicates the presence of adequate amounts of estrogen and, therefore, basically normal pituitary gland, ovaries, and uterus. Further diagnostic studies must then be done to determine any condition that might produce temporary reversible failure of ovulation with normal ovarian production. If no withdrawal bleeding occurs, either estrogen or the normal endometrial response to estrogen is absent. Next, a combined estrogen-progesterone preparation is given in a cyclic regimen. Endometrial failure is indicated by absence of bleeding. If bleeding results, a 24-hour pituitary gonadotropin urinary excretion test can be done. High levels

Table 13-7. Causes of primary amenorrhea

I. With normal feminization and female secondary sex characteristics; normal hypothalamic-pituitary-gonadal axis
   A. Congenital obstruction
      1. Cryptomenorrhea
      2. Imperforate hymen
      3. Cervical stenosis
   B. Congenital absence of uterus (failure of müllerian duct development)
   C. Testicular feminization
II. Without normal feminization and absent secondary sex characteristics; failure to produce estrogen; sexually infantile
   A. Gonadal dysgenesis; normal pituitary with low level estrogen (e.g., Turner's syndrome)
   B. Failure of gonadotropin secretion; amenorrhea-galactorrhea syndromes such as Chiari-Frommel
   C. Panhypopituitarism
III. Virilization or abnormal secondary sexual development; excessive androgen present
   A. Adrenal tumor or congenital hyperplasia
   B. Stein-Leventhal syndrome
   C. Ovarian tumor
   D. Mixed gonadal dysgenesis

suggest primary ovarian failure, low levels pituitary failure, and normal levels hypothalamic difficulties (Green, 1977). Appropriate treatment is directed at the cause of the symptom, amenorrhea.

Many of the causes of primary amenorrhea are not curable, particularly in regard to fertility. In the client who has underdeveloped secondary sex characteristics, hormonal therapy is desirable to provide as normal an appearance as possible. Surgery to correct anatomic defects is indicated when possible.

Secondary

Secondary amenorrhea is considered to exist when a woman who has previously menstruated normally develops amenorrhea lasting more than 3 months. The most common cause of amenorrhea in a woman between the ages of 18 and 45 who has a previously benign history is pregnancy. If the client has been well and suddenly stops menstruating, pregnancy must be ruled out. A careful menstrual history and exploration of possible sexual exposure is indicated. Any associated symptoms, such as breast tenderness, nausea and vomiting, or fatigue, should be noted. A pelvic examination may confirm a diagnosis of pregnancy if gestation is at least 10 to 12 weeks. A rapid pregnancy test on a first voided specimen should confirm pregnancy in a woman who is 42 days past her last menstrual period.

If pregnancy has been ruled out, then a malfunction of the hypothalamic-pituitary-ovarian axis is considered.

Table 13-8. Secondary amenorrhea

Galactorrhea: Prolonged lactation; Chiari-Frommel syndrome following normal delivery, not necessarily associated with breastfeeding; pituitary tumor associated with headache, heaving, or visual losses; del Castillo syndrome (occurs in nulligravidas)

Systemic disease: tuberculosis, hyperthyroidism, diabetes mellitus, mitral stenosis

Cushing's syndrome: Amenorrhea associated with hirsutism, hypertension, diabetes, trunk and facial obesity

Medications: Oral contraceptives; tranquilizers (especially phenothiazine and chlorpromazine groups)

Sheehan's syndrome: Postpartum pituitary necrosis following severe postpartum hemorrhage (symptoms include axillary and pubic hair loss, loss of libido, loss of breast tissue, dry vaginal mucosa, muscle weakness, possibly premature aging and hot flashes)

Ovarian cysts: Persistent graafian follicle that does not rupture and continues to release estrogen

Nutritional disorders: Anorexia nervosa; weight loss and obsessive concern with diet and weight control may cause stress-related anovulation; obesity: anovulation may be the result of increased conversion of androstenedione to estrone by adipose tissue

Systemic illnesses and other organic causes of secondary amenorrhea are summarized in Table 13-8.

Amenorrhea may mean many things to a woman; her self-concept may be threatened in several ways. She may feel she is not really a woman, that her "marriage-ability" is threatened, and her ability to conceive and bear children is compromised. She may feel concern about appearance and peer acceptance or approval. The nurse can help the client to acknowledge and work through these feelings. Some may be reality based; she may indeed be infertile. In these instances the client will need to gain acceptance of this fact and develop a self-concept that is not based on childbearing functions. Sexual issues frequently surface and must be examined. The nurse will need a thorough understanding of how she herself views the feminine role and what constitutes "female identity" before she can assist the client in exploring and resolving these issues.

Oral contraceptives can cause amenorrhea by their effect on both the hypothalamic-pituitary-ovarian axis and the uterine endometrium. The hypothalamic release of FSH and LH is suppressed by provision of a continuous exogenous source of progesterone and estrogen. Endometrial build-up is atypical in that it does not reach the thickness of normal endometrium. Occasionally, endometrial increase is not sufficient for sloughing following hormonal withdrawal and there is only slight spotting or amenorrhea. A small but significant number of women experience "post-pill" amenorrhea; menstrua-tion is not reestablished for up to 12 months following discontinuation of oral contraceptives. It is thought that high levels of endogenous estrogen in a rebound effect suppress FSH and LH release. Additionally, following the removal of exogenous estrogen, it may take time for estrogen levels to rise sufficiently to trigger the LH surge necessary for ovulation.

Hypothalamic amenorrhea, or lack of menses in the absence of systemic illness or organic cause, is often thought to be emotional in origin. Emotional disturbances of various types can lead to amenorrhea through their effect on the hypothalamus. Common examples of such stressors are marital discord, fatigue, travel, examinations, nervous tension, chronic anxiety, or concern over pregnancy. During chronic stress, the increased adrenal function provides estrogen precursors. This may result in a constant unchanged estrogen feedback state that is comparable to "constant estrus," causing loss of gonadotropic cyclicity. If, while talking with the woman, the nursing practitioner perceives that these factors may be operant, they should be specifically explored. Exploration of these factors and assistance with resolution are appropriate therapeutic measures. The progesterone and estrogen-progesterone withdrawal tests described earlier will assist in diagnosis of hypothalamic causes.

Spotting

Spotting may be a symptom of a relatively innocuous or benign condition or it can be an indication of a serious, possibly life-threatening situation. Typical examples of problems that are often first indicated by spotting are spontaneous abortion, ectopic pregnancy, hydatidiform mole, cervical erosions, various gynecologic infections, and malignancy.

Spontaneous abortion

Spontaneous abortion is the natural termination of a pregnancy before the fetus is considered to be viable. As many as one pregnancy in five ends in a spontaneous abortion. The majority occur in the first trimester of pregnancy and often before the woman is aware she is pregnant. It may be that her period is somewhat delayed and when it begins the flow is heavier than usual but she does not identify this as an early spontaneous abortion. It has been suggested that every woman who is sexually active will experience at least one spontaneous abortion in her reproductive lifetime. Abortions can occur for many reasons; however, in as many as 50% of all cases the causative factor is never identified. When a cause can be identified it is in one of three categories: abnormalities of the ovum, abnormalities of the female reproductive tract, or maternal host factors. There can be imperfections of the ovum or sperm, defects of the zygote, imperfections in the implantation of the products of conception due to faulty intrauterine environment, or defects of the placenta. In these cases the fetus dies and is expelled by the uterus as a foreign body. Uterine anomalies, malposition of the uterus, and incompetent cervix may also result in spontaneous abortion. Maternal infections, hormonal imbalances or inadequacies, malnutrition, and some systemic diseases may be incompatible with fetal life.

Spontaneous abortion is classified by clinical symptoms. *Threatened abortion* is indicated by vaginal spotting, which may be accompanied by cramps and backache. This can last for several days or weeks. About half or less of the women who experience this will lose the pregnancy. No treatment has been shown to definitely affect the outcome. Usually, activities are restricted. If bleeding develops, cramping increases, and the cervix begins to dilate, abortion becomes *inevitable.* The process continues and all or part of the products of conception are expelled. Abortion is considered *incomplete* when only part of the products of conception are expelled. In this case bleeding may be profuse. Supportive measures such as transfusions and removal of retained tissue by dilatation and curettage are done immediately. Occasionally, a *missed abortion* will occur, in which the fetus dies but remains in utero for 8 weeks or longer. Most missed abortions terminate spontaneously; if they do not, oxytocin or prostaglandin stimulation of the uterus is instituted. If a woman experiences three or more spontaneous abortions she is considered to have *habitual abortions.* This is a serious problem with complex etiology.

A spontaneous abortion is a crisis situation for the woman and her family. Vaginal bleeding always produces anxiety. This may compound the view that loss of pregnancy is a threat to a woman's femininity as well as her life. Habitual abortion is even more threatening for the woman who desires to bear children and raise a family. The nurse must assess the client's physical status and psychologic functioning. Monitoring of vital signs; assessment of amount and type of bleeding; and determination of the character, type, and location of pain are specific aspects of nursing assessment. The client's feelings about her pregnancy loss, her coping behaviors, the amount of anxiety and depression experienced, her present stage in the grief process, and stage of loss exhibited should also be noted. The nurse supports both physiologic and psychologic functioning. The woman needs time to mourn, to verbalize her feelings, and explore verbally what has happened to her. Successful grief work will be facilitated by return to healthy physical status. The nurse should allow the client to progress through the stages of mourning at her own pace; this is not the time to focus on possible future pregnancies with happier outcomes.

Ectopic pregnancy and hydatidiform mole

Spotting may be present when a client has an ectopic pregnancy (see p. 246). Hydatidiform mole may first be recognized when the woman experiences a brownish, watery discharge beginning in the tenth to twelfth week of pregnancy. It may be scant and intermittent or possibly continuous. The uterus will be enlarged out of proportion to the estimated week of gestation. There are no fetal heart tones, high levels of serum human chorionic gonadotropin (HCG), and often signs and symptoms characteristic of pre-eclampsia. Treatment is evacuation of the contents of the uterus. Follow-up care is mandatory because of the increased possibility of the development of choriocarcinoma following a hydatidiform mole. The woman who experiences this condition not only has to cope with the loss of her pregnancy but with the fear that she may develop cancer at some later date.

Chronic cervicitis and cervical erosion

Chronic cervicitis or cervical erosions frequently cause spotting, and this may be the first indication of the condition. The primary symptom of acute cervicitis is discharge, usually purulent and profuse; it is most often caused by gonorrhea. From 90% to 95% of all parous women have some evidence of chronic cervicitis (Romney, 1978). The cause is usually cervical laceration incurred during delivery and infection, resulting in ectropion. In this condition a considerable amount of endocervix is exposed to the acid pH and bacterial flora of the vagina. The condition is often asymptomatic and may only be diagnosed during a pelvic examination.

The most common clinical manifestation is cervical erosion or a zone of infected tissue surrounding the cervical os that has a granular, angry appearance (see Chapter 7). The symptoms of chronic cervicitis are vaginal discharge that is thick, yellow-white, and tenacious and postcoital or postdouching spotting or bleeding. The endocervical epithelium is often swollen, edematous, and exposed; it is easily traumatized so that the client may say she is experiencing slight irregular intermenstrual bleeding. She may also experience backache and urinary urgency and frequency.

The most important consideration in the diagnosis of chronic cervicitis is exclusion of malignancy. Papanicolaou smears and biopsies of suspicious areas should be obtained. Treatment should not be started until the final reports of cytologic smears and tissue biopsy are available. Treatment is both preventive and curative. Prevention of recurrent infection and trauma during labor and delivery will decrease the incidence of cervicitis and erosion. Cauterization or cryosurgery is used to change the edematous, friable cervix to one that more nearly resembles that of a nulliparous woman. When a client undergoes cauterization she should be told that she will smell the odor of burning tissue and there will be slight bleeding. There should be no discomfort. Various vaginal infections may also cause spotting; these were discussed earlier in this chapter. Mittelschmerz may also be associated with spotting (see p. 244).

Malignancy

Spotting may be a signal of malignancy of the reproductive tract. Unfortunately, spotting does not usually occur until metastasis has begun. In this case it is a symptom of potentially life-threatening magnitude. (For a thorough discussion of reproductive malignancies see Chapter 16.)

Alterations in cyclic bleeding

Women may seek health care for a variety of alterations in their normal cyclic patterns of bleeding. These concerns are usually associated with amount, duration, interval, or irregularity. Often a woman will worry about menstruation that is short or in small amount or that occurs too frequently. It is important to determine whether this pattern is cyclic or noncyclic. Cyclic bleeding implies an ovulatory cycle, while irregular flow is more probably associated with anovulatory cycles.

Short, scant menstruation that is cyclic may be the normal pattern for some women and usually indicates normal, frequent ovulations. This can be determined by assessing whether or not the woman is ovulating by monitoring basal body temperature and testing for ferning and spinnbarkeit of cervical mucus (see Chapter 22). If the tests demonstrate ovulation, the woman can be reassured as to the normalcy of her periods. Explaining about the wide variation in the normal experiences of women at all ages of their reproductive lives can be helpful.

Scanty flow is most commonly caused by oral contraceptives; at times amenorrhea may also be experienced. Decreased duration is also characteristic of women who are taking oral contraceptives. It should be noted that "implantation bleeding," or spotting that occurs about the time of implantation of a pregnancy, occurs about the time of an expected menstrual period and may be mistaken for one of short duration. A few women continue to have menses after conception and these are lighter and shorter than usual. Short menstrual cycles in a woman who is not ovulating may indicate infertility or endometrial hyperplasia. Beck and associates (1972) make the point that unopposed estrogen is the cause of endometrial hyperplasia and that the woman who does not ovulate has unopposed estrogen. Further, all endometrial cancer occurring in women 30 years of age or younger is in women who have been consistently anovulators (Beck, 1975). Among clients in the reproductive and premenopausal age group who have frequent anovulatory cycles, there is a much greater chance

that the cause is organic disease, particularly when a change in pattern is involved. This must be evaluated and treated.

Menorrhagia, or excessive menstrual flow, can cause grave distress and inconvenience. A single episode of heavy bleeding may occur or a woman may regularly experience flooding as a pattern during which she may soak tampons or pads every few hours for 7 to 9 days. A single episode of heavy bleeding can indicate spontaneous abortion or ectopic pregnancy. Occasionally, a woman with an IUD or taking oral contraceptives will experience an episode of heavy bleeding. This is thought to be associated with anovulation and subsequent excessive endometrial proliferation. Endometrial build-up is under the influence of estrogen and endometrial sloughing is not regulated by progesterone. This bleeding tends to be sudden and profuse and to last longer than normal menses.

Hypermenorrhea associated with an IUD may be caused by erosion into an endometrial vessel by the IUD or chronic endometritis; these explanations are speculative, however. Women who have experienced conizations or cautery of the cervix may experience profuse bleeding, which may be interpreted as hypermenorrhea if it coincides with the menstrual period.

Fibroids and adenomyosis are common causes of menorrhagia. Submucous fibroids are usually associated with bleeding; heavy bleeding is caused by ulceration, hyperplasia, or venous dilation and congestion of the endometrium. The cause of abnormal bleeding associated with adenomyosis is not known. The degree of disability and discomfort associated with these conditions will influence treatment. The presence of anemia should be determined. Conservative treatment consists of hormonal therapy, usually progestins in the latter half of the cycle, or myomectemy if childbearing function is desired. Hysterectomy is often done, particularly if severe anemia is present, severe pain is associated with the fibroids, considerable disruption of life-style is occurring, and future childbearing is not desired.

Systemic diseases of nonreproductive origin can cause hypermenorrhea. Blood dyscrasias and hypothyroidism are examples. Medications may also cause abnormal bleeding. Anticoagulants, thiazide diuretics, anticholinergics, hypothalamic depressants, and phenothiazines have all been associated with excessive flow. Chronic iron-deficiency anemia has been implicated in hypermenorrhea. It is thought that a clotting defect is caused by decreased activity of the cytochrome oxidase system, which decreases uterine muscle contractility (Romney, 1978).

Women from 30 to 35 years of age may experience longer menstrual periods that differ in type of bleeding. There may be 2 to 3 days of spotting, followed by 1 to 2 days of steady bleeding, or there may be regular menses followed by 2 to 3 days of spotting. This is characteristic of degenerating corpus luteum function. Instead of the smooth hormonal withdrawal in the latter half of the menstrual cycle, there is "staircase" withdrawal, which results in intermittent sloughing and spotting.

Dysfunctional uterine bleeding

Dysfunctional uterine bleeding (DUB) is associated with menstrual irregularities, most often excessive bleeding of some type: too frequent flow, too heavy flow, too prolonged flow, or irregularities. DUB is a result of a functional derangement of the hypothalamic-pituitary-ovarian-endometrial axis. It most often occurs at the extremes of the reproductive years; approximately one half of these women are in their fifties and 20% are adolescents (March, 1977). These are the ages during which anovulatory cycles are most common. High rates of infertility have been reported in women who experienced DUB as teenagers; a common cause of infertility is persistent anovulation.

Dysfunctional uterine bleeding is diagnosed only when any other local or systemic conditions that might cause abnormal bleeding have been ruled out. The most common cause of DUB is prolonged estrogen stimulation of the endometrium following long periods of anovulation secondary to faulty neuroendocrine and/or ovarian function. The steady estrogen stimulation produces a

continuously proliferating endometrium that can (1) outgrow its blood supply, (2) lose nutrients because of the persistence of acid mucopolysaccharides, (3) have asynchronous development of stroma, glands, and blood vessels, and (4) have an overdeveloped Golgi lysosomal complex capable of releasing hydrolytic enzymes in excessive amounts. Any of these can lead to the irregular endometrial shedding that is characteristic of dysfunctional uterine bleeding (March, 1977).

Dysfunctional bleeding that is ovulatory occurs secondary to dysfunction of the corpus luteum. A variety of conditions or problems may appear to be dysfunctional uterine bleeding and should be excluded before the diagnosis can be made. Table 13-9 summarizes these.

Once the diagnosis has been determined, therapy is begun following these principles: (1) control of bleeding, (2) prevention of recurrences, (3) preservation of fertility, (4) correction of any coexisting conditions, and (5) establishment of ovulation in those women who wish to have children. No one method is effective; approaches consist of observation; surgical measures such as dilatation and curettage, ovarian wedge, myomectomy, and hysterectomy; and medical management such as ovulation inhibitor, estrogens, progesterones, androgens, ovulation induction, ergot derivatives, and thyroid preparations. Table 13-10 lists treatment guidelines.

The prognosis with intermenstrual and irregular bleeding depends on etiology, whether or not other gynecologic or systemic conditions exist, and whether or not fertility is desired. A careful history and diagnostic work-up followed by treatment specific to the problem are most likely to resolve an acute episode and prevent recurrences.

Postmenopausal bleeding

Any bleeding that occurs in postmenopausal years must be considered to be a serious symptom. The incidence of carcinoma in women with postmenopausal

Table 13-9. Conditions causing abnormal bleeding

1. Pregnancy (should always be considered first)
   a. Intrauterine (abortion, hydatidiform mole)
   b. Extrauterine (ectopic)
2. Malignancy
3. Endometritis (chronic)
4. Uterine myoma or polyp
5. Cervical erosion, polyp
6. Vaginal infection, trauma, foreign bodies
7. Ovarian dysfunction
   a. Polycystic ovarian disease
   b. Luteal phase defects
   c. Neoplasms
   d. Cysts (functional)
8. Systemic disease
   a. Blood dyscrasia
   b. Thyroid disease
   c. Severe nutritional deficiencies
   d. Cardiac, renal, liver failure
9. Iatrogenic
   a. Steroids (oral contraceptives, androgens, anabolic agents, menopausal agents)
   b. Other medications (anticoagulants, psychoactive drugs)
   c. Mechanical (IUD)
10. Psychogenic (depression, chronic anxiety, emotional shock)

Table 13-10. Treatment guidelines for dysfunctional uterine bleeding

Symptoms	Treatment
One bleeding episode without anemia	Observe for recurrence, exaggeration, or alleviation of symptoms
Repeated bleeding episodes without anemia	Hormonal
Repeated bleeding episodes with anemia	Hormonal and supportive
One or more bleeding episodes with hypovolemia	Transfusion; curettage
Over 35 years of age	Curettage
Failed hormonal therapy	Curettage

bleeding is 30% to 40%. Malignancy must be a prime suspect in this age group and must always be ruled out. (See Chapter 16.) Another common cause of postmenopausal bleeding is injudicious use of estrogen replacement therapy. Postmenopausal estrogen therapy is being questioned more and more, as more evidence is amassed pointing to an increase in endometrial cancer in women taking replacement estrogen. (See Chapter 18.)

SUMMARY

The symptoms of gynecologic discharge and itching, pain, and bleeding are common to women and cause discomfort, interference with life-style, and distress, both physical and emotional. The nursing practitioner can effectively alleviate these adverse effects through intervention. Client education to facilitate self-care activities and intervention that supports specific diagnosis and treatment measures are appropriate nursing roles. Permeating all nursing endeavors should be a relationship of mutual trust that enhances an honest communication and support of the client.

REFERENCES

Adams, H. G., and others: Genital herpetic infection in men and women: clinical cause and effect of topical application of adenine arabinoside, J. Infect. Dis. 133:A151-A159, 1976 Supp.

Abraham, G. E.: Primary dysmenorrhea, Clin. Obstet. Gynecol. 21(1):139-145, 1975.

Annon, J. S.: The behavioral treatment of sexual problems, brief therapy, New York, 1976, Harper & Row, Publishers.

Arnas, G., Breen, J. L., and Levy, D.: Cooling down pelvic inflammation, Patient Care 8(21):90-99, 1974.

Aydar, G. K., and Coleman, B.: Treatment of primary dysmenorrhea, J.A.M.A. 192(11):1003-1005, 1965.

Bardwick, J. M.: Psychology of women, New York, 1971, Harper & Row, Publishers.

Beck, W. W., and others: When a youngster bleeds vaginally, Patient Care, pp. 56-70, Nov. 1, 1973.

Beck, W. W., and others: Diagnosis and treatment during the child-bearing years, Patient Care, pp. 20-60, Oct. 15, 1972.

Beck, W. W., and others: When abnormal bleeding is the problem, Patient Care, pp. 104-116, Dec. 1, 1975.

Beck, W. W., and others: When the postmenopausal women bleeds, Patient Care, pp. 70-93, Dec. 1, 1977.

Benedick, T. F.: Sexual functions in women and their disturbances. In Seite, S. A., editor: American handbook of psychiatry, New York, 1959, Basic Books, Inc.

Berger, J. A., and others: Endometriosis: new virus, new therapies, Patient Care, pp. 24-96, Nov. 15, 1978.

Bhattacharyra, M. N., and Jephcott, A. E.: Diagnosis of gonorrhea in women, Br. J. Ven. Dis. 50:109-112, 1974.

Carey, H. M.: Dysmenorrhea, Med. J. Aust. 2:349-352, 1975.

Center for Disease Control: VD fact sheet, 1975, ed. 32, DHEW Pub. No. (CDC) 76-8195, Atlanta.

Cox, D. J.: Behavioral treatment parameter with primary dysmenorrhea, presented at the Menstrual Cycle Conference, May 26, 1978.

Dalton, K.: The premenstrual syndrome, London, 1964, Heineman.

Dan, A. J.: Behavioral variability and the menstrual cycle, presented at American Physiological Association meeting, Washington, D.C., Sept. 1976.

Darrow, W. W.: Changes in sexual behavior and venereal diseases, Clin. Obstet. Gynecol. 18:255-267, 1975.

Edwards, M. S.: Venereal herpes: a nursing overview, J. Obstet. Gynecol. Nurs. 7(5):7-15, 1978.

Fleischauer, M. L.: A modified Lamaze approach in the treatment of primary dysmenorrhea, J. Am. Coll. Health Assoc. 25:273-275, 1977.

Fleury, F. J.: Vulvovaginal infections. Postgraduate seminar family planning nurse practitioners lecture, 1978, University of North Carolina.

Golub, S.: The magnitude of premenstrual anxiety and depression, Psychosom. Med 38(1):4-12, 1976.

Gonorrhea infection: discussing complications, Contemp. OB/GYN 5:36-48, 1975.

Green, T. H.: Gynecology: essentials of clinical practice, ed. 3, Boston, 1977, Little, Brown & Co.

Guerriero, W. F., and others: Pelvic pain, gynecic and nongynecic: interpretations and management, South. Med. J. 64(9):1043-1048, 1971.

Halbert, D. R.: Dysmenorrhea and prostaglandin, Obstet. Gynecol. Survey Supp. 31(1):77-81, 1976.

Heczey, M. D.: Effects of biofeedback and autogenic training on dysmenorrhea, presented at the Menstrual Cycle Conference, Apr. 1977.

Ledger, W. J.: Relationship of pelvic infection to various types of contraception, Clin. Obstet. Gynecol. 17(1):79-91, 1974.

Lennane, K. J., and Lennane, R. J.: Alleged psychogenic disorders in women—a possible manifestation of sexual prejudice, N. Engl. J. Med. 288(6):288-292, 1973.

Lovesky, J.: Menstruation: alternatives to pharmacologic therapy for menstrual distress, J. Nurse Midwifery 23:34-44, 1978.

Maddox, H. C.: Menstruation, New Canaan, Conn., 1975, Today Publishing Co., Inc.

March, C. M.: Management of dysfunctional bleeding, Female Pat. pp. 54-59, Oct. 1977.

Martin, L.: Health care of women, Philadelphia, 1978, J. B. Lippincott Co.

McGaffery, M.: Nursing management of the patient in pain, Philadelphia, 1972, J. B. Lippincott Co.

McGuire, L. S.: Chronic vaginitis masking serious affective disorders: an illustrative case, J. Obstet. Gynecol. 7(2):13-16, 1978.

Meckler, J., and Jordan, J.: The relationship of life change events, social supports, and symptoms of dysmenorrhea, unpublished Masters report, University of North Carolina–Chapel Hill, 1980.

Meeker, C. I.: Candidiasis—an obstinate problem, Med. Times 106 (12):26-32, 1978.

Nahmias, A. J.: Herpes simplex virus infection—present status of diagnosis and management, South. Med. J. 68:1191-1194, 1975.

Parlee, M. B.: The premenstrual syndrome, Psychol. Bull. 80(6):454-465, 1973.

Parsons, L., and Sommers, S. C.: Gynecology, vol. 1, ed. 2, Philadelphia, 1978, W. B. Saunders Co.

Phipps, W., Long, B. C., and Woods, N.: Medical-surgical nursing, St. Louis, 1979, The C. V. Mosby Co.

Ranney, B.: The prevention, inhibition, palliation, and treatment of endometriosis, Am. J. Obstet. Gynecol. 123(8):778-785, 1975.

Romney, S., and others: Gynecology and obstetrics, New York, 1978, McGraw-Hill Book Co.

Ruble, D. N.: Premenstrual symptoms: a reinterpretation, Science 197:291-292, 1977.

Schwartz, A.: Primary dysmenorrhea, Obstet. Gynecol. 44(5):709-712, 1974.

Steiner, M., and Carroll, B. J.: The psychobiology of premenstrual dysphoria: review of theories and treatment, Psychoneuro. 2:321-335, 1977.

Taylor, D.: Endometriosis—a gynecological enigma, Nurs. Mirror **147**(9):30-32, 1978.

United States Department of Health, Education, and Welfare: Criteria and techniques for the diagnosis of gonorrhea, United States Department of Health, Education, and Welfare, Center for Disease Control, 1975.

United States Department of Health, Education, and Welfare: Factsheet for Gonorrhea, 1975, United States Department of Health, Education, and Welfare, Center for Disease Control, 1975.

Voogd, C. E., Van Derstei, J. J., and Jacobs, J. A.: The mutagenic action of nitromidazales—I. Metronidazole, Nemorazole, Demetridazole and Ronidazole, Mutat. Res. **26**:483-490, 1974.

Ylibarkala, O., and Dawood, M. Y.: New concepts in dysmenorrhea, Am. J. Obstet. Gynecol. **130**(7):833-847, 1978.

Zabrowski, M.. Cultural components in responses to pain. In Jaco, E. G., editor: Patients, physicians and illness, New York, 1958, The Free Press.

ADDITIONAL REFERENCES

Adolescent gynecology: sorting out the causes of amenorrhea, Patient Care, pp. 93-102, Dec. 1, 1975.

Altcheck, A.: Dysfunctional uterine bleeding in adolescence, Clin. Obstet. Gynecol. **20**(3):633-650, 1977.

Asch, H., and Greenbladt, R. B.: Primary and membranous dysmenorrhea, South. Med. J. **71**(10):1247-1249, 1978.

Barnett-Connor, E., Conger, K. B., and Lucas, J. B.: Keeping up with gonorrhea guidelines, Patient Care, **9**(2):72-87, 1975.

Beloff, S., and others: When vaginitis keeps coming back, Patient Care, pp. 44-77, Sept. 15, 1974.

Blount, J. H., Darrow, W. W., and Johnson, R. E.: Venereal disease in adolescents, Ped. Clin. North Am. **10**:1021-1033, 1973.

Culbertson, C.: Monistat: a new fungicide for treatment of vulvovaginal candidiasis, Am. J. Obstet. Gynecol. **120**(47):973-976, 1974.

Davis, J., Frerdenfeld, J. H., and Goddard, J. L.: Comparative evaluation of Monistat and Mycostatin in the treatment of vulvovaginal candidiasis, Obstet. Gynecol. **44**(3):403-406, 1974.

Denness, R. G.: Vaginal bleeding, Nurs. Times, pp. 998-1000, June 30, 1977.

Engel, G. L.: Conversion symptoms. In MacBryde, M. C. M., and Blacklow, R. S., editors: Signs and symptoms, ed. 5, Philadelphia, 1970, J. B. Lippincott.

Fleury, F. J.: Clinical management of genital herpes, Cont. Obstet. Gynecol. **7**:36-40, 1976.

Friedrich, E. G.: The viral infections—an increasing problem, Med. Times **106**(12):53-57, 1978.

Gardner, H. L.: Infections of the vagina and vulva, Med. Times **106** (12):21-24, 1978.

Gardner, H. L., Graves, W., and Peudon, T. F.: Managing the rising risk of herpes genitalis, Patient Care **VIII**(19):140-153, 1974.

Grederick, J. A.: Psychological aspects of chronic pain, Clin. Obstet. Gynecol. **19**(2):399-406, 1976.

Greenbladt, R. B.: Recent advances in endometriosis, New York, 1975, Excerpta Medica.

Kreutner, A., Kessler, K., and Hollingsworth, D. R.: Adolescent obstetrics and gynecology, Chicago, 1978, Year Book Medical Publishers, Inc.

Miller, A. W.: Gynecological symptoms, Br. Med. J., pp. 456-458, May 20, 1972.

Nahmias, A. J., and others: Genital herpetic infection—the old and the new. In Catterall, R. D., and Neol, C. S., editors: Sexually transmitted diseases, New York, 1976, Academic Press.

Nahmias, A. J.: Herpes simplex virus infection—present status of diagnosis and management, South. Med. J. **68**:1191-1194, 1975.

Nahmias, A. J., and others: Prenatal risk associated with maternal genital herpes simplex virus infection, Am. J. Obstet. Gynecol. **110**(6):825-837, 1971.

Pherfer, T. A., and others: Nonspecific vaginitis, N. Engl. J. Med. **298**(26):1429-1434, 1978.

Primary amenorrhea: why haven't her menses started? Patient Care, pp. 74-82, Oct. 15, 1972.

Quirk, B., and Huxall, L. K.: VD, the equal opportunity disease, J. Obstet. Gynecol. Nurs. **4**(1):13-22, 1975.

Secondary amenorrhea: why has she missed six cycles? Patient Care, pp. 64-71, Oct. 15, 1970.

Shuster, E., and Giulian, K. A.: A new drug for vulvovaginal candidiasis in pregnancy, Obstet. Gynecol. **14**:13-15, 1976.

Steele, S. J.: Amenorrhea, Nurs. Mirror, pp. 46-48, Oct. 5, 1978.

Wentz, A. C., and Jones, G.: Off. Gynecol. **60**(1):161-164, 1970.

14

Infertility

Nancy Fugate Woods

Infertility may seem an insignificant health problem in the context of increasing concern for world population growth, rapid utilization of expendable natural resources, and the hunger and poverty experienced by children in all parts of the world, including many urban areas of the United States. Yet to the infertile couple, infertility may constitute a life crisis. In the course of acknowledging and investigating their inability to conceive and give birth to a living child, the infertile couple confronts feelings about control, self-image, self-esteem, and sexuality. Questions about personal adequacy arise as do concerns about the exploration of the most intimate aspects of their sexual relationship. Not only can infertility be emotionally and economically stressful, but also assessment and management can be physically painful.

Health professionals who interact with infertile individuals are likely to do so at times that are especially stressful for the clients. Often clinicians do not have the same degree of preparation or insight regarding infertility that they have with respect to family planning. Yet family planning in its broadest sense includes being able to choose whether or not to have children, how many, and when. For many infertile persons, the option to have their own biologic child may be in question or nonexistent. Health professionals can assist infertile persons to explore the cause of their problem; to seek appropriate therapy for those problems that can be treated medically or surgically; to choose from alternatives such as remaining childfree, adopting, or attempting further therapies; and to work toward acceptance of their diagnosis as a couple or with others in a supportive group.

The purpose of this chapter is to provide the nursing practitioner with a knowledge base from which to assess, promote, and maintain the health of the infertile individual, especially the female client. An introduction to the problem of infertility will include definitions of fertility, infertility, and sterility; a description of the prevalence and known determinants of infertility; and a discussion of the sociocultural milieu in the United States as it influences the infertile woman and her partner. Next,

the approaches currently used for health assessment of the infertile couple will be reviewed. Finally, health maintenance and promotion strategies will be discussed, with an emphasis on those self–health care activities believed to be especially helpful for infertile individuals and couples. Because the focus of this text is on the health of women, primary emphasis will be given to the etiology, assessment, and treatment of the infertile woman.

DEFINITIONS

Fertility has been defined as the ability for a woman to conceive and give birth to a living infant or the ability for a man to impregnate. By definition, fertility can only be known after conception occurs. Fertility is usually presumed until it becomes evident that the individual is *not* fertile. Although there is currently available technology to effectively prevent pregnancy, as Menning (1977) states, "fertility is not a life force that may be turned on at will." (p. 4)

Infertility is regarded as the involuntary reduction in one's reproductive ability and is defined by most health professionals as the inability to conceive after a year or more of regular sexual intercourse. Some also include the inability to carry pregnancies to a live birth in the definition of infertility.

Infertility may be either primary or secondary. *Primary* infertility describes infertility in couples when there is no previous history of pregnancy. *Secondary* infertility implies that a couple has conceived at least once previously.

Sterility denotes the incapacity to conceive. It is usually reserved for the description of an individual who has some absolute known factor preventing procreation. Infertility is a relative term; sterility indicates an absolute.

INCIDENCE OF INFERTILITY

Although the incidence of infertility has not been systematically documented for the population of the United States, it is estimated that between 10% and 15% of all

257

couples are involuntarily infertile (Speroff et al., 1978; Menning, 1977). This represents as many as one of every six couples of childbearing age, or approximately 10 million Americans. Although these statistics may seem overwhelming, it is also estimated that about half of the couples who are evaluated and treated in major infertility clinics are likely to become pregnant. About 10% to 20% of the individuals who are determined to be medically healthy (that is, have a problem that cannot be diagnosed by current technologies) will remain infertile (Speroff et al., 1978).

Some attempts are being made to form infertility data registries. These data bases will allow evaluation of the techniques used for management of infertility (Rosenfeld et al., 1978).

DETERMINANTS OF INFERTILITY

In order to examine the determinants of infertility, it is important to recognize the processes essential for pregnancy as well as determinants of fertility. These topics will be explored prior to a discussion of the determinants of infertility.

Processes essential for pregnancy

There are several processes that appear to be essential for pregnancy to occur. The woman must ovulate a normal, fertilizable ovum, which has access within a few hours to a patent oviduct. The man must be able to produce sufficient numbers of normal, mature, motile spermatozoa that can be ejaculated from the urethra through patent pathways (i.e., the vas) into the woman's vagina. The spermatozoa must then survive the vaginal milieu as they travel to the cervix, pass through the cervical mucus, and ascend through the uterus into the oviduct at the time of the menstrual cycle appropriate for fertilization. The spermatozoa must also be able to penetrate and fertilize the ovum. After fertilization, the ovum must be able to move into the uterus, implant in a prepared endometrium, develop normally, and produce a glycoprotein gonadotropin capable of rescuing the corpus luteum (Warren, 1975).

Fertilization

Fertilization depends on the integration of a complex series of physiologic mechanisms that involve several structures. Three of the physiologic mechanisms that are especially important to consider when making infertility evaluations include: (1) ovum and sperm transport, (2) sperm capacitation, and (3) fertilization.

Ovum and sperm transport

Once ovulation has occurred, the egg adheres to the ovarian surface by means of the follicular cells until it is picked up by the fimbriae of the fallopian tube. The cilia of the fimbria move the ovum into the tube. The follicular cells appear necessary for the cilia to move the ovum effectively. Processes from the follicular cells also extend through the zona pellucida to the vitelline membrane of the ovum, possibly providing a mechanism for transfer of nutrients.

Sperm transport

Shortly after ejaculation semen forms a gel, but then is liquefied by prostatic enzymes in 20 to 30 minutes. The sperm are protected from the acid pH of the vagina by the alkaline pH of the semen; this, however, is transitory and within 2 hours most sperm left in the vagina are immobilized. The more motile sperm enter the cervical mucus; indeed, sperm have been noted in the cervical mucus within 90 seconds of ejaculation. Sperm have been found in the tubes 5 minutes after insemination. There is a substantial attrition of sperm from the vagina to the tube with fewer than 200 of the 200 million to 300 million ejaculated reaching close to the egg. The major loss occurs with expulsion of semen from the vaginal introitus, although sperm also are digested by vaginal enzymes, phagocytized along the reproductive tract, and even lost into the peritoneal cavity (Speroff, et al., 1978).

Sperm capacitation

Not only must sperm be motile and capable of surviving in the vaginal environment, they must also be capable of penetrating ova. Capacitation is a process that appears to alter the surface characteristics of the sperm such that there is decreased stability of the plasma membrane and the outer acrosomal membrane. In the vicinity of the ovum or follicular fluid, these membranes break down and merge, allowing the enzyme contents of the acrosome to be freed. It is believed that these enzymes, which include hyaluronidase, a neuramidinase-like factor, corona-dispersing enzyme, and a protease (acrosin), influence sperm penetration of the egg. While the sperm of some mammals must spend some hours in the female reproductive tract before they are capable of penetrating ova, this does not appear to be the case for humans (Speroff et al., 1978).

Fertilization

Usually fertilization occurs in the ampulla of the tube. Adherence of sperm to the egg is followed by their rapid passage through the zona. Enzymes appear to mediate the cell membrane fusion that permits the egg to engulf the sperm. When the sperm penetrates the egg, meiosis is completed and the zona becomes impervious to penetration by a second sperm. Transport of the egg from the fimbria to the junction of the ampulla and the isthmus may take only a few minutes to a few hours and is actively accomplished by segmental contractions of tubular musculature. Cilia in the tubes appear to play an important part in ovum transport. Usually the ovum passes into the uterus within 60 to 70 hours after ovulation.

The control mechanism for ovulation and ovum transport is thought to depend on fine tuning of estrogen and progesterone levels such that estrogen could cause the ovum to be maintained in the tube until the endometrium is in an advanced secretory state, and progesterone could trigger the release of the ovum into the uterus at the time that it also causes the endometrial morphology to change. The importance of the sympathetic nervous system and prostaglandins in ovum transport is yet to be elucidated (Speroff et al., 1978).

The ovum is not merely a passive participant in the process. Indeed, even prior to ovulation it is actively involved in protein synthesis. After fertilization the embryo produces a protein or other product that signals to the uterus to initiate implantation. The trophoblast appears to adhere independently of the participation of maternal tissues (Speroff et al., 1978).

Factors influencing fertility

There are several factors influencing the fertility of any couple. These include the age of the female, the age of the male, the frequency of intercourse, and the duration of exposure.

Age of the female. The woman's age is an important determinant of her fertility. At very young ages fertility is low, but it peaks at about 24 years of age and then declines, with rapid fall ensuing after age 30. These statistics probably reflect the patterns of the culture since this is the period when most persons establish their families. It is rare for pregnancy to occur after the woman is 50, and infertility is anticipated after menopause.

Age of the male. In men fertility reaches its peak at age 25 and declines thereafter. Fertility in aging males has been documented as late as the eighth and ninth decades but usually declines rapidly after age 40. Again, this may reflect cultural influences on the timing of pregnancy.

Frequency of intercourse. It appears that frequency of intercourse (with ejaculation) enhances fertility up to a point. Frequent ejaculation seems to enhance the potential fertility of semen inasmuch as it improves the degree and quality of motility of sperm. When age is held constant, the proportion of conceptions rises with frequency of intercourse. The optimal frequency for persons attempting conception appears to be four or more times per week. At this rate about 80% of couples who are 25 years of age are likely to conceive in a 6 month period (Warren, 1975). Yet most married couples report a frequency of intercourse less than this (about twice per week). There may be a frequency of intercourse that is excessive, depleting the number of available sperm

more quickly than it can be replenished. However, this has not been well documented.

Duration of exposure. As the duration of exposure increases, so does the likelihood of pregnancy, but again only to a point. Average couples who are not using contraceptive measures might expect to conceive at the following rates given varying durations of exposure (Behrman and Kistner, 1973):

Duration of exposure	Rate
1 month	25%
6 months	65%
9 months	75%
12 months	80%
18 months	90%

Couples who have not conceived after 4 or more years, even in the absence of demonstrable pathology, have a poor prognosis (Speroff et al., 1978).

Causes of infertility

There are many causes of infertility, some of which affect only men or women, and others that affect the couple as a unit. It is estimated that male factors account for about 40% of infertility problems, failure of ovulation for 10% to 15%, and tubal pathology for another 20% to 30%. In 5% a cervical factor can be implicated. In 10% to 20% of couples there will be no known cause for infertility (Speroff et al., 1978).

Causes in women

A summary of the causes of infertility in women is given in Table 14-1. Causes of infertility for women can be attributed to developmental anomalies, endocrine disturbances, and diseases of the genitals. In addition, infertility may be attributable in some instances to general factors such as nutritional disorders as well as to antispermatozoan antibody formation. The *processes* that most commonly interfere with female fertility include those that create a mechanical barrier to prevent union of the ovum and sperm; cause structural defects in the cervix or uterus; or interfere with the neuroendocrine events of the menstrual cycle. The role of stress in infertility remains unclear. Those causes of infertility most common in women will be discussed in greater detail.

Infection. Infection appears to be the leading cause of infertility in women; infectious processes lead to the formation of scar tissue and adhesions that can involve the uterus, tubes, ovaries, and peritoneal cavity. Pelvic inflammatory disease,* which can be caused by bacteria from internal as well as external sources, as well as syph-

---

*PID may be iatrogenic, as seen in women who contract pelvic infections attributable to an IUD.

Table 14-1. Causes of infertility in women

Tubal obstruction or dysfunction	Ovulation factors	Uterine factors	Cervical factors	Vaginal factors

Pelvic inflammatory disease
Tuberculosis
Puerperal infection
Endometriosis
Congenital anomalies
Peritonitis (from ruptured appendix or viscus or from surgery)
	Anovulation
	Inadequate corpus luteum
	Amenorrhea with low estrogen production
	Production of pathologic ova
	Ovarian tumors, Stein-Leventhal syndrome
	Ovarian endometriosis
	Genetic absence of follicular tissue
		Myomas
		  polyps,
		Developmental anomalies of the endometrial cavity
		Synechiae
		  Congenital absence of uterus
		  Endometritis
		Endometriosis
		Insufficient transformation of endometrium
		Neoplasms
		Infections
		Pelvic inflammatory disease
			Obstruction or stenosis of cervix from surgery or neoplasms
			Destruction of endocervical glands from surgery
			Chronic cervicitis
			Inadequate cervical mucus
				Congenital absence of vagina
				Imperforate hymen
				Vaginismus
				Vaginitis
				Hyperacidity of vaginal secretions

illis, may lead to problems similar to those created by gonorrhea (e.g., adhesions). Gonorrhea is highly destructive inasmuch as it is often asymptomatic in women. *T. mycoplasma* creates an asymptomatic infection that appears to interfere with fertility by a mechanism not well understood. Tuberculosis can lead to infertility, although it is not a common cause in the United States. Monilia and trichomoniasis do not appear to cause infertility.

Endometriosis. Endometriosis is a disease process in which endometrial cells that have become implanted in pelvic organs other than the uterine endometrium stimulate differentiation of the peritoneal lining cells into endometrial type tissue. This tissue responds to cyclic hormonal changes as does the endometrium of the uterus; because it bleeds at the normal time of menstruation it creates scarring and adhesions. It is most common in women past age 30 and may be accompanied by dysmenorrhea or dyspareunia (Warren, 1975).

Tubal factors. Obstruction or dysfunction of the tubes can be caused by postoperative pelvic adhesions and infectious processes, or surgical trauma such as that incurred with ectopic pregnancy.

Ovulatory problems. Ovulatory problems are manifested in three general classes: (1) ovulation failure in the presence of normal levels of estrogen; (2) amenorrhea with low estrogen and either low or high gonadotropin levels; and (3) inadequate corpus luteum. Although women may experience regular menstrual cycles, at times they do not ovulate at all or ovulate only irregularly. Ovulation failure is often marked by a history of erratic bleeding episodes, a monophasic basal body temperature (BBT) curve, and findings of a proliferative endo-

metrium just before the onset of menstrual bleeding. Hypoestrogenic, low gonadotropin amenorrhea is associated with a history of no bleeding, a flat BBT curve, little or no response to progesterone, a maturation index indicating little or no estrogen production, and a low-grade proliferative or atrophic endometrium on biopsy. The woman with an inadequate corpus luteum has a luteal phase that lasts about 10 days instead of 14, and an endometrial biopsy that shows the endometrium to be about 4 days behind its expected development at the onset of the menses. The woman who has low estrogen, high gonadotropin amenorrhea probably has ovaries that are bereft of follicles and therefore is likely to be sterile.

Women with polycystic ovaries encased in a tough fibrotic covering ovulate only irregularly or not at all, and have increased daily production of both estrogen and androgens.

Pituitary and hypothalamic tumors may lead to improper neurohormonal control mechanisms. Ovarian dysgenesis, or Turner's syndrome, occurs in women who receive only one half of their sex chromosome complement (X rather than XX). This is associated with congenital absence of the ovaries. Women with Turner's syndrome do not develop secondary sex characteristics or menstruate without hormonal therapy (Warren, 1975).

Uterine factors. In addition to endometriosis, which may affect the tubes, ovaries, and uterus, fibroid tumors, congenital malformation of the uterus, and extreme malposition may be associated with infertility. Minor flexion forward or backward is common and is not usually a cause of infertility. Retroversion of the uterus accompanied by adhesions that limit its mobility may, along with congenital malformations of the uterus, interfere

Table 14-2. Causes of infertility in men

Decreased production of spermatozoa	Abnormal semen	Ductal obstructions	Failure to transport spermatozoa to vagina
Varicocele	Volume low	Epididymis, postinfection	Ejaculatory disturbances
Testicular failure	Necrospermia and agglutination	Congenital absence of vas deferens	Hypospadias
Endocrine disorders	High viscosity	Postvasectomy	Sexual problems such as impotence
Cryptorchidism	Autoimmunity	Ejaculatory duct postinfection	
Other causes—stress, smoking, heat, systemic infections			

with pregnancy, but not usually with fertility. Lesions that distort or obliterate the endometrial cavity are most likely to cause infertility (Warren, 1975).

Cervical factors. Cervicitis, hostile or thick cervical mucus, or cervical obstruction from polyps or stenosis can be factors in infertility. The usual response of cervical mucus to the hormonal changes of the menstrual cycle was described in Chapter 6. Relaxation of the muscles around the cervix (sometimes referred to as cervical incompetence) has been implicated in second trimester abortion, although no evidence exists for a relationship between first trimester abortions and this problem.

Vaginal factors. Congenital absence of the vagina is often associated with absence of the uterus, although some women may have rudimentary uterine and endometrial tissue. Usually, the woman has normal ovaries and develops secondary sex characteristics. An artifical vagina can be constructed, which permits coitus. Imperforate hymen can be easily treated surgically. Vaginismus is treated by means of dilators and desensitization (see Chapter 9) (Warren, 1975). Hyperacidity of vaginal secretions may or may not be implicated in infertility (douching may alter the pH). Some forms of vaginal infection or lack of vaginal lubrication may limit the desire for intercourse because of discomfort.

Antibody problems. Antibodies can cause spermatozoa to be either immobilized or agglutinated. Sexual abstinence or intercourse with the use of a condom appears to lower the antibody titer in the serum of women who have positive results to sperm agglutinating tests.* There is some doubt as to the specificity of the sperm agglutinating antibodies; some believe the tests for immobilizing antibodies provide better estimates of immunologic reactions against sperm (Beer and Neaves, 1978; Speroff et al., 1978).

Causes in men

Causes of fertility disturbances in men are summarized in Table 14-2. Male fertility can be impaired by

*All contact with sperm, even oral genital contact, must be avoided for this to be effective.

processes that (1) interfere with spermatogenesis or maturation of sperm, (2) decrease the motility of the sperm, (3) obstruct transport of sperm from the testicles through the urethra, or (4) interfere with ejaculation of the sperm into the vagina.

Varicocele. Varicocele is a varicose vein usually occurring next to the left testicle. It is believed to interfere with sperm production because it causes the temperature in the testis to rise. An alternative explanation is that reflux blood flow from the adrenal inhibits sperm production and maturation. Ligation of the left internal spermatic artery leads to improved sperm count and motility in about 80% of cases.

Mumps. In adult males mumps is associated with testicular inflammation in more than half of the men who contract it. Bilateral atrophy from orchitis leads to sterility.

Infections. Infection of the prostate and epididymis can cause reduced sperm production. Venereal disease is more likely to be symptomatic in males than in females and thus more readily treated, although it is estimated that about 50% of males do not experience symptoms of urethritis with gonorrhea. However, damage to the ejaculatory ducts may occur as a result of the venereal diseases. Tuberculosis may damage the epididymis or vas. *T. mycoplasma* can be transmitted sexually.

Other causes. Febrile diseases, such as hepatitis and mononucleosis, can dramatically depress sperm production. Fortunately, this is a temporary phenomenon. *Cryptorchidism* (undescended testicles) can lead to permanent impairment of testicular function if not repaired prior to puberty. *Heat exposure* also impairs sperm maturation but usually can be reversed within 3 months after removal of the heat source. Saunas, steam baths, athletic supporters, long hot showers, and prolonged sitting, (e.g., office workers, truck drivers) may be heat sources.

Men also appear to produce *antibodies* against their own sperm, and this is believed to occur as a consequence of a trauma, vasectomy, or infection that permits sperm to enter surrounding tissues and precipitate an antigen-antibody reaction.

Table 14-3. Causes of infertility in both men and women

Stress
    Severe physical stress
    Severe psychic stress
    Long-standing psychiatric problems
Nutritional deficiencies
    Malnutrition
    Fat, mineral, or vitamin deficiencies
Exposure to toxic substances
    Chronic alcoholism
    Nicotine poisoning
    Metal poisoning (e.g., arsenic, lead)
    Dye poisoning (e.g., aniline)
    Drugs such as morphine, cocaine, quinine, some antineoplastic agents and hormones
    Radiation
Congenital anomalies
    Chromosomal aberrations (e.g., Klinefelter's and Turner's syndrome)
Immune responses
Disease processes
    Pituitary disturbances
    Thyroid malfunction
    Adrenal dysfunctions
    Severe cardiac disturbances
    Chronic nephritis
    Diabetes
    Anemia
Infectious processes
    Gonorrhea
    Tuberculosis

Causes of infertility in both men and women

Nutritional deficiencies, stress, exposure to toxic substances, congenital anomalies, disease processes, and immune and infectious processes are capable of interfering with fertility in both men and women. Some of the suspected correlates of infertility are given in Table 14-3.

Causes of infertility in the couple

There are approximately 20% of couples in which the problem leading to infertility cannot be attributed solely to the man or woman but to the couple. In some instances the problems affecting each individual are minor, but as a couple the individual problems are magnified, resulting in infertility. In other instances the problem arises because of interaction between the individuals. In the first instance, the woman who ovulates randomly may have a partner with a desire for infrequent sexual intercourse. A woman with thick cervical mucus might have a partner whose sperm has low motility. In the second instance the couple may experience immunologic reactions, for example, the woman may

Table 14-4. Causes of infertility in the couple

   I. Magnification of individual problems
  II. Couple problems
     A. Immunologic reaction
     B. Sexual problems
        1. Infrequent sexual intercourse
        2. Unconsummated relationship
        3. Sexual dysfunction
        4. Nonoptimal sexual technique

produce agglutinating or immobilizing antibodies to her partner's sperm.

Sexual problems may also interfere with fertility. The most obvious problem is that of infrequent sexual intercourse. For a number of reasons couples may not be optimizing their chances to conceive. Some will "save up sperm" until the time of the rise in BBT, thus missing the optimal time for fertilization. Others simply have such a low frequency of intercourse that conception becomes very unlikely. Intercourse on alternate days around the suspected time of ovulation probably gives optimal changes of conception.

In some instances the relationship may be *unconsummated.* This may be attributable to lack of information on the part of the couple or to sexual dysfunction in either partner. Vaginismus, a spasming of the muscles surrounding the introitus, and inability to attain an erection (impotence) or ejaculating so quickly that penetration is impossible are sexual dysfunctions that can be treated with a combination of psychotherapeutic techniques.

Nonoptimal sexual techniques for impregnation may include a wide range of behaviors. Position for intercourse may be a factor. The preferred position to facilitate conception in a woman with a normally positioned uterus is the woman supine with the man astride. The woman's thighs are flexed and her hips can be slightly elevated on a pillow. Having the man discontinue thrusting and keeping his penis inside the woman's vagina after he ejaculates is also recommended. The woman is often counseled to remain in bed with her hips elevated for about 30 minutes following intercourse. It is believed that this practice delivers the maximal number of sperm to the area around the cervix. Women who have a sharply flexed or tilted uterus may need to use other positions (e.g., having the man make entry with his penis from behind the woman). In some instances insemination using the husband's semen is necessary (Menning, 1977).

The use of lubricants such as petroleum jelly, jellies, or creams are discouraged because they all have slightly spermicidal effects. Saliva is an excellent natural lubricant that is readily available. The woman's own vaginal lubrication is usually quite adequate, providing that she receives appropriate stimulation.

The woman should not arise to urinate or douche for at least an hour after intercourse on days when conception is being attempted. Causes of infertility in the couple are summarized in Table 14-4.

SOCIOCULTURAL PERSPECTIVES

It is impossible to fully appreciate the infertile individual's experience without an awareness of how society and culture shape our expectations about fertility, parenting, family planning, and related issues. The popular myths about infertility reflect the influence of society and culture as well as religious influences.

Myths and misconceptions about infertility

There are a number of myths about infertility that are prevalent in the United States. Despite the fact that the causes of infertility are distributed about equally between men and women, it is often assumed that infertility is the woman's problem. Even in the face of evidence attributing most infertility to physical problems, many assume that a psychologic factor is at fault. Some believe that infertility is incurable or a sexual disorder, yet infertile couples are frequently able to eventually conceive, and most infertile people are able to experience the same range of sexual pleasure and physical response as fertile people. Finally, some believe that in view of the world's population problems it is irresponsible to attempt to have a child in spite of being infertile. "Zero population growth" implies that two people have a right to replace themselves; just as raising a single child or remaining childfree is a choice, infertility represents a denial of the right to choose for those couples desiring a child (Menning, 1977).

Religious influences

Earliest forms of worship directed their attention to mother-goddesses. Woman's ability to bear children and suckle and raise young, as well as her mysterious monthly cycles, caused her to be held in awe. Even after it was determined that men played an important role in reproduction, worship of a mother-goddess persisted.

In some religions there is an obvious connection between fertility and worthiness. Infertility was seen as a punishment from a vengeful god and subsequent pregnancy a favor of the deity.

Some religions that were influenced by more recent moral codes about sexuality prohibit intercourse with a lawful wife if conception is in any way prevented. The Roman Catholic Church not only prohibits some means of birth control as well as abortion, but it also prohibits homosexuality, masturbation, and donor insemination. Orthodox Judaism takes a firm stand on some of these practices as well. Sexual pleasure, though sinful, apparently can be vindicated if a child is produced.

Some religions teach that childbirth is necessary for a woman's salvation; in some a marriage can be annulled if the woman proves infertile, although the reverse is not the case if the man proves infertile (Menning, 1977).

It is easy to see how the religious influence on fertility can account for many of the attitudes toward a childless couple.

Sociocultural influences

Culture is the body of transmittable patterns for living or normative standards that guide social behavior. The culture into which we are born and the culture in which we live our adult lives have a pervasive influence on our values and attitudes. Institutions are influenced by the culture and thereby transmit important elements of the culture to society. The influence of culture and society in the infertile individual or couple is significant.

Public opinion, the law, education, customs, art, literature, and psychoanalytic psychology all appear favorable to motherhood and "the family" as well as fostering dual sets of expectations for girls and boys (Menning, 1977).

Pronatalism

The belief that everyone should have children is widely held in American society. Most of the social structure is family-centered, with a great deal of emphasis being placed on the "normal" family, consisting of a mother, father, and child. Parenthood is held out as an ideal, but simultaneously regarded with awe and perhaps dread. There is pride in having produced a child, yet admonitions abound regarding parenthood being a "time to settle down."

In cultures everywhere there have always been symbols and rites celebrating fertility. Although the current symbols are perhaps more subtle than the phallic symbols or fertility dolls used to enhance fertility in other cultures, they are nevertheless present. In addition, there are still rituals connected with fertility. Though not as apparent a fertility ritual as those celebrating the fertility of the harvest or the birth of a child, the custom of throwing rice at the bride and groom is a vestige of an old fertility custom. The cigars passed out by a new father as well as the baby showers held in anticipation of the child's birth are contemporary ways of celebrating fertility. Last but not least is the image of motherhood—not worshipped as an icon as in the ancient cultures, but paid homage in the communications media of the United States.

Contraception mentality

This is the era of the "planned family." Couples or singles now commonly choose when to be fertile. Because of the contraceptive technology now available, individuals can regard their fertility as a phenomenon under their control, to be activated at the desired time. Imagine the response by the couple who carefully used contraceptive methods for several years, waiting until the moment when they felt ready to be parents, as they discover they are infertile:

I had religiously taken the pill for 5 years, rarely missing a day. I had fantasized that as soon as I quit taking the pill I would get pregnant. For the first few cycles I was not too surprised when my menstrual period started. After about six months I began feeling more and more disappointed. It was beginning to occur to me that I might be unable to become pregnant, to have a child. After all those years of rigorous prevention that was quite a shock! We had planned things so that we would be well established in our careers and on solid ground financially before having any children. I was angry that our plans were not fulfilled, guilty that it might be my fault, and sad about my inability to be a parent.

I never imagined this would happen to us. I was always busy worrying how to avoid a pregnancy. When I finally felt ready to be a father, fatherhood was much more elusive than I ever imagined.

The family planning mentality not only affects infertile couples, it also pervades most of their social network. It is often assumed by others that not being a parent is a decision made voluntarily. As a result most people are not sensitive to the feelings of the infertile individual or couple, particularly when they are unaware of their infertility. Having a menstrual period has very different meanings for the woman who is infertile compared with the woman who is actively practicing contraception; for the first woman the event may elicit despair, for the latter, relief. It is not surprising that it may be difficult for one to feel empathy for the other.

HEALTH ASSESSMENT OF THE INFERTILE COUPLE

A thorough assessment of the couple who has been unable to conceive after a year of regular intercourse with no contraception should be initiated at their request. For couples who are over 30 years of age, such an investigation might be warranted earlier. The purposes of the infertility assessment are to determine the diagnosis, establish a prognosis, and provide a basis for medical intervention and a plan for health promotion and maintenance acceptable to the infertile individuals.

An important component of an infertility assessment is provision of adequate information to the couple so that they are able to make well-informed choices. Such information is essential in view of the general misinformation and mythology about infertility. Another component of the assessment process is obtaining a data base for counseling the individual or couple regarding when

further investigation will not be useful, and at what point alternatives to having their biologic child need to be considered.

Although women are likely to seek assistance from a gynecologist or nurse practitioner in dealing with infertility, it is essential that the male partner involve himself in the assessment process and plans for medical therapy as well as plans for health promotion and maintenance. Usually, the assessment phase is lengthy, lasting from 6 months to a few years. Although this may often mean a lengthy and expensive course of assessment procedures and attempts at treatment, it also affords the couple and the clinician the opportunity to interact over a long time period. The importance of the helping relationship between a nurse and clients cannot be underestimated.

The initial contact
Establishing rapport

The initial interview of an infertility assessment is frequently initiated by the woman. Many health professionals prefer to begin their relationship with the *couple* and recommend that the male partner be included in the initial interview if at all possible. The male partner not only can contribute information but also will realize that he and his female partner are *both* involved in the assessment and consequently may be less reluctant to request information or participate in the assessment and treatment.

This interview is likely to be a particularly stressful episode for the individuals involved. Initiating contact with a health professional often is the first opportunity the individual has for confronting his or her feelings about being infertile. It is not uncommon for the woman seeking an infertility assessment to share a waiting room with obstetric clients who are very obviously pregnant. Therefore, for a number of reasons, the infertile individual or couple may approach the first interview with anxiety.

In order to pursue the questions essential for a complete infertility assessment, it is important that the clinician attempt to establish a working relationship with the couple. A few minutes devoted to getting to know them as individuals is necessary before proceeding wtih an interview that deals with highly personal and emotionally laden issues. Assurance of privacy for the interview and confidentially can make this part of the assessment comfortable.

Data collection

The data obtained during the first clinic visit are likely to include information obtained at the interview as well as the results of a physical examination of one or both partners. During the initial interview the couple will be requested to provide data about their sexual knowledge and practices, their past sexual, contraceptive, reproductive, and urogenital history, exposure to environmental agents that may cause infertility, and their psychosocial status.

The interview. Some of the same guidelines used in interviewing a client with a sexual concern might profitably be applied to the conduct of the initial interview with the infertile couple, since both types of interviews deal with intimate and emotion-laden information (see Chapter 9). Provision of privacy and confidentiality are important. The individuals may benefit from being interviewed privately, especially when it is necessary for one individual to discuss feelings he or she is unable to share with the partner. Progressing from less threatening to more threatening topics allows the couple to feel comfortable with the clinician before revealing intimate information. An outline of the types of data obtained in the interview is found in Table 14-5.

Throughout the interview, infertility is regarded as a *symptom.* The purpose of the interview and subsequent portions of the assessment is to elicit abnormalities in the anatomy or physiology of the reproductive systems of either or both partners. At the same time, the clinician seeks an appraisal of behavioral causes of infertility, such as the clients' sexual practices, and the couple's ability to cope with their problem.

The first portion of the history format includes identifying data that give the clinician some insights about the client as an individual within relevant family, community, and social systems. The statement of the problem is obtained in the client's own words. Of special importance are the client's notions about the cause and maintenance of the problem and attempts at therapy. Some clients are especially well informed and can provide a wealth of data regarding observations they have made about their own health. On the other hand, the individual's attempts at self-help may be based on misinformation. Data on past physical health emphasize the gynecologic and obstetric history for the female and urogenital history for the male. These data do not, however, preclude a careful assessment of general health.

Table 14-5. Data obtained during the initial interview for assessment of infertility

I. Identifying information: name, sex, age, education, marital status, occupation, religion, family composition or significant others, community, ethnocultural influences, environmental exposures

II. Statement of the problem
   A. Client's description in own words
   B. Onset and duration of the problem
   C. Clients' concept of the cause and maintenance of the problem
   D. Past attempts at therapy
      1. Self-treatment
      2. Professional assistance
   E. Precipitating events that led client to seek assistance at this time
   F. Current expectations of treatment and goals for treatment

III. Data on past related physical health
   A. Female
      1. Gynecologic history
         a. Menstruation: menarche, interval, duration, last menstrual period, regularity of menstrual periods, symptoms associated with menstrual cycle phase (e.g., mittelschmerz, dysmenorrhea, watery vaginal discharge at midcycle, prodromal signs of menstruation, cramping)
         b. Contraceptive history:
            (1) Use of oral contraceptives, intrauterine devices, etc., duration and patterns of use
            (2) Effectiveness of contraception
            (3) Complications of contraceptive methods (e.g., infection)
         c. History of infectious diseases involving the pelvis, vagina, cervix:
            (1) Pelvic inflammatory disease
            (2) Venereal diseases
            (3) Peritonitis (e.g., from ruptured appendix)
         d. Awareness of other gynecologic problems
            (1) Congenital anomalies
            (2) Endometriosis
            (3) History of surgery to the reproductive organs (e.g., hysterectomy, cervical surgery)
      2. Obstetric history
         a. Past history of pregnancies: number, dates, outcomes, spontaneous abortions, miscarriages, stillborn infants
         b. Responses to obstetric events (e.g., satisfaction with living children, grief over abortions or stillbirths)
         c. Obstetric complications (e.g., infections, obstetric lacerations)
         d. History of elective abortions: dates, reasons for abortions, complications of the procedure, feelings about abortion
   B. Male: urogenital history
   C. Assessment of general status (may be done by referring professional) including:
      1. Past therapies
         a. Surgeries
         b. Hospitalizations
         c. Drug reactions, allergies, and immunizations (especially rubella if titer warrants it)
      2. Family history of disease, cause of death

Continued.

Table 14-5. Data obtained during the initial interview for assessment of infertility—cont'd

---

   3. Other systems
     a. Cardiovascular and hematopoietic
     b. Respiratory, including mouth, throat, larynx
     c. Gastrointestinal
     d. Urinary
     e. Endocrine
     f. Musculoskeletal
     g. Nervous
     h. Integumentary
     i. Mental health
IV. Environmental exposure
  A. Personal exposure
    1. Alcohol
    2. Nicotine
    3. Other drugs (see Table 14-3)
  B. Hazards of the work environment or iatrogenic exposure
    1. Metals (e.g., arsenic)
    2. Dyes (e.g., analine)
    3. Drugs
    4. Radiation
  C. Stress
    1. Physical
    2. Psychic
V. Sexual practices and knowledge
  A. Sexual information (where obtained, from whom, how adequate?)
  B. Influence of religious, educational, and social factors on sexual value system
  C. Current sexual practice
    1. Frequency of intercourse
    2. Duration of exposure
    3. Use of lubricants
    4. Positions used

    5. Postcoital activities (e.g., douching, arising immediately after intercourse)
    6. Satisfaction with sexual relationship; ability to discuss desires with one another
    7. Areas of concern about sexual relationship (e.g., anorgasmic or partner impotent)
  D. Sexual involvement with other partners; pregnancies; other outcomes
  E. Awareness of sexual practices that are optimal for conception
    1. Frequency of intercourse
    2. Duration of exposure
    3. Timing of intercourse to coincide with ovulation
    4. Use of lubricants discouraged
    5. Use of female supine position
    6. How to deal with deadlines (e.g., when to have intercourse)
VI. Coping with infertility
  A. Perception of problem
    1. Meaning of ability or inability to have a child
    2. Beliefs and values; motivations for pregnancy; expectations for childbearing and childrearing from the couple's parents
  B. Response to infertility
    1. Emotional
    2. Problem-solving
  C. Factors influencing ability to cope with infertility
    1. Usual coping mechanisms (e.g., denial, try harder, intellectualize)
    2. Support systems
     a. Partner
     b. Family
     c. Significant others
     d. Attachments to supportive groups

Careful documentation of environmental exposures and personal habits influencing fertility is followed by a sexual history and assessment of sexual knowledge. Coping with infertility is of primary concern to the individuals seeking help. An extremely important component of the health assessment includes the client's perception of the problem, response to infertility, and factors influencing the client's ability to cope not only with infertility but also with the assessment and therapy to follow.

Although the data base described here may appear unnecessarily extensive, obtaining a complete data base at the initial interview may prevent unnecessary testing later. For example, being aware of simple sexual problems such as misinformation about the timing of intercourse may make further procedures unnecessary.

Physical examination. A physical examination usually follows the initial assessment. Of special interest during the physical examination are:

1. General health state
2. Development of secondary sex characteristics
3. Presence, size, position, and condition of the reproductive organs
4. Signs of infection or other disease processes related to infertility

Examination of the woman. The infertile woman will have many pelvic examinations. An assessment of her previous experiences may be helpful in determining positive approaches for her. The first examination she has can set the stage for her future experiences. Ensuring that the woman has the opportunity to be in control during the first examination is extremely important. The practitioner can share control by extending options to the woman such as: use of drapes, presence of a chaperone during the examinations, use of a lighted speculum and mirror so the woman can observe, presence of her partner, and position of the table (e.g., whether she would prefer to have the head of the table elevated). The woman can also be informed that at any time she can ask that the examination be interrupted for questions or because of discomfort.

At the first examination, the practitioner can explain the examination to the woman while she is dressed, and only then proceed with the pelvic examination. Adequate time should be allowed after the examination for discussion of findings. The woman needs to be advised that other practitioners may be examining her during the course of the assessment, especially if this is a teaching institution. She should also be aware that she can share her preferences with other practitoners. A summary of the pertinent physical findings for the female client is given in Table 14-6.

Examination of the man. The physical examination for the male client includes a similar emphasis on the male reproductive organs, endocrinopathy, other secondary sex characteristics, and congenital anomalies. This examination may be performed by a urologist from another clinic or practice. In this instance coordination of the diagnostic processes is especially important.

Further assessment of the infertile couple

As shown in Fig. 14-1, the assessment of infertility in the female has been much better refined than that for the male as indicated by the number of tests that have been developed for screening the woman. Unless there is obvious pathology in the male partner, infertility assessment is limited to evaluation of sperm production and viability and ascertaining the presence or absence of obstructions in the male reproductive tract that could interfere with ejaculation.

Assessment of the male partner

The first step in an infertility assessment should be a semen analysis. It is a relatively simple, low-risk procedure and may preclude the unnecessary exposure of the female partner to higher-risk procedures.

Semen analysis. The total ejaculate is usually collected by means of masturbation or coitus interruptus. The semen is collected into a clean, dry, glass container. Prior to obtaining the semen specimen, the man is usually instructed to abstain from intercourse for a period corresponding to his usual frequency of intercourse. Usually, the specimen must be kept at body temperature and examined as soon after ejaculation as possible (preferably no longer than 2 or 3 hours later). This may cause the male partner to experience difficulty, even inability, to have an erection because of anxiety about timing. It is not usually acceptable for the specimen to be brought to the laboratory except during business hours, and it is sometimes impossible for the man to masturbate to ejaculation in the examining room of the clinic.

Table 14-6. Summary of physical findings useful in assessment of infertile female client

1. General health status
   a. Habitus and contours
   b. Thyroid size
   c. Hair distribution
   d. Abdominal scars
2. Vagina
   a. Presence or absence of vagina; imperforate hymen
   b. Vaginismus
   c. Presence of a vaginal septum
   d. Signs of vaginitis
3. Cervix and uterus
   a. Presence or absence of cervix
   b. Evidence of previous surgery
   c. Presence or absence of cervical mucus, adequacy
   d. Cervix open at midcycle
   e. Presence or absence of uterus
   f. Size, shape, position, fixation of uterus
   g. Evidence of unknown or forgotten IUD
   h. Presence of tender uterosacral nodules on rectovaginal examination (possible sign of endometriosis)
4. Tubes
   a. Tubal enlargement
   b. Tenderness on palpation
5. Ovaries
   a. Size
   b. Mobile or fixed

The ejaculate will be inspected for sperm motility. At least 40% of the sperm should demonstrate good forward progression, and 60% should be motile. The sperm should be greater than 20 million per milliliter. The semen volume should range from 2 to 5 ml; 60% to 80% of the sperm heads in the count should be normal in appearance. The semen should liquefy within 10 to 45 minutes.

Other tests. At times a split ejaculate may be required. Semen is collected in the same way as described before, except that the first portion of the ejaculate is collected in one container and the second portion in another container. This is done because seminal emission entails discharge of sequential fractions, some of which come from the urethral and bulbourethral glands, prostatic secretions, testicular and epididymal secretions, and seminal vesicle secretions. The specimens are analyzed to determine if ejaculation shows a normal sequence, sperm concentration, and levels of citric acid, nucleic acid, acid phosphatase, and fructose.

Male clients may also require testicular biopsy if they are azoospermic; urethral calibration, cystourethroscopy, and vasography may also be done. Evaluation of the male client who requires more extensive assessment than a semen analysis is commonly conducted by a urologist. Currently, studies of sperm penetration of mammal

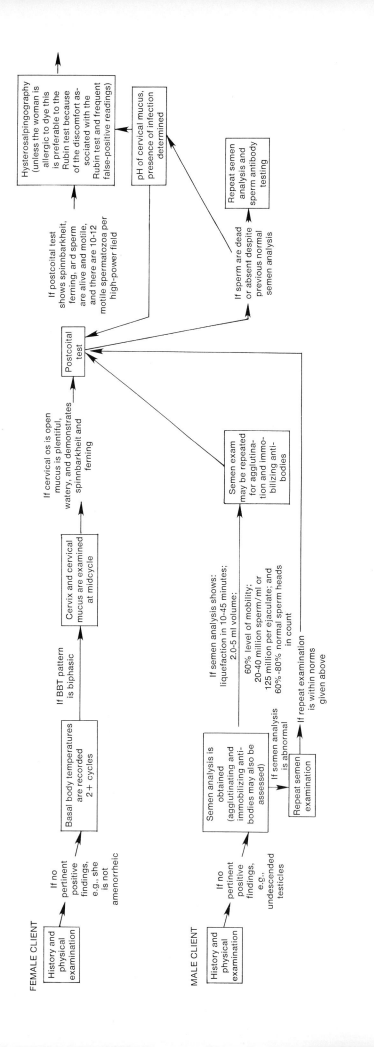
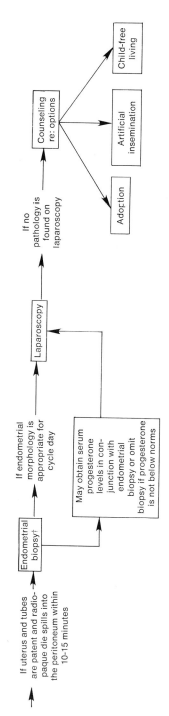

Fig. 14-1. An approach to assessing the infertile couple.

FEMALE CLIENT

History and physical examination

If no pertinent positive findings, e.g., she is not amenorrheic

Basal body temperatures are recorded 2+ cycles

If BBT pattern is biphasic

Cervix and cervical mucus are examined at midcycle

If cervical os is open mucus is plentiful, watery, and demonstrates spinnbarkheit and ferning

Postcoital test

If postcoital test shows spinnbarkheit, ferning, ard sperm are alive and motile, and there are 10-12 motile spermatozoa per high-power field

Hysterosalpingography (unless the woman is allergic to dye this is preferable to the Rubin test because of the discomfort associated with the Rubin test and frequent false-positive readings)

pH of cervical mucus, presence of infection determined

If sperm are dead or absent despite previous normal semen analysis

Repeat semen analysis and sperm antibody testing

MALE CLIENT

History and physical examination

If no pertinent positive findings, e.g., undescended testicles

Semen analysis is obtained (agglutinating and immobilizing antibodies may also be assessed)

If semen analysis shows: liquefaction in 10-45 minutes; 2.0-5 ml volume; 60% level of mobility; 20-40 million sperm/ml or 125 million per ejaculate; and 60%-80% normal sperm heads in count

Semen exam may be repeated for agglutination and immobilizing antibodies

If semen analysis is abnormal

Repeat semen examination

If repeat examination is within norms given above

If uterus and tubes are patent and radiopaque die spills into the peritoneum within 10-15 minutes

Endometrial biopsy†

If endometrial morphology is appropriate for cycle day

May obtain serum progesterone levels in conjunction with endometrial biopsy or omit biopsy if progesterone is not below norms

Laparoscopy

If no pathology is found on laparoscopy

Counseling re: options

Adoption

Artificial insemination

Child-free living

ova are underway. This assay may provide another assessment method for infertile men. For further discussion of therapy see Amelar and Dubin, 1973; Behrman and Kistner, 1975; and Kremer, 1977.

Assessment of the female partner

The options for further assessment of the woman who presents with infertility are more numerous and refined than those for the male. The reason for this is perhaps because more is known about the processes necessary for pregnancy to occur in the woman than is known about spermatogenesis and transport in the male; also, the fact that infertility is often assumed to be a problem of the female may be responsible for this phenomenon. The approach to assessment described in Fig. 14-1 assumes that the woman is menstruating. If she has amenorrhea, then hormonal analysis would be done to determine if she has normal estrogen levels and low or high gonadotropin levels.

Basal body temperature (BBT) charting. The basal body temperature chart is the most common means of initial assessment of fertility in the woman. It requires little risk, is inexpensive, and contributes some evidence about the woman's ovulatory status. The woman is usually instructed to take an oral temperature every day before rising at about the same time. (Some practitioners may recommend a rectal measurement because of its greater accuracy.) During an ovulatory cycle the body temperature should be lowest during the immediate postmenstrual period, and drops to its lowest point at the time of ovulation; this is followed by a rise of nearly 1° during the ovulatory phase, which is maintained during the premenstrual phase of the cycle, though it may dip slightly before the onset of menstruation.

The use of the BBT is helpful inasmuch as it provides indirect confirmatory evidence of ovulation. It does not, however, pinpoint the exact day of ovulation. Usually, a significant increase in temperature is not noted until about 2 days after the LH peak, coinciding with a rise in peripheral levels of progesterone. It is believed that physical release of the ovum probably occurs on the day prior to the time of the first temperature elevation. If an approximate time of ovulation can be determined from temperature charts, the couple is instructed to attempt coitus every other day for 3 to 4 days before expected ovulation, and for 2 to 3 days after ovulation. It is estimated that sperm retain their ability to fertilize for 24 to 48 hours and that an ovum is fertilizable for 12 to 24 hours. For some individuals, the scheduling of coitus precipitates sufficient anxiety to inhibit sexual behavior or interfere with pleasure.

Examination of the cervix and cervical mucus. Often the practitioner will suggest examination of the cervix and cervical mucus at midcycle. This can be carried out in conjunction with the pelvic examination. The purpose of this examination is to obtain additional documentation suggestive of follicular development and ovulation as well as to determine that cervical factors are adequate. Women who are currently involved in the self–health care movement or who are interested in learning to examine their own cervix may prefer to be involved in this examination. Use of a mirror and a light source can permit the woman to visualize her cervix and cervical mucus and allow her to contribute further information to the practitioner. For example, women who perform their own pelvic examinations have baseline data about the usual appearance of the cervix and can inform the practitioner about any observed deviations from the usual appearance. At midcycle the cervical os should be open, sometimes described as pouting. The cervical mucus should be thin, watery, and plentiful. Inspection of the mucus for spinnbarkheit is usually performed (see Chapter 6). In addition, the clear, watery, abundant cervical mucus characteristic of midcycle should demonstrate a ferning or arborization pattern when dried on a slide (Fig. 5-21, p. 88). The cervical mucus contains chains of glycoproteins that line up in parallel at midcycle to create channels through which sperm can migrate. The Ovutimer, a device that quantifies the viscosity of cervical mucus, may be available soon and can be used for timing ovulation.

Postcoital test. The postcoital test is a low-risk kind of assessment that provides information about both male and female factors. The couple is told to abstain from intercourse for 48 hours before the test and to have intercourse within 8 hours of the test. The woman may shower but should not take a tub bath between the time she has intercourse and the test. The test is usually performed about the expected time of ovulation as determined by previous BBT charts or from the length of prior menstrual cycles. Cervical mucus is removed with a nasal polyp forceps within 3 to 24 hours after intercourse (but ideally not longer than 8 hours after intercourse has occurred) and is subsequently examined for macro- and microscopic characteristics. If sperm are found in the cervical mucus, it probably indicates that coital technique is adequate and the pH of the cervical mucus is supportive to sperm; the pregnancy rate is likely to be higher than if all the sperm are immotile. If there are more than 20 sperm, the man is likely to have a sperm count above 20 million per milliliter.* If the mucus is clear and abundant with good spinnbarkheit, the woman has a better chance for pregnancy than if it were thick and sparse (Speroff et al., 1978).

Hysterosalpingography. The tubal insufflation test

---

*The postcoital test is not advocated as a substitution for the semen analysis, since the morphology of sperm found in the cervical mucus is usually less abnormal than those in the total ejaculate.

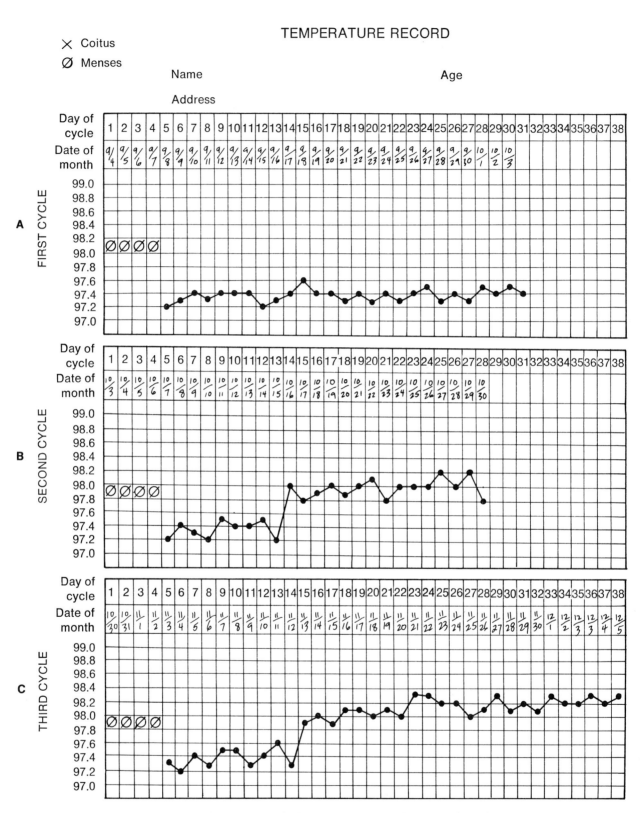

Fig. 14-2. A, Monophasic BBT; **B,** biphasic BBT; **C,** BBT chart showing early pregnancy.

(Rubin test), a procedure in which carbon dioxide gas is passed through the cervix to the uterus and tubes, has become a less preferred method for determining tubal patency because of the discomfort associated with it and also because of frequent false positive readings. The Rubin test, however, is more convenient than hysterosalpingography because it can be performed in the clinic and does not require the patient to be exposed to radiation.

Hysterosalpinogography is used for those women who are not allergic to the dye used for the X-ray study. The study is performed 2 to 6 days following menstrual flow and thus decreases the possibility of flushing a fertilized ovum out of the tube and into the peritoneal cavity. A water-soluble radiopaque substance (iodine) or oil medium is injected through a cannula inserted into the cervix, through the uterus and tubes, and spills into the peritoneum within 10 to 15 minutes. Usually, only three films are necessary: one before injection of the dye, one showing spill of the dye from one or both of the tubes, and a later film to show spread of the dye through the peritoneal cavity. Only 3 to 6 ml of dye is needed, but if the woman complains of cramping, the injection can be stopped for a few minutes and the fluoroscopy may be temporarily discontinued. Some speculation exists about the potential therapeutic effects of hysterosalpingography. It may:

1. Mechanically lavage the tubes, dislodging mucous plugs
2. Straighten the tubes and break down peritoneal adhesions
3. Stimulate the cilia of the tubes
4. Improve the cervical mucus
5. Exert a bacteriostatic effect on the mucous membranes (from the iodine) (Speroff et al., 1978)

Whatever the therapeutic effects of the procedure, it requires the woman to come to the radiology department rather than the clinic, and perhaps to be premedicated. After the procedure the woman may experience shoulder pain, indicative of subphrenic irritation from the dye. This may be acute, but it usually subsides with change of position and should disappear within 12 to 24 hours. The woman should be cautioned that the pain and/or premedication may interfere with her ability to drive an automobile. Therefore, she will require someone to transport her home from the clinic. Because some of the dye is not absorbed, the woman can be given a perineal pad after the hysterosalpingogram to prevent staining of her clothing.

Endometrial biopsy. Endometrial biopsy is obtained late in the menstrual cycle, just prior to menstruation, to assess the function of the corpus luteum and the state of the endometrium for implantation. It may be done during dilation and curettage with general anesthesia, or preferably a specimen may be taken by means of mini-curette in the clinic. A small piece of endometrium is removed for examination and assessment for presence of tuberculosis, but more commonly the influence of progesterone on the corpus luteum. The procedure is painful, and usually the woman experiences cramping during the biopsy and for a few minutes thereafter. Many infertility specialists obtain a plasma progesterone level instead of the endometrial biopsy. To prevent inadvertent abortion, couples can be instructed to abstain from intercourse during the "fertile" period of the woman's cycle.

Laparoscopy. Laparoscopy is often the final diagnostic procedure in an infertility assessment. If results of the hysterosalpingogram are normal, some specialists recommend waiting for 6 months to do a laparoscopy in order to allow time for any fertility-enhancing potential of the X-ray procedure to take effect. The laparoscopy is done during the luteal phase of the cycle, but women taking clomiphene or other ovulation-induction therapy may have the laparoscopy performed on day 14 or 15 to assess whether ovulation occurred. The laparoscope is inserted through a small incision made near the umbilicus. Another stab wound is made above the pubic area to allow carbon dioxide insufflation of the peritoneal cavity. Although general anesthesia may be used, the procedure has successfully been carried out using local anesthesia in conjunction with muscle relaxants and minimal premedication. During the laparoscopy, methylene blue dye can be passed through the cervix, uterus, fallopian tubes, and into the peritoneal cavity if the reproductive tract is patent. Laparoscopy permits direct visualization of cysts, endometriosis, adhesions, tumors, and other obstructions or abnormalities. Ovarian and endometrial biopsies may be taken at the same time. Lysis of some adhesions can be accomplished with local anesthesia, though more involved surgery would warrant general anesthesia. Laparoscopy is not without risk, and complications may include subcutaneous dissection of carbon dioxide, perforation of a viscus, intraabdominal hemorrhage, and cardiac arrhythmias. Following laparoscopy, the woman usually requires a small dressing over both incisions.

Hormone analysis. Serum progesterone levels have been used to confirm the presence of ovulation and normal corpus luteum function. Estrogen levels and FSH and LH determinations may be made to assess whether the woman is hypoestrogenic and has high or low gonadotropin levels. Assessment of urinary 17-ketosteroids and 17-hydroxycorticosteroids is also done to determine endocrine function.

Assessment of couple factors

There are three factors that could be considered "couple" factors rather than exclusively male or female factors. These include: immunologic incompatibilities,

T. mycoplasma infections, and sexual behavior patterns.

Immunologic incompatibilities. Of couples with no demonstrable cause of infertility, a high proportion have evidence of circulating antibodies to sperm. Sexual abstinence or use of a condom by the husband for 2 to 6 months can lower the antibody titer. Sperm antibodies can be present despite postcoital testing that demonstrates adequate numbers of motile sperm. There appear to be antibodies present in cervical mucus, and possibly cervical and endometrial tissue. Agglutination of sperm in semen caused by autoimmunity is seen rarely, and there does not seem to be any effective treatment (Speroff et al., 1978).

T. mycoplasma. *T. mycoplasma* is found in the cervical mucus and semen of infertile men and women as well as in couples having habitual abortions more frequently than it is found in fertile couples. This is a new area of investigation and therapy with doxycycline is still controversial (Speroff et al., 1978).

Sexual behavior patterns. Some sexual behavior patterns that contribute to infertility may not be disclosed during the initial interview. The woman may feel comfortable discussing dyspareunia or vaginismus in a later interview. Inability to have an erection, ejaculation into the bladder rather than through the urethra (retrograde ejaculation), depressed libido, and increased or decreased frequency of intercourse may interfere with the male partner's fertility. Impotence may be triggered by anxiety regarding testing procedures that demand performance at a prescribed time. Retrograde ejaculation is associated with some metabolic and neurologic disorders. Depressed libido can be associated with any number of life stressors, drugs, or diseases. Alcohol may be used for "relaxation," but it may cause the male partner to experience difficulty in having an erection. Sometimes a couple will purposefully avoid intercourse in order to "save up sperm" for the ovulatory phase of the woman's cycle. This practice may have deleterious effects on the motility of sperm because of the increased proportion of older sperm. However, if intercourse occurs daily or more frequently, sperm counts may be depressed because of frequent ejaculation.

The "normal" infertile couple

The "normal" infertile couple, according to Behrman and Kistner (1973), "are not normal or they would not have an infertility problem, yet they are the most poorly managed patients. They must, then, *not be allowed to leave the office with the impression that they are normal.*" (p. 3) The infertile couple for whom no *medical* diagnosis can be made should not be given inflated hopes for fertility. In the zealous attempt to convey this information, however, health professionals need not deemphasize the health of these individuals, for most are quite well in every other aspect.

Table 14-7. Interferences with fertility inferred from diagnostic tests

1. Findings suggestive of follicular development, ovulation
   a. BBTs are biphasic
   b. Elevation of BBT persists for 12 days
   c. Cervical mucus is copious, watery; demonstrates spinnbarkheit and arborization
   d. Endometrial biopsy shows secretory endometrium
   e. Laparoscopic documentation of follicular development
2. Findings suggestive that cervical factors are supportive of pregnancy
   a. Cervix open at midcycle and cervical mucus is copious and demonstrates good spinnbarkheit and arborization
   b. Postcoital test is satisfactory
3. Findings suggestive that tubal and uterine factors are supportive of pregnancy
   a. Hysterosalpingography demonstrates spill of radiopaque dye into peritoneum
   b. Laparoscopic documentation rules out peritubal adhesions, silent endometriosis
4. Findings suggestive that luteal phase is supportive of pregnancy
   a. Plasma progesterone levels during luteal phase are at levels consistent to sustain early pregnancy
   b. Endometrial biopsy consistent with day of cycle
5. Findings suggestive of normal sperm production
   a. Ejaculate contains adequate numbers of sperm
   b. Sperm morphology is normal
   c. Sperm are motile
6. Findings suggestive of normal sperm transport
   a. Postcoital test demonstrates adequate numbers of live, motile sperm
   b. Semen sample demonstrates adequate numbers of true, motile sperm

One disastrous consequence of an undiagnosed cause for infertility is the assumption by the clinician, significant others, and the couple themselves that their problem must be of psychologic origin. Visible signs of anxiety, depression, and frustration are often imputed to be the cause of infertility. Yet the assessment process and the problem itself is likely to elicit these same emotions as responses! Some psychotherapists interpret the "normal" infertile couple situation as caused by their subconscious wish to avoid pregnancy. If this were the case, unwanted pregnancies could be prevented by mere volition! At times, the frustrations of the clinicians who work with infertile couples interfere with their objectivity. Clinicians (who are human also) sometimes tend to deal with their own frustrations by avoiding discussion of the psychosocial aspects of infertility, such as the couple's feelings, or by "blaming the victim" rather than merely stating that they have been unable to define a cause of infertility and therefore can offer no treatment. The admission of inability to diagnose and treat requires that the clinician admit that at the current state of the art she or he cannot help the couple.

Just as the clinician might have difficulty ending the quest for a diagnosis, so may the couple. Often these couples need to be supported in deciding that they have had enough cycles of hope and despair and that the time has come to experience their loss and grieve. Sometimes the most difficult step is saying "Enough!"

Data analysis

The results of the diagnostic tests used for infertility assessment are reviewed to determine what, if any, interferences with fertility are present. The inferences that can be made from the various tests are summarized in Table 14-7.

HEALTH PROMOTION AND MAINTENANCE
Prevention of infertility

Prevention of infertility can be achieved in some measure through integration of information about infertility in the school curricula as well as at home and in the church. Menning (1977) specifies that such information might include:

1. Necessity of immediate treatment of infection of the reproductive tract in either the male or female; gonococcal cultures every 6 months for women who have multiple partners (to diagnose asymptomatic gonorrhea).
2. Immunization of prepubescent boys for mumps to prevent orchitis.
3. Avoidance of birth control pills for women who do not have already established normal menses or who have irregular menstrual cycles; also, use of birth control pills for more than 2 years should be avoided.
4. Use of an IUD should be carefully monitored. It should not be inserted in the presence of an infection and should be removed if infection develops.
5. Abortion decisions should be made carefully. Laminaria wicks can be used to cause cervical dilation when the cervix is tight and firm. Postabortion symptoms of infection need prompt treatment.

Available treatment methods for women
Induction of ovulation

Clomiphene. Induction of ovulation is currently managed with drug therapy. Clomiphene citrate (Clomid) is the current mainstay of ovulation induction therapy. It is administered if there appears to be adequate endogenous estrogen and follicular function, but inadequate cyclic stimulation by pituitary gonadotropins. Clomiphene does not competitively inhibit the action of estrogen at the level of estrogen receptors but modifies the hypothalamic activity by affecting the concentration of intracellular estrogen receptors. This keeps the hypothalamus from perceiving or acting upon the true en-

dogenous estrogen level in the circulation, thus activating the homeostatic negative feedback relationship between estrogen and the gonadotropins. Subsequent ovulation occurs as a manifestation of the hormonal and morphologic changes produced by growing follicles. Clomiphene does not directly stimulate ovulation but initiates a sequence of events that are the features of a normal cycle by causing an appropriate FSH discharge (Speroff et al., 1978).

Absent or infrequent ovulation is the main indication for clomiphene administration. Pituitary, adrenal, and thyroid disorders should be ruled out before using clomiphene, since it requires the woman's own endocrine tissues to respond, and it should not be administered without a complete history and physical examination. Clomiphene is contraindicated in the presence of an ovarian cyst, and side effects include vasomotor flushes, breast discomfort, abdominal distension, pain, bloating or soreness, abnormal ovarian enlargement, multiple ovulations, spontaneous abortion, nausea and vomiting, increased weight gain, mittelschmerz, headache, visual disturbances, and dryness or loss of hair.

In order to evaluate the size and consistency of the ovaries, a pelvic examination is performed before each course of clomiphene therapy. Significant ovarian enlargement is more common with periods of treatment longer than 5 days. If the woman has symptoms of ovarian enlargement, further pelvic examinations, intercourse, and undue physical exercise are contraindicated because of fragility of the enlarged ovaries. In order to avoid cyst formation, clomiphene therapy is withheld when ovarian enlargement is encountered. Because of the increased chance of abortion during the first treatment cycle, some clinicians recommend that the couple do not try to conceive during this time. This, at best, requires the couple to make a major change in their thinking. About 75% of women respond during the first three cycles with clomiphene therapy.

Clomiphene therapy is begun on the third to fifth day of a cycle following spontaneous or induced bleeding with an initial dose of 50 mg per day. If ovulation is not achieved in the very first cycle of treatment, dosage can be increased to 100 mg for the next cycle, and thereafter increased in staircase fashion by 50-mg increments to a maximum of 200 mg daily. The highest dose is pursued for 3 or 4 months before discontinuing therapy (Speroff et al., 1978).

Basal body temperatures are required for evaluation of the response to climiphene therapy. When an inadequate luteal phase is evident, the clomiphene dosage is increased to the next level. If the woman is already receiving the 200-mg daily dose, human chorionic gonadotropin (HCG) may be added to the clomiphene to improve the midcycle surge of LH; 10,000 units of HCG are administered intramuscularly on the seventh to tenth day after clomiphene therapy when follicular maturation is likely to be at its peak. Determining the quantity and ferning of cervical mucus can allow the precise timing of HCG administration. If HCG is given in the morning, intercourse is advised for that night and for the next 2 days (Speroff et al., 1978).

The presence of a biphasic temperature does not necessarily indicate the physical extrusion of the ovum. Luteinization of follicle cells without ovulation has been invoked as an explanation for the discrepancy between the apparent ovulatory rates and the pregnancy rates seen in response to clomiphene. About 70% of patients who are appropriate candidates for therapy can be expected to ovulate and about 40% become pregnant with clomiphene therapy. Multiple pregnancy rates are about 8%, with most being twins. About 30% of the women who have estrogen production but do not respond to clomiphene become pregnant when treated with human menopausal gonadotropin.

Human menopausal gonadotropins (HMG). HMG is recommended for use following failure of clomiphene therapy. HMG is a purified preparation of gonadotropins extracted from the urine of postmenopausal women and is available as Pergonal, containing 75 units of FSH and 75 units of LH. It is an expensive form of therapy, with treatment costing from $200 to $900 per cycle for the drug alone, depending on the dosage used. It is administered by intramuscular injection. Ovarian competence must be demonstrated before the administration of Pergonal, for without ovarian function the drug is useless. High serum gonadotropins with a failure to demonstrate withdrawal bleeding indicates ovarian failure, and these women should not be treated with ovulation induction therapy.

The purpose of HMG therapy is to achieve follicular growth and maturation. Follicle stimulation is achieved with continuous administration of HMG for 7 to 14 days, starting with 2 ampules daily. The response to HMG is assessed by the amount of estrogen produced by the growing follicles. The quantity and quality of the cervical mucus can also be used as an indication of estrogen production. Twenty-four hour urinary excretion of total estrogens or the plasma estradiol level is also used to monitor the effectiveness of therapy. When the cervical os opens and when cervical mucous changes that reflect a normal midcycle pattern are achieved, the woman is given an ovulatory stimulus of 10,000 units of HCG as a single intramuscular dose. The woman is advised to have intercourse the day of the HCG injection and for the next 2 days. However, because of the fragility of hyperstimulated ovaries, further intercourse and strenuous physical exercise are contraindicated by some physicians.

Estrogen measurements are used to prevent hyperstimulation and to determine the correct time for the administration of the HCG ovulatory dose. Blood and urinary levels of estrogen are a source of controversy, with the recommended levels for blood estrogens being between 1000 and 1500 pg/ml for estradiol measured by radioimmunoassay and between 100 μg but less than 200 μg per 24 hours in the urine. The range between the dosage that does not induce ovulation and the dosage that produces hyperstimulation is extremely narrow. Therefore, close supervision and experience in the administration of HMG are essential (Speroff et al., 1978).

Counseling of the couple is important, since a thorough understanding of the need for daily treatment and observation is necessary before therapy can be initiated. The husband may be taught to administer the injection, and daily recording of the BBT and body weight are important. The couple needs to be informed about the need for scheduled intercourse and should know that multiple courses of treatment may be necessary. They have a right to know the expense associated with the therapy, and also must be aware that there is no guarantee that the therapy will work. More than 90% of women with competent ovaries will ovulate in response to HMG-HCG, and a pregnancy rate of between 50% to 70% is likely to occur. Two to five therapeutic cycles are usually required to achieve pregnancy (Speroff et al., 1978).

Hyperstimulation of the ovaries may be a life-threatening consequence of HMG-HCG therapy. In mild cases there is ovarian enlargement, abdominal distention, and weight gain. With a severe hyperstimulation syndrome, a critical condition may develop that includes ascites, pleural effusion, electrolyte imbalance, and hypovolemia with hypotension and oliguria. The ovaries are tremendously enlarged, and may have multiple follicular cysts, edema of the stroma, and many corpora lutea.

The pathophysiology of the hyperstimulation syndrome is given in Fig. 14-3. Hyperstimulation causes a shift of fluid from the intravascular space into the abdominal cavity. The consequences are hypovolemia, ascites, and hemoconcentration. These lead to low blood pressure and a decreased central venous pressure, which in turn may lead to complications of increased coagulability and decreased renal perfusion. The woman may become oliguric because of decreased renal perfusion and may retain both water and sodium. Hyperkalemic acidosis may result from this as well as an increased blood urea nitrogen.

The woman who gains more than 20 pounds, has a hematocrit over 50%, is oliguric or dyspneic, or demonstrates postural hypotension must be hospitalized. Pelvic and abdominal examinations are contraindicated because of the possibility of hemorrhage from ovarian rupture. Ovarian rupture is a danger and can be monitored by serial hematocrits. The falling hematocrit in the pres-

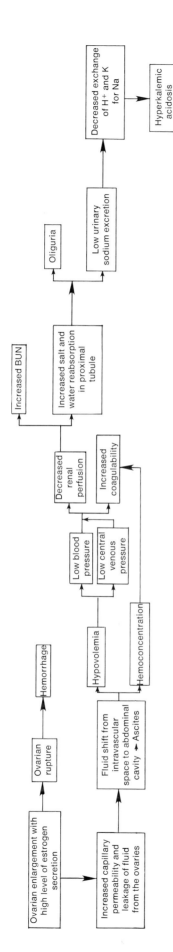

Fig. 14-3. Pathophysiology of the hyperstimulation syndrome.

ence of diuresis, however, is a sign of resolution. Intravenous fluids, plasma expanders, albumin, and potassium exchange resins may be necessary. Mannitol is used to maintain urinary output. Diuretics are ineffectual and dangerous since diuresis may produce hypovolemic shock or thrombosis (Speroff et al., 1978).

Combination therapy. Two new methods for induction of ovulation include a combination of clomiphene and HMG in sequence and therapy with gonadotropin-releasing factors. Ergot alkaloids inhibit pituitary secretion of prolactin and can be used to return ovulatory function in women who have hyperprolactinemia as well as some anovulatory patients with normal prolactin levels, but at this writing, bromocryptine has not been approved for treatment of infertility because it is not known whether it produces birth defects (Speroff et al., 1978).

Ovarian wedge resection. Wedge resection of the ovaries is performed to remove a significant amount of steroid-producing tissue. It has been demonstrated that there is a sustained reduction of testosterone following wedge resection, suggesting that the barrier to ovulation is the atresia-promoting effects of high testosterone levels. Some women return to ovulation permanently, most return to their anovulatory state, and some do not respond at all. Formation of adhesions is one risk of therapy in addition to the operative risk.

Correcting structural anomalies

Relaxation of the cervix. The woman who has relaxation of the cervix (sometimes called cervical incompetence) may be able to conceive but unable to carry a pregnancy to the point of fetal viability. She has a history of midtrimester abortions, and dilation of the cervix can be noted on hysterography. Circlage of the cervix may be performed. Nonabsorable Dacron mesh may be placed around the cervix, which will necessitate delivery by cesarean section; or temporary polyethylene tubules, which can be severed at the thirty-seventh to thirty-eighth week of gestation to permit vaginal delivery, can be placed after 14 weeks of gestation to avoid the securing of a pregnancy resulting from an imperfect ovum.

Congenital anomalies of the uterus. The bicornuate, septate, or double uterus may require surgical reconstruction. The couple is advised to avoid conception until 8 to 12 months after the surgery. Surgery is indicated when no other cause of infertility is revealed and when there is a history of spontaneous abortions.

Tubal reconstruction. When the tubes are nonpatent and diagnostic studies reveal normal male fertility and normal female function, tuboplasty may be considered. Closed tubes may be delineated by means of the Rubin test and X-ray studies such as the hysterosalpingogram. The oviducts are usually lavaged before tuboplasty is attempted. Variations of tuboplasty are used for several types of defects of the oviduct. The formation of adhesions following this surgery is a major deterrent to achieving pregnancy postoperatively.

Therapy of endometriosis. Endometriosis often progresses slowly over the years and regresses at menopause. The degree of intervention depends on the severity of the disease and the desire to preserve or promote childbearing function. The cause of endometriosis is believed to be retrogade menstrual flow causing a spread of endometrial cells into the pelvis where they implant or set up irritative foci to stimulate differentiation of peritoneal lining cells into endometrial-type tissue. Diagnosis of endometriosis is made on the basis of progressively severe dysmenorrhea, dyspareunia, or pain on defecation. The pain from endometriosis is most severe during the menses, but is also present throughout the cycle. This pain is attributed to stretching of the peritoneal or fibrous bands following bleeding into cavities created by the endometrial implants. The pain is not necessarily proportional to the pathology, and low back pain may also be attributable to endometriosis.

The pelvic examination may show no abnormality, but with more extensive disease there will be enlargement of the ovaries. The uterus may be fixed and retroverted. Beading, nodularity, and tenderness of the uterosacral ligaments can be determined on rectovaginal examination and are characteristic of endometriosis.

Women with minimal symptoms are followed carefully without therapy. With more severe symptoms, ovarian enlargement, fixation of a retroverted uterus, and nodular tender uterosacral ligaments, and if indication of endometriomas or pelvic adhesions to the adnexae are found on laparoscopy, surgery is indicated. After 6 to 8 weeks of noncyclic hormonal therapy with oral contraceptive pills to suppress endometrial growth, surgery is performed. Conservative surgery can include lysis of adhesions, endometrioma excision, fulguration of implants of endometriosis, suspension of the uterus, appendectomy, and peritonealization. A 40% to 80% pregnancy rate can be expected postoperatively depending on the extent of the disease. If pregnancy does not occur within 2 years of the surgery, it is usually best for the couple to consider adoption or remaining childfree (Speroff et al., 1978).

When limited areas of endometriosis are identified on laparoscopy in the cul-de-sac, on the uterosacral ligaments, or on the surface of the ovary, hormonal therapy is attempted with continuous noncyclic use of oral contraceptives for 6 to 9 months. It has not been determined how minimal endometriosis interferes with fertility, or what percentage of these women can attain pregnancy without treatment.

Testosterone may be used to reduce pelvic pain and dyspareunia from endometriosis, and it does not eliminate ovulation. Although relief of symptoms is sometimes impressive, relief of infertility is not as successful. Danazol, a synthetic steroid, has antigonadotropin and slight androgenic activities. It is administered in doses of 800 mg daily for 3 to 9 months to reduce the symptoms of endometriosis. Suppression of gonadotropins supposedly diminishes steroid hormone stimulation of endometriosis to allow spontaneous healing and atrophy to occur. Its effects on infertility are only now being established. Unfortunately, in some women there is a rapid return of symptoms and pelvic abnormalities after Danazol is discontinued. In addition, side effects include amenorrhea, hot flushes, weight gain, acne, and increased oiliness of the skin. Periovarian adhesions have also been noted following Danazol and laparoscopic biopsy. The risks of such therapy have not yet been fully evaluated.

Prevention of endometriosis can be achieved by avoiding tubal insufflation, hysterosalpingography, and cervidilation during menstrual flow so that the endometrial cells will not be forced out through the tubes. Pregnancy at an early age may be preventive. The use of progestin contraception with the protective effect of decidualization may be the best method of prevention.

Available treatment methods for men

Treatment methods for men include those directed toward improving semen quality and those for correcting structural anomalies.

Improving semen quality

A number of pharmacologic agents are used in an attempt to influence the quality of the semen. Drug therapy may be used to improve the general health status (for example, to treat obesity, allergy, general or recurrent infection, or hypo- or hyperthyroidism). Cytomel (L-liothyronine) may be given to subfertile men with thyroid dysfunction. Testosterone-propionate is sometimes used to suppress gonadotropin function in order to produce a rebound of large amounts of gonadotropins after the drug is discontinued. HMG or HCG may be administered to stimulate spermatozoa and to elevate the sperm concentration in men with oligospermia. Gonadotropin-releasing factors may also be used to stimulate secretion of gonadotropins. Clomiphene therapy has been associated with some improvement in sperm count.

Correcting structural anomalies

Surgical correction of undescended testicles, hypospadia, epispadias, congenital chordee, and deformities of the penis is usually best performed at an early age.

Urethral strictures, fistulas, and diverticula can be corrected to improve sperm transport through the ductal passages. Varicocelectomy has been performed to improve semen quality, especially sperm motility. In the case of obstruction, vasovasotomy or vasoepididymostomy is necessary. Testicular transplantation and grafts of the vas deferens have also been attempted to improve male fecundity.

Available treatment methods for couples

Methods available for treatment of the infertile couple include those directed at improvement of coital technique, interrupting immunologic interferences with fertility, and artificial insemination.

Improvement of coital technique

Couples can be counseled with respect to the optimal time of the menstrual cycle to achieve a pregnancy, the optimal frequency of sexual intercourse, and the most appropriate positions to use. The woman is instructed not to arise, urinate, or douche for at least 30 minutes after intercourse.

For men who have subfertility, it is recommended that the penis be withdrawn from the vagina after intravaginal deposition of the first portion of the ejaculate, with the remaining semen being deposited outside of the vagina. The reason for this technique is that in subfertile men (men with high semen volumes and good semen quality in the first fraction of the semen specimen), sperm concentration, motility, morphology, and viability are greater in the first portion of the ejaculate.

Interrupting immunologic interferences with fertility

When immunologic problems such as sperm agglutination or immobilization have been documented, the woman is instructed to avoid all contact with her partner's sperm. This usually means using a condom for a period of months to a year, avoiding orogenital sex, or perhaps even abstaining from intercourse for a period of time.

Artificial insemination

Artificial insemination may be accomplished with the partner's sperm, that of a donor, or a combination. The semen is collected by masturbation into a sterile container and is administered in either a fresh or thawed state (if frozen originally). Artificial insemination is timed to coincide with signs of ovulation as indicated by BBT and spinnbarkheit. Semen specimens with low counts do not tolerate freezing well, since freezing and thawing depress sperm motility to some extent. There are several methods of artificial insemination, which may involve injecting semen into the cervical canal,

into the vaginal vault, directly into the uterus (which is painful), or placing semen in a plastic cap fitted over the cervix and left in position for at least 8 hours. To encourage fertilization, the woman is sometimes placed in a Trendelenberg position for 30 minutes following the insemination. Some couples may wish to be together during this procedure, and the woman may find it comforting for her spouse to be present, even though he may not be in the same room. Two to three inseminations may be done per cycle, and the procedure is usually not done for longer than 12 months. About 90% of the women who will become pregnant from artificial insemination will do so within 6 months.

Because artificial insemination is morally objectionable to some individuals, the procedure is kept confidential, and the couple is often counseled not to discuss the procedure with family and friends.

Both homologous and heterologous insemination may be performed. Homologous insemination (artificial insemination husband or AIH) may be indicated when the sperm count is adequate, but the volume of ejaculate is low; when the sperm count is low normal, but the volume of semen is adequate, or when normal coitus is not possible (e.g., paralysis).

Artificial insemination donor (AID) is performed for azoospermia, after unsuccessful homologous insemination, when the male is a carrier of a serious hereditary disease, and for couples with Rh immunologic incompatibility. AID donors are carefully screened for health problems and semen analysis. The ethnic background and physical characteristics can be matched to the male partner's as closely as possible, and the same donor and recipient are maintained. The spouse's semen may also be mixed with the donor's, if not medically contraindicated. This procedure has the advantage that the spouse's semen may be responsible for a resulting pregnancy.

For some couples there are advantages of AID over adoption, including the full experience of pregnancy, a more private process, and a greater chance that the child will look like the parents. Fears that the birth parents will reclaim an adopted child are also eliminated. The couple must sign a contract indicating their comprehension of the procedure and indicating that resulting offspring are their legitimate legal heirs. Couples who conceive with AID are referred to other professionals for obstetric care to eliminate legal problems such as perjury with respect to legitimacy in signing the child's birth certificate or to avoid conflict of interest.

Future approaches to infertility therapy

In vitro fertilization. In vitro fertilization has the potential ability to circumvent many problems that interfere with fertilization. Louise Brown, the first baby to be born following fertilization outside the mother's body, was born July 25, 1978. It is believed that her birth resulted from a procedure similar to that described below.

Preovulatory oocytes are obtained from the ovaries 33 to 34 hours after the woman is given an HCG injection to prepare the follicles. The oocytes are removed surgically during laparoscopy under general anesthesia. Other hormones may be administered to facilitate preparation of the uterus for implantation. Sperm are diluted, then placed in a saline solution to cause capacitation. Droplets of the sperm solution are then put into a petri dish filled with inert oil. The droplets sink to the bottom and each preovulatory oocyte is pipetted into one of the droplets; this procedure keeps the ova and sperm in a small volume. A few hours later fertilization occurs. Twelve hours later the embryo is transferred to a solution designed for embryonic growth; it is kept in an atmosphere of low oxygen tension with some carbon dioxide. After 2 days the embryo is an eight-celled organism and by 4 days it is about a 100-celled blastocyst. The developing 2- to 4-day-old embryo is inserted into the uterus through a plastic cannula and may implant (Kolata, 1978). The first clinic in the United States to use in vitro sterilization is scheduled to begin treatment of patients in 1980.

Table 14-8. Agencies and services for adoptive parents

Agency	Services	Agency	Services
Adoption Resource Exchange of North America (ARENA) 67 Irving Place New York, NY 10003 (212)254-7410	Information about adoption in North America, especially for children with "special needs"	Friends of Children, Inc. 4325 Memorial Drive Suite 1 Decatur, GA 30032	Assists with international adoptions (e.g., India, El Salvador, Indonesia, Colombia, Ecuador, Guatemala, Honduras)
AASK (Aid to Adoption of Special Kids) 3530 Grand Avenue Oakland, CA 94610	Agency providing adoptive services for children who are mentally, emotionally, or physically handicapped, older children, and siblings	Holt Adoption Program P.O. Box 2420 Eugene, OR 97402	Agency dealing with international adoptions, primarily in South Korea
Children's Home Society of Minnesota 2230 Como Ave. St. Paul, MN 55108	Adoption services for Korean children and older children, especially Amerasians	Kuan Yin Foundation, Inc. 533 Brant, Suite 4 Burlington, Ontario Canada L7R 2G6	International adoptions of children from India between 4 and 16 years old
Committee for Single Adoptive Parents Box 40704 Washington, D.C. 20015	Information source for single persons interested in adoption of domestic or foreign children	OURS (Organization for a United Response) 3148 Humboldt Avenue, South Minneapolis, MN 55408 (612)827-5709	Adoptive parent organization with a wealth of experience, especially in international adoptions; excellent bimonthly newsletter filled with adoption information
Crossroads, Inc. 4901 West 77th St., office 124b Minneapolis, MN 55435	Can only place children in Minnesota, but can provide information about adoption of children from agencies in Korea, Colombia, El Salvador, Thailand, and India	World Family Adoptions, Ltd. 5048 Fairy Chasm Road West Bend, WI 53095	International adoption agency
Dillon Family and Youth Services 2525 East 21st St. Tulsa, OK 74115	Adoption services for Korean children, mostly infants	Local agencies: Catholic Children's Services Children's Home Society Jewish Family and Child Services Latter Day Saints Social Services Regular Baptist Child Placement Agency State Department of Social Services Superior Court of each State and county Traveler's Aid Society	These agencies offer services which vary from one locale to another, but may provide home studies, have custody of children, and place children
Families for Children, Inc. 10 Bowling Green Pointe Clare 720 Quebec, Canada	Resources for several types of international adoptions		
Foreign Adoption Resources 911 Cypress Drive Boulder, CO 80303	Information source regarding international adoptions		

Alternatives to pregnancy

There are two alternatives to pregnancy available to the infertile couple: adoption and childfree living. Both require adjustments on the part of the infertile couple.

Adoption

Availability of birth control, new abortion legislation, and the fact that the majority of single women choose to keep their babies have contributed to the reduced supply of infants for adoption. The waiting period for healthy infants varies from less than a year to over 5 years in some locations. Although healthy infants and preschoolers are in short supply, there are other children who must wait for homes. Children of all races with special needs include children of school-age and older; sibling groups of two or more children; and children with serious medical handicaps, mental retardation, or special emotional or learning disorders. Unfortunately, in some instances these adoptions are unsuccessful. Infants and children from other countries often can be adopted through international agencies.

The adoption process can reactivate old feelings of loss of control as well as anger over the helplessness of infertility. Although adoption can give the couple a chance to be parents it does not eradicate their infertility. Thus it is important for the couple to understand that infertility and adoption are two separate issues; their infertility cannot be "cured" by adopting a child. Indeed, the notion that adoption will precipitate a subsequent pregnancy is a myth.

The couple considering this option may need continued support; some peer support groups provide information about adoption services as well as counseling about a variety of aspects of the experience. A list of resources for persons who are considering adoption is given in Table 14-8.

Childfree living

Infertile couples can reconsider their desire for parenthood and decide to remain childfree. Infertility gives couples a chance to reexamine their motives for pregnancy and parenting. One organization to support persons who choose childfree living is the National Organization for Non-Parents (806 Reistertown Road, Baltimore, Md. 21208). Founded by Ellen Peck, author of *The Baby Trap* and co-author with Judith Senderowitz of *Pronatalism: The Myth of Mom and Apple Pie*, the organization attempts to provide support for persons who are childfree in a society that encourages couples to have children. There are limitless ways in which childfree individuals can have contact with children if they so desire. The infertile couple should be helped to feel that it is acceptable to choose this alternative at any point in their workup.

INFERTILITY AS A LIFE CRISIS

Infertility has been described as a developmental crisis. Failure to reproduce may be seen as the failure to achieve a developmental milestone. It has even been suggested that failure to reproduce interferes with achieving generativity, an important stage of adult development in Erikson's schema (Menning, 1977).

Meaning of the diagnosis

The meaning of a diagnosis of infertility to the couple is likely to reflect their motivations for parenthood. Becoming a parent may be motivated by a desire to conform to societal pressures, to experience the rites of passage to adulthood, to relive a childhood of one's own, to compete with one's own parents, or to fulfill sex-role expectations. And some people desire parenthood because they *like* children! Some women desire the experience of pregnancy (or the chance to recapitulate a previous pregnancy) or to breastfeed. Some men may desire pregnancy as proof of their virility. The couple may also desire genetic continuity (Menning, 1977).

Responses to infertility

Responses to infertility may be feelings of surprise, denial, isolation, anger, guilt and unworthiness, depression, and grief. Because many persons perceive their infertility as stigmatizing, they isolate themselves from others who might be able to provide support or allow them to share their feelings. Because from adolescence onward, we assume that we have the ability, if not the obligation, to regulate our fertility, it is not surprising that a common response is denial and surprise. The surrender of control to health workers who conduct the infertility assessment often provokes feelings of helplessness and anger. Guilt and feelings of unworthiness may be precipitated by amorphous events or by past history, such as having had venereal disease or an abortion. If the individual is unable to link these feelings to the present circumstances, he or she may experience confusion. Depression is reflected in feelings of sadness, despair, lethargy, or vague symptoms of distress. It is a natural part of moving toward acceptance of a loss. The infertile couple who reaches the end of a workup with no hope of pregnancy may actually grieve for their loss of fertility, the loss of future children, and the loss of the pregnancy experience (Menning, 1977).

Menning points out that this is a unusual kind of grief because it is for a potential rather than a real loss. She also suggests that grief may fail to occur because there may be no recognized loss or the loss may be so "unspeakable" that the infertile couple cannot share it with those in their social support system. For others, there may be uncertainty about the loss. Some couples may find that infertility is negated as a loss by others in their social milieu, such as those who do not value parenting or who minimize the importance of infertility by comparing it to a fatal illness. In some instances there may be no support system available to the infertile couple to help them deal with their grief.

Resolution

Resolution occurs when the couple can discover or name their feelings about infertility, talk about them, and feel relief or that the feelings are subsiding. A block in resolving any of the powerful feelings aroused by infertility can result in pathologic depression (Menning, 1977).

Often the couple facing an obstacle to fulfillment of a life goal find themselves in a situation in which their usual coping mechanisms are not adequate. Fortunately, most crises move toward resolution. There are variable outcomes associated with crisis: the relationship may remain stable; it may move to a less stable level of functioning; or it may grow. Nurses in infertility treatment centers can help the couple to learn new ways of coping. This crisis can be growth-producing.

A concept of crisis

For some individuals, the crisis precipitated by a diagnosis of infertility cannot be readily resolved, and the clinician may be requested to provide crisis counseling for the individual or couple. Walkup's (1977) concept of crisis provides a useful framework for nursing practitioners who care for infertile clients. Her concept of crisis is presented in a serial order of emergent behaviors (Walkup, 1974):

1. A change occurs to a client (individual or couple) in dynamic equilibrium.
2. The client perceives the change as a disruption of balance of internal needs and external demands.
3. The client mobilizes habitual problem-solving energies, (internal resources) and desires situational support from external resources to attempt resolution of the imbalance.
4. Internal and external resources fail to resolve the demands of the client's problems.
5. Feelings of helplessness and ineffectiveness experienced by the client result in behavioral disorganization.

Walkup also outlines a structure for obtaining information about the specific problem as well as structure for crisis resolution. Table 14-9 includes an example of the application of Walkup's concept of crisis to the care of a woman who experienced disorganization following the diagnosis of her husband as azoospermic. The serial order of emergent behaviors is described, followed by a description of the assessment and interventions incorporated in providing nursing care.

Coping with infertility

If the assessment and therapy for infertility do not induce a crisis, they at least constitute a stressor impinging on the couple's relationship. For example, sexual intercourse can become prescribed by the temperature chart rather than enjoyed by the couple in synchrony with their feelings. Some couples find it useful to redefine their situation, setting aside a few days for reproductive sex, but maintaining a "recreative" orientation to the remainder of their sexual experiences. Some find it helpful to "take vacations" from the temperature chart.

The temptation to "blame" one member, particularly when that individual is the one diagnosed as infertile, may lead to marital conflict. Even when blame is not verbalized, the infertile partner may feel faulty or worthy of blame. To help decrease the feelings of blame that the infertile partner may experience, the couple can attempt to share solutions to their problem. For example, the female partner can help the male partner to produce a semen specimen, or the woman can receive her injection from the man with whom she shares the problem of infertility.

Infertile couples are confronted with the need to communicate about their sexual relationship. For some persons this is stressful inasmuch as they regard discussing sexuality as taboo. The sensitive nature of the assessment may create anxieties, precipitate sexual dysfunction, and initiate the discussion of powerful and conflicting expectations for the resolution of the infertility assessment. The professional can help couples by modeling effective communication about sexuality and other powerful feelings. Sometimes the nurse will find it useful to help couples say things aloud—to verbalize feelings they cannot deal with in the context of their relationship. At times the couple may not have the words to express their concerns—not an unusual situation in a society in which sex is often discussed in euphemistic or derogatory terms.

At the very time the couple is faced with many anxiety-provoking issues, they must also learn how to collect specimens, time ovulation, and so on. Their anxiety level may actually prevent them from comprehending or retaining important information when it is presented only in one mode. The nurse providing instructions can reinforce verbal messages with pictures and written instructions that can be reviewed at a later time.

To complicate matters, the couple may discover their ambivalence about childbearing or how important it is to them in the midst of their workup. They may discover their expectations about parenting are unrealistic. They may need to face (both as individuals and as a couple) changes in the way they perceive themselves—body image, self-concept—and one another. They may need

Table 14-9. Illustration of Walkup's concept of crises with infertile clients

Serial order of emergent behaviors	Assessment	Interventions
A and W find that after 5 years of marriage and planning for a child that they are infertile. W has azoospermia. A had always planned to have a family after initially working for a few years to provide some financial security. Religious orthodoxy keeps the couple from considering AIH or artificial insemination donor (AID).	In this instance A and W face a totally unanticipated change in their life plans. They have been accustomed to planning carefully for the future and find that their past experiences offer them no preparation for this event. They fell helpless and out of control.	The clinical specialist (CS) in the infertility clinic met with A and W during their final assessment conference with the gynecologist and urologist. She also arranged to meet with them privately after the team conference. During this time A and W registered shock and surprise. They both attempted to minimize the importance of their problem to one another, but A had tears in her eyes and W kept swallowing hard and didn't talk much. At this point the clinical specialist was able to help A and W verbalize that the change they were experiencing was a mismatch between their expectations of having a child and finding that they were unable to conceive. A and W defined their immediate problem as not knowing what to do and feeling helpless.
A is experiencing inability to sleep at night, is tired during the day, and has missed work frequently over the last 3 weeks since the diagnosis was made. Yet she feels compelled to present her "best side" to W in order to help him along. She has been able to focus on reassuring W for the last few weeks, and has not let him know her real feelings. She "cannot ask him to support me as he's too depressed." A feels that she "is trapped" and "has no options" and "no one to turn to."	A has been denying her feelings in order to help W, but now finds she can no longer contain her sadness. She feels she has no alternatives.	The clinical specialist arranged to see the couple at the end of the week. She shared with them that they might both feel sad and disappointed. A kept the appointment but W cancelled at the last minute. The clinical specialist observed to A that she seemed to be protecting W from feeling sad about his infertility yet was not allowing herself an opportunity to vent her own emotions. The CS also suggested that A's sleeping problem might be associated with her response to the diagnosis. The CS attempted to help A identify external resources to help her such as friends or clergy.
A has a close woman friend whom she can confide in. Her friend, however, recently had an abortion and is still very involved with her own feelings about the procedure. A thinks that this would be a poor time to make demands on her friend and that sharing her bad news might make her friend feel worse. A has found that praying helped her cope with problems in the past. She decides to talk with her clergyman about her problem.	A's close friend cannot be a support for A at this time; A does have internal resources and has used prayer in the past to cope with other problems. She has access to a clergyman.	A's plan to seek support from clergy and to use her own resources were reinforced by the CS. A did not appear comfortable confiding in her parents or siblings. A was encouraged to return to the clinic when she felt she needed to talk.
A's prayers do not help her feelings disappear. Her clergyman tells her that if she "only has enough faith, she will be able to cope with her problem" and that her first responsibility is "to help her husband since sterility for a man is hard to accept."	Although A was able to express her problems to her clergyman, his response was not perceived as supportive. A could not suppress her feelings through her prayers, although she felt that prayer helped "put things in perspective."	A was initially attempting to deny herself her feelings, and was later able to share them with her clergyman. Because the clergyman was unable to help A, the CS tried to help A identify other situational supports and to explore alternatives. A was not able to identify other supports and was encouraged to maintain telephone contact with the clinic or to return to see the CS when necessary. A did not feel she was ready to be involved in a mutual support group.

Continued.

Table 14-9. Illustration of Walkup's concept of crises with infertile clients—cont'd

Serial order of emergent behaviors	Assessment	Interventions
A finally is unable to see children in the neighborhood without crying. She finds herself avoiding her pregnant friends and occasionally finds that she is angry with them for no apparent reason. Because of her inability to sleep and the necessity to miss work she realizes her job is in jeopardy. She realizes that she needs some help and comes back to the Clinic to talk to the clinical specialist.	At this point A perceives she is losing control and feels helpless.	Although A's behavior is disorganized she does not have any suicidal thoughts. The CS arranges for daily telephone contacts for continued support for A. A will encourage W to come to the clinic when he feels ready. When A feels ready the CS will offer her a referral to a support group of infertile couples.
After daily telephone contacts with the CS, A expresses she "feels more together" and thinks she could benefit from the support groups' help. W still does not believe that anybody can do much to help him.	A is expressing readiness and willingness to broaden her support network. W is continuing to deal with his feelings alone. With some assistance from the group, A can cope with her activities of living, and perhaps at a later date deal with her relationship with W.	A was referred to the peer support group. She was given the option to maintain contact with the CS if necessary.

support to acknowledge their feelings. It may be necessary for the professional to accept their feelings of ambivalence and to help the couple own these feelings.

One or both partners may demonstrate coping mechanisms that are not optimal. To deny that one is infertile after 3 years of attempting a pregnancy and 2 years of assessment and therapy would not be conducive to a successful resolution of the problem. Yet optimism is necessary to cope with the expensive, intrusive, and sometimes painful assessment and therapy. Prolonged grief and depression also interfere with resolution, and persons experiencing these responses may require psychotherapy as well as other forms of support. Some couples find they are unable to plan ahead because they do not know what their childbearing status may be. While this may be an anticipated outcome of the uncertainty they feel with respect to their infertility, it would significantly impede readjustment of their life plans should it persist indefinitely. Sometimes allowing a definite period of time for the workup is useful. The couple may be willing to attempt a pregnancy for a period of a few years, but have a contingency plan in mind if they have not become pregnant within the period of time they allot.

One or both partners may be lacking in support from significant other persons. This is a special problem for individuals or couples who perceive their infertility as stigmatizing. Reluctance to share their situation with others may lead the couple to intensify the demands they make of one another for support at a time when each is in need of support. Thus the anxiety that one

individual experiences becomes intensified as one also is expected to support one's partner. Recognition of the need for support from others and the need to share feelings about the experiences associated with infertility led Barbara Eck Menning to form Resolve, Inc., a support group, in 1973. The group started as a small group of women who were experiencing infertility; now several chapters of Resolve exist around the United States.

Another model for peer support has recently evolved in King County, Washington, that incorporates both information dissemination techniques and peer support. A series of four infertility awareness seminars sponsored by the Seattle Infertility Peer Support Group included presentations of the following topics: (1) medical aspects of infertility, (2) psychosocial aspects of infertility, (3) adoption and other alternatives for infertile couples, and (4) lobbying for improved health care, insurance coverage, etc. Anticipated outcomes of the first four seminars include an ongoing peer support group, increased patient assertiveness, enhanced awareness of the diagnostic and treatment processes as well as awareness of others' emotional responses to their infertility, and consumer advocacy of better health care and improved insurance coverage. Such groups can provide infertile persons with a knowledge base to help them in problem-solving, emotional support from others who share the same problem, and activities such as advocacy, which might be a creative way for infertile people to deal with their dilemma.

REFERENCES

Amelar, R., and Dubin, L.: Male infertility, Urology, pp. 1-30, Jan. 1973.

Amelar, R. D., and Dubin, L.: A coital technique for promotion of fertility, New York, New York, Urology, Vol. 5, No. 5, Feb. 1975.

Ansbacher, R.: Artificial insemination with frozen spermatozoa, Fertil. Ster. 29(4):375-379, 1978.

Asch, R. H.: Laparoscopic recovery of sperm from peritoneal fluid in patients with negative or poor Sims-Huhner test, Fertil. Steril. 27(9):1111-1114, 1976.

Beer, A. E., and William B. N.: Antigenic status of semen from the viewpoints of the female and male, Fertil. Steril. 29(1):3-22, 1978.

Behrman, S. J., and Kistner, R.: Progress in infertility, ed. 2, Boston, 1975, Little, Brown and Co.

Breitenecker, G., Friedrich, F., and Kemeter, P.: Further investigations on the maturation and degeneration of human ovarian follicles and their oocytes, Fertil. Steril. 29(3):336-341, 1978.

Bronson, R. A.: Tubal pregnancy and infertility, Fertil. Steril. 28(3):221-228, 1977.

Canales, E. S., and others: Infertility due to hyperprolactinemia and its treatment with ergocryptine, Fertil. Steril. 27(11):1335-1336, 1976.

Canales, E. S., and others: Induction of ovulation with clomiphene and estradiol benzoate in anovulatory women refractory to clomiphene alone, Fertil. Steril. 29(5):496-499, 1978.

Check, J. H., and Rakoff, A. E.: Treatment of cervical factor by donor mucus insemination, Fertil. Steril. 28(1):113-114, 1977.

Cockett, A. T. K., and Urry, R. L., editors: Male infertility: workup, treatment, and research, New York, 1976, Grune and Stratton, Inc.

Cohen, M. R.: Office gynecology: diagnostic survey of the infertile couple; special aspects of primary care, Postgrad. Med. 62(4):201-205, Oct. 1977.

Dodson, K. S., MacNaughton, M. C., and Coutts, J. R. T.: Infertility in women with apparently ovulatory cycles. Comparison of their plasma sex steroid and gonadotropin profiles with those in the normal cycle. Br. J. Obstet. Gynaecol. 82:615-624, 1975; 82:625-633, 1975.

Dor, J., Homburg, R., and Rabau, E.: An evaluation of etiologic factors and therapy in 665 infertile couples, Fertil. Steril. 28(7):718-722, 1977.

Fredricsson, B., and Bjork, G.: Morphology of postcoital spermatozoa in the cervical secretion and its clinical significance, Fertil. Steril. 28(8):841-845, 1977.

Garcia, J., Jones, G. S., and Wentz, A. C.: The use of clomiphene citrate, Fertil. Steril. 28(7):707-715, 1977.

Glass, R. H., and Golbus, M. S.: Habitual abortion, Fertil. Steril. Vol. 29, No. 3, Mar. 1978.

Hammons, C.: The adoptive family, Am. J. Nurs. 76(26):251-257, 1976.

Heritage, D. W., and others: Cytogenetics of recurrent abortions, Fertil. Steril. 29(4):414-417, 1978.

Huggins, G. R.: Contraceptive use and subsequent fertility, Fertil. Steril. 28(6):603-612, 1977.

Jones, G. S.: The luteal phase defect, Fertil. Steril. 27(4):351-356, 1976.

Kistner, R. W., Siegler, A. M., and Behrman, S. J.: Suggested classification of endometriosis: relationship to infertility, Fertil. Steril. 28(9):1008-1010, 1977.

Kolata, G. B.: In vitro fertilization: is it safe and repeatable? Science 201(4357):698-699, 1978.

Koninckz, P. R., and Brosens, I. A.: The 'gonadotropin-resistant ovary' syndrome as a cause of secondary amenorrhea and infertility, Fertil. Steril. 28(7):926-931, 1977.

Koninckz, P. R., and others: Delayed onset of luteinization as a cause of infertility, Fertil. Steril. 29(3):266-269, 1978.

Kremer, J.: Infertility: Male and female. I. Male aspects of fertility. In Money, J., and Musaph, H., editors: Handbook of sexology, Amsterdam, 1977, Elsevier/North-Holland Biomedical Press.

Lenton, E. A., Weston, G. A., and Cooke, I. D.: Long-term follow-up of the apparently normal couple with a complaint of infertility, Fertil. Steril. 28(9):913-919, 1977.

Lenton, E. A., Weston, G. A., and Cooke, I. D.: Problems in using basal body temperature recordings in an infertility clinic, Br. Med. J. 1:803-805, 1977.

Mai, F. M., Munday, R. N., and Rump, E. E.: Psychiatric interview comparisons between infertile and fertile couples, Psychosom. Med. 34:431-440, 1972.

Marik, J., and Hulka, J.: Luteinized unruptured follicle syndrome: a subtle cause of infertility, Fertil. Steril. 29(3):270-274, 1978.

McGuire, L.: Psychologic management of infertile women, Postgrad. Med. 57(6):173-176, 1975.

Menning, B. E.: Resolve—a support group for infertile couples, Am. J. Nurs. 76(2):258-259, 1976.

Menning, B. E.: Infertility: A guide for the childless couple, Englewood Cliffs, N.J., 1977, Prentice Hall, Inc.

Mitchell, C.: The infertile family. In Armstrong, M. E., et al., editors: Blakiston's handbook of clinical nursing, New York, 1979, McGraw-Hill Book Co.

Moghissi, K. S.: Postcoital test: physiologic basis, technique, and interpretation (modern trends), Fertil. Steril. 27(2):117-129, 1976.

Moore, D. E., Thompson, R. S., and Israel, R.: Recovery of midcycle human follicular histology, Fertil. Steril. 29(5):518-522, 1978.

Nakano, R., and others: A schematic approach to the work-up of amenorrhea, Fertil. Steril. 28(3):229-236, 1977.

Peck, E.: The baby trap, New York, 1971, Bernard Gies Associates, Inc.

Peck, E., and Senderowitz, J.: Pronatalism: the myth of mom and apple pie, New York, 1974, Thomas Y. Crowell and Co.

Rakoff, A. E.: Ovulatory failure: clinical aspects, Fertil. Steril. 27(5):473-492, 1976.

Renne, D.: There's always adoption: the infertility problem, Child Welf. 56(7):465-470, 1977.

Romney, S., et al.: Gynecology and obstetrics: the health care of women, New York, 1975, McGraw-Hill Book Co.

Rosenfeld, D. L., Garcia, C., and Bullock, W.: An infertility data registry, Fertil. Steril. 29(1):112-114, 1978.

Rosenfeld, D. L., and Garcia, C.: A comparison of endometrial histology with simultaneous plasma progesterone determinations in infertile women, Fertil. Steril. 27(11):1256-1266, 1976.

Seki, K., and others: Effect of clomiphene citrate on serum prolactin in infertile women with ovarian dysfunction, Am. J. Obstet. Gynecol. 124(2):125-128, 1976.

Shivers, C. A., and Dunbar, B. S.: Autoantibodies to zona pellucida: a possible cause for infertility in women, Science 197:1082-1087, 1977.

Shulman, S., and others: Immune infertility and new approach to treatment, Fertil. Steril. 29(3):309-313, 1978.

Speroff, L., Glass, R. H., and Kase, N.: Clinical gynecologic endocrinology and infertility, ed. 2, Baltimore, 1978, The Williams & Wilkins Co.

Steiman, R. P., and Taymor, M. L.: Artificial insemination homologous and its role in the management of infertility, Fertil. Steril. 28(2):146-150, 1977.

Sulewski, J. M., Eisenbert, F., and Stenger, V. G.: A longitudinal analysis of artificial insemination with donor semen, Fertil. Steril. 29(5):527-531, 1978.

Thompson, P. E.: Stress in the adoption process: a personal account, Social Work, 1978.

Toaff, R., and others: Role of androgenic hyperactivity in anovulation, Fertil. Steril. **29**(4):407-413, 1978.

Toppozada, M., and others: Aberrant uterine response to prostaglandin E, as a possible etiologic factor in functional infertility, Fertil. Steril. **28**(4):434-439, 1977.

Tsapoulis, A. D., Zourlas, P. A., and Comninos, A. C.: Observations on 320 infertile patients treated with human gonadotropins (human menopausal gonadotropin/human chorionic gonadotropin), Fertil. Steril. **29**(5):492-495, 1978.

Walkup, L. L.: A concept of crisis. In Hall, J., and Weaver, B., editors: Nursing families in crisis, Philadelphia, 1974, J. B. Lippincott Co.

Warren, J. C.: Reproductive failure. In Romney, S., and others: Gynecology and obstetrics: the health care of women, New York, 1975, McGraw-Hill Book Co.

Weed, J. C., and Holland, J. B.: Endometriosis and infertility: an enigma, Fertil. Steril. **28**(2):135-155, 1977.

Whelan, E. M.: A baby? . . . maybe, Indianapolis, 1975, The Bobbs-Merrill Co.

REFERENCES FOR CLIENTS

Adoption

Anderson, D. C.: Children of special value, New York, 1971, St. Martins Press.

Berman, C.: We take this child, New York, 1974, Doubleday and Co. Inc.

DeHartog, J.: The children, New York, 1969, Atheneum Publishers.

Dywasuk, C. T.: Adoption—is it for you? New York, 1973, Harper & Row Publishers.

Klibanoff, S., and Klibanoff, E.: Let's talk about adoption, Boston, 1973, Little, Brown and Co.

MacNamera, J.: The adoption advisor, New York, 1975, Hawthorne Books, Inc.

OURS: The unbroken circle; carry it on (International and interracial adoption). Available from OURS, Inc., 4711 30th Ave., Minneapolis, MN. 55406.

Sorosky, A. D., Baran, A., and Pannor, R.: The adoption triangle, New York, 1978, Anchor Press/Doubleday.

Childfree living

Peck, E.: The baby trap, New York, 1971, Bernard Geis Associates, Inc.

Peck, E., and Senderowitz, J.: Pronatalism: the myth of mom and apple pie, New York, 1974, Thomas Y. Crowell and Co.

Whelan, E. M.: A baby? . . . maybe, Indianapolis, 1975, The Bobbs-Merrill Co.

Infertility

All about that baby, Newsweek **92**:66-72, Aug. 7, 1978.

Boston Women's Health Book Collective: Our bodies, ourselves, New York, 1976, Simon & Schuster.

Brody, J. E.: New hope for infertile couples, Woman's Day, pp. 24-28, Feb. 3, 1978.

Consumers Union of the U.S.: The Consumers Union report on family planning, ed. 2, Mount Vernon, N.Y., 1966, Consumers Union.

D'Aulaire, E., and D'Aulair, P. O.: New hope for the childless, Read. Dig. **111**:197-200, Dec. 1977.

Decker, A., and Loebl, S.: Why can't we have a baby? New York, 1978, Dial Press.

First test tube baby, Time **112**:58-59, July 31, 1978.

Good news for couples who can't have babies, Good Housekeeping, p. 4, May, 1978.

Harrison, M.: Infertility: a couples' guide to its causes and treatments, New York, 1977, Houghton Mifflin Co.

Humphrey, M.: Hostage seekers: A study of childless and adopting couples, Studies in Child Development, 1969.

Kaufman, S. A.: New hope for the childless couple, New York, 1970, Simon & Schuster.

Kolata, G.: Infertility: promising new treatments, Science **202**:200-203, Oct. 13, 1978.

Lane, R. M.: The specter of sterility, Esquire, pp. 30-33, April 11, 1978.

Martin, K.: Infertility: how one couple faced it and found new expectations, Glamour **76**:184-185, Mar. 1978.

Masters, W. H., and Johnson, V. E.: Advice for women who want to have a baby, Redbook. **144**:701, Mar. 1975.

McCauley, C. S.: Pregnancy after 35, New York, 1976, E. P. Dutton and Co.

Menning, B. E.: Infertility: A guide for the childless couple, New York, Prentice-Hall, 1977.

Morrone, W. W.: Facts and fictions about becoming pregnant that every woman should know, Glamour pp. 100-101, Dec. 1975.

My husband couldn't give me a child, Good Housekeeping **183**:36, Nov. 1976.

Phillipp, E.: Overcoming childlessness: its causes and what to do about them, New York, 1975, Taplinger Publishing Co., Inc.

Roberts, N.: I want to have a baby—and can't, Mademoiselle, pp. 116-117, Oct. 1978.

Sarrel, P., and Sarrel, L.: Why some couples can't conceive, Redbook, p. 55, Nov. 1978.

Selber, S. J.: How to get pregnant, New York, 1980, Scribner.

Skrocki, M. R.: Infertility: the loneliest problem, McCalls, **105**:68-69, Aug. 1978.

Test-tube baby heralds (brave) new medical era, Med. World News, pp. 10-11, Aug. 7, 1978.

15

Reproductive surgery

Deitra Leonard Lowdermilk

Practitioners in both primary and secondary health care settings are often involved in care of the woman who is having gynecologic surgery, but nursing information that would aid the nurse in providing adequate care for these women is sparse. Until now the nurse has had to rely on medical texts to find out about surgical procedures, and there have been few sources of information about nursing care.

Perhaps because of the woman's health movement there is increased interest in providing consumers as well as practitioners with information about reproductive surgery. There is concern about the number of hysterectomies being performed, and many people question whether all of these are necessary. New surgical and diagnostic techniques have been introduced by the medical profession that may be used instead of major surgery, thereby reducing the potential of needless operations for women.

The purpose of this chapter is to acquaint the nurse with reproductive surgery, using the nursing process. Assessment data include identification of clients at risk at different periods in the life span. Diagnostic measures that may be used prior to surgery are explained. Information that will help the client as she makes her decision is also included so that the nurse can act as a client advocate. Management strategies of the most common gynecologic surgical procedures are explained, and the physiologic and psychosocial components of pre- and postoperative nursing care are described. Criteria for evaluation of care are presented to help the nurse assess whether or not the client's needs were met.

The chapter focuses mainly on hysterectomy because it is the most common major surgery performed on women today. This discussion includes information of patients at risk, reasons for surgery, the different procedures and alternatives, pre- and postoperative care, the use of estrogen therapy, and sexual, cultural, and emotional implications.

Surgery related specifically to gynecologic oncology (vulvectomy, pelvic exenteration) is discussed in Chapter 16.

ASSESSMENT

The nurse must recognize women who are at risk for reproductive surgery and the factors that influence this at-risk state. The practitioner can use this knowledge to inform clients of the potential risk and to counsel them about the ways in which the health care system can meet their needs.

Age. Women are at risk for different reproductive problems throughout the life cycle. Apart from pregnancy and the related operative procedures that may be used, the childbearing years may involve a number of surgical procedures. The number of sterilizations performed on women ages 25 to 35 years who wish to limit the number of children in their families is high. Surgery for infertility problems is also prevalent in this age group. Women are at risk in young to mid-adulthood (20 to 40) for problems related to menstruation and cancer of the cervix. This might lead to dilatation and curettage or hysterectomy. There is a high incidence of pelvic surgery in the 60 to 69 year age groups. This fact is correlated with the increased longevity of the female (Martin, 1978; Mattingly, 1977) and the concomitant increased risk of cancer and pelvic relaxations.

Functional disturbances. Symptoms related to functional or metabolic disturbances can also be identified as risk factors. Dysfunctional uterine bleeding may or may not be a significant pathologic problem. Abdominal pain may indicate an enlarging pelvic tumor (see Chapter 13). Pregnancy-related conditions such as pelvic relaxation may become more symptomatic with advanced age (Maeck et al., 1975).

Screening. Regular health screening to identify any existent health problems is an essential part of the care of women. The nurse should be alert to problems related to obstetric and gynecologic conditions that may require surgical intervention. The use of the problem-oriented record is encouraged. This information collection process includes identification of the chief complaint, client profile, history of the present illness, past medical history, a review of systems, and findings related to the physical examination and laboratory data.

A list of current problems is identified that can be updated periodically as problems are resolved (see Chapter 7 for specifics on assessment).

DIAGNOSIS

The health care team analyzes data concerning the problems presented by the client in order to make a diagnosis. Certain diagnostic procedures that may be used prior to surgery for the client with a reproductive problem should be explained by the nurse. This explanation will facilitate the client's decision-making and allow her to be an active participant in treatment.

Diagnostic measures that should be explained, when appropriate, are: diagnostic radiology including x-rays, intravenous pyelograms, barium studies, cystography, and ultrasonography; and culposcopy.

Diagnostic radiology now plays an important role in diagnosis of pelvic problems. Previously, the gynecologist relied on bimanual examination, exploratory laparotomy, or laparoscopy to obtain the information needed to make a diagnosis. However, because there are alternatives to the more radical procedures, including microsurgery, an accurate assessment is essential. Better assessment also means there are fewer disadvantages to the woman.

X-rays have only a minor role in diagnosis of pelvic conditions. Routine chest X-ray is most frequently done when there is the possibility of malignancy.

Intravenous pyelogram is a very important diagnostic procedure in gynecology. The demonstration of the anatomy of the uterus is an integral part of the preoperative assessment of any large pelvic tumor or any patient with cancer of the cervix. It also is important in diagnosing urinary incontinence.

Barium studies, such as the barium enema, are important for diagnosing problems in the left lower quadrant of the abdomen. Sigmoidoscopy is often used in association with barium enemas. Cystography plays an important part in the evaluation of stress incontinence (Howkins and Hudson, 1977).

Ultrasonography is especially useful in women of childbearing age because it does not have the harmful effects of radiation and can be used to diagnose problems during pregnancy, such as placental problems or ectopic pregnancy, and other problems such as fibroids, ovarian cysts, and benign and malignant tumors. The abdomen is scanned with high frequency soundwaves, that can be displayed on an oscillograph (Schram and Bretcher, 1975).

Culposcopy enables the operator to study cervical epithelial changes undetectable by the naked eye. A more detailed discussion of the use of culposcopy can be found in Chapter 16, Reproductive Malignancies.

Each client should be told what to expect during each procedure, why it is being done, what preparations she can expect (i.e., dietary restrictions, enema), where the procedures are performed (clinic, physician's office, hospital), the cost, and whether or not insurance or Medicaid/Medicare will pay for the procedures.

CONSULTATION

The woman should be aware of her right to consult other health care providers prior to consenting to surgery. Factors for the client to consider when contemplating a second opinion include the urgency of the indications for surgery and the quality of life she can expect after surgery (ACOG, 1977).

MANAGEMENT STRATEGIES

The client's decisions concerning treatment and nursing care are two areas that need the nurse's attention when considering management strategies. Once the diagnosis is made, the physician discusses the disease or condition requiring surgery. It is important that this discussion be thorough, include family members if possible, and be done at the client's level of understanding. The role of the nursing practitioner is to complement the physician's explanation by making sure the woman understands what has been said to her, by re-emphasizing important points, and making further explanations when necessary. At all times the nurse should emphasize the woman's right to control her body and the right to make informed decisions.

The indications for surgery, including the risks, should be discussed. Alternatives to the surgery as well as reasons why the physician has chosen a particular treatment should be mentioned. The predicted outcome of the surgery as well as the side effects or complications must be included. The wishes of the woman regarding future childbearing are very important. She should be informed if the surgery will end her ability to bear a child.

Whether or not the surgery will alter sexual performance is another area to be discussed. Often clients have misconceptions, which should be cleared up prior to surgery. The discussion should also include information about anesthesia, hospitalization, convalescence, and costs. There should be time for the woman to ask any questions she has concerning the surgery. The nurse is often the health worker who is available for discussion of further concerns and she should be directed to the woman who has unanswered questions (Ridley, 1974; T. J. Williams, 1974).

After the decision for surgery has been made, the nursing care needed by the client pre- and postoperatively must be planned. In the following discussions of surgical procedures attention is given not only to the techniques but also to the physical and emotional needs of women undergoing the procedures, and criteria for evaluation of the nursing care.

OPERATIVE PROCEDURES

Certain operative procedures can be used as diagnostic tools or as alternatives to other surgical procedures when it is desirable to retain childbearing ability. There are alternative sterilization procedures, and infertility surgery often uses the same operative procedures as diagnostic surgery. Hysterectomy can be performed vaginally or abdominally and with or without the removal of tubes and ovaries. There are alternatives even to this surgery. The rest of this chapter focuses on specific reproductive surgical procedures, their uses, complications, nursing care, emotional implications, and sexual implications.

Dilatation and curettage

Indications

Dilatation of the cervix and curettage of the endometrium (D & C) is currently one of the most frequently performed operative procedures on the uterus. Indications for this procedure include diagnosis of uterine malignancy, control of dysfunctional uterine bleeding, complications of an incomplete abortion, therapeutic abortion, evaluation of causes of infertility, and relief of dysmenorrhea. The diagnostic purpose of endometrial curettage is to differentiate bleeding related to hormonal dysfunction from bleeding related to uterine malignancy. The therapeutic value of curettage is to control abnormal bleeding by removing the endometrium (Mattingly, 1977).

Technique

Dilatation and curettage may be done as an outpatient procedure or the woman may be admitted to the hospital. The client is prepared in the usual way for a vaginal operation. She is usually given general anesthesia but epidural, spinal, or local anesthetic agents may be used. The woman is placed in a lithotomy position. A bimanual examination is done to determine the position of the uterus. A speculum is inserted into the vagina to expose the cervix. A sound is introduced into the uterus for measurement of the uterine cavity, and then the uterus is dilated gradually with metal dilators. The curet is then introduced into the uterine cavity and the endometrium scraped away. Suction curettage may be used as well. All material is sent to a pathology laboratory for analysis and confirmation of the preoperative diagnosis.

Complications

Secondary hemorrhage develops occasionally during the second postoperative week. It is treated by vaginal packing. Lacerations of the cervix may cause bleeding; treatment varies according to the degree of laceration. Perforation of the uterus is unusual (approximately 1 in 500 cases) although it may occur in cases of adenocarcinoma of the endometrium and during abortion. If perforation occurs in a clean operation, no treatment is required except careful observation. The only real danger is the possibility of uterine rupture in subsequent labor. There is always a risk of infection, which may take the form of peritonitis or septicemia (Howkins and Hudson, 1977).

Nursing care

Preoperative. The client may or may not have a perineal shave, an enema, or a vaginal douche depending on the surgeon's preference. Usually the patient has nothing by mouth past midnight the day of surgery.

Postoperative. The nurse should check vital signs every 15 minutes until stable. She should also check the amount of vaginal bleeding and keep a pad count. Mild analgesics may be given for pain. Diet is usually as tolerated by the client.

The nurse should make sure the client knows what to expect, especially if she is to be discharged the same day. Information to be given to the client includes the following:

1. After the first hour, pads should not be changed more than once an hour for the first postoperative day. Keep a pad count and notice if pads are soaked through. A few small clots may be passed. Bleeding is excessive if more than one pad (changed hourly) is saturated in 8 hours.
2. Spotting is normal up to 8 weeks after spontaneous abortion.
3. Abdominal cramping is not unusual the first few days. This can usually be relieved by taking mild analgesics (aspirin, Tylenol) every 4 hours as needed or by placing a heating pad or hot water bottle on the abdomen.
4. Tampons are not usually worn for at least 1 week after curettage.
5. Temperature should be taken every 4 hours for 2 days. Notify the physician if the temperature rises over 100° F.
6. There should be no intercourse for 2 weeks.*

Cryosurgery

Cryosurgery is used in the treatment of chronic cerliving tissue.

---

*Based on instructions given patients at North Carolina Memorial Hospital, Chapel Hill, N.C.

Indications

Cryosurgery is sued in the treatment of chronic cervicitis, endocervicitis, erosions, and nabothian cysts. It is also used as a preventive measure to treat dysplasia and can be used for palliative reduction of inoperable and recurrent carcinoma (Disaia, 1975).

Technique

Cryosurgery is best performed 1 week after the end of the menstrual period to avoid freezing a uterus with an early pregnancy and to permit the most active phase of cervical regeneration to take place prior to the onset of the next menstrual period. Treatment is usually performed in the physician's office or clinic without anesthesia. A speculum as large as the patient can tolerate is inserted into the vagina. The refrigerant (nitrous oxide) is circulated through a special cryoprobe, which is placed in the area to be frozen. This local freezing causes necrosis (frostbite) of the affected or diseased tissue, which then sloughs off. The remaining healthy tissue then heals cleanly (Howkins and Hudson, 1977).

Complications

Occasional spotting and cervical stenosis have been reported. Injuries to normal tissue occur if the probe touches vaginal epithelium.

Nursing care

The nurse's role is to make sure the client is informed about the treatment and the effects she can expect afterward. An explanation of the procedure prior to treatment will help the client tolerate the uncomfortable position for the length of time it takes to freeze the tissue. (Sudden movements could cause damage to normal tissues.) An explanation of side effects is also helpful. A profuse watery discharge may be present for 2 to 3 weeks following cryosurgery. Sanitary pads, maxi or mini, may be necessary. Some authorities recommend avoiding sexual intercourse, douching, swimming, or use of tampons for 2 weeks because cervix is somewhat friable. Occasionally, a woman will have spotting or bleeding after she has intercourse, but this should not be heavy. Showers are recommended although tub bathing is allowed if the tub is cleaned well first.

Biopsy

Abnormal appearance of the cervix is a frequent finding in gynecologic examinations; some of these changes are indicative of a malignancy, others are not.

Indications

A cervical biopsy is recommended whenever there is a need to investigate suspicious cervical tissue in order to diagnose or rule out cervical cancer in its earliest stages. Decisions about treatment are usually dependent on the histopathologic examination of biopsy specimens. Endometrial biopsy is widely used in infertility clinics to ascertain whether ovulation has occurred. Conization is the treatment of choice for the majority of women with marked dysplasia or carcinoma in situ. Diagnostic conization is indicated if atypical squamous cells are repeatedly found in cytology smears and colposcopy examinations, biopsies, and curettage are negative.

Techniques

The three techniques usually used for obtaining histopathologic specimens for examination are punch biopsy, excision biopsy, and conization.

Punch biopsy. Punch biopsy forceps are used to remove pieces of tissue from the cervix, vagina, and vulvar region. The procedure is almost painless and is used in the outpatient setting.

Excision biopsy. Cervical specimens are excised with a scalpel. The excision usually extends into normal tissue, which means the specimen is larger than a punch biopsy and bleeding is more frequent. Sutures may be necessary, making the procedure painful and necessitating the use of an local anesthetic agent. If vulvar biopsy is necessary, anesthesia is always used (Kolstad and Stafl, 1977).

Conization. The size and length of the core of tissue to be removed from the cervix are determined by the extent of the lesion on the ectocervix and in the endocervix. Colposcopy is used to localize the lesion prior to the operation. Local or general anesthesia may be used, and the procedure can be performed in outpatient as well as inpatient settings. Suturing the side ligaments of the cervix may prevent postoperative bleeding. A scalpel is usually used to remove the cone of tissue (Kolstad and Stafl, 1977).

Endometrial biopsy. The patient is not anesthetized for endometrial biopsy. It is usually performed in the physician's office or other outpatient setting. The procedure is used to scrape the endometrium during the last premenstrual phase of the menstrual cycle. A small curette or small suction device (Vibra aspirator) is used.

Complications

After conization and often with curettage the next two or three menstrual periods may be prolonged or profuse with a dark brown premenstrual discharge. Usually there is no specific treatment for this. Secondary hemorrhage is a risk for all cervical operations; the bleeding is usually controlled by vaginal packing for 24 to 48 hours. Stenosis is a rare complication and is usually treated by dilatation. Infection can occur after conization but it is usually controlled by the use of antibiotics.

Endocervical granulations may occur after conization but they usually require no treatment.

Extensive conization affects subsequent pregnancy and childbirth by increasing the incidence of abortion (13.6%) and premature labor (18%). If cervical atresia occurs, a cesarean section may be necessary (Howkins and Hudson, 1977).

Nursing care

The nurse should know about these biopsy procedures so that she can tell the client what to expect during the procedure and postoperatively. It is helpful to tell the client which procedures may be painful so that she will know that pain is a normal sensation. The client should be informed that she may have profuse or prolonged menstrual periods for several cycles following the procedure. If procedures such as conization are performed for treatment of carcinoma in situ or cervicitis, the client should be informed that she should continue to have frequent examinations, usually at 4- to 9-month intervals. Possible effects on subsequent pregnancy and childbirth should be explained especially if childbearing is desired. Close observation for postoperative bleeding is important both by the nurse and the client to prevent complications of hemorrhage.

Biopsy surgery can also have emotional effects on the woman. If the histopathologic examination of the tissue removed is negative for malignancy, the woman will be relieved. If the diagnosis is cancer the woman will need support from the nurse in coping with the diagnosis and implications for future treatment.

Laparoscopy

Laparoscopy is a procedure by which the pelvic organs are visualized and examined by the insertion of a laparoscope through the abdominal wall. A local anesthetic is injected prior to insertion of the instrument (Phipps, Long, and Woods, 1979).

Indications

Laparoscopy may be diagnostic or therapeutic. It can be used instead of an exploratory laparotomy to make a diagnosis in a client with chronic pelvic pain, an abdominal mass, indications of abdominal cancer or metastases, or ectopic pregnancy. Laparoscopy is also valuable in infertility evaluations. Tubal patency as well as ovulation can be determined; endometriosis can be diagnosed; biopsies can be obtained and peritubal adhesions can be removed. Laparoscopy is also used as a method of tubal sterilization.

Technique

Laparoscopy may be performed as an inpatient or outpatient procedure. Short-acting general anesthesia is most commonly used although local and regional anesthetic agents can be employed. Local agents are not preferred because the woman then requires more sedation and is not able to leave the clinic as quickly as when general anesthesia is used. Usually clients are able to go home within 2 hours postoperatively.

The woman is placed in a head-down position. A small incision is made in the skin of the lower rim of the umbilicus. A needle is inserted and is converted to the insufflation apparatus. Carbon dioxide or nitrous oxide is used to distend the abdomen and separate the organs. The endoscope is then inserted for visualization. Often a second instrument is needed to visualize the whole pelvic cavity and to perform the operative procedure. The usual site for this is lower than the umbilicus, above the symphysis pubis. When the surgery is completed, as much gas as possible is expelled. Clips or sutures are used to close the puncture sites.

Contraindications

A woman with any preexisting cardiovascular or respiratory condition that precludes insufflation or the Trendelenburg position should not undergo laparoscopy. Obesity and abdominal adhesions may also be considered contraindications.

Complications

Transient shoulder pain resulting from the insufflation is a common occurrence. Blood vessels may be punctured by the sharp instruments. Insufflation can be associated with embolism, emphysema, and other cardiovascular and respiratory problems. Infection is always a risk. If diathermy is used, burns to abdominal and bowel tissue can occur, which can lead to necrosis and peritonitis (Howkins and Hudson, 1977).

Nursing implications

Preoperatively, the client usually has nothing by mouth past midnight. Cathartics or enema are optional, as are skin preparation (shaving), depending on the physician's instructions. The nurse should see if the woman has questions about the procedure and give information as needed.

Postoperatively, vital signs are taken frequently the first hour or until stable. If the client is having the surgery as an outpatient, she will be taken to a recovery area until she is ready to leave. She may have fluids and light snacks if desired. Prior to discharge the woman should be told what to expect with regard to convalescence. She should know that she may have a sore throat from intubation and a sore chest from insufflation, which will gradually disappear, usually within 48 hours. She can engage in sexual intercourse within a week or less if she desires. The scar will be barely noticeable; this may be important to a woman concerned with body image. Her recovery should be fast and easy.

Tubal sterilization

Sterilization and infertility procedures are the primary reasons for tubal surgery. Tubal sterilization as a method of contraception is discussed in Chapter 22. The focus of the discussion here is on assessing women who may choose this method of contraception in order to advise them concerning which procedure might best meet their needs. Information about reversal and microsurgery is included because of the increased requests for these procedures.

Counseling

The nurse must have current information on the prerequisites or guidelines for sterilization used by the medical profession. As of February 1978, guidelines set up by the Department of Health, Education and Welfare included the following:

1. A full explanation to the client of the procedures, including risks and benefits
2. A statement to the client about the permanent nature of the surgery
3. At least a 72-hour wait between signing the papers and the surgery (a 30-day period is required if federal funds are used)
4. Knowledge on the client's part that refusal of the procedure may be made at any time

The American College of Obstetricians and Gynecologists no longer stipulates the number of children a woman must have before a sterilization can be performed. Sterilization is treated like any other surgical procedure. A husband's consent is not legally required in most states; however many physicians discourage potential legal actions by getting the husband's consent whenever possible (Moukhtar and Romney, 1974).

Before a decision for tubal sterilization is made, factors such as the number of previous pregnancies, family size desired, cultural influences, and personal preferences should be considered and discussed. The changing status of women in society, especially with regard to women's rights and independence, has resulted in more single women requesting sterilization. The decision to sterilize a woman should be made independently of her age and marital status as long as she understands the effects of the surgery and is sure of her desire for the procedure (Moukhtar and Romney, 1974).

It is the responsibility of any health professional serving women who are considering sterilization to provide counseling and information and obtain informed consent. Counseling should be thorough and include information on available alternatives, likelihood of reversibility, degree of permanence, and risks and complications. Counseling should be done with both partners if possible. The counselor should be on the lookout for the woman who thinks sterilization will solve all her problems. Psychologic side effects have been noted in women with a history of menstrual problems, unstable marriage, sexual problems, and somatic complaints.

Methods and selection of procedures

There are several techniques for tubal sterilization and the choice for each woman depends on her life situation and specific needs. Pomeroy tubal ligation is usually performed soon after delivery. Sterilization combined with therapeutic abortion can include laparoscopic sterilization after vacuum aspiration, or vaginal tubal ligation after dilatation and curettage. Laparoscopy is usually used as an interval tubal sterilization because it can be done on an outpatient basis and is highly effective and convenient (Porter and Hulka, 1975).

Traditional surgical approaches: abdominal approach. A number of techniques have been developed to interrupt ovum transport through the fallopian tube. The major variations are related to the portion of the tube involved: isthmic (Irving technique), interstitial (cornual resection), ampullar (Madline and Pomeroy techniques), and fimbriated end (Aldrich technique) (Meeker and Gray, 1975).

Abdominal Pomeroy tubal ligation is the most commonly used method of postpartum sterilization. It can be done under local or general anesthesia and takes about 20 minutes. Most procedures are performed within 24 to 48 hours after delivery when the fallopian tubes are near the surface of the abdominal wall and can be reached easily through a small incision. A loop is formed in the midportion of the tube, which is ligated and resected. Infection and bleeding are the principal complications; the reported failure rate is less than 1%. The second traditional abdominal method is the Irving technique, which is usually used after cesarean section. The fallopian tubes are cut in the isthmic portion and ligated. The ends nearest the uterus are imbedded in the uterine musculature and the distal ends are buried in the broad ligament. This procedure takes 5 to 10 minutes and is almost 100% effective (Porter and Hulka, 1975).

Vaginal approach. Vaginal tubal ligation is usually performed using the Pomeroy procedure for the fimbriectomy. Failure rates are slightly higher for the vaginal approach; this may be the result of problems in identification of the tubes through a colpotomy incision. A fimbriectomy includes the ligation of the distal portion of the tubes with excision of the fimbriated ends. Reversibility for fimbriectomy is almost nil because the fimbriae have been removed. Vaginal tubal sterilization can be performed in 10 to 15 minutes. It is cosmetically advantageous because there is no external incision.

However, it is contraindicated if the uterus is fixed, if there are pelvic adhesions, or if the woman is extremely obese. Complications include infection and bleeding (Porter and Hulka, 1975).

Endoscopic approaches. Laparoscopy, culdoscopy, and hysteroscopy can be used as sterilization procedures without major surgery and hospitalization. Either general or local anesthesia can be used. The procedure for laparoscopy has been described earlier in this chapter. The tube can be cauterized or clips can be applied. Complications are the same as previously mentioned. Pregnancy rate is less than 1%.

Culdoscopy sterilization involves a transvaginal approach. The woman is placed in the kneechest position and local anesthesia is used before a trochar is inserted in the peritoneal cavity. A culdoscope is inserted. The fallopian tube is pulled through the incision, ligated and cut or clipped and replaced in the peritoneal cavity. Complications include infection and hemorrhage.

Experimental hysteroscopic techniques for sterilization are being studied. Local anesthesia is used and the cervix is dilated in order to insert the hysteroscope. The uterotubal junctions are cauterized causing formation of scar tissue, which blocks the tubes (Porter and Hulka, 1975).

Reversibility

It can be expected that a certain proportion of the decisions for tubal sterilization are based on personal and social rather than medical reasons and are later regretted. There is currently an increased number of requests for tubal reconstruction. Most of these requests are from women who have been divorced and remarried and who desire to have a child by their new spouse.

The clip method has the greatest potential for successful reversibility because this method causes less interference in the tubal blood supply than cauterization or ligation. Fimbriectomy usually cannot be reversed. In general, the shorter the tube is after reanastomosis, the smaller the chance of pregnancy.

Microsurgery is a recent technique for reversal. This technique involves keeping the tissues continuously soaked in saline, removing the dead tissue, and reanastomosing the tube. Microsurgery offers the best opportunity to restore tubal patency. However, it is so recent that there are few long-term results of this type of treatment. One study reports a 50% to 60% pregnancy rate after microsurgery (Diamond, 1977).

Nursing implications

The nurse should explain to the client the physical and emotional changes that will occur following sterilization. The woman should be informed that she will continue to menstruate and that the menstrual period may vary in length of cycle, duration of flow, or amount of blood loss. These changes will probably be mild, if present at all, and will seldom require treatment. The woman will still ovulate and there is no physiologic effect on hormones, weight, or sexual response.

Emotional reactions may occur if the woman has a poor sexual or mental adjustment. She may also have problems if she thought the surgery would alleviate menstrual difficulties. When there are no predisposing factors there are usually few psychologic problems.

There are some general psychologic considerations or implications that the nurse may want to assess in regard to tubal sterilizations (Swenson, 1974):

- Cultural implications. Areas to assess include cultural variations in the role of the woman, the importance of childbearing, attitudes toward surgery, and fears of body mutilation.
- Timing of procedure in relation to childbearing/ abortion. Many women are dissatisfied initially after a postpartum sterilization if they had not made the decision antepartally. They did not have enough time to adjust to and accept the decision. Many women are dissatisfied after sterilization following an abortion for the same reasons.
- Tubal vs hysterectomy sterilization. A study by Barglow (1965) reports more dissatisfaction among women who had a hysterectomy for sterilization than among those choosing tubal sterilization. Women having a tubal sterilization still felt like women because they had the uterus and still menstruated. The unrealistic fantasy that the woman could still get pregnant after the tubal ligation was also reported.
- Marital status. From 75% to 95% of married women have no regrets.
- Reason for procedure. There are reports of more dissatisfaction when sterilization is done for medical reasons rather than as an elective procedure.

Operative treatment for infertility

Several previously discussed procedures may also be used for infertility treatment. Dilatation and curettage is used to open a rigid cervical canal and evaluate the luteal phase of the menstrual cycle. This procedure is frequently combined with a laparoscopic examination of the ovaries and tubes, which may demonstrate occlusions and ovulation (Mattingly, 1977). Tuboplasty or correction of tubal obstruction usually is performed for four major areas of disease: (1) peritubal adhesions, (2) occlusions of the distal end of the tube, (3) proximal tubal obstruction, and (4) segmental obstruction.

Success is directly related to the degree of damage that can be corrected. The most common problem after surgery is the reformation of adhesions. The use of hydrotubation following tubal surgery has been helpful in maintaining patency and preventing adhesion formation. An important fact is that a woman who has tubal surgery is at risk (5% to 10%) to have an ectopic pregnancy (Menning, 1977).

Microsurgery has recently been applied to tubal surgery with much success because of the more accurate reanastomosis of the ends of the tubes. This procedure should increase the success of tubal surgery and pregnancy rates. See Chapter 14 for a more detailed discussion of surgical procedures related to treatment of infertility.

Hysterectomy

Within the medical profession there is tremendous controversy over hysterectomy. It is second only to tonsillectomy as the most frequently performed major operation. There has been an increase in the incidence of hysterectomy to where an estimated 25% of the women over age 50 in the United States have had one (Silverberg, 1977). At the current rate, more than one half of the women in the United States will have had the uterus removed before they are 65 years old (Boston Women's Health Book Collective, 1976). Numerous reports have concluded that at least one third of the hysterectomies performed are unnecessary and that other procedures would have been as good as or better than removing the uterus (Rodgers, 1975). The use of hysterectomy as a form of elective sterilization or abortion (instead of simple procedures such as tubal ligation or vacuum aspiration) has been presented as an unnecessarily extreme measure (Rebutting charges, 1976).

In spite of the adverse publicity and controversy, women are still receptive to having a hysterectomy. Because the number of hysterectomies being performed is large, the nurse needs knowledge about the physiologic and psychologic changes that may occur so that she can give comprehensive care. This section provides information on the indications for hysterectomy, alternatives, the procedure involved including treatment for urinary stress incontinence, pre- and postoperative care, and psychosocial responses. A method for evaluating using outcome criteria concludes the discussion.

Indications

Although there is some disagreement among physicians about the absolute indications for hysterectomy, certain conditions are usually treated with this type of surgery. The primary care nurse should be alert for women who may need hysterectomy, to get them into the health care system.

Usually, cancer of the uterine endometrium or ovary is treated with hysterectomy. Premalignant conditions such as severe cervical dysplasia may also be treated with hysterectomy (Howkins and Hudson, 1977).

Leiomyomas or fibroids are the most common benign tumors of women. They are more common in nulliparas and five times more prevalent in blacks than whites. In women in their forties and fifties, bleeding is usually the first sign of a fibroid. Depending on the size of the fibroid, symptoms are usually pain and discomfort, increased menstrual flow, or irregular bleeding. Abdominal hysterectomy may be performed if the tumor is large (12 week gestational size) or there is persistent bleeding or no further childbearing is desired. Myomectomy is usually the treatment of choice especially in younger women who desire further childbearing (Romney et al., 1975).

Hysterectomy is an acceptable method of treatment of *endometriosis* when menorrhagia and dysmenorrhea are the dominant symptoms and when no further childbearing is desired.

Other conditions that may be treated by abdominal hysterectomy are chronic pelvic infections, life-threatening hemorrhage, and rupture of the uterus if suturing is not possible. Hysterectomy is also done following septic abortion that does not respond to treatment. Abdominal procedures are done in women who have had multiple pelvic operations and for women who will have their ovaries removed along with the uterus.

Indications for vaginal hysterectomy include uterine prolapse (which usually occurs in the older woman), pelvic relaxation when bladder supports need to be repaired (which is more common in multiparous women), dysmenorrhea or dysplasia; it is also used as a method of sterilization for women in their thirties and forties. Many physicians consider hysterectomy unjustifiable as a method of elective sterilization in women without pelvic pathology, but it is a totally acceptable procedure for sterilization.*

In recent years there has been a shift from anatomic to functional indications for hysterectomy. Reproductive, endocrine, and sexual function are the primary considerations today. The client's desires are important in the function approach, and today many women share in the decision-making process with the physician. For example, a woman with carcinoma in situ may choose to have therapeutic conization rather than a hysterectomy if she still desires to have children (Burchell, 1974).

The woman must understand all options for treatment. Preoperative counseling should include information about whether or not alternative procedures would be as beneficial and information about hospital admission, the procedure, anesthesia, side effects, postoperative care, convalescence, and resumption of activities. If ovaries are to be removed, an explanation of surgical

---

*Burchell, 1977; Higgins, 1971; Novaks et al., 1975; T. J. Williams, 1974.

menopause should be given as well as information about estrogen replacement therapy if warranted (Steele and Goodwin, 1975). With this information the woman can make an intelligent decision and give informed consent for the procedure. Making sure the woman is fully informed is a step toward eliminating unnecessary hysterectomies.

Myomectomy. For patients who want to maintain their childbearing potential, myomectomy may be the treatment of choice for fibroids causing discomfort or infertility. However it is usually not recommended for women over 35 years of age because of increased incidence of complicated pregnancies. Preservation of a nonfunctioning uterus with large fibroids is usually unjustified.

Myomectomy is a major procedure with all the risks of such surgery. Preoperative preparations are similar to those for abdominal hysterectomy. Surgery should be performed in the proliferative phase of the menstrual cycle to minimize blood loss. This also avoids the possibility of unsuspected pregnancy.

The procedure should include removal of all fibroids and reconstruction of the uterus without compromising tubes and ovaries. A minimal number of incisions into the uterus should be made; incision into the uterine cavity should be avoided except for removal of fibroids.

Postoperative hemorrhage is a significant problem because the incised uterus can bleed into the peritoneal cavity. Mortality rates can be higher than for abdominal hysterectomy for benign conditions (T. J. Williams, 1974).

Contraindications

Vaginal hysterectomy. Absence of pelvic relaxation increases the morbidity of vaginal procedures and should be considered as a contraindication. Other contraindications include the presence of pelvic inflammatory disease, ovarian tumors, an enlarged uterus (up to a 12 to 14 weeks gestational size), previous abdominal procedure, previous pelvic radiation therapy, and conditions that limit the mobility of the uterus, such as endometriosis, cervical cancer, and a narrow, fixed vagina. Women who have vascular and orthopedic problems should not have a vaginal hysterectomy because it requires prolonged suspension of the legs in the stirrups.

Abdominal hysterectomy. There is no contraindication for abdominal procedures other than the usual contraindications to surgical procedures (Barter, 1974).

Techniques

Abdominal procedures account for 70% of all hysterectomies, and total hysterectomies account for 95% of all procedures. Subtotal hysterectomy, in which the cervix is not removed, are infrequently performed because of the danger of cancer of the cervix. In a radical hysterectomy, the lymph nodes are dissected and they may be removed along with the upper vagina and parametrium (Barter, 1974).

The choice of abdominal or vaginal hysterectomy is based on many factors, including indications and contraindications, advantages and disadvantages, and morbidity and mortality.

In both the abdominal and vaginal hysterectomy, the procedure consists of removing the uterus from its supporting ligaments. These ligaments (broad, round, and uterosacral) are attached to the vaginal cuff so that normal depth of the vagina is maintained.

"Panhysterectomy" refers to removal of the uterus, tubes, and ovaries. Total abdominal hysterectomy with bilateral salpingo-oophorectomy means the same thing and is often seen on charts abbreviated "TAH-BSO." The fate of the ovaries—whether to leave them in or take them out—is an important question to be decided by the physician with input from the woman.

Usually, the ovaries are not removed in premenopausal women because oophorectomy causes surgical castration and menopause, leading to decreased libido and decreased lubrication and sensation in the lower vaginal tract (Amias, 1975). On the other hand, some physicians argue that there is a risk of ovarian cancer if the ovaries are left in, although the incidence of cancer in ovaries retained after hysterectomy is difficult to determine (Howkins and Hudson, 1977).

The variables that must be considered in deciding whether or not to perform oophorectomy include the extent and nature of pathology; the age, emotional stability, and general health of the woman; and the difficulty of extra surgery. The ovaries should not be removed routinely; the woman should always be included in the decision-making process.

Advantages and disadvantages

Vaginal hysterectomy has advantages over abdominal procedures, especially for the poor-risk elderly woman. The procedure can be done quickly with little anesthesia, which keeps respiratory complications to a minimum. Early ambulation is possible, there is less postoperative discomfort, and fewer problems with bowel functions result than with abdominal hysterectomy. It is also advantageous for the obese woman with pelvic relaxation.

One disadvantage of vaginal hysterectomy is that there is a greater risk of postoperative infection. Difficulties with surgery or unexpected complications with surgery are better controlled if the abdominal procedure is chosen, because every structure is visualized directly and there is a wider opening. There is less chance of overlooking problems with the bowel, adnexa, or pelvic lymph nodes if the abdominal hysterectomy is done (Barter, 1974). Low midline abdominal incisions are best for large tumors or intestinal complications. Transverse incisions are stronger and more cosmetic (T. J. Williams, 1974).

Anterior and posterior repairs. As noted earlier, uterine prolapse and pelvic relaxation are two major indications for vaginal hysterectomy. Repair of the anterior and posterior vaginal walls is included when there is displacement of one or more of the pelvic organs, including the urethra, bladder, uterus, and rectum. Displacement of these organs usually results from weakening of the pelvic supporting structures by repeated childbearing or obstetric injury. Complaints include a heaviness in the pelvis and a bearing down sensation. There is usually strong familial history of these disorders, and they are more frequently seen in whites than in blacks. Obesity increases the symptoms (Stander, 1975).

A specific complaint related to weakening of bladder support is loss of urine whenever there is increased intra-abdominal pressure such as laughing or coughing (stress urinary incontinence). Weakening of the rectal wall causes constipation and difficult defecation.

These symptoms are distressing and women are often embarrassed to relate them to their physician. An alert nurse can assess these problems during history-taking and physical examination. The history should include the nature and severity of the problem, onset, and association with urinary tract infections, if the problem is urinary incontinence. Physical examination should include some means to reproduce the symptom. Having the woman cough or bear down with a full bladder is an easy way to assess incontinence.

The surgical treatment for stress urinary incontinence is usually the Marshall-Marchetti procedure, which is major surgery. Before surgery is chosen as treatment, the risks, anesthesia, and recovery should be weighed against the degree of distress. Alternative treatments for mild cases of stress urinary incontinence include the use of Kegal exercises to increase pelvic muscle tone, the use of vaginal tampons or pessaries to support the bladder neck, especially in the elderly woman, and weight reduction in the obese woman. Fecal incontinence is relieved only by surgical repair (Martin, 1978; Ulfelder, 1975).

Nursing care

Preoperative. The nurse in the gynecologic or surgical hospital setting is responsible for physiologic and psychologic preparation of the preoperative hysterectomy patient. Preoperative teaching can be done individually or in groups. The preoperative class described by Menhatz (1977) is designed to answer questions about procedures and to give reassurance to the women. The nurse can be a positive leader of the discussion group by encouraging ventilation of feelings and concerns. One way to get discussion started in a quiet group is to bring up old wives' tales. The nurse can expect the group to bring up common concerns including sexuality, cancer, anesthesia, and pain (Menhatz, 1977).

When a woman is given the information about hysterectomy prior to surgery, she will be less anxious and better able to cope in the postoperative period (Barter et al., 1975, Carbary, 1975). The nurse should make sure the woman has an adequate explanation of pre- and postoperative procedures, when they are done, why they are done, and what to expect. A general guide for the preoperative check list includes the following:

- Consent signed: the nurse should make sure this is informed consent
- Laboratory work: CBC, hemoglobin, hematocrit, type and cross-match of blood, urinalysis, chest X-ray, electrocardiogram
- Physical examination and history
- Surgical preparation: abdominal-perineal shave
- Soapsuds edema
- Vaginal douche
- pHisoHex shower
- Sedation night before surgery
- NPO past midnight
- Preoperative medication
- Removal of dentures, glasses, etc.
- Removal of makeup, nailpolish, jewelry
- Identification bracelet in place

Prophylactic antibiotics may be given 6 to 8 hours prior to surgery, at the time of the surgery, and for several doses after surgery.

Postoperative. Postoperative care begins in the operating room immediately after surgery, and continues until convalescence is complete. Miller and Avery (1965) describe four progressive stages of nursing responsibilities. The *first stage* begins in the operating room. The staff transfer the client to the recovery room without causing injury. The *second stage* is managed by the recovery room staff who stabilize the client. The *third stage* is managed on the nursing floor until the woman is discharged. The *fourth stage* is managed at home by the woman's family and primary care providers until she has fully recovered. The quality of care in these stages will determine the rate of recovery.

Vital signs are usually taken every 15 minutes postoperatively for the first hour, every ½ hour until stable, then every 4 hours. Deviation from the base line data should be reported to the physician.

An unobstructed airway must be maintained and the woman's head should be turned to one side to prevent aspiration. Turning, coughing, and deep breathing should be done at frequent intervals (every 2 hours) for the first 24 hours. If the woman has had an abdominal hysterectomy she may need to support her abdomen with a pillow on her hands when she coughs.

Circulation is stimulated by leg exercises (passive and active), administration of heparin, and the use of anti-embolism stockings. These actions will help prevent thrombophlebitis.

Checking for signs of bleeding that may lead to hemorrhage is done by assessing the amount of drainage on abdominal dressings and/or perineal pads. It is normal to have a moderate amount of vaginal bleeding. A drop in blood pressure or signs of shock should be regarded with concern and reported to the physician.

The amount of *pain relief* needed will depend on the type of operation and the woman's pain tolerance. Analgesia (narcotics) and sedation are usually ordered liberally the first 24 hours. By this time the degree of discomfort lessens and by the third or fourth day medications are reduced in amount and strength. Nursing measures for pain relief such as a back rub should be utilized along with medication. Simple measures such as ambulation or application of heat to the abdomen may relieve discomfort of gas.

Fluid intake is usually accomplished by intravenous methods immediately after surgery. Ice chips are offered by mouth before other clear liquids especially for the client who has had an abdominal hysterectomy, who will probably be nauseated. Maintenance needs as well as replacement of fluids lost are ordered by the physician, and intake should be carefully recorded.

Urinary output is also measured carefully to assess achievement of fluid balance. Foley catheters are usually discontinued by 48 hours for hysterectomy patients. After surgery for prolapse with repairs, retention of urine is a problem and often a catheter (Foley or suprapubic) is left in for 7 days. Urinary infection occurs in many women after repair surgery; therefore, nitrofurantoin may be administered prophylactically (Miller and Avery, 1965).

Care of the bowels usually consists of administration of mild laxatives as necessary until a bowel movement occurs. Enemas are not given unless the woman fails to respond to laxative treatment.

Early ambulation is advantageous for improving venous circulation, muscle tone, lung expansion, and bowel function. Hysterectomy clients are encouraged to be out of bed at least by the first postoperative day. If the surgery has been extensive or complicated ambulation should be delayed until the woman's condition is satisfactory. Women having gynecologic surgery should always be treated individually in regard to ambulation. The nurse may need to assist the woman to get out of bed without straining. To do this, the woman is told to roll on her side, bring her knees up so that her thighs are at right angles to the abdomen, put her feet over the side of the bed, push up on her elbow, and sit up (Holm, 1976; Howkins and Hudson, 1977).

The *diet* usually progresses from clear liquids to full liquids to soft diet to regular diet. The progression should depend on the woman's desires and ability to eat. Sugar in foods and liquids tends to cause gas production and may need to be kept at a minimum for hysterectomy clients, who usually have problems with gas.

Abdominal dressings are changed as needed to keep them dry and intact. Superficial drains (Hemovacs) may be present the first 24 to 48 hours. Sutures are usually removed after the fifth day.

Vaginal sutures may be absorbable and not removed. Sitz baths and perineal care with warm water aid in keeping the vaginal wound clean. Vaginal packing to control oozing and hematoma formation is usually removed in 24 to 48 hours (Howkins and Hudson, 1977).

Postoperative complications

The nurse should be aware of the woman who is at risk for postoperative complications. Advanced age is correlated with the severity of all complications, especially pulmonary embolism; risk of infection is increased in the premenopausal woman. Obese women are at risk, especially for thrombophlebitis. Women who have a history of medical problems such as diabetes or cardiac or pulmonary problems are at a higher risk for complications. Women from low socioeconomic backgrounds are also more at risk than other clients (Macasaet and Nelson, 1974).

Hemorrhage. Hemorrhage may be immediate (within 24 hours) or late (10 to 30 days postoperatively). Hemorrhage is more frequent in vaginal hysterectomy. The nurse should watch for signs of internal as well as external bleeding.

Urinary tract complications. Urinary tract infections, such as cystitis or pyelitis, or urinary retention occur more frequently with vaginal hysterectomies. Usually, a temperature of 100° F for 2 to 3 days postoperatively signals an infection (Macasaet and Nelson, 1974). Urinary problems may appear even 6 months after surgery. In her study of adjustment to hysterectomy, Chynoweth (1973) found difficulty in urination in 20% of subjects, incontinence in 39%, infection in 20%, and impaired bladder sensation in 13%.

Infection. Wound infection is more frequent after vaginal hysterectomy. An elevated temperature is often the first sign, with redness and swelling of the wound area also noted. Treatment is usually with antibiotics or draining of hematomas if these are the problem (Macasaet and Nelson, 1974).

Intestinal obstruction or paralytic ileus. This is a more common complication after abdominal hysterectomy. The chief symptoms are constipation and vomiting, with distension a late symptom. Bowel sounds are absent with paralytic ileus. The usual treatment is deflation of the bowel with a nasogastric tube (Levin, Miller, Abbott, etc.) that is connected to suction.

Thromboembolism. Thrombophlebitis is a late complication involving the deep veins of the lower extremities, and it is more common after abdominal hysterectomy. Preventive treatment described in the postoperative care section is instituted along with rest in bed with the leg elevated.

Pulmonary. Pulmonary complications occur more often after abdominal hysterectomy. They include atelectasis, pneumonitis, and pulmonary embolism. Early ambulation and respiratory therapy are preventive measures for these complications.

Evisceration. Wound dehiscence occurs more often with abdominal hysterectomies. Secondary closure of the wound is required.*

Preparation for convalescence

The nurse should be aware of the information needs of the woman postoperatively. The physician should provide the client with information relevant to recovery both physically and emotionally, and the nurse should be available to answer questions or clarify as needed.

The following information should be given regarding physical changes and recovery (Barter, 1974; M. A. Williams, 1976):

- Discharge from hospital will usually be in 7 days
- Postoperative check-up will be in 4 to 6 weeks
- Avoid sitting for long periods, which could cause pelvic congestion
- Defer vacuuming, hanging out clothes, picking up heavy objects for at least 1 month
- Weakness and fatigue are normal
- Driving may be resumed before 2 weeks after discharge if the car is automatic and all "power" (some sources say the client can drive when she feels like it)
- Resume intercourse in 6 to 8 weeks although 3 to 4 weeks may be suggested; hysterectomy should not affect sexual enjoyment or response
- With anterior and posterior repair intercourse may be painful because of tightening of the vaginal walls
- There will be no more pregnancy
- There will be no more menstruation
- Masculinization, weight gain, etc., are merely old wives' tales
- Surgical menopause occurs if ovaries are removed
- Estrogen replacement therapy may be instituted (see below)
- Emotional changes may occur

---

*See Mattingly, 1977; Miller and Avery, 1965, Novaks et al., 1975.

Estrogen replacement therapy

Currently there is controversy both within the medical profession and among the general public about the use and misuse of estrogen. This discussion will be limited to the use of estrogen following hysterectomy with removal of the ovaries.

Estrogen is often prescribed for the premenopausal woman who has undergone surgical menopause. This is based on reports in the literature that the incidence of cardiovascular disease and osteoporosis is higher when estrogen therapy is not instituted. Estrogen is administered in low doses (1.5 mg daily) on a cyclic basis of 5 days on and 2 days off until the average age of menopause (age 50). The interrupted use of estrogen avoids excessive stimulation to the estrogen target tissues, particularly the breast; long-term use avoids unnecessary deprivation of estrogen in bone and lipid metabolism (Mattingly, 1977).

A study of the long-term effects of estrogen use (Byrd et al., 1977) with 1016 women who were placed on estrogen therapy for an average of 13½ years found a decrease in the death rate from heart attacks and cancer, an increase in breast cancer (but a decrease in death from breast cancer), and a decrease in the incidence of osteoporosis. The nulliparous woman was found to be at a high risk (two to three times higher than other women) for breast cancer in the first 10 years of therapy. The woman over 55 years of age and the woman experiencing late menopause were also in a high-risk category for breast cancer. Recommendations of the study were to give special consideration to these women before prescribing estrogen.

Some gynecologists do not give estrogen therapy after surgery for endometrial cancer or other malignancy. Estrogen replacement therapy, is recommended by some gynecologists for the postmenopausal woman following hysterectomy-oophorectomy. This hormone treatment is said to be beneficial in providing a feeling of well-being, but it is usually not a long-term treatment. Estrogen cream or suppositories are recommended for senile vaginitis (Barter, 1975).

The nurse's role in estrogen replacement therapy is to assess the woman's knowledge of the treatment, including risks and advantages, so that she can make an informed decision about its use. The nurse should also know about administration of the drug in order to assess effects and side effects.

Cultural responses to hysterectomy

It is important for the nurse to assess a woman's response to having a hysterectomy. Ethnically derived meanings that hysterectomy has for the woman and her family need to be identified when planning nursing interventions. Most research studies do not use ethnicity as a variable and most do not indicate the educational level or social background of the woman in the sample. One study reported by M. A. Williams (1973) that did compare women of two different ethnic groups (Mexican-American and Anglo) suggests that cultural patterning of the feminine role is an important variable in a woman's view of the hysterectomy experience. For example, old wives' tales and misinformation were reported by both groups: the Mexican-American woman reported that changes in sex life would occur after hysterectomy while the Anglo woman felt that emotional changes would occur.

More studies of the cultural response to hysterectomy in women of other ethnic groups are needed before conclusions can be made about how ethnocultural concepts of femininity affect the outcome of this procedure. In the meantime, however, the nurse should be alert for the woman who may be fearful or anxious about hysterectomy because it threatens her concept of the feminine role.

Psychologic responses to hysterectomy

An association between the uterus and psychologic problems has been posed for hundreds of years. Both the ancient Greeks and Egyptians ascribed the conduct of an unstable woman to her "discontented womb" (M. A. Williams, 1973). In more recent times—since the late 1870s—studies on the effects of gynecologic surgery have been carried out and emotional reactions after hysterectomy have been reported in both the nursing and the medical literature. There is still no positive proof, however, the hysterectomy causes the emotional disorders that have been associated with the procedure. Even so, the gynecologic nursing practitioner should know what research studies have identified as responses to hysterectomy and the factors affecting these responses, including high-risk categories and adjustment responses. Armed with this knowledge the nurse can carry out pre- and postoperative nursing assessments, identify problems, and intervene accordingly.

Reported reactions to hysterectomy. Depression is the most frequently reported symptom of the hysterectomy client. In 1941, Lindemann reported that depression was more frequent following pelvic surgery than after upper abdominal surgery. Drellich and Bieber (1958), in a study of twenty-three premenopausal women who had undergone hysterectomy, found that depression was related to concerns about the feminine role. Wolfe (1970) also reports depression relating to the feminine role but notes that depression is higher in women of lower socioeconomic groups. Budd (1977) has found that femininity is related to postoperative depression but also that housewives are less depressed than others—a finding that differs from most studies.

Kroger's 1962 study reported an incidence of postoperative depression as high as 40% and indicated factors that help to identify the woman at risk for experiencing postoperative depression. Women who may develop depression postoperative are those who are overanxious, indifferent, or who have had repeated surgery. Melody (1962), in a study of 267 hysterectomy clients, found that 4% who expressed fears before surgery experienced postoperative depression. The depression was precipitated by a traumatic social event perceived by the woman as rejection or devaluation by her spouse. Patterson et al. (1960) reported that depression is related to the concept of body wholeness being dependent on external appearances rather than internal intactness. In a study of 200 women, Richards (1973) reported an incidence of depression of 36.5% and concluded that women who have had a hysterectomy are four times more likely than other women to have depression within 3 years and need follow-up during this time. Chynoweth (1973) reported a study of 100 women in which one third expressed anxiety, depression, and irritability postoperatively. She also concluded that postoperative follow-up should be as long as 1 to 2 years.

Factors affecting emotional responses to hysterectomies. The following factors have been cited as having a potential negative relationship to prognosis after hysterectomy: poor feminine self-concept, including gender identity and body image; previous adverse reactions to stress, especially depression; a family history of depression or other mental illness; a history of multiple physical complaints or numerous surgeries or hospitalizations; age of less than 35; unfinished childbearing; fears of loss of sexual interest; husband's negative attitude; marital instability; cultural or religious objections to hysterectomy; and lack of vocation or other outside interests (Drellich and Bieber, 1958; Roeske, 1978). Barker (1968) in a study of 729 women cites several factors related to emotional illness. These include the absence of pelvic disease, previous psychiatric referrals, marital disruption, lack of preoperative anxiety, presence of misconceptions, and removal of the ovaries (Chafetz, 1971).

Feminine self-concept. The importance of the uterus to menstruation, pregnancy, and childbearing is reflected in the attitudes and perceptions of gender function and body image in women (Wolf, 1970). The response of a woman to a hysterectomy is based on biologic, psychologic, and sociocultural factors. The way a woman perceives herself after surgery is most crucial. Although the physical changes are not readily apparent to others, they can alter the concept of self and body image (Woods, 1979).

Female sexual desirability contributes to the woman's ability to carry out biologic function. In our culture many women have tended to find their identity through femininity (attractiveness and the ability to bear children); given this orientation to self-worth, the uterus becomes essential for a positive self-concept (Polivy, 1974). Drellich and Bieber (1958) equate the uterus with femininity. Their list of functions of the uterus includes reproduction, excretion, regulation of body processes, expression of sexuality, and maintenance of strength, youthfulness, and attractiveness. Newton and Barron (1976) report that a hysterectomy removes two aspects of femininity: fertility and menstruation. They report that younger women are more unhappy about loss of fertility than older women and ambivalent about the loss of menses. Menses are regarded as a cleansing process as well as a mood regulator. Fears about attractiveness to men are also reported to result from hysterectomy (Newton and Barron, 1976).

The response to hysterectomy is related to the degree of *emotional investment* in the uterus (Green, 1973). Conscious and unconscious ideas about the uterus, which may or may not be realistic, determine the fears that occur when the uterus has to be removed (Hackett and Weisman, 1960). If a woman is unable to change her self-concept to a nonproducer she will be more likely to experience depression after hysterectomy (Cornish, 1976).

Assessment of psychodynamic dimensions. The gynecologic nursing practitioner must recognize the psychodynamic dimensions of the hysterectomy client and relate these to her own psychodynamics. *Intrapersonal dimensions* for the client include inner experiences of herself as a person, societal attitudes, perceptions, conflicts, symptoms, and pain. For the practitioner the intrapersonal dimensions include her attitude toward the sterilized woman. *Interpersonal* dimensions are encounters between the client and nurse that bring comfort or compliance. The woman has to adjust to a new set of societal expectations during hospitalization while the nurse needs to react to what the woman wants, not what the nurse thinks she needs. *Impersonal dimensions* include the nature of the surgery, which may force the woman to change from established routine to new patterns of adaptation. For the nurse the impersonal dimension is the lack of choice about caring for the woman (Hackett and Weisman, 1960). Knowing these dimensions facilitates implementation of effective nursing care.

SEXUAL RESPONSE AFTER GYNECOLOGIC SURGERY

Sexual concerns are common before and after gynecologic procedures. The following discussion is presented to assist the nurse in providing help or information to women who have undergone gynecologic surgery.

Abdominal hysterectomy. Sexual intercourse is usually restricted for 6 weeks; however it may be 3 to 4 months before the woman is comfortable because of soreness in the abdomen and a temporary shrinking of the vagina, which makes it feel narrow and short. Reassuring the couple that coitus will help stretch the vagina is a necessary support measure.

If sexual maladjustment persists the cause may not be the surgery. Factors to be considered are these: the hysterectomy may be performed at a time of life when there is a reduction in sexual drive; the woman may be suffering from emotional reactions to the hysterectomy; a realistic view of sexual function will decrease disappointment that "all is not better" after surgery; and finally, the woman may use the hysterectomy as an "escape route" to keep from having to have intercourse (Amias, 1975).

Vaginal hysterectomy. Recovery from vaginal hysterectomy is quicker than from abdominal surgery. Sexual intercourse can be resumed in approximately 3 weeks.

Prolapse surgery. Sexual functioning is poorly preserved in repair surgery; therefore, prior to surgery the woman should be assessed to ascertain her wishes with regard to coitus and the amount of atrophy already present. Anterior repairs are the most common procedures. These cause narrowing of the vagina and some shortening. Posterior repairs are the major cause of vulval and vaginal stenosis. Resumption of intercourse in 6 weeks will help keep postoperative stenosis to a minimum. Dilators and lubricants may relieve some of the vaginal tightness. Despite these measures many women practice intercourse infrequently with discomfort or stop all together after prolapse surgery.

Oophorectomy. When ovaries are removed surgical castration results causing decreased libido, decreased lubrication, and decreased sensations in the lower vaginal tract. Estrogen replacement therapy may be used as a coital lubricant although water-soluble jellies work just as well (Woods, 1979). A study by Dennerstein et al (1972) demonstrated that estrogen administration decreased dyspareunia but was not related to enjoyment or desire.

In general, couples who have engaged in sexual intercourse less than once a week have more sexual deterioration postoperatively than those couples who had intercourse more than once a week. Preoperative anxiety about sexuality also is related to sexual deterioration postoperatively. Masters and Johnson (1970) have described the three main causes of dyspareunia after hysterectomy with oophorectomy. These are:

1. *Psychologic:* the woman who has negative expectations will have poor outcome; this is a self-fulfilling prophesy
2. *Hormonal:* estrogen therapy has not been found beneficial for decreased libido but the data in the literature are conflicting

3. *Organic:* 47% of women have decreased vaginal lubrication that is organic or psychologic; very little production of lubrication is cervical in origin

SUMMARY

This chapter has attempted to provide the nurse with a broad knowledge base to use with gynecologic client in the areas of preventive teaching and counseling, technical nursing skills, and restorative physiologic and psychologic care. More research is needed in the area of gynecologic nursing, and, hopefully, as more practitioners become engaged in clinical practice in this area the knowledge base will expand.

Nursing process

The observational and assessment skills of the gynecologic nurse are important in identifying problems and implementing nursing care. The following data collection for assessment is suggested (Budd, 1977):

I. Preoperative assessment
  A. Significance of loss of the uterus
    1. Loss of reproductive function
    2. Loss of sexual function related to the uterus
      a. Loss of attractiveness, reliance on physical attributes
      b. Loss of husband's love or fear of rejection
    3. Cultural implications related to femininity
  B. Coping mechanisms with previous surgery or in other crisis situations
  C. Knowledge of surgical procedures
    1. Effects on body, hormones
    2. Anesthesia
    3. Physiologic preparation: skin, bowel, etc.
    4. Postoperative expectations: IVs, dressings, etc.
  D. Emotional support systems
    1. Family
    2. Friends
  E. Misconceptions about hysterectomy
II. Postoperative assessment
  A. Signs of depression
    1. Agitation
    2. Insomnia
    3. Crying spells
    4. Weakness
    5. Anorexia
    6. Withdrawal
  B. Interest in appearance
III. Interventions
  A. Preoperative
    1. Discussion of fears about hysterectomy
    2. Expression of feelings
    3. Exploration of expectations concerning outcome of surgery

4. Anticipatory guidance to prevent or lessen severity of depression
5. Identification of high-risk woman: overanxious, casual attitude, previous mental health problems, marital instability, absence of disease, presence of misconceptions, age below 40, self-image and femininity equated to uterus, family not completed
  B. Postoperative interventions
    1. Discussion of sexual relations
    2. Expression of feelings
    3. Provision of privacy and time to work through feelings
    4. Counseling and teaching as needed
    5. Referral or followup after discharge
IV. Evaluation
  A. Measurable criteria
    1. No signs of depression
    2. Positive self-concept; no fears or doubts about femininity or body image
    3. No misconceptions
  B. Collaboration with referral sources for continued assessment and identification of potential problems

REFERENCES

ACOG Statement of Policy on Consultations Prior to Gynecologic Surgery. Issued May 7, 1977. Executive Board of American College of Obstetricians and Gynecologists, Chicago.

Amias, A. G.: Sexual life after gynecologic operations. I and II. Br. Med. J. 2(5971):608-609, 1975.

Barglow, P., and others: Hysterectomy tubal ligation: a psychiatric comparison, Obstet. Gynecol. 25:520-527, 1965.

Barter, R. H.: Vaginal versus abdominal hysterectomy. In Reid, D. E., and Christian, C. D., editors: Controversy in obstetrics and gynecology. II. Philadelphia, 1974, W. B. Saunders Co.

Barter, R., and others: Hysterectomy—the kindest/most unkindest cut of all, Patient Care. 9:75-90, 1975.

Boston Women's Health Book Collective: Our bodies ourselves, ed. 2, New York, 1976, Simon & Schuster.

Budd, K.: Variations of response to hysterectomy—basis for individual care to women. In Lytle, N. A.: Nursing of women in the age of liberation, Dubuque, Iowa, 1977, William C. Brown Co.

Burchell, R. C.: Decision regarding hysterectomy, Am. J. Obstet. Gynecol. 27(2):113-117, 1977.

Burchell, R. C.: Gynecologic surgery in women desirous of further childbearing. In Reid, D. E., and Christian, C. D.: Controversies in obstetrics and gynecology, Philadelphia, 1974, W. B. Saunders Co., p. 438.

Byrd, B. F., Burch, J. C., and Vaughn, W. K.: The impact of long term estrogen support after hysterectomy, Ann. Surg. 185(5):574-579, 1977.

Carbary, L.: The hysterectomy patient, Nurs. Care, 8(2):8-12, 1975.

Chafetz, M. E.: Hysterectomy and castration—an emotional look alike, Med. Insight, p. 44, Jan. 1971.

Chynoweth, R.: Psychiatric complications of hysterectomy, Aust. N. Zeal. Psych. 7:102-104, 1973.

Cornish, J.: Psychodynamics of the hysterectomy experience. In McNall, L. K., and Galeener, J. T., editors: Current practice in obstetrical and gynecologic nursing, St. Louis, 1976, The C. V. Mosby Co.

Cryocautery. North Carolina Memorial Hospital, Chapel Hill, NC.

Deets, C., and Schmidt, A.: Outcome criteria based on standards, AORN J. **127**(2):220-222, 1978.

Dennerstein, L., Wood, C., and Burrows, G.: Sexual response following hysterectomy and oophorectomy, Obstet. Gynecol. **49**(1): 92, 1972.

Diamond, E.: Microsurgical reconstruction of the uterine tube in sterilized patients, Fertil. Steril. **28**:1203, 1977.

Disaia, P. J.: The cervix. In Romney, S., and others: Gynecology and obstetrics—the health care of women, New York, 1975, McGraw-Hill Book Co.

Drellich, M. G., and Bieber, I.: The psychologic importance of the uterus and its functions, J. Nerv. Mental Dis. **126**:322, 1958.

Greene, R. L.: The emotional aspects of hysterectomy, South. Med. J. **66**(4):442, 1973.

Hackett, T., Weisman, A.: Psychiatric management of operative syndromes: psychodynamics factors in formulation and management, Psychosom. Med. **22**:356-359, 1960.

Higgins, J. R.: More hysterectomies—fact, fantasy or fad? Can. Nurse, **62**:33-35, 1971.

Holm, L. A.: Nursing care of patients having a hysterectomy, Can. Nurse **62**:36-37, July 1971.

Howkins, J., and Hudson, C. N.: Shaw's testbook of operative gynecology, ed. 4, Edinburgh, 1977, Churchill Livingston.

Instruction for patients after dilatation and curettage. North Carolina Memorial Hospital, Chapel Hill, NC.

Kolstad, P., and Stafl, A.: Atlas of culposcopy, Baltimore, 1977, University Park Press.

Kroger, W. S., editor: Psychomomatic obstetrics, gynecology and endocrinology, Springfield, Ill., 1962, Charles C Thomas Publishers.

Lindemann, E.: Observations on psychiatric sequela to surgical operations in women, Am. J. Psych. **98**:132, 1941.

Lytle, N. A.: Nursing of women in the age of liberation, Dubuque, Iowa, 1977, Wm. C. Brown Co.

Macasaet, M. A., and Nelson, J. H.: Vaginal versus abdominal hysterectomy. In Reid, D. E., and Christian, C. D., editors: Controversy in obstetrics and gynecology. II. Philadelphia, 1974, W. B. Saunders Co.

Maeck, J. V., and others: In Romney, S., and others: Gynecology and obstetrics—the health care of women, New York, 1975, McGraw-Hill Book Co.

Martin, L. L.: Health care of women, Philadelphia, 1978, J. B. Lippincott Co.

Masters, W. H., and Johnson, V. E.: Human sexual inadequacy, Boston, 1970, Little, Brown & Co.

Masters, W. H., and Johnson, V. E.: Human sexual response, Boston, 1971, Little, Brown & Co.

Mattingly, R. F.: TeLinde's operative gynecology, ed. 5, Philadelphia, 1977, J. B. Lippincott Co.

McNall, L., and Galeener, J.: Current practice in obstetrical and gynecological Nursing, St. Louis, 1976, The C. V. Mosby Co.

Meeker, C. I., and Gray, M. J.: Birth control, abortion and sterilization. In Romney, S., and others: Gynecology and obstetrics—the health care of women, New York, 1975, McGraw-Hill Book Co.

Melody, F. G.: Depressive reactions following hysterectomy, Am. J. Obstet. Gynecol. **83**:410, 1962.

Menhatz, R.: Preoperative teaching for gyn patients, Am. J. Nurs. **74**(6):1072-1074, 1974.

Menning, B. E.: Infertility: a guide for the childless couple, Englewood Cliffs, N.J., 1977, Prentice-Hall Inc.

Miller, N. F., and Avery, H.: Gynecology and gynecological nursing, Philadelphia, 1965, W. B. Saunders Co.

Moukhta, M., and Romney, S. L.: Preferable medical and surgical methods of conception control. In Reid, D. E., and Christian, C. D., editors: Controversy in obstetrics and gynecology. II. Philadelphia, 1974, W. B. Saunders Co.

Newton, N., and Baron, E.: Reactions to hysterectomy: fact or fiction? Primary Care **3**:781, 1976.

Novaks, E. R., Jones, G. S., and Jones, H. W.: Novaks textbook of gynecology, ed. 9, Baltimore, 1975, The William & Wilkins Co.

Patterson, R. M., and others: Social and medical characteristics of the hysterectomized and nonhysterectomized psychiatric patients, Obstet. Gynecol. **15**:209, 1960.

Phipps, W., Long, B., and Woods, N.: Medical surgical nursing: concepts and clinical practice, St. Louis, 1979, The C. V. Mosby Co.

Polivy, J.: Psychological reactions to hysterectomy: a critical review, Am. J. Obstet. Gynecol. **18**:417, 1974.

Porter, C. W. J., and Hulka, J. F., Female sterilization in current clinical practice, Nurs. Digest, pp. 32-36, Sept/Oct 1975.

Rebutting the changes of unnecessary hysterectomy, Contemp. Ob/Gyn. **8**:100-109, 1976.

Reid, D. E., and Christian, C. D.: Controversy in obstetrics and gynecology. II. Philadelphia, 1974, W. B. Saunders Co.

Richards, D. H.: Depression after hysterectomy Lancet, **2**:430-432, 1973.

Ridley, J. H.: Gynecological Surgical Errors, Safeguard Salvage, Baltimore, 1974, The Williams & Wilkins Co.

Rodgers, J.: Rush to surgery, New York Times Magazine, Sept 21, 1975.

Roeske, N.: Quality of life and facts affecting the response to hysterectomy, J. Fam. Pract. **7**(3):484, 1978.

Romney, S., and others: The uterus. In Romney, S., and others: Gynecology and obstetrics—the health care of women, New York, 1975, McGraw-Hill Book Co.

Romney, S., and others: Gynecology and obstetrics—the health care of women, New York, 1975, McGraw-Hill Book Co.

Schram, S. H., and Bretscher, J.: Ultrasonic diagnosis in obstetrics and gynecology, New York, 1975, Springer-Verlag.

Silverberg, S. G.: Surgical pathology of the uterus, New York, 1977, John Wiley & Sons.

Stander, R. W.: Pelvic insecurity and incontinence. In Romney, S., and others: Gynecology and obstetrics—the health care of women, New York, 1975, McGraw-Hill Book Co.

Steele, S. J., and Goodwin, M. F.: A pamphlet to answer the patient's questions before hysterectomy, Lancet, pp. 492-493, Sept. 13, 1975.

Swenson, I.: Psychological implications of female sterilizations, J. Nurse. Midwif. **19**(4):12-17, 1974.

Ulfelder, H.: Disorders of pelvic supporting structures. In Romney, S., and others: Gynecology and obstetrics: the health care of women, New York, 1975, McGraw-Hill Book Co., p. 61.

Williams, M. A.: Cultural pattering of the feminine role, Nurs. Forum **12**(4):378-387, 1973.

Williams, M. A.: Easier convalescence from hysterectomy, Am. J. Nurs. **76**(3):426, 1976.

Williams, T. J.: Abdominal hysterectomy, myomectomy, and presacral neurectomy with management of bladder injury and attention to thromboembolic disuse. In Ridley, J. H.: Gynecological surgical errors, safeguard, salvage, Baltimore, 1974, The Williams & Wilkins Co.

Wolfe, S. R.: Emotional reactions to hysterectomy, Postgrad. Med. **47**:77-79, May 1970.

Woods, N. F.: Human sexuality in health and illness, ed. 2, St. Louis, 1979, The C. V. Mosby Co.

16

Reproductive malignancies

Deitra Leonard Lowdermilk

The incidence of cancer of the uterus has dropped substantially in the last 24 years. Death rates from uterine cancer are now 65% less than 40 years ago. Still, uterine cancer is the fourth highest cause of cancer death in women today. Ovarian cancer death rates have increased slightly in the last 25 years, although 5-year survival rates have shown a slight gain from 25% in the 1940s to 34% in the 1970s. The National Cancer Institute's Third National Cancer Survey estimated 45,000 new cases of uterine cancer and 11,000 deaths in 1978. About one third of these people will be alive 5 years after treatment. With earlier diagnosis and prompt treatment, one half might be saved (American Cancer Society, 1977).

Nursing practitioners can be vital in assessment and early detection of reproductive cancers, which can then be treated promptly by surgery, radiation, chemotherapy, or a combination of these methods. To carry out this role the nurse will need sound knowledge of gynecologic oncology and an ability to apply nursing interventions in community and hospital settings.

This chapter will focus on seven reproductive cancers; discussion of each will include epidemiology, classification and staging, symptoms and detection, diagnosis and treatment, prognosis, and prevention. Current concepts of management including radical surgery, such as vulvectomy and pelvic exenteration, are discussed, with emphasis on nursing care and psychologic implications. Radiation, chemotherapy, and immunotherapy are described along with physiologic and psychologic effects of treatment, nutritional aspects, and nursing management. General nutritional considerations including hyperalimentation are also presented.

Psychosocial problems are ever present with cancer patients, and gynecologic clients are no exception. Concerns about the emotional impact of gynecologic cancer or its treatments, especially in relation to body image and sexuality, are identified in the discussion, and suggestions are given for appropriate nursing interventions. Terminal care is discussed in relation to the client's needs, palliative treatments, the family's reactions, and the nursing staff's feelings.

The conclusion of the chapter summarizes the nurse's role in gynecologic oncology and lists nursing objectives in providing care.

Disease processes

CANCER OF THE CERVIX
Epidemiology and etiology

Cancer of the cervix is ranked third after breast cancer and colon and rectal cancer in incidence in women. It has been estimated that 2% of all women will develop cancer of the cervix by the time they are 80 years old (Romney et al., 1975). The American Cancer Society estimates that 20,000 new cases of cancer of the cervix and 7,400 deaths occurred in 1978. Cancer of the cervix occurs most often in women ages 40 to 49; the average age is 35 for preinvasive cancer and 45 for invasive cancer (Romney et al., 1975).

Social factors associated with a high incidence of cancer of the cervix (and therefore considered high-risk factors) include low socioeconomic status, early age of first coitus, early marriage, early age of first pregnancy, and multiparity. A history of multiple sex partners, a positive history of venereal disease, and prostitution are also risk factors. There is a low incidence in nuns and Jewish women. This latter fact has been considered by several authors as an indication of some type of relationship to coitus (American Cancer Society, 1977; Romney et al., 1975). Some sources even label cervical cancer as a "venereal disease" (Disaia et al., 1975; Romney et al., 1975). Other women at high risk include those whose husbands have prostatic or penile cancer, wives of unskilled laborers (Martin, 1978), those with poor care during and immediately following pregnancy (American Cancer Society, 1977), and black or Mexican-American women (Romney et al., 1975).

Adenocarcinoma of the cervix has also been found in virgins and women with a history of herpesvirus type II (Romney et al., 1975).

Assessment
Screening

When a woman is told she has an abnormal Pap smear, she may react in different ways. She may express fear that she has cancer. She may deny that there is any problem or say there was a mistake in the report (Martin, 1978). If she reacts in a positive manner the woman will seek further information and medical assessment. One method used to evaluate a woman with an abnormal Pap smear is recommended by Disaia and associates (1975) and is demonstrated diagrammatically in Fig. 16-1. This evaluation and treatment plan includes colposcopic examination, which significantly increases the accuracy of the diagnosis when combined with re-

peated cytology. Accuracy of the Pap smear is only about 95% for detection of cervical cancer (Romney et al., 1975).

Colposcopy

Colposcopy was first introduced in 1925 by Hans Hinselmann in Germany as a practical method for comprehensive examination of the cervix and vaginal vault. It has become popular in the United States only since the 1960s and is now recognized as an adjunctive treatment with cytology in the investigation of epithelium. Colposcopy is based on the study of the transformation zone, which is simply that area of cervix and/or vagina that was initially covered with columnar epithelium and through the process of metaphasia has been replaced by squamous epithelium. The wide range of variations in the zone is the subject of the science of colposcopy (Romney et al., 1975).

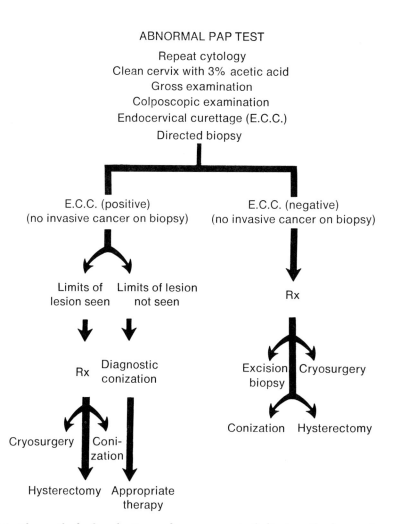

Fig. 16-1. The method of evaluation and management of clients with abnormal cytology. (From Disaia, P. J., Morrow, C. P., and Townsend, D.: Synopsis of gynecologic oncology, New York, 1975, John Wiley & Sons.)

The colposcope is a stereoscopic binocular microscope with low levels of magnification, ranging from ×6 to ×40.

Procedure. The woman is placed in a lithotomy position with the cervix exposed with a vaginal speculum. The colposcope is focused at the external os at a distance of approximately 20 cm. The cervix is gently swabbed to remove mucus, and the cervix is viewed before and after application of 2% aqueous acetic acid solution. This solution removes mucus and enables the viewer to see the epithelium with more clarity (Howkins and Hudson, 1977). A green filter is then placed between the light source and the tissue to accentuate vascular patterns and color tone differences (Romney et al., 1975). The last step of the examination is to soak the cervix with Schiller's iodine solution to differentiate glycogen-filled cells from glycogen-free cells, although some believe that this is still a nonspecific test and biopsies must be done to detect cancer in situ (Kolstad and Stafl, 1977).

Findings. Diagnosis is made with reference to five observable features (Kolstad and Stafl, 1977):

1. Vascular pattern
2. Intercapillary distance
3. Surface pattern
4. Color tone and opacity
5. Clarity and demarcation

After evaluation of these features, the findings are divided into four groups (see Table 16-1). Normal findings usually indicate no significant pathology. Abnormal findings are followed by directed punch biopsies. White epithelium usually reveals dysplasia or carcinoma in situ. It can also be found in young women exposed to DES. Irregular punctuation or mosaic can indicate carcinoma in situ. Atypical vessels are found only in invasive cancer (Kolstad and Stafl, 1977).

Use of colposcopy increases the accuracy of diagnosis, decreases the necessity for biopsies, and can lead to more focused treatments for women with abnormal Pap smears. For example, if a lesion covering less than 25% of the cervix is found, only 15% will need a diagnostic conization (Herbert et al., 1976). Colposcopy is also useful in evaluation of DES-exposed women because these women have an extended transformation zone. The use of colposcopy for malignant conditions is especially important in cancer of the cervix because almost all lesions arise at the squamocolumnar junction (transformation zone). Colposcopy is also used to assess vulvar disease and vaginal lesions (Disaia et al., 1975).

The nurse's role with colposcopic examinations is to prepare the woman, who may be very anxious. The procedure should be explained and the scope shown to her. The woman should be told that the examination will probably take from 5 to 10 minutes and that it

Table 16-1. Colposcopic findings*

A. Normal colposcopical findings
  1. Original squamous epithelium
  2. Columnar epithelium
  3. Transformation zone
B. Abnormal colposcopical findings
  1. Atypical transformation zone
    a. Keratosis (leukoplakia)
    b. White epithelium
    c. Mosaic
    d. Punctation
    e. Atypical vascular pattern
  2. Suspect invasive carcinoma
C. Unsatisfactory (indecisive) colposcopical findings (squamo-columnar junction not visible)
D. Miscellaneous colposcopical findings (inflammatory changes, atrophic changes, true erosion, condyloma, papilloma, etc.)

*From Disaia, P. J., Morrow, C. P., and Townsend, D. E.: Synopsis of gynecologic oncology, New York, 1975, John Wiley & Sons.

will be similar to a pelvic examination, with the scope never inserted into the vagina. If the woman is to have a biopsy, she should be told she may experience a stinging or pinching sensation. Relaxation techniques such as slow mouth breathing are often helpful (Herbert et al., 1976).

Staging and classification

The majority of cancers are epidermoid or squamous epithelial cell arising from the endocervical canal. Dysplasia or the presence of individual atypical epithelial cells can be divided into three categories: mild, moderate, and severe. As one progresses from mild to severe, development of carcinoma in situ becomes more likely (Romney et al., 1975). Adenocarcinoma makes up approximately 5% of cervical cancers and also originates in the endocervix.

In the early stages of cervical cancer, the cancer is a small lesion near the external os, which appears as a hard granular area. Moderately advanced types are usually on the lip of the cervix and appear as exophytic (everting) or entophytic (inverting) growths. Advanced lesions are ulcerating, bleeding, and usually exophytic growths. Metastasis can occur to any organ (Novaks et al., 1975).

The TNM classification (T = primary *t*umor, N = regional *n*odes, and M = *m*etastasis) is used to identify the anatomic extent of disease. Staging further defines and describes tumors based on the classification system and clinical evaluation. Treatments are then planned according to the findings of the staging process. The staging is also useful in estimating the patient's progress (Jackson and Armenaki, 1976). The staging classification used here are the groupings adopted by the International Federation of Gynecology and Obstetrics (FIGO) in 1970.

Stage 0　Carcinoma in situ
Stage I　Carcinoma confined to the cervix
　　Stage IA1: Early stromal invasion
　　Stage IA2: Occult cancer
　　Stage IB: All other cancers limited to the uterus
Stage II　Cancer involves the vagina but not the lower third, in infiltrates the parametrium but not out to the sidewall
　　Stage IIA: Cancer involves the vagina but there is no evidence of parametrial involvement
　　Stage IIB: Infiltration of the parametria but not out to the sidewall
Stage III　Cancer involves the lower third of the vagina or extends to the pelvic sidewall
　　Stage IIIA: Cancer involves the lower third of the vagina but is not out to the pelvic sidewall if the parametria are involved
　　Stage IIIB: Involvement of one or both parametria out to the sidewall
　　Stage III (urinary): Obstruction of one or both ureters on intravenous pyelogram without the other criteria for stage II disease
Stage IV　Cancer extends outside the reproductive tract
　　Stage IVA: Involvement of the bladder or rectum
　　Stage IVB: Distant metastasis or disease outside the true pelvis

Symptoms

One of the earliest signs of cancer of the cervix is a thin, watery, blood-tinged vaginal discharge, which is frequently unrecognized by the woman as unusual. The classic symptoms are painless, abnormal intermenstrual bleeding, which begins as spotting, often after intercourse or douching. As a malignancy enlarges, the bleeding becomes heavier, more frequent, and of longer duration. If no treatment is begun, the bleeding will become continuous. Late signs or signs of recurrence include weight loss; pain in the pelvis, back, or abdomen; or referral pain to the flank or leg secondary to ureteral, pelvic wall, or sciatic nerve involvement. Dysuria, hematuria, rectal bleeding, or constipation may occur if there is metastasis to the bladder or rectum. Persistent leg edema occurs when there is lymphatic or venous blockage. Coughing or hemoptysis can occur with lung involvement. Preterminal signs include massive hemorrhage or uremia (Disaia et al., 1975, Martin, 1978; Romney et al., 1975).

Diagnosis

Once invasive carcinoma has been identified, the woman undergoes routine studies as part of the staging workup prior to planning treatment. Diagnostic procedures that are acceptable for arriving at a staging classification include physical examination and laboratory studies: CBC, platelets, BUN, creatinine, protein, SGOT, SGPT, bilirubin, electrocardiogram (if the woman is over age 35), intravenous pyelogram, barium studies of the lower colon, X-ray studies of the chest, cystoscopy, sigmoidoscopy, and colposcopy. Lymphangiograms and pelvic examinations performed under anesthesia are often included in staging workups, although not in all institutions (Disaia et al., 1975; Romney et al., 1975).

To diagnose recurrent carcinoma of the cervix, tissue biopsies, cytology, X-rays of the skeleton, radioisotope scans of the liver, bones, and brain, and exploratory laparotomy are added to the above studies to identify the spread and extent of the disease process (Disaia et al., 1975).

Treatment

After the diagnosis is confirmed and invasive carcinoma of the cervix is established, specific treatment is planned based on the woman's general health, age, the extent of the cancer, and presence of abnormalities. The information from the staging workup gives the gynecologist/oncologist and the radiotherapist complete information for the treatment plan.

Carcinoma in situ. Carcinoma in situ can be treated with a cone biopsy or total hysterectomy (with or without removing the ovaries), depending on whether or not further childbearing is desired. If a hysterectomy is performed, the cure rate is almost 100% (Rudolph, 1974).

Stages I to IIA. Lesions of limited extent are curable by local radiation treatment. Intracavitary radium therapy (IRT) is the basic method used because the accessibility of the cervix makes it possible to place radium close to the lesion. External radiation therapy (ERT) is added to irradiate regional nodes. Large bulky tumors may first be treated with external radiation to shrink the tumor before internal therapy is instituted (Disaia et al., 1975).

Surgery can also be done for stage I and IIA tumors, although controversy about this has existed for years. The cure rates for stage I cancer of the cervix are about the same whether treated with surgery or with radiation. Radiation is usually instituted because it is applicable to almost all women, whereas approximately 20% of these woman cannot undergo surgery (Disaia et al., 1975). Surgery is often reserved for young women who wish to retain ovarian function. Other reasons for choosing surgery are occurrence of cancer of the cervix during pregnancy, presence of pelvic inflammatory disease, and client preference (Romney et al., 1975).

Stage IIB. Stage IIB is usually treated with ERT to

Table 16-2. Radiation treatment of invasive cervical cancer—suggested maxima*

Stage	Whole pelvis (rads)	Radium (mg/hours)	Parametrial (rads)
Ia micro-invasive	0	8,000 (2 appl.)	0
Ib (small)	2,000	8,000 (2 appl.)	2,000
Ib (large)	4,000	6,000 (2 appl.)	0
IIa	2,000	8,000 (2 appl.)	2,000
IIb	4,000	6,000 (2 appl.) 7,000 (2 appl.) *or*	0
IIIa	4,000	4,000 (1 appl.) and inter-stitial im-plant	0
IIIb	5,000-6,000	4,000 (1 appl.) 5,000 (2 appl.)	Possible 1,000 rad boost on in-volved side
IVa	6,000	4,000 (1 appl.) 5,000 (2 appl.)	Possible 1,000 rad boost on in-volved side
IVb	1,000 rad pulse 2 times, 1 week apart	Palliation	

*From Disaia, P. J., Morrow, C. P., and Townsend, D. E.: Synopsis of gynecologic oncology, New York, 1975, John Wiley & Sons.

shrink the tumor prior to IRT. Treatments are usually fractioned over several weeks to achieve maximal shrink-age of the tumor, optimal dose distribution, and im-proved tolerance of the normal tissue (Disaia et al., 1975).

Stages III and IV. Stages III and IV are usually treated with ERT for a more uniform dose throughout the pelvic. (See Table 16-2 for suggested radiation dosages for cancer of the cervix.) Pelvic exenteration (to be discussed later) may also be performed on women with recurrence cancer that is still localized in the pelvis. Other forms of treatment for recurrent cancer of the cervix that has metastasized outside the pelvic are often only palliative. These treatments may include irradia-tion to bone metastases to decrease pain and chemo-therapy for recurrent unresectable pelvic wall tumors and interactable pain (Disaia et al., 1975).

Cancer of the cervix and pregnancy. Treatment for women with cancer of the cervix during pregnancy depends on the stage of cancer, duration of pregnancy, and desire for children. If carcinoma in situ is diag-nosed, the woman is usually allowed to complete preg-nancy and is treated 2 to 3 months postpartum with a cone biopsy if further childbearing is desired. For in-vasive carcinoma abortion is recommended up to 24 weeks. After 24 weeks therapy is delayed until fe-tal viability at which time a cesarean section is per-formed. ERT or a hysterectomy is the treatment of choice in the postpartum period (Disaia et al., 1975). Pregnancy does not seem to alter the prognosis (Ru-dolph, 1974).

Adenocarcinoma of the cervix. Adenocarcinoma is often treated with IRT and a hysterectomy because en-largement of the endocervix places disease in the myo-metrium, too far away for the radium sources to treat the cancer adequately alone (Disaia et al., 1975).

Prognosis and spread

Cancer of the cervix is spread by direct extension to the vaginal mucosa, lower uterine segment, parame-trium, pelvic wall, bladder, and rectum (Martin, 1978). It spreads from the paracervical lymph nodes to the most commonly involved lymph nodes and can metastasize in distant organs, although it is prone to remain localized in the pelvis (Meigs, 1968).

In 1975 Romney reported 5-year survival figures from two large studies, one involving women treated with surgery alone and the other involving women treated with radiation. One was Currie's study of 552 radical operations for cancer of the cervix, which reported a survival rate of 86.3% and 75% for stages I and IIA, re-spectively. The other was Fletcher's (1968) study of 2000 women treated with radiation therapy, which reported a survival rate of 91.5% and 83.5% for stages I and IIA. These studies demonstrate comparable survival rates for the two treatment procedures (Romney, 1975).

Recurrent cancer of the cervix

The survival rates for recurrent carcinoma are 15% for 1 year and 5% for 5 years. Fifty percent of the re-currences occur in the first year after treatment and 75% occur in the first 2 years. Common sites for re-currences are (Disaia et al., 1975).

Vagina, cervix, uterus, parametrium, bladder, rectum
Pelvic wall
Paraaortic nodes
Peripheral lymph nodes
Lungs
Lower vagina
Axial skeleton

Women who have been treated for cancer of the cervix are encouraged to have frequent examinations to diag-nose recurrence before it spreads too far. The following schedule is suggested by Disaia and associates:

1. Examination every 2 months for 2 years; every 4 months for 3 years; and every 6 months for 5 years
2. Pap smear at every visit
3. Chest X-ray every 6 months
4. Intravenous pyelogram every 6 months for 2 years

Prevention

Most sources agree that yearly Pap smears* for sexually active women under 21 years of age and all women over 21 years of age would greatly reduce cancer of the cervix as a cause of death (Martin, 1978; Romney et al., 1975; Rudolph, 1974). Other prevention procedures include having Pap smears done every 6 months for women in their forties and fifties since these are the ages of highest risk. Women over 35 years of age who have abnormal bleeding should report it promptly to their physician. Women who have had a hysterectomy should have Pap smears taken every 2 years to screen for vaginal cancer.

The nursing practitioner should be aware of women who may be in the high-risk categories and encourage these women to have Pap smears done regularly. In all clinical settings the practitioner can teach good personal hygiene and the danger signs of cervical cancer.

CANCER OF THE OVARY

An enlarged ovary is one of the most frequent and potentially serious conditions in gynecology. The exact nature of the enlargement and the threat it poses to the woman's life and reproductive function need to be determined.

Cancer of the ovary is fifth among the leading causes of cancer death in women. It has been estimated that in the United States one woman in every one hundred will develop ovarian cancer, and 5% to 7% of American women are at risk for developing this cancer; 1978 statistics reported by the American Cancer Society (1977) estimate an incidence of 5% or 17,000 new cases of ovarian cancer and 6% or 10,800 deaths for the year.

Incidence is infrequent under age 35 and most frequent in the women between the ages of 40 and 65 years. The average age at diagnosis is 52. Identified high-risk factors include a history of breast cancer, occupational exposure to asbestos, and familial history of ovarian cancer. Social class and race have not been considered etiologic factors, although Fisher and Young (1978) cite a high incidence in white women and Disaia and associates (1975) cite a higher incidence associated with a rise in social class.

There is higher incidence in nulliparas and older primiparas than in other women (Fisher and Young, 1978). Death rates are higher for single women. Wynder and associates (1969) report a higher incidence of ovarian cancer in women who have dysmenorrhea and heavy menstrual flow.

There is no known cause of ovarian cancer, although

Disaia and associates (1975) report speculations of hormonal involvement based on the fact that few ovarian cancers occur before puberty, and there is a high rate of occurrence after menopause. They also report that ovarian cancer is common in women with certain genetic diseases such as Peutz-Jegher syndrome.

Assessment

Palpation of a pelvic mass is the only consistent clinical screening method of detecting ovarian cancer. A Pap smear of the vagina will occasionally detect cancer of the ovary in the early stages and will detect it in 20% to 30% of advanced cases (Romney et al., 1975). At present there is no practical, accurate, or cost-effective method of mass screening for ovarian cancer although there is hope for development of a reliable laboratory test (Disaia et al., 1975).

Table 16-3. Histogenetic classification of ovarian neoplasms

1. Neoplasms derived from celomic epithelium
   Serous tumor
   Mucinous tumor
   Endometrioid tumor
   Mesonephroid (clear cell) tumor
   Brenner tumor
   Undifferentiated carcinoma
   Carcinosarcoma and mixed mesodermal tumor
2. Neoplasms derived from germ cells
   Teratoma
      a. Mature teratoma
       Solid adult teratoma
       Dermoid cyst
       Struma ovarii
       Malignant neoplasms secondarily arising from mature cystic teratoma
      b. Immature teratoma (partially differentiated teratoma)
   Dysgerminoma
   Embryonal carcinoma (endodermal sinus tumor)
   Choriocarcinoma
   Gonadoblastoma
3. Neoplasms derived from specialized gonadal stroma
   Granulosa-theca tumors
      a. Granulosa tumor
      b. Thecoma
   Sertoli-Leydig tumors
      a. Arrhenoblastoma
      b. Sertoli tumor
   Gynandroblastoma
   Lipid cell tumors
4. Neoplasms derived from nonspecific mesenchyme
   Fibroma, hemangioma, leiomyoma, lipoma, etc.
   Lymphoma
   Sarcoma

---

*In their most recent guidelines, The American Cancer Society recommends a Pap smear every 3 years for women ages 20 to 65.

Staging and classification

Because of the variety of ovarian cancers, numerous systems of classifications have been devised. Currently, the most popular system is based on the histogenesis of the ovary. In this system the cancers are divided into four major groups according to their origin (Table 16-3). From 60% to 70% of all ovarian neoplasms are derived from the celomic epithelium, 15% to 20% are of germ cell origin, and 10% to 20% derive from specialized and nonspecific gonadal stroma (Disaia et al., 1975).

Malignant tumors of the ovary derived from celomic epithelium account for 85% of all ovarian cancers. All types are usually differentiated as serous, mucinous, endometrioid, or mesonephroid. Serous carcinoma is the most common cancer of the adult female and occurs in about 50% of all epithelial malignancies. This tumor tends to grow rapidly with early spread in the peritoneal cavity. Mucinous carcinoma accounts for 15% of epithelial malignancies. It is usually confined to one ovary. Endometrioid carcinoma comprises 15% of ovarian carcinomas and has a slow growth rate. Mesonephroid, or clear cell, carcinoma accounts for 5% of ovarian carcinomas (Disaia et al., 1975).

Germ cell tumors are second only to epithelial tumors in occurrence, but most are benign or rare and therefore they will not be discussed here. Specialized gonadal stroma neoplasms are associated with adenocarcinoma of the ovary and are usually low-grade malignancies. Fibromas and lymphomas are the most common nonspecific gonadal stroma neoplasms (Disaia et al., 1975).

The extent of ovarian cancer is usually expressed in terms of stages. Table 16-4 shows the FIGO stages for cancer of the ovary.

Table 16-4. FIGO stage-grouping for primary carcinoma of the ovary (1974)

Stage I	Growth limited to the ovaries
	Stage Ia: Growth limited to *one* ovary; no ascites
	(i) No tumor on the external surface; capsule intact
	(ii) Tumor present on the external surface or/and capsule ruptured
	Stage Ib: Growth limited to *both* ovaries; no ascites
	(i) No tumor on the external surface; capsule intact
	(ii) Tumor present on the external surface or/and capsule(s) ruptured
	Stage Ic: Tumor either Stage Ia or Stage Ib, but with ascites* present or positive peritoneal washings
Stage II	Growth involving one or both ovaries with pelvic extension
	Stage IIa: Extension and/or metastases to the uterus and/or tubes
	Stage IIb: Extension to other pelvic tissues
	Stage IIc: Tumor either Stage IIa or Stage IIb, but with ascites* present or positive peritoneal washings
Stage III	Growth involving one or both ovaries with intraperitoneal metastases outside the pelvis and/or positive retroperitoneal nodes. Tumor limited to the true pelvis with histologically proven malignant extension to small bowel or omentum.
Stage IV	Growth involving one or both ovaries with distant metastases. If pleural effusion is present there must be positive cytology to allot a case to Stage IV.
	Parenchymal liver metastases equals Stage IV.
Special category	Unexplored cases which are thought to be ovarian carcinoma.

*Ascites in peritoneal effusion which in the opinion of the surgeon is pathological or/and clearly exceeds normal amounts.

Symptoms

Ovarian tumors have similar characteristics. Enlargement of the tumor causes compression of surrounding pelvic structures, which may cause urinary frequency, pelvic discomfort, abdominal swelling, dyspareunia, pain, and abnormal bleeding. Gastrointestinal symptoms such as heartburn, nausea, anorexia, and abdominal pain may be associated with ovarian cancer. Ascites, which is a late symptom, is often mistaken for a symptom of liver disease. Malignant tumors are seldom found in asymptomatic women, probably because of the rapid tumor growth (Disaia et al., 1975).

Diagnosis

Diagnosis and treatment of ovarian cancer are ultimately dependent on surgical exploration. The preoperative evaluation should be individualized to the woman's symptoms, medical condition, and physical findings. Procedures that are usually included in a staging workup are a complete history and physical examination, laboratory tests including CBC and urinalysis, IVP, upper and lower Gl series, X-rays of chest and abdomen, liver studies if ascites is present, endometrial biopsy for bleeding, breast examination to rule out breast cancer, and an exploratory laparotomy to define cell type, origin of malignancy, and area of spread (Romney et al., 1975; Rudolph, 1974). The incision should be made above the umbilicus in order to adequately stage the cancer (Fisher and Young, 1978).

Treatment

Surgery, radiation, and chemotherapy all play an important role in the treatment of ovarian cancer. Because the cancers are often detected only in advanced stages, these management procedures have not improved survival rates.

Stage I. A total hysterectomy with bilateral salpingo-oophorectomy is recommended for all women with stage I ovarian cancer. Postoperative treatment with pelvic and abdominal irradiation or chemotherapy with an alkylating agent for 12 to 18 months or intraperitoneal isotope therapy is initiated immediately because of the rapidly growing malignancy (Disaia et al., 1975; Romney et al., 1975).

Stage II. A total hysterectomy with bilateral salpingo-oophorectomy is recommended for stage II tumors. Radiation therapy followed by chemotherapy is strongly advised (Disaia et al., 1975).

Stage III. Removal of as much tumor as possible as well as a total hysterectomy and bilateral salpingo-oophorectomy is recommended, with radiation therapy followed by chemotherapy (Rudolph, 1974). Following treatment, a drastic response with disappearance of cervical tumor masses may occur. "Second look" laparotomies are advocated to evaluate the results of the therapy and often to remove the remaining tumor, which is surgically resectable (Disaia et al., 1975).

Stage IV: Often a biopsy is all that can be done, but removal of as much tumor as possible is advocated. Irradiation of the abdomen may be useful. Chemotherapy is useful for palliative therapy. Intestinal obstruction is a frequent complication and may require surgical management if medical management is not successful (Rudolph, 1974). Conservative management (unilateral salpingo-oophorectomy) to preserve childbearing potential in young women is acceptable when the tumor is a low-grade malignancy and confined to one ovary (Romney et al., 1975).

Cancer of the ovary and pregnancy. Most ovarian cancers discovered in pregnancy are stage IA. The risk to the fetus primarily results from treatments, which is the same as for the nonpregnant woman.

Prognosis and spread

Ovarian malignancies initially grow locally, invading the capsule and mesovarium. Adjacent organs are involved by contiguous growth and lymphatic spread. When the malignancy reaches the external surface of the capsule, cells and tissue fragments are exfoliated into the peritoneal cavity where they are able to implant or any serosal surface. Local and regional metastasis can occur in the uterus, fallopian tubes, and pelvic lymph nodes. Spread to the aortic nodes occurs via the lymphatic drainage of ovarian vessels (Romney et al., 1975). It is generally reported that ovarian cancer remains confined to the abdomen and pelvis, although liver, lung, and bone metastases have been reported (Disaia et al., 1975).

The volume of tumor and extent of disease spread at the time of diagnosis are the most important variables influencing prognosis. Aure and associates (1971) report in a large study of ovarian cancer cases the following 5-year survival rates:

Stage I	63%
Stage II	30%
Stage III	12%
Stave IV	8%

Griffiths and coworkers (1972) report a 19% full-year survival rate for stage II with surgery alone, as compared to 42% for surgery with postoperative radiation.

Prevention

The only known method of prevention is surgical castration (Disaia et al., 1975), but since the risk of a woman developing ovarian cancer in her lifetime is only 1%, this prophylactic surgery cannot be considered a good solution.

CANCER OF THE ENDOMETRIUM

Endometrial carcinomas account for approximately 7% of all cancers affecting females, with 90% of these being adenocarcinomas. Many authors report that endometrial cancer is on the increase especially in industrialized countries. The American Cancer Society (1977) reports an estimated 28,000 new cases for 1978 and 3,300 estimated deaths from endometrial cancer.

Endometrial cancer is most common in the age range of 50 to 70 years and is primarily a postmenopausal tumor more frequently seen in white women. Obesity, diabetes, and hypertension have been associated with endometrial cancer, and arthritis, arteriosclerotic heart disease, and fibryocystic disease of the breast have also been cited as risk factors, although documentation is poor. Other risk factors associated with endometrial cancer are infertility, nulliparity, tall stature, anovulatory cycles associated with ovarian pathology, abnormal postmenopausal bleeding, a history of dilatation and curettage for abnormal bleeding problems early in life a history of endometrial cancer in the immediate family background, hyperplasia, and prolonged, sustained estrogen stimulation, especially postmenopausally with estrogen replacement therapy.*

Etiology

There is little evidence that a virus is responsible for the development of endometrial cancer. It is likely that malignancy is triggered by metabolic abnormalities associated with impaired glucose metabolism and pituitary

---

*Disaia et al., 1975; Gray et al., 1977; Greenwald et al., 1977; Mack et al., 1976; Romney et al., 1975; Rudolph, 1974; Smith et al., 1975; Ziel and Finkle, 1975.

hyperactivity and with a background of prolonged drug-induced estrogen stimulation (Benjamin et al., 1963). However, there is continuing debate concerning whether or not estrogen is carcinogenic, especially in endometrial cancer (Disaia et al., 1975; Romney et al., 1975).

Screening

At present there is no practical or accurate method for mass screening of women for endometrial cancer. The Pap smear is ineffective in detecting this carcinoma; most authors report only 40% or lower reliability (American Cancer Society, 1980). Women who are at a high risk for endometrial cancer should have endometrial biopsies done at least yearly. Any postmenopausal woman reporting abnormal uterine bleeding should have a diagnostic dilatation and curettage (Gusburg, 1973).

Staging and classification

Clinical staging of carcinoma of the endometrium is not as definite as staging of cervical cancer because the spread of the cancer is more difficult to determine. However, approximately 75% are classified as stage I. The following is the staging description adopted by FIGO in 1977:

Stage I   The carcinoma is confined to the corpus.
        Stage Ia: The length of the uterine cavity is 8 cm or less.
        Stage Ib: The length of the uterine cavity is more than 8 cm.
        Stage I cases should be subgrouped with regard to the histologic type of adenocarcinoma as follows:
           G1: Highly differentiated adenomatous carcinomas.
           G2: Differentiated adenomatous carcinomas with partly solid areas.
           G3: Predominantly solid or entirely undifferentiated carcinomas.
Stage II   The carcinoma involves corpus and cervix.
Stage III   The carcinoma extends outside the corpus but not outside the true pelvis (it may involve the vaginal wall or the parametrium but not the bladder or the rectum).
Stage IV   The carcinoma involves the bladder or rectum or extends outside the pelvis.

Symptoms

The most common symptom of endometrial cancer is abnormal uterine bleeding in the menopausal and postmenopausal woman. The presence of uterine polyps is also associated with endometrial cancer (Rudolph, 1974). Low abdominal and back pain are frequent symptoms, especially as the malignancy progresses. An enlarged uterus is often a sign of advanced disease (Disaia et al., 1975).

Diagnosis

A complete history, including menstrual history and hormone ingestion, is important in the assessment process. A pelvic examination, including a bimanual examination to determine the position and size of the uterus, and palpation of the parametria are essential to diagnosis and staging. The diagnosis is established by endometrial biopsy or fractional curettage (Romney et al., 1975). Fractional curettage involves scraping of individual sections of the uterus: the endocervix, each wall of the uterine cavity, and the fundus (Gusburg, 1973).

Since many women with endometrial cancer are elderly and need optimal preparation, a thorough preoperative evaluation is important. This workup should include a chest X-ray, electrocardiogram, and serum electrolytes. A staging workup can also include cystoscopy, sigmoidoscopy, and intravenous pyelogram to rule out spread to other organs.

Procedures that are useful but not routinely used include lymphography, hysterography, hysteroscopy, arteriography, and venography (Rudolph, 1974).

Treatment

The plan of treatment depends on an accurate diagnosis and location of the carcinoma, the condition of the woman, and selection of the therapy best suited to the client. The best planning involves collaboration by the medical team—the gynecologist/oncologist, radiologist, and pathologist (Romney et al., 1975).

Hysterectomy is the treatment of choice for endometrial cancer, with radiation and chemotherapy used as adjunctive therapy to increase survival rates and decrease recurrence. Treatment by stage includes:

Stage I: Total abdominal hysterectomy/bilateral salpingectomy and oophorectomy (internal radiation therapy); external radiation therapy pre- or postoperatively

Stage II: External or internal radiation therapy followed in 4 to 6 weeks by total abdominal hysterectomy

Stage III: External and internal radiation therapy

Stage IV: External radiation and hormone treatment

Recurrences are treated with hormones, usually progestins, which are used palliatively to treat pain and give comfort (Rudolph, 1974).

Prognosis and spread

Survival rates are high because approximately 75% of the women with endometrial cancer are diagnosed with localized disease (Romney et al., 1975). For stage I tumors the 5-year cure rate is over 80% when treated with surgery and radiation. Stage II cancers have survival rates of approximately 50%; stage III carcinomas 25%; and with stage IV tumors extending beyond the uterus less than 10% (Disaia et al., 1975).

Endometrial cancer is a slow-growing neoplasm characterized by premalignant stages (hyperplasia, carcinoma in situ) and ultimately a definite invasive neoplasm (Romney et al., 1975). In carcinoma in situ the lesion occurs on the average 10 years prior to invasive cancer. The line of spread of invasive carcinoma of the endometrium includes spread to the lymph nodes, myometrium, cervix, vagina, other pelvic structures including broad ligaments, fallopian tubes, and ovaries, and distant metastasis. Metastasis sites include the abdominal serosa, para-aortic nodes, inguinal nodes, supraclavicular nodes, and lungs.

Prevention

All women at menopause and after should have a yearly pelvic examination as well as a Pap smear. Women at high risk for endometrial cancer should have an endometrial tissue sample examined as well. Postmenopausal bleeding should be checked by a physician. The use of estrogen during and following menopause should be carefully monitored, and the risks and benefits should be seriously considered until there is more evidence concerning the association of estrogen therapy and endometrial cancer.

The practitioner should be aware of women who may be in the high-risk categories and recognize that the menopause is a time of life when these women can be identified.

Carcinomas of the cervix, endometrium, and ovary make up 90% of female reproductive system neoplasms. The remainder occur infrequently and will be discussed only briefly.

CANCER OF THE VULVA
Epidemiology

Cancer of the vulva accounts for 3% to 5% of female genital carcinoma. It is primarily a disease of older women, in the age range of 50 to 70 years; the average age is 62. Risk factors include a history of leukoplakia, venereal disease, kraurosis, diabetic vulvitis, and other primary malignancies, cancer of the cervix being the most common (Parsons, 1968; Rudolph, 1974).

Assessment

Since the lesion is located on the external genitalia, clinical detection usually occurs when the woman seeks help, although women tend to delay seeing a physician for the problem.

Staging

Approximately 95% of vulvar carcinomas are squamous cell; the rest are adenocarcinomas, Paget's disease, malignant melanomas, and sarcomas.

Many attempts have been made to stage and classify vulvar cancer, but none has been internationally accepted. The TNM classification is well suited for this kind of tumor because metastasis is primarily to the inguinal nodes. The system adopted by the FIGO in 1970 for cancer of the vulva is as follows:

T Primary tumor
T1 Confined to vulva, 2 cm or less
T2 Confined to vulva, more than 2 cm
T3 Tumor of any size with adjacent spread to the urethra and/or vagina/anus and/or perineum
T4 Tumor of any size infiltrating the bladder mucosa or rectal mucosa or both

N Regional lymph
N0 No nodes palpable
N1 Nodes palpable in either groin, not enlarged, mobile; not suspicious of neoplasm
N2 Nodes palpable in either or both groins; enlarged, firm, and mobile; suspicious of neoplasm
N3 Fixed or ulcerated nodes

M Distant metastasis
M0 No clinical metastasis
M1a Palpable deep pelvic lymph nodes
M1b Other distant metastasis

Stage I:	T1 N0 M0
	T1 N1 M0
Stage II:	T2 N0 M0
	T2 N0 M0
Stage III:	T3 N0 M0
	T3 N1 M0
	T3 N2 M0
	T1 N2 M0
	T2 N2 M0
Stage IV:	T1 N3 M0
	T2 N3 M0
	T3 N3 M0
	T4 N3 M0
	T4 N0 M0
	T4 N1 M0
	T4 N2 M0

All other conditions containing M1a or M1B.

Symptoms

The most common symptom reported is a lesion on the vulva. Other less common symptoms include pruritis, discharge, bleeding, and pain.

Diagnosis

Biopsy of suspicious lesions is the diagnostic procedure of choice. Pelvic examination is also useful (Romney et al., 1975).

Treatment

Since the location of the lesion makes it suitable for excision, the treatment of choice is a radical vulvectomy with or without lymphadenectomy. The need for node removal is debatable (Disaia et al., 1975; Romney et al., 1975). Advanced disease with bladder and rectal involvement may require an exenteration. (Both surgical procedures are discussed in the management section of this chapter.) Surgery must be individualized since many of the women are elderly and may have multiple medical problems complicating the treatment plan.

Because of the radiosensitivity of the vulvar area, radiation is unsuitable as a method of treatment, but it may be used palliatively in advanced disease (Rudolph, 1974).

Prognosis and spread

Five-year survival rates with vulvectomy and lymphadenectomy are reported at approximately 65%. Recurrence as well as distant metastasis may appear in the first 2 years (Romney et al., 1975). When lesions are diagnosed in an advanced stage with node involvement the survival rate is only 8% to 10%.

Vulvar carcinoma has a slow growth rate and remains localized for long periods. Seventy percent are located in the labia, primarily the labia majora. Another 13% are located on the clitoris. Areas of local spread are the urethra, vagina, anus, and rectum. Lymphatic spread, both bilateral and contralateral, is common. The direction of spread is to inguinal, femoral, and pelvic nodes and finally periaortic nodes. Distant metastasis is uncommon. Death usually occurs from widespread metastasis, uretral obstruction, uremia, hemorrhage, or sepsis.

Prevention

All women need to be informed that they should promptly report any lesion on the genitalia. Yearly pelvic examinations are encouraged.

CANCER OF THE VAGINA
Epidemiology

Cancer of the vagina is extremely rare, accounting for 1% to 2% of all female carcinomas. The age range affected is usually 50 to 70 years; 60 is the average age. Cancer of the vagina is rare in blacks and almost nonexistent in Jewish women. Possible but not proved predisposing factors include repeated pregnancies, syphilis, use of a pessary, uterine prolapse, leukoplakia, and leukorrhea. Maternal ingestion of diethylstilbestrol (DES) has been associated with adenocarcinoma of the vagina in daughters who are usually past menarche but less than 30 years of age (average age is 17½) (Disaia et al., 1975; Romney et al., 1975; Rudolph, 1974).

Assessment

In situ lesions can be found by using Pap smears, and lesions can be identified during the pelvic examination.

Table 16-5. Staging and classification adopted by FIGO (1970)

Stage I	Carcinoma is limited to the vagina.
Stage II	Carcinoma has involved the subvaginal tissue but has not extended onto the pelvic wall.
Stage III	Carcinoma has extended onto the pelvic wall.
Stage IV	Carcinoma has extended beyond the true pelvis or has involved the bladder or the rectum. Bullous edema or tumor bulge into the bladder or rectum is not acceptable evidence of invasion of these organs.

Staging and classification

Staging is similar to that used for other pelvic malignancies in which the primary lesion and involvement of adjacent structures are considered. Table 16-5 shows the staging classification.

Symptoms

Painless vaginal bleeding is the most frequent symptom reported. Other symptoms common to vaginal cancer are vaginal discharge, spotting, pruritus, presence of a lesion, and pain. Bladder symptoms such as pain and frequency occur with compression of the bladder by the tumor (Disaia et al., 1975; Romney et al., 1975).

Diagnosis

Vaginal examination and biopsy are essential in diagnosing vaginal cancer. Colposcopy is also useful in noting the extent of the changes in the vagina and cervix (Romney et al., 1975; Rudolph, 1974). Lack of staining when Lugol's solution is applied to the lesion is used to identify areas that are suspect. Unfortunately, these lesions are often well advanced before symptoms appear and lesions are often misdiagnosed or missed altogether.

Treatment

Radiation therapy and surgery are the methods of treatment for vaginal cancer. Radiation is most often the treatment of choice even though there are technical difficulties in getting enough radiation dosage to the tumor. Surgical approaches are often radical and the clients who are usually elderly are poor surgical risks.

External radiation therapy is used in all stages of vaginal cancer. Internal radiation is used in stages I and II in conjunction with external radiation. Interstitial implantation with radium needles allows for a more effective dose to be obtained than when the vaginal applicator is used (Disaia et al., 1975). The difficulty of applying radiation to the vagina without harming other radiosensitive tissues such as the bladder and rectum has led some physicians to prefer a surgical approach. For stage I or IIA, a radical hysterectomy, lymphadenectomy, and vaginectomy are used. Exenteration is used for more advanced tumors where there is bladder and/or rectal involvement (Romney et al., 1975).

Prognosis and spread

Clients with lesions limited to the upper third of the posterior vagina have a better prognosis than those with lesions in the lower vagina. The 5-year survival rates are dependent on the stage of the cancer, although the American Cancer Society reports an overall cure rate of 35%, with one half of the patients dying within 18 months after diagnosis. Reasons for this low survival rate include the rarity of the cancer, which makes it difficult to perfect a reliable treatment, the advanced stage of the disease at diagnosis, and the difficulty in treating the cancer with radiation or surgery (Romney et al., 1975; Rudolph, 1974).

The vagina is a thin-walled structure with rich lymphatic drainage, which can lead to early metastasis. Most lesions appear in the upper third of the vagina, and the posterior wall is the most common site for the carcinoma, which generally spreads like cancer of the cervix. Tumors in the lower portion spread like cancer of the vulva. Death is usually the result of urinary tract obstruction with uremia or infection (Romney et al., 1975).

Adenocarcinoma of the vagina

Even though this cancer is one of the rarest reproductive malignancies, mention here is important because of the increased number of reported cases since 1971. As of 1973, 200 confirmed cases had been registered with the national registry. They were established by investigators who carried out an epidemiologic study showing an association of adenocarcinoma with maternal ingestion of diethylstilbestrol (DES) (Herbst, 1974). This drug was commonly used from 1945 to 1960 in the treatment of threatened or habitual abortion and other high-risk pregnancy problems (Green, 1977).

Systematic examinations of DES-exposed daughters has revealed that at least 60% have vaginal adenosis, although adenosis has not been established as a precursor to adenocarcinoma. Even so, all DES-exposed women should have a gynecologic examination at least twice a year beginning at menarche or age 14, whichever comes first. The examination should include visual inspection of the vagina and cervix before and after staining with Lugol's solution. Cytology should include scrapings from the cervix and any suspicious area in the vagina. Colposcopy is useful for identifying areas for biopsy.

Stilbestrol and related drug compounds must not be taken during pregnancy (Disaia et al., 1975).

CANCER OF THE FALLOPIAN TUBE
Epidemiology

Carcinoma of the fallopian tube makes up less than 1% of genital tract cancers. The age range is 45 to 60 years; 50 years is the average. High-risk factors identified include infertility and nulliparity (Rudolph, 1974).

Assessment

Cancer of the fallopian tube is rarely if ever picked up during a routine health examination. Vaginal cytology is reported to be of no value, although some cases have been reported with a positive Pap smear (Disaia et al., 1975). At present there is no practical or accurate method for mass screening.

Staging

No official staging has been established. The following is suggested as a classification system. It parallels ovarian cancer because of the similarity of the diseases (FIGO, 1971):

Stage 0	Carcinoma *in situ.*
Stage IA	One tube involved—no serosa.
Stage IB	Both tubes involved—no serosa.
Stage IC	One or both tubes involved with ascites or positive peritoneal fluid cytology.
Stage IIA	Involvement of tubal serosa.
Stage IIB	Involvement of ovaries, uterus, or pelvic wall.
Stage III	Extension of tumor beyond the pelvis but limited to abdominal cavity.
Stage IV	Extension outside the abdominal cavity.

Symptoms

Two thirds of the women with carcinoma of the fallopian tube have pain, vaginal discharge, and adnexal mass. The pain is described as cramp-like abdominal pain. Vaginal discharge can be clear yellow or amber and watery.

Diagnosis

Diagnosis is seldom made preoperatively. A diagnostic laparotomy is usually performed.

Treatment

Hysterectomy and bilateral salpingo-oophorectomy are the usual treatment. Postoperative radiation is frequently used, but effectiveness has not been proved. Chemotherapy, especially with the progestins and alkylating agents, has been used but there are little data about the benefits (Disaia et al., 1975).

Prognosis

Five-year survival rates range from 50% if the disease is limited to the tube to 25% and less if spread is outside the tube.

Prevention

There is no known prevention for carcinoma of the fallopian tube.

GESTATIONAL TROPHOBLASTIC DISEASE

Three pathologic forms of the human trophoblast are *hydatidiform mole*, *invasive mole*, and *choriocarcinoma*. These maternal neoplasms are unique in that they are derived from fetal tissue, are able to produce human chorionic gonadotropin, and can undergo spontaneous regression, although this is rare for choriocarcinoma.

A classification system for trophoblastic neoplasms was developed by the Union Internationale Centre de Cancer in 1969 (Disaia et al., 1975).

I. Clinical diagnosis
  1. Nonmetastatic
  2. Metastatic
    a. Local (pelvic)
    b. Extrapelvic (specify location)
  3. Other required information
    a. Evidence
      (i) Morphologic
      (ii) Nonmorphologic
    b. Antecedent pregnancy (specify duration)
      (i) Normal
      (ii) Abortal
      (iii) Molar
    c. Previous treatment
      (i) Untreated
      (ii) Treated (specify)
II. Morphologic diagnosis
  1. Hydatidiform mole
    a. Noninvasive
    b. Invasive
  2. Choriocarcinoma
  3. Uncertain
  4. Other required information
    a. Diagnostic basis (specify)
      (i) Curettage
      (ii) Excised uterus
      (iii) Necropsy
      (iv) Other
    b. Date of diagnosis (with respect to date of onset of treatment)
    c. Subsequent change in morphologic diagnosis. Specify diagnostic basis as in II,4a

Hydatidiform mole
Epidemiology

Hydatidiform mole occurs in 1 in 2000 deliveries in the United States and 1 in 25 in Taiwan. The occurrence is more frequent in women over 40 and under 20 years of age, and the risk of developing a second mole is four to five times greater than an initial molar pregnancy. The frequent occurrence of trophoblastic disease in the Orient suggests a nutritional etiology, with folic acid deficiency being suspected. Other causative factors that have been considered are racial susceptibility, fetomaternal histocompatibility, and infectious agents (Disaia et al., 1975).

Symptoms and diagnosis

Hydatidiform mole should be suspected in any woman with bleeding during the first half of pregnancy, toxemia before 24 weeks gestation, or hyperemesis gravidarum. Physical examination often reveals a uterus that is large for the gestational age and an absence of fetal heart tones or fetal parts.

A determination of urinary chorionic gonadotropin (HCG) titers may be helpful. The normal pregnancy values are 100,000 IU in 24 hours; hydatidiform mole values are over 500,000 IU in 24 hours. Amniocentesis and ultrasonography are also used in diagnosing hydatidiform moles.

Treatment

Termination of the molar pregnancy should be done as soon as the diagnosis is confirmed. Suction curettage is the method of choice, although hysterectomy is acceptable for women desiring sterilization.

Invasive mole

About 15% of all molar pregnancies will invade the myometrium. Hemorrhage and tissue necrosis accompany the invasion. Invasive mole has all the characteristics of a malignant tumor except that it is self-limiting and will involute spontaneously if no hemorrhagic complications occur.

Choriocarcinoma

Choriocarcinoma will occur in approximately 3% of hydatidiform mole cases. It is a highly malignant tumor, symptoms of which can imitate other disease processes such as ectopic pregnancy or threatened abortion.

Diagnosis is by determination of chorionic gonadotropin titers. After a hydatidiform mole has been removed, a program for follow-up should be established to monitor the presence or absence of invasive mole or choriocarcinoma. Procedures that should be performed include chest X-rays; pelvic examinations every 2 weeks until the human chorionic gonatotropin (HCG) level is normal, then monthly; oral estrogen-progestin contraceptives for 12 months; and HCG determinations (weekly until three consecutive normal values [25 IU/L] are obtained, then monthly for 6 months, and then every 2 months for another 6 months).

During the follow-up, treatment is instituted if there is a tissue diagnosis of invasive mole or choriocarcinoma. Other indications for treatment initiation are rising HCG values, presence of metastasis, or elevation of HCG values after the normal level has been reached.

Treatment

Choriocarcinoma is the only disseminating solid tumor that can be cured by chemotherapy alone. Methorexate and actinomycin D are superior to other cytotoxic agents in treating nonmetastatic trophoblastic disease. These agents are administered in cycles with at least a 7-day rest in between cycles. Chemotherapy is continued until three consecutive weekly HCG titers are normal (usually three to four cycles). Titers are obtained monthly for 6 months, every 2 months for the next 6 months, and every 6 months thereafter. Oral contraceptives are recommended to suppress gonadotropin and to prevent pregnancy in the first year of follow-up.

A hysterectomy can be performed if the woman requests sterilization or if the disease is resistant to chemotherapy. Irradiation is used for metastatic disease.

Prognosis and spread

The rate of cure for women with nonmetastatic disease is almost 100% when treated with chemotherapy. Clients with poor prognosis are women with brain or liver metastasis or with metastatic disease that is resistant to single-agent chemotherapy.

Choriocarcinoma is predisposed to hematogenous spread. The organs involved in metastasis are the lung, lower genital tract, brain, liver, kidney, and gastrointestinal tract (Romney et al., 1975).

Special management considerations

Gynecologic nursing practitioners must be able to prepare and care for women undergoing any treatment chosen by the physician. In order to do this, practitioners must have a thorough understanding of the three major treatment choices for gynecologic cancer—surgery, radiation, and chemotherapy—and should also be informed about immunotherapy, although this mode of treatment is not commonly used in gynecology at present.

This section describes the different types of surgery, radiation, and chemotherapeutic agents used in treating gynecologic cancer and discusses nursing management of patients undergoing these treatments. Emphasis is on nutrition, pain management, psychosocial aspects, and terminal care. Finally, education of the general public about gynecologic cancer is discussed with emphasis on community resources.

SURGERY

Discussion of types of surgery will be limited here to the more radical procedures: radical hysterectomy, vulvectomy, and exenteration. Whereas hysterectomy is the most common surgical procedure employed, it has been discussed in Chapter 15 and the description will not be repeated here.

Radical hysterectomy and vaginectomy

Invasive cancer of the cervix, stages I and II, can be treated with radical hysterectomy. This procedure includes removal of the uterus, combined with excision of paracervical and paravaginal tissue as well as the upper one third to one half of the vagina.

Risks of a radical hysterectomy are postoperative infection, hemorrhage, fistulation of urine or feces, and problems with voiding. Usually the recovery time is longer than for a conventional hysterectomy, although nursing care is essentially the same (see Chapter 15).

The advantages of the radical hysterectomy are: (1) there can be no recurrence in organs removed, (2) the ovaries need not be removed, which benefits younger women, and (3) there is no exposure of normal organs to irradiation. The disadvantages are that not all clients are suitable for surgery, the surgery has a high risk of death from complications, the vagina is shortened, and urinary and rectal fistulas occur more frequently than after radiation therapy (Romney et al., 1975).

Vulvectomy

A simple or radical vulvectomy can be done depending on the woman's medical status and extent of the lesion. A simple vulvectomy includes surgical excision of the vulva with a wide margin of skin. Radical vulvectomy entails excision of tissue from the anus to a few centimeters above the symphysis pubis (skin, labia majora and minora, and clitoris) (Fig. 16-2). Bilateral superficial groin and deep inguinal, femoral, iliac, hypogastric, and obturator node dissection may be done as well (Avery et al., 1974).

Preoperative nursing care

The client must be prepared for the postoperative procedures that will be performed, for preoperative procedures, and for the surgery itself. The nurse should explain the following to the client to prepare her for surgery:
1. Abdominal perineal shave
2. Nothing by mouth after midnight
3. Enema and douche

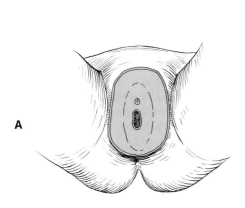
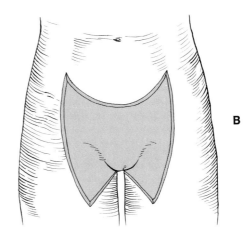

Fig. 16-2. A, Simple vulvectomy; **B,** radical vulvectomy.

4. Intravenous fluid
5. Foley catheter

The extent of the surgical procedure and the appearance of the wound should be clearly explained, given the mutilating aspects of the surgery.

Postoperative procedures that should be explained prior to surgery to help the client be prepared are these (Serviatius, 1975):

1. Vital signs will be taken at regular intervals.
2. Respiratory therapy (blow bottles, IPPB) techniques used to prevent respiratory complications should be demonstrated.
3. A Foley catheter will remain in place 1 to 2 weeks to prevent wound contamination and to accurately measure urinary output.
4. Pain and nausea medications are ordered every 3 to 4 hours as necessary.
5. Intravenous feedings will be used the first 2 postoperative days. The diet then progresses to clear liquids, then to solid foods.
6. Hemovacs will be inserted into the incision to remove drainage.
7. Antiembolism stockings will be worn to prevent leg edema and thrombophlebitis.
8. A footboard will be on the bed to encourage leg exercise and prevent circulatory problems.
9. An air mattress will facilitate comfort and prevent pressure sores.
10. A bed cradle may be used to keep the bed linens away from the incision.

Emotional support should begin preoperatively and continue until discharge. Often the woman has guilt feelings, especially if she has postponed treatment because of embarrassment. The fear of disfigurement or loss of a body part may precipitate a grief reaction accompanied by crying, depression, or withdrawal. The nurse must be accepting of these moods and allow venti-lation of feelings while helping the family understand these actions so it can be supportive.

Fear of death because of the diagnosis of cancer is frequently expressed. By allowing the client to work through her feelings about death and dying while providing information on 5-year survival rates based on the extent of regional involvement, the nurse can help the woman deal realistically with her situation.

Sexuality is also a concern of the woman whether she is married, single, widowed, divorced, young, or old. The woman may feel that she will no longer be feminine or that she will be sexually inadequate after surgery or that her sexual partner will no longer find her attractive. The practitioner can tell the woman that sexual activity can usually be resumed within 3 months, depending on the extent of surgery and the healing process.

Postoperative nursing care

The woman will return from the operating room with dressings on the perineum and groin. These dressings should be changed frequently because there is a lot of drainage and wet dressings increase the risk of infection. A strong vaginal odor is present, which can be controlled with frequent perineal care and room deodorizers. Perineal care and/or sitz baths are also done after voidings and bowel movements to decrease the risk of contaminating the incision. The warm solutions promote healing by increasing circulation and decreasing discomfort.

Wound care consists of the use of hydrogen peroxide for debridement; antibacterial solutions may be used also. Solutions can be applied with an asepto bulb syringe or by using a Water-Pic machine to squirt the solution into the wound. A heat lamp or a hairdryer is used after the irrigation to promote drying and healing of the wound area. Wound care is important because infection and necrosis are the most common postoperative complications. If the wound opens, healing must take place by granulation and this will prolong the healing process for as long as 6 months.

The indwelling catheter will remain in place for 7 to 14 days to prevent urethral stenosis and urinary incontinence. After the catheter is removed, the urine stream may be deflected to the leg because of edema. The woman can be encouraged to stand while urinating to decrease strain on the sutures.

Postoperative pain is usually controlled with parenteral analgesics given every 3 to 4 hours the first day or two after surgery. Then mild analgesics are all that is needed. Fecal softeners can decrease discomfort of bowel movements.

Leg edema is common postoperatively and is treated with the continued use of elastic stockings.

Because vulvectomies are disfiguring procedures, the woman must deal with body image changes. Her first reaction to the disfigurement may be at the first dressing change or with the first sitz bath. Adaptation to the body change will depend on her coping abilities, the responses of her family and friends, and support of the health team. Women need time to adjust to the fact that they are permanently changed, and this adjustment is often preceded by depression and introspection.

The sexually active woman needs special counseling and reinforcement of the preoperative information about sexual activity. She should be informed that intercourse may be unsatisfactory because of the loss of the fatty pads of the mons pubis, the loss of the clitoris, and decreased lubrication from the vulvar glands. Water-soluble lubricants can be used during intercourse. The loss of pubic hair and the scarring are upsetting to some women. Sexual partners may have a traumatic emotional reaction to this surgery, which needs to be considered. A discussion of alternative methods of achieving sexual satisfaction may help.

Discharge instructions should include wound care and how to detect abnormal changes in the healing process. Frequent follow-up visits are necessary until healing is complete (Dyche, 1975).

Pelvic exenteration

The most common indication for pelvic exenteration is recurrent cancer of the cervix (Hamilton and Schlapper, 1979), although fewer than 5% of these clients are suited for surgery. Other indications include colorectal cancer, recurrent cancer of the endometrium, extended cancer of the vulva or vagina, and radiation necrosis (Dwyer, 1976).

Pelvic exenteration is usually done as a "last ditch" effort to control pelvic cancer and is only done if there is a good chance for cure. It cannot be used if the cancer has spread outside the pelvis or if the woman is massively obese or very elderly (Dyche, 1975).

There are various degrees of exenteration (see Fig. 16-3), and the procedure chosen depends on the extent of the disease at the time of surgery. The patient is told that an exploratory laparotomy will be done first; if there is no metastasis an exenteration will be done. A total exenteration includes the removal of all pelvic reproductive organs and lymph nodes, the bladder and the distal ureters, the rectum and distal sigmoid colon, the perineum, and pelvic floor, peritoneal, and levator muscles. An anterior exenteration will exclude the bowel, whereas the posterior exenteration will exclude the bladder. The 4- to 9-hour procedure involves making an artificial bladder from a resected section of ileum or sigmoid and anastomosing the ureters to the bowel forming a conduit, which usually is placed on the right side of the abdomen. A colostomy is also performed, and the stoma is usually on the left side of the abdomen.

After the organs are removed, the small bowel drops down and fills the empty pelvis. An opening is left where the vagina has been, which permits drainage.

Preoperative care

Along with the physical and medical indications for exenteration as a mode of treatment for advanced pelvic cancers, emotional and social indications should be assessed. Selection of candidates for the procedure should include assessment of emotional capability to withstand the surgery, the long recovery, and the body image changes; physical strength to endure the diagnostic workup and surgery; and the woman's social and financial situation, including support systems.

Preparation for the procedure begins on admission to the hospital and should include mental and physical preparation. Preoperatively, clear and complete explanations of procedures should be given to reduce the woman's anxiety. The woman is often devastated to learn that cancer is again suspected. She may deny the need for surgery; she may agree that surgery is necessary but be horrified about body changes so that she may or may not agree to the procedure; or she may express relief that some hope of a cure remains and agree to the procedure.

When the decision has been made to go ahead with the surgery, the woman may need to become dependent on the nursing staff and family; this behavior should be noted by the nurse who is assessing coping mechanisms.

Prior to the surgery the woman undergoes a barrage of diagnostic tests to rule out metastasis outside the pelvis. These tests include blood studies, urinalysis, chest-X-ray, barium studies, physical examinations, cystoscopy, IVP, and proctoscopy.

Physical preparation for the surgery begins 3 to 5 days before the operation. Extensive bowel preparation, which consists of enemas, laxatives, and antibiotic instillations, is started 4 to 5 days prior to surgery. The

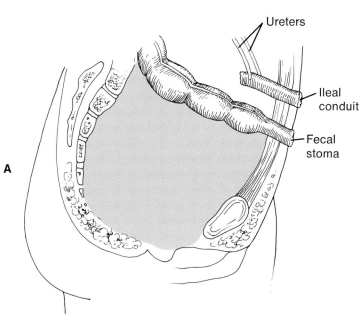

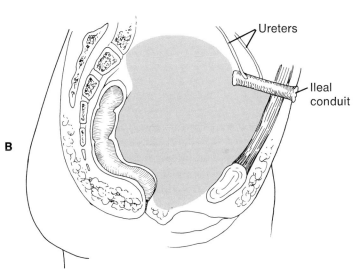

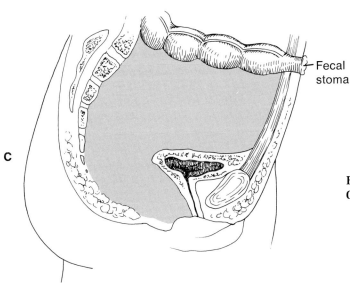

Fig. 16-3. A, Total exenteration; **B,** anterior exenteration; **C,** posterior exenteration.

woman is usually placed on a low-residue diet on admission that is changed to clear liquids for 48 hours postoperatively. An intestinal tube is passed nasally into the ileum 24 to 48 hours preoperatively. An enterostomy therapist will mark the sites for stoma placement the day before surgery. The night before surgery an abdominal perineal shave is done, and a subclavian catheter may be inserted if the patient has poor veins.

Anxiety is highest in the patient and the family immediately prior to the operation; therefore, the nurse should provide support and explanations as necessary.

Postoperative care

The patient usually spends the first 3 to 4 days of the postoperative period in an intensive care unit because of the high morbidity and mortality rates and the need for frequent observations for shock, cardiac changes, and kidney failure. In addition to the usual postoperative care, these aspects should be stressed by the practitioner:

1. Ambulation should begin in the first 24 to 48 hours postoperatively.
2. Respiratory therapy (IPPB) and deep breathing should be encouraged.
3. Passive leg exercises and the use of elastic stockings will improve circulation and prevent thrombosis.
4. Fluid and electrolyte balance must be maintained. Protein is lost in the first 2 postoperative weeks and should be replaced. Albumin is given to decrease edema. Sodium and clorides are lost through gastrointestinal fluid loss and must be replaced. Potassium is usually replaced in intravenous fluids. Close observation of intake and output is essential.
5. The patient is kept NPO until peristalsis returns (in 4 to 6 days). The nasogastric tube remains in place, and low suction is used until signs of bowel function are demonstrated. The tube is clamped for 24 hours and clear liquids are given; if no distention occurs, the tube is removed and diet is advanced as tolerated.
6. Serosanguineous drainage from the perineal opening should be checked for signs of infection. This drainage will continue for 1 to 12 months, and the woman should be advised to wear minipads or beltless sanitary pads in order not to interfere with the stomas. Bowel obstructions and infections are the most frequent physiologic complications.

Emotional needs. The woman is usually dependent the first day or two postoperatively. About the fourth day she begins to express grief over mutilation of her body. She may go through three phases of recovery: she may deny the change by not looking at the wound or stoma sites, become depressed, or withdraw; then she may attempt reality testing by becoming angry and hostile with the staff, by questioning staff about care, and moving on to observe the staff do the wound care; finally she will adapt to the body changes by becoming independent in her physical care and planning for her discharge. The patient will have emotional fluctuations and the practitioner should always be alert to mood changes (Disaia et al., 1975; Hamilton and Schlapper, 1979).

Sexual considerations. The woman will no longer be able to engage in vaginal intercourse unless an artificial vagina is constructed in a later procedure. This procedure involves making a vagina from segments of colon or ileum or skin grafts, which are placed over a tent. If the clitoris is not removed the patient can still have clitoral stimulation, and alternate methods of sexual gratification such as oral sex can be utilized to achieve orgasm.

The nurse should assess the need for sexual counseling and listen for clues concerning feelings about the body changes. She should also allow for private times between the woman and her partner.

Problems related to colostomy and ileal conduit

Physical considerations. Breakdown of skin resulting from irritation by caustic intestinal fluid is a common problem. Treatment of the area depends on the severity of the breakdown. For skin that is only reddened or irritated, washing with soap and water and drying is the first step. Then an application of an antacid such as Maalox and a light coating of karaya powder before the appliance is fitted should be all that is necessary. If the skin is excoriated, the nurse or client should wash and dry the area and apply Kenolog spray or nycostatin powder to the area before fitting the appliance.

For a severe breakdown the area should be exposed to air for 30 minutes several times a day. Aluminum hydroxide paste and karaya powder should be used in fitting the appliance.

Another problem to be considered is odor control. The patient can avoid odorous foods such as asparagus, onions, fish, eggs, and cheese. Bismuth subgallate tablets or aspirin can be placed in the ostomy bag for odor control.

Other problems related to food intake that should be avoided include skipping meals, which causes gas problems, eating fibrous foods, which are difficult to digest, and eating foods that may cause diarrhea such as strong tea, bananas, applesauce, and peanut butter.

Problems related to the ileal conduit are similar to those of the colostomy. The skin must be protected from leaking urine. Encrustations in the bag result from alkaline urine pooling in the bag and can be avoided if the bag is changed frequently. Crystal deposits in the bag can be dissolved with vinegar. For odor problems, the woman can increase her intake of fluids, especially cranberry juice, and increase ascorbic acid intake (Brown et al., 1972).

Psychologic considerations. Adjustments to the ileal conduit and colostomy are related to the adjustments to mutilation and desexualization. In a study of fifteen women reported by Brown and associates in 1972, 40% reported changes in their social habits, 80% had changed jobs, and 66% were enjoying activities such as dancing, swimming, and horseback riding. Some of the women also reported dreams with sexual content, and others reported ileostomal masturbation or autoerotic sexual experiences.

In an earlier study Dyk and Sutherland (1956) reported that women who had colostomies had decreased sexual activity, decreased libido, and increased depression.

Appropriate assessment and intervention by the nurse are important in the adjustment of the woman who has had radical surgery. Observations, discussions, and perceptions must be used to identify problems. In planning care the nurse must involve the client and teach self-care of the colostomy and ileal conduit. Privacy should be provided as necessary. Finally, the nurse should help the client maintain her feminine role while she learns to accept her new image (Murray, 1972).

RADIOTHERAPY

Both internal and external irradiation are commonly used for patients with gynecologic cancers. The treatments are determined by the stage of disease, the extent of the disease process, and the shape of the pelvis, which must allow for radium application.

The purpose of intracavitary radium therapy (IRT) is to irradiate the local tumor around the cervix and intrauterine cavity. External radiation therapy (ERT) irradiates the lateral extension of the disease in the parametrium and pelvic wall nodes.

Depending on the extent of the disease, ERT is given over a 4- to 6-week period with pre- or posttreatments of IRT for a total dose of 2,000 to 7,000 rads. IRT usually consists of two radium applications at intervals during the treatment period, for the purpose of increasing normal tissue tolerance and increasing the shrinkage of the tumor between insertions (Hilkemeyer, 1967).

The radiation source for ERT is usually supplied by megavoltage machines such as cobalt, betatron, or linear accelerators. These machines given homogeneous doses of radiation to the pelvis and cause little injury because the rays pass through the skin with little absorption (Romney et al., 1975).

The source for IRT is usually cesium, which is implanted in the cervix or vagina in needles or applicators. The discussion of IRT here will focus on the fixed radium application with intrauterine tandems and vaginal colpostats used with the afterloading system (Disaia et al., 1975). The Fletcher-Suit afterloading system is advantageous and widely used in the United States today because of its flexibility and safety. It is safe because only the applicator is inserted in the operating room; the cesium is inserted in the client's room, which decreases exposure of hospital personnel. The flexibility of the system is based on the fact that the cesium can be placed more accurately by using X-rays after surgical placement of the applicator.

Successful radiation therapy depends on the ability of the treatment to kill malignant cells while doing little damage to normal cells. Since the reproductive organs are highly radiosensitive, time must be allowed for normal tissues to recover after irradiation. For this reason ERT is given over a period of 4 to 7 weeks with only four to five treatments per week. The client must be in good physical condition for optimal success with radiation therapy. This success is measured clinically by disappearance of the tumor, rate and degree of tumor regression, and survival rates.*

Nursing care

General emotional support should be given throughout the radiation therapy. Many clients have fears about death, being burned by the radiation treatments, disfigurements, pain, sterility, and loss of sexual function. Careful assessments should be made to determine if the woman has these fears and to determine if she has misconceptions or needs more explanations about the treatments. Assessments of the socioeconomic situation should be made to determine the need for financial assistance, transportation to treatments, or help at home (Hilkemeyer, 1967).

Preparing the client for IRT

Clients are usually admitted the day before the insertion. Preoperative procedures include the following:
1. Soapsuds enema until clear to clean the intestinal tract
2. Betadine douche to clear the vaginal tract
3. Low residue diet to decrease bowel motility
4. NPO past midnight
5. Usually no skin preparation except for a bath or shower
6. Anesthesia workup including on call medications

The nurse should give thorough explanations of what is to be done and what to expect.

The radium applicator is inserted in the operating room with the woman under general anesthesia. After

---

*Disaia et al., 1975; Romney et al., 1975; Rotman, 1976; Rubin, 1974.

the woman is reactive she is taken to the X-ray department for X-rays to localize exact placement of the radium source. She then returns to her room where the radium source is placed in the applicator.

Postoperative care

Positioning. The woman should be placed on her back with the head of the bed flat or elevated no more than 10 to 15 degrees. She should restrict her movements to prevent dislodgement of the radium. She should not turn from side to side but if she must be turned, "log-rolling" should be employed. To do this, a pillow is placed between the knees and the woman is assisted to roll to one side with her body in straight alignment. The client may perform active range of motion exercises on her arms and use a footboard to do foot and leg exercises. An air mattress is recommended to prevent pressure sores.

Vital signs. Vital signs are taken every 4 hours; an increase in temperature over 100° F the first evening is not unusual.

Skin care. A complete bath every day is unnecessary. Bathing below the waist need not be done unless the client is soiled. Partial back rubs are appreciated. The skin should be checked for any rashes or evidence of dehydration.

Elimination. The woman will have a Foley catheter inserted during surgery, and this will be attached to straight drainage. The tube should be placed under the client's leg to decrease the possibility of infection. To reduce trauma to the bowel and prevent bowel movements and diarrhea, the patient is usually on a low-residue diet and is given drugs such as Lomotil, 2 mg, four times a day. If the client has a bowel movement she should not be raised onto a regular bedpan because of the likelihood of displacing the applicator. A fracture pan or emesis basin may be used.

Fluids. The client usually returns from the operating room with an intravenous infusion. This may be continued until she is taking clear liquids well. Fluids should be encouraged because IRT patients can become dehydrated easily.

Medications. Pain medications are given according to need. Mild analgesics such as Darvocet-N (100 mg) and stronger medications such as codeine (0.03 mg to 0.06 Gm) or Demerol (50 to 100 mg) are ordered every 3 to 4 hours as needed. Sedatives such as pentobarbital (60 mg) or chloral hydrate (0.5 Gm) are given at bedtime if needed. Antiemetic drugs such as prochlorperozine (Compazine) (10 mg) or phenergan (25 mg) are given for nausea (Breeding and Wollin, 1976; Hilkemeyer, 1967).

Special precautions

In order to minimize radium exposure of the staff, three factors should be considered in planning nursing care: distance, shielding, and time.

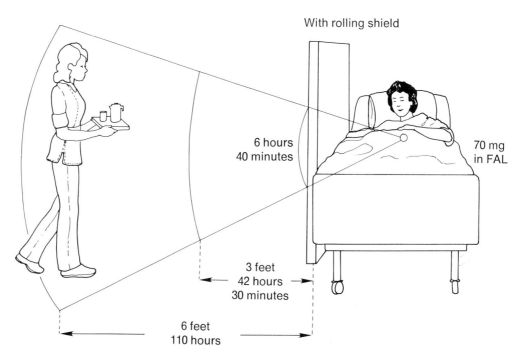

With rolling shield

6 hours
40 minutes

70 mg
in FAL

3 feet
42 hours
30 minutes

6 feet
110 hours

Fig. 16-4. Approximate times nurse can safely spend at distances from client with radiation source in place.

Distance. Personnel should work as far away from the radium source as possible. The intensity of the radiation is decreased by the square of the distance between the source and the practitioner.

Shielding. A lead shield should be kept between the radium source and nurse at all times. Many shields are movable and allow the nurse to change the position as she cares for the client.

Time. The less time a nurse spends at the bedside, the less radiation received. The practitioner must work as effectively as possible and have care well organized before entering the room. The client should be told why the nurse is limiting time in the room. Fig. 16-4 illustrates the approximate time a nurse can safely spend at certain distances from the patient.

The cumulative dose a person receives from radiation is measured in millirems (MREM). By United States law a person can only receive 1250 MREM every 3 months. One way to keep track of the dosage received is by wearing a film badge. This is simply a piece of unexposed film in a holder, which will turn dark when exposed to ionizing radiation. The badge is turned in at monthly intervals, the film is developed, and the amount of radiation is noted. Another device for calculating radiation dosage is the pocket dosimeter, which can be held up to the light and read immediately.

Other special considerations are the following:
1. The client should be assigned to a single room that is not in a heavy traffic area. If a private room is not available, a semi-private room can be used if the other patient is postmenopausal or has had her ovaries removed.
2. A precaution sign should be on the door.
3. Pregnant nurses should not be assigned to these clients if possible.
4. Pregnant women and children under 18 should not be allowed to visit.

Radium removal

The radium source is removed after 48 to 72 hours. The client is given a soapsuds enema and a Betadine douche and is assisted with a shower or bath. She is allowed out of bed as desired and given a regular diet. She is usually discharged the next morning.

Discharge instructions should include the following:
1. Sexual intercourse may be resumed within 7 to 10 days depending on the reaction of the cervix and vagina to radiation. The client should be told that vaginal atrophy may cause stenosis and she may need to use a plastic rod for prevention.
2. Vaginal discharge will be present and the woman may douche daily if necessary
3. She should avoid direct sunlight to the areas exposed to radiation

4. Use of an emollient cream may alleviate the itching of pruritus

Caring for the client on ERT

ERT can be managed on an outpatient or inpatient basis depending on the proximity of the client's home to the treatment center, availability of motel units or boarding rooms near the hospital, and the client's financial and physical condition.

Suggestions for women having ERT include no sunbathing, no lotions or creams to the irradiated areas, no soap or water on the site of treatments because markings will wash off, and watching for signs of skin breakdown. The woman is usually on a low-residue diet. A big consideration for client's on ERT who are in the hospital is boredom. Nurses should encourage these women to become involved in activities such as recreational or occupational therapy. Encouragement of interactions among the ERT clients on the unit can provide these women with a group in which they can express their concerns about treatment or any other subject and receive support from each other.

Complications of radiation therapy

The vast majority of radiation injuries involve the pelvic structures. Areas that have a low tolerance to radiation because of excessive moisture and warmth such as the perineum and buttocks can have mild to severe skin reactions. Erythema can precede desquamation like second-degree or severe third-degree burns. Treatments include keeping the skin dry and well aerated and applying cornstarch, baby powder, or steroid creams to the affected areas.

Cystitis is another complication that is usually controlled by increasing fluid intake and giving antispasmodics and analgesics.

Proctosigmoiditis is manifested by diarrhea and cramping. It usually responds to a low-residue diet, steroid suppositories, or antispasmodics. Belladonna or opium suppositories are also effective.

Enteritis is usually associated with nausea, cramping, and diarrhea. A low-residue diet and low lactose intake can usually control the diarrhea. Elemental diets are also useful, although because of their high osmolarity they must be given at reduced strength at first. They should also be served very cold and sipped slowly to avoid cramping. Antiemetics and antispasmodics are also employed.

Delayed reactions can occur 6 to 24 months after therapy has been discontinued. Proctitis is characterized by pain, diarrhea, constipation, and rectal bleeding. A low-residue diet and administration of Metamucil and antispasmodics are effective treatments.

Rectal fistulas are one of the most common injuries.

Surgical intervention to provide for a proximal diverting colostomy is necessary. Sigmoiditis is caused by very high doses of radiation. A right transverse colostomy is the usual treatment. Small bowel injuries, although not common, are usually in the terminal ileum. Symptoms are similar to an incomplete bowel obstruction: cramps, pain, diarrhea, nausea and vomiting, bloating, and weight loss. Surgical intervention such as resection and anastomosis may be necessary (Disaia, 1975; Rotman, 1976).

Nutritional problems associated with radiation therapy

There are many problems related to radiation therapy. Nursing goals should be to prevent these problems when feasible or to minimize the effects through early interventions. The nurse should include in the nutritional assessment information concerning the client's normal dietary intake, her likes and dislikes, her mealtime patterns or number of meals per day, and cultural and social information that may influence intake.

The biggest problem to consider is malnutrition related to decreased calcium intake, hypermetabolism, anorexia, a negative nitrogen balance, and clinically apparent edema. The loss of interest in food results from taste alteration that occurs in the first 2 weeks of therapy and stabilizes by the third week. Decreased taste perception (hypogeusesthesia) with a perverted sense of taste (dysgeusia) will cause some foods to taste spoiled or rancid. Many foods will taste salty, bitter, sour, or metallic. If dysgeusia is not present, foods tend to be tasteless.

Many patients develop an aversion to protein. This tends to be selective and progressive. The greatest dislike is for beef, then pork. Poultry, fish, eggs, and cheese follow in descending order of aversion. Often a change in seasoning will help make these foods more tolerable (Schrieier and Lavenia, 1977).

Anorexia usually increases as the day progresses. The nurse should encourage the client to get at least one third of the day's protein and calories at breakfast time. Another way to increase protein and calorie intake is to offer milkshakes, custards, eggnog, or commercial supplements. Food should be served at room temperature, although cold foods are soothing if the client has a sore mouth. Fruits and fruit sauces can be used for clients with dysgeusia.

If mastication becomes difficult, foods can be chopped or blended. If swallowing becomes difficult, gravies or sauces may help. Viscous lidocaine can also be given prior to eating. Tube feeding is implemented only if and when the interventions mentioned here have ceased to provide the client with adequate nutrition (Rose, 1978).

Palliative radiation treatment

Radiation is employed to provide pain relief when there is bone pain caused by metastasis or to stop bleeding, to decrease pressure on vital organs, or to stop or slow down tumor growth (Rotman, 1976).

CHEMOTHERAPY

Five chemotherapeutic agents are commonly used for gynecologic malignancies: alkylating agents, antibiotics, antimetabolites, hormones, and plant alkyloids. These agents are used: when the client is not suited to surgery or radiation; for recurrent cancer of the cervix, endometrium, or ovary; to eliminate lesions predisposed to cancer when surgery or radiation is impossible; for persistent gestational trophoblastic disease; and in combination with surgery and radiation (Wall and Blythe, 1976).

Mode of action

Chemotherapeutic agents work by interfering with the normal life cycle of cells and exerting cytocidal effects. The main purpose of chemotherapy is to provide maximal destruction of cancer cells with minimal toxicity. A brief review of cellular biology and the cell cycle is included here as background for understanding the action of specific chemotherapeutic agents.

Normal cell cycle. A cell is the fundamental unit of living tissue, the metabolic and biologic activities of which are controlled and directed by genetic data incorporated into nuclear deoxyribonucleic acid (DNA).

DNA molecules are made up of two strands wound in a double helix. These two chains are joined by chemical bonds between the two base pairs. Each chain is comprised of a polymer of nucleotide subunits made up of deoxyribase, a purine or pyrimidine base, and a phosphate group. At the time of cell division or DNA replication, the double helix uncoils and adds complementary purine and pyrimidine bases to each strand. The new cell thus has one new chain and one old chain. An additional function of DNA is controlling protein synthesis, which will determine cell structure and function. Information stored in the pyrimidine and purine units is transcribed to ribonucleic acid (RNA). The following diagram illustrates the relationship of DNA and RNA to protein synthesis (Disaia, 1975).

$$DNA \xrightarrow{\text{Transcription}} RNA \text{ Cell information transfer}$$

$$\xrightarrow{\text{Translation}} \text{Protein}$$

Replication. Malignant cells go through the same life cycle phases for replication as do normal cells. The following is a description of the four stages of the cell cycle.

The time interval between the phases of mitosis and

synthesis (G₁) and synthesis and mitosis (G₂) is called the G₀ interval and is a resting phase (the letter G stands for "gap"). The cell will remain at rest until triggered by cell death or other cell activity. It will then move into the G₁ phase where RNA and protein are synthesized. Duration of the G₁ interval is related to the proliferation activity of the tissue, and this proliferative capacity is the principal consideration in planning chemotherapy because cancer cells are very sensitive during division.

The cell then enters the DNA synthesis (S) phase lasting 4 to 6 hours, where the DNA complement is duplicated. After the S phase the cell moves into the second gap interval (G₂). This phase is fairly quiet with some RNA and protein being synthesized. The cell moves from G₂ to mitosis (M) where cell division is completed, producing two daughter cells. These cells can repeat the cycle or go into a G₀ phase and wait for activation.

The time for completion of the cycle from mitosis to mitosis is called generation time. This time can be hours, days, weeks, months, or even years (Wall and Blythe, 1976). Fig. 16-5 illustrates the cell cycle.

The main problem in chemotherapy is the presence of drug-resistant resting or noncycling cells. Also, cells must be well nourished to be maximally affected by chemotherapeutic agents, which means that clients must be well nourished to get the best response to therapy (Bingham, 1978).

Various agents work in different ways to interrupt the cell cycle. Generally, agents that affect the cells during specific phases are antimetabolites, which interfere with DNA synthesis; plant alkyloids, which inhibit mitosis; and L-asparaginase, which inhibits movement from G₁ to S phase. Cycle nonspecific agents act independently of phases. These agents include most of the alkylating drugs and antibiotics (Fig. 16-6).

The nurse should be familiar with the five commonly used agents in gynecologic oncology, including the indications for use, dosage and administration, side effects, nutritional problems, and nursing considerations. The following section presents this information.

Agents used against gynecologic cancers
Alkylating agents

The most common single agents used for squamous cell carcinoma of the ovary, cancer of the cervix, and vaginal cancer are the alkylating agents. The most commonly used drugs are chlorambucil, melphalan (Alkeran), cyclophosphamide (Cytoxan), nitrogen mustard, and thiophosphoramide (Thio-Tepa). Table 16-6 presents the dosage and route of administration, side effects including nutritional problems, and nursing considerations for these drugs. Approximately 85% of the patients receiving alkylating agents will develop resistance to the drugs

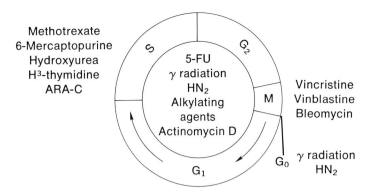

Fig. 16-5. The cell cycle.

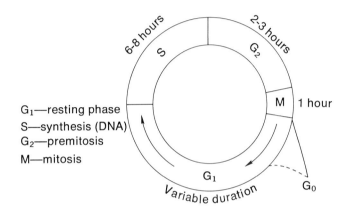

Fig. 16-6. Drug activity related to phases of cell cycle.

after 16 months. Multiple drug therapy may be initiated at this time. Two popular combinations are incristine, actinomycin D, and Cytoxan or actinomycin D, Cytoxan, and 5-fluorouracil. The purpose of this multiple therapy is to attack the cell cycle at different phases and kill more cancer cells. Approximately 43% of patients will respond to this triple therapy (Wall and Blythe, 1976).

Antibiotics

Actinomycin D interferes with the S phase of the cell cycle and is used to treat ovarian cancer and persistent gestational trophoblastic disease, for which there is a potential 100% cure rate with low-risk clients. Bleomycin is used for recurrent squamous cell carcinoma, and adriamycin is used for uterine sarcoma.

The following table shows the dosage, route of administration, side effects, and nursing considerations for these three drugs.

Text continued on p. 328.

Table 16-6. Alkylating agents used in the treatment of gynecologic cancers

Agent	Usual dosage and route	Side effects	Nursing considerations
Melphalan (Alkeran, L-phenylalanine mustard, L-PAM)	6 mg/day PO for 2-3 weeks; rest for 3-4 weeks; then 2-4 mg/day for maintenance; may be given IV	Usually well tolerated Thrombocytopenia and leukopenia Nausea and vomiting, especially if fasting at time of dose	Thrombocytopenia and leukopenia: Protect client from injury; observe for bleeding or signs of infection Nausea and vomiting: Give antiemetics at earliest sign of nausea Cyclophosphamide: Give antiemetics prior to IV treatment since client will become nauseated 3-4 hours after treatment
Chlorambucil (Leukeran)	0.1-0.2 mg/kg/day or 0.4-0.8 mg/kg/day every 2 weeks PO; rest for 2 weeks	Permanent bone marrow depression with prolonged use Nausea and vomiting Anorexia Dermatitis with large doses Hepatotoxicity	Anorexia: Small, frequent feedings; decrease sights and sounds contributing to nausea Diarrhea and gastrointestinal disturbances: Observe stools for consistency, number, and color; give low-residue diet; replace fluid and nutritional losses; treat with paregoric or atropine sulfate (Lomotil)
Cyclophosphamide (Cytoxan, Endoxan, CTX)	50-100 mg/day PO or 20-40 mg/kg every 3 weeks IV; give IV push or into running IV; be sure crystals are dissolved	Alopecia Hemorrhagic cystitis Hepatotoxicity Bone marrow depression Nausea and vomiting Anorexia Stomatitis	Dermatitis: Calamine lotion and Benadryl Hepatotoxicity: Assess for jaundice Alopecia: May use scalp tourniquet; suggest use of scarves, caps, wigs; hair will grow back in 3-6 months Hemorrhagic cystitis: Force fluids to 3 liters/day; encourage frequent voiding Stomatitis:
Nitrogen mustard (Mustargen, HN$_2$, mechlorethamine HCl)	0.4 mg/kg/day, 3-30 mg into rapidly running IV Intracavitary for effusions Avoid extravasation	Pain Fever Diarrhea and gastrointestinal disturbances Nausea and vomiting (severe 30-60 minutes after administration) Anorexia Vesicant	Avoid irritating foods such as fruit, hot foods, etc.; use soft toothbrush; avoid strong mouthwashes; use peroxide; increase protein and calorie intake; give bland diet; cool foods are soothing; use lidocaine viscous before meals to decrease discomfort Pain: Give pain medications as ordered Pain at injection site:
Triethylenethiophosphoramide (Thio-Tepa)	0.8-1 mg/kg/day IV at 2 week intervals; rest for 2 weeks Give directly and rapidly into IV	Pain at injection site Thrombocytopenia and leukopenia Nausea and vomiting (occasional)	Keep drug refrigerated; use local anesthesia to decrease pain Fever: Observe for temperature elevation Vesicant: Avoid skin and eye contact; inject slowly in rapidly running IV; use gloves to mix; use immediately after mixing; *sodium thiosulfate is antidote* for skin contact and infiltration

Table 16-7. Antibiotics used in the treatment of gynecologic cancers

Agent	Usual dosage and route	Side effects	Nursing considerations

Actinomycin D (dactinomycin, Cosmegan)	0.015 mg/kg/day for 5 days every 2-4 weeks
	IV: inject into tubing or scalp vein needle
	Avoid extravasation
		Leukopenia and thrombocytopenia
		Nausea and vomiting 3-4 hours after injection
		Stomatitis
		Diarrhea
		Paralytic ileus
		Alopecia
		Dermatitis, acne
		Mental depression
		Malaise
		Fever
		Hepatic dysfunction
		Extremely corrosive
			Thrombocytopenia and leukopenia:
			  Protect client from injury; observe for bleeding or signs of infection
			Nausea and vomiting:
			  Give antiemetics at earliest sign of nausea
			Actinomycin: Give antiemetics prior to IV treatment since client will become nauseated 3-4 hours after treatment
			Anorexia:
			  Small, frequent feedings; decrease sights and sounds contributing to nausea
			Diarrhea and gastrointestinal disturbances:
			  Observe stools for consistency, number, and color; give low-residue diet; replace fluid and nutritional losses; treat with paregoric or atropine sulfate (Lomotil)

Bleomycin (Bleoxane, Bleo)	15-60 mg/kg/week in divided doses IV, IM, or SC	Pulmonary fibrosis: *Observe for fibrosis or pneumonitis if dose exceeds 300 mg/sq. meter (major toxicity)*
		Alopecia
		Fever or skin blisters; other allergic reaction
		Stomatitis
		Nausea and vomiting
		Anorexia
			Paralytic ileus:
			  Observe for distension; may need to pass Levin tube and apply suction
			Stomatitis:
			  Avoid irritating foods such as fruit, hot foods, etc.; use soft toothbrush; avoid strong mouthwashes; use peroxide; increase protein and calorie intake; give bland diet; cool foods are soothing; use lidocaine viscous before meals to decrease discomfort

Adriamycin (Adria, (Doxorubicin, Doxyrubicin)	60-75 mg/sq. meter once every 3 weeks up to total dose of 550 mg/sq. meter
	IV: inject by IV push, avoid extravasation
	or
	20-30 mg/sq. meter IV for 3 days every 3 weeks to total dose of 450 mg/sq. meter
		Fever
		Bone marrow depression
		Alopecia (severe)
		Nausea and vomiting
		Stomatitis
		Diarrhea and gastrointestinal disturbances
		Red urine (hematuria) up to 12 days after treatment
		Drug will reactivate radiation site
		Fatal cardiomyopathy; premature ventricular contraction and congestive heart failure
		Local tissue necrosis at injection site
			Fever:
			  Observe for temperature elevation
			Bone marrow depression:
			  Watch for signs of bleeding and infection; implement precautions such as protection from injury, careful mouth care
			Dermatitis:
			  Calamine lotion and Benadryl
			Hepatotoxicity:
			  Assess for jaundice
			Alopecia:
			  May use scalp tourniquet; suggest use of scarves, caps, wigs; hair will grow back in 3-6 months
			Mental depression:
			  Assess for depression and malaise
			Local tissue necrosis at injection site:
			  Avoid extravasation; apply warm compresses to site as needed
			Cardiomyopathy:
			  Watch for shortness of breath, edema; listen for rales; watch daily weight; tachycardia and EKG changes are first signs of toxicity
			Hematuria:
			  Caution patient about this effect to decrease anxiety
			Allergic reaction *(Bleomycin):*
			  May want to skin test prior to first dose or give test dose prior to therapeutic dose; have Benadryl and Adrenalin on hand.

Table 16-8. Antimetabolites used in the treatment of gynecologic cancers

Agents	Usual dosage and route	Side effects	Nursing considerations
Methotrexate (Aminopterin, MTX)	2.5-10 mg/day PO 30 mg/sq. meter IV or IM at 2 week intervals Large doses: 500 to 1500 mg IV for 2 weeks followed by "Leucovorin rescue"	Bone marrow depression Fever Hepatic and renal dysfunction (not usually given if renal function impaired) Photosensitivity Alopecia Dermatitis Stomatitis and GI ulcerations Diarrhea (may lead to hemorrhagic enteritis and perforation Nausea and vomiting Anorexia Drug incompatibilities	Thrombocytopenia and leukopenia: Protect client from injury; observe for bleeding or signs of infection *Methotrexate:* If platelets drop below 100,000 stop treatment until platelets recover If WBC below 3,000 stop treatment; if count below 1,000 client should be on reverse isolation and antibiotics Nausea and vomiting: Give antiemetics at earliest sign of nausea Anorexia: Small, frequent feedings; decrease sights and sounds contributing to nausea
5-Fluorouracil (5-FU, Fluorouracil)	500 mg/10 cc vial PO with water IV doses are variable: 12 mg/kg for 5 days/month *or* 10-15 mg/kg/week, not to exceed 1 Gm Give IV push or infusion Avoid extravasation	Bone marrow depression 9-14 days after treatment Alopecia Dermatologic effects: Darkening of veins with prolonged use, especially in blacks Nausea and vomiting Diarrhea 2-3 days after treatment Stomatitis 5-8 days after treatment Anorexia	Diarrhea and gastrointestinal disturbances: Observe stools for consistency, number, and color; give low-residue diet; replace fluid and nutritional losses; treat with paregoric or atropine sulfate (Lomotil) Fever: Observe for temperature elevation Bone marrow depression: Watch for signs of bleeding and infection; implement precautions such as protection from injury, careful mouth care
Imidazole carboxamine (DTIC, DIC)	150-250 mg/sq. meter for 5 days every 2 weeks IV push	Bone marrow depression (rare) Hepatotoxicity (mild) Nausea and vomiting after infusion, worse the first 2 days of each treatment Flu-like symptoms for up to 10 days Metallic taste on injection	Stomatitis: Avoid irritating foods such as fruit, hot foods, etc.; use soft toothbrush; avoid strong mouthwashes; use peroxide; increase protein and calorie intake; give bland diet; cool foods are soothing; use lidocaine viscous before meals to decrease discomfort Dermatitis: Calamine lotion and Benadryl Hepatotoxicity: Assess for jaundice Alopecia: May use scalp tourniquet; suggest use of scarves, caps, wigs; hair will grow back in 3-6 months Photosensitivity: Protect from bright light Drug incompatibilities *(methotrexate):* Incompatible with sulfonamides Avoid vitamins, tetracycline, chloramphenicol, Dilantin, alcohol Give Leucovorin calcium for toxicity

Table 16-9. Hormones used in the treatment of gynecologic cancers

Agent	Usual dosage and route of administration	Side effects	Nursing considerations
Megestrol acetate (Megace)	40 mg/day PO	Usually no acute toxicity Thrombotic disorders (phlebitis, CVA) Fluid retention, hypocalemia (if diuretics used)	Give diuretics Monitor weight Observe for hypertension
Medroxy progesterone acetate Depo-Provera Provera	200-600 mg twice a week IM 100-200 mg/day PO		
Hydroxyprogesterone caproate (Delalutin)	1 Gm 1-2 times/week IM		

Table 16-10. Plant alkyloids used in the treatment of gynecologic cancers*

Agent	Usual dosage and route	Side effects	Nursing considerations
Vincristine (Oncovin, VCR)	0.5-2 mg/sq. meter every 1-2 weeks IV push or scalp vein needle Used with actinomycin and cyclophosphamide (Cytoxan): 1.5 mg/sq. meter week IV Avoid extravasation	Neuromuscular disorders: weakness, neuritis, ataxia, paresthesias, mental depression; first sign is paresthesia of fingertips; *stop drug if reflexes diminish* Alopecia (20%) Bone marrow depression Constipation Abdominal pain Diarrhea Nausea and vomiting Stomatitis	Thrombocytopenia and leukopenia: Protect client from injury; observe for bleeding or signs of infection Nausea and vomiting: Give antiemetics at earliest sign of nausea Diarrhea and gastrointestinal disturbances: Observe stools for consistency, number, and color; give low-residue diet; replace fluid and nutritional losses; treat with paregoric or atropine sulfate (Lomotil) Constipation: Increase fluid intake
Vinblastine (Velban, VLB)	5-15 mg/sq. meter for 2 weeks IV push or infusion Avoid extravasation	Leukopenia and thrombocytopenia 5 days after treatment Alopecia (occasionally) Anorexia Stomatitis Diarrhea Constipation Nausea and vomiting (mild) Neurotoxicity in high doses: paresthesias, loss of deep tendon reflex, paralytic ileus, mental depression	Abdominal pain: Increase roughage; give cathartics and stool softeners Anorexia: Small, frequent feedings; decrease sights and sounds contributing to nausea Alopecia: May use scalp tourniquet; suggest use of scarves, caps, wigs; hair will grow back in 3-6 months Bone marrow depression: Watch for signs of bleeding and infection; implement precautions such as protection from injury, careful mouth care Stomatitis: Avoid irritating foods such as fruit, hot foods, etc.; use soft toothbrush; avoid strong mouthwashes; use peroxide; increase protein and calorie intake; give bland diet; cool foods are soothing; use lidocaine viscous before meals to decrease discomfort

*Data from Disaia (1975); Hildebrand (1978); Marino and LeBlanc (1976); Mourad and Donahue (1978); Wall and Blythe (1976); Winick (1977).

Antimetabolites

Three antimetabolites are presently used in gynecologic oncology: methotrexate, 5-fluorouracil, and imadazole Carboxamide (DTIC). Methotrexate is used mainly for treatment of gestational trophoblastic disease. 5-Fluorouracil is used in the treatment of recurrent ovarian cancer and usually in combination with actinomycin D and Cytoxan, DTIC is a relatively new drug that acts during the S phase of the cell cycle and is used with adriamycin or vincristine in the treatment of uterine sarcomas (Wall and Blythe, 1976).

Table 16-8 gives the dosage and administration, toxicity, and nursing considerations for these three drugs.

Hormones

Hormones presently used in gynecologic oncology are the progesterones such as medroxy progesterone (Depo-Provera), hydroxyprogesterone caproate (Delalutin), and megestrol (Megace). They are used for stage I adenocarcinoma of the endometrium or stage II, III, or IV of other gynecologic malignancies (Wall and Blythe, 1976).

Table 16-9 gives the dosage and administration, side effects, and nursing aspects of these hormones.

Plant alkyloids

Vinca alkyloids are derived from the periwinkle plant and affect the M phase of the cell cycle. Vincristine is most frequently used in gynecologic oncology for the treatment of recurrent ovarian cancer (Wall and Blythe, 1976).

Table 16-10 contains information on dose and administration, side effects, and nursing considerations for vincristine and vinblastine.

General considerations about toxicity

If toxicity occurs with the first treatment, the dose can be decreased by 25% for the next course and by 50% if side effects are severe. The high point of toxicity usually occurs 1 to 3 weeks after administration. If the patient shows signs of toxicity during the treatment, this is usually considered ominous (Disaia, 1975).

Immunotherapy

Immunotherapy is the treatment of malignant disease by altering the immune status of the patient. Most human malignancies possess tumor-associated antigens or molecules that can be recognized by the individual's host defense mechanism as nonself and to which the person has an immunologic response. This response produces lymphocytes that can directly or indirectly affect the malignant cells, although the immunoglobins produced are not consistently capable of destroying those cells (Disaia, 1975).

There are three broad approaches to immunotherapy:
1. *Active:* Specific cancer antigens are used to stimulate a specific response in the host. These antigens are tumor cells from another person with a similar tumor and are usually irradiated cells. Use of live cells is limited because a new tumor may develop.
2. *Passive:* Antiserum from another person who has been immunized against a tumor-specific antigen is used.
3. *Nonspecific:* The person's immune response is increased by using a substance known to stimulate the immune system such as BCG (bacillus Calmette-Guerin) (Dominick, 1978).

All are experimental today and are seen as adjunctive therapy rather than primary treatment. Further research is needed to identify tumor-associated antigens that can lead to early diagnosis and maximal curability (Silverstein and Morton, 1973).

NUTRITIONAL ASPECTS OF GYNECOLOGIC ONCOLOGY

Most patients will experience some change in their nutritional status both because of the cancer itself and as an effect of treatment. Nurses should be knowledgeable about nutritional effects of the tumor or the treatment so that problems can be assessed early and interventions implemented appropriately.

The effects of the tumor on nutritional status include weight loss and emaciation, which occur because the tumor makes increased demands on the body while also causing the client to have a decreased appetite. Anorexia and cachexia occur because the sense of taste is lost or altered because of a zinc deficiency and a lowered rate of renewal of taste bud cells (Anderson, 1977). The client also has an increased metabolic rate secondary to increased tumor destruction, which causes loss of protein and body fat; abnormal carbohydrate metabolism; decreased sensitivity to insulin; water and electrolyte disturbances including decreased sodium, serum albumin, and blood volume; and increased extracellular fluid, which causes fluid retention and edema (MacFadyen et al., 1977).

Treatments for gynecologic cancer also cause nutritional problems. For example, the consequences of radiation therapy include bowel damage resulting in acute and chronic diarrhea, malabsorption from the Gl tract, stenosis, and obstruction. Chemotherapy also causes nausea and vomiting, diarrhea, stomatitis, and anemia. Surgical procedures usually lead to weight loss from protein and calorie malnutrition (Goodhart and Shils, 1973). If clients are not in optimal nutritional condition at the time of surgery, there is a higher morbidity and mortality rate. Those who are grossly overweight or underweight or who have pancreatic insufficiency, celiac disease, massive bowel resections, or alcoholism are at a higher risk for complications. Clients who have been on 5% dextrose intravenous solutions for 2 or more weeks are at a high risk, as are those with higher metabolic requirements secondary to fever, trauma, pregnancy, fistulas, or abscesses. Clients who are unable to eat a 1,500 calorie, eighty Gm protein diet after 10 days of relative starvation are also included in this high-risk group (MacFadyen et al., 1977).

Diet therapy for specific problems

The client's nutritional status must be assessed at time of diagnosis and before treatment is initiated. The woman should be at a normal nutritional level prior to any treatment in order to experience maximum benefit. Interventions to assess nutritional status during treatment include regular determination of the client's height, weight, triceps skin fold measurements, upper arm circumferences, hair and nail growth, and serum albumin levels.

Protein. Several interventions can help increase protein intake for gynecologic cancer patients. All methods of oral feeding should be tried before initiating parenteral feedings. When problems arise, the nurse should try to control the symptoms that interfere with eating. For example, protein intake can be increased by serving foods cold or at room temperature. Foods such as cheese, luncheon meats, tuna, egg, or chicken salad, deviled eggs, ice cream, milkshakes, or puddings may be more acceptable forms of protein than beef and pork dishes. Meats can be made more acceptable by using marinades such as soya sauce, fruit sauces, or sweet wines, especially for clients with altered sense of taste. Protein intake can also be boosted by adding meats to soups, and cheese, eggs, or powdered milk to other foods (MacFadyen, 1977).

Fat intake. To keep cholesterol levels down, fat intake should be limited; however, if increased calories are needed, butter and sour cream can be added to foods. Peanut butter, mayonnaise, and whipped cream can also be added to the diet to increase calorie intake.

Vitamins and minerals. Deficiencies should be replaced. Most gynecologic clients are given multivitamin and iron supplements daily. Potassium is also a frequent addition to the diet.

Nausea and vomiting and diarrhea. To prevent nausea and vomiting, foods should pass through the stomach as quickly as possible. Sweet starchy foods can be given at frequent intervals. Little or no fluid should be given with meals. The head of the bed should be elevated during and after meals. Sourball candy can reduce the bitter taste in the mouth.

To prevent diarrhea, foods should be served warm, not hot. A low-residue diet with no milk can also be given (Anderson, 1977).

Liquid diets

Elemental diets or high caloric nutritious liquid formulas, such as Ensure or Sustagen, can be given to supplement protein intake orally. These solutions contain a balanced mixture of amino acids, fats, and carbohydrates as well as vitamins, electrolytes, and minerals for protein anabolism. Solutions should be given in a diluted form at first to avoid diarrhea caused by high osmolarity of the solution.

An alternative to oral feeding is tube feeding using nasoesophageal, esophagostomy, or gastrostomy tubes. Vivonex is the most frequently used diet formula. Aspiration can be a serious problem; to reduce the possibility of this complication, the feeding should be at a slow rate and the patient should be sitting no lower than at a 30 degree angle for feeding and for a short period afterward (Ross Laboratories, 1978).

Hyperalimentation

The next alternative is parenteral feeding. Total parenteral nutrition (hyperalimentation) should be initiated as a last resort. Hyperalimentation is intravenous therapy that provides adequate carbohydrate and positive nitrogen balance in cancer patients who cannot take nutrients orally. It is usually initiated for gynecologic patients with bowel obstruction, G1 fistulas, or renal failure (Borgen, 1978). It does not appear to stimulate malignant cell growth.

The solution is hypertonic dextrose, which usually supplies 1,000 calories per liter and contains all essential proteins (amino acids), electrolytes, vitamins, and trace elements.

The first liter is usually infused over a 24-hour period because the solution is six times the concentration of blood and faster infusion may cause hyperglycemia and hyperosmolarity. By the third day the client usually receives 1 liter every 8 hours. The infusion rate should be constant, and a constant-rate IV infusion machine is often used. The infusion rate should never be increased even if the rate is behind because of the danger of convulsions or coma (Disaia et al., 1975; Woods and DeCosse, 1977).

The solution is usually administered through the subclavian vein to the superior vena cava. The left side is safest and easiest to use. The internal jugular vein can also be used. Nursing considerations to be implemented are listed on the following page.

1. Test urine for sugar and acetone every 6 hours.
2. Weigh client daily.
3. Take vital signs every 4 hours.
4. Record intake and output accurately at least every 8 hours.
5. Change tubing with each bottle or at least every day.
6. Change dressing over administration site every 48 hours or 3 times a week.
7. Use line only for hyperalimentation.
8. Protect solution from bright light.

Complications that may occur are related to the metabolic process or catheter care. Metabolic problems are related to the highly concentrated glucose infusion, which may cause acidosis (nonketotic or ketotic) in the diabetic client or hypocalcemia. Catheter-related problems are caused by infections or incorrect placement of the line. Most of these complications can be avoided by strict metabolic surveillance and strict adherence to the principles of catheter care (Borgen, 1978).

Fat emulsion. The high caloric value of fat and its potential advantage for parenteral nutrition have been recognized for years. However, it has been difficult to produce a medically acceptable solution to use. At present a 10% emulsion of fat (Intralipid) is available for intravenous administration. This solution is isotonic; therefore, it can be administered peripherally and can be used to supplement hyperalimentation. Since this solution is a high energy source in a small volume of fluid, it is advantageous to use with clients who are not able to tolerate large amounts of fluid (Woods and De-Cosse, 1977). Nursing considerations for administration are: (Borgen, 1978)

1. Give solution through a separate line that joins the hyperalimentation solution just before the line enters the vein.
2. Give no more than 2.5 Gm per day.
3. Give 500 ml in at least 4 hours.
4. Do not give a mixture that is separated.
5. Shake the bottle at intervals during administration to keep in solution.

MANAGEMENT OF PAIN WITH MEDICATIONS

Cancer pain comes from the pathologic changes directly related to the infiltration of nerves, blood cells, and the lymphatic system by the tumor cells. Pain is also derived from mechanical pressure of the tumor on blood or lymph vessels, invasion of the tumor into the periosteum, or inflammatory or necrotic tissue changes.

In assessing the pain of a client with a gynecologic malignancy, the practitioner must understand what the woman is experiencing—the ,location, intensity, and sensation of pain—to determine the physical nature of the pain and to evaluate the effect of the pain on the client. The nurse also must consider the influence of psychologic factors such as emotional state, personality, past experiences, and previous coping mechanisms (Benoliel and Crawley, 1974; Parsons, 1977).

Once the presence of pain is assessed, the nurse can initiate pain relief measures including the use of medications. The nurse should neither withhold drugs because of the fear of addiction nor give medications without instituting other relief measures first (Mastrovito, 1974).

Narcotic drugs should not be used until nonnarcotic agents no longer give adequate relief. A fixed dose schedule, although commonly used, should not be established. Instead, medications should be given based on the client's needs. Utilizing drugs in this manner can delay buildup of tolerance to the drugs and reserve higher doses for terminal care (Drakontides, 1974).

Bromptom's cocktail. One drug that has gained popularity for use with terminal patients, especially after other medications have failed to control pain, is Bromptom's cocktail. This drug is a potent oral liquid containing morphine, cocaine, and aromatic elixir of orange, lemon, corriander, and anise oils in a simple syrup mixture and 22% alcohol. These drugs cause a synergistic reaction that potentiates the effectiveness of the medication.

Bromptom's cocktail is popular because it can be titrated to meet each client's needs and it does not cause the side effect of a clouded sensorium, which occurs with high doses of other narcotics.

The drug should be given every 3 to 4 hours to *prevent* rather than to treat pain. Until Bromptom's cocktail provides an adequate blood level the woman may require a narcotic injection as well (Davis, 1978).

Chemotherapy, surgery, and radiation therapy are used as palliative measures to remove or decrease tumor size, which may be causing pain.

PSYCHOSOCIAL ASPECTS OF CANCER TREATMENT
The meaning of cancer

Cancer often is equated with severe pain and death by gynecologic clients. Cancer is feared because the treatments or the disease may affect physical attractiveness or usefulness. Cancer is seen as one of the lowest status diseases and is described as a loathsome disease by many people. Cancer may be seen as a punishment, especially when the reproductive system is involved (Donovan and Pierce, 1976; Bard, 1973). Certain psychosocial principles can be used in caring for the woman who has a gynecologic malignancy.

During the *prediagnostic phase* the client seeks reassurance that the symptoms are not indicative of cancer. She may deny the problem because of her fears about cancer. The role of the nurse during this phase is to encourage the woman to seek medical advice about her symptoms and to provide support and a listening ear when the client is undergoing diagnostic tests.

In the *diagnostic phase* the nurse should first find out if the woman has been told her diagnosis and if so how long she has known. Most clients want to know the diagnosis; after this information has been given by the physician, the nurse can provide further explanations as needed. The client will usually let the nurse know how much of the details she wants to hear.

The woman should be encouraged to ventilate her feelings about the diagnosis. How the woman copes with the diagnosis will depend on her basic personality and her previous coping behaviors. The nurse is most helpful when she relates to the client honestly and realistically.

The initial reaction to the diagnosis is often disbelief; after this reaction, the client may become angry or hostile, depressed and anxious, or withdrawn. She then moves into a more accepting stance and can openly discuss her disease and begin to adapt in a positive manner. The nurse may have to use crisis intervention therapy if the client does not make a healthy adaptation.

The impact of the diagnosis is also felt by the family. The family members usually experience shock, anxiety, and despair when they first learn of the diagnosis. The nurse can help family members by telling them that a person can live with cancer and by giving hope that the treatment will be successful.

The family may experience some disruption because the hospital vigil may replace former responsibilities. Role changes in household management, child care, or leadership may occur. There is the problem of isolation when family members are separated because of hospitalization. The nurse can foster cohesion and help the family set priorities.

The issue of who to tell about the diagnosis is another problem the family must solve. Often the family closes ranks and keeps to themselves. The nurse can encourage open communication. The feeling of helplessness is often expressed by families. The nurse can involve them in caring for the patient and foster problem-solving for family needs.

The *treatment phase* often involves a crisis because of the effects of the treatment. Radical surgery is viewed as a severe stress situation because of possible mutilation or death. It is also permanent and complete. The anatomic and physiologic changes resulting from surgery and the client's adaptation to these changes may be disrupted by unrealistic and irrational conceptions about the effects of surgery.

Clients usually express a grief reaction to the change in their body image. The feelings of loss may depend on the visibility of the loss, the function, and the amount of emotional investment. Adaptation to the change in body image must include a change in value systems, accep-

tance of the limitations of the effects of the disability, and a regard for the change as an asset rather than a liability. The nurse may need to implement crisis intervention in helping the client adapt to the body changes. She can also involve the woman in planning and implementing self-care.

Reactions to radiation therapy treatment vary. The treatments are mysterious; there is nothing to see or feel during the therapy. The client's greatest distress is at the beginning of treatment and at the end when the results are still unknown.

Clients having chemotherapy need information about the side effects before treatments begin. Alopecia is disconcerting (to say the least) to any woman who has an interest in her appearance.

During any of the treatments some clients react pessimistically even when the outcomes are good. This behavior may be a way of protecting oneself from disappointment if the outcome is not favorable.

The next phase the client may experience is the *follow-up phase*. In this period the client is hoping to pass the 5 year mark without recurrence. The family is also waiting and is anxious that no symptoms appear. A return to normalcy within the family is attempted.

If there is recurrence of the tumor the client goes into the *recurrence and retreatment phase*. The woman may not acknowledge the first signs of recurrence, and this may be apparent when she begins to miss appointments. The client may express grief and hostility about the recurrence and may be very skeptical about treatments now that a cure is not likely.

The family also reacts to the recurrence of the tumor, and is fearful that other catastrophes may strike them. The family must begin to think about the death of the client and to reorganize the family unit. Role obligations must be redistributed so that family goals can be met. The nurse should be supportive to family members and encourage them to begin to make time to remember the woman's life so that after death the memories will remain.

When the client is near death she will enter the *terminal-palliative phase*. The nurse's role is to keep the woman comfortable and to foster death with dignity.

The family experiences separation and mourning during this phase. The nurse should provide privacy and encourage the expression of grief. If the family is able to work through this period of mourning they will accept the death as inevitable but not insurmountable and will begin to reestablish social contact with other people.*

---

*Barkley, 1973; Crayton, 1974; Donovan and Pierce, 1976; Drelich et al., 1974; Francis, 1973; Giacquinta, 1977; Schmale, 1974.

SUMMARY

Education of the client is the primary role of the practitioner. This teaching includes prevention and detection as well as principles of treatment and rehabilitation. Other nursing objectives include (Crayton, 1974; Shepherdson, 1972):

1. Helping the client to accept treatments
2. Protecting the client from complications
3. Providing for physical and psychologic comfort of the client and family
4. Helping the client deal with anxiety and maintain hope
5. Teaching the client and her family the skills that will help her remain independent
6. Helping the client to learn to live with a disability or body image change if necessary
7. Helping terminally ill patients to die with dignity and helping the family cope with the death
8. Carrying out medical orders

These goals can be met by using the team approach in caring for the woman with gynecologic cancer. Physicians, dietitians, occupational, recreational, and physical therapists, the clergy, and social workers as well as nurses must share their observations and ideas about the client to meet all her needs. Continuity of care is also important, not only around the clock on all shifts in the hospital but through community services as well (Madden, 1977).

Gynecologic practitioners have an important role in the prevention, detection, care and counseling, teaching, and rehabilitation of oncology clients, and through their knowledge of gynecologic oncology they can provide the best care possible. However, nurses must continue to add to this knowledge by participating in research and by in all aspects of cancer care nursing, thereby discovering new and better methods of prevention, detection, and nursing care.

REFERENCES

American Cancer Society: 1978 Cancer facts and figures, New York, 1977, The Society.

American Cancer Society: 1980 Cancer facts and figures, New York, 1979, The Society.

Anderson, J. J. B.: Nutrition and cancer: a self-instructional program, Health Sciences Consortium, Chapel Hill, 1977, p. 16.

Aure, J. C., Hoeg, K., and Kolstad, P.: Clinical and histologic studies of ovarian cancer: long-term follow-up of 990 cases, OB-GYN 37 (1):1-94, 1971.

Avery, W., Gardner, C., and Palmer, S.: Vulvectomy, Am. J. Nurs. 74(3):454, 1974.

Ball, B., editor: Easing the shock of a radical vulvectomy, Nursing 75, pp. 27-31, August 1975.

Bard, M.: The psychological impact of cancer and cancer surgery. In American Cancer Society: Proceedings of the American Cancer Society National Conference on Human Values and Cancer, Atlanta, Ga., 1973, pp. 24-26, 1973.

Barkley, V. B.: The crisis in cancer. In Browning, M. H., and Lewis, E. P. editors: Nursing the cancer patient, Am. J. Nurs. pp. 133-137, 1973.

Benjamin, F., Caspar, D. J., Sherman, L., and Kolodny, H.: Growth hormone secretion in patients with endometrial carcinoma, N. Engl. J. Med. 281:1448-1451, 1963.

Benoliel, J., and Crawley, D. M.: The patient in pain: new concepts. In American Cancer Society: Proceedings of the National Conference on Cancer Nursing, Sept. 10, 1973, pp. 70-78, 1974.

Bingham, C. A.: The cell cycle and cancer chemotherapy, Am. J. Nurs. 78(7):1200-1205, 1978.

Borgen, L.: Total parenteral nutrition in adults, Am. J. Nurs. 78(2): 224-228, 1978.

Breeding, M. A., and Wollin, M.: Working safely around implanted radiation sources, Nursing 76, p. 62, May 1976.

Brown, R. S., Haddox, V., Posada, A., and Rubio, A.: Social and psychological adjustment following pelvic exenteration, AJOG 114: 163, 1972.

Crayton, J. K.: The nurse in cancer care. In Rubin, P., editor: Clinical oncology for medical students and physicians, a multidisciplinary approach, ed. 4, 1974, American Cancer Society, University of Rochester, Rochester, N.Y., pp. 216-252.

Davis, J. J.: Brompton's cocktail: making good byes possible, Am. J. Nurs. 78(1):610-612, 1978.

Disaia, P. J., Morrow, C. P., and Townsend, D. E.: Synopsis of gynecologic oncology, New York, 1975, John Wiley & Sons, Inc.

Dominick, N. P.: The methanol extract residue of bacillus calmette-Guerin in cancer immunotherapy, Nurs. Clin. North Am. vol. 13 (2):69-80, 1978.

Donovan, M. I., and Pierce, S.: Cancer care nursing, New York, 1976, Appleton-Century-Crofts.

Drakontides, A. B.: Drugs to treat pain, Am. J. Nurs. 74(3):508-513, 1974.

Drelich, M., Bieber I., and Sutherland, A.: Adaptation to hysterectomy. In Psychological impact of cancer, Professional Education Publication, American Cancer Society, 1974, pp. 88-94.

Dwyer, J. M.: Human reproduction, Philadelphia, New York, 1976, F. A. Davis Co.

Dyche, M. E.: Pelvic exenteration: a nursing challenge, J. Obstet. Gynecol. Nurs. 4(6):11-19, 1975.

Dyk, R. B., and Sutherland, A. B.: Adaptation of the spouse and other family members to the colostomy patient, Cancer, 9:123, 1956.

Fisher, R. I., and Young, R. C.: Initial diagnosis and treatment of ovarian cancer, Female Patient 3(4):75-77, 1978.

Giacquinta, B.: Helping families face the crisis of cancer, Am. J. Nurs. 77(10):1583-1588, 1977.

Goodhart, R. S., and Shils, M. E.: Modern nutrition in health and disease, ed. 5, Philadelphia, 1973, Lea & Febiger.

Gray, L. A., Sr., Christopherson, W. H., and Hover, R. N.: Estrogens and endometrial carcinoma, Obstet. and Gynecol. 48(4):385-389, 1977.

Green, T. H., Jr.: Gynecology—essentials of clinical practice, Boston, 1977, Little, Brown and Co.

Greenwald, P., Capito, T. A., and Wolfgang, P. E.: Endometrial cancer after menopausal use of estrogens, Obstet. Gynecol. 50(2): 239-243, 1977.

Griffiths, C. T., Grogan, R. H., and Hall, T. C.: Advanced ovarian cancer: primary treatment with surgery, radiotherapy, and chemotherapy, Cancer, 29(1):1-7, 1972.

Gusburg, S. B.: An approach to the control of cancer of the endometrium, New York, 1973, American Cancer Society.

Hamilton, M. S., and Schlapper, N. B.: Pelvic exenteration, Am. J. Nurs. 76(2):266-272, 1976.

Herbert, P., Welch, H., and Jackson, B.: Coloscopy—what is it? J. Obstet. Gynecol. Nurs. May-June 1976, pp. 29-32.

Herbst, A. L.: Current data from the clear cell adenocarcinoma registry. Presented at the Fifth Annual Meeting of the Society of Gynecologic Oncologists, Key Biscayne, Fla., Jan. 9, 1974.

Hildebrand, B. F.: Nursing process and chemotherapy for the woman with cancer of the reproductive system, Nurs. Clin. North Am. 13(2):351-368, 1978.

Hilkemeyer, R.: Nursing care in radium therapy, Nurs. Clin. North Am. 2(1):83-94, 1969.

Howkins, J., and Hudson, C. N.: Shaw's textbook of operative gynecology, ed. 4, Edinburgh, 1977, Churchill-Livingston.

Jackson, B., and Armenaki, D. W.: A tumor classification system, Am. J. Nurs. 76(8):1330, 1976.

Kolstad, P., and Stafl, A.: Atlas of colposcopy, Baltimore, 1977, University Park Press.

Mack, M. T., and others: Estrogen and endometrial cancer in a retirement community, N. Engl. J. Med. 294:1262, 1976.

Madden, B.: Rehabilitation principles, philosophy, practice, Nurs. Dig. 5(2):35-39, 1977.

Marino, E., and LeBlanc, D. H.: Cancer chemotherapy, Nurs. 76, pp. 22-33, Nov. 1976.

Martin, L. L.: Health care of women, Philadelphia, 1978, J. B. Lippincott Co.

Mastrovito, R. C.: Psychogenic pain, Am. J. Nurs. 74(3):514-519, 1974.

Mattingly, R., editor: TeLindes operative gynecology, ed. 5, Philadelphia, 1977, J. B. Lippincott Co.

Meigs, J. V.: Cancer of the cervix. In Cancer: a manual for practitioners, ed. 4, Boston, 1968, American Cancer Society.

Mourad, L. A., and Donahue, M. P.: Guide to the administration of IV chemotherapeutic agents, Columbus, Ohio, Ohio State University, 1978.

Murray, R. L.: Principles of nursing interventions for the adult patient with body image changes, Nurs. Clin. North Am. 7:697, 1972.

Novaks, E., Jones, G. S., and Jones, H. W.: Novak's textbook of gynecology, ed. 9, Baltimore, 1975, The William & Wilkins Co.

Parsens, J. B.: Needs of the cancer patient, Nurs. Dig., Vol. 5, No. 2, Summer 1977.

Parsons, L.: Cancer of the vagina and the vulva: In Cancer: a manual for practitioners, ed. 4, Boston, 1968, American Cancer Society.

Romney, S., Gray, M. J., Little, A. B., and others, editors: Gynecology and Obstetrics: the health care of women, New York, 1975, McGraw-Hill Book Co.

Rose, J. C.: Nutritional problems in radiotherapy patients, Am. J. Nurs. 78(7):1194-1196, 1978.

Ross Laboratories: Nutrition—a helpful ally in cancer therapy, Columbus, Ohio, Jan. 1978.

Rotman, M.: Supportive and paliative radiation treatment, CA 26(5): 292-294, 1976.

Rudolph, J.: Cancer of the female genital tract. In Rubin, P., editor: Clinical oncology for medical students and physicians, a multidisciplinary approach, ed. 4, Rochester, N.Y., 1974, University of Rochester, American Cancer Society, pp. 249-250.

Rubin, P., editor: Clinical oncology for medical students and physicians—a multidisciplinary approach, ed. 4, Rochester, New York, 1974, American Cancer Society.

Schmale, A. H.: Principles of psychosocial oncology. In Rubin, P., editor: Clinical oncology for medical students and physicians, a multidisciplinary approach, ed. 4, Rochester, N.Y., 1974, American Cancer Society.

Schnieder, H., Anderson, C., and Coursin, D., editors: Nutritional support of medical practice, 1977, Harper & Row.

Schreier, A., and Lavenia, J.: The nurses role in nutritional management of radiotherapy patients, Nurs. Clin. North Am. 12(1):173-181, 1977.

Serviatius, D., and others: Easing the shock of a radical vulvectomy, Nursing '75 5:26-31, 1975.

Shepherdson, J.: A team approach to the patient with cancer, Am. J. Nurs. 72(3):488-491, 1972.

Silverstein, M., and Morton, D. L.: Cancer immunotherapy, Am. J. Nurs. 73(7):1178-1181, 1973.

Smith, D. C., Prentice, R., Thompson, D. J., and Herrman, W. L.: Association of exogenous estrogen and endometrial carcinoma, New Engl. J. Med. 293:1164-1167, 1975.

Wall, T. P., and Blythe, J. G.: Chemotherapy in gynecological malignancies and its nursing aspects, J. Obstet. Gynecol. Nurs. 15(5): 9-13, 1976.

Winick, M., editor: Nutrition and cancer, New York, 1977, John Wiley & Sons.

Woods, J. H., and DeCosse, J. J.: Hyperalimentation. In Mattingly, R., editor: Te Lindes operative gynecology, ed. 5, Philadelphia, 1977, J. B. Lippincott Co.

Wynder, E. L., Dodo, H., and Barber, H. R.: Epidemiology of cancer of the ovary, Cancer 23:359, 1969.

Ziel, H. K., and Finkle, W. D.: Increased risk of endometrial carcinoma among users of conjugated estrogens, New Engl. J. Med., 293:1167-1170, 1975.

17

Problems of the breast

Sally K. Graham
Barbara Hansen Kalinowski

Because society has placed such significance on the breast as a symbol of femininity, a discussion of the breast, its problems, and the associated health care from a nursing perspective is especially pertinent. Preventive and self-care aspects of breast care will be described, and common types of breast disorders and possible treatments will be presented. Because breast cancer is the leading cause of cancer in females today, the last part of this chapter will focus mainly on caring for the woman who has breast cancer, from the biopsy experience to the long-term treatment of the woman with metastatic breast disease.

We have attempted to present the most current concepts in early detection, diagnosis, and treatment of breast disease. Some of the material is controversial, particularly the surgical approach to breast cancer. We urge the reader to explore all facets of treatment in light of current research, considering the individual nature of each woman's disease.

In this chapter, the terms "practitioner" and "primary nurse" are interchangeable and describe the nurse who is primarily responsible for assessing the client and planning, implementing, and evaluating nursing care in inpatient, outpatient, and community settings.

Prior to interacting with any woman experiencing a possible dysfunction of or insult to the breast, it is helpful for health care personnel to be aware of factors, conscious or subconscious, that may influence the woman's reaction to this potential crisis. Underlying her perception of the event are fundamental issues dealing with self and body image. The breast, in psychoanalytic and other schools of thought, is considered to be the one obvious physical attribute that denotes femininity. To threaten the breast is to shake the very core of . . . feminine orientation (Renneker and Cutler, 1952).

In American society, the importance the breast has played in determining beauty and sexuality has varied throughout the years, but, as Margaret Mead (1949) states, "the female breast has been idealized in the U.S.

so that it has become a primary source of identification with the female role." Stehlin (1979) emphasizes that ours is a breast-oriented society, stating that, for the average woman, the breast is an important part of her allurement to charm her male. To a man, the breast is a source of excitement and erotic stimulation. Certainly, the number of magazines displaying the female nude, X-rated movies, and the popularity of topless clubs and revealing fashions enhance women's perception of the breast as a primary factor in identifying themselves as feminine and sexual beings. The upsurge of awareness and rebellion by women against identification as sex objects—largely resulting from the women's movement—has probably helped to decrease some of the cultural emphasis on the size and shape of the breast, but the threats to body image, femininity, and function still remain paramount.

Other factors also affect a woman's reaction to breast dysfunction. For example, attempts have been made to predict the severity of the woman's reaction to potential injury (mastectomy in particular) based on her position in the life cycle (Renneker and Cutler, 1952). During childbearing years, the woman may view the injury as a threat to her nurturing role as a mother as well as to her sexual self. The menopausal woman may perceive the injury as a threat to her femininity in addition to the hormonal changes and loss of reproductive functions she is experiencing. Fear of pain, surgery, and potential change or loss of support systems may also influence a woman's reaction to breast dysfunction. The past experience of the woman with any facet of the experience may also influence her later reaction and attitude. Care must be taken by health professionals to identify as clearly and as early as possible the meaning the potential threat has for that individual.

Certainly, other factors affect the woman's perception of the meaning of her breasts and the reactions evoked by a threat to them. The woman's care-seeking behavior will be influenced by such factors. By understanding breast disease and the issues involved, a nurse can work with the woman and help educate her to practice preventive health care, to recognize when specialized assistance is indicated, and, if necessary, care for and support the woman during and after treatment.

BREAST DISEASES

Because breast cancer is the leading source of cancer in females today, abnormal breast findings are particularly anxiety producing for most women. Although statistically the majority (75% to 80%) of breast masses are symptomatic of benign disease, any woman who has discovered a lump can relate the feelings of fear and anxiety that followed her discovery. The five most common breast diseases are presented here in order of frequency of occurrence, to aid the practitioner in distinguishing one from another and to aid in the education of her patients concerning their disease.

Cystic hyperplasia (fibrocystic disease, chronic mastitis)

Cystic hyperplasia is the most common of all breast diseases. It occurs between the ages of 20 and 25 years and often subsides with menopause. It is characterized by multiple and often bilateral lumps. The breasts are frequently painful and tender, with tenderness increasing just prior to the menstrual period. The lumps are firm, mobile, and regular in shape. They are most commonly found in the upper outer quadrants of the breasts and may increase or decrease rapidly in size. A nipple discharge is rare. The diagnosis may involve observation of the lump(s) throughout one or more menstrual cycles and/or aspiration for the typical gray-green fluid that fills such cysts.

Treatment of cystic hyperplasia is primarily based on the amount of pain the client experiences as a result of the disease. Bilateral or unilateral subcutaneous mastectomies with the insertion of implants may be presented as an alternative for those women whose pain interferes with normal, daily functioning. The question as to whether cystic disease is a premalignant disease—thus placing these women at higher risk for breast cancer—is controversial. According to some authors, the risk for breast cancer is four to five times greater for women with cystic disease (Haagenson, 1971). Others emphasize the difficulty in diagnosing breast cancer for these women, since the cystic disease may interfere with diagnostic techniques such as palpation and mammography.

Breast cancer

Breast cancer is one of the three most common causes of breast lumps in women and is the leading cause of cancer incidence and death for females in the United States today. The statistics are frightening: one of thirteen women will develop breast cancer. In 1978 there were an estimated 91,000 new cases in the United States, and there is evidence that the incidence is slowly rising (American Cancer Society, 1978). Several factors are associated with an increased risk of breast cancer. The most notable of these are a family history of breast cancer, a history of breast cancer in one breast, and age—risk increases over the age of 40 years. Other factors are listed in Table 17-1.

The most common symptom of breast cancer is a breast mass, felt usually as a single focus in one breast. This mass is typically firm, dense, and may be irregular in shape. The upper outer quadrant is the most frequent site of occurrence, with 38% of breast cancers found in this location. Symptoms including nipple retraction, nipple discharge, palpable lymph nodes, skin changes—such as dimpling and orange-peel appearance—and ulceration may be indicative of advanced disease.

Breast cancer is not a single disease. The term refers to a heterogenous group of diseases with differing rates of growth and thus of potential malignancy (Henderson and Cannellos, 1980). The two most common types, comprising approximately 65% of all breast cancers, are ductal carcinomas (originating in the ductal system) and adenocarcinomas (originating in the breast glands). Much of the professional controversy and the public's confusion concerning the treatment of breast cancer stems from the lack of understanding of the multifocal nature of this disease. By the time a breast cancer is palpable (1 cm in diameter), most physicians believe that micrometastases are certainly present (Cooperman

Table 17-1. Patients at high risk for breast cancer*

Women.
Those over 40 years of age.
Patients with a familial history of breast cancer.
Nulliparous women or those with first parity after age 34.
Patients with a previous cancer in one breast.
Those with a precancerous mastopathy type of fibrocystic disease.
Women with an adverse hormonal milieu.
Patients with lowered immunological competence.
Those with excess exposure of the breast to ionizing radiation.
Patients exposed to carcinogens.
Those with other organ cancers, especially the endometrium.
Patients with high dietary intake of fat.
Patients with chronic psychological stress.
Those living in the Western hemisphere or a cold climate, belonging to the upper socioeconomic group and of the white race.

*From Leis, H. P., Jr.: The diagnosis of breast cancer, Cancer **27**(4): 213, 1977.

and Esselstyn, 1978). It is estimated that a breast tumor requires from 90 to 270 days to grow to that size (Haagensen, 1971). The natural history of the disease involves early invasion of the surrounding tissue, growing through the fat, fascia, and the ductal system. As the disease progresses, the cancer may not only continue to grow locally, but also may metastasize through the ductal system, lymph channels, and circulatory system. Distant metastatic sites resulting from spreading through these routes most frequently include the bones, liver, and lungs. On a local basis, the cancer ultimately invades the skin, causing immobility of the skin overlying the tumor, and dimpling, redness, and eventually ulceration.

Because of the metastatic nature of this disease, public and professional education focuses on early detection and treatment. The extent of the disease at time of diagnosis is the most important factor influencing survival. Breast cancer is staged at the time of diagnosis and/or treatment and further medical management is based on this information. In the United States, mastectomy remains the treatment most physicians would recommend for breast cancer (Henderson and Canellos, 1980), yet there is increasing interest in exploring alternative therapies.

Fibroadenoma

Fibroadenoma is a benign disease of young women, most frequently occurring between the ages of 15 and 60 years, with a median age of 20 years. It is often referred to as a disease of the childbearing years. Typical symptoms include a mobile, firm, solid, well-delineated mass. This lump is usually painless and is multiple and bilateral in 14% to 25% of cases. Unlike the masses of cystic hyperplasia, these do not change in size or character with the menses. The nipple remains normal without evidence of discharge. Treatment of this problem involves simple enucleation of the tumor. Because the mass is encapsulated and separate from surrounding tissue, removal of additional tissue is not usually necessary.

Interductal papilloma

Interductal papilloma most frequently occurs in women between the ages of 35 and 45 years. The primary symptom is a serous or serosanguineous nipple discharge. Usually no mass or tumor is palpable. If a mass is present, it is soft and poorly delineated from the surrounding breast tissue. This disease may cause moderate pain and discomfort. Treatment for interductal papilloma includes excision of the involved ductal system by wedge resection.

Mammary duct ectasia

Duct ectasia commonly occurs near or at the menopause. The presenting symptom is frequently a sticky, multicolored, nipple discharge. Pain, itching, and redness around the nipple may also be evident. A mass may be palpable, either soft or firm, and usually poorly delineated. Because of the nonspecific nature of the symptoms, distinguishing duct ectasia from malignant disease is often difficult. Therefore, open biopsy of the mass may be recommended.

BREAST EXAMINATION

It is estimated that approximately 90% of women seeking medical attention for breast lumps discover their masses through self-examination. Factors such as the women's movement and the American Cancer Society's efforts encouraging women to be knowledgeable consumers of the health care system and to become more familiar with their own bodies have encouraged a trend toward more effective self-detection. However, the high percentage of masses that are self-discovered should not lead to false assumptions regarding the prevalence of the practice of breast self-examination (BSE). Other figures raise questions as to whether most lumps are discovered as a result of regularly practiced breast examination or simply by chance (for example, while bathing) or as the result of an overt symptom. In 1974 a Gallup poll showed that although 77% of the 1,007 women surveyed had heard of BSE, only 18% of the total sample actually performed regular monthly self-examinations. A 1978 study indicated that of the women who performed BSE, only 51% did so on a regular basis (Grunwald et al., 1978). The women surveyed in the 1974 Gallup poll felt that monthly breast self-examinations would produce anxiety rather than reassurance.

These statistics point out the discrepancy between the major rationale for encouraging BSE and women's beliefs and actual behaviors. Cooperman and Esselstyn (1978) found that most women with breast cancer noted the signs and symptoms themselves. However, the average diameter of the breast lump was 5.1 cm; of those lumps that were malignant, 60% had metastasized to the lymph nodes, indicating advanced rather than early disease. These facts are distressing considering that the goal of BSE is to detect *early* lesions that are palpable as small as 1 cm, since at this stage, the survival rate is greatly improved.

The rationale for health professionals and agencies to encourage BSE is based on its low cost (free); the fact that a lump is the major presenting symptom in the majority of breast cancers; and that the effectiveness of treatment and cure increases significantly the earlier the lump is discovered. The most recent data also indicate that breast cancers discovered by BSE are *smaller* in diameter than previously documented and are associated with more favorable clinical stages and fewer axillary lymph node metastases (Foster et al., 1978).

Why then, even when presented with these facts, are

Table 17-2

Condition	Age	Pain	Nipple discharge	Location	Consistency mobility	Diagnosis	Treatment
Cystic hyperplasia	20-49 years; median age 30; may subside with menopause	Yes	No	Upper outer quadrant	Bilateral multiple lumps with menstrual cycle	Needle aspiration; observation; biopsy with unresolved mass or mammography changes	Aspiration; bilateral or unilateral subcutaneous mastectomy with implants
Breast cancer	40-71 years; median age 54	No	No	Upper outer quadrant	Unilateral mass, irregular, poorly delineated, decreased mobility	Mammography; xeromammography; surgical or needle biopsy	Controversial, depends on stage; mastectomy most common; lumpectomy followed by radiation, chemotherapy
Fibroadenoma	15-39 years; median age 20	No	No	No specific location	Mobile, firm, smooth, well-delineated	Mammography; xeromammography; surgical or needle biopsy	Enucleation of tumor
Interductal papilloma	35-55 years; median age 40	Yes	Serous or serosanguineous; usually unilateral from one duct	No specific location	Usually soft, poorly delineated	PAP smear of nipple discharge; biopsy	Wedge resection
Duct ectasia	35-55 years; median age 40	Burning around nipple	Sticky, multicolored; usually bilateral	No specific location	Retroareolar mass with advanced disease	Open biopsy	Local excision of diseased portion of breast

women so reluctant to practice BSE? Fear seems to act as a negative motivator. Most women believe that the majority of breast masses are malignant. This belief may be based on the fact that only in the past 5 years has the subject of breast cancer and its treatment been openly discussed. Previously, the fact that a woman had breast cancer was revealed only at the time of her death. Women who were treated and cured usually told few people about their surgery; therefore, the only association with breast cancer was with death, not cure. This phenomenon seems cyclical. As fear and anxiety increase treatment may be delayed. Because of the delay, the tumor at time of treatment may be larger, thus more likely metastasized. The woman has engaged in a self-fulfilling prophecy as the outcome becomes more likely to be what she feared originally. In addition, because the most widely practiced treatment is the radical mastectomy, often the fear of the treatment is greater than fear of the disease itself. Although the subject is treated more openly today, these beliefs persist.

Related to fear and lack of accurate knowledge of breast disease is the use of denial as a defense mechanism against the possibility of discovering a lump. This is exemplified by such thinking as, "If I have a lump I'd rather not know about it," or "What I don't know can't hurt me," or "What difference will knowing about it make? It's more likely to be malignant and then I'll die anyway." This process also results in discouraging BSE.

In addition to these factors that deter women from practicing BSE, other research has shown deterrents to include a lack of knowledge regarding both BSE technique and normal findings, financial factors related to the expense of health care, religious and cultural taboos discouraging self-manipulation of the sexual organs, an overall neglect of self–health care, and a lack of confidence in available treatments or with the health care system in general. It is the health professional's obligation not only to instruct women in proper technique for BSE, but also to help them ventilate and overcome these barriers to this relatively simple and effective health practice.

Self-examination

Because it is not feasible for women to be screened for breast cancer by health professionals on a regular basis (at least every 3 months), it is essential that women be taught breast self-examination. Not only is verbal instruction of the technique important, but also a careful explanation of the usefulness and necessity of the procedure is vital. At the same time the woman should be allowed to ask questions and to ventilate concerns or fears. Women who have actually had the procedure demonstrated and are allowed to return the demonstra-

tion to a professional have higher practice rates than those who just receive an explanation.

Some feminist health teaching groups advocate demonstrations on breast examinations, using oneself as a model. This might be the most explicit and effective method of all, but it is not yet common practice.

The woman should be instructed to perform BSE once a month. Premenopausal women should do the examination several days after the menstrual period when breast swelling is minimal; menopausal women should do the examination at the same time every month. It may be helpful for these women to correlate this with another event, such as a regularly scheduled appointment or social event. A cursory examination for more obvious lumps is possible during and after bathing or showering, while the skin is slippery. Throughout this instruction, it should be stressed that only 10% to 15% of breast masses are malignant and that 90% of the breast cancers confined to the breast are curable (Tyrer and Ganzig, 1975).

The first step in BSE is a visual examination of the breasts. When doing this, the nurse instructs the woman to observe her breasts in a mirror for differences in shape (keeping in mind that breasts are normally somewhat asymmetrical), for skin puckering and orange-peel appearance (an area of small, pitting holes), a reddened or inflamed area, or change in contour or size of a breast. The nipples should also be examined for discharge, flattening, bleeding, or retraction. This is best done by observing the breasts with the arms at the side and then with the arms raised above the head. Any changes in contour, skin dimpling, or the nipple should be noted. Next, the woman should place her hands on her hips, pressing firmly to cause flexing of the chest muscles. She should check for skin dimpling or retraction. Particular points to emphasize when teaching visual examination are: (1) normally, the breasts are not perfectly symmetrical, and (2) any nipple change, even the smallest amount of discharge or bleeding, or skin change requires medical attention.

The next step in BSE is manual palpation of the breasts. The importance of using a systematic, thorough method should be emphasized. It may be useful to remind the client that the purpose of BSE is to detect abnormalities, especially those that are very small. Palpation is most effectively done lying down. The woman should be shown how to place a folded towel or small pillow under the side of the chest being examined. This distributes the breast tissue evenly over the chest wall and is especially important for women with large breasts. She should also be taught to place the hand on that side behind her head (Fig. 17-1). With her free hand, fingers flat, she should begin manual palpation beginning at the midline upper point (12 o'clock of the breast) and mov-

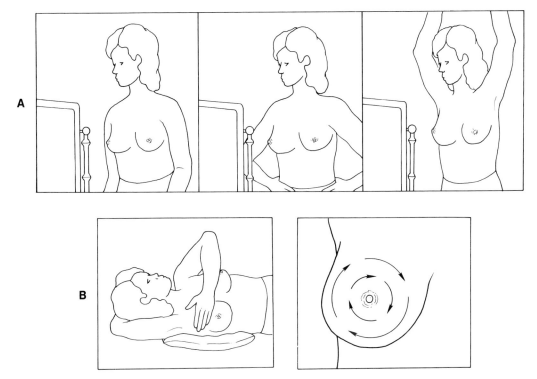

Fig. 17-1. A, Visual examination of breasts. Woman observes breasts in mirror for deviations in size or shape, puckerings or "orange peel" appearance, reddening or inflamed area. The nipples are examined for discharge, flattening, bleeding, or retraction. This should be done not only by observing with arms at the side, but also with arms raised above the head. The woman should also place her hands on her hips, pressing firmly to flex chest muscles to check for skin dimpling or retraction. **B,** The next step in breast self-examination (BSE) is manual palpation of the breast, done most effectively lying down with a pillow or towel under the side of chest being examined. Palpation should begin at the midline upper point and move in circles around the breast toward the nipple.

ing in circles around the breast slowly moving in toward the nipple.

Many women are timid and afraid to press the breast firmly lest they damage the breast tissue. They should be assured that firm palpation will not damage breast tissue and that trauma is not a causative factor in breast cancer. Practice with a commercial breast model used to teach BSE may reinforce the technique and the importance of deep palpation.

Finally, the woman should be taught to squeeze the nipple gently between her thumb and forefinger for evidence of discharge. As previously mentioned, any discharge, nipple abnormality, or lump should be brought to the physician's attention.

As stated above, one of the major reasons why women do not practice BSE is the use of denial. These same women, once a lump is discovered, tend to delay long periods before seeking the advice of a physician. These women are also apt to ignore written literature (such as the American Cancer Society's folders on BSE) or films demonstrating the BSE technique. Therefore, it is important that the health professional not only demonstrate BSE, using herself or a model, but also allow the woman to examine herself as the professional guides and explains the procedure. This enhances the learning process and also reduces associated anxiety and fear since the woman can ask questions and verbalize her feelings about BSE and her fears of finding a lump during the practice. The importance of regular breast self-examination should be stressed for those women at increased risk for breast cancer.

Examination by the practitioner

In addition to teaching breast self-examination, every woman having a physical examination should have a thorough breast examination by the practitioner. Before beginning the examination, the practitioner should assure privacy and warm her hands. This will help decrease embarrassment and encourage the woman to return for regular care. The examination begins with a visual inspection of the breasts, with the woman sitting on the edge of the table or bed, facing the examiner. She should be asked first to raise her hands above her head, then to press them against her hips, flexing her chest muscles. The breasts should be inspected for size and symmetry, signs of dimpling, masses, changes in the skin such as reddening, subcutaneous vein dilation, and edema. The nipples also should be inspected noting the size and shape, presence of retraction, and reddened or broken areas. While the client is sitting, the axillae should be palpated for the presence of any abnormal nodes. (It should be remembered, however, that women who have recently experienced infection, particularly in the corresponding hand or arm, will normally have enlarged nodes.) Palpation should be performed in a gentle, systematic manner.

The woman then should be asked to lie on the examining table with a pillow placed under her chest on the side being examined. For palpation of the medial aspect of the breast, the woman's arms are positioned above her head. The examiner should begin below the clavicle and palpate gently from the nipple toward the sternum, moving in transverse steps down the breast until inferior to the inframammary fold. For palpation of the lateral breast, the woman places her arm down by her side. Again, the examiner should move from the midaxillary line toward the nipple, moving downward by small increments until below the inframammary fold.

When examining any woman's breasts, it is important to remember that each woman acts as her own standard control. Indeed, this is one of the major advantages of BSE, as women learn what is normal vs abnormal for themselves. It is difficult for the practitioner to evaluate what is normal, especially for women with large breasts. There are wide variations in the consistency or elasticity of the breast, depending on the woman's age, and in the lobularity and density of the breast. There are also differences for the same women according to the phase of the menstrual cycle. These changes include fullness, tenderness, and nodularity.

The final step, providing the breast has been found to be within normal parameters, is an examination of the nipple and the subareolar area. The nipple and the surrounding skin area should be palpated and the nipple expressed for the presence of discharge.

While performing the breast examination, any findings the practitioner believes might be useful for the woman to be aware of for BSE should be pointed out to her. She should also be allowed to palpate these herself under the examiner's guidance. For example, the inframammary fold or ridge, which is a ridge of dense tissue at the junction of the mammary tissue to the chest wall fascia, is often palpable. This may be mistaken by the woman to be a tumor. Much fear can be avoided if this is demonstrated and explained to the woman at the time of examination. Pointing out normal findings is useful for all women, but especially for those with cystic breast

disease, since many masses are followed by a physician over a period of months for changes in size and consistency and should also be followed by the woman herself.

Screening

The purpose of any screening program is to identify those people who appear well but have covert signs or symptoms suggesting the presence of disease. Breast cancer screening methods have included clinical examination, mammography, xeromammography, and thermography. Because approximately 10% of breast cancers become apparent within a year following a negative examination by these methods, women are advised to practice breast self-examination regularly between visits (Strax, 1978).

Mammography is the only test capable of detecting nonpalpable breast cancers so, like BSE, its use is based on the fact that early detection results in improved survival rates. Indeed, breast cancers detected by mammography tend to be very early and offer very high cure rates (American Cancer Society, 1980). The largest program, The Breast Cancer Detection Demonstration Projects, was funded by the National Cancer Institute and involved 280,000 women. Of the 2,379 cancers found, 44% were detected by mammography and were not clinically palpable. Seventy-seven percent of these women were without nodal involvement, placing them in the stage 0 or stage 1 classifications. In the Health Insurance Plan study, 78% of patients with early cancers detected by mammography had a 10-year survival rate (Shapiro, 1978).

In spite of the effectiveness of these programs, concern and controversy have arisen among professionals and the public over potential risks and costs of mammography, particularly for women under the age of 50. Recommendations proposed by the American Cancer Society are based on the increased accuracy of mammographic techniques and the fact that the radiation exposure involved only decreases the net beneficial effect in terms of mortality to be less than 1%. These recommendations are that women under 20 years perform BSE monthly (as should all women), women 20 to 40 years have a breast examination every 3 years, women over 40 have a breast examination every year, and women over 50 have a low-dose mammogram every year. In addition, women with risk factors such as personal or family histories of breast cancer should consult their physicians concerning the need for additional examinations or mammography prior to the age of 50 (American Cancer Society, 1980).

Examination of a breast mass or abnormality

If through BSE, physical examination, or detection at a breast cancer detection clinic a breast mass or abnormality is discovered, a more thorough physical examination by a physician is usually necessary. Before this is performed, however, a careful history should be obtained. The woman should be questioned as to when and how the lump was discovered, changes in size and consistency since its discovery, presence of pain, related symptoms such as skin and nipple changes, past history of breast disease, family history of breast disease, and her menstrual and reproductive history. Included in the latter are time of first menses, number of children and age of the woman at pregnancy, breast-feeding history, and age at menopause. This information, together with findings from the physical examination, helps to identify women at risk for breast cancer. In addition, this can be a time for teaching and ventilation of feelings. Many women who have delayed coming for medical advice after discovering a lump are extremely anxious as to what effect this delay will have on the outcome of their potential illness. Other women may use this time to seek information regarding the possible cause of the mass, the meaning of related or unrelated symptoms, and what studies may be necessary.

Once a history is obtained, the breasts should be examined as described previously, but with special attention to the suspicious area. The size of the mass, if palpable, should be estimated in terms of centimeters, using a ruler if necessary. The shape should also be described. The mass should be gently palpated and its consistency and involvement with surrounding tissue evaluated. The examiner should attempt to gently move the lump, assessing its fixation to the underlying tissue. Finally, any overt symptoms should be noted. The skin of the affected breast should be carefully inspected for edema, which presents as either an abnormal fullness or an orange-peel (peau d'orange) appearance and skin dimpling, sometimes more evident when the chest muscles are flexed. Signs of venous prominence should also be noted. The practitioner should look for any abnormal contours of either the breast or nipple, which may become apparent if the woman sits and raises her hands over her head and then leans down, facing the practitioner. The axillae and subclavicular areas should then be palpated for the presence of any abnormal lymph nodes. Using these findings and information from the history, the practitioner makes a decision concerning the necessity of further diagnostic workup. Certainly, for the practitioner not experienced in the examination of the breasts and breast masses, the discovery of any lump indicates the need for referral to a specialized clinician.

If the physical findings or the woman's history indicates a need for further diagnostic studies, radiologic studies may be ordered. These include mammography, xeromammography, and thermography. When preparing the woman for these tests, the nurse should explain that they are painless and similar to having a chest X-ray taken. It may be helpful to discuss not only the purpose of the procedure and the client's participation, but also to explain that the amount of radiation from a mammogram is less than that from a dental X-ray examination. It should be stressed that the controversy surrounding mammography involves its use as a routine, periodic screening method for young women over a period of many years. There is no disagreement about its use for high-risk women nor for those with a breast mass.

With the additional information obtained from these studies, a decision is made concerning whether or not further diagnostic procedures are needed. If the physician believes that the findings suggest the possibility of malignancy or if the woman's level of anxiety is extreme, a biopsy, either surgical or by aspiration, may be performed. Despite the fact that diagnostic procedures to this point are usually painless and noninvasive, the woman's anxiety is likely to be at an extremely high level, regardless of how much has been explained by her physician regarding the possibility or probability of the mass being malignant.

DIAGNOSIS

The anxiety and fear surrounding diagnostic biopsy of a breast lump may be overwhelming for a woman confronted with this situation. The intensive support and care provided by nursing personnel during this time may help alleviate fears and provide an outlet for verbalization.

The initial nursing assessment, which is done soon after the woman is admitted to the hospital, includes a general health and family history. In addition, assessment of the woman's perception and past experience with hospitalization, surgery, and breast cancer is important so that nurses can enhance support as the hospital course evolves. Identification of the client's past coping mechanisms and present support systems is also necessary (Aguilera and Messick, 1974).

The assessment can lead to a meaningful dialogue between the nurse and woman and may help form a firm base for a trusting relationship for the duration of the woman's hospitalization.

Biopsy

Definitive diagnosis of a suspicious breast lump, beyond the noninvasive preliminary techniques previously described, always involves a biopsy of some kind, either by aspiration or incision. An aspiration biopsy is done by inserting a large bore needle into the tumor to withdraw a core of tumor cells or cystic fluid for microscopic evaluation (Haagensen, 1971). Incisional biopsy includes direct examination of a portion of the tumor by frozen section. Local or general anesthesia is re-

Table 17-3. Clinical staging for breast cancer

Columbia

Stage A: No skin edema, ulceration, or solid fixation to chest wall; axillary node clinically negative

Stage B: As in A, clinically involves nodes not more than 2.5 cm in transverse diameter; nodes not fixed to skin or deeper structures palpable

Stage C: Presence of any *one* of five grave signs:
1. Edema of the skin of limited extent (involves less than one third of the breast surface)
2. Skin ulceration
3. Solid fixation to chest wall
4. Massive axillary nodes (more than 2.5 cm transverse diameter)
5. Fixation of axillary nodes to skin or deep structures

Stage D: Includes all the more advanced carcinomas:
1. Any combination of two or more grave signs
2. Extensive edema (more than one third of breast surface)
3. Satellite skin nodules
4. Inflammatory carcinoma
5. Clinically involved supraclavicular nodes
6. Parasternal tumor of internal mammary nodes
7. Edema of the arm
8. Distant metastases

TNM*

T Primary tumors

TX Tumor cannot be assessed

T0 No demonstrable tumor in breast

TIS Preinvasive carcinoma (carcinoma in situ), noninfiltrating intraductal carcinoma, or Paget's disease of the nipple with no demonstrable tumor

NOTE: Paget's disease associated with a demonstrable tumor is classified according to the size of the tumor.

T1† Tumor 2 cm or less in its greatest dimension

T1a With no fixation to underlying pectoral fascia and/or muscle

T1b With fixation to underlying pectoral fascia and/or muscle

T2† Tumor more than 2 cm but not more than 5 cm in its greatest dimension

T2a With no fixation to underlying pectoral fascia and/or muscle

T2b With fixation to underlying pectoral fascia and/or muscle

T3† Tumor more than 5 cm in its greatest dimension

T3a With no fixation to underlying pectoral fascia and/or muscle

T3b With fixation to underlying pectoral fascia and/or muscle

T4 Tumor of any size with direct extension to chest wall or skin

NOTE: Chest wall includes ribs, intercostal muscles, and serratus anterior muscle, but not pectoral muscle

T4a With fixation to chest wall

T4b With edema (including peau d'orange), ulceration of the skin of the breast, or satellite skin nodules confined to the same breast

T4c Both of the above

T4d Inflammatory carcinoma

N Regional lymph nodes

NX Regional lymph nodes cannot be assessed clinically

N0 No palpable homolateral axillary nodes

N1 Movable homolateral axillary nodes

N1a Nodes not considered to contain growth

N1b Nodes considered to contain growth

N2 Homolateral axillary nodes considered to contain growth and fixed to one another or to other structures

N3‡ Homolateral supraclavicular or intraclavicular nodes considered to contain growth or edema of the arm

NOTE: Edema of the arm may be caused by lymphatic obstruction; lymph nodes may not then be palpable

M Distant metastasis

MX Not assessed

M0 No evidence of distant metastasis

M1 Distant metastasis present

Specify sites according to the following notations:

Pulmonary	PUL
Osseous	OSS
Hepatic	HEP
Brain	BRA
Lymph nodes	LYM
Bone marrow	MAR
Pleura	PLE
Skin	SKI
Eye	EYE
Other	OTH

---

*Revised clinical staging system for carcinoma of the breast, American Joint Committee for Cancer Staging and End Results Reporting Clinical-Diagnostic Classification.

†Dimpling of the skin, nipple retraction, or any other skin changes except those in T4b may occur in T1, T2, or T3 without affecting the classification.

‡Homolateral internal mammary nodes considered to contain growth are included in N3 for surgical evaluative classification and postsurgical treatment classification.

quired for an incisional biopsy, and a small scar at the site of the incision results from this procedure. Surgical biopsy may take place in an outpatient or inpatient setting. Initial diagnosis of the tumor by the pathologist may be immediate if a frozen section of the tumor is used for diagnosis, but careful examination of a permanent tissue specimen usually takes several days.

If the tumor is benign (noncancerous) and problems with wound healing are not anticipated, no further treatment is necessary except symptomatic relief of pain from the incision, removal of stitches, and monthly BSE with half-yearly or yearly physical examination.

The physical experience of a breast biopsy is generally not extremely traumatic or painful and healing is usually quite rapid. The emotional component of this experience, however, with the implications of possible malignant disease and mutilating surgery, are often overwhelming for the woman and her family. Alternatives for treatment, should the biopsy prove to be malignant, are presented to the woman and family during this time of severe emotional upheaval.

Other diagnostic tests

If the tumor is malignant or cancerous, the next phase of treatment depends on the results of several tests to determine if the disease is local (confined to the breast) or if it has metastasized to other organs of the body. These tests are important to help determine the stage of the disease and ultimately will influence the recommended treatment.

Tests performed on a woman who has suspected or proved early breast cancer are: a full physical examination to include size of the tumor and presence and location of involved lymph nodes, chest X rays and lung scan to determine lung involvement, and studies of blood samples (primarily serum alkaline phosphatase) and liver and bone scans to detect liver or bone marrow involvement (Rubin, 1974). Other tests may be performed if the disease is suspected to be in a late stage. These will be discussed later in the section on treatment of advanced breast disease.

These tests may be performed either before or after a biopsy has been done. The test results plus the biopsy findings allow staging or classification of the tumor to be done in order to specifically and statistically determine the most beneficial treatment for this particular woman.

Staging

Staging or classification is based on a set of parameters agreed on by physicians across the country. There are two systems for staging breast cancer widely used in the United States today. The Columbia staging system was developed by Haagensen; the TNM (tumor, node, metastasis) system is used in Europe and has become

Table 17-4. Clinical stage-grouping in carcinoma of the breast

TIS Carcinoma in situ		
Invasive carcinoma		
Stage I	T1a N0 or N1a	} M0
	T1b N0 or N1a	
Stage II	T0 N1b	} M0
	T1a N1b	
	T1b N1b	
	T2a or T2b N0, N1a or N1b	
Stage III	T1a or T1b N2	} M0
	T2a or T2b N2	
	T3a or T3b N0 or N1 or N2	
Stage IV	Any T4 Any N Any M	
	Any T N3 Any M	
	Any T Any N M1	

more widely accepted in the United States. The details of both systems are presented in Table 17-3.

Recommended treatment for each stage may vary according to physician and current research results. Treatment for stages I and II (TNM) and A and B (Columbia), range from lumpectomy to extended radical mastectomy and may include radiation treatment or chemotherapy following surgery. Radiation and chemotherapy are usually the initial treatments of choice for stages III and IV (C and D). Hormonal manipulation, either surgically or medically, and local excision of the breast mass are often included in the treatment plan for these tumors.

TREATMENT OF MALIGNANT BREAST DISEASE

In the following section, various methods of primary treatments for malignant breast disease and the nurse's role in the care of the woman will be discussed.

Breast surgery
Procedures

The most widely used procedures for the initial surgical treatment of breast cancer range from simple removal of the tumor to total resection of chest wall muscles and axillary contents.

Radical mastectomy. Radical mastectomy was hailed as the first successful treatment of breast cancer. Introduced by W. Halstead in 1890, the procedure involves removal of all of the breast tissue, removal of associated muscles including pectoralis major and minor and the latissimus and serratus, and complete dissection of the axilla and removal of lymph nodes. This procedure removes large quantities of tissue and skin and usually re-

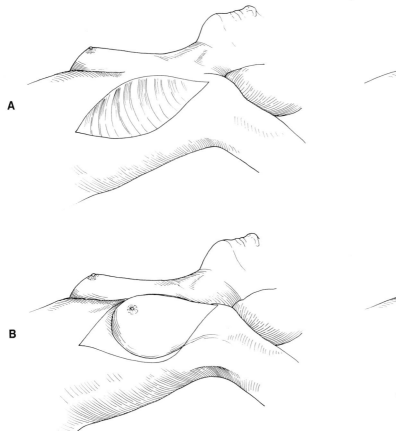

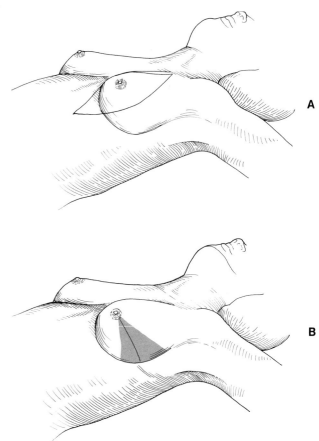

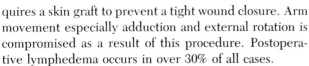

Fig. 17-2. A, Radical mastectomy; **B,** modified radical mastectomy.

Fig. 17-3. A, Simple mastectomy; **B,** segmental excision.

quires a skin graft to prevent a tight wound closure. Arm movement especially adduction and external rotation is compromised as a result of this procedure. Postoperative lymphedema occurs in over 30% of all cases.

Modified radical mastectomy. A modified procedure involves removal of all of the breast tissue and skin through a horizontal or vertical incision and removal of most or all of the axillary lymph nodes, sparing the pectoralis muscle. Recent studies of large numbers of women who have undergone this procedure reflect as good a survival rate as for those women who underwent radical mastectomy for the same disease stage (Hermann and Steiger, 1978; Leis, 1980). The modified radical mastectomy is becoming a preferred mode of treatment for breast cancer because, compared with the radical procedure, there are fewer complications, is shorter, and survival data are just as optimistic.

Simple mastectomy. A simple mastectomy, or removal of breast tissue alone, is often used when a large breast mass, which has been documented to have metastasized, is likely to enlarge to become an ulcerating, draining lesion.

Tylectomy/lumpectomy (Fig. 17-3). Lumpectomy is the removal of the breast lump along with large margins of breast tissue, but leaving the breast and axilla intact. Good survival rates in stage I (TNM) and A (Columbia), especially when combined with radiation therapy have recently been reported (Atkins et al., 1972). Critics of this technique have as their major argument the multicentric nature of carcinoma (Haagensen, 1971), but the protocol that includes radiation after surgery theoretically eradicates microscopic metastases if they exist.

Subcutaneous mastectomy. Subcutaneous mastectomy with or without immediate implantation of a silicone prosthesis, is a procedure that removes all of the breast tissue and may involve some dissection of the axilla but leaves the breast skin and areola. Silicone implants are inserted (either immediately or during a second procedure) to fill the space left by the removal of the breast tissue. This procedure is considered only when the tumor does not involve the areola or tissue close to and including the skin.

Breast reconstruction. Immediate reconstruction of the breast is a plastic surgical intervention. It involves

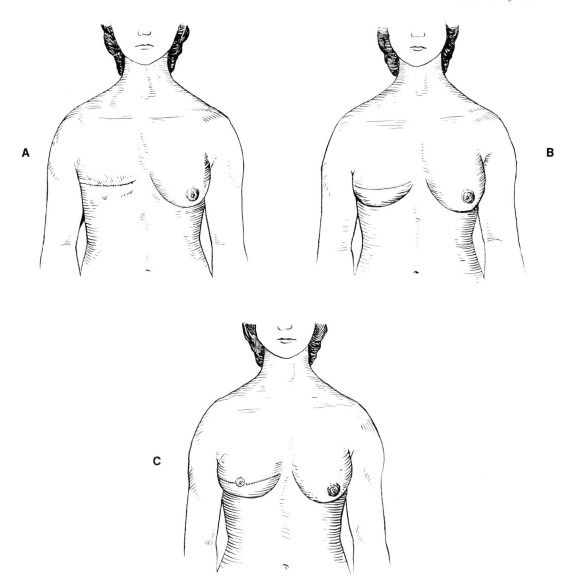

Fig. 17-4. Breast reconstruction.

implantation of a silicone prosthesis after a radical, modified radical, or subcutaneous mastectomy. A small prosthesis is placed under the skin of the chest wall. At the same time, the nipple of the affected breast, if it is not invaded by tumor, may be grafted to a separate area of the body to be brought back to the breast at a later time. The reconstruction of the breast after mastectomy usually occurs in stages. The small silicone implant is usually replaced by a larger implant about 2 months after the initial mastectomy. The nipple may be grafted back to the breast at this time. If the nipple was not able to be saved at the first surgery, a new one may be created from other tissue, usually from the labia or the other areola (Georgiade, 1976).

One-stage vs two-stage procedures

Depending on the position, size, and other findings of the disease, the surgeon determines which approaches are most appropriate and then presents the data to the woman and her family for deliberation. Hopefully, all possible alternatives and their risks and benefits will be explored by the surgeon and woman to determine which procedure will be most appropriate for her should the tumor prove to be malignant.

There is controversy concerning the timing of the biopsy and any indicated surgery. As previously stated, tests to determine stage of the disease prior to curative surgery are highly recommended but not always performed in the preoperative phase. In some cases, the biopsy may be the first procedure performed, especially if the surgeon determines from the physical examination and the woman's history that there is a great chance of the lump being benign or very early cancer. Before the biopsy is actually done, the physician will discuss the possibilities of the lump being malignant and will present the various treatments available, taking into consideration the risk factors involved, the woman's health history, and her preference.

At this time it must be decided whether the procedure will be done in one stage or two (Schain, 1976). A *one-stage* procedure means that the woman is taken to the operating room and is anesthetized (locally or with general anesthesia) for a breast biopsy. A section is taken and examined immediately by a pathologist; if the tumor is malignant, the mastectomy or lumpectomy will be performed as agreed on prior to surgery. In a *two-stage* procedure the biopsy and any further surgery are done at separate times. The tissue specimen is examined by the pathologist; if the tumor is malignant, the method of treatment will be decided upon later.

Whether a one- or two-stage procedure is used depends on several factors: risk of anesthesia, the woman's age and physical condition, her preference, and the likelihood that the tumor is malignant. Advantages of the single-stage method are: a single risk of anesthesia and no waiting period between diagnosis and treatment. A disadvantage of this method is that the woman consents to surgery not knowing what will be done. The effect of waking up and finding a breast gone may retard or upset the grieving and rehabilitation processes. A second disadvantage of this method is that the diagnosis of a malignancy is made only on the *frozen section* of tumor rather than on a permanent specimen, which may take several days to prepare.

Benefits of a two-stage procedure include prior knowledge of the extent of surgery the woman is to undergo with no unexpected results. If further treatment is required after biopsy, she can then begin to cope with the crisis before it occurs. Although the end result is as traumatic as with a one-stage procedure, the woman will have had a chance to begin coping with the reality of the situation before it actually happens. A disadvantage of the two-stage procedures is undergoing the risk of anesthesia twice, although the biopsy is often performed under local anesthesia. A second aspect of this two-stage procedure has recently been under discussion: once the malignant tumor has been violated by biopsy, the cells may travel and the cancer will possibly spread faster. Research indicates that a waiting period of 5 to 7 days is safe and, hopefully, will not result in unnecessary spread (Cammarata et al., 1978).

Preoperative care

The period before surgery is the optimal time for the nurse to help prepare the woman for what is to come, both physically and emotionally. Generally, anxiety is high among patients preoperatively regardless of the type of surgery to be performed. Fears about anesthesia, pain, and recovery are common, regardless of whether or not the tumor is likely to be malignant. For the woman facing possible malignancy, these fears of surgery are heightened and may be overshadowed by the potential diagnosis of cancer. During this preoperative period, useful information that should be available to the woman includes physical self-help measures, such as coughing, deep-breathing exercises, and range of motion exercises. Careful assessment by the nurse of the woman's anxiety level prior to surgery is imperative in order to correctly gauge her level of understanding to prevent giving too much or too little information at this time. The nurse needs to be particularly perceptive and empathetic during this period to allow ventilation of fears and questions, yet encourage and familiarize the woman with the surgical routine of the hospital.

Women facing breast biopsy and possible mastectomy are concerned about what they will look like following surgery and how family members will react. Obviously, questions about these concerns cannot be answered precisely, but they may be clues to unspoken fears. These types of difficult questions are often ignored by health professionals, perhaps because of their own discomfort with this potentially emotional situation. The primary nurse, who has built a trusting relationship with the client, can use this opportunity to help her explore her feelings about the decision, her fears about surgery and how she will look and feel afterward, and any other concerns apparent at this time. There is no specific way to approach a woman prior to biopsy except with a caring attitude and a willingness to listen. As in all aspects of nursing, individualized care is of the utmost importance.

All women do not exhibit the same reaction to breast surgery and, therefore, should not be cared for in the same way. Coping mechanisms useful to the woman in the past can be supported by nursing staff. The nurse might ask, "What can we do to help you through these next few days?" Responses vary from "Tell me everything about what is going to happen," to "I don't want to know what is going on." The woman may want to keep busy, have quiet visits with her family, or read by herself. Coordination of other supportive services at this time is an important part of the nurse's responsibility in helping to prepare the woman for surgery. Chaplains are usually available, and a preoperative visit from a Reach to Recovery volunteer may be helpful for the woman who will definitely undergo mastectomy.

Suggestions for exercises after a mastectomy

1. *Hand grips:* Squeeze a ball (size of a lemon) or a rolled-up bandage in your hand on the operated side. This helps strengthen the muscles in your hand and forearm and improves circulation. You can start this the day after surgery.
2. *Hair brushing:* Sit beside a night table. In the beginning rest your arm on a few books. Brush your hair with your affected arm gradually working around your entire head.
3. *Arm lifting:* Start with your arm at your side, lift your arm straight out in front of you then gently swing it to the side, then relax. Always keep elbow straight. Repeat several times.

You can start Nos. 1 to 3 in the hospital. Check with your physician about Nos. 4 and 5.

4. *Walking the wall:* Stand facing the wall, with toes as close to the wall as possible, feet apart. Place palms on the wall at shoulder level. Slowly "walk" your fingers up the wall. Slide palms back to shoulder level. Repeat several times. Each day, try to "walk" your fingers a little higher. You goal is to be able to extend your arms straight above your head and full length with elbows straight.

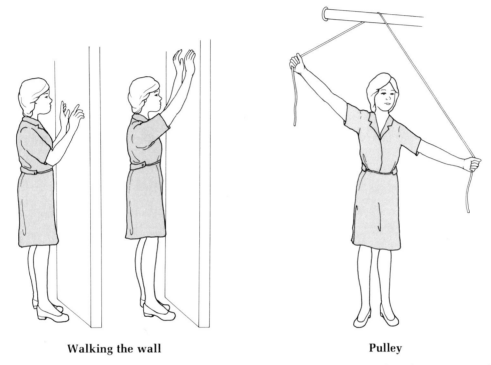

Walking the wall   **Pulley**

5. *Pulley:* Toss a 6-foot rope or bandage over a rod (e.g., shower curtain). Stand as nearly under rope as possible. Grasp an end in each hand and extend arms straight and away from body. Pull left arm up by tugging with right arm and continue this see-saw motion.

Teaching self-care measures and describing the routines related to surgery are important functions of the primary nurse. Depending on the needs of the woman, the nurse should set time aside, ideally over several days, to introduce, demonstrate, and observe the return demonstration of measures to prevent postoperative complications. Coughing and deep-breathing exercises to help prevent atelectasis and pneumonia, leg and ankle exercises to prevent thrombophlebitis, and turning and moving in bed after surgery should be explained and demonstrated to the woman. During this time a discussion of the progression of events (room to holding area to operating room to recovery, etc.) average time involved, and where family and friends should wait should be explained.

Expected equipment and procedures, such as intravenous lines, oxygen masks, dressings, and drains, should be discussed as should the routine diet and activity progression usually suggested in the institution. Two important areas to emphasize are pain at the incision site and early mobilization of the affected arm. The discomfort and pain experienced after surgery is subjective and highly individualized. The woman should know that she may have pain medication on a regular basis if she requests it. It should also be made clear that the medication does not usually eliminate the pain, but lessens its intensity while promoting relaxation. Use of the hand and arm after surgery will be encouraged. The woman usually starts by squeezing a bandage roll or small ball about ten times an hour as soon as she is able. The rationale for early mobility, including decreased joint stiffness, minimal or no lymphedema, and a faster return to normal functioning, should be given to enhance compliance with these activities. Range of motion exercises (see box on p. 347) may be taught at this time. If possible, family members or friends who will be with the woman after surgery should be included to help alleviate some of their fears and questions about procedures and to enhance reinforcement of self-help measures. As has been mentioned, this preoperative period usually is marked by a high level of anxiety; reinforcement and repetition of information by the nurse is necessary and should be incorporated in the plan of care.

Documentation in both the permanent record and the care plan is necessary in order to keep associate nurses and other personnel aware of the progress and to allow them to reinforce and add meaningful information as appropriate during this period.

Postoperative care

If the lump is determined to be benign, great relief is felt by all. Routine postoperative nursing care, including hydration, monitoring of vital signs, and management of pain is important during this time. Hospitalization usually lasts a day or two after the biopsy with a return appointment to the physician in 1 or 2 weeks for suture removal. Discharge teaching by the nurse emphasizes or reinforces monthly breast self-examination and care of the incision.

If the tumor is found to be malignant and some type of surgery was agreed upon prior to biopsy, the woman will need all aspects of physical and emotional care immediately following surgery. Generally, the woman returns to the surgical unit from the recovery room still experiencing effects of the anesthesia. A large dressing covers almost half of the chest wall, and drains are usually used (hemovac or wall suction) to prevent fluid and lymph from accumulating under the skin flap. Depending on the procedure and the woman's response to surgery, early activity and/or ambulation is encouraged as well as oral fluids and elimination. The amount of pain

experienced from this surgery differs greatly among women and depends upon the extent of surgery, as well as individual factors such as pain threshold and cultural influences. Observations important during this immediate postoperative phase are monitoring of vital signs, temperature, and intake and output. The condition of the dressing and/or wound is also important. The nurse should check for swelling in the immediate area and the amount of drainage apparent in hemovac or wall suction, to help determine the patency of drains and occurrence of hemorrhage. The level of the woman's awareness needs to be assessed continuously and protective measures should be taken (e.g., side rails up) until the woman has sufficiently recovered from anesthesia.

Arm care. If the surgery included axillary dissection and removal of lymph nodes, precautions must be taken to protect the affected arm and prohibit invasive or constrictive procedures to occur on that extremity. *Blood pressures, injections, and venipunctures should not be performed on the affected arm*, and reminders should be visible in the room and on the chart.

Psychologic aspects of care

As the immediate postoperative period passes, the woman will begin to realize the extent or seriousness of surgery. Whether mastectomy, lumpectomy, or biopsy was the chosen procedure, the diagnosis of cancer and the implications this has for the woman, and her family, and significant others now must be dealt with.

The woman who has had a mastectomy has undergone radical surgery. She has undergone a major insult; her body boundaries have been invaded. Reactions to surgery vary from person to person and are influenced by many factors including whether or not the surgery was expected or unexpected. Reactions run a full spectrum from relief to be rid of the cancer to feelings of anger at the violation of the body. Grief and sadness over the loss of the body part are an expected and healthy reaction to this surgery. Whether these emotions or "grief work" are experienced during the initial hospitalization depends on the woman and also the primary nurse. The amount of freedom the woman feels to express her initial feelings of grief depends largely on the needs of the woman and the relationship between the nurse and woman. Grieving a loss takes time, from months to years. The primary nurse can help start this process by sanctioning expression of emotion; she may help the woman bear the reality of the amputation by being with her when she first looks at the incision.

Self-help/rehabilitation: discharge teaching

Range of motion exercises. Because of the location of surgery and the possibility of major muscle and nerve injury, arm range of motion (ROM) exercises should be

---

Some suggestions for care of the hand and arm after a mastectomy

Breast surgery may include removal of some of the lymph nodes or glands (that normally drained fluid from arm) in the armpit. The absence of lymph nodes will not affect your general health, but your arm may have a tendency to swell. This swelling may be slight or severe. Presence of infection in the hand or arm can make the swelling worse. The following suggestions will help you avoid unnecessary swelling, injury, infection, or discomfort after your surgery.

1. Avoid having blood pressure or blood taken from the arm on the side that surgery was performed. Avoid vaccinations or injections on that side. This decreases chance of infection or decreased circulation.
2. Protect your hand and arm by:
   a. Wearing gloves when injury is a possibility (gardening, yard work)
   b. Wearing thimble when sewing
   c. Avoiding burns by wearing a mitt when cooking and being careful about cigarette burns
   d. Wearing rubber gloves when hands are in water for a prolonged period of time
   e. Pushing rather than cutting cuticles
   f. Avoiding excessive exposure to the sun on the affected side
3. If injury does occur:
   a. Wash open area immediately with soap and water, apply antiseptic cream, and protect from dirt
   b. Notify your physician if signs of infection develop (redness, heat, pain, swelling, or fever)
4. Help prevent swelling by:
   a. Keeping arm elevated when sitting (put it right up on the back of a sofa or chair)
   b. Keeping jewelry, sleeves, and watch band loose on operated side
   c. Not carrying heavy handbags in crook of elbow on operated side
   d. Not carrying heavy objects on operated side

---

done. These can be demonstrated by the nurse during hospitalization and can be incorporated into a daily exercise program in the hospital and at home to enhance recovery. Vigorous exercise need not be started during hospitalization since the tissues are healing, stitches are still in, and unnecessary pain may be experienced. Consultation with the physician prior to initiating active exercises is usually necessary to determine an appropriate, individualized course of arm exercises. Because various procedures include skin grafts and resection of muscles, no one exercise program is correct for every woman. Useful exercises include hair brushing, straight arm raising, and "walking the wall" (see p. 347). Gentle range of motion should be encouraged, stopping with any sensation of pulling or pain.

Arm and hand care. Care of the arm and hand on the affected side is a second important area for teaching because of the potential for lymphedema (swelling caused by lymph fluid) if lymph nodes were removed from the axilla. The arm on the affected side will always have the potential to swell (Rudolph, 1979), but certain measures can help the woman avoid unnecessary discomfort (see accompanying box).

Care of the incision. A third area in which the nurse can help the woman further her self-care is teaching care of her incision. Basic good hygiene—washing with soap and water, avoiding use of heavy lotions, medications, or creams on the incision—and inspecting the healing

scar daily are to be encouraged. Signs and symptoms of infection should be explained to help the woman recognize when additional assistance may be needed.

Range of motion exercises, hand and arm care, and care of the wound are all important measures that the woman can be responsible for both in the hospital and at home. The primary nurse should be certain that the woman has access to the information she needs to be able to care for herself knowledgeably.

Sexual concerns. Although sexual concerns may not be verbalized at this time, the nurse should include this in teaching prior to discharge without expecting the patient to initiate the discussion. The client may fear cessation of the nurse's concern by bringing up a potentially uncomfortable subject. The importance of the nurse's initiation of the discussion about sexual activity following discharge is stressed by Graf (1977). She found that 50% of the women studied felt the nurses' attitudes precluded initiation of a discussion of sexual concerns; however, 63% felt that had the nurse initiated the subject, they would have to be willing to discuss their concerns. Between 17% and 32% of mastectomy patients report that their surgery has adversely affected their sexual lives (Graf, 1977; Morris et al., 1977).

Nursing interventions depend upon the individual woman's situation and response to her surgery. The meaning of the loss of the breast to a woman's sexuality depends on several factors that should be assessed prior to counseling. Because the partner acts as a major determinant of the woman's sexual activity and identity, he or she should be included in the discussions if possible. One of the first questions usually asked is when sexual intercourse can be resumed following discharge. The advice, "When you feel up to it," is too vague to be helpful. The woman and her partner should be encouraged to begin as soon as possible depending on her physical status (e.g., wound healing, pain at the operative site). This is not recommended for the sake of the act itself but because intercourse may help the woman to confront her loss. More importantly, she will be shown that her partner still considers her desirable, lovable, and feminine (Witkin, 1973).

To decrease anxiety about resumption of sexual activity, specific suggestions may be offered. The first issue related to sexuality is that of confronting the change in physical appearance. Looking at the incision may be as difficult for the partner as it is for the client. He or she should be encouraged to see the incision prior to discharge with an explanation of its appearance and support provided by the nurse. The couple should be encouraged to share their feelings concerning the change resulting from surgery. Feelings such as anxiety, shock, and relief should be openly expressed and explored. Positive and negative feelings on the part of each partner may be present and need to be dealt with.

Suggestions regarding positions for intercourse involve consideration for protection of the chest wall from trauma, decreasing attention to the absence of the breast, and the woman's physical tolerance for activity. A face-to-face position, partner superior supported by knees and elbows, may be preferred (Witkin, 1973). If, because of the woman's physical condition, intercourse is not immediately possible, the partner should be encouraged to express feeling of desire, thereby not only demonstrating his or her continued physical attraction, but also enhancing the woman's acceptance of herself, both sexually and emotionally.

Reach to Recovery. An important source of support for many women who have undergone mastectomy is Reach to Recovery, organized by Terese Lasser in 1953. This organization consists of women who have undergone mastectomy and is a service function of the American Cancer Society. The members provide support and empathy to women who have had breast surgery and provide useful, practical information regarding prostheses, exercises, and clothing. The primary nurse is in an excellent position to suggest to the physician that a Reach to Recovery volunteer visit the woman while she is in the hospital. If this is not possible, the woman may contact the organization herself. Depending on the client's needs and the availability of volunteers in the community, a volunteer may visit the woman in the hospital or at home. For many women, this initial contact with another woman who has undergone a similar surgical procedure is a positive, enlightening encounter. It may be a vehicle to provide further contact with women in the community after discharge for support and sharing of feelings.

Prosthesis. Information regarding a prosthesis is extremely important for the woman to have prior to discharge. A general rule is that a permanent prosthesis may be worn from 4 to 6 weeks after surgery (to allow tissues a chance to heal), but a soft form may be made out of cotton or gauze and pinned into a bra for use during the initial postoperative period. Information about the varieties of prostheses available and where to buy them may be obtained from a local chapter of Reach to Recovery, the American Cancer Society, or local department stores. Some large medical centers have their own prosthetic departments, and fittings for the breast prosthesis may take place during follow-up visits to the surgeon. The types of prostheses available include air-filled pillows of vinyl, fluid-filled sacks of plastic, and silicone pouches. The weight of the prosthesis varies as does color and price. Every woman should be encouraged to obtain some kind of permanent prosthesis. Many insurance companies include this as a medical expense.

Emotional support. During the early rehabilitative phase, which usually begins in the hospital, other sources of support for the woman should be identified by the primary nurse and included, if possible, during teaching and question sessions. As in the preoperative period, including supportive family members or friends may help alleviate their discomfort and answer their questions as well as serve to reinforce teaching and encourage self-care activities.

Discharge planning and teaching must encompass not only the physical but also the emotional needs of the woman. Fears about what to say to friends and family, especially children, may be expressed. It may be helpful for her to role play explanations to these people with the primary nurse. Communication between nurse, physician, social worker, and other members of the health care team is essential prior to discharge so that plans can be made to meet the client's needs after discharge.

Quint (1963) suggests contact with some supportive person or service for at least 1 year after surgery. She bases this recommendation on reports from women that family and friends become impatient or weary of hearing about the surgery after the initial recovery period at home. The primary nurse may be in a setting where it is possible to see the woman when she comes back for follow-up care by the surgeon. This type of continuity is important and extremely helpful in assessing the client's needs and status after discharge from the hospital.

Often during these initial outpatient visits, further treatment may be prescribed. Access to a support group of other women may be especially helpful after surgery.

In the following sections, radiation therapy, chemotherapy, and hormonal treatment will be discussed relative to breast cancer, as well as nursing support of the client undergoing these therapies. Although the following sections on radiation and chemotherapy are aimed at supporting the woman with early primary disease, the principles of support and teaching are applicable when caring for a woman undergoing these therapies in any stage of the disease.

Radiation therapy as primary treatment

A woman may choose radiation therapy as the primary form of therapy of a malignant breast tumor. Several studies have been published advocating the use of radiation as a primary treatment for stages I and II breast cancer (Prosnitz et al., 1977; Wallner et al., 1976; Weber and Hellman, 1975).

Levine and associates (1977, 1978) have presented statistics that show comparable survival rates at 5 years for surgically treated cases and those treated by radiation. However, care must be taken when comparing these modalities of cancer treatment to make sure that the results really are similar, particularly with regard to staging of the disease and numbers in the sample.

Radiation, for many reasons, has been slow to become a first choice in the treatment of early breast disease. Because radical surgery so drastically changed the length of survival of women with breast cancer, physicians have been reluctant to change or experiment with an unproved method of treatment. As a result, only women who refused surgery or those with very late-stage breast cancer were treated with radiation, hardly adequate samples to compare effectiveness of treatment. As the understanding of the physics of radiation increased and machines capable of finer direction and intensity of beams were developed, this form of treatment has become more acceptable in treating early breast cancer.

There is still a great deal of controversy over the use of radiation for primary treatment of breast disease. One main objection to this treatment is that radiation may alter or damage the body's immune response and thus render it susceptible to micrometastases, which ordinarily would be kept in control by an intact immune system. Another objection is that although an excisional biopsy is performed, axillary lymph node sampling or dissection is frequently not done, making staging according to the accepted standards (TNM or Columbia) impossible. This makes comparison of the treatments highly speculative and often means prescribing treatments based on incomplete data. Much work has yet to be done in this area, particularly regarding adequate statistical comparison of radiation with other forms of therapy. If this occurs, a treatment for early breast cancer that may be physically and esthetically more tolerable may enjoy greater acceptance in the health profession.

The purpose of external radiation therapy in early breast cancer is to cure, as opposed to external and internal radiation aimed at palliation in advanced cancer of the breast. It is considered to be a local treatment, like surgery, in that it only affects the area it directly touches. The desired outcome of radiation therapy is to promote tumor cell death. The radiation alters the composition of the cellular water and damages the nucleus of the cell (DNA and RNA), rendering it incapable of reproduction and promoting cell death (Horton and Hill, 1977).

The more rapidly growing cells are those most affected by radiation. Cancer cells characteristically divide rapidly and theoretically are sensitive to destruction by radiation. Normal body cells that rapidly divide (such as mucous membrane, bone marrow, and skin) are also affected by radiation and are destroyed with the cancer cells.

The dose of radiation determined to be therapeutic for a particular tumor is fractionated—given over a period of time in small doses. The rationale for dividing the dose is based on the theory that normal cells have a greater ability to recuperate from radiation damage than do abnormal or cancer cells, thus helping to sustain the life of the healthy tissues while creating a hostile environment for tumor growth (Leahy et al., 1979). The dose of radiation for breast cancer after excisional biopsy or removal of the tumor is between 5,000 and 6,500 rads (the measurement of radiation absorbed by the body) divided into doses of about 200 rads per day. The biopsy site and axilla may receive additional doses of radiation.

Increased knowledge of the physics of radiation and development of sophisticated equipment capable of delivering precise amounts of radiation to specific parts of the body have helped increase acceptance of this therapy both in the medical world and from an esthetic viewpoint. The most frequent untoward side effects from breast irradiation are lung and skin involvement and general malaise. Radiation effects on lung tissue is decreased by judicious placement of protective wedges and careful aiming of the energy beams. The response of the lung to radiation is inflammatory in nature (radiation pneumonitis) (Ogi, 1978) and may be manifested by respiratory distress and shortness of breath. Depending on the amount of radiation delivered to the lung, the fibrosis resulting from alveolar damage may or may not be reversible (Horton and Hill, 1977).

The effect of radiation on skin is a reddening or sunburn-like reaction. The reaction can range from mild erythema to severe skin necrosis. Because of new developments in many areas of radiation therapy, especially "skin sparing," drastic skin damage is not as common as in the past.

General malaise or radiation sickness resulting from radiation therapy is thought to be caused by the increase in bodily waste products from the cellular breakdown (Ogi, 1978). A program of rest, antiemetics, and adequate nutrition is usually all that is needed when this phenomenon occurs.

Care of the woman undergoing external radiation therapy

As with any aspect of nursing care, in order to support a woman's decision for a particular treatment, the nurse must understand the options and relate to each person as an individual. Care includes the previously described pre- and postoperative nursing as well as teaching the woman about the radiation treatments, including details of the procedure, the tumoricidal effects, and the later reaction of the body.

The procedure. Prior to the onset of therapy, the nurse needs to assess the woman's level of knowledge and perceptions about the therapy. Based on this assessment, teaching should include an explanation of the basic principles of radiation, the physical environment she will encounter, time involvement per day, and expected reactions from the radiation. If at all possible, the primary nurse should include family or significant others to help reinforce the teaching and answer their questions. Although the environment is different from institution to institution, the nurse can explain that once the woman has been properly positioned by the radiologist or technician in the treatment room, all of the staff will leave but will stay in voice and visual contact through windows and microphones. Portals or boundaries that have been mathematically calculated will be marked on the skin with gentian violet or some other marking material. This outlines the area to be irradiated and must be left on the skin until the entire treatment course (over a period of weeks) has been completed. Since it is often an unspoken fear, the woman should be reassured that she will not be radioactive after the treatments.

Reactions to therapy. As in preoperative teaching, it is important for the woman to know what to expect following treatment to help decrease anxiety and to provide her with some means of control of her situation. One of the most important areas to be planned by the primary nurse and woman is an optimal activity/rest schedule. Fatigue and malaise may occur during the treatment regimen as a result of increased metabolic demands, and although they are temporary, these reactions need to be considered. Care of the skin during and after treatment should be discussed and reinforced during this

period. Lotions, creams, or oils should not be used on the irradiated skin during the time radiation therapy is being given. Mild soap and warm water may be used on the site, taking care not to wash off portal markings. A soft, nonconstrictive, cotton bra should be worn to avoid irritating irradiated skin. If blisters or desquamation of skin should occur after treatments are completed, the physician should be consulted regarding treatment, or lanolin or Vaseline may be applied after gentle cleansing with water or half-strength hydrogen peroxide.

Susceptibility to respiratory infections increases with damage to the lung from radiation. Other manifestations of lung involvement range from shortness of breath to fibrotic changes. Signs and symptoms of pulmonary infections should be discussed, as well as early medical intervention to prevent overwhelming infection from developing. Comfort measures to ease dyspnea, or shortness of breath, may be discussed, emphasizing the need for frequent rest periods during the active phase of treatment.

Since radiation therapy often takes place on an outpatient basis, it is important that the primary nurse teach the woman and her family about the treatment as soon as is feasible. The nurse and the woman should collaborate to plan the best potential schedule for the woman, considering her responsibilities and normal routines prior to radiation. The nurse should encourage communication with the woman even while she is receiving therapy on an outpatient basis for continued support and revisions in the plan for care.

Adjuvant chemotherapy

Recent research has indicated that, in addition to local treatment to remove the breast tumor, survival rates have improved with some form of systemic therapy (Henderson and Canellos, 1980). The concept of adjuvant chemotherapy, or therapy to enhance medical treatment, is aimed at eliminating micrometastases (Rubens, 1978). Many studies have been done in search of the ideal drug or drugs and the most optimal sequence for their use. A study by Bonadona (1976) compares the survival of women after surgery combined with chemotherapy (Cytoxan, Methotrexate, and 5-FU) versus surgery only. After 2 years, three times as many women who had not received the chemotherapy had relapsed as those who had taken the drugs. After further analysis of the results it was determined that only premenopausal women showed any significant improvement in the length of the disease-free interval. This may show that the cytotoxic drugs affect ovarian function (which the tumor may depend upon to grow), or that tumors in premenopausal women are more susceptible to the specific drugs than tumors in postmenopausal women (Carter et al., 1977). A study by Fisher and associates (1977) also shows a reduction of treatment failures in premenopausal women with L-phenylalanine (L-PAM) is used for 2 years after surgery.

The action of cytotoxic agents on cancer cells is similar to radiation in that it impairs or destroys the cells' ability to replicate. The effect chemotherapy has on rapidly dividing normal cells (bone marrow, mucous membrane, hair, etc.) may determine the amount of the drug prescribed and the length of treatment.

Preventive measures to help lessen the undesirable side effects of chemotherapy are presented in Table 17-5. The primary nurse should discuss these measures with the woman and include visual material if appropriate to help reinforce the teaching. In addition to general information about chemotherapy, information about specific drugs the woman is to receive should also be discussed.

Table 17-6 describes the most common chemotherapeutic agents used in adjuvant therapy for breast cancer. It includes dosages, toxic effects, and special teaching considerations. For additional information and more detailed descriptions of the mechanism of cytotoxic drugs, the reader is referred to texts dealing specifically with cancer and cancer therapy.

Psychologic support: continuing care

Chemotherapy, hormonal therapy, and radiation treatments generally are carried out on an outpatient basis over a period of time. After initial teaching has been done by the primary nurse, contact should be maintained for supportive purposes with some member of the health care team. A nurse-to-nurse referral from the inpatient to outpatient or clinic setting is usually appropriate and will help to assure continuity of care during this phase of treatment.

The meaning of breast cancer for each woman usually is not realized during the diagnostic or immediate treatment period. As the woman returns periodically for follow-up visits or further therapy, assessment of her needs and ability to cope should be ongoing, with additional intervention from nurses or other supportive personnel if necessary. Issues the woman may face during this time period range from dealing with distressing physical symptoms from drug therapy or radiation to the incorporation and integration of the diagnosis of breast cancer and all that may mean for her life and relationships (Warren, 1979; Woods and Earp, 1978).

Care of the woman with advanced breast disease

Complaints of bone pain, difficulty breathing, or discovery of a lump may be the first signs a woman brings to the health practitioner that signal recurring or advanced breast malignancy. Recurrences of breast cancer primarily occur through lymph channels, exhibited by tumors of the axillae, supraclavicular area, and the mediastinum; and through blood channels affecting primarily bone, lungs, and liver (Horton and Hill, 1977). Less common but sometimes affected are the central nervous system, endocrine glands, pericardium, the abdominal cavity, and the eye. After carefully performing the diagnostic tests previously described (bone scan, X-ray studies, liver scan, liver function tests, and biopsies of any lump), the results are evaluated and presented to the woman to begin the process of planning treatment from this point forward.

Generally, hospitalization is required for the series of tests needed to evaluate the disease as various preparatory medications and periods of fasting may be necessary. The primary nurse can begin to develop a trusting, open relationship with the woman during this time, of anxiety and waiting. This hospitalization may have various meanings for the woman. The waiting period may now be over as metastasis is confirmed. The hopefulness after surgery, that the tumor is gone, may now be replaced by fears of what lies ahead. Individual perceptions and past experiences with other family members

Table 17-5. General considerations for people receiving chemotherapy

Effect on	Preventive measures
Mouth	Perform scrupulous mouth care every 4 hours. Use mouthwash (½ strength commercial brand, mild salt solution, warm water; avoid those containing alcohol), use soft toothbrush or swab. Make sure dentures fit properly. Remove dentures at night, clean thoroughly. See a dentist regularly. Inspect mouth daily for white or red patches, sores. Notify physician if these are present.
Appetite and diet	Try to eat high-protein high-calorie foods (meat, cheese, beans, fish, chicken, peanutbutter, nuts, eggs). Drink extra amounts of fluids, about double usual intake. Eat six small snacks or meals instead of three large ones.
Colon	Prevent constipation or diarrhea. Eat balanced meals, include bran, vegetables, fruits, peanut butter, prunes, apples. *For constipation:* take a mild laxative, stewed fruits, fruit juices, water. *For diarrhea:* take a binding or antispasmodic medicine if severe, eat cheese, milk, bread. Avoid rough vegetables (lettuce, broccoli, cabbage).
Bone marrow	Prevent infection; know early signs and symptoms. Daily inspection of skin, hands, feet. Daily mild exercise in fresh air if possible. Prevent bleeding; avoid cuts, bruises. Use electric razor, put pressure over venipuncture sites for 5 minutes. Do not take aspirin. Notify physician if bruises, bleeding from bowel, bladder, mouth, or nose develops or tiny red spots appear on arms or legs.

Table 17-6. Chemotherapeutic agents commonly used in adjuvant therapy for breast cancer

Drug	Classification	Route/dose	Side effects/toxicities	Nursing considerations
Cyclophosphamide (Cytoxan)	Alkylating agent	50-200 mg/day PO 3.5-5.0 mg/kg/day IV for 10 days	Nausea, vomiting, bone marrow depression, possible alopecia, hemorrhagic, cystitis, amenorrhea	Take oral dose on an empty stomach, encourage 2000-3000 ml fluids per day to prevent irritation of kidneys and bladder by drug
Methotrexate (Amethopterin)	Antimetabolite	2.5-5.0 mg/day PO 0.4 mg/kg IV 1-2 times per week	Stomatitis, bone marrow depression, chills, fever, nausea, vomiting, photosensitivity	Consistent mouth care regimen every 4 hours, do not use aspirin, vitamins, tetracycline, or Dilantin (they interfere with drug); encourage use of sunglasses, sunscreen
5-Fluorouracil	Antimetabolite	12 mg/kg/day IV for 3 days	Stomatitis, bone marrow depression, nausea, vomiting, anorexia, diarrhea	Encourage adequate hydration (at least 2000 ml/day); teach mouth care and encourage every 4 hours
Melphalan (Alkeran, L-PAM)	Alkylating agent	0.1 mg/kg/day PO for 7 days 2-4 mg/day for maintenance	Some bone marrow depression, nausea and vomiting, stomatitis	Stomatitis may be an indicator toxic dose has been reached
Adriamycin (Doxorubricin)	Antibiotic	50-75 mg/sq. meter every 3 weeks	Nausea, vomiting, definite alopecia, possible cardiac toxicity leading to congestive heart failure, extreme extravasation reaction, bone marrow depression	Red urine for a period after administration due to drug excretion; monitor cardiac status prior to administration; dosage is limited to 550 mg/sq. meter; consider premedication with antiemetic prior to administration
Oncovin (Vincristine)	Plant alkaloid	1-2 mg/m² IV weekly	Bone marrow depression, possible peripheral neuropathy (range from mild to severe), constipation, possible extravasation reaction	Prevent constipation, encourage mild exercise, teach signs and symptoms of neurotoxicity

and friends who were treated for advanced cancer greatly influence the woman's emotional state during this time. Helping people express their concerns and past experiences may be one of the most therapeutic maneuvers a nurse can perform to clarify misconceptions and update old information. False reassurance is not useful (Klein, 1971) and generally inhibits further expression of feelings and concerns. Assessment of coping mechanisms is useful during this time and should be documented in the nursing plan of care as to how nursing staff and other support services can help the woman cope with this ordeal.

After the diagnostic tests have been performed and results have been collected and evaluated, the primary physician along with other members of the health care team will present possible options of treatment to the woman for discussion and consideration. In addition to the previously described therapies of radiation and chemotherapy that are also used to treat metastatic disease, hormonal therapy may be used. It is important to be aware that factors affecting the decisions concerning the choice of therapy include stage of the disease, physical status of the woman, findings of current research, and the desires of the woman based on her understanding of risks and benefits of the treatment.

Hormonal therapy

Approximately 40% of women experiencing recurrent or metastatic breast cancer will benefit from hormonal therapy. The accuracy in predicting potential effectiveness of hormonal therapy on individual tumors has increased with the ability to determine estrogen receptor (ER) status. Two thirds of tumors containing estrogen receptors will respond to hormonal therapy (Kennedy, 1978). For premenopausal women who are designated ER positive, removal or blockage of the estrogen effect may decrease disease progression. This is usually achieved through surgical procedures such as bilateral salpingo-oophorectomy or the use of antiestrogen compounds such as the drug Tamoxifen. Although the mechanism is poorly understood, for postmenopausal women who are ER positive, the administration of estrogen hor-

Text continued on p. 359.

Plan of care for the woman undergoing mastectomy

Assessment

1. General health history
2. Family history
3. Perception of the event
   a. How lump was found
   b. Emotional response
   c. Intellectual response
4. Support systems available (family, friends, significant others)
5. Coping mechanisms or patterns (elicit information on how she has dealt with hospitalization, events of this nature in the past)
6. Life-style profile
7. Position in family, job status, recreational activities, other physical demands

Potential problem	Behavioral objective/ desired outcome	Nursing interventions
Preoperative period		
Anxiety caused by lack of information regarding biopsy, surgery, testing procedures	Client verbalizes rationale for various tests, states routines of hospital (before biopsy and surgery).	1. Explain rationale for tests (i.e., blood test, bone scan, mammograms). 2. Explain routines and procedures of biopsy and surgery pertinent to client's hospital course (i.e., shave and preparation, NPO, recovery room, postoperative pain medication, dressing, Hemovac, early ambulation, respiratory and arm exercises, diet).
Anxiety caused by change in body image, possible cancer.	Verbalizes fears and concerns. Nonverbal behavior demonstrates decreased anxiety.	Encourage ventilation preoperatively. Clear misconceptions if possible: 1. Use diagrams to discuss surgical approach. 2. Discuss possible prosthesis if mastectomy is possible or planned. 3. Demonstrate prosthesis if client requests or it seems necessary. 4. Discuss postoperative activity and potential function with client. 5. Provide information and encourage ventilation related to malignancy of breast cancer.
Postoperative period		
Potential hemorrhage resulting from surgical interruption of circulatory system.	Adequate circulation and perfusion as indicated by: 1. Stable BP, pulse 2. Dry, warm skin 3. Surgical dressing dry and intact, minimal wound drainage 4. Urine output >30 ml/hr	Check blood pressure q1h × 8 then q4h or as ordered 1. Inspect dressing q1h × 12 then q2h × 12 2. Check for S/S shock 3. Empty wound drainage device and record output 4. Maintain potency of system
Potential infection resulting from bacterial invasion (wound, urinary tract).	Absence of infection indicated by: 1. No elevation of temperature 2. Absence of purulent drainage from wound 3. Suture line pink, not swollen 4. Urine clear, no foul odor	Check temperature q2h × 8 then q4h or as ordered 1. Assess wound every shift (plus 1st dressing change), notify physician of signs and symptoms of infection. 2. Change dressing using sterile technique. 3. Antibiotics as ordered. 4. Teach client catheter or perineal care. 5. Encourage fluids to 3000 ml when able to take orally. 6. Instruct to not allow BP venipunctures, or injections to be done on affected side. Place sign in client's room to emphasize this.

Continued.

Plan of care for the woman undergoing mastectomy—cont'd

Potential problem	Behavioral objective/ desired outcome	Nursing interventions
Postoperative period —cont'd Pain and discomfort resulting from tissue damage from surgical insult.	Verbalizes minimal discomfort. Nonverbal behavior demonstrates lack of pain.	Assess pain/discomfort and possible reasons for it: 1. Check position of affected arm for correct alignment, possible swelling. 2. Check bandages and drains for pulling or binding. 3. Medicate for pain per physician's order. 4. If appropriate, initiate alternative measures of pain relief (back rub, heat, distraction, therapeutic touch). 5. Assess client's anxiety level and need for emotional support or ventilation.
Advanced postoperative period Potential contracture of affected arm resulting from immobility or pain postoperatively.	Exhibits full range of motion of elbow and shoulder joints 1 month after discharge.	Teach beginning range-of-motion 1. Encourage gentle exercises twice per shift. 2. Encourage gradual use of affected arm in ADLs postoperative. 3. Discourage protection of surgical incision by holding affected arm over chest. 4. Encourage upright posture when ambulating: shoulders back, back straight.
Potential lymphedema resulting from interrupted lymphatic drainage from removal of axillary lymph nodes.	Absence of swelling/discomfort of affected arm 2 weeks postoperatively.	1. Assess affected arm every shift for signs of swelling. 2. Instruct client to squeeze ball of bandage roll. Start immediately postoperatively and continue throughout hospitalization. 3. Elevate affected arm on two pillows when in bed. 4. Instruct client on arm care beginning 2 to 3 days postoperatively.
Altered body image resulting from loss of breast.	Verbalizes feelings about change in body, implications for life-style, relations with significant others Looks at surgical scar prior to discharge.	1. Provide quiet time to talk with client and/or others about thoughts and feelings. 2. Provide and interpret information where appropriate (i.e., surgical procedure, biopsy report, pain, phantom breast sensation, pain, phantom breast sensation, numbness or tingling under affected arm, prosthesis, Reach to Recovery). 3. Consult with other support services when appropriate, (i.e., volunteer, chaplain, physical therapy).
Discharge planning phase Contracture of elbow and limited range of motion of shoulder leading to decreased functional use of affected arm.	Full range of motion of shoulder and elbow 6 to 8 weeks following surgery.	1. Instruct client on arm exercises and activity for postdischarge period: a. Pendulum swings: facing back of chair, bend at waist and grasp chair with unaffected arm. Slowly swing affected arm in circles from shoulder. b. Forward arm lifting: with arm held straight in front of body, slowly lift until sensation of pulling is felt. Lower and repeat.

Plan of care for the woman undergoing mastectomy—cont'd

Potential problem	Behavioral objective/ desired outcome	Nursing interventions
Discharge planning phase —cont'd		
		c. Lateral arm lifting: with arm held straight to side of body, slowly raise until pulling sensation is felt. Lower and repeat.
		d. Wall climbing: face wall with feet apart. Raise both arms in front of body, elbows straight, fingers touching the wall. "Walk" hands up wall until pulling sensation occurs. Lower slowly, repeat.
		2. Encourage upright posture, back straight, shoulders back, both arms hanging by sides when ambulating. Discourage patient from carrying affected arm. Avoid heavy lifting of objects with affected arm (less than the weight of a grocery bag; i.e., 10 lbs). Begin driving as energy level permits. Warn patient of continued fatigue following discharge. Inform woman of any community programs related to exercise programs for mastectomy patients.
Lymphedema resulting from interrupted lymph drainage; potential lymphedema resulting from infections or injury of affected arm.	Absence of swelling or edema and of symptoms of infection or injury.	1. Explain relationship between injury and infection and lymphedema. Teach arm care precautions including: a. Not having blood drawn, injections given, or blood pressures taken from the affected arm without physician's permission. b. Wearing a mitt when cooking to avoid burns. c. Using a lanolin-based cream to keep cuticles soft rather than cutting them. d. Protecting the affected arm and hand during other activities such as gardening, sewing, or washing dishes. e. In the event of injury to the arm, washing it immediately with soap and water. f. Avoiding excessive exposure to the sun. 2. Instruct client to notify physician if pain, swelling, and redness, with or without fever, are noticed. Encourage patient to maintain arm at shoulder level or higher when possible (i.e., resting arm on the back of the sofa or chair when sitting).
Disrupted or delayed healing of incision secondary to infection, hematoma, or swelling.	Incision heals without signs of swelling, redness, increased heat, drainage, pus, or fever.	1. Encourage client to look at incision prior to discharge. Explain expected appearance first and during session. Avoid phrases such as, "It looks good" but use instead "It is healing well." Teach client to look at incision daily for signs of infection or drainage collection under skin flap. Instruct her to avoid use of any medications or creams unless prescribed by physician. Avoid use of deodorant under affected arm. May bathe or shower if wound is healed completely. Provide any special information related to individual incision care.

Continued.

Plan of care for the woman undergoing mastectomy—cont'd

Potential problem	Behavioral objective/ desired outcome	Nursing interventions
Discharge planning phase —cont'd		
		2. Warn client that feeling of numbness over chest wall, incision, and occasionally the affected arm may occur. Duration is individual but incisional numbness is usually permanent. Instruct to call physician if signs of infection or swelling occur.
Altered body image from loss of breast results in depression.	Maintenance of positive body image.	1. Assess meaning of breast to each client. Provide opportunities for ventilation of feelings related to change in body structure. Instruct about prosthesis: a. Light, temporary breast prosthesis can be worn with nonbinding, wireless bra until incision is completely healed (6 to 8 weeks). b. Health professional should advise when swelling is subsided sufficiently for proper fitting of permanent prosthesis. c. Permanent forms, made of heavier weight materials and fitted to the individual, can be obtained through department stores, specialty shops, and medical supply facilities. These should be fitted by trained personnel. Most insurance companies cover the majority of the cost of the first prosthesis. 2. Early observation of the incision by the woman and appropriate family members and early resumption of sexual activity enhance acceptance of changed body image. Inform woman and obtain physician's and client's consent for visitation by a Reach to Recovery volunteer.
Decreased sexual activity causing disruption in interpersonal relationships with significant others.	Return to preoperative pattern of sexual activity.	Inform woman and partner that sexual activity can be resumed when energy level permits. Provide information regarding suggested position: face to face, man on top supported by elbows to avoid trauma to chest wall. If sexual activity is not possible, encourage expression of partner's feelings of sexual desire. Sexual or marriage counseling may be indicated for selected individuals.
Noncompliance with follow-up medical treatment resulting in decreased survival rate and increased recurrence of disease.	Complies with medical regimen by keeping appointments, self-administering medications, and contacting physician when appropriate.	Collaborate with physician regarding plans for planned postoperative therapy. Teach about prescribed medications such as chemotherapy. Provide information about: 1. Purpose of drug. 2. Side effects and related precautions and methods of avoiding or minimizing these. 3. Symptoms related to side effects necessitating physician's attention. 4. Methods, times, and dates of administration. Teach about other possible therapies such as radiation, immunotherapy, or hormonal manipulation.

mones, such as diethylstilbestrol produces an objective response rate exceeding 35%. Other types of hormonal therapies, which are considered second-line, include hypophysectomy, bilateral adrenalectomy, androgens, progestins, corticosteroids, and aminoglutethimide.

Treatment of advanced primary disease

Treatment of advanced or recurrent breast disease may include surgery, chemotherapy, hormonal therapy, and radiation. Factors influencing the type of treatment modality include the effectiveness of the primary treatment, menopausal status, because of the possibility of hormonal manipulation, and the desire for control of uncomfortable or intolerable symptoms of metastasis. If a tumor is causing pain or is draining, a simple mastectomy may be performed. If hormone receptors are available and the tumor is dependent upon estrogen, antiestrogens may be administered or oophorectomy or other endocrine surgery may be performed. If the woman does not respond to endocrine therapy or is not a candidate for it, chemotherapy may be instituted using single agents or combinations as described previously. Radiation may be used to control pain and shrink recurrent nodules or the breast tumor itself. Treatment of recurrent breast disease is highly individualized with emphasis on the longest remission possible with the selected treatment modality. The course of recurrent breast disease has periods of exacerbations and remissions and over time any or all of the described treatment modalities may be instituted.

Emphasis for nursing care at this time should be on helping the woman identify and manage the symptoms of advancing disease and the side effects of the various therapies. Since the most common sites of metastases are bone and lung, bone pain, pathological fractures, pleural effusions, and other respiratory complications may be present. Other sites of metastases include brain and viscera and involvement of these organs may also be present (McCorkle, 1973). While awaiting response from the selected therapy, the goal of nursing care should be to support the woman and help control distressing symptoms by whatever means are possible, such as, pain medication, respiratory hygiene, chest tubes, and dressing changes. At the same time, side effects of treatment need to be managed (nausea, stomatitis, diarrhea, fatigue, etc.).

A larger issue—facing death—may also be present when interacting with the woman with advanced breast disease and her family, and it needs to be addressed during this time. For in-depth examination of this topic see Moos (1977) and Weisman (1979).

Caring for the woman with advanced breast disease may at times appear to be overwhelming and the nurse may need to identify personal support systems to be able to maintain a therapeutic relationship with the woman and her family. Understanding the needs of the woman with advanced breast disease is essential for the primary nurse in both the inpatient and outpatient setting. A relationship can be established that enhances self-care and promotes well-being of the woman and her family.

SUMMARY

As prevention of breast cancer becomes a possibility and early detection a reality, the role of the nurse in these endeavors cannot be overemphasized. Because of her knowledge base as well as teaching ability, the nurse is an invaluable resource to a community interested in promoting health maintenance.

The controversy over appropriate treatment of breast cancer will continue probably for years to come because of the individual nature of the disease as well as the lengthy clinical investigation time needed to gather results about the effects of various therapies. The nurse may act as advocate for the woman confronted with this vast amount of sometimes confusing information. She may accept the responsibility in the community or inpatient setting to work with the woman and her significant others during all the phases of prevention, detection, and treatment. The nurse must be familiar with current medical and nursing research to implement important new findings in her practice.

Awareness of the nurse's own feelings toward the treatment of breast disease is an important prerequisite to successfully intervening with women who must make decisions regarding their disease.

REFERENCES

American Cancer Society: Cancer facts and figures '79, New York, 1978, The Society.

American Cancer Society, **30:**224-232, 1980.

Aguilera, D., and Messick, J.: Crisis intervention: theory and methodology, St. Louis, 1974, The C. V. Mosby Co.

Atkins, H., and others: Treatment of early breast cancer: a report after ten years of a clinical trial, Br. Med. J. 2:423-429, 1972.

Bonadona, G.: Combination chemotherapy as a adjuvant treatment in operable breast cancer, New Engl. J. Med. **294:**405-410, 1977.

Cammarata, A., Rosen, P., and Leis, H. P., Jr.: Breast biopsy: surgical aspects and the role of frozen sections and specimen radiography. In Gallager, H. S., and others, editors: The breast, St. Louis, 1978, The C. V. Mosby Co.

Carter, S., and others: Chemotherapy of cancer, New York, 1977, John Wiley & Sons.

Cohen, L.: Radiation response and recovery: radiobiological principles and their relation to clinical practice. In Schwartz, E. E., ed.: The biological basis of radiation therapy, Philadelphia, 1966, J. B. Lippincott, Co.

Cooperman, A. M., and Esselstyn, C. B.: Breast cancer: an overview, Surg. Clin. North Am. **58:**659-665, 1978.

Fisher, B., and others: L-phenylalanine mustard in the management of primary breast cancer, Cancer 39(6):2883-2901, 1977.

Foster, R. S., and others: Breast self-examination practices and breast cancer stage, New Engl. J. Med. **299:**265-270, 1978.

Gallup Organization: Woman's attitudes regarding breast cancer, Princeton, N.J., Nov. 1974.

Georgiade, N.: Reconstructive breast surgery, St. Louis, 1976, The C. V. Mosby Co., 1976.

Graf, M. S.: Sexual adjustment following mastectomy. Unpublished research paper, Milwaukee, 1977, Marquette University.

Greenwald, P., and others: Estimated effect of breast self examination and routine physician examinations on breast cancer mortality, New Engl. J. Med. **299**:271-273, 1978.

Haagensen, C.: Diseases of the breast, Philadelphia, 1971, W. B. Saunders Co.

Henderson, C., and Canellos, G. P.: Cancer of the breast—the past decade, New Engl. J. Med. **302**:17-30, 1980.

Hermann, R., and Steiger, E.: Modified radical mastectomy, Surg. Clin. North Am. **58**(4):743-753, 1978.

Gallup Poll. In Gallager, H. S., editors: Early breast cancer—detection and treatment, New York, 1975, John Wiley & Sons.

Horton, J., and Hill, G.: Clinical oncology, Philadelphia, 1977, W. B. Saunders.

Kaahe, S., and Johansen, H.: Simple mastectomy plus postoperative irradiation by the method of McWhirter for mammary carcinoma.

Kennedy, B. J.: New role of endocrine therapy in breast cancer. Radiation, Oncology, Biology, Physics **4**:469-472, 1978.

Klein, R.: A crisis to grow on, Cancer, December 2-7, 1971.

Leahy, I., and others: The nurse and radiotherapy, St. Louis, 1979, The C. V. Mosby Co.

Leis, H. P.: Current concepts in the surgical management of breast cancer, J. Reprod. Med. **24**:159-166, 1980.

Levene, M., and others: Primary radiation therapy for operable carcinoma of the breast, Surg. Clin. North Am. **58**(4):767-776, 1978.

Levene, M., and others: Treatment of carcinoma of the breast by radiation therapy, Cancer **39**(6):2840-2845, 1977.

McCorkle, R.: Coping with physical symptoms in metastatic breast cancer, Am. J. Nurs. **73**(6):1034-1038, 1979.

McGuire, W., and others: Current status of estrogen and progesterone receptors in breast cancer, Cancer **39**:2943-2947, 1977.

Mead, M.: Male and female: a study of the sexes in a changing world, New York, 1949, William Morrow and Co., Inc.

Moore, D. H., and Charney, H.: Breast cancer: etiology and possible prevention, Am. Sci. **63**:159, 1975.

Moos, R., editor: Coping with physical illness, New York, 1977, Plenum Medical Book Co.

National Cancer Institute and American Cancer Society Statement on X-ray Mammography in Screening for Breast Cancer, U.S. Department of Health Education and Welfare, Bethesda, Md., August 23, 1976.

Ogi, S.: Radiotherapy, cancer and the nurse. In Burkhalter, P., and Donley, D., editors: Dynamics of oncology nursing, New York, 1978, McGraw-Hill Book Co.

Prosnitz, M., and others: Radiation therapy as initial treatment for early stage cancer of the breast without mastectomy, Cancer **39**:917-923, 1977.

Renneker, R., and Cutler, M.: Psychological problems of adjustment to cancer of the breast, J.A.M.A. **148**:833, 1952.

Rubin, P., editor: Clinical oncology for medical students and physicians: a multidisciplinary approach, Rochester, 1978, American Cancer Society.

Rudolph, B.: Lymphedema following a radical mastectomy, Oncol. Nurs. Forum **6**(2):13-17, 1979.

Schain, W.: Psychological impact of the diagnosis of breast cancer on the patient. In Vaeth, J., editor: Frontiers of radiation therapy and oncology, vol. II, Basel, Switzerland, 1976, Zeitung.

Shapiro, S.: Evidence on screening for breast cancer in a randomized trial, Cancer **39**:2772-2782, 1977.

Stehlin, J. S., and others: Treatment of carcinoma of the breast, Surg. Gynecol. Obstet. **149**:911-922, 1979.

Strax, P.: Evaluation of screening programs for the early diagnosis of breast cancer, Surg. Clin. North Am. **58**:667-679, 1978.

Tryer, L. B., and Granzig, W. A.: Instructing patients in self-examination of the breast, Clin. Obstet. Gynecol. **18**:175-195, 1975.

Wallner, P., and others: Subtotal mastectomy and radiation therapy in the definitive management of localized breast malignancy, Am. J. Roentgen. **127**:505-507, 1976.

Warren, B.: Adjuvant chemotherapy for breast disease: the nurse's role, Cancer Nurs. **2**(1):32-37, 1979.

Weber, E., and Hellman, S.: Radiation as primary treatment for local control of breast carcinoma, J.A.M.A. **234**:608-611, 1975.

Weisman, H.: Coping with cancer, New York, 1979, McGraw-Hill Book Co.

Witkin, M. H.: Sex therapy and mastectomy, J. Sex Marital Ther. **1**:290-304, 1973.

Woods, N. F., and Earp, J.: Women with cured breast cancer, Nurs. Res. **27**(5):279-285, 1978.

UNIT FOUR

Women and health

18

Aging

Janet Larson Gelein
Pamela Heiple

What is the first thought that comes to mind when you think about growing older? Some women look to old age as the time to explore opportunities they never had time to initiate in the past. Others see it as a time when responsibilities toward others are lessened, leaving more energy for creativity, introspection, and self-development. However, because of our value systems, many American women look toward aging with ambivalence, if not with sorrow or rebellion. The high value American society places on youthful attractiveness makes women fear the aging process; for some women in our society, aging and beauty are mutually exclusive. The feelings women have about their bodies and lives as they age influence their attitudes toward health.

Because so many of our negative attitudes about aging are based on myths and stereotypes, expansion of our knowledge base about the normal process of aging will help us view this process more realistically. In this chapter, we will consider aging women and describe the change, loss, and growth experienced by females as they grow older. The first sections in this chapter will consider the meaning of midlife changes for women, and the last part will examine the challenges of the later years. In both the middle and later years there are biologic, social, and psychologic factors that influence the experiences of women in health and illness. Until recently we have had very little reliable data about these factors.

Much of the past research and literature on older women and health, and a great deal of what exists today, has been biased by ageism and sexism. Even though older women have long outnumbered elderly men and use health care services more frequently, there are few resources, basic research, or health care services that consider or provide for the special needs of older women. There is practically nothing written on preventive health care for elderly females; most of the literature from the women's health movement focuses on the reproduction issues of young women, and there is a significant lack of research on chronic illnesses in females.

This lack of services combined with the negative values associated with aging create a double challenge for older women and health care providers: ageism and sexism. As women, we are long overdue in accepting this challenge; it is time to consider the health status of older women and mechanisms for change. The number of older women in America is rapidly increasing. In 1900 there were approximately 3.1 million people aged 65 and over in the United States. In 1975, there were 24.4 million; the projections for year 2000 are 30.6 million and by the year 2030, there may be as many as 51.6 million elderly (Census, 1970). The majority of these elderly will be females, as they are today. This accelerating number of older women will increasingly demand quality health care, which is their right. To enhance our work with older women to maintain and improve their health, this chapter considers individual change in the middle and later years of women's lives and describes strategies that women may use individually or collectively to promote health as they age.

IMAGES AND STEREOTYPES OF MIDDLE-AGED WOMEN

Today's middle-aged menopausal women became wives and mothers during the era of the "feminine mystique" (Friedan, 1968). Following the insecurity and fear caused by World War II, the values of domestic and family life were at a premium. Staying home, raising a large family, and vacuuming the rugs while wearing stockings and heels were attributes of the ideal "feminine" women. About this same time psychologic theories of childrearing came into vogue and women were advised that they were directly responsible for the integrity of their children's personalities. These societal values and pressures, along with a general lack of opportunity, influenced many women to devote their energies to domestic and maternal responsibilities.

These women were also influenced by experiences with their mothers and grandmothers. Many of them grew up thinking menstruation was "the curse"; consequently, it was difficult for them to conceive of its initiation or termination (menopause) as a healthy, normal process. These images of menopause are reinforced by attitudes of health care providers, medical textbooks, and popular media.

We are all familiar with the media's stereotype of the middle-aged, menopausal woman. She is portrayed as red faced, emotionally labile, and in need of some kind of medicatior either tranquilizers or estrogen. This stereotype is used to the advantage of drug companies, which promise that their products will help return the irritable, possibly more assertive, menopausal woman back to her old self—passive, docile, and pleasing.

One of the many messages middle-aged women receive from this kind of image is that growing older is a process to be prevented, not enjoyed. Popular books on the market reinforce this image when they promise eternal youth in return for the price of a paperback. In addition, magazines that many middle-aged women read are full of advertisements for various methods of retaining "youthful attractiveness." Middle-aged women are usually portrayed as worrying about constipation or hemorrhoids, rarely are they viewed having fun.

Perpetuation of negative stereotypes in the media has several effects on women as consumers. Today's women are relatively psychologically minded; they have ready access to literature that prepares them for the "midlife crisis" and the "empty nest syndrome." It should be noted, however, that preparing someone for a developmental life event by labeling it a crisis may influence the person's perception of the event—in effect, creating anticipation of stress and possibly precipitating an actual crisis. Women who have been looking forward to the departure of children in the hope that they will be able to have more time for themselves may be confused by hearing that they are expected to experience the "empty nest syndrome." The actual scientific data regarding menopausal changes are so scanty that many women must rely on rumors and folklore for this information, the nature of which usually tends to be negative. The result of these stereotypes and images is that they tend to promote a self-fulfilling prophecy: the "midlife crisis."

In many ways, health professionals also perpetuate these myths. A glance through a leading gynecologic textbook (Novak, 1977) reveals that the chapter on the process of menopause is given the title, "The Management of the Menopause." Implications of this are twofold: (1) The menopause is equivalent to a disease process requiring treatment and (2) menopausal women have no control over changes during menopause and therefore must be "managed." The terms often used in texts in relation to menopause include such terms as "deficiency," "symptom," and "sexual decline." They all imply that menopause is something less than healthy,

that it is a disease process. Contrary to popular belief, menopause is a normal physiologic process—one phase of normal, healthy aging, as we will review in the following section.

PHYSIOLOGIC PROCESSES OCCURRING IN MIDLIFE

The climacteric (derived from the Greek word meaning "rung of the ladder") is the transition phase between reproductive and nonreproductive ability in the woman. During this phase a variety of physiologic changes occur, and the menopause, the actual cessation of the menses, is one part, usually occurring somewhere in the middle of the climacteric. The onset of menopause, similar to menarche, varies from woman to woman. While the age of onset for the majority of women is about 47, a natural menopause may start as early as age 35 or as late as age 60. The average age of menopause—absence of menstruation for one year—is 51 years. The popular belief that an early menarche predisposes to a late menopause is not substantiated. Various factors have been implicated in causing an early menopause. In addition to oophorectomy, excessive exposure to radiation, poor general health, prolonged breast-feeding, hypothyroidism with serious obesity, inadequate spacing between pregnancies, frequent abortions or miscarriages, and hard manual labor have been cited as determinants of early menopause (Boston Women's Health Book Collective, 1976).

Physiology of climacteric

The physiologic events of the climacteric can be divided into three phases: premenopausal, menopausal, and postmenopausal (Botella-Llusia, 1973). In the premenopausal phase the woman is still menstruating, but the menses may become irregular. The fertility index rapidly declines because of the progressive disappearance of corpus luteum activity. This results in gradual atresia of the ovarian follicles. This change is reflected in turn in the endometrium by a persistent state of proliferation, leading to the tendency of women in this phase to develop uterine fibroids and endometriosis. This phase corresponds to the beginning of estrogen decline.

In the menopausal phase, the ovaries' inability to respond to gonadotropins results in the cessation of the menses with resultant infertility. It will be recalled that menstruation is dependent on a negative feedback system, which acts in a rhythmic fashion (Fig. 18-1). The estrogen and progesterone secreted by the corpus luteum exert negative feedback on the hypothalamic adenohypophyseal complex. Progesterone acts specifically to suppress luteinizing hormone (LH), while estrogen regulates follicle-stimulating hormone (FSH). Because

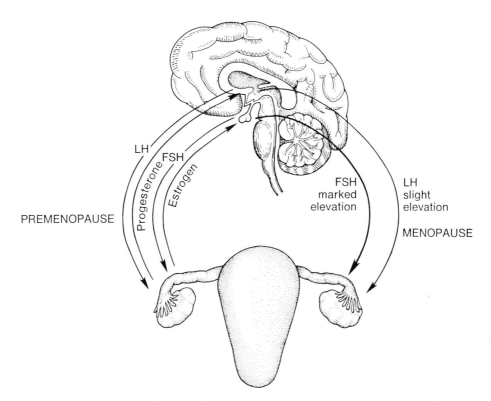

Fig. 18-1. A comparison of neuroendocrine mechanisms during premenopause and menopause. (Adapted from Hertz, R., and Kase, N.: Estrogen for postmenopausal women? Patient Care **2**[3]:56-66, 1972.)

of the decline in ovarian hormone production, estrogen and progesterone levels drop and gonadotropin production is no longer inhibited. Consequently, the pituitary becomes overactive and FSH and LH are produced in large quantities.

It is thought that this hyperactivity and a possible increase in ACTH activity result in stimulation of the interstitial tissue of the ovary and the adrenals giving rise to a compensatory production of steroids (Botella-Llusia, 1977). The ovaries become unable to respond to the FSH and LH and the hyperactivity soon ceases. However, it is evident that some menopausal women produce estrogen in the absence of a functioning corpus luteum. If some women can maintain normal hormonal levels, why then does the bleeding cease? Although vascular phenomena and the level of estrogen synthesis determine menstrual bleeding, menstruation is precipitated by the sudden drop in the estrogen level. It is not the quantity of estrogen activity that regulates menstruation, but the fluctuations in estrogen levels. Although the menopausal woman may still be producing estrogen, the alternating rhythmicity in estrogen synthesis is lost.

Menstruation does not always cease abruptly. Although hormone withdrawal deflections become less abrupt, they may be of sufficient magnitude to reach the menstrual threshold and cause bleeding. Eventually, the deflections plateau to below threshold level and the bleeding stops. In the postmenopausal stage of the climacteric the majority of women appear to have lost all trace of ovarian activity and signs of estrogen decline may be present.

Effects of estrogen decline

While the loss of progesterone primarily affects the woman's fertility, estrogen decline can have systemic effects, perhaps disrupting the physiologic equilibrium of the entire body. The list of estrogen-related disorders occurring among older women varies from source to source, reflecting the present state of knowledge. Much research is presently being done to explore the effects of estrogen decline and subsequent replacement therapy. However, at this time there are no studies on middle-aged women that examine the multifaceted parameters of health, including the impacts of social, psychologic, and physiologic changes, to determine the interrelationships of all these dimensions of health. Consequently, we are forced to examine each of these separately, recognizing that each woman responds individually to these changes. It is the combined impact of these changes and their interrelationships that determine the level of health maintained or achieved during this period of life.

Much of the research on estrogen decline is inconclusive, yet there is general agreement that vasomotor instability (hot flashes) and atrophic vaginitis are menopausal disorders. Some investigators believe that joint and muscle pain, urinary frequency, painful micturition, cardiovascular disorders, and osteoporosis also have a relationship to estrogen decline. We believe it is premature to attribute all these disorders to menopause. In the following section we will examine the role decreased estrogen levels may play in selected disorders and describe the therapeutic and self-help measures that may alleviate or prevent discomfort associated with these changes.

Vasomotor instability

"Hot flashes" are the sensation of overwhelming heat suddenly spreading from the chest upward over the neck, face, and arms. They usually last from several seconds to a minute; they occur most often at night and may disturb sleep. The skin of the affected areas may become flushed, and the woman may perspire excessively. There may be increased pulse and respiration rates. Excitement, exercise, intake of alcohol, eating, and other situations of increased heat production tend to provoke hot flashes.

Although the precise mechanism responsible for menopausal vasomotor instability is unknown, there is some indication that women who have experienced marked premenstrual changes are most disturbed by flashes and night sweats in later life. On the basis of these data, the cause of vasomotor instability has been attributed to a delicate balance in the relationship between feedback from the ovaries and activity of the hypothalamus and pituitary gland (specifically, the high levels of FSH that result from pituitary overactivity). Others suggest that estrogens may cause vasomotor instability by "sensitizing" the autonomic nervous system (Detre et al., 1978). Hot flashes stop once the woman's body adjusts to the new levels of estrogen. Although not every woman experiences hot flashes, it is one of the two physiologic phenomena most characteristic of the menopause (the other being atrophic vaginitis) and therefore deserves more attention by researchers.

Exogenous estrogens are sometimes prescribed for the relief of hot flashes and are discussed in the section dealing with estrogen replacement therapy (ERT). The following nutritional measures may be helpful to the woman who is troubled with hot flashes and who cannot or chooses not to risk the side effects associated with ERT.

Ginseng. Ginseng is the common name for several species of herbs that have been used in Oriental healing practices for centuries. It has been found to have a general "normalizing" action on the body and apparently is particularly helpful in facilitating adaptation to heat stress (Seaman and Seaman, 1977). It is believed that ginseng eventually changes the metabolic rate; however, its precise mechanism of action is unknown. Although there has yet to be a scientifically controlled study exploring the effects of ginseng on menopausal discomfort, many women have found that it either cures or diminishes the intensity of their hot flashes. Although untoward effects have not as yet been reported from the use of ginseng (because we know so little about it), its use in the absence of symptoms or stress is not recommended (Seaman and Seaman, 1977). Ginseng has a positive effect on energy levels and, therefore, it may overstimulate women with hyperactive tendencies. The exact dosage of ginseng varies with body weight. There are many types of ginseng currently on the market (in health food stores) and care must be taken to determine the authenticity of the product.

Vitamin B complex. Vitamin B complex aids in the detoxification and elimination of FSH and LH by the liver. While adding supplements of this nutrient to the diet may not eliminate hot flashes, it may aid in their control (Tyson, 1978). Wheat germ, yogurt, whole grains, brewer's yeast, liver, and milk are good sources of the B vitamins.

Vitamin E. Women taking vitamin E for menopausal discomfort have reported that it promotes energy and feelings of well-being, alleviates leg cramps, and relieves hot flashes (Seaman and Seaman, 1977). Increases in FSH and LH production have been related to vitamin E deficiency. Because the body's requirement for E increases during periods of general stress or extra demands on the reproductive system, menopausal women may be deficient, leading to increased FSH production, which is thought to be the cause of hot flashes.

Vitamin E takes longer to relieve hot flashes than does estrogen replacement (ERT) (about 2 to 4 weeks) and may be contraindicated in women with diabetes, hypertension, or rheumatic heart conditions. High doses may cause gastric distress, which abates when the vitamin is taken in its dry, powdered form. Seaman and Seaman (1977) reported that the effectiveness of a combination of vitamin E and ginseng almost equals that of ERT in alleviating hot flashes.

Dosages of E vary according to the nutritional status of the woman (women who smoke and eat a large amount of processed foods are more likely to be deficient). It has been recommended that women who are having marked hot flashes start with 100 IU and gradually increase the dose over a period of weeks or months until relief is obtained (Seaman and Seaman, 1977). This does not apply to the woman with hypertension, diabetes, or heart disease, who should consult a physician before supplementation is started. Dietary sources of E include vegetable oils, wheat germ, soybeans, peanuts, and spinach.

Changes in genital tissue

Vulva. The skin of the perineum is particularly responsive to estrogen decline. The epidermis thins, causing the labia majora and minora to become flatter. The introitus tends to shrink and dyspareunia may result. Lubrication such as K-Y jelly can be used during intercourse to prevent discomfort.

Vagina. The vagina loses elasticity and becomes shorter and narrower because of the increase in submucosal connective tissue. The usual rugosity is also lost. Thinning of the vaginal epithelium makes it prone to bleeding. The lack of estrogen causes the usually acidic vaginal secretions to become more alkaline, thus predisposing to infections. This increased susceptibility to irritation and vaginal infections may produce symptoms of atrophic vaginitis, which usually respond well to the local application of a vaginal cream. Some women have reported that vitamin E supplements over a long period of time alleviate dryness of the vaginal tissues.

One of the most important things a woman can do to maintain pliability of vaginal tissue is to continue an active sex life. Although the media often portray women experiencing menopause as asexual, a survey among menopausal women found that 65% of those questioned maintained that their sexuality had remained unchanged by the menopause. One half of the remaining women thought sexual relations become more enjoyable after menopause; the other half, less than 20% of the total, stated that sexual activity became less important (Neugarten and Kraines, 1965).

The supporting connective tissue and muscular supports of the vagina and the surrounding organs may also be subject to estrogen-related atrophic changes. This may lead to the development of uterovaginal prolapse, rectocele, and cystocele. Perineal exercises such as Kegel exercises improve muscle tone and may be helpful.

Uterus. The progressive decrease in the thickness of the myometrium causes a marked decrease in size and weight of the uterus after menopause. The cervix shrinks and becomes pale. Relaxation of the uterosacral ligaments may fail to keep the uterus in the usual anteroflexed position. As discussed earlier, as women approach the menopause, the pattern of the menses changes and becomes more irregular. Abnormal (excessive or prolonged) bleeding should always be investigated. The timing and cause of the bleeding should be assessed. For example, postmenopausal bleeding (occurring 6 months to 1 year after the last menstrual period) is more serious than perimenopausal bleeding (occurring around the time of menopause) (Notelovitz, 1978).

Ovaries. During the menopause, the ovaries gradually decrease in size and are normally nonpalpable. Follicular activity is rare in women past the age of 50, and an increase in fibroblasts and connective tissue replaces the follicles. However, the ovarian stroma remains functional and capable of synthesizing androgens and, to a lesser extent, estrogens. Although there is a marked decrease in fertility during the climacteric, because ovulation occurs sporadically up to the time of the menopause (and sometimes after), it is advisable for menopausal women to continue using contraception for one year after the last menstrual period. Because oral contraceptives are associated with an increased risk of venous thrombosis and myocardial infarction in women over age 40, menopausal women should be encouraged to use other methods, such as the vaginal diaphragm or a condom and foam (Notelovitz, 1978).

Urinary frequency and painful micturition

There is no evidence that estrogen directly affects the bladder itself. However, it has been shown that estrogen decline in postmenopausal women may result in atrophic distal urethritis and stricture formation. This affects bladder function by producing obstruction, raised residual urine, and ascending infection with symptoms of urinary frequency and dysuria (Smith, 1976). Women can be advised to maintain or increase their fluid intake to decrease urine concentration and bacterial multiplication. A number of drugs in various combinations may also be therapeutic in some situations.

Effects on skin

Skin is a major target for estrogenic action. At the menopause, estrogen decline causes a negative nitrogen balance with diminution of muscle, which is then replaced by fibrous tissue (Cope, 1976). The epidermis becomes thin, and subcutaneous fat atrophies and loses elasticity, which accounts for the tendency of the breasts to sag and for the previously described changes in vaginal tissue. Exogenous estrogen, taken internally, is usually helpful in treating dryness and menopause-related changes in the vaginal epithelium; however, its beneficial effects on facial skin have not been scientifically demonstrated.

These changes, which present no physiologic malfunction or disorder, are often the most threatening to aging women because they represent the visible loss of youth. A recent study demonstrated that women's concern about facial attractiveness is highest during middle age. While women who are younger or older can separate their appearance from their activities, interests, and feelings, middle-aged women, especially those between 45 and 55 years, are less able to do so. It has also been found that middle-aged women, significantly more than any other age/sex group, equate attractiveness with youthfulness (Nowak, 1977). The cosmetics industry uses this concern of middle-aged women to its advantage.

Cardiovascular disorders

The relationship of estrogen to coronary heart disease is uncertain. The premise that estrogens protect premenopausal women from heart disease was based on two observations: (1) the sex advantage that younger women possess (death rates from coronary artery disease are five to eight times greater in men than in women ages 25 to 55) disappears after the menopause, and (2) estrogen administration reduces serum levels of low-density lipoprotein and cholesterol, which correlate with increased risk for coronary heart disease in both sexes. However, double blind clinical trials based on this premise show that instead of protecting male survivors of myocardial infarctions, estrogen administration results in a dose-related increased risk of recurrence (Ryan, 1976). Data from the Framingham study further complicate our understanding of the role estrogen decline plays in heart disease in women. In a cohort of 2873 women followed for 24 years, the incidence of coronary heart disease increased, along with the severity of presenting symptoms. Postmenopausal women taking estrogen replacements were found to have a double risk of coronary heart disease (Gordon et al., 1978).

As the general death rate from coronary artery disease increases with age in both sexes, middle-aged menopausal women are a target group for preventive counseling (Ryan, 1976). Cigarette smoking, hypertension, stress, hyperlipidemia, and obesity are all risk factors over which women may have some control.

Musculoskeletal disorders

Both osteoporosis and joint and muscle pain have been attributed to estrogen decline. Both men and women reach peak bone mass at about age 35. After this, either a plateau is maintained or loss begins. It has been demonstrated that the rate of loss is greater for women and statistically associated with the menopause.

Bone loss starts earlier in oophorectomized women, indicating that time after menopause is more strongly related to bone loss than is age (Heaney, 1976). The symptomatic manifestations of osteoporosis (incidence of fracture) are usually present about 10 years after the cessation of menses in 25% of postmenopausal women (Martin, 1978). Over the past three decades there have been numerous contradictory theories about the cause

and treatment of osteoporosis. We will only consider some of these involving the role of estrogen.

It is now believed that estrogen acts on bone by suppressing the activation of the mesenchymal process involved in bone remodeling, the net effect of which is the reduction of bone resorption and thin bone formation (Heaney, 1976). When this stabilizing influence is lost with menopausal decline in estrogen, there is an increased loss of bone substance caused by resorption resulting in a decrease in mass. Pain occurs secondary to fracture and is most common in the thoracic and lumbar spine, the femoral neck, or the distal radius and ulna. These fractures are usually associated with mild stress.

Recent evidence has identified the homeostatic balance between calcium and phosphorus as a causative factor in osteoporosis. A number of mechanisms act to maintain normal serum calcium levels; exchange of calcium between blood and bone is most likely responsible for minute-to-minute regulation, whereas long-term calcium homeostasis is maintained by the activity of osteoblasts and osteoclasts (Jowsey, 1978). These processes are complex and involve the parathyroid glands, vitamin D, the kidneys, and the intestine. Parathyroid hormone acts directly on the kidney to decrease renal excretion of calcium and also increases intestinal absorption of calcium in a process involving vitamin D. This is significant to the development of osteoporosis because if the intestines absorb a lesser amount of calcium than the kidneys excrete, bone is lost to make up the deficit. When serum levels of calcium fall, parathyroid hormone secretion is stimulated and osteoclastic bone resorptive activity increases, thus maintaining a normal serum calcium level (Jowsey, 1978).

Data from recent research indicate that imbalance in the calcium:phosphorus ratio may be the most significant factor in the development of osteoporosis. The ratio of calcium to phosphorus in the adult should approximate 1. However, factors such as the increased ingestion of foods with a high phosphorus content (bread, cereal, soft drinks, and foods high in phosphate-based preservative) and the reduced ability of older people to absorb calcium from the intestines contribute to an imbalance in the relationship caused by phosphorus excess. The ingestion of foods with a high phorphorus content causes a rise in serum inorganic phosphorus concentration, which stimulates parathyroid hormone release. This has the effect of releasing calcium from bone to equalize the serum calcium-phosphorus balance, thus producing a phosphate-induced bone loss over time.

Prevention of osteoporosis has several nutritional implications. Women should be encouraged to select foods high in calcium and avoid those having a high phosphorus content. The calcium requirement for the postmenopausal woman is 1.4 Gm per day, which is higher than the minimum daily requirement (Jowsey, 1978). Unfortunately, most foods that are high in calcium, such as dairy products, are also high in phosphorus. The few foods that contain a large amount of calcium and little phosphorus (sesame seeds, seaweed, turnip greens) are not part of the average woman's diet. Therefore, some authorities recommend that calcium supplementation be started at age 25 and continued throughout the life span. It has been demonstrated in persons with osteoporosis that calcium supplements effectively suppress secretion of parathyroid hormone (Jowsey, 1976). While this practice may have some value as a preventive measure, some women may prefer just to decrease their intake of soft drinks and other high-phosphate foods while increasing their intake of cheddar cheese, milk, sesame seeds, and other foods with a high calcium content.

Other nutritional aspects of osteoporosis include the effects of vitamin D, fluoride, and protein excess. Vitamin D deficiency is rare in the United States; however, elderly women with poor dietary practices may be subject to vitamin A deficiency, which could cause bone loss by interfering with calcium utilization.

Both fluoride and calcium are necessary for bone density; however, fluoride alone causes bone disease by removing calcium from bone in the process of mineral exchange. It is difficult to approximate daily individual intake of fluoride because of the variability of fluoride content in drinking water and other fluids.

It has also been suggested that diets high in protein can result in bone loss (Martin, 1978). High nitrogen levels resulting from metabolism of excessive proteins require increased calcium for the kidney to buffer the acidic waste products. Because of the lack of supply to meet this increased demand (calcium absorption does not increase), calcium is taken from the bones and negative calcium balance ensues.

Another factor found to be significant in the development of osteoporosis is lack of exercise. The amount of calcium deposited in the bone is determined by the load the bone must carry; therefore, the more the bone is used, the denser it becomes. It has been found that the incidence of osteoporosis is lower in populations who exercise regularly throughout the life span. Exercise, or lack of it, may also play a part in the joint and muscle pains that some menopausal women experience. Although the actual relationship to estrogen decline is unclear, it is thought that these pains result from a decrease in muscular strength with a reduced ability to disperse the build-up of lactic acid after exercise. Laxity of the ligaments is also a factor (Cope, 1976). Animal studies have shown that exercise increases the strength of the ligamentous structures, thereby decreasing the

chance of fracture resulting from minimal trauma (Seaman and Seaman, 1977).

Along with its beneficial effects on bone and muscle, regular exercise can help the menopausal woman maintain her body weight (frequently a problem because of decreased caloric requirements) and improve circulation. Exercise also can promote feelings of well-being. Of course, any exercise program should be initiated gradually. Women who have disk problems or osteoarthritis of the spine should avoid jogging; however, brisk walking, swimming, bicycling, and gardening are enjoyable and beneficial (Tyson, 1978). Many women find muscle stretching exercises or yoga helpful (Page, 1977).

Behavioral effects of estrogen decline

Is there a relationship between estrogen decline and psychologic symptomatology, or do we look for these disturbances because they validate our stereotype of the middle-aged, menopausal woman?

Some of our behavioral stereotypes of the menopausal woman originate from psychoanalytic theories. Benedek (1952), a psychoanalyst, has proposed that a woman responds to estrogens with an increased tendency for heterosexual activity, and heterosexual desire increases and reaches its height at the time of ovulation. Then the progestins take over and the woman's emotional interest turns toward herself, pregnancy, and children. According to Benedek, a woman must have a personality that permits her to be passive and to be cared for so that she can "give in" to her physiologic needs with pleasure. She describes the woman's desire to have control over her destiny as a "conflict of feminine development" that generates emotional tension. This tension is neutralized by hormonal function during the years of sexual maturity; however, at menopause this tension may become manifest because of the decline of these "hormonal tranquilizers," and the woman may become irritable, angry, and ultimately depressed.

Because of the lack of definitive research, our knowledge about the relationships of hormones to behavior in menopausal women is too scanty to make a fair judgment as to the validity of psychoanalytic theories. Other theories suggest that the autonomic nervous system develops a sensitivity to estrogen and therefore becomes dependent upon it for balance. The estrogen decline in menopause causes disruption of this balance, which is then reflected in the body systems that are under the control of the autonomic nervous system. Some suggest that the hypothalamus is involved and that dysfunctions in the relationship between the hypothalamus and the central nervous system cause the psychologic symptoms of irritability, anxiety, confusion, and depression (Bardwick, 1971).

Table 18-1. Estimates of estrogen use*

Study	Population	Results (incidence)	Duration
Stadel and Weiss (1975)	Women in King and Pierce Counties, Wash.	51% of the women reported estrogen use for more than 3 months	Median use was over 10 years
Pfeffer (1977)	Postmenopausal women living in a retirement community	15% used estrogens: use continued into 7th, 8th, and 9th decades, but use declined after age 70	Mean duration was 10.5 months for most recent continuous use

*From Woods, N. F.: The hormone controversy. Presented to the Women's Information Center, University of Washington, Seattle, 1979.

Recent data suggest that there may be a relationship between estrogen decline and depression in menopause. A significant positive correlation has been found between total estrogen concentration and the level of free tryptophan in the plasma (Alyward, 1976). Tryptophan is the precursor of serotonin, a biogenic amine thought to be related to depression. A decreased level of free plasma tryptophan has been found in some depressed people. Research indicates that natural estrogens act to increase the availability of free plasma tryptophan for synthesis of serotonin (Alyward, 1976). Therefore, as estrogen levels decrease, the amount of available tryptophan would decrease causing a biologic state that predisposes to depression. Studies have been done to test the effect of exogenous estrogen in alleviating depression in middle-aged women; however, most of them have failed to control for intervening variables and therefore are inconclusive.

While the possibility of a hormonal basis for some behavior changes occurring in menopause cannot be discounted, the effects of the other physiologic changes must be considered. It is reasonable to propose that a woman who has her sleep constantly disturbed by hot flashes and night sweats will be tired and irritable. Headaches may also result from fluid retention. Women at this age are also adjusting to several major role changes, all of which may increase stress and contribute to feelings of well-being or illness. Each woman needs to be assessed from social, psychologic, and biologic frameworks.

Estrogen replacement therapy (ERT)

The consideration of menopause as an "estrogen deficiency disease" has lead to the use of exogenous estrogens to treat menopausal changes. It was formerly thought that estrogen's "magical" youth-preserving properties would help women stay "feminine" forever. However, aside from the fact that this claim has proved false, research has shown that treatment of the menopausal woman with exogenous estrogens may present serious risks.

The most serious potential risk is that of endometrial carcinoma. In a retrospective study, Smith et al (1975) compared 317 women having adenocarcinoma of the cervix with matched controls and found that the risk of endometrial cancer was 4.5 times greater among women who had been receiving ERT. When other variables (e.g., obesity, hypertension, age) were controlled, it was found that the risk is greater for women who had no other predisposing factors.

Another retrospective study performed by Zeil and Finkle (1975) used ninety-four patients matched with 188 controls to examine the relationship of duration of ERT to risk of cancer. They found that the risk ratio for women who used ERT from 1 to 4.9 years was 5.6 times higher than the normal population. When the length of exposure to ERT was increased to 7 or more years, the relative risk increased to 13.9. Another study indicates that ERT users have a chance of developing endometrial cancer eight times greater than women who do not use exogenous estrogens. When the relationship between dosage of ERT and risk was examined, it was found that as the dosage increases, so does the risk (Mack et al., 1976). On the basis of these results and other studies, the United States Food and Drug Administration has recently modified the labeling of exogenous estrogens to inform the user of the risk of endometrial cancer. As Table 18-1 indicates, estrogen use is common in women of menopausal age. One study shows that despite the fact that only 26% of the women interviewed reported severe trouble with hot flashes, nearly 50% had used estrogen for 3 or more months. Although women not at risk for endometrial cancer (e.g., women who had had a hysterectomy) were included among the estrogen users, there still was a substantial difference between the percentage of women using estrogens and those with discomfort from flushing. A later study indicates that estrogens are used well into later life (Pfeffer, 1977).

The relationship between breast cancer and ERT also is presently under investigation. Although one study reports an increased risk of breast cancer among ERT users, it has come under criticism for failing to provide an adequate control group (Hoover et al., 1976).

The cardiovascular effects of exogenous estrogens in male heart patients were discussed in a previous section. Kase (1976) concludes that there is strong evidence of an increased risk of thromboembolic disease, strokes,

Table 18-2. Association between exogenous estrogen and endometrial carcinoma*

Study	Population	Results
Smith et al. (1975)	317 patients with adenocarcinoma of the endometrium were compared with 317 patients who had other gynecologic neoplasms, matched for age at diagnosis and year of diagnosis	Risk of endometrial cancer was 4.5 times greater among women exposed to estrogen therapy than in women not exposed to estrogen
Ziel and Finkle (1975)	94 patients with endometrial cancer from the Kaiser Permanente Medical Center in Los Angeles were each compared with 2 controls selected from the health plan and matched for date of birth and zip code	Risk of endometrial cancer was estimated to be 7.6 times greater among women exposed to estrogen than among women not exposed. Risk increased with duration of exposure: $\widehat{RR} = 5.6$ for 1-4.9 years $\widehat{RR} = 13.9$ for 7 or more years
Mack et al. (1976)	All (N = 63) residents of an affluent retirement community who had endometrial cancer were compared with women from the same community without endometrial cancer (matched on age, martial status)	Risk of developing endometrial cancer for women taking estrogens was 8 times greater than the risk for women not taking estrogens, risk was greater at higher doses of estrogen
Antunes et al. (1979)	451 women with endometrial cancer were compared with 888 women patients without endometrial cancer and from services other than gynecology or psychiatry; were matched by hospital, age, race, and date of admission	Risk of developing endometrial cancer for women taking estrogens was 6 times that for women not taking estrogens. Risk associated with cyclic use was as great as that for continuous use

*From Woods, N. F.: The hormone controversy. Presented to the Women's Information Center, University of Washington, Seattle, 1979.

and coronary artery disease with ERT. These risk are known to increase with age. Estrogen replacement therapy also has been known to contribute to the risk of hypertension, gallbladder disease, disturbed lipid metabolism, and decreased glucose tolerance.

What are the advantages of ERT? Do they outweigh the risks? Exogenous estrogens can help to alleviate the discomfort of hot flashes and atrophic vaginitis. Some believe that ERT is helpful in the prevention of osteoporosis. It is thought that ERT restores positive calcium balance by decreasing the elevated plasma calcium and phosphate levels found in menopausal women and by decreasing the tubal resorption of phosphate. However, to be effective in preventing osteoporosis ERT must be instituted early, before serious loss of bone density (Kase, 1976).

Women who choose to take ERT should be given the lowest effective dose. Since the discovery that the presence of estrone may be linked to endometrial cancer, controversy has ensued regarding the type of estrogen that should be given. It has been discovered that estrone is synthesized in the adipose tissue of menopausal women; therefore, it may be preferable to use estriol or estradiol preparations to keep the level of estrone at a minimum (Notelovitz, 1978b).

Estrogen is usually taken in 3-week cycles. Because of the recent association of endometrial hyperplasia with atypical adenomatous hyperplasia, many physicians are presently encouraging the use of a progestin during the last week of estrogen administration to initiate shedding of the endometrium. Women on this type of regimen should be prepared for the continuation of their monthly menses.

Absolute contraindications to ERT include diseases of the liver, gallbladder, and pancreas; sickle cell anemia; history of deep venous thrombosis and pulmonary embolism; cerebrovascular disease; history of myocardial infarction; and estrogen-dependent tumors of the breast and uterus (Lauritzen, 1978). Since obesity, diabetes, and hypertension have been found to increase the risk for endometrial cancer, women with any of these risk factors should be carefully monitored.

A thorough physical examination should be performed before the initiation of ERT. The examination should include measurement of weight and blood pressure, thorough breast and pelvic examinations, Pap smear, and endometrial biopsy. Fasting plasma levels of glucose, cholesterol, and triglyceride should be determined in addition to serum antithrombin III levels. Follow-up at 3 and 9 months after the initiation of ERT is recommended (Notelovitz, 1978a).

The decision the woman makes to initiate ERT must be an informed one. The risks and benefits of ERT should be fully explored and alternatives, such as nutritional supplementation and exercise programs presented. Some women may have severe discomfort that can be alleviated only by exogenous estrogens. However, it is our hope that support and knowledge of sound health practices can prevent or alleviate much of the menopausal woman's discomfort.

Women's perceptions of menopause

We have explored some of the menopausal changes thought to have a physiologic basis. How do women experience these changes? What is their perception of the process of the menopause and its implications?

Neugarten and Kraines (1965) were among the first to directly seek information from women about the reality of menopausal changes and their attitudes toward them. Their sample of 460 women included women aged 18 to 54 divided into five age groups. The women between the ages of 45 and 54 were divided into two groups: those who were either pre- or postmenopausal, and those who were experiencing the menopause at the time of the study. The subjects were given a checklist consisting of twenty-eight somatic, psychosomatic, and psychologic symptoms and were asked to indicate which symptoms they had recently experienced.* Results indicate that adolescents and menopausal women had the largest number of symptoms, while postmenopausal women had the fewest. Adolescents tended to have more psychologic symptoms (crying spells, feelings of fright) while menopausal women generally reported more somatic symptoms (hot flashes, weight gain). On the basis of these results, Neugarten and Kraines concluded that the stress experienced by women during adolescence and menopause is related to endocrine changes. Over the years, the middle-aged woman develops more effective means of coping with biologic stress, which is reflected in her tendency to report fewer psychologic symptoms.

How do women feel about the process of menopause? In another study, Neugarten et al (1968) found that there were no significant differences in the views of middle-aged women classified as premenopausal, menopausal, or postmenopausal. As a group, these women tended to minimize the significance of menopause; only four of 100 women viewed it as a major source of worry. Fear of their husband's death, cancer, and just getting older were the main concerns of the women. In this study, severity of menopausal symptoms was correlated with more negative experiences in the areas of menstruation, first sexual experience, pregnancy, and childbirth.

In another, more recent survey, the members of the Boston Women's Health Collective (1976) mailed out questionnaires inquiring about attitudes and menopausal symptoms to women aged 25 to 60 years. Of the 484 respondents, most were living in large cities or suburbs, three fourths had children, and about three fourths of the menopausal and postmenopausal women worked outside the home (volunteer work included). The results

of the survey indicate that younger women generally feel more fearful and negative about menopause than do older women. As in Neugarten's study, postmenopausal women indicate a general lack of concern regarding menopausal changes. Respondents were also asked to complete a symptom checklist (all of the symptoms were associated with the menopause; however, hot flashes and vaginal dryness were not included). Results show that more symptoms were checked more frequently by women in the 25 to 40 age group: the fewest symptoms were checked by women over 60. (It would have been interesting to see if employed women had more or fewer symptoms than those who were unemployed.) These women were also asked to describe menopausal changes as they experienced them. Responses range from "relief" and "delight that childbearing years were coming to a close" to "tearfulness" and "unexplainable period of nervousness and irritation." Generally, about two thirds of the menopausal and postmenopausal women feel neutral or positive about menopausal changes, while one third feel clearly negative. Ninety percent feel either neutral or positive about the loss of childbearing ability.

The results of these studies lead one to question the popular image of the middle-aged, menopausal woman. Although many women do experience some degree of physiologic discomfort, the menopause does not seem to be as much of a problem for women as the media portray. It is interesting that younger women have the most negative attitudes, while women who have experienced the menopause view it more positively. Perhaps younger women view the menopause as an undeniable indicator of aging, a process that society identifies as undesirable. The knowledge that severity of menopausal symptoms is correlated with other negative reproductive and sexual experiences has important implications for prevention. Perhaps if these "high-risk" women were identified early, counseling and teaching about self-help measures could prevent some of their discomfort.

ROLE CHANGE IN MIDLIFE

We have explored the physiologic changes that women may experience in midlife. For many women, midlife also is a time of role change and a chance for growth. Changes in maternal role expectations are incurred with the "launching" of the children. Many women choose to assume the role of worker or student at this time and experience the process of "re-entry." For some women, changes in the role of daughter ensue because of the illness or death of a parent. Also, women who are married may experience changes in the marital relationship as a result of their own role change or that of their spouse.

This section will explore the nature of these changes

---

*Since most studies use the term "symptom" to describe menopausal changes, we will use this term in discussing their results.

as women have experienced them. Since one of our images of the midlife woman is derived from the notion that she "falls apart" when children leave home, the majority of this section will be spent discussing changes in the maternal role.

Changes in the maternal role

Does the departure of the children indeed precipitate the crisis of the "empty nest syndrome"? It is interesting that the term "empty nest," a term used indiscriminately to refer to this period in midlife, was initially defined as "the temporal association of *clinical depression* with the cessation of childrearing" (Deykin, 1966). The continued use of this term in reference to the midlife change in maternal role expectations perpetuates the idea that this process constitutes a crisis for women. Whether or not a crisis occurs depends on how the outcome of the change is perceived. Some women indeed may be highly invested in the maternal role and unable to cope with the changes in role behaviors and expectations incurred by the departure of the children; they consider loss to be the outcome of this change. These women may experience a crisis at this time. However, many women are able to utilize successful coping mechanisms in adapting to this role change. They see the outcome as a gain—they have more time for themselves or can pursue a career.

Many variables influence a woman's ability to cope successfully with this role change and reap the benefits of having more time for herself. This section will explore the variables of personality style and sociocultural factors as they relate to the woman's ability to adapt.

Personality style

Proponents of the "empty nest" theory believe that it is a woman's intense identification with the mothering role that predisposes to adjustment problems when the children leave. Psychoanalytic theorists believe that this identification is biologically (hormonally) determined, while more contemporary theorists believe it is a result of sex-role socialization. A woman's sense of identity and self-esteem have been linked to her ability to successfully perform the traditional mothering role (Bardwick, 1971). This would seem to indicate that women who hold traditional role stereotypes and live in traditional role settings will have more difficulty than nontraditional women adjusting to the changes in the mothering role that occur in middle age. However, cross-cultural studies have shown that women identified as "traditional" and "liberated" adapt better to midlife changes than women in a transitional kind of life-style (Williams, 1977). It has been suggested that a key factor in how the woman adapts to changes at this time may be the "fit" between her personality and social role (Livson, 1976).

Livson obtained data on the patterns of adjustment of twenty-four "psychologically healthy" women between the ages of 40 and 50 years and found two distinct styles of adjustment. The "traditionals" were women who at 50 were conventional, sociable, and nurturing. They placed high value on closeness with others and were considered to possess the traditional attributes of femininity, having minimal conflict between their personalities and social role. Their way of coping with midlife changes was to continue to invest themselves in interpersonal relationships. The second group, the "independents," were women who at 50 were described as intellectual, achievement-oriented, and unconventional. As opposed to the "traditionals," who since adolescence had placed a high value on socializing, these women valued achievement and "doing." There was less of a match between their personalities and social roles; consequently, these women experienced conflict and, by age 40, they were depressed and unable to use their intelligence or creativity in an adaptive way. However, when the children left home, they were freed from the constraints of the traditional role and able to reacquaint themselves with their intellectual interests and ambitions.

This study points out that a woman's individuality must be taken into account when helping her to prepare for and cope with midlife role changes. Women who fit the "traditional" pattern may find support groups or involvement in organizations that encourage the formation of interpersonal relationships to be particularly helpful. Promoting adaptation for "independent" women at this time may consist of supporting a return to work or school.

How likely is it that the need for mobilization of coping resources will arise with the departure of the children? What does research actually reveal about women's responses to this event? Table 18-3 is a summary of the "empty nest" research gathered thus far. These studies show great variation as to design, indices of measurement, and characteristics of the sample. Part of the difficulty in attempting to identify actual changes that women experience in the "empty nest" or "postparental" period* is caused by the variations in definitions of this time period. For example, in one study "empty nest" was defined as total cessation of childrearing in the past 10 years, while "empty nest" criteria for another study was considered to be the departure of just one child from the home. It is also evident from the table that most studies using nonhospitalized women as subjects demonstrated overall high satisfaction during this period. However, when the results are examined more carefully, differences begin to emerge. For example, the findings

---

*Bart (1971) suggests that the term postparental is used by those who tend to see this period as not being problematic.

Table 18-3. Summary of research on the postparental period*

Author and year	Purpose	Characteristics of sample	Definition of postparental period	Measure	Findings and interpretations
Axelson (1960)	Explore theory that mothers and fathers have severe adjustment problems in this period	390 men and 461 women (no ages reported) who had a child under 25 years marry within 2-year period	Had 2 categories: 1. Quasi postparental: still having 1 or more single children under 18 remaining at home 2. True postparental: those with no child under 18 at home	Mailed questionnaires measuring present degree of satisfaction in 7 basic life areas involving family income, house, recreation, relationships to children and spouse, daily work, and the community in which they lived	No significant difference between women in both groups; 62.4% of women in true postparental period indicate satisfaction in 7 life areas, 61.6% of women in quasi-postparental period were satisfied Significant loneliness reported by women in true postparental period, women indicate greater concern about health than men *Interpretation:* No basis for assumed correlation between mental disorder and postparental period
Deutscher (1964)	Attempt to describe quality of postparental life	21 men and 28 women between ages of 40 and 65	Husband and wife alive and living together having had from 1 to 4 children, all of whom had been launched	Interviews: questions asking about the quality of postparental life in relation to other parts of the life cycle	50% of women say that postparental life is better than preceding phases; a larger percent of women evaluate the postparental life more favorably than men *Interpretation:* "This is crucial time of life for the woman and it is being clearly resolved one way or the other as far as she is concerned." (p. 267)
Deykin et al. (1966)	Identify conflict between depressed "empty nest" women and their adult children	16 lower middle class women hospitalized for depression who were mothers of adult children and no longer had childrearing functions; median age, 59 years	Had ceased childrearing in the past 10 years	Hospital records, charts, social work interviews	Identified overt conflict in 7 of the women; latent conflict in 7; no conflict in 2 *Interpretation:* Related depression in women in later middle age to their ability to deal successfully with termination of childrearing
Neugarten (1970)	Can this life event be considered a crisis? Does this role change have an effect on woman's well being?	100 "normal" women aged 43 to 53 from working class and middle class backgrounds, all married and living with husbands; all mothers of at least one child	1. "Intact" stage: no child had left home 2. "Transitional" stage: 1 or more had left 3. "Empty nest": all children had left	Life satisfaction questionnaire; questions dealing with role change behaviors	1. Women in empty nest stage had higher life satisfaction than women in the other phases 2. Satisfaction was highest in home- and community-oriented women; lowest in work-oriented *Interpretation:* Departure of children only causes a crisis when it occurs "off time" (in a different phase of the life cycle)
Bart (1971)	Is maternal role loss associated with depression in middle age?	533 women in psychiatric hospital with various diagnosis of depression; ages from 40 to 49 years	Maternal role loss recorded when at least one child was not living at home	Demographic data; projective biography test; unidentified questionnaires	Homemakers with maternal role loss who have overprotective or overinvolved relationships with their children have highest (82%) rate of depression

Author	Purpose	Sample	Sample/Definitions	Measure	Results/Interpretation
					"mothers" who have adhered most rigidly to prescribed sex-role behavior are most likely to have adjustment problems
Lowenthal and Chiriboga (1972)	Is there a midlife crisis caused by the empty nest?	27 men age 51; 27 women age 48	Sample was *approaching* empty nest stage; youngest child was about to graduate from high school	Life evaluation chart (subjects rate each year of their lives on scale of 1-9)	1. For women the present period was more likely than early middle age to include high points 2. No woman singled out the pending departure of the youngest child as a current problem *Interpretation:* Contrary to the "crisis theory," the pre–empty nest women are looking forward to establishing a complex life-style and the effect of children leaving home on morale is favorable
Glenn (1975)	Does the child's leaving home have a negative effect on the mother's well being?	From national surveys Gallup: 1963, 1966; ages 40 to 59 Roper, 1971; ages 35 to 69 National Opinion Research Center, 1972, 1973; ages 40 to 59	For Gallup survey: postparental period is defined only on the basis of whether or not anyone under 21 in household; therefore, this category contains people who never had children For Roper survey: only reported children under 17; thus a good many of postparental people were really in the launching stage For NORC: data allows exclusion of persons with children but does not allow separation of postparental people from those who had children 18 or older still at home	Questions differ among surveys: Gallup: "In general, how happy would you say you are—very happy, fairly happy, not happy." Roper: Asked respondents to rate themselves according to what proportion of time they enjoyed themselves. NORC: "Taken all together, how would you say that things are these days: very happy, pretty happy, not too happy."	Split up ages; all surveys show greater happiness or enjoyment of life in postparental category as compared to other ages Only Gallup data for people 50 to 54 show higher psychological well being in parental than postparental category *Interpretation:* Children leaving home does not lead to decline in psychologic well being of mothers
Harkins (1978)	Study effects of "empty nest" on well-being over time; identify characteristics of women who may find "empty nest" most disturbing; explore women's definitions of this period	318 women divided into three groups: pre–empty nest, empty nest, post–empty nest	*Pre–empty nest* —children still in high school *Empty nest* —last child graduated from high school within 18 months *Post–empty nest* —last child graduated over 2½ years ago	Affect Balance Scale (ABS); Cornell Medical Index (CMI)	Objectively defined "empty nest" transition has no effect on psychologic well-being as indicated by ABS; neither does age nor menopause Empty nest women report more CMI symptoms than pre– and post–empty nest In subjectively defined empty nest, transitional women reported more well-being than the other groups *Interpretation:* "The empty nest transition has, at most, a rather slight effect on psychological well-being and essentially no effect on physical well-being of mothers" (p. 555)

*From Heiple, P.: A study of women's responses to midlife changes. Unpublished Masters Thesis, University of Rochester, School of Nursing, 1979.

of Neugarten (1970) and Lowenthal and Chiriboga (1972) indicate that women in the earlier part of the middle years (when the launching of the children has not yet taken place but is anticipated) tend to have lower life satisfaction than women in later middle age. This suggests that the initial phase of readjustment in maternal role expectations may be the most crucial for women and require the greatest mobilization of individual coping resources.

Sociocultural factors

Cultural practices and attitudes, availability of other roles, extent of the role loss, and especially the degree of emotional investment in the maternal role have been suggested as factors influencing a woman's ability to cope with changes in this role. The tendency for some women to gain their entire sense of identity from heavy investment in the nurturing role has been discussed previously.

Bart (1971) has extensively studied this high cathexis of women to the role of nurturer using a sociocultural feminist model. This model describes the culture as containing certain "props" necessary for individuals to successfully perform their roles and become inegrated into societal structure. When the woman's "props" of domestic and maternal roles are no longer available to her, she becomes "unintegrated" and loses her defined place in society which results in a situation of anomie. The woman must change her expectations at this time to deal with the anomic situation that is created when maternal role changes; however, this is difficult partly because there are neither guidelines nor rites of passage to facilitate the woman's role transition. The discomfort the woman feels at this time is compounded by feelings of anger toward her children because of her perception that they no longer need her. Because of our culture's taboo against showing hostility to one's children, the woman turns this anger inward and becomes depressed.

Bart (1971) conducted extensive studies and interviews that included projective tests. Her results indicated that housewives with the greatest sense of loss are those with overprotective or overinvolved relationships with their children. These women are most likely to get depressed. In this study housewives had a higher rate of depression than working women, and middle class housewives displayed higher rates of depression than working class housewives. These results indicate that depression or other negative reactions, if they occur during the climacteric, may be a by-product of cultural expectations and restrictions on women's roles.

The interrelationship of societal expectations and negative reactions to the climacteric is depicted in Table 18-4. It can be seen that American society at the present time reinforces a female value pattern conducive to midlife depression.

Table 18-4. Model for negative reactions during climacteric*

The society	The woman
Socializes girls to wife-mother role	Aspires to wife-mother role as fulfillment
Youth oriented, values females as sex objects	Self-esteem based on sexual attractiveness and maintenance of youthful beauty
Denies or discourages other or additional roles for women	Leaves job in first pregnancy; no career involvement of her own; promotes and supports husband's career
Child-centered, nuclear family	Dedicated mother; children are primary concern
Values passivity, humility, and self-sacrifice in women	Subjugates her own needs to family's; puts self-interest last
Values masculine, competitive model of achievement	Identifies vicariously with achievements of husband and child
Male oriented; women seen as inferior	Sees self and other women as inferior; ready to blame self, feel guilty
Transitional; both traditional and modern life-styles in evidence	Matriarchal role not available; has neither desire nor necessary skills for "liberated" role
Double standard of aging for men and women	Fears aging with its loss of status, loneliness, isolation

*Reproduced from *Psychology of women: A behavior in a biosocial context*, by Juanita H. Williams, by permission of W. W. Norton & Co., Inc. Copyright © 1977, 1974 by Juanita H. Williams.

Changes in role of worker

Women have a pattern of participation in the labor force very different from men's. Since 1890, the proportion of very young women in the labor force has increased, contrary to the trend for young men. However, differences are most striking in the middle years: from 1890 to 1966 the proportion of working women from age 35 through 44 increased from 12% to 47%. The percentage increased from 11% to 52% for women between the ages of 45 and 54 years. Females tend to enter the labor force earlier and retire later than men. Age 47 is when the proportion of women in the labor force is at its highest. This is the average age of menopause, and the time when women are most likely to have children leave home. After children leave home some women may decide to put their energy and creativity, previously consumed by maternal responsibilities, into a career.

Upon returning to the labor force, employment may have a positive effect on a woman's sense of self-esteem and feelings of satisfaction. One study found that college-educated "empty nest" women, employed full-time, had significantly fewer psychiatric symptoms than women not employed outside the home (Powell, 1978). Some have suggested that as the number of employed mothers increases, the "empty nest syndrome" will become something of the past (Fuchs, 1977).

The women's movement may be having a two-fold effect on the increase in female labor force participation at this time—one positive and the other possibly negative. While the women's movement has facilitated society's receptivity of women workers, misrepresentation of the goals of the movement by the media may lead some middle-aged women to feel that they must be employed to be considered worthwhile. Unfortunately, this is far from the truth; the real message of the women's movement is that every woman should have the freedom to do whatever she chooses.

The woman who chooses to enter or re-enter the work force may encounter several obstacles. The double standard for men and women is alive and well in the labor force. Some employers may be reluctant to invest in the middle-aged woman because she is considered an "older worker." These same employers consider middle-aged men to be in their prime. The middle-aged woman may also find that her experience and skills are outdated and that there is a lack of jobs for which she is qualified. Some women are out of the labor force for so long that they do not have the "connections" or resources available to others. Women's career centers, re-entry workshops, and support groups have been formed in various communities to help meet the special needs of the middle-aged woman seeking employment.

The married or single woman who has never left the labor force may also experience changes in the worker role. During the middle years, awareness of time left before retirement increases and re-evaluation of personal goals takes place. If reaching these goals seems to be an unrealistic expectation, the woman may need to change her goals or her job.

Changes in role of spouse

Although early studies showed the middle years to be a time of marital disenchantment, more recent research has found that after the children leave home, the majority of middle-aged couples experience the same level of satisfaction that they had as young expectant parents. However, the early part of the launching phase is identified as the most troublesome for marital relationships (Rollins and Feldman, 1970). Note the similarity between this finding and those from "empty nest" research: there seems to be a brief period at the onset of role change when parents experience difficulty. Again, this has implications for assessment and working with middle-aged women.

Stress in the marital relationship at this time may occur for several reasons. First, if the couple has based their relationship around their parental roles, the departure of children may leave them with little in com-

mon. This can lead to boredom—or to an exciting process of mutual rediscovery. Second, if the couple has chosen to assume traditional roles, the changes in role expectations may increase the woman's need for support from her husband. However, this is a time when many men become preoccupied with their careers, and they may have a diminished amount of energy available to put into this type of relationship.

Another potential stressor in the midlife marital relationship is sexual relations. It has been found that for many reasons the incidence of sexual dysfunction (impotence) increases sharply for men past the age of 50. However, this is a time when many women experience an increased interest in sex; they no longer have to worry about pregnancy and their energy is no longer expended in childrearing. If couples are able to resolve these issues, it contributes to the strength of the marital relationship and increases their satisfaction with each other.

Changes in the daughter role

As her parents age or become ill the woman experiences changes in her role as daughter. She may need to make a decision regarding institutionalization, taking one or both parents into her home, or assuming more responsibility for helping them maintain their independence. Studies show that it is usually the middle-aged daughter or daughter-in-law who assumes supportive care for aging family members during illness and at the time of bereavement and adjustment to widowhood (Treas, 1975). The middle-aged woman who is a mother may experience conflict as her children's dependence on her decreases at the same time as her parents' dependence increases.

Eventually, the woman will have to deal with the death of her parents. It has been suggested that research exploring the effect of the death of one's parents on adults is too threatening a topic for middle-aged social scientists (Kimmel, 1974). We do know that when one of our parents dies, our sense of safety and security is threatened as we confront our own mortality.

Experiencing the death of a mother may be particularly stressful for the middle-aged woman. Nancy Friday (1977), who has sensitively written about the mother-daughter relationship, states, "There are two times in women's lives when the unconscious drive to become the mother we dislike speeds up. The first is when we become mothers ourselves. The second is when our mother dies" (p. 402). The death of a mother may bring to the surface old, resolved, mother-daughter conflicts that complicate the process of bereavement.

In this section, we have explored the varied opportunities for growth catalyzed by midlife role changes. The middle-aged woman's perception of herself changes as she integrates the changes in her body and the changes in her roles and relationships with others into an acceptable self-image. Data presented in this section challenge our stereotype of the "midlife crisis." Adaptation to midlife changes is an individualized task and cannot be generalized. Women's responses to these changes reflect their past experiences and in some ways determine their responses to future experiences. In the next section, we will explore the opportunities for growth that changes in the later years bring.

CHALLENGES OF THE LATER YEARS

What we believe about older women—their capabilities, desires, and interests—influences how we behave toward them. Likewise, our behavior and caring about them affect their image of themselves. Sometimes in our caring we are afraid to look too closely; the appearance of older women reflects on our own approaching old age and mortality. In this section on the last years of a woman's life, we will examine the social, psychologic, and biologic aspects of aging to acquire insights into the multifaceted nature of being old and female in American society.

In the first part of this chapter, we explored the means by which societal expectations influence a woman's perception of herself during the middle years. We have seen that focusing on the negative rather than positive outcomes of midlife role changes can result in the self-fulfilling prophecy of the "midlife crisis." Women in the later years also feel the impact of this "looking glass self." We will attempt to analyze some of these intervening variables that influence health outcomes as we consider the loss, growth, and change experienced during the last part of the life cycle.

Attitudes toward aging

Since prehistoric times, cultures have employed various rituals and ceremonies to maintain youth and ward off old age and death. There were, and still are, rites that serve to wipe out the past and free life from the weight of years—to begin anew. Feasts at the beginning of a new year or season endow that time with the significance of a cosmic rejuvenation. This idea of regeneration explains one of the Shinto customs in Japan, where at stated intervals temples are entirely rebuilt and their furnishings and decorations completely renewed. Their rebuilding symbolically prevents time from weakening the bond between the individual and the world as a whole. At another time old women were symbolically used to expel old age from a community. In Italy, France, and Spain, on the fourth Sunday in Lent, there was a "sawing of the old woman," in which community members symbolically cut an old woman in two. In other cultures, images representing old men were burned, again to protect villagers and their institutions from weakening, aging, and dying and to maintain and renew the perpetual vigor of youth (de Beauvoir, 1972).

Our concern for maintaining the vigors of youth and postponing the inevitability of aging and death has contributed to the lack of knowledge about older people. Many myths and stereotypes surrounding women and old age can be explained in part by insufficient research and limited contacts with a wide variety of elderly people. Some of the common myths and stereotypes surrounding old age may be found in the following health care provider's description of an encounter with an 85-year-old woman.

Ms. J. cannot learn to give her own insulin. I have worked with her for some time now and she will never change. She moves and thinks so slowly and dislikes innovation and new ideas. She seems only concerned with the past and is not willing to look forward. Like most elderly she is becoming increasingly egocentric and demands more from the environment than she is willing to give to it. Her multiple diseases restrict her activities of daily living, influence her desire for food and feelings of well-being. As her body has aged and shrunk the blood flow to her brain has decreased. I really don't believe it is safe to teach her responsibility for her own health. Furthermore, I don't think she could learn even if she wanted to; she is too tied to her own personal traditions and growing conservatism.

This sketch not only closely approximates the picture of old women held by some health professionals, but also it more than likely comes near to the perception of old age imagined by many Americans. A number of our current views of old age represent confusions, misunderstandings, and lack of knowledge about the facts and experiences of aging.

Myths and realities about the old

The elderly are often depicted as rigid, egocentric, demanding, restricted in their activities, interested only in their past, and unable to learn. Stereotypes about aging will be examined in various sections of this chapter. Here we will consider how negative attitudes contribute to ageism. We will review one national study that reveals some of the realities and myths about aging.

Myths and stereotypes contribute to deep and profound prejudice against the elderly, referred to as ageism. Ageism is a process of systematic stereotyping of and discrimination against people because they are old. Just as sexism and racism accomplish stereotyping and discrimination because of gender and skin color, ageism achieves the same because of age. Ageism allows younger generations to see older people as different from themselves; thus they may select to subtly cease to identify with their elders as human beings (Butler and Lewis, 1973). It makes it easy to accept negative images about aging and to ignore the true experience of being older.

The National Council of Aging (NCOA) in conjunction with Louis Harris and Associates, Inc., conducted an extensive study of American attitudes toward aging, older Americans' views about themselves, and personal experiences of old age. This study provides definitive data about many of the myths and realities of aging. The study reveals that most older people have the desire and potential to be productive, contributing members of society. While the young prefer to picture older people as spending their time sleeping, sitting and doing nothing, or nostalgically dwelling on the past, older people are unwilling to accept this relegated role of passivity. Three out of four people aged 65 and over prefer to spend their time with people of all different ages and they are interested in a variety of activities. A number of older people in this study felt they have specific skills they could use if given the opportunity in a working environment. In addition, 15% (over 3 million) of the people aged 65 and over indicate an interest in learning new skills or participating in job training programs for different jobs. While the public at large tends to underestimate the effectiveness, open-mindedness, and alertness of most people aged 65 and over, the older public have confidence in their own abilities. They have as much confidence in their abilities as do the young, and a lot more confidence in themselves than the public has in them (NCOA, 1975).

Like the young people in the NCOA report, older people as a group make up a very heterogenous entity. Measures of the experience of older people in their later years indicate that there is no such thing as a "typical" older person. Instead, the same type of social, economic, and psychologic factors that influence individuals when they are young also affect them as they grow older. Even though older individuals may share the same chronological age, factors more powerful than age alone determine the experiences and conditions of their later years. The following sections of this chapter will consider some of these factors. Selected aspects of the social system as well as individual biologic and psychologic factors will be explored as they influence the process of aging.

Processes of aging

The biologic, psychologic, and social aspects of aging present numerous difficulties in conceptualization. We are only beginning to appreciate the multifaceted nature of aging, and each of these three areas has special difficulties of its own. Aging, as we observe and experience it, affects the coordinated activities of a number of individual cells, tissues, organs, and organ systems. These changes, which range from the way cells respond to increased metabolic demands to the manner in which organ systems function in an integrative fashion, influence adaptation of aging women to environmental demands. Likewise, these biologic changes of aging affect older women's perceptions of themselves. This interaction of biologic, sociologic, and psychologic changes influences a woman's adaptive potential; how she copes with these changes determines successful aging. In this section we will first explore selected facets of social and biologic aspects of aging as they may influence older women and then examine the psychology of aging.

Even though each of these will be considered separately, the interaction of all biopsychosocial phenomena in aging determines the adaptive responses of women and thus ability to cope with growth, loss, and change.

Sociology of aging

Studies on social and psychologic aspects of aging generally concern themselves with three problems: (1) variables that affect the adult personality with aging; (2) variables that influence the social situation of persons in their later years; and (3) normative concepts concerning degrees of adaptation, adjustment, or success in the process of aging (Williams and Loeb, 1968). We will consider each of these, beginning with selected aspects of the social situation of older women.

Economic status of older women. In our society, at every age and every stage, women are more vulnerable to poverty than men, especially when they function in the dual role of family head and homemaker (Arshansky, 1974). Many older women have grown old functioning in this dual role, and as elderly females they are far more likely than older men to be poor.

Even though poverty is largely a situation of aged women, especially widows, the special concerns of older women and their economic status has been largely ignored in research on aging. Statistics confirm the increasing percentage of elderly females in our population, but this differential is not significantly reflected in either the theory or practice of gerontology or the public policies that influence aging women. Some of the problem areas that need further research and action to improve the status and economic condition for older women are unemployment, nonpaying work, earnings, retirement benefits, Social Security, and the relationships between physical and mental health in employed and unemployed older women.

Unemployment. Even though older women outnumber older men and large numbers of women would like to work if they could find a job, unemployment figures for older women are consistently higher than they are for older men. Table 18-5 provides data on the employment status of older men and women. As shown in the table, 6% of men and 13% of women aged 18 to 54 define themselves as unemployed. In the "preretirement" decade, ages 55 to 64, 5% of the men and 14% of the women are unemployed, a ratio of almost three to one. In the 65 and over age bracket, the disparity between males and females rises to eight to one. These discrepancies reflect a greater difficulty for older women in the job market. They also provide evidence of the economic dependency of many older women.

Table 18-5. Current employment status by age and sex*

Employment status	Age 18-54		Age 55-64		Age 65 and over	
	Male	Female	Male	Female	Male	Female
Employed full-time	74%	28%	60%	19%	5%	2%
Employed part-time	8%	13%	8%	13%	12%	7%
Retired	3%	1%	27%	10%	82%	50%
Unemployed	6%	13%	5%	14%	1%	8%

* From *Aging in America: implications for women,* published 1976 by the National Council on the Aging, Inc., Washington, D.C. 20036. Based on the NCOA Louis Harris & Associates public opinion survey, *The Myth and Reality of Aging in America,* published by the National Council on the Aging, Inc., Washington, D.C. 20036, 1975.

A large number of older women are former home-makers. Encouraged to raise families and stay at home in their younger years, as older women they are penalized for not having "worked." Our retirement system does not provide a viable mechanism for retired home-makers, except as dependents. Ironically, when considering the economic plight of older women, one could say that women are punished for doing what society expected them to do (Sommer, 1974).

Social security. Society, through the social security laws, has created another inequity for older women. Initially planned in 1935 as a compromise between the insurance principle and society's responsibility for the aging, social security benefits were designed for dependents at retirement, disability, or death of the wage earner. A person needs at least 10 years of "creditable work" to meet the requirements for fully insured status. This creates an inequity and a double bind for many older women.

An older single woman may wish to work but is unable to find employment; thus she is not eligible for Social Security at a later date. An employed married woman, on the other hand, may receive more income as a dependent of her husband than through employment because of the pay differential between sexes. Married women also receive nothing for their extra contributions. If divorced, they may be left out entirely.

Nonpaying work. Even though the role of homemaker is basic to the well-being and economy of our nation, the homemaker's contribution is systematically ignored by society. Just as homemaking is overlooked as a contributing factor to our economy, another service provided by elderly women that is conveniently ignored in the realm of statistics and policy-making is nonpaying work. Older people perform services for their children and grandchildren that represent substantial monetary savings for the young (Harris, 1976). These free services of older family members, with women giving more service hours than men, are largely taken for granted, even though they provide significant economic contributions to those served. In addition to homemaking services,

Table 18-6. Percent of elderly men and women in various living arrangements, 1970

Living arrangement	Men	Women
Family	79	59
Head of household	71	10
Wife is head of household	—	33
Other relative is head of household	8	16
Alone or with nonrelative	17	37
Head of household	14	35
Living with a nonrelative	3	2
Institution	4	4

older women provide many unpaid services to community organizations. Perhaps if more opportunities were available for employment, increased numbers of older women would be paid for their work.

Living environments. The context in which many older people live significantly determines how they behave. We have ample statistics on the living arrangements of elderly women but we have very little information on health-engendering environments for these same females.

Older women, because of their increased longevity and fewer available potential mates for remarriage, are more likely than men to live alone after being widowed or divorced, as depicted in Table 18-6.

Even though older women may live alone, their connectedness to other family members is substantial. The majority of elderly women (59%) live in family situations or in their own homes. Only 4% of the aged are institutionalized. The tendency for older people to maintain their own households has increased over the past decade. However, information on the types of households or living environments and their effects on the well-being of the aging woman is sadly lacking.

Some of the so-called effects of aging may, in fact, be the result of society creating an environment that is built for younger people. Consequently, performance levels for aging women are lowered as they deal with social designs and demands developed for young and middle-aged adults. More attention to environments that engender health could affect both competence and functioning of older women.

Biology of aging

Is the end of life built into its very beginning? Many hypotheses about the cellular basis of aging exist. Several theories of aging are concerned with aging at a cellular level: the error hypothesis, wear-and-tear theory, the theory of damage to the DNA molecule, deprivation and accumulation theories, the cross-linkage theory, and free-radical theory (Finch and Hayflick, 1977). The view that we are programmed to die, that death is built into the beginning of life, arises primarily from two areas of biologic research on dying. One is concerned with somatic mutation in DNA as the cause of aging; the second arises from the speculation that aging occurs through defects in the control of genetic programs (Sinex, 1977). It is not certain that a person is programmed to age; however, it is possible that in later life our programs are inadequate to deal with aging injury because of defects in tools of biochemical repair. On a cellular level, biochemical adaptation seems to slow with aging. The ability to initiate adaptive activities in a large number of enzymes is impaired as well as the ability to integrate various mechanisms in response to stress. This breakdown in the integrative mechanisms may produce more of the actual changes we see in aging than the changes in individual cells, tissues, or organs (Shock, 1977).

Organ system integration. The integrative processes and mechanisms involved in adaptation require the coordinated activities of a number of organ systems. Since research in aging on the interactions between cells, organ systems, and control mechanisms has only recently been explored by physiologists, we know how some of these integrative processes are influenced by aging; however, we know very little about those processes that may be unique to women. We do know that the female of any species generally lives longer than the male (Rockstein, 1958); we do not know what combination of intrinsic, genetic attributes and external environmental variables nurtures this longevity. If more research on aging examined and compared organ system integration of females we might find some answers to their superiority in longevity. Since this research is not available, we will consider system integration through the examination of studies on both aging men and women. Age decrements in performance and an indication of the role of integrative mechanisms in age can be seen in Fig. 18-2 in which the age decrements are compared with the mean performance of 30-year-old subjects, considered to be at peak 100% performance levels.

It can be seen that the maintenance of internal envi-

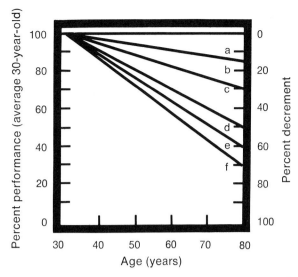

Fig. 18-2. Age decrements in physiologic functions in males. Mean values for 20- to 35-year-old subjects are taken as 100%. Decrements shown are schematic linear projections: *a*, fasting blood glucose; *b*, nerve conduction velocity and cellular enzymes; *c*, resting cardiac index; *d*, vital capacity and renal blood flow; *e*, maximum breathing capacity; *f*, maximal work rate and maximal oxygen uptake. (From Schock, N.: Systems integration. In Handbook of the biology of aging, editors: Caleb E. Finch and Leonard Hayflick. © 1977 by Litton Educational Publishing, Inc. Reprinted by permission of Van Nostrand Reinhold Co.)

ronmental variables under resting conditions is not altered with age (see curve *a* for fasting blood glucose or pH of blood). Nerve conduction velocity shows an average decrement of about 15% between the ages of 30 and 80 years. The resting cardiac index decreases about 30%, and vital capacity and renal blood flow in 80-year-olds are only about one half the average values for 30-year-olds. The performances that require integrated activity of the cardiovascular, nervous, muscular, and respiratory systems—the maximum breathing capacity and maximum cardiac uptake—fall 60% and 70%, respectively (Shock, 1972). These data are based on cross-sectional studies, which emphasize age differences rather than age changes in any one individual over time. Longitudinal data are not yet available to measure these same physiologic characteristics in one individual over time. Even though these age decrements are observed when comparing the elderly with those at peak performances, it is generally accepted that these changes with age are gradual and compensated for by a slower life pace. These changes do become accentuated when the individual is stressed, but behavioral and biologic intervention strategies may reverse some of the decrease in performance observed in old people.

Physiologic age functions may not be fixed and inevitable. Recent research indicates selected physiologic functions may be maintained and decline reversed (Woodruff, 1975). One study on aging women has shown that age-related losses in physiologic variables important to performance are more highly related to decreased habitual activity level than to age itself (Wessel and Van Huss, 1969). The term "hypokinetic disease," has been created for a spectrum of somatic and mental derangements induced by inactivity (Kraus, 1961). It raises the question of how much of the observed losses in function are the result of long-term deconditioning and increasingly sedentary life patterns with aging.

Physiologic patterns: the loss of youth. Physiologic changes have been documented with aging, and it is their resultant alterations in the appearance of older women that represent the threat of lost youth and beauty. At the same time that hair whitens and becomes thin on the head, it appears in new places, such as on the face. Supportive tissue becomes dehydrated with less elasticity, resulting in thin, wrinkled skin giving the appearance of excess skin over the eyelids and hollows under the eyes. The upper lip grows thinner and the ear lobes enlarge. Skeletal structures change resulting in decreased height, spinal disks compress and bend the spine, the pelvis broadens, and shoulders and chest become narrower. These visible changes in a woman's body over time are perceived as a loss of youthfulness and attractiveness, since in our society one is not attractive if one is not young. To be old and to look old are two very uncomplimentary things, especially for women (Troll et al., 1977). Even though both men and women experience common physiologic and physical changes as they age, middle-aged women are most distressed with the physiologic "damages" of old age.

Research reveals that a middle-aged woman's anticipation of these "damages" is far worse than the actual changes as experienced by older women. Looking old and unattractive in comparison to societal standards of youthfulness and beauty are among the least of concerns that elderly women have. While some investigators attribute this lack of concern to "denial" of growing older, others support this as a true lack of concern for stereotypic worries. The anticipation of lost youth and beauty and the perceived transition into "old age" experienced by women in midlife prompt confusion and disillusionment. It seems that once a middle-aged woman accepts her own aging, she can then continue to grow and consider herself attractive (Nowack, 1977).

In some ways aging is much more a social judgment than a biologic eventuality. When older women overcome the "possession" of their imaginations that growth is beauty and to be old is bad, they are free to imagine themselves (Sontag, 1976).

Psychology of aging

The psychology of aging considers many aspects of individual changes throughout the life cycle. We will consider only selected aspects of these changes as they seem to influence the health and adaptation of older women. In this section we will examine behavioral processes and basic needs that contribute to successful aging.

Behavioral processes. A number of behavioral processes influence the aging patterns of women. We will concentrate on two of these, cognitive abilities and personality changes. We will also consider several sociopsychologic theories of aging that help to explain some of the behaviors related to longevity.

Cognitive abilities. The changes in cognition associated with old age involve a range of capacities: motivation, short- and long-term memory, intelligence, learning and retention tasks, and a host of factors that seem to facilitate or impede cognitive capacities.

Most of the studies on cognitive abilities in older people have been cross-sectional in design; consequently, it has been difficult to attribute change in function to a process of aging. Most studies of learning favor the abilities of the young adult over older learners. Although research reveals many elderly people function as well as they did when they were young, the young of today function at a much higher level than did those who were young 50 years ago (Schaie, 1975). Rather than concentrating on the differences in abilities of young and older learners, a number of recent studies have identified variables that improve or impair learning performance in older people. More geropsychologists are considering alternatives to the traditional notion of an irreversible decrement of intelligence in the elderly.

There may be a good deal more plasticity to intelligence in old age than has been acknowledged thus far. A study on training and intelligence in elderly women reveals that cognitive strategy training riases the intellectual performance of females on certain component skills. Rather than de-emphasizing competent behavior and fostering dependency and helplessness, these researchers stress the role that environmental variables may play in modifying performance levels of the elderly (Labouvie-Vief and Gonda, 1976). Others have found that an environment designed to bring about more favorable self-appraisals in older women enhances optimal functioning (Bellucci and Hoyer, 1975). In this regard, there is also evidence that supportive instructions facilitate performance (Labouvie-Vief and Gonda, 1975). In addition to studies that emphasize environmental variables to enhance learning, there are a number of other procedures that may facilitate cognitive capacities of older women. These will be discussed in the last section of this chapter under strategies for coping and intervention.

Personality and patterns of aging. The Kansas City Study of Adult Life, over the past several decades, has concluded that personality organization and coping style are the major factors in life adjustment of individuals as they grow older. Throughout the life span adaptation to aging is related to changes in the structure and function of the human body and changes in the social environment. It seems that when there is a close "fit" between the social environment and the physical organism, adaptation is relatively easy and aging is successful. In general, this close "fit" is maximized when the personality is strong and flexible, the social environment is supportive, and the body is vigorous. This is not the case for all older women; consequently, we see a variety of patterns of aging and personality dimensions.

Four major personality types were defined in the Kansas City Study of Adult Life: (1) integrated, (2) armored-defended, (3) passive-dependent, and (4) unintegrated personalities. Patterns of aging behavior were further refined in this study through analyzing personality, role activity, and life satisfaction. From this analysis eight patterns of aging were established and predictable by middle age. Table 18-7 classifies these eight personality patterns in aging.

For some of the elderly, as the level of activity decreases, so does the feeling of contentment and life satisfaction. Others, who are more disengaged from this obligations, seem to enjoy relatively inactive lives. Of the three dimensions studied (personality, role activity, and satisfaction) personality was the pivotal dimension that predicted relationships between activity and life satisfaction.

Another approach to considering personality and

adaptation has been taken by Lieberman (1975). He has described the qualities of grouchiness or combativeness as "adaptive paranoia" in old age, and his findings reveal that these qualities have a survival asset. These same patterns have been found to enhance survival in men in various preliterate societies.

Results from a variety of projective tests and questionnaires reveal consistent age differences in the following dimensions: (1) a change from active to passive mastery styles in relating to the environment, and (2) an inner-world orientation with less ego investment in social roles. These findings tend to support one of the major theories of aging, the disengagement theory.

Disengagement theory postulates a mutual withdrawal between the elderly person and society. When disengagement is complete there is an increased sense of freedom as the individual feels less controlled by norms governing everyday behavior. Fully disengaged persons have transferred much of their cathexis to their own inner life; their memories, fantasies, self-image are those of someone who was something and accomplished something (Cumming and Henry, 1961). This view seems to contradict other assumptions about older people keeping active to ward off failure, loss, and deterioration.

The *activity theory* of aging advocates successful aging through continuing the interests, activities, and attitudes of middle age. From this framework, if older people can find substitutes for activities they must give up, adjustment and successful aging will be enhanced. In other words, the elderly individual who ages optimally is one who stays active and manages to resist the shrinkage of his or her social world.

The conceptions of disengagement and activity related to successful aging are both incorporated in the concept of styles of life, developed empirically by Williams and Wirths (1965). Their research on 168 older men and women, observed over a 5½-year period, reveals that the style of life that an older person has established throughout life contributes to successful aging. Six primary life-styles are delineated in their study: familism, couplehood, living fully, world of work, living alone, and easing through life with minimal involvement. Both those who aged successfully and nonsuccessfully were found in all six life-styles. Some oldsters were active and others were disengaged. Their past style of living contributed to the extent of involvement and activity or inactivity maintained in old age.

Basic needs. Several basic needs must be satisfied to maintain and promote stability in aging women. Only three will be considered here: nutrition, activity and rest, and sexuality.

Nutrition. The ideal nutritional requirements for older women in good health should not differ significantly

Table 18-7. Personality patterns in aging*

Personality types	Role activity	Life satisfaction
Integrated		
Reorganizers	High	High
Focused	Medium	High
Disengaged	Low	High
Armored-defended		
Holding on	High or medium	High
Constricted	Low or medium	High or medium
Passive-dependent		
Succorance-seeking	High or medium	High or medium
Apathetic	Low	Medium or low
Unintegrated	Low	Medium or low
(disorganized)		

*Adapted from Havinghurst, R.: A social-psychological perspective on aging, Gerontologist 8(2):67-71, 1968.

from those of younger women, assuming that caloric intake is proportional to energy expenditure. However, since total daily metabolic requirements decline with age because of reduced physical activity, the caloric energy requirements for an over age 65 woman weighing 55 kg is approximately 1800 calories, compared to 2100 calories for a 45-year-old woman (Winick, 1976).

In order to assess the total nutritional status of the older population, several national surveys have been conducted to examine dietary intake and nutritional problems of the aged. Nutritional status is influenced by factors other than aging, especially socioeconomic status and income.

The standards developed in 1974 by the National Center for Health Statistics reveals the following guidelines for classifying and interpreting daily dietary intake of women aged 60 years and older: protein, 1.0 Gm/kg; calcium, 600 mg; iron, 10 mg; vitamin A, 3,500 IU; and vitamin C, 55 mg. Utilizing these standards, several national surveys have found that recommended dietary allowances are met in high socioeconomic groups, although some marginal deficiencies exist. However, as income decreases and reaches or goes below poverty levels, nutritional deficiencies and health impairments become more frequent and severe. Those nutrients most deficient in this group are protein, niacin, thiamine, iron, calcium, and vitamins A and C. Therefore, it seems that both nutritional intake and status of the elderly are more related to health and poverty than they are to age per se (Barrows and Roeder, 1977).

Activity and rest. Several changes occur in the sleep and rest patterns of women as they age. Deep sleep (stage four) virtually disappears, and there is a decrease in the proportion of sleep spent in rapid eye movement and slow wave stages. Compared to younger people it generally takes older people a longer time to fall asleep, sleep is lighter, and there are more frequent awakenings (Kahn and Fisher, 1969). These normal changes are also accompanied by an alteration in the distribution of sleep over the 24-hour cycle. Several naps are usually taken during the daytime, which range from 15 to 60 minutes. This normal pattern of sleep with less deep sleep, frequent awakenings, and naps during the day should be encouraged and not disturbed with sleeping medication that enforces 8 hours of sleep at night and less daytime rest (Pfeiffer, 1977).

Along with adequate sleep and rest, exercise promotes health. Exercise contributes both to the utilization of oxygen with less noticeable fatigue and to the restoration and improvement of muscles, body mechanics, and posture. Fitness parameters reveal five dynamic target variables appropriate for physical fitness programs. These components are: (1) body composition, (2) muscle strength, (3) body flexibility, (4) body balance, and (5) circulorespiratory endurance. Research on each of these components indicates that regular participation in exercise programs has a positive effect on the well-being and quantitative dimensions of aging (Piscopo, 1977). A number of studies on older women indicate that those who participate in physical training programs also show improvement in work performance and physiologic response to exercise (Adams and deVries, 1973).

Sexuality. Older women are capable sexual partners and competent physiologically and psychologically to establish meaningful sexual relationships. However, there are a number of factors that influence their sexual abilities: normal physiologic changes of aging, established behavioral patterns, illness, the availability of a satisfactory mate, and societal values. If a healthy elderly female has remained sexually active, is not inhibited by societal stereotypes and myths against sex with advanced age, and has a partner who has maintained sexual interests, it is likely that she will have continued satisfactory sexual relationships.

It is difficult to separate the physiologic, psychologic, and social factors that affect an older woman's sexuality, since they are all so closely intertwined. However, we can briefly examine each one, consider how they may influence older females, and make some speculations for aging women of tomorrow.

Many older women today are the products of a Victorian value system; they grew up believing that desire, pleasure, and orgasm were to be avoided since they supposedly interfered with conception. Sexual intercourse was acceptable only for procreation. Females were encouraged to be passive and submissive. Chastity, continence even in marriage, self-control, and denial of sexual desires were the prevailing messages (Haller and Haller, 1974). This value system not only influenced their sexual functioning as younger women, but also has contributed to a lack of sexual interest and drive. In fact, Masters and Johnson (1966) believe that women who found little satisfaction with sexual relationships in young adulthood may use advancing age as a culturally acceptable excuse for decreasing or eliminating sexual functions with advancing years. For women not inhibited by this Victorian value system, sexual activity and interest may continue well into old age.

Several longitudinal studies on sexuality and aging indicate that for some healthy older people sexual activity remains the same or may even increase with aging (Pfeiffer, 1969). For the older females, the regularity of sexual expression and the availability of an interested partner are two key variables influencing continued sexual gratification. A significant decrease in sexual activity for women is noted following the loss of a spouse (Newman and Nichols, 1960) or the lack of interest or capacity for intercourse in the husband (Pfeiffer et al.,

Table 18-8. Phase-specific changes in the sexual response cycle of aging women*

Target tissue	Phase of sexual response			
	Excitement	Plateau	Orgasm	Resolution
Breast	Vasocongestive increase in size less pronounced, especially in more pendulous breasts	Engorgement of areola less intense	—	Loss of nipple erection slowed
Skin	Sex flush does not occur as frequently	Sex flush does not occur as frequently	—	—
Muscle	Degree of myotonia decreases with age	Degree of myotonia decreases with age	—	—
Urethra and urinary bladder	—	—	Minimal distention of meatus†	—
Rectum	—	—	Contraction of rectal sphincter only with severe tension levels	—
Clitoris	—	—	—	Retracts rapidly; tumescence lost rapidly
Labia majora	No women past age 51 demonstrated flattening, separation, and elevation of labia majora	—	—	
Labia minora	Vasocongestion reduced	Labial color change (sex skin) usually pathognomonic of orgasm decreased in frequency among women 61 years of age and older	—	—
Bartholin's glands	—	Reduction in amount of secretions and activity, especially among postmenopausal women	—	—
Vagina	Rate and amount of vaginal lubrication decreased; lubrication occurs 1 to 3 minutes after stimulation; vaginal expansion in breadth and width decreases	Inner two thirds of vagina may still be expanding during this phase; vasocongestion of orgasmic platform reduced in intensity	Postmenopausal orgasmic platform contracts 3 to 5 times versus 5 to 10 times in younger women	Rapid involution and loss of vasocongestion
Cervix	—	—	—	Dilation of cervix not noted
Uterus	Uterine elevation and tenting of transcervical vagina develops more slowly and is less marked	Uterine elevation and tenting of transcervical vagina develops more slowly and is less marked	Some women report painful contractions with orgasm	—

*Summary of findings from The aging female. In Masters, W., and Johnson, V.: Human sexual response. Boston, 1966, Little, Brown & Co., pp. 223-247.

†Mechanical irritation of urethra and bladder may occur as a result of thinning of vagina, which minimizes protection of these structures during thrusting.

1972). Women with younger spouses tend to have higher coital rates than those with older spouses (Christenson and Gagnon, 1965). The frequency of sexual expression also seems to be a factor. Despite the recognized physiologic changes with aging, Masters and Johnson (1966) found three women over age 60 who consistently lubricated the vagina effectively. These women had maintained a regular pattern of coitus at least once or twice a week during their adult lives.

The physiologic changes in elderly women and their relationship to the phases of the sexual response cycle are summarized in Table 18-8. In older women, the intensity and duration of physiologic response to sexual stimulation are diminished. These changes, primarily associated with steroid changes, do not necessarily interfere with sexual satisfaction. The pleasure and stimulation of sexual expression may be prolonged in an elderly couple, since older men can maintain erections longer before orgasm. The pleasure involved with orgasm, even though it is over more quickly in older women, is still fulfilling and satisfying. In addition, as people age, the intimacy of the sexual act, the sharing, closeness, and caressing have a meaning that is exquisitely real. To some aged the achievement of orgasm may be largely symbolic (Glover, 1977).

Another sexual practice that may be gratifying for older women is self-pleasuring (masturbation). If older women can overcome the sexual taboos that have existed about this form of expressing their sexuality, they can learn to enjoy this source of pleasure. Especially for those who are widowed, have no sexual partner, or are physically incapacitated, self-stimulation may be a satisfactory sexual outlet. It resolves sexual tensions, keeps sexual desires alive, is good physical exercise, and promotes tissue circulation and lubrication (Butler and Lewis, 1976).

Women today are more aware of their sexuality and less inhibited in their responses to sexual expression than was true in the past. Perhaps this awareness and their motivation to promote the health and well-being for womankind will nurture the culture of tomorrow to be more tolerant and open in their support for sexuality throughout the life cycle. Because of our efforts today, sexuality in aging women tomorrow will be even more of an integral part of their self-concept, body image, and self-esteem.

Loss, change, and growth

Older women, as in other phases of the life cycle, experience losses, changes, and growth. However, there are some circumstances in the later years that are likely to create more discontinuity, precipitating either a crisis and despair or innovation. Those changes having the potential for promoting loss and growth are physiologic alterations in health, retirement, the death of loved ones, and the eventual preparation and acceptance of one's own death. Each of these requires time to assimilate an altered structure and meaning in life.

Health alterations

In our studies of aging women and health alterations we have moved from disorder and disease to order and health. Not long ago aging was seen as a chronic disease: if biologic functions could be controlled we would not "catch" old age (Glover, 1977). Geriatrics, the study of diseases of old age, is still perceived by some as the science that will eventually eliminate the "disease" of old age through prophylactic measures (Rosenfeld, 1976).

Only recently have we advocated aging as a natural process.

Gerontology, the science of aging that considers aging as a process that involves numerous interrelated biologic, psychologic, and social elements, has significantly contributed to the concept of health and aging. Gerontologists have helped us see that the assessment of health in the elderly must be considered from both a subjective and objective perspective. Objectively, a much larger proportion of older women suffer from chronic disabling conditions than do those under age 65. In addition, such disabilities usually last longer and are more severe. Heart disease, arthritis, and rheumatism afflict more of the elderly than do any other chronic conditions. The aged consult physicians more frequently and are hospitalized more often than are those under age 65 (Health of Older Persons, 1978). Even though we have abundant data on these more objective measures of health alterations (data on mortality, morbidity, cure rates, days of hospitalization, discharge and admission rates), we are just beginning to consider the subjective, self-perceived limitations of health alterations in the aged. Those studies done by gerontologists on the subjective self-assessments of health in the elderly reveal a very different perspective.

One study on self-assessment of health in the aged found that to a considerable degree, even when disease is present, aged persons consider themselves healthy and function that way (Stenbeck et al., 1978). Another cross-national study of elderly in the United States, Denmark, and Great Britain demonstrates that the majority of old people say they are in good health for their age. Men in this study were more likely than women to say their health was good (Shanas et al., 1968) Aged persons' ratings of their own health have been demonstrated to be better indications of future health status than physicians' ratings of health predictions (Maddox, 1964). What older people are capable of doing and what they think they will be able to do are useful indicators of how healthy they are and may serve as a guide for predicting the type of resources that will be required (Maddox, 1976).

A definition of health alterations in older women must move beyond the absence or presence of disease and pathology to incorporate an overall assessment of individual perceptions—strengths as well as weaknesses. Each woman makes an accommodation to loss and changes in health with aging. Some women become health pessimists and report their health as poor when objective indices reveal otherwise; others are health optimists and insist, even when facing overwhelming distress, that their health is better than others'. This task of regarding one's body and interpreting a state of health has been described by Robert Peck (1956). He considers that one of the greatest developmental tasks facing older people is the choice between body transcendence and body preoccupation. For those women who perceive pleasure and comfort predominantly in terms of physical well-being, declining health may be the gravest insult. They become preoccupied with their bodily states. Others, who also suffer pain and physical disabilities, still enjoy life greatly. In their value system, social and mental sources of pleasure along with self-respect seem to transcend physical comfort. Attitudes about health and conceptions of physical well-being are most relevant when we consider alterations in the health of aging women.

Retirement

Until recently, the plethora of studies on retirement has totally excluded females. Formerly, the work role was seen as a major source of identity for males only, the implicit assumption being that working roles for women were unimportant and retirement an insignificant state for females. As more women enter the labor force, the realities of work and retirement on their adaptation in old age are being clarified.

The work life expectancy of women climbed from 6.3 years in 1900 to 22.9 years in 1970. The most recent projections indicate that between 1975 and 1990, nearly 12 million women will be added to the labor force. By 1990, over 48.5 million women are projected to be in the labor force, somewhat more than 1 of every 2 in the population 16 years old and over (USDL, 1977). These trends mandate a closer examination of women's adjustment to the loss of a working role and the changes in social and personal resources as well as psychologic and physical well-being.

One analysis of cross-sectional data from a national probability sample of 2398 women aged 65 and over reveals that employed women have a higher morale than retirees, with the exception of women with annual incomes of $5,000 or more; among these, retirees have better morale than workers. Women classified as never having worked have the lowest morale. Group differences in morale stem in part (but not entirely) from the fact that working women are somewhat younger, healthier, and financially better off. Those who had never worked tended to be the oldest, poorest, and in poorest health (Jaslow, 1976). Employment may provide the older woman with a source of dignity, self-esteem, and an opportunity for social participation. When this role is lost through retirement, there may be deleterious social and psychologic ramifications.

The few studies that have examined women's retirement suggest that it may be a difficult transitional period in old age. Atchley (1976), who compared men and women retirees, found that women report taking longer to get used to retirement and are more lonely and depressed than men. Another study on middle class women retirees reveals that retirement appears to lower feelings of psychologic well-being by reducing income and the overall number of people women associate with daily. Perception of poor health and lower "affect balance" were also characteristic of retired women in this sample (Fox, 1977). Additional research is needed to clarify the relationships between retirement and measures of women's health.

One theory on the socialization process of women, the *readjustment theory*, maintains that because women have had considerably more experience than men in adjusting to age-linked changes (roles of worker, housewife, mother; children leaving home; menopause; the greater likelihood of widowhood) they are more accustomed to change and impermanence. Thus role discontinuity and change in life situations make adaptation to old age and associated loss easier for women. If this theory is correct, women should adapt more easily than men to retirement and more easily re-engage in new and meaningful activities (Kline, 1975).

Death: coping with the loss of others and self

One of the losses for older women often requiring great changes in life-style is the loss of a spouse. Along with the death of friends, family, and other relatives, most aging females will eventually cope with widowhood. The average woman will spend the last 7 years of her life alone. One fifth of the female population between the ages of 55 and 64 is widowed, and this proportion doubles for women aged 65 to 74 years; at 75 and over nearly three fourths of all women are widowed (Health of Older Persons, 1978). Thus conjugal bereavement and widowhood have become almost natural components of aging women's lives. The forms of adjustment to this loss are varied. Some of the factors that seem to influence the outcome are social class, education, and the extent to which identity must be reconstructed during widowhood.

There seems to be great variation in the amount of modification required in women's reconstruction of identity following a husband's death. One study of 301 older widows reveals that 46% felt that they themselves and their social lives were unaffected by their husband's death. The degree of disorganization depends upon the pervasiveness of the role of wife. Least affected were women who had not been living with their husbands at the time of the husband's death. Those separated through external circumstances (armed services or occupational assignments) vary in their responses, depending upon the extent they had built an independent life for themselves. Those with the greatest degree of disorganization are the women dependent upon the role of wife.

Other researchers have found that less educated, lower class females live in a sex-segregated world, often with little communication with their husbands. The more educated middle and upper class females usually live couple-companionate lives. Less educated women also seem unaccustomed to conscious construction and reconstruction of their social world and self-identity in marriage and widowhood (Lopata, 1973a). Because of these variations in women's relationships with their spouses we may observe different patterns of bereavement.

Even though patterns of bereavement do not generally follow a neatly structured sequence, there is a series of events with which older women must cope or experience subsequent problems and crises. The process of bereavement and the tasks associated with different phases of this reconstruction of identity may roughly be classified into three stages: impact, recoil, and recovery (Tyhurst, 1958). The initial impact of death is often accompanied by a numbness and disbelief with a tendency to deny reality. Strong emotions, various physical symptoms, and a state of panic may ensue as the woman finds she is unable to get her mind off the loss of her spouse. Overwhelming feelings of guilt and preoccupation with images of the deceased, including visual hallucinations, may occur. Hostile reactions toward the husband who has left her alone and unreasonable anger and jealousy toward those couples still living may ensue. Anger may be directed toward doctors and nurses, who may be blamed for the husband's death. The loss of usual patterns of living and contact with others may compound incapacitating feelings of sadness and loneliness. Along with these common psychologic reactions the widow may not have the energy or psychic strength to cope with the initial tasks of this period of impact: arranging for the funeral, determining financial affairs, and starting legal estate processing.

The recoil stage usually begins with the aftermath of the funeral, when friends and relatives depart and the woman begins her life alone. Tasks at this stage include resuming household duties, adjusting to the loneliness and role of widow, and making plans for her future life.

The final phase, recovery, begins anywhere from 3 months to 2 years following the death of a spouse and includes the following tasks: learning to live alone and make decisions with full responsibility for the outcomes; establishing a new identity and developing a viable philosophy of life; finding a meaningful emotional life with activities that provide satisfaction; deciding on suitable living arrangements; and adjusting to a new standard of living along with a changed status. Unless the couple has planned appropriately for old age and living alone, inadequacy of income is a major contribution to problems of adjustment of widows. Income may be the major intervening variable in morale through its influence on the mobility and social interaction of widows (Lopata, 1971).

Coping with the loss of a spouse and friends and relatives in some ways contributes to the final task in the lives of older women: death. The awareness of death and the recognition of a limit to life is a necessary condition of living. This value orientation is most prevalent in the elderly, whom Erikson (1963) has described as achieving the developmental task of integrity. The basic task in this phase of a woman's life involves the acceptance of one's own life cycle; in such final consolidation, death loses its sting.

We have considered several losses experienced by older women: health alterations, retirement, the loss of others, and preparation for one's own death. With most losses, if elderly females are given time to assimilate changes from these experiences, there is potential for growth. The role of health care providers is to be aware of those circumstances that initiate change and to assist older women as they confront loss, giving them the opportunity to react, to articulate their ambivalent feelings, and to work out their own sense of meaning. Growth from these losses occurs when older women impose new purpose on circumstances, giving meaning to life and relationships that did not exist prior to these changes.

SUCCESSFUL AGING: STRATEGIES FOR COPING

As we have reviewed in this chapter, aging involves the process of loss, growth, and change. Success in this process depends on characteristics of the woman, her access to resources that promote health, and her ability to facilitate strategies for coping with loss and change. The strategies we will focus on in this section will first consider individual strategies that may facilitate successful aging and then collective group resources that may promote health.

Individual strategies

Coping with the changes that accompany aging involves some losses that may not be anticipated; however, many of the normal psychologic and physiologic changes that affect older women may be predicted. If women are educated about such changes and given time to assimilate and plan a meaningful structure to the process of transition from one phase of life to the next, the outcome of successful aging will be enhanced. Humans strive for adaptive compromise that not only preserves them as they are, but also permits them to grow and increase their autonomy.

To promote growth and optimal aging, women must secure adequate information about themselves and factors in their environment that will promote health; they must maintain satisfactory internal physiologic and psychologic conditions for processing information, decision-making, and action; and they must maintain autonomy and freedom to facilitate their goals. Since earlier sections of this chapter considered many of the internal physiologic and psychologic conditions for the promotion of health, this last section will focus on acquisition of information, and autonomy and freedom as prerequisites for successful aging.

Acquiring information

The information that older women need to facilitate successful aging may be classified according to Clark and Anderson's (1967) five adaptive tasks for older persons. These tasks represent a model for adjustment to aging; with information about these tasks women may continue or begin to plan for aging.

The first adaptive task of aging is to admit that *aging involves limitations.* In many ways these limitations are relative, since they depend so much on the individual's life-style. However, in spite of this variation, there are limitations to some degree in most aging women's lives, as there are in other phases of the life cycle. As a result, each women can decide which activities provide the most meaning to her life and conserve her energies to participate in these activities. Second, once an older woman perceives the reality of aging and makes choices about the activities that nurture her life-style, *alterations in social roles and physical activities* must be designed to match the reality of these limitations and decisions. These adjustments may involve changes in outside commitments, personal goals, physical exercise, financial expenditures, and social relationships.

In addition to changing activities and roles during the process of aging, the elderly female must *find new ways to fulfill needs,* the third adaptive task. This is most evident when aging women are required to find new identities and activities following their children's departure from home or the loss of a husband to death. This adaptive task is closely related to social obstacles that influence old age, such as inadequate income, limited transportation services, prejudice against remarriage, and stereotypes about aging. Because of these social obstacles it is difficult for some women to fulfill their needs, even when they recognize altered roles and activities.

A national sample of older people's opinions reveals the following steps should be taken to prepare for the later years of life. In order of priority, the elderly in this sample feel aging would be enhanced through: (1) making sure medical care is available, (2) preparation of a will, (3) building savings, (4) learning about pensions and social security benefits, (5) buying their own home, (6) developing hobbies and other leisure-time activities, (7) deciding on a move or permanent residence, (8) planning new or part-time jobs, (9) talking to other older people about what it's like to grow old, (10) enrolling in retirement counseling or preparation programs, and (11) moving in with other relatives or children. Many of the elderly in this sample had considered and made preparations for altered roles and activities in aging. Consideration and planning for these steps are likely to promote success with aging.

The fourth adaptive task that the elderly must cope with is the *development of new criteria for self-evaluation.* Changing activities and roles, along with finding new ways to fulfill one's needs, all require new measures for reinforcing one's self-worth. This demands the ability to find satisfaction and meaning in activities for their own personal value. This is difficult for some older women in our society, since success is usually equated with the fulfillment of some productive role. They should begin early in their lives to create activities and roles that provide gratification based on an internal criterion of success. Along with reinforcement from others, there is a basic need to believe in oneself and satisfy internal goals and desires.

The final task for successful aging is the *need to establish new values and goals in life.* Only in old age do people experience a personal sense of the entire life cycle, a finding of the self in a larger scheme of things. This sense of satisfaction is not separated from continued growth, curiosity, creativity, and the capacity to change. To maintain a sense of wonder and expectation, to share and cultivate friendships during the process of achieving goals, is to counter disillusionment and cynicism. This fifth task of establishing new goals and values in life can be found in many older women. In fact, it may be the first time one becomes creative as previous burdens and responsibilities decrease. Many older women find satisfaction in creating something that will survive them and contribute to the lives of others.

Maintenance of autonomy

With adequate information about themselves and their environment to promote health, along with maintenance of internal physiologic and psychologic conditions for the promotion of actions and decisions, older women are in a position to maintain and facilitate autonomy for achieving goals.

Autonomy is the factor of first priority in Williams and Wirths' (1965) general theory of optimal aging. Their theory was derived empirically from the careful analysis of 168 elderly men and women observed and interviewed over 5½ years. In this study an autonomy-dependency continuum was designed to ascertain how much energy an older person contributed to significant others in his or her social system. The older person was in balance with respect to the amount of energy exchanged in the environment if he or she was not receiving more than was given to others. If there was more energy given than received a person was said to be autonomous. To be autonomous an individual must have contributed to the values and goals of others. Within this framework, if an older woman is autonomous and develops a clear style of living, successful aging will be enhanced. This approach to optimal aging may be developed early in a woman's life, so that as she grows older she becomes deeply entrenched in autonomy, develops a clear life-style, uses action energy in optimal ways, and learns to be flexible. All of these measures enhance successful aging (Williams and Wirths, 1965).

Older women together

Who will be the primary source of support to women as they age? We have seen that women usually outlive their husbands or male partners; consequently, this source of support will not be available to all elderly women. Can older women depend upon their families for continued support as they age, now and in the future? In the past, it was traditional for women in the household to provide care for elderly parents, despite the fact that elderly women often preferred to care for themselves. Today, however, with the social roles of young and middle-aged women changing, we see an alteration in this traditional pattern.

Women are increasingly working outside the home setting. In 1940 11.1% of the married women between the ages of 45 and 54 worked outside the home; in 1970, 47.8% of the women in this age group were employed. In addition, compared to their predecessors, more women who have responsibility for supporting elderly parents also have husbands and children (Treas, 1977). Working women spend more time on household tasks than their husbands, an average of *at least* 6 more hours a week (U.S. National Commission, 1977). With these additional responsibilities, will working women be able to continue to support aged parents, especially if there is an alteration in their parents' health?

One study on adults providing care to aged parents in their home demonstrated that two fifths of those studied devoted time to care of their parents that was equivalent to a full-time job (Newman, 1976). As more women assume full-time responsibilities outside the home, some in addition to their roles as wife and mother, other sources of support will continue to play an increasingly important role as resources to older women. Kith and organized sources of social support will be important social networks for aging women.

Natural support systems

Support systems have been described as enduring patterns of continuous or intermittent ties that play a sig-

nificant part in maintaining psychologic and physical integrity of individuals over time. They provide persons with feedback and validate their expectations about others, which tends to balance deficiencies that may exist in the larger community context. This type of support may be continuous or intermittent. The type of support most of us are familiar with is family, or *kin*. The other form, which older women will have to nurture more in the future for support, is referred to as *kith*.

Kith are natural support systems that include such persons as friends, neighbors, and other acquaintances. Like kin, kith support systems provide three functions: they share tasks, provide supplies (money, skills, tools, etc.), and they offer cognitive guidance for the promotion of problem-solving. Along with kin they also provide another essential characteristic: they deal with the individual as a unique person worthy of respect and affection. This characteristic is believed to buffer stress and protect the individual against disease.

A number of studies on psychosocial support indicate that the presence of such support has a protective effect upon the person experiencing stressful stimuli (Kaplan et al., 1977). Biologic and pyschosocial theories have been proposed to explain the health conditioning qualities of social support systems. For the aged, research is beginning to yield findings that further unravel the relationships between stress and adaptation (Lowenthal and Chiriboga, 1973). The results consistently suggest that relatively healthy aged individuals successfully cope with stressful life situations (Eisdorfer and Wilkie, 1977). What we do not yet know is what influence repeated stressors over time have on the health outcomes of aging persons. Since we can predict that older women will more than likely be relying on kith sources of support in the future, additional research and practice models need to consider the conditioning effect these various forms of social support have on the health of aging women. Some of these networks of social support are currently being evaluated and will be briefly considered in this final section on collaboration for change.

Collaboration for change

Older women are beginning to organize and develop strategies for promoting change. Much of the research and education on aging has not involved the aged themselves. They have important contributions to make and need to participate. As Margaret Kuhn (1977) recently commented in a conference on aging, for too long old people have been objects of social inquiry—like mice in laboratories and butterflies in cases; they need to be viewed as living, breathing collaborators in and contributors to society's understanding of aging. Action and strategies for aging women should not be designed *for* them, rather they must be done *with* them.

Some national movements are emerging that emphasize the collaboration and contributions of old people. One such movement involves the Gray Panthers, an organization that distinguishes itself from other "senior citizens" groups (a euphemism they reject) by the following three characteristics: it is an action coalition of young and old people working for change; it is concerned with all forms of injustice and oppression; and it is experimenting with new, flexible structures and multiple leadership. The long-range goals of the Gray Panthers involves social change in the direction of a more humane, just society to liberate all persons oppressed and powerless, among them the nonwhites, aged, and women (Kuhn, 1977).

Another example of an innovative strategy for promoting adaptation among older women is described in "The Unexpected Community," a group of forty widows who developed their own kind of extended family in their housing unit. Other communities are planning to develop cooperative nonprofit living arrangements that would house young and old adults (Hochschild, 1973). In addition to these supportive housing arrangements, several highly successful consciousness-raising groups (Feldman, 1976) and advocacy training sessions for older persons are promoting new life-styles for the elderly (California Project, 1971).

Aging individuals are showing signs of increasing activism with the intent of improving the quality of life for the aged of today and tomorrow. An agenda for activism has been designed by Robert Butler (1976) that includes many specific activities that older women can conduct under their own leadership. This agenda provides information about political activity and community and legal actions that may be taken to improve the quality of life for older people. Along with grievance, surveillance, resistance, and protective activities, older women have a ready access to a number of strategies for advocacy with aging. Kerschner (1976) describes the issues and experiences of advocacy by and for the elderly along with vehicles and strategies for promoting change.

The political power of the women's movement is still another vehicle that can be used by aging women collectively. A coalition between older women and the women's movement would be mutually beneficial for changing the stereotypes about older women originating from ageism and sexism. For the most part, women's liberation has ignored older women, even though the oppression that women have experienced throughout the years makes aging a feminist issue (Butler, 1972). It is time to change these patterns and work together. Through working together women can strive to improve the quality of life for older women today and also for themselves as the older women of tomorrow (Streib, 1976). The quality of life for older citizens in the future will depend upon the leadership of women because older women are healthier, they live longer, and they have special abilities for organizing, socializing, and caring. It will be to the advantage of all women to begin to examine what they can do for themselves and each other collectively that will make their aging more successful.

This chapter has focused on women in the later years of their lives. It has examined women both in middle and old age along with the attitudes, images, and stereotypes that influence their perception of this phase of the life cycle. We have considered physiologic processes and physical and psychologic changes that affect health; all of these are modified by sociocultural factors that combine either to promote or hinder adaptation, growth, and change in the lives of aging women. Successful aging for women may be enhanced through individual behavior and action, or collective collaboration with other women by organizing and promoting strategies for change. Through exposing and challenging the stereotypes that perpetuate ageism and sexism women will appreciate that aging can be a basis for hope, rather than a reason for despair. Through understanding the process of normal aging we can begin to dispel the myths that cloud the beauty of aging. By working together and by maintaining mental openness and enthusiasm for learning, older women will enjoy the discovery of a completed life cycle; as they age they will find there is time to greet the true reasons for living. The full maturity of old age captures the unique experiences of each life cycle: if we look closely we will find that in the final phase of life there is more to see than we first imagined. To be old is to be beautiful!

REFERENCES

Adams, G., and deVries, H.: Physiological effects of an exercise training regimen upon women 52 to 79, J. Gerontol. **28**:50-55, 1973.

Antunes, C., and others: Endometrial cancer and estrogen use, N. Engl. J. Med. **300**(1):9-13, Jan. 1979.

Alyward, M.: Estrogens, plasma tryptophan levels in perimenopausal patients. In Campbell, S., editor: The management of menopause and post menopausal years, Baltimore, 1976, University Park Press.

Atchley, R.: Selected social and psychological differences between men and women in later life, J. Gerontol. **31**:204-211, 1976.

Axelson, L. S.: Personal adjustments in the post parental period, J. Marr. Fam. Liv. **22**:66-70, 1960.

Bardwick, J.: Psychology of women, New York, 1971, Harper and Row, Publishers.

Barrows, C., and Roeder, L.: Nutrition. In Finch, C., and Hayflick, L., editors: Handbook of the biology of aging, New York, 1977, Van Nostrand Reinhold Co.

Bart, P.: Depression in middle aged women. In Gornick, V., and Maran, B. K., editors: Women in a sexist society, New York, 1971, Basic Books, Inc.

Bellucci, G., and Hoyer, W.: Feedback effects on the performance and self reinforcing behavior of elderly and young adult women, J. Gerontol. **30**(4):456-460, 1975.

Benedek, T.: Psychosocial functions in women, New York, 1952, Ronald Press Co.

Bogomolets, A.: The prolongation of life, New York, 1946, Duell, Sloan and Pearce.

Booth, P.: We can still yell. An interview with Maggie Kuhn, Women and Aging, New York, 1976, A Journal of Liberation Co.

Boston Women's Health Book Collective: Our bodies, ourselves, New York, 1976, Simon and Schuster.

Botelia-Livsia, J.: Endocrinology of women, Philadelphia, 1973, W. B. Saunders Co.

Butler, R.: Why survive? Being old in America, New York, 1975, Harper and Row, Publishers.

Butler, R., and Lewis, M.: Why is women's lib ignoring older women? Aging Hum. Devel. 3:223-232, 1972.

Butler, R., and Lewis, M.: Aging and mental health: positive psychosocial approaches, St. Louis, 1973, The C. V. Mosby Co.

Butler, R., and Lewis, M.: Love and sex after sixty, New York, 1976, Harper and Row, Publishers.

California Rural Legal Assistance Senior Citizens Project: Training older Americans in America, San Francisco, 1971, The Project.

Caplan, G.: Support systems and community mental health, New York, 1974, Behavioral Publications.

Christenson, C. V., and Gagnon, J. H.: Sexual behavior in a group of older women, J. Gerontol. 20:351-356, 1965.

Clark, M., and Anderson, B.: Culture and aging, Springfield, Ill., 1967, Charles C Thomas, Publisher.

Cope, E.: Physical changes associated with the post menopausal years. In Campbell, S., editor: The management of the menopause and post menopausal years, Baltimore, 1976, University Park Press.

Cumming, E., and Henry, W.: Growing old, New York, 1961, Basic Books Inc.

deBeauvoir, S.: The coming of age, New York, 1972, G. P. Putnam's Sons.

Detre, T., and others: Management of the menopause, Ann. Int. Med. 88:373-378, 1978.

Deutscher, I.: The quality of post parental life. In Neugarten, B., editor: Middle age and aging, Chicago, 1968, University of Chicago Press.

Deykin, E., and others: The empty nest: psychosocial aspects of conflicts between depressed women and their grown children, Am. J. Psych. 122:1422-1426, 1966.

Eisdorfer, C., and Wilkie, F.: Stress, disease, aging and behavior. In Birren, J., and Schaie, W., editors: Handbook of the psychology of aging, New York, 1977, Van Nostrand Reinhold Co.

Erikson, E.: Childhood and safety, New York, 1963, W. W. Norton and Co.

Feldman, H.: Consciousness raising as a new life style for the elderly. In No longer young: the older women in America. Proceedings of the 26th Annual Conference on Aging, Institute of Gerontology, Wayne State University, 1976.

Finch, C., and Hayflick, L., editors: Handbook of the biology of aging, New York, 1977, Van Nostrand and Reinhold Co.

Fox, J. H.: Effects of retirement and former work life on women's adaptation in old age, J. Gerontol. 32:196-202, 1977.

Friday, N.: My mother, myself, New York, 1977, Delacourte Press.

Friedan, B.: The feminine mystique, New York, 1968, Dell Publishing Co.

Fuchs, E.: The second season, New York, 1977, Onchat Press, Doubleday.

Glenn, N.: Psychological well-being in the post parental stage—Some evidence from national surveys, J. Marr. Fam. 36(part 1):105-110, 1975.

Glover, B.: Sex counseling of the elderly, Hosp. Pract. 12(6):101-112, 1977.

Gordon, T., and others: Menopause and coronary heart disease, J. Int. Med. 89:157-161, 1978.

Gutman, D. L.: Dependency, illness and survival among Navajo men. In Palmore, E., and Jeffers, F., editors: Prediction of life span, Lexington, Mass., 1971, Health Lexington.

Haller, J. S., and Haller, R. M.: The physician and sexuality in Victorian America, Urbana, Ill., 1974, University of Illinois Press.

Harkins, E.: Effects of empty nest transition of self report of psychological and physical well being, J. Marriage Family 40(3):549-556, 1978.

Havighurst, R.: A social-psychological perspective on aging, Gerontologist 8(2):67-71, 1968.

Health of older persons, Statistical Bull. 59(1):14-15, 1978.

Heaney, R. P.: Estrogens and postmenopausal osteoporosis, Clin. Obstet. Gynecol. 19(4):791-804, 1976.

Heiple, P.: A study of women's responses to midlife changes. Unpublished Master's thesis, University of Rochester, School of Nursing, 1979.

Hochschild, A.: The unexpected community, Englewood Cliffs, N.J., 1973, Prentice-Hall, Inc.

Hoover, R., and others: Menopausal estrogens and breast cancer, N. Engl. J. Med. 295:401-405, 1976.

Jaslow, P.: Employment, retirement and morale among older women, J. Gerontol. 31:212-218, 1976.

Jowsey, J.: Why is mineral nutrition important in osteoporosis? Geriatrics 33(8):39-52, 1978.

Jowsey, J.: Osteoporosis—its nature and the role of diet, Postgrad. Med. 60(2):75-79, 1976.

Kahn, E., and Fisher, C.: The sleep characteristics of the normal aged male, J. Nerv. Ment. Dis. 148:477-494, 1969.

Kaplan, B., and others: Social support and health, Medical Care 15:47-58, 1977.

Kase, N.: Yes or no on estrogen replacement therapy—a formulation for clinicians, Clin. Obstet. Gynecol. 19(4):825-833, 1976.

Kerschner, P., editor: Advocacy and age, University of Southern California, Los Angeles, 1976, The Ethel Percy Andrus Gerontology Center.

Kimmel, D.: Adulthood and aging, New York, 1974, John Wiley & Sons.

Kline, C.: The socialization process of women, Gerontologist 15:486-492, 1975.

Komarovsky, M.: Blue-collar marriage, New York, 1967, Random House.

Kraus, H., and Radbi, W.: Hypokinetic disease, Springfield, Ill., 1961, Charles C Thomas, Publisher.

Kuhn, M.: Learning by living, Int. J. Aging Hum. Devel. 8:359-365, 1977-1978.

Labouvie-Vief, G., and Gonda, J.: Cognitive strategy training and intellectual performance in the elderly, J. Gerontol. 31(3):327-332, 1976.

Lair, C. V., and Moon, W. H.: The effects of praise and reproof on the performance of middle aged and older subjects, Aging Hum. Devel. 3:279-284, 1972.

Lauritzen, C.: Management of the patient at risk, estrogen therapy, frontiers of hormone research, 5, Basel, 1978, S. Karger.

Lieberman, M. A.: Adaptive processes in late life. In Datan, N., and Ginsberg, L., editors: Life span developmental psychology: normative life crises, New York, 1975, Academic Press, Inc.

Livson, F.: Patterns of personality development in middle aged women: a longitudinal study, Int. J. Aging Hum. Devel. 7(2):107-117, 1976.

Lopata, H.: Self identity in marriage and widowhood, Soc. Quart. 14:407-418, 1973a.

Lopata, H.: Widowhood in an American city, Cambridge, Mass., 1973b, Schenkman.

Lopata, H.: Widows as minority groups, Gerontologist 11:67-76, 1971.

Lowenthal, M., and Chiriboga, D.: Social stress and adaptation: toward a life course perspective. In Eisdorfer, C., and Lawton, P., editors: The psychology of adult development and aging, Washington, D.C., 1973, American Psychological Association.

Lowenthal, M. E., and Chiriboga, D.: Transition to the empty nest, Arch. Gen. Psych. **26**(1):8-15, 1972.

Mack, T. M., and others: Estrogens and endometrial cancer in a retirement community, N. Engl. J. Med. **294**:1265-1267, 1976.

Maddox, G.: Aging, health and health resources. In Binstock, R., and Shanas, E., editors: Handbook of aging and social sciences, New York, 1976, Van Nostrand Reinhold Co.

Maddox, G.: Self assessment of health status: a longitudinal study of selected elderly subjects, J. Chron. Dis. **17**:449-460, 1964.

Martin, L.: Health care of women, Philadelphia, 1978, J. B. Lippincott Co.

Masters, W., and Johnson, V.: Human sexual response, Boston, 1966, Little, Brown & Co.

National Council on the Aging, Inc. and Louis Harris and Associates, Inc.: The myth and reality of aging in America, Washington, D.C., 1975, The Council.

Neugarten, B.: Adaptation and the life cycle, J. Geriat. Psych. **4**(1): 71-87, 1970.

Neugarten, B., and others: Women's attitudes towards the menopause, In Neugarten, B., editor: Middle age and aging, Chicago, 1968, University of Chicago Press.

Neugarten, B., and Moore, J.: The changing age status system. In Neugarten, B., editor: Middle age and aging, Chicago, 1968, University of Chicago Press.

Neugarten, B., and Haines, R. J.: Menopausal symptoms, Psychosom. Med. **271**(3):266-273, 1965.

Newman, G., and Nichols, C.: Sexual activities and attitudes in older persons, J.A.M.A. **173**:33-35, 1960.

Newman, S.: Housing adjustments of older people: a report from the social phase, Ann Arbor, 1976, Institute of Social Research.

Notelovitz, M.: Gynecologic problems of menopausal women. Part 1. Changes in genital tissue, Geriatrics **33**(8):24-32, 1978a.

Notelovitz, M.: Gynecologic problems of menopausal women. Part 2. Treating estrogen deficiency, Geriatrics **33**(9):35-38, Sept. 1978b.

Nowak, C.: Does youthfulness equal attractiveness? In Troll, L., and others, editors: Looking ahead—a woman's guide to the problems and joys of growing older, Englewood Cliffs, N.J., 1977, Prentice-Hall, Inc.

Novack, E., Jones, G. S., and Jones, H., editors: Novak's textbook of gynecology, Baltimore, 1975, The Williams & Wilkins Co.

Orshansky, M.: Federal welfare record and the economic status of the aged poor, Staff Paper No. 17, Washington, D.C., 1974, Office of Research and Statistics, U.S. Social Security Administration.

Page, J.: The other awkward age, Berkeley, 1977, Ten Speed Press.

Peck, R.: Psychological developments in the second half of life. In Anderson, J., editor: Psychological aspects of aging, Washington, D.C., 1956, American Psychological Association.

Piscopo, J.: Fitness after fifty, Health Values **1**(5):211-217, 1977.

Pfeffer, R.: Estrogen use in postmenopausal women, Am. J. Epidemiol. **105**(1):21-29, 1977.

Pfeiffer, E.: Sexual behavior in old age. In Busse, E., and Pfeiffer, E., editors: Behavior and adaption in late life, Boston, 1969, Little, Brown & Co.

Pfeiffer, E.: Psychopathology and social pathology. In Birren, J., and Schaie, K. W., editors: Handbook of the psychology of aging, New York, 1977, Van Nostrand Reinhold Co.

Pfeiffer, E., Verwoerdt, A., and Davis, G.: Sexual behavior in middle life, Am. J. Psych. **128**:1262-1267, 1972.

Population Reference Bureau, Inc.: Administration on Aging, facts and figures on older persons, No. 5, Washington, D.C., 1975, Department of Health, Education and Welfare, Publication OHD 74-20005, pp. 4-6.

Powell, B.: The empty nest, employment and psychiatric symptoms in college-educated women, Psychol. Women **2**:35-43, Fall 1977.

Rockstein, M.: Heredity and longevity in the animal kingdom, J. Gerontol. **13**:7-12, 1958.

Rollins, B., and Feldman, H.: Marital satisfaction over the family life cycle, J. Marriage Family **32**(1):20-28, 1970.

Rosenfeld, A.: Prolongevity, New York, 1976, Alfred A. Knopf.

Ryan, K. J.: Estrogens and atherosclerosis, Clin. Obstet. Gynecol. **19**(4):805-816, 1976.

Salvatore, J., and others: Nutrition in the aged: review of the literature, J. Am. Geriat. Soc. **17**(8):790-806, 1969.

Schaie, W.: Age changes in adult intelligence. In Woodruff, D., and Birren, J., editors: Aging: scientific perspectives and social issues, New York, 1975, D. Van Nostrand Co.

Seaman, B., and Seaman, G.: Women and the crisis in sex hormones, New York, 1977, Rawson Associates.

Shanas, E., and others: Old people in three industrial societies, New York, 1968, Atherton Press.

Shock, N.: Systems integration. In Finch, C., and Hayflick, L., editors: Handbook of the biology of aging, New York, 1977, Van Nostrand Reinhold Company.

Sinex, M.: The molecular genetics of aging. In Finch, C., and Hayflick, L., editors: Handbook of the biology of aging, New York, 1977, Van Nostrand Reinhold Co.

Smith, P. J.: The effects of estrogen on bladder function in the female. Management of the menopause and post menopausal years. In Campbell, S., editor: The management of menopause and post menopause years, Baltimore, 1976, University Park Press.

Smith, D., and others: Association of exogenous estrogen and endometrial carcinoma, N. Engl. J. Med. **293**(23):1164-1167, 1975.

Sommers, T.: Aging in America—implications for women. Based on the NCOA Louis Harris and Associates Public Opinion Study, The Myth and Reality of Aging, Washington, D.C., The National Council on Aging, 1975.

Sommer, T.: The compounding impact of age on sex, Civil Rights Digest **7**:2-9, 1974.

Sontag, S. The double standard of aging. In No longer young: the older woman in America. Proceedings of the 26th Annual Conference on Aging, The Institute of Gerontology, University of Michigan, Wayne State University, 1976.

Stadel, B., and Weiss, N.: Characteristics of menopausal women: a survey of King and Pierce counties in Washington, 1973-1974. Am. J. of Epidemiol. **102**(3):209-216, 1975.

Stenback, A., and others: Illness and health behavior in septuagenarians, J. Gerontol. **33**:57-61, 1978.

Streib, G.: Mechanisms for change viewed in a sociological context. In No longer young: the older woman in America. Proceedings of the 26th Annual Conference on Aging, The Institute of Gerontology, Wayne State University, 1976.

Treas, J.: Aging and the family. In Woodruff, D., and Birren, J., editors: Aging: scientific perspectives and social issues, New York, 1975, Van Nostrand Co.

Treas, J.: Family support systems for the aged: some social and demographic considerations, Gerontologist **17**:486-491, Dec. 1977.

Troll, L., Israel, J., and Israel, K., editors: Looking ahead—a woman's guide to the problems and joys of growing older, Englewood Cliffs, N.J., 1977, Prentice-Hall, Inc.

Tyhurst, J.: The role of transitional states including disasters. In Mental illness, Walter Reed Symposium on Preventive and Social Psychiatry, Washington, D.C., 1958, U.S. Government Printing Office.

Tyson, M. C.: Let's talk about menopause, Nursing '78 **8**(8):34-36, 1978.

U.S. Bureau of the Census: Census of Population, 1970. Subject reports, final report PC (2)-6A, Employment Status on Work Experience, Washington, D.C., 1973, U.S. Government Printing Office.

U.S. Bureau of the Census: Demographic aspects of aging in the

United States, current population reports, Series PC-23, No. 59, Washington, D.C., 1976, U.S. Government Printing Office.

U.S. National Commission for UNESCO: Report on Women in America, Department of State Publication 8923, Nov. 1977.

U.S. Department of Labor: U.S. working women: A databook, Washington, D.C., 1977, Bureau of Labor Statistics.

Wessel, J. A., and Van Huss, W. D.: The influence of physical activity and age on exercise adaptation of women aged 20-69, J. Sport Med. 9:173-180, 1969.

Widows in the United States, Statistical Bull. 58:8-10, 1977.

Williams, J.: Psychology of women, New York, 1977, W. W. Norton and Co.

Williams, R., and Wirths, C.: Lives through the years, New York, 1965, Atherton Press.

Williams, S. R., and Loeb, M.: The adult's social life space and suc-cessful aging: some suggestions for a conceptual framework. In Neugarten, B., editor: Middle age and aging, Chicago, 1968, University of Chicago Press.

Winick, M., editor: Nutrition and aging, New York, 1976, John Wiley & Sons.

Woodruff, D.: A physiological perspective of the psychology of aging. In Woodruff, D., and Birren, J., editors: Aging: scientific perspectives and social issues, New York, 1975, D. Van Nostrand Co.

Woods, N. F.: Human sexuality and the healthy elderly. In Brown, M., editor: Readings in gerontology, St. Louis, 1978, The C. V. Mosby Co.

Ziel, H., and Finkle, W.: Increased risk of endometrial carcinoma among users of conjugated estrogens, N. Engl. J. Med. 293(23):1167-1170, 1975.

19

Exercise

Patricia Holleran Cotanch
Nancy B. Alexander

For too long women have ignored the need to exercise and be physically active. Physical fitness and sport have been viewed as desirable attributes for men but not women. Biologically the differences between the exercise abilities of males and females are few and the similarities are many. Surmounting the social and cultural determinants has been the greatest barrier for women.

Physical fitness for women and men is considered a positive health criterion, thus the link between exercise and health maintenance is clear. Data are currently being collected on the psychologic benefits derived from regular physical activity. The terms "health" and fitness" must, therefore, be the sum of the psychologic and physical states of an individual. Health promotion and illness therapy must logically be directed toward both entities. If the results of exercise are shown to be beneficial to total health, it is likely that exercise may be viewed not only as a recreational activity but as a means for health promotion.

EXERCISE AS STRESS

The benefits of exercise as a recreational activity have been recognized for many years; however, the health benefits both physiologically and psychologically are only currently being realized. The concept of stress is a useful way to examine how the health benefits are derived from exercise.

Present day life has many stressors, both physiologic and psychologic. All life stressors result in the release of stress hormones. The effect of the stress hormones on the body cannot be separated from the effect on the mind, whether the stress is physical or psychologic. One only has to recall the many somatic sensations experienced when something has gone awry in daily living.

It is postulated that exposure of the body to a controlled stressor like exercise results in the development of an adaptation that enables the body to handle that and possibly other stressors. Exercise may act as a stabilizer for the homeostatic balance of the stress response by providing a means of equalizing the physiologic aspects of emotional stressors.

According to Hans Selye (1950), stress is the nonspecific systemic response of the body to any demand made on it. The nonspecific factor is important to recognize since the physiologic response to either a positive or negative stimulus has been shown to be identical. Selye has described the general adaptation syndrome (GAS) as a triphasic process through which the organism either adapts to the stressor or does not. He explains the differences between "superficial" and "deep" adaptation to stress. Superficial stress, in small quantities that are encountered occasionally, requires a given amount of energy that is rapidly regenerated, but the deep stress reactions such as the gnawing, exhausting effort one puts forth under ongoing excessive emotional strain results in irreparable degeneration of the organism. Selye believes the wear and tear of an excessively stressful life (deep stress adaptation) is actually responsible for a shortened life span.

Exercise may be considered as a stressor; in fact, physical exercise was one of the first research models used by physiologists to test and reproduce the typical stress response.

The physiologic response to a stressor is coordinated by the neural and endocrine centers that form the main defense mechanisms of the body. Through activation of the autonomic nervous system and the adrenal cortex, the ability to withstand a stressor is present. If a stressor is repeatedly encountered, conditioning against that stressor may occur, such that a type of resistance may develop. The development of resistance can be supported physiologically by findings of adrenal hypertrophy in animals repeatedly exposed to various stressors (Selye, 1975). The significance of adrenal hypertrophy is the increase in adrenocortical hormones, which decreases the stimulation threshold thereby decreasing the time needed to adjust to or resist the stressor. Exercise, by activating the autonomic nervous system and the adrenal cortex, affects the inherent defense mechanisms of the body. If the body's defense mechanism could be developed as a result of regular exercise, there would be a more efficient reaction to stress. Regular exercise, as a stressor, may improve the efficiency of the stress response, thereby conditioning the individual against the detrimental effects of stress.

Physical exercise of sufficient intensity and duration elicits all the major characteristics of the GAS (Selye, 1976). For example, the initial period of exercise parallels the alarm phase when sympathetic activity is increased to meet the systemic needs incurred by muscular work. Mediated by neural and hormonal processes, exercise stimulates secretion of epinephrine (adrenaline) and ACTH (adrenal corticotropic hormone). ACTH stimulates the adrenal cortex to produce glucocorticoids, which causes an increase in gluconeogenesis. Through the process of gluconeogenesis the blood glucose level and the liver glycogen concentrations are increased. The adrenal cortex also produces mineralocorticoid, causing the retention of sodium and excretion of potassium. The cumulative effect of the alarm stage is to prepare the individual to resist a stressor. In this case, the stressor is exercise.

If Selye's theory of stress is tenable then the conditioning against nonspecific stressors is a physiologic conditioning characterized by increased adrenal sensitivity. As mentioned previously, the ability to adapt to stress is influenced by the available physiologic mechanisms, thus the advantage of exercise is the stimulation of the inherent defense mechanisms. Since the defense mechanisms are activated by both physiologic and psychologic stressors, exercise may possess a degree of protection against both physical and emotional threats to health. Just as rest and sleep can restore resistance and promote adaptation, regular exercise can increase adaptation and enhance resistance.

The effects of regular exercise have been studied extensively in relation to cardiac disease and found to be a valuable therapeutic approach. However, cardiac rehabilitation represents only one way exercise can be used. The context in which exercise is used must be expanded to include health promotion and maintenance as well as restoration. Use of this conceptual approach allows one to look at stress and exercise as holistic phenomena that influence health—irrespective of gender. Women and men encounter many stressors throughout the life cycle; some are similar and others are not. Physiologically, the stress response is nearly identical; behaviorally, the responses vary based on individual expectations, perceptions, and societal role proscriptions.

DEFINITIONS
Muscle action

There are two types of skeletal muscle contractions, each with significant characteristics. These are isotonic and isometric muscle contractions.

Isotonic. When activated, the muscle varies in length with concomitant joint movement. Isotonic muscle contraction is also called dynamic exercise when there is total body involvement. The important element of dynamic exercise is the rhythmic, alternating contraction and relaxation of the involved muscles, which enhances arterial flow in the muscle bed and venous return to the right atrium (Bruce, 1977). Since blood flow is facilitated by alternating muscular contractions, the oxygen stores in the muscle are repeatedly depleted and replenished (Astrand and Rodahl, 1977). Dynamic exercise benefits the circulatory system and does not exceed aerobic capabilities. Examples of isotonic exercise include walking, bicycling, jogging, running, and swimming.

Isometric. In this type of skeletal muscle contraction, there is no joint movement and the muscle length is constant (i.e., sustained contraction against a fixed resistance). Isometric, also called static, exercise has significant local and systemic effects. Locally, the blood vessels dilate during muscle contraction; however, the blood flow through the muscle is limited since the inflow is impeded by the compression of the small arteries by the contracting muscles.

Circulatory responses to static exercise are significant, and include elevated systolic and diastolic pressures and elevated heart rate and cardiac output. The circulatory response to static work often exceeds the aerobic capabilities of the involved muscles (Bruce, 1977; Andersen et al, 1978). Examples of isometric exercise include weight-lifting and water-skiing.

Both isotonic and isometric contraction may occur simultaneously in different muscle groups in the same individual. An example is an individual who is walking while carrying a heavy load in her arms.

Metabolism

There are two types of metabolic processes that operate in the body to produce the needed energy for cellular fuel. These are aerobic and anaerobic metabolism.

Aerobic. Aerobic metabolism requires the presence of oxygen to oxidize specific nutrients for energy to be used by active muscle cells. Use of the term "aerobic," which refers to a metabolic system for energy production, has gradually evolved into "aerobic" exercise. The latter term implies an exercise activity that involves efficient use of oxygen. Examples of aerobic exercise are those activities that involve total body motion, such as those cited as dynamic exercise.

In recent years the terms "dynamic" and "aerobic"

exercise have been used interchangeably. Aerobic exercise may be defined as that form of exercise that demands a substantial increase in oxygen consumption and utilization for task completion" (Brammell and Niccoli, 1976). Thus the relationship between aerobic metabolism and dynamic exercise is the presence of adequate oxygen and efficient utilization of oxygen to meet cellular requirements. The intermittent muscle relaxation and contraction permits arterial flow and a supply of oxygen. The aerobic oxidative capabilities are developed through habitual dynamic exercise. The ability to use oxygen efficiently is called aerobic capacity.

Anaerobic. The anaerobic metabolic process does not utilize oxygen to produce energy for muscular work. Energy for cellular use can be produced by anaerobic oxidation, but the energy is in a limited quantity. This process can and does operate in both isotonic and isometric muscular work. Anaerobic metabolism often functions in the very early stages of dynamic exercise, when immediate energy is needed and the oxygen supply is too limited to permit aerobic energy production. The energy supplied by anaerobic means is for a short duration. If aerobic mechanisms are not adequate, exercise will be terminated because of cellular depletion of ATP, which is manifested as muscle fatigue and exhaustion (Morehouse and Miller, 1976).

PSYCHOLOGIC EFFECTS OF EXERCISE

The benefits of regular exercise have been associated with improvement in physiologic parameters such as circulation, muscular strength, and motor skills, which in turn promotes efficiency with less fatigue caused by physical exertion. While the physiologic parameters have been studied widely, prior to 1953 comparatively little data had been compiled on the psychologic effects of regular exercise. Early reports of the euphoria and positive sense of well-being after physical activity have been considered subjective, unreliable, and lacking scientific basis. Since 1953 the research data on the psychologic effects have multiplied. Research studies have attempted to operationalize and measure specific behavioral and personality variables associated with individuals who engage in some form of regular exercise. The major limitations of the research include the diversity of tools used to measure the psychologic variables, limited use of experimental design, and the paucity of longitudinal studies. In addition, there are few studies using women who exercise as subjects. With increased awareness of the psychologic effects of exercise on stress and the active female, investigations exploring specific relationships should proliferate. As the quantity and quality of research increase, the ability to draw definitive conclusions about the psychologic benefits of exercise on the overall health status of women will increase.

It is important to recognize the potential impact of exercise on the psychologic well-being of active individuals. Reports of extraordinary psychic changes occurring during and after exercise were common in the literature as early as 2000 years ago and continue in the present time. Thus the mind-body concept of unity and interrelatedness is not a new idea and is easily applied to the psychologic effects of physical activity. A timely example of the mind-body concept is the "runner's high," which has been popularized in the lay literature.

Factors such as elevated cerebral oxygenation, increased levels of thyroid-stimulating hormone (TSH), and increased sympathetic activity have been proposed as possible explanations for the reports of positive psychologic states during exercise. The increased metabolic rate could account for the positive psychologic state that occurs during and immediately after the exercise periods. The direct effects of the hormonal and neural processes could also explain the short-lived "runner's high" phenomenon; however, the longer lasting psychologic benefits are not as easily explained. For example, the frequently reported positive sense of well-being is not attributed to increased metabolic activity. Since the positive affective response does not diminish after the exercise period (as do the hormonal and neural levels), another explanation is needed. A more tenable explanation is that the positive affect may be a product of satisfaction with perceived body image, which has been altered as a result of weight loss or redistribution achieved through regular exercise. This approach suggests that exercise, as a physical activity, does affect the psyche (i.e., mind-body interplay).

Given that mind-body unity means a two-way interplay of mind and body, the focus has interestingly been directed toward somatic changes produced by psychologic factors. It is now accepted that physical ailments can be the result of psychic stress (psychosomatic). For example, the type A personality is viewed as a risk factor for coronary heart disease. In contrast, the notion that a psychologic state can be directly affected by a somatic variable is less popular (somatopsychic). The terms psychosomatic and somatopsychic have evolved in an effort to delineate causation and the etiologic factor (Harris, 1973). It is from the somatopsychic viewpoint that exercise will be described.

This approach does not infer cause and effect, but rather it is an attempt to illustrate the psychologic benefits of exercise. Research on the psychologic effects of physical activity began in 1953 when Cureton studied the psychologic correlates of exercise in 2500 adults. He followed the subjects over a 10-year period through varied physical conditioning programs. He reported that "nervous tension" decreased or disappeared in those individuals who exercised regularly. Cureton (1963) has proposed that physical inactivity has a negative effect on tension release whereas physical activity provides a mechanism for release of tension. DeVries (1968) used surface electromyography to measure tension and observed a 58% decrease in physiologic tension (neuromuscular activity) in individuals after exercise periods.

Layman (1974) reviewed the literature on the psychologic effects of physical activity with particular emphasis on perception, body image and self-concept, aggression, and anxiety. While she accomplished an impressive and thorough literature review, the research data are less than clearcut. The relationship between physical activity and psychologic variables is complicated by many factors inherent in the subjects or the environment. Nevertheless from these studies some commonly accepted statements have been derived:

1. Basic personality structure does not change as a result of improved fitness.
2. Physical fitness has been correlated with changes in mood variables; a large amount of data exists on the relationship between fitness and self-concept.
3. Work efficiency seems to benefit from increased physical fitness.
4. Individuals who are least physically and psychologically fit will show the most improvement; however, further increases in physical fitness will not necessarily increase psychologic fitness.
5. Cultural expectations are different concerning the female's participation in sport and exercise. Not only are women consistently less physically fit, but women have been found to be less "psychologically fit" as compared to the male of the same age.

Current consideration is being given toward exercise as a mechanism to promote psychologic adaptation to stress. Certainly, stress is a rather global concept that must be operationalized to be useful. For the woman, stress could be related to enactment of multiple social roles, participation in predominantly male social roles, or confinement to traditional female roles. Stress also occurs as the result of intrapsychic conflict, such as low self-esteem, discrepancy between perceived self and ideal self, distorted body image, or suppression of aggressive impulses. In reference to aggression, there is no data on the effect of participation in athletics on the aggression traits in women (Layman, 1974).

Data have shown that self-concept is influenced by physical fitness. In an experimental study, Biles (1968) measured self-concept changes in 102 college women enrolled in a physical education course. Women in the experimental group had less of a discrepancy between perceived self and ideal self, thereby decreasing dissatisfaction with self. Harris (1965) found college women with low fitness levels demonstrate greater feelings of inferiority than those with high fitness levels. Schultz (1961) studied highschool girls and found that those girls with high physical fitness have significantly higher body image scores than do those girls with low fitness. Hellison (1969) concluded that improvement in attitudes toward self is a product of intensity and frequency of activity rather than the actual physical fitness changes. While this is an interesting finding, Hellison's subjects were college men and the intensity/frequency variables might be attributed to past cultural experience in athletics.

Measurement of state anxiety has been valuable in clarifying confusion about multiple definitions of anxiety, as well as operationalizing psychologic stress resulting from situational and intrapsychic conflict. Since *state anxiety* is a more transitory state, as opposed to *trait anxiety*, which is a personality trait, state anxiety is expected to be influenced by physical activity to a greater extent than trait anxiety. The tools commonly used to measure anxiety, however, have largely measured *trait* anxiety. Confusing, indeed! Despite the confusion, some conclusions can be drawn from the research studies on anxiety as summarized by Layman (1974):

1. Trait anxiety may be influenced by physical activity if individuals begin with relatively high anxiety, if the exercise activity is of long duration and high intensity, and if the individual must adjust to high-intensity activity.
2. The decline in trait anxiety is greater in men than in women.
3. There is a significant inverse relationship between state anxiety and physical fitness.

Interpretation of these findings again is difficult because of the limited data on women. The differences in female-male state and trait anxiety may reflect the social role expectations. The role of women has not been consistent with vigorous activity. The low activity pattern for females has been societally reinforced, whereby girls and women who have engaged in vigorous activity may experience negative associations and psychologic discomfort. Of course, this explanation is speculative; however, culture and sex-role patterns have been shown to affect activity pattern in males and females throughout the life cycle. For example, girls ages 9 to 12 years have considerably less energy expenditure than boys of the same age (Andersen et al, 1978).

Ogden (1977) measured fourteen personality traits in women with varied levels of activity. She found that the participants' personality characterisitcs were related to the individuals' cultural definition of the activity. Since the cultural value of athletic participation for the female is different from that for the male, the woman participates for different reasons. These reasons, according to Ogden, reflect traits typical of the female. Whether there are characteristic personality traits of active women is still inconclusive.

Because of recent changes in the cultural roles for women, younger women who exercise could be expected to experience more congruence between self-concept and social identity than older women who have had to overcome the negative associations of women and vigorous activity. To speculate even further, if a woman develops a life-style that includes regular exercise, will she be involved in more nontraditional female roles than the woman who does not exercise? Will an active woman have a more positive and integrated self-concept such that there is increased satisfaction with marital, parental, and professional roles?

These questions are still unanswered; however, there is heightened awareness of the limited research studies done *by* women and *about* women.

PHYSIOLOGIC EFFECTS OF EXERCISE
Metabolism

Aerobic exercise is a near-total body activity, yet the actual energy production that permits physical activity occurs at the cellular level. In order to effect any movement, millions of muscle cells require energy in the form of adenosine triphosphate (ATP). ATP is crucial for cellular functioning whether the body is at rest or involved in physical activity. During exercise the demand for ATP increases and must be provided if exercise is to continue. The metabolic requirements of skeletal muscle cells may increase as much as 50% to 100% during strenuous exercise (Morehouse and Miller, 1976; Astrand and Karre, 1977). This enormous increase necessitates acceleration in production of ATP as well as the removal of heat and metabolites. Energy for cellular use is liberated by breaking the covalent bonds of the ATP molecule. (ATP $\rightleftharpoons$ ADP + pi + Energy). The resynthesis of ATP occurs continuously in order to meet the cellular demand for energy. It is important to note that ATP is regenerated by both aerobic and anaerobic pathways; however, there are distinctive characteristics of aerobic metabolism that have significant advantages for the exercising individual. These advantages include: efficient use of oxygen and food sources, increased ATP production, and production of nontoxic metabolites (Table 19-1).

Organic compounds serve as the energy sources for the resynthesis of ATP needed for cell function during exercise. The organic compounds (three food sources) are converted from complex molecules to simpler molecules in several steps, which involve various enzymatic reactions. These chemical reactions occur within the living cells of the body and, as stated previously, may occur with or without oxygen. The organic compounds that serve as energy-producing fuel are carbohydrate in the form of glycogen and fatty acids in the form of acetylglycerols (triglycerides). Because protein is complexly metabolized and contributes minimally to the skeletal

Table 19-1. Characteristics of aerobic and anaerobic metabolism

Aerobic	Anaerobic
Presence of oxygen	Absence of oxygen
Use of CHO, fat, protein	Use of CHO only
1 mole glucose = 38 mole ATP	1 mole glucose = 3 mole ATP
CO_2, H_2O excreted	Lactic acid accumulation

muscle during exercise (Astrand and Rodahl, 1977), discussion of protein metabolism will not be included. The breakdown of fatty acids is solely an aerobic process; however, the breakdown of glycogen and glucose (carbohydrate) may occur either aerobically or anaerobically. Thus in muscle cells functioning anaerobically, carbohydrate is the only available energy-yielding foodstuff, whereas aerobically-functioning cells have access to both carbohydrate and fatty acids as potential energy sources.

The presence of oxygen for use by the cells is, overall, the critical factor in determining the metabolic processes that occur in the active muscles during exercise. The presence of oxygen also determines, in part, the food sources used for ATP resynthesis. For this reason nutrition and diet are important factors affecting metabolism during exercise. Additional variables, such as state of physical conditioning, current health status, and the type of exercise, also determine whether fats, carbohydrates, or proteins will be utilized.

The cellular mitochondria are the sites of the aerobic oxidation of carbohydrates and fatty acids. Through a series of chemical reactions, carbohydrate and fatty acids are converted to a compound called acetyl coenzyme A (CoA), which enters the Krebs citric acid cycle and the electron-transport chain. ATP is formed during the transport phase by a process known as oxidative phosphorylation and is stored in limited quantity in the cell as readily available energy.

The oxidation of glucose and glycogen (carbohydrate) to pyruvate is identical for both aerobic and anaerobic processes; however, the similarities end here. When oxygen is available the pyruvate is chemically modified and able to enter the Krebs cycle. In anaerobic metabolism, the pyruvate is ultimately converted to lactate through a series of enzymatic reactions. In the absence of oxygen the Krebs cycle and the electron transport chain are not functional; however, ATP is still resynthesized but in smaller quantity. The energy production of ATP for one molecule of glucose varies considerably between aerobic and anaerobic oxidations: aerobic yields thirty-eight molecules of ATP as compared to three molecules from the anaerobic reaction. It should be apparent that the anaerobic process severely limits the ATP needed for exercise. Since there are limited glycogen stores in the body, these stores will be depleted thirteen times faster in the muscles that are functioning anaerobically rather than aerobically (Astrand and Rodahl, 1977).

Energy yield from fatty acid metabolism plays a significant role in the cellular resynthesis of ATP as well. As a solely aerobic process, the various fatty acids are altered and prepared for oxidation in the Krebs cycle and respiratory chain (fatty acid → CoA esters → acetyl CoA → Krebs cycle and respiratory chain → CO_2 H_2O). The energy yield will vary depending on the type of fatty acid oxidized; however, for one molecule of palmitate, a fatty acid, about 129 molecules of ATP are produced (Astrand and Rodahl, 1977).

Lactate or lactic acid, as the end-product of anaerobic metabolism, is not as easily excreted as are the aerobic end-products, water and carbon dioxide. Lactic acid accumulates in the cell, diffuses into the blood and, if generalized, will lower the blood pH. Lactic acidosis, as seen by elevated blood lactate levels (Wilmore, 1977) and a lowered blood pH, serves as an index of anaerobic metabolism during exercise (Astrand and Rodahl, 1977). The aerobic metabolites (CO_2, H_2O) are nontoxic and readily transported by the capillary network to be excreted by skin, kidneys, and lungs (Morehouse and Miller, 1976).

In relation to exercise, the combined effects of decreased production of ATP from limited glycogen stores and lactate accumulation limit the overall ability of an individual to exercise. In contrast, the development of the aerobic oxidative pathways permit quantitative changes in an individual's exercise intensity and duration. Regular exercise, which stresses the cardiopulmonary systems develops aerobic capacity or the ability to utilize oxygen efficiently.

Repeated exposure of the body to aerobic activities such as swimming and running progressively alters the metabolism from anaerobic to aerobic oxidation. This is achieved as a result of an increased functional capacity of the oxidative enzyme systems of the skeletal muscle mitochondria (Neill, 1977). Kiessling et. al. (1973) found that the endurance training increases both the size and number of mitochondria in skeletal muscle. Whether endurance training affects the enzymes involved in anaerobic metabolism is unclear (Morgan et al., 1973; Gollnick et al, 1973). Therefore, skeletal muscles in the conditioned individual utilize oxygen more efficiently during exercise than the muscles in the unconditioned individual. Because aerobic exercise is a near–total body activity the oxidative enzyme potential is widely developed throughout the active muscles of the body. Other subsystems are important in facilitating aerobic exercise and derive similar benefits from it as well. The increased physiologic efficiency is significant for the development of exercising ability; however, the ability to perform usual daily activities with greater ease and less fatigue is a significant health benefit for both women and men.

The development of the oxidative ability of an individual can be improved with regular aerobic activity and can be quantified as aerobic capacity. Aerobic capacity (VO_2max) is the best criterion of cardiorespiratory fitness and represents the ability of the body to use the available oxygen in cellular metabolism (Wilmore, 1977). Aerobic capacity can be defined as "the highest oxygen uptake an individual can attain during physical work while breathing air at sea level" (Astrand and Rodahl, 1977). The amount of oxygen consumption is measured by indirect calorimetry and expressed as liters of oxygen used per minute and milliliters of oxygen per minute per kilogram of body weight (Morehouse and Miller, 1976). Development of an individual's aerobic potential is associated with improvement in the functional efficiency at the cellular level and of the oxygen transport mechanism, specifically the cardiac and peripheral circulatory system. VO_2max is achieved through cardiac activity (increase in maximal cardiac output) and increased oxygen extraction in the peripheral circulatory circuit (Morehouse and Miller, 1976). The significance of the VO_2max is that it represents the maximal energy produced by aerobic oxidation and the level of functioning of the circulation. The circulatory aspects will be discussed later; however, there is a direct relationship between maximal cardiac output and maximal aerobic capacity (Astrand and Rodahl, 1977). Because of individual differences and other variables that contribute to VO_2, it is difficult to cite a "normal" aerobic capacity. The oxygen uptake for an average woman running at 5.5 mph is approximately 2.1 liters/minute. With physical training, the VO_2 may increase to levels as high as 6.0 liter/minute. It is important to note that the maximal aerobic capacity can be achieved at a workload that is not necessarily maximal or exhausting (Astrand and Rodahl, 1977).

VO_2max is influenced by many factors such as age, body size, level of fitness, and sex. Before puberty, girls and boys have approximately the same maximal aerobic capacity; after puberty women's capacity declines to about 70% to 75% of men's of the same age (Andersen et al., 1978; Drinkwater, 1973). Both sexes reach peak aerobic potential at 18 to 20 years of age. Astrand and Rodahl (1977) found that the maximal oxygen uptake for the average 65-year-old man is approximately equal to an average 25-year-old woman. Certainly, natural endowment and other individual qualities contribute to the variance.

It has been demonstrated that the VO_2max of the

average woman is less than that of the average man of the same age. At first glance, the sex factor might be the easy explanation of the female-male differences. However, several reasons have been proposed to explain why women have a lower VO₂max than do men. Women do have a lower hemoglobin level than men, thus the oxygen-binding capacity of the blood is lower. The decreased binding capacity of hemoglobin for oxygen could explain how less oxygen would be available for cellular use (Astrand and Rodahl, 1977).

The female hormones, specifically estrogen, affect body composition such that there is a higher percentage of body fat in the female after puberty. The higher ratio of fat to muscle tissue in women may limit aerobic capacity since adipose tissue is metabolically inactive, thus unable to enhance oxygen use (Andersen et al., 1978). In the male, who has a greater muscle than fat distribution, the potential to develop the aerobic oxidative patterns is greater. When comparing the aerobic power of women and men in relation to lean body mass (weight of adipose tissue subtracted from body weight), women have approximately the same VO₂max as men.

Another explanation of the sex variance in VO₂max may be related to the habitual activity pattern of females and males. Increasing sedentary habits over the past decades in both work and leisure activities may have contributed to decreased fitness in our society. In terms of energy expenditure, boys' motor activity increases with age, and overall they have a greater total energy expenditure than girls, especially after puberty. Girls' energy expenditure peaks at age 11 years, stabilizes, and may even decline with age. Energy expenditure for adolescents indicates that boys spend 13% of the day (24 hours) in moderate to heavy activity while adolescent girls spend 11% of the day in similar levels of activity (Andersen et al., 1978). These differences in activity levels between female and male throughout the life cycle lead to differences in the oxygen transport mechanism and the metabolism in muscle cells, subsequently in aerobic capacity.

An international study was done with adolescents from nonindustrialized, hunting and nomadic communities to determine if sex roles with the role-prescribed activity patterns could explain the differences in aerobic capacity between males and females. The results showed that there are similar female-male differences at puberty compared to adolescents in the United States. These results would suggest that the differences are of a biologic origin rather than cultural or socioenvironmental; however, the data are not definitive (Andersen et al., 1978).

Admittedly, data are lacking about the aerobic capacity of women involved in moderate physical activity. Hopefully, as more women become physically active, data will increase quantitatively and qualitatively.

Circulation

As the individual moves from the resting to the exercising state, (whether aerobically fit or not) various circulatory processes occur that are directed toward delivering oxygenated blood to active tissues and removing waste products. The increased demand for oxygen delivery and the necessity to use oxygen efficiently are contingent upon the physiologic ability to circulate oxygenated blood selectively. Clearly, during exercise the circulation-oxygenation interrelationship is apparent. In order to explicate the interactions these processes will be examined separately.

The circulatory system responds to the stress of exercise in an orderly manner in an effort to maintain a dynamic physiologically steady state. The elements of the circulatory process include the cardiac and the peripheral circulatory factors, which are both operational during aerobic exercise. The increased oxygen demand of the exercising individual is dealt with in two ways: by changes in cardiac activity through increased cardiac output and by changes in peripheral circulation through increasing vascular resistance and selective shunting of blood. The oxygen demand occurs in all exercising individuals; however, the ability to utilize oxygen more efficiently is unique to the aerobically conditioned person. This will be examined later.

The increase in cardiac output, mediated by sympathetic activity, is the key factor in the circulatory adaptation to exercise. The cardiac output (CO), as a dynamic process, is the product of heart rate (HR) and stroke volume (SV), which is represented by the equation $CO = HR \times SV$. The cardiac output in the resting state is approximately 4 to 6 liters/minute as compared to a possible cardiac output of 20 liters/minute (unconditioned) and 30 liters/minute (conditioned) during strenuous exercise. The increase in cardiac output during exercise is seen in all individuals irrespective of conditioning; however, the maximal cardiac output is increased in the conditioned individual. The differences in levels of aerobic fitness are apparent when examining how the cardiac output is regulated. The factors regulating cardiac output are heart rate and stroke volume, thus an increased cardiac output can be attained by elevating heart rate, stroke volume, or a combination of the two.

As exercise is initiated, the heart rate increases to compensate for exertional demands (workload). The relation between heart rate and workload is a linear progression, so that as workload increases the heart rate will similarly increase and plateau at a maximal level. This process occurs in both the short- and long-term adaptive processes. For the aerobically fit individual, the distinctive difference is in the greater exercising capacity. The increase in heart rate during maximal exercise is about equal for both, yet the unconditioned person will reach the maximal heart rate sooner. The fit individual will be able to perform a greater workload at the same heart rate as the average individual. From another perspective, the fit individual can perform the same workload (submaximal) as the episodic exerciser at a lower heart rate. The difference is that the fit individual can accomplish the task through a greater capacity to increase stroke volume (Morehouse and Miller, 1976).

The ability of the heart rate to return to a normal level after exercise is contingent upon the intensity of exercise, the condition of the individual, and certain other physiologic factors. As expected, intense activity will require a longer recovery period, as will the poorly conditioned individual who exercises. Other physiologic factors that influence heart rate recovery include decreased blood pH, elevated body temperature, and blood pooling in dilated muscles (Morehouse and Miller, 1976).

At rest, the aerobically fit individual's heart rate differs from the average individual's heart rate. Resting heart rates of 40 to 50/minute for conditioned individuals are commonplace, whereas the average individual has a resting heart rate of 80 to 100/minute. In addition to the level of aerobic fitness, there are other variables that influence heart rate. The resting heart rate may be somewhat decreased with advancing age, as well as decreased in the supine body position. In contrast, the heart rate is increased to compensate for oxygen demand incurred in elevated environmental temperatures and at high altitudes. Heart rate is closely related to the emotional state of the individual as well (Astrand and Rodahl, 1977).

Measurement of heart rate is a significant parameter in monitoring the workload of the heart. The linear relationship between heart rate and oxygen consumption at submaximal levels of exercise makes heart rate a reliable estimation of work intensity. In addition, the myocardial blood flow and oxygen consumption are highly correlated with heart rate; therefore, myocardial work can be kept constant if the exercise intensity is monitored. Exercise at submaximal levels (50% to 80% of total endurance capacity) produces optimal conditioning effects if intensity is maintained within the individual's range for 20 to 40 minutes. Determination of the optimal exercising heart rate should be done individually, especially for those with decreased endurance capacity caused by age or disease. The heart rate derived from a standardized table has a large variance (± 10/minute) and does not consider the sex of the individual or the individual with a decreased cardiac capacity (Wilmore, 1976).

As stated previously, an elevated stroke volume is a means of increasing cardiac output. Rushmer (1976) states that the increased cardiac output is attained almost exclusively by an increased heart rate. For the average individual, there is a small increase in stroke volume during exercise. The disadvantage to the unconditioned individual is that the tachycardia may not efficiently elevate cardiac output and exhaustion will follow. In addition, the chronotropic activity increases the myocardial oxygen consumption considerably. The significance of this is apparent in individuals with ischemic heart disease, when the myocardium has a decreased reserve and less resilience to lowered myocardial oxygen tensions.

When discussing stroke volume it is important to consider the relationship that exists between stroke volume and body position. Recent research has verified that the stroke volume (at rest and during exercise) is influenced by body position; however, earlier inattention to measurement of stroke volume in various body positions has yielded confusing data about the stroke volume in the exercising individual. Much of the data on stroke volume was obtained from the supine exercising individual, a position not representative of typical exercise. For meaningful data it is critical to consider resting-exercising parameters in the same body position.

In an upright sitting or standing position at rest, the stroke volume and cardiac output (CO) decrease (CO by 30% to 40%) relative to the supine position. This decrease is attributed to the hydrostatic pressure effects caused by peripheral pooling of blood and a decrease in venous return. The lower stroke volume baseline in the upright-rest yields a larger net increase in stroke volume during maximum exercise than the stroke volume increase from supine-rest to maximum exercise. However, the maximal stroke volume attained during exercise is nearly equal or slightly higher than the supine-rest. In a review of eight studies, Rushmer (1976) found that the stroke volume changed minimally when average individuals performed a wide range of exercise levels (oxygen consumption was used to grade workload). Exercise in the supine position, even when strenuous, produced little if any increase in stroke volume. Another mechanism must exist to compensate for the increased metabolic rate (heart rate) incurred by exercise in the unconditioned individual in the supine position.

As stated previously, the maximal heart rates for fit and unfit individuals is nearly equal; therefore, the greater increase in cardiac output seen in the aerobically fit is attributed to the capacity to increase stroke volume (Morehouse and Miller, 1976). The stroke volume at rest, at submaximal, and maximal levels of exercise is increased as a result of aerobic conditioning (Wilmore, 1977). Aerobic exercise does increase the maximal stroke volume, so that a given cardiac output is reached through less of a chronotropic effect, thereby increasing the efficiency of the heart's pumping action.

The conditioned individual's greater capacity for CO is related to actual myocardial changes. Heart volume and weight increase as an adaptation to the regular stress of exercise (Wilmore, 1977). In addition to cardiac hypertrophy, there is an increase in the metabolic rate of the heart (Penpargkul and Scheuer, 1970). Whether physical training promotes the growth of collateral circulation in the normal or diseased myocardium has not been determined; however, no quantitative method to measure collateral flow in humans has been developed (Barmeyer, 1976).

It is important to note that cardiac muscle does not increase its aerobic capacity with regular exercise. This can be explained by the fact that the heart is an aerobic organ and normally endowed with a very high aerobic capacity (Barnard, 1975).

Peripheral circulation

Aerobic exercise involving the large muscle groups puts an increased demand on the oxygen transport mechanism. The peripheral circulatory response to the oxygen demand is through an increased total blood flow to active tissues and more complete oxygen extraction (Rushmer, 1976). The oxygenation of active muscles must be accomplished but not at the expense of vital functions. Oxygen requirements of the myocardium during exercise are increased and blood flow through the lungs must be maintained at specified flow rates to permit gas exchange. Similarly, cerebral blood flow must be kept at a constant level. Conversely, the splanchnic and renal circulation can be reduced through vasoconstriction irrespective of the level of exertion. Renal blood flow has been reported as low as 50% to 80% of normal flow (Morehouse and Miller, 1976).

Blood flow to all tissues is not constant, but dependent on the tissue needs. During exercise blood is shunted from areas of decreased metabolic activity (i.e., kidney, stomach, intestines) to the active, contracting muscles. The amount of blood flow shunted to active muscles is correlated with increased metabolic activity of the muscles (Rushmer, 1976) and varies with the type and intensity of activity. The sympathetic nerve fibers are responsible for vasodilation of the arterioles supplying active muscle, whereas compensatory vasoconstriction controls inactive arterioles. Rushmer (1976), however, contends that blood vessels in inactive muscle are constricted because of their intrinsic tone rather than being dependent on nervous control. The vasodilation necessary to deliver oxygen commensurate with need is achieved by neural, chemical, and mechanical factors. As mentioned, the sympathetic fibers are activated; the increase in temperature and metabolites in active muscles also stimulates vasodilation. It is proposed that local hypoxia, with increased lactic acid and carbon dioxide levels is responsible for chemical changes. The shunting mechanism combined with the increased cardiac output

increases total blood flow to active tissues so that the oxygen uptake level is increased from resting state values. The oxygen uptake at rest (measured in milliliters of oxygen used per 100 Gm of muscle per minute) is approximately 0.16 compared to 12 during exercise, the difference representing a 75-fold increase (Morehouse and Miller, 1976).

The vascular beds of the skin and abdomen contain large amounts of blood as represented by the following distribution of the cardiac output (5.4 liters/minute) in the normal resting woman: abdominal organs, 2.8 liters/minute; skin, 0.5 liters/minute; skeletal, 0.8 liters/minute; and other organs, 1 liter/minute (Morehouse and Miller, 1976). During exercise, constriction of abdominal vasculature adds volume to the active circulation. The vascular beds contained in the skin initially constrict, but as heat is increasingly produced by contracting muscles, dilation occurs to facilitate heat loss. The skin and active muscles receive increasing amounts of blood flow as workload increases. However, a long exercise period and/or elevated environmental temperatures will decrease blood flow to the muscles and redirect blood flow to the periphery (skin) to accelerate heat dissipation and metabolite loss (Wilmore, 1977).

Long-term adaptations to aerobic exercise are related to the improved shunting efficiency and the increased peripheral blood flow caused by increased capillary density in active muscles. The increase permits improved perfusion and a greater volume of blood flow during maximal exercise (Wilmore, 1977). The widened arterial-venous oxygen difference (A-VO$_2$ diff) seen in aerobically fit individuals signifies a greater oxygen extraction ability attributed to the increased capacity of the oxidative enzyme systems of skeletal muscle. The metabolic process is changed from anaerobic to aerobic energy production, a process that is more oxygen efficient. Regular aerobic activity, such as running or swimming, which involves near–total body musculature, increases the metabolic capacity of the specific skeletal muscles only. The circulatory benefits of the trained muscle groups are nontransferable to nontrained muscles (Neill, 1977); for example, a runner will not have the same metabolic capacity in her upper extremities as a long distance swimmer who has aerobically developed her arm and upper trunk muscle groups.

Alterations in peripheral resistance caused by shunting during exercise will have concomitant effect on blood pressure (BP = cardiac output × total peripheral resistance). Systolic pressures are elevated with increased levels of exercise while diastolic values remain unchanged. The long-term impact of aerobic exercise on blood pressure is inconclusive due, in part, to the difficulty in obtaining a reliable reading during exercise without using an invasive technique. However, the blood pressure of the normotensive individuals who have been studied remains unchanged. The hypertensive person may experience a decrease in blood pressure resulting from the effects of aerobic exercise (Wilmore, 1977).

The woman with some degree of cardiac dysfunction (e.g., coronary artery disease) will not equally derive the same skeletal muscle and peripheral circulatory benefits as the normal woman. With normal myocardial function the oxygen demands are met by coronary dilation and increased coronary blood flow, whereas in angina the myocardial oxygen needs are not met because of interrupted coronary blood flow (manifested by chest pain). Therefore, exercise must be stopped prematurely, which prevents development of skeletal muscle aerobic capacity and increased coronary blood flow. In fact, any increase in the peripheral circulatory process would demand further myocardial work in the face of an already decreased oxygen supply. The individual with angina can benefit from aerobic exercise in many ways, one being the increased workload capacity without onset of anginal pain (Neill, 1977).

Temperature regulation

As mentioned earlier, circulation in the peripheral areas is directly related to heat conservation and dissipation. Core body temperature must be maintained within a 7° F range and is accomplished by constriction or dilation of superficial blood vessels (Claremont, 1976), and by sweat secretion. The amount of superficial blood flow and the amount of sweat secreted are under control of the temperature-regulating center located in the preoptic anterior hypothalamus. Neurons in the hypothalamic region, sensitive to thermal conditions, respond to changes in blood temperature by sending impulses to superficial vessels to either dilate or constrict. Similarly, impulses to the secretory nerve fibers either stimulate or inhibit sweat gland production. In either situation the purpose is to maintain body temperature (Morehouse and Miller, 1976).

For the woman exerciser cold acclimatization is less problematic than adjustment to heat, since the human body is far better equipped to handle cold. Energy production even at slow running speeds (5 to 5.5 mph) is adequate to maintain body temperature even in subzero weather. The body's protective mechanism to increase metabolic heat production in cold climates includes voluntary and involuntary (shivering) movement. The vasoconstriction of the surface vessels diverts blood away from the periphery resulting in a lower skin temperature. The decrease in skin temperature serves as insulation for the body to prevent heat loss by convection and radiative heat transfer (Claremont, 1976). In addition, the female exerciser has an increased per-

centage of subcutaneous tissue that contributes to the insulative effect.

The potential dangers of cold are associated with the sudden drop in internal body temperature causing physiologic disturbances and even death. In such situations, hypothermia results from excessive heat loss to the environment without concomitant metabolic heat production. Fatigue or injury are conditions of concern when exercising in cold weather, since if exercise intensity is reduced thermal balance cannot be maintained. Clothing with insulative qualities is important in order to maintain the microclimate immediately surrounding the individual. Except in extreme situations (i.e., subzero temperature with wind chill factor, poor clothing quality, fatigue or injury) the thermoregulatory process is largely concerned with heat dissipation. As exercise intensity or duration increases, heat production secondary to increased metabolism occurs and must be eliminated to prevent overheating. Heat loss caused by evaporation of perspiration maintains the body temperature within a functional range.

Adjustment to elevated environmental temperature is not accomplished as easily and is more hazardous to the exerciser than cold weather. Any thermal stress whether caused by increased environmental temperature or intense physical activity or both causes an increased body temperature, which will continue to rise until hypothalamic activity brings modes of heat dissipation into operation (Nadel, 1977). Since a great deal of energy is released in the form of heat during physical exertion, the temperature-regulating mechanisms are twice stressed by exercise in excessive environmental heat (Daniels et al, 1978). The heat generated during exercise may be up to thirty times greater than at rest (Morehouse and Miller, 1976) and must be dissipated through the body's compensatory mechanisms: peripheral vasodilation, increased heart rate, and perspiration. Because ambient air is quite warm, the peripheral vasodilation and tachycardia responses are usually not adequate heat loss mechanisms, especially if exercise intensity continues to increase. Perspiration occurs as a result of plasma volume shifts into interstitial spaces and to the skin by way of the sweat glands. Sweat production in itself does not cause heat loss from the body. Cooling occurs when heat is transferred to the environment through evaporation of sweat. Evaporative heat loss is inhibited when humidity is elevated (70% relative humidity) and the water from perspiration cannot be taken up by the already saturated atmosphere. The result of decreased evaporation is a rise in core body temperature, which may contribute to early exhaustion.

Other heat-related problems, such as heat exhaustion, heat stroke, and dehydration, occur quite often in hot weather. In these cases fluid loss is marked causing hemoconcentration. Hemoconcentration of red blood cells and plasma proteins can be harmful if the fluid loss is excessive, since this alters blood viscosity and electrolyte levels. These heat-related conditions can be minimized if sensible precautions are instituted. These include avoidance of high heat periods during the day, modifying exercise intensity to match heat and humidity conditions, adequate hydration, and absorptive clothing.

The process of heat acclimatization will decrease the chances of developing heat-related problems. Becoming acclimatized to a warm or hot environment occurs fairly quickly—in 4 to 7 days with 2 to 4 hours of daily work in the heat (Morehouse and Miller, 1976). Acclimatization results in more efficient control of fluid loss (less sweating) and a lower concentration of electrolytes in the sweat. Once acclimatization occurs, individuals maintain a lower internal temperature while exercising and develop increased plasma and interstitial fluid volumes, which contribute to cardiovascular stability because of a greater blood volume. The lower body temperature results from the increased responsiveness of the sweating mechanism (earlier onset and a greater volume of sweat production) and a greater capacity for cutaneous vasodilation (Morehouse and Miller, 1976). Sweat production in the acclimatized individual occurs at a lowered temperature threshold, thus permitting heat dissipation at an early point in the exercise period.

For the female, the heat acclimatization process poses no greater problems than for the male counterpart. While women do have a larger number of active sweat glands, Wynaham et al (1965) report that women have a lower total body sweat rate than men when working in a hot environment. The greater percentage of adipose tissue in the female is an asset in cold weather but in hot weather the reverse may be operational since adipose tissue may inhibit heat dissipation.

Proposed differences in heat adaptation between males and females are inconclusive largely because of the small number of studies comparing the male and female exerciser. While the heat-acclimatized male has been found to have a marked increase in total body sweat, thereby facilitating heat dissipation, no evidence has been reported to support this process in the female. One investigator suggests that women may have more efficient regulation of body temperature and fluid loss than men because of their ability to achieve the same outcomes with less water loss (Wynaham et al., 1965).

Oxygenation

The process of oxygenation can be considered as internal and external. The internal processes are concerned with the transfer of respiratory elements, oxygen and carbon dioxide, to the active tissues. (Internal respiration is described in detail in the sections on

metabolic and circulatory adaptations to exercise.) External respiration deals with the functional exchange of of oxygen from the environment to the lungs, and the actual diffusion of oxygen across the alveoli-capillary membrane into the circulating blood. Since carbon dioxide production is approximately parallel to oxygen consumption, the elimination of CO_2 is also considered in external processes (Wilmore, 1977).

During rest, external respiration is based on pressure-volume changes that occur in the lungs and is the result of the action of the ventilatory muscles (the diaphragm, intercostal and accessory muscles.) Boyle's law states that volume and pressure are inversely related, so that as the lung volume increases during inspiration, the intrapulmonary pressure decreases and is less than atmospheric pressure, thus air flows into the lungs. At rest, expiration is a completely passive process, involving only relaxation of the ventilatory muscles. However, during exercise, respiratory rate, tidal volume, and other ventilatory patterns are increased, and respiration itself becomes an active process requiring increased energy expenditure (Daniels et al., 1978).

The respiratory rate, normally 12 to 18 breaths/minute, may increase to 40 or 50/minute and the tidal volume increases from the average 500 ml to 2 to 3 liters/minute during strenuous exercise. Pulmonary ventilation, which is expressed as the minute volume (minute volume = respiratory rate × tidal volume) is approximately 6 liters at rest, but may rise to 100 liters/minute during exercise (Wilmore, 1977). The element of aerobic conditioning is important in establishing and maintaining a pulmonary ventilation pattern, since a linear relationship exists between pulmonary ventilation and an individual's exercise capacity. Beyond a certain point, which is usually 60% to 90% of the individual's exercise capacity, the onset of anaerobic processes prompts rapid increases in pulmonary ventilation. In an effort to maintain a given minute volume, the respiratory rate is higher compared to the depth in the unconditioned individual (Daniels et al, 1978). Consider the following example:

Two female runners during submaximal exercise each have a vital capacity of 4.0 liters. Runner A breathes 22 times per minute at a depth of 3.0 liters per breath, which yields a minute volume of 66 liters (22 × 3.0 = 66 liters). Runner B takes 33 breaths per minute with a resulting minute volume of 66 liters (33 × 2.0 = 66 liters). Since the minute volume is equal for both women, the same amount of air is being moved per minute; however, runner B's energy expenditure is greater. The increased energy expenditure is attributed to the increased work necessitated to breathe at the rate of 33 per minute. In addition runner B's tidal volume (2.0 liter) is less than runner A's (3.0 liter), so that runner A is able to more widely ventilate her lungs and effectively exchange oxygen and carbon dioxide.

The vital capacity and other lung volume measurements have wide variability, which are dependent on factors such as body size, age, sex, and lung compliance. Often these factors occur concomitantly in individuals so that isolating the significant factor is difficult. Therefore, one should be cautious in attributing differences in female-male pulmonary abilities to the sex factor. Lung volumes in women are about 10% smaller than those of men of the same size and age. Differences are attributed to the hormonal regulation of tissue composition, organ size, and possible past sedentary characteristics of the women tested.

Common to both the female and male are the effects of aging on the respiratory functions. Lung volumes are altered significantly with age in both women and men because of the changes in lung elasticity. However, a longitudinal study by Astrand et al. (1973) suggests that lung deterioration can be prevented with regular exercise that stresses the respiratory system. In his findings, Astrand reports that certain lung volume parameters, namely vital capacity, remain unchanged in the women and men tested at ages 20 years and 45 years. During the interim years these individuals maintained a regular exercise pattern. The idea that life-long exercise may be beneficial physiologically is supported by longitudinal studies such as Astrand's.

The effect of aerobic conditioning on external respiration appears to be of much less importance than the circulatory and metabolic adaptations involved in internal processes of oxygenation. For example, the vital capacity is not normally altered as a result of aerobic activity, although the respiratory pattern may change to decrease the work of breathing (Morehouse and Miller, 1976). The respiratory pattern assumed by an individual may be modified by aerobic conditioning; however, it is best to allow each person to assume the breathing pattern most comfortable for her. A rhythmic pattern is often developed with time and conditioning; this pattern is often naturally adapted to the motions of the specific activity. Runners and bicyclists have wide variations in respiratory patterns, whereas a swimmer's pattern is more fixed and closely associated with the arm movements. The question of nose versus mouth breathing is usually resolved naturally, as well. The increased demand for oxygen during strenuous activity and the increased air resistance when nose breathing make mouth breathing a naturally advantageous alternative (Astrand and Rodahl, 1977).

Although not an external respiratory process as such, there are additional factors that affect respiration. Inhalation of certain elements such as smoke, dust particles, and noxious gases is detrimental to the respiratory function of any individual on a short-, and possibly long-term, basis. These elements initiate a reflex response in the bronchial tree; bronchoconstriction is the protective response. Because of the decreased lumen of the bronchi and bronchioles, there is increased airway resistance and increased energy expenditure to breathe. Individuals who exercise outdoors are exposed to one or more of these substances, which may necessitate an increased effort to maintain oxygen levels. As expected, exercise activity may be prematurely terminated because of fatigue or unpleasant reaction to the substances. Long-term effects on the pulmonary system are unclear, but Astrand and Rodahl (1977) suggest prolonged exposure to certain pollutants is toxic to lung tissue.

Direct inhalation of cigarette smoke causes increased airway resistance, which interferes with aerobic ability. The effects are not observable at rest, but during exercise an individual who smokes has marked limitations in endurance activities. Shortness of breath, light-headedness, early exhaustion, and tachycardia occur early in the exercise period. Nicotine is not the causative agent, rather, the minute particulate matter and carbon monoxide affect respiratory function. The small particles interfere with the sensory receptors causing increased secretion in the respiratory passages, thereby increasing airway resistance. Hemoglobin has an increased affinity to carbon monoxide (200 to 300 times greater than to oxygen), which is contained in tobacco smoke (and exhaust fumes from automobiles). The result is increased carboxyhemoglobin, which may appreciably decrease the oxygen transport processes during exercise. During strenuous exercise there is no way to remedy the oxygen deficit except by terminating the activity (Astrand and Rodahl, 1977).

The effects of environmental pollutants should be considered when selecting a site or time to exercise. Avoiding busy thoroughfares and heeding pollution alerts minimizes exposure to carbon monoxide from exhaust fumes, particulate matter, and noxious industrial wastes. In addition, avoidance of these hazards will make exercise activity more pleasant and healthful.

As mentioned above, bronchoconstriction is the protective response to an irritant in the respiratory tract. However, the increased sympathetic tone characteristic of physical exercise may counteract the bronchoconstriction; that is, bronchodilation may occur. It is not clear if bronchoconstriction caused by environmental irritants is minimized by the sympathetic stimulus. It has been speculated that the increased sympathetic tone may counteract or minimize the bronchoconstriction of asthma. The literature does not directly address this assumption; however, statements from individuals with asthma discount the belief that exercise promotes asthma attacks. These self-reports indicate that the exercise activity has helped to control the asthma, as well as allergic reactions. If the asthma results from an allergic response to pollen, etc., outside activities may desensitize the allergic individual. Although research data do not support these ideas, some individuals with allergies and asthma will attest to them.

Fat and muscle distribution

It is a well-known fact that lack of physical exercise leads to excess body fat. This will occur even if the person's weight is unchanged. A number of cross-sectional studies done on men (no studies have been done specifically on women) have shown that body weight reaches a maximum around age 45. Between the ages of 45 and 65, body weight remains constant or decreases but the skin-fold thickness does not change; it is the body's lean tissue that decreases with age. For many women, increasing age not only means a decrease in lean tissue, but also an increase in body weight with the weight being stored as fat. The simple relationship that explains the change in body composition is input = output + storage.

The normal upper limit of body fat for women is 28% of total body weight; for men it is 18%. There are no minimal levels of body fat for men or women. If a person receives adequate nutrition it is impossible to be too lean (Astrand et al., 1977). Actual body weight is a common method of interpreting the fat content of a person, but body weight is not a good measure since it does not distinguish between body fat and lean body tissue (Morehouse and Miller, 1976).

Lean body weight can be determined by measuring skin-fold thickness on the abdomen, thigh, and upper aspect of the upper arm. A double fold of skin and subcutaneous tissue has a thickness of 2 to 3 mm if the tissues immediately under the skin are free of fat. In North America, the average skin fold thickness is 14 to 22 mm for women and 11 to 15 mm for men.

Lean body weight can be measured in several ways. A formula for the estimation of body weight in women that does not require special equipment was developed by Wilmore and Behnke (1962). Lean body weight (LBW) is computed from measuring nude weight. Then, while the woman is standing, the wrist diameter is measured at the level of the styloid process along with the maximal abdominal protrusion inferior to the umbilicus, hip circumference at the maximum protrusion of the gluteals, and forearm circumference at the maximum girth just below the elbow with the arm extended and forearm supinated. The equation is LBW in kg = 8.987 + 0.732 (wt kg) + 3.786 (wrist diameter in centimeters) − 0.157 (maximal abdominal circumference in centimeters) − 0.249 (hip circumference in centimeters) + 0.434 (forearm circumference in centimeters). LBW in kg is converted to pounds by multiplying by 2.2. The amount of fat in pounds is determined by subtracting LBW from weight (weight − LBW = fat). Fat percentage is then computed by dividing fat by weight (fat/weight = % fat).

Another method of determining lean body weight is to apply Archimedes' principle of density and water displacement. This procedure requires special equipment but it gives a fairly accurate measurement of body fat composition. The person is weighed in water and body density is determined by comparing body weight in air and body weight in water. Appropriate corrections must be calculated to correct for normal intestinal and lung gases. Since fat is lighter than water, fat content is inversely related to body density.

If lack of physical exercise causes an increase in body fat, it stands to reason that increase in physical exercise results in a decrease of body fat. When total body weight remains constant the following changes occur in body composition in response to physical activity: (1) an increase in lean muscle tissue at the expense of fat, and (2) an increase in the bone mass because of an increase in the compressional load on the bones used in the physical activity. It has been shown that people who participate in aerobic running will develop considerably heavier bones than sedentary people, since physical stress stimulates osteoblastic deposition of bones.

The alteration of bone composition and deposition in the woman who exercises regularly is likely to prevent or at least delay the most common of all bone diseases, osteoporosis. Osteoporosis results from abnormal organic matrix rather than abnormal bone calcification. The osteoblastic activity in the bone is less than normal and consequently the rate of bone deposition is reduced. The two most common causes of osteoporosis are (1) lack of use of the bones; and (2) the aging process in which many of the protein anabolic functions are slowed so that bone matrix cannot be satisfactorily deposited. In addition to change in bone architecture, conditioning results in a thickening of articular cartilages and in an increase in the tensile strength of affected tendons. The extent to which exercise alters body fat/muscle distribution is directly proportional to the intensity, duration, and frequency of participation in the exercise activity.

Underlying the gross physiologic change of increase in lean tissue to decrease in fat tissue are some remarkable biochemical adaptations to regular exercise. Exercise elicits a mild stress reaction, which results in a release of epinephrine with resultant sympathetic activity. The blood glucose concentration tends to decrease and this causes an increase in glucagon secretion. The increased glucagon, in turn, results in glucose being mobilized from the liver to be used by the muscles. Increased muscle activity increases the transport of glucose into the muscle cell even in the absence of insulin. This is the reason why people with diabetes can decrease their need for exogenous insulin when they participate regularly in exercise (Morehouse and Miller, 1976).

Both epinephrine and, to a lesser extent, glucagon mobilize fatty acids from adipose tissue. The fatty cells of adipose tissue are modified fibroblasts capable of storing almost pure triglycerides. The oxidation of triglyceride and other fatty acids for the production of ATP takes place in the mitochondria. The number of mitochondria increases in the muscles of a person who exercises regularly. The increase in mitochondria, coupled with an increase in mitochondrial enzymes (succinic dehydrogenese for pyruvate oxidation, phosphofructokinase for glucose breakdown, phosphorylase-A, and synthetase I and D for glycogen synthesis and breakdown) provides faster synthesis and more sites for the production of ATP (Morehouse and Miller, 1976). The increase in tissue enzymes also facilitates the use of fat as a muscle fuel, thus sparing glycogen for bursts of anaerobic activity. Consequently, trained muscles (1) have the ability to maintain tension when repetitively stimulated; (2) the greatest endurance ability, and (3) increased reserve capacity. Muscle contraction in a trained muscle is both faster and stronger when compared to muscle contraction in a less well-trained muscle (Morehouse and Miller, 1976). It has been demonstrated that at the neuromuscular junction cholinesterase activity increases with endurance training. This is the enzyme responsible for the breakdown of acetylcholine released at the nerve terminals, preventing prolonged contraction and promoting more effective muscle contraction (Astrand and Radahl, 1976).

Some women have been concerned about developing bulging muscle and have consequently been reluctant to participate in regular physical activity. Muscle hypertrophy does not result from aerobic type activity. It takes high resistance, low repetition exercise (e.g., heavy weight-lifting) over a period of time to cause muscles to hypertrophy. Muscle hypertrophy has nothing to do with endurance fitness. In fact, it could have negative results because muscle hypertrophy results in a reduction of the oxygen diffusion surface area/per unit volume of muscle fibers. This results in a reduction in the O_2 supply to muscle fibers, and often a reduction in efficiency. Consequently, body builders are not necessarily physically fit.

Female sex hormones

The effects of exercise on the female sex hormones has generally been investigated using female athletes as subjects rather than females involved in moderate levels of activity. Even these studies have reported conflicting results as will be cited later. There is very little in the literature about the effects of exercise on the female nonathlete. Information on the effect of exercise as a means of attaining physical fitness shows there are no long-term adverse physiologic effects on the female who participates even in vigorous physical training. In fact, improved physical conditioning has been shown to actually improve regularity of the menstrual cycle and bring relief to women who experience dysmenorrhea (Gendel, 1978). Still, it is of interest to health care professionals to gain some understanding of how participation in exercise may be affected by the cyclic changes of estrogen and progesterone.

The results of most research indicate that the resting heart rate is not noticeably affected by the various menstrual cycle phases. Other studies have reported an increase in heart rate before ovulation and a decrease in heart rate before menses. Some investigators have found the blood pressure slightly elevated a few days before menses, but others have found it to be lower. During the middle of the progesterone phase (18 to 20 days of a 28-day cycle) hemoglobin levels are highest. At the onset of menses, the hematocrit and hemoglobin are at the lowest levels of the cycle (Gendel, 1976). The alterations in hemoglobin and hematocrit are rarely noticed by female athletes in training, so that these alterations should not elicit any difficulties to women who are participating in exercise for improved general health. Many women notice the changes in body weight that result from the cyclic effects of estrogen. In some women, body weight increases during the premenstrual phase probably because of sodium retention. Body temperature and metabolism are slightly increased during the luteal phase. Maximal weight is reached on the second day of menstruation and then begins to decrease until the eighth day of the cycle. The high levels of estrogen present during the follicular phase causes subtle changes in capillary permeability and osmotic pressure. Other subtle physical changes documented during the follicular phase are increases in heart rate, cardiac contractility, glucose release from liver, and a decrease in urinary output. High arousal levels that may accompany the follicular phase may be conducive to more alertness and keener sensory perception. Therefore, as far as the female athlete is concerned, there may be a greater ability to detect and respond to environmental stimuli, which is important in competition events (Gendel, 1976).

Studies have shown that in the premenstrual phase women have a slower reaction time. During this phase some athletes try to avoid competition or artificially alter the menstrual cycle to prevent the premenstrual phase from coinciding with the competitive event. Some reports have indicated that physical performance is best in the estrogen phase, fair to good in the progesterone phase, and poorest during the menstrual phase (Gendel, 1976).

Menstrual extraction

Some women have elected to use menstrual extraction to eliminate the inconvenience of blood flow during training and/or competition. Menstrual extraction is performed at the first sign of bleeding. There are several kits available. Some require cervical dilation and others do not. Usually the kits include a double-walled soft cannula that is inserted vaginally. With limited negative pressure, extraction of the products of menstruation ensues. With the use of the menstrual extraction kit, within 7 to 15 minutes the uterus is emptied and no further bleeding occurs. Data on this procedure, as it is carried out by women, are difficult to obtain. It is not known what happens in terms of microscopic or macroscopic changes in the uterine living with repeated endometrial evacuation. Gendel (1976) reports on two uterine perforations as a result of performing menstrual evacuations.

While menstrual evacuation will eliminate the "inconvenience" of bleeding, it is likely that it does not alter the systemic effects of the menstrual cyclic hormones. The relationship of menstrual extraction to hormonal balance and to the ongoing physiologic functioning of women is unknown because there have been no comprehensive, controlled studies carried out. Until more scientific knowledge is accumulated, menstrual extraction must be considered as an invasive technique with possible hazards and should be used judiciously, if at all.

Altering the menstrual cycle

Other methods of altering the menstrual cycle have been used by women athletes. Birth control pills with follicular hormones will postpone menstruation. This is of little advantage to the female athlete since, according to some studies, it is the premenstrual phase that is the least advantageous time for physical competition. Also, follicular hormones as well as progesterone result in sodium and water retention, which may make performance more difficult for the female athlete.

Another method of altering the menstrual cycle is to bring it on prematurely. This can be accomplished by taking oral contraceptives for 13 or 14 days instead of the usual 21 days. Withdrawal menstrual bleeding will usually occur 2 to 3 days after the last pill has been taken. Progesterone, without the oral contraceptive, may be administered for 3 to 5 days and then suddenly stopped. Depending on the time of the cycle, this may precipitate a menstrual flow but it is less reliable than oral contraceptives.

Women who are seriously competing in athletics may feel it is necessary to alter the menstrual cycle to improve their performance; and health professionals need to be aware of the methods available to accomplish this.

The female athlete and the health professional need to be completely informed on the possible risks and benefits of the various interventions. For example, if the female athlete is sexually active, rearranging the schedule of taking oral contraceptives may result in an unwanted pregnancy. Other methods of birth control need to be instituted. *It has not been shown to be necessary to alter the menstrual cycle in the majority of women who are participating in physical activity to improve their general health state.* Indeed, amateur women runners have participated in marathons while in all phases of the menstrual cycle and female Olympic participants have won gold medals in all phases of the menstrual cycle.

Dysmenorrhea

In the past, specific therapeutic exercises were prescribed for women who experienced dysmenorrhea. Many of these exercises were based on the assumption that dysmenorrheaic pains were caused by the shortening of pelvic nerves. Bending and stretching exercises were prescribed to stretch these nerves and relieve the pain. Current views do not support such a simple explanation for dysmenorrhea. Most authorities agree that any exercise will help relieve dysmenorrhea and the more strenuous the exercise the more helpful.

While this correlation is frequently described in literature on exercise, controlled studies have not been done. In one study of 160 college freshmen, women were classified as those who had regular exertion and those who had minimal physical exertion. Those who were the most active had the fewest complaints when compared with those who were less active. According to Gendel (1978), the study does not address whether the passive women just did not participate and consequently had problems or whether they did not participate because of their discomforts.

Faulty posture and poor body mechanics are suspected causes of dysmenorrhea. It is believed that sedentary habits and poor muscle tone contribute to weak uterine supports (Hitchcock, 1976).

More research needs to be done on the effects of exercise and phases of the menstrual cycle. Data to promote scientific understanding and dispel the folklore of the menstrual mystique need to be collected. This is especially important since the enforcement of Title IX is having an impact on women's sports and physical fitness facilities in schools and colleges.

Menstrual dysfunction

The effect of increased strenuous physical activity on the menstrual cycle has been studied by a small number of investigators. Erdelye (1962) studied 557 female athletes and found that strenuous training had no effect on the menstrual cycle in 83% of the cases; 5% appeared to have a slightly favorable effect (more regularity, decrease in dysmenorrhea); and an adverse effect was experienced by 12% of the women (increased irregularity, amenorrhea, and oligomenorrhea).

Another study was done on 168 women who were divided into three groups: runners (over 30 miles per week), joggers (5-30 miles per week), and controls (no running) (Dale, Gerlach, and Wilhite, 1979). The subjects were evaluated for serum levels of pituitary and ovarian hormones and determination of changes in total body weight and percentage of body fat. In addition, the participants filled out a questionnaire concerning information on age, height, weight, past and present sports participation, and menstrual data (menarche, gravidity, interval, duration, and character of menses), and contraceptive information. There were significant differences among the three groups with the female long distance runners showing the greatest drop in total body weight and percentage of body fat. They also had the lowest serum hormone levels and the highest incidence of oligo/amenorrhea. Although it is not firmly documented, it appears that the severity of physical exertion (judged by miles per week) is directly proportional to the degree and incidence of menstrual dysfunction. Dale et al. (1979) found an inverse relationship between prior gravidity and subsequent development of exercise-induced oligo/amenorrhea. They conclude that intense training schedules, competitive events (and associated psychologic stress), and loss in percentage of body fat and total body weight may possibly be the mechanism for oligo/amenorrhea. They postulate that the dysfunction is associated with the low normal range of pituitary gonadotropin and ovarian hormone production and that the menstrual dysfunction is reversive and amenable to therapeutic measures such as discontinuing training and/or gaining weight.

While the study presents some interesting correlations, it must be kept in perspective. Dale et al. (1979) warn that the people who respond to and participate in studies of this nature might be the same people who are likely to have menstrual problems and therefore the results may be skewed.

Other investigations (Garlick and Bernauer, 1968; Zhanel, 1971) have shown that no consistent relationship exists between physical exercise and menstrual dysfunction.

Pregnancy

The idea of exercising during normal pregnancy is currently supported by the majority of health professionals. This was not always the case. In fact, it has only been in the last 20 years that the importance of maintaining activity throughout pregnancy has been strongly encouraged. In the early 1900s, it was likely that women participated in daily activity that was adequately strenuous and additional activity was unnecessary. In the early part of this century, physicians and midwives noticed that working class women seemed to have less difficult labors and deliveries than the upper class, sedentary women. The physicians deduced from this observation that inadequate muscle fitness and tone led to more complicated childbirth. They began to prescribe physical exercises as part of childbirth preparation. In the 1940s, basic exercises were suggested to help women become adequately physically fit so that they would not be left exhausted by labor and delivery. In the 1950s, labor was viewed as a demanding muscular feat, and a calisthenic exercise program for pregnant women was recommended by some obstetricians. Also in the 1950s, Lamaze supported the need for specific muscle development in pregnant women so that they would be able to regulate their bodies and actively participate in the childbirth process. Even into the 1960s vigorous exercise aimed at improving total physical condition was not formally documented in the popular literature.

The traditional approach to exercise during pregnancy is now changing. Emphasis is being placed more on total aerobic conditioning in addition to the more common calisthenic and toning exercises. The general rule for the pregnant woman who wants to participate in physical activity is to listen to her body. Many physiologic changes take place when a woman is pregnant. These changes will affect how she responds to physical activity. Increased body weight causes increased cardiopulmonary demands. The cardiac output is increased up to 40% to meet the needs of greater body volume, increased metabolic rate, and fetal growth needs. The increased cardiac output is brought about by an increase in heart rate and stroke volume. Yet, in the pregnant runner, both endurance and VO_2max may be reduced. There are reasons for the possible slight decrease in performance. One is that the uterus as a "low resistance shunt organ." Blood will always pass through to the uterus before supplying other muscles and organs. Another reason for decrease in endurance during exercise in the pregnant state is that blood constituency is changed. There is an increase in both plasma and erythrocytes, but plasma increase in proportionately higher. This results in a relative or physiologic anemia with a lower hematocrit and hemoglobin level. The oxygen dissociation curve is the same for mother and fetus; the result is a slight decrease in endurance.

Usually during pregnancy a woman is able to continue participation in any activity that she had participated in before pregnancy. Some physicians have reservations about women beginning new physical activity during pregnancy. There are many testimonials from women who began new physical activities while being pregnant and experienced no difficulties. One woman stated she began taking snow skiing lessons when she was 4 months pregnant and continued to ski through the eighth month. This occurred while she was living in England. Upon her return to the United States, her obstetrician felt her European physician had been negligent. She concluded that in America, pregnancy is considered to be more serious and clinical (Gendel, 1976).

There are few studies done on the effects of pregnancy and the woman athlete and even fewer are available concerning the effects of pregnancy on women desiring better physical condition during exercise. Erdelye (1976) reported on 172 female athletes with 184 pregnancies and deliveries. Two thirds of the athletes continued sports activities in the first 2 or 3 months. Many stopped during the fourth month because their performance began to drop, but not because of any physical discomfort. Threatened abortion occurred in 6.5% of the pregnant athletes. In 90% of these cases the bleeding was not connected with the physical exercise (Gendel, 1976).

Erkkola and Rauramo (1976) reported on the correlation of maternal physical fitness during pregnancy with maternal and fetal pH and lactic acid at time of delivery. They found that the more physically fit mothers and their babies had higher blood pH values at the time of birth. The higher pH values possibly resulted from a more capable oxygenation system with more elimination of CO_2 in physically fit women. Physically fit mothers may be more capable of producing energy through the oxygenative process and therefore may require less anaerobically produced energy. Consequently, there is a lower production of acid metabolites during the second stage of labor. It has also been shown that newborns of physically fit mothers have higher blood pH levels than newborns of less physically fit mothers. This results either from lower concentrations of acid metabolites in the mother to transfer to the fetus or from better uterine and placental circulation, which results in efficient elimination of CO_2 from the fetal blood. The latter idea is supported by findings that the placentas of physically fit women are significantly heavier than those of unfit women (Erkkola and Rauramo, 1976).

Women who are physically fit are at an advantage throughout pregnancy and during labor and delivery. Some studies show women athletes have a longer first stage of labor. This may be the result of the rigidity of the uterine muscle and the strong abdominal muscle tone of sportswomen. It is also suspected by some investigators that there is a general lack of flexibility of the soft parts of the birth tract in sportswomen. The second stage of labor is much shorter for athletes than nonathletes. It is believed that the shorter second stage results from the strong abdominal pressure generated by the athletic women (Zaharieva, 1972).

It is generally believed that childbirth among athletes as compared to nonathletes is more frequently associated with perineal ruptures. Zaharieva's study reports no substantial differences between the two groups, but states that ruptures of the perineum were more frequent among leading women athletes than among ordinary sportswomen (Zaharieva, 1972).

There are many physical advantages to remaining in good physical condition during pregnancy. Regular physical activity will improve venous circulation and decrease leg swelling and the resultant bloated feeling. Back muscles and pelvic floor muscles are strengthened by most aerobic activity (Kegel exercises should still be employed). Regular physical activity has been shown to decrease constipation by improving general muscle tone and circulation resulting in more efficient peristaltic activity.

FOCUS ON WOMEN AND EXERCISE
How it was then

In any society where the ability to merely survive depends on maximal physical output, the concept of physical exercise is meaningless. There is little reason to expect that either men or women would have the time, energy, or need to participate in physical activities outside of those necessary for survival.

In the past 30 years many technologic advances have been made that take the physical labor out of many tasks. It is very likely that even less physical effort will be required to fulfill the future activities of daily living. Improved automation has made many labor-saving devices readily available and has resulted in drastic changes in physical effort required for work on the farm, in industry, in the office, at home, and even in leisure.

As mentioned earlier, in the past total effort was required by both sexes to survive, but as leisure time became available it was the men who were first to participate in physical activity for recreation. A brief review of sports history describes the limited number of women who physically participated.

It is known that in the sixth century BC girls participated in running races and Spartan women participated in wrestling. Little is known about women's private lives as far as exercise and physical activity are concerned because Greek literature deals almost exclusively with public life. It is interesting to note that in ancient Greece, the Olympic games were open to all spectators with the exception of married women.

Throughout the ages, women have not participated in physical activity or sports anywhere near the degree that men have. This point is illustrated in reviewing women's participation in the modern Olympics. No women participated in the first 1896 Olympics, six women participated in the 1900 Olympics, and none in the 1904 event. In 1932, 4.1% of all contestants were women and in 1968, only 13.9% of the Olympic contestants were female. The most recent Olympics held in 1980 had only 33.3% of women contestants.

In the near future more women will be active participants in athletics. This will be ensured because of regulations under Title IX of the Education Amendment of the 1972 US Department of Health, Education and Welfare, which allows for the withdrawal of federal funds from schools that discriminate against women in any activity including athletics. Title IX requires that all schools receiving federal aid offer comparable sports programs to both females and males. The schools must establish separate teams or have teams that are open to both sexes. However, there is a loophole in Title IX because the schools are *not* required to give *equal funds* to the women's programs. People interested in school sports activities must be assertive to assure that the female athletic programs get their fair share of funds.

Cultural biases against women and physical activities are many and subtle. It will take more than Title IX to acculturate women to the necessity and advantages of physical exercise. From early childhood, females are discouraged from participating in strenuous activities. Fortunately, the outlook for women and exercise is changing. This is evidenced by the various advertisements that now picture women participating in strenuous recreational activity and successfully handling jobs that previously were held by men. It is hoped that the media will help expose women to the idea of exercise and activity, and yet not succeed making women feel they need a certain sanitary napkin before they can start exercising!

How it is now

Presently, more women than ever before have a greater need for physical activity. Not only is less activity needed to carry out activities of daily living, but we consume many processed foods that are often high in calories. In addition, presentday life, whether urban or rural, for homemaker or employee or both, is laden with stress. Our life-style is essentially nonconducive to increasing one's physical strength and endurance. At the same time, with the extension of civil rights legislation, women have succeeded in opening a number of jobs that require physical exertion and until now have been performed only by men. There are deeply ingrained beliefs that physiologic differences between sexes will affect job performance, but there is little scientific evidence to support a position one way or the other.

There are many prevalent myths that surround the concept of women and exercise. Some have been dispelled, others are still firmly ingrained. As mentioned earlier, the myths surrounding menstruation, pregnancy, and lactation are still prevalent.

Another common myth that shrouds the development of women in exercise and athletics is the increased susceptibility of women athletes to injuries. Studies show that only three types of injuries appear to be more likely to happen in women, (1) dislocation of the patella, (2) shin splints, and (3) joint sprains. The wider female pelvis increases the angle between the femur and tibia, which permits the patella to move laterally when the leg is flexed and tends to lead to dislocation of the patella. This increases the possibility of chondromalacia because the quadriceps muscles are frequently weaker in women than in men. The laxed quadricep mechanism probably results from inadequate conditioning and could be corrected with proper training.

Shin splints and joint sprains occur because of the looseness of female joints. It is this increased flexibility that enables the female to move with a fluid, agile, graceful motion, and with proper training and equipment women are at no greater risk of injury in sports or exercise than men.

It is recognized by authorities that women can play faster and harder and participate more vigorously than they believed possible (Zaharieva, 1972). This has been demonstrated by the training results of women in the military academies and women's responses to regulation sports. For example, there are no longer specific regulations for women's basketball teams.

EXERCISE GROUPS

Health professionals are becoming increasingly involved in various aspects of exercise as a means to attaining better physical and mental health. The health professional can be the organizer of a therapeutic exercise group or a participant in an exercise group. Health professionals are frequently singled out as knowledgeable group members and asked technical questions about the effects of exercise. Consequently, it is important to be aware of the qualities that make a good formal or informal group leader.

First is belief in self. One must have the self-assurance that what is offered in the group is beneficial. Ambiguity is easily perceived by group members and leads to uncertainty on the part of clients. Along with belief in self comes belief in exercise as a means of improving psychophysiologic well-being. This requires the group leader to be an active, enthusiastic participant in exercise. Otherwise, group members will sense a lack of sincerity, which may hinder their full participation. If the leader is sincerely convinced of the benefits of exercise and displays a life-style conducive to attaining high levels of physical fitness, group members will benefit more from participating in the group.

The literature is replete with examples of placebo

effects and researcher bias effects that alter the outcome of controlled studies. A dramatic example reported by Beecher (1961) explains the different results obtained from surgical treatment of peptic ulcers. Surgeons who were skeptical of the ulcer operation obtained only half as many 5-year cures as those surgeons who were enthusiastic about the procedure. The sharing of personal experiences helps to maintain an open line of communication. A person who has experienced muscle discomfort, the discouragement with beginning a program, and the difficulty of establishing an exercise habit will be more credible and effective as an exercise group leader.

An effective group leader has to be aware of the group members' fears and problems associated with exercise. Group members are more likely to continue their exercises if they believe the person helping them is aware of the struggles associated with beginning and continuing in an exercise program. The leader should provide explicit explanations about what is going to be done and what the purpose is. It is also important to state what discomforts and benefits are likely to be experienced. A group that does not share knowledge and experience is likely to be less cooperative.

Finally, successful group leaders must allow for individual group members to make their own decisions about exercise. If choices are made for participants, they can transfer the blame to the leader if expected results are not obtained. This makes it easier to quit when the program gets difficult, because the members are not quitting on themselves—they are quitting on the leader (Whitehouse, 1977).

It is likely that women (especially older women) may experience more difficulty in making decisions about participation in exercise because of learned sociocultural taboos. The health professional can assist women in following through with an exercise program by establishing a flexible teaching plan for each person. This can be accomplished by collaboratively setting forth a competency-based objective for an exercise—health maintenance program (Borgeman, 1977). An example of a set of objectives is given below.

The participant in the exercise program should be able to:

1. Express a personal concept of health
2. Examine personal views in relation to exercise and health maintenance
3. Express personal likes and dislikes concerning exercise
4. Recognize exercise as an important factor in health maintenance
5. Identify community resources for an exercise program
6. Plan a schedule that includes a set time for exercise

7. Recognize types of exercises that are appropriate for his or her lifestyle
8. List personal habits that facilitate participation in exercise
9. List personal habits that hinder participation in exercise
10. Recognize adaptations that need to be learned, such as diet management, cessation of smoking, overcoming inhibitions to exercising in public
11. Describe suitable clothing to wear during exercise
12. Explain the concept of aerobic exercise
13. Explain the importance of warm-up and cooling down periods
14. Demonstrate monitoring of his or her pulse before, during, and after exercise
15. Maintain personal exercise log to compare progress over time
16. Value personal improvements gained from exercising

GETTING STARTED IN AN EXERCISE PROGRAM

First, the individual must become aware of her safe exercise levels. If a woman is overweight, has a tendency toward hypertension, or a family history of heart disease, a physical examination (preferably with a stress test) is recommended. Some health authorities recommend a stress test for anyone over age 40 who wants to begin an exercise program. Many beginners believe they have a good idea of their fitness level and decide not to have a medical stress test. For beginners who want to further qualify their fitness level, an easy and acceptable method of evaluating fitness level is with the Harvard step test.

The only equipment needed to perform the Harvard step test is a sturdy stool or bench and a watch with a second hand. Benches of different heights are required depending on the height of the woman. The following is recommended:

Height of woman	Height of bench (inches)
5 feet and under	12
5 feet to 5 feet, 3 inches	14
5 feet, 3 inches to 5 feet, 9 inches	16
5 feet 9 inches to 6 feet	18
Over 6 feet	20

The Harvard step test should not be done after eating a full meal and comfortable flat shoes and clothing should be worn. Place the bench on a sturdy, level surface. Step from the floor onto the bench and down again thirty times/minute for 4 minutes. A metronome can be used to keep time, but timing can also be accomplished using the second hand of a watch. If the woman experiences fatigue and cannot continue for the 4 minutes, she should stop. This will, of course, result in a lower score. As soon as the woman has finished she should sit quietly and count her pulse or have someone else take it for 30 seconds, 1 minute after completing the step test. The pulse is taken again at 2 minutes and at 3 minutes (for 30 seconds each time). Record each pulse reading. To compute a recovery index (RI) the following formula is used:

$$RI = \frac{\text{Duration of exercise in seconds} \times 100}{\text{Sum of pulse counts} \times 2}$$

Rates of RI are: 60 or less   Poor
61 and 70   Fair
71 and 80   Good
81 and 90   Very good
91 or more   Excellent

The test itself is very strenuous and should be done using caution. If a woman is out of shape, she should not overstress herself. At the onset of any adverse symptoms such as headache, vertigo, difficulty in breathing, or chest pain the test should be stopped immediately. The Harvard step test is recommended by the American Medical Association's Committee on Exercise and Physical Fitness. How the woman scores on the Harvard step test will determine how hard the beginning exercise should be. The important rule is to "listen to your body." Workouts should be limited at first and gradually increased until they reach approximately 30 minutes for most aerobic sessions.

General rules apply to most common types of aerobic activities such as cycling, running, walking, and swimming.

Warming up

It is advisable to spend from 10 to 15 minutes participating in limbering activities before starting exercise. Warm-up stimulates the circulation and raises the body temperature, which enhances the efficiency of muscle contraction. Warm-up is especially important in middle-aged and older people because some reports show degrees of myocardial ischemia at the onset of strenuous exercise not preceded by a warm-up period. Also, muscles tighten noticeably as a person ages unless they are frequently stretched.

Warm-up should consist of 10 to 15 minutes of stretching and flexing exercise. Stretching and flexing is especially important for running activities because running does not promote flexibility as much as do swimming or cycling. Almost all runners will develop tight posterior leg muscles unless they do stretching exercising. Tight leg muscles may cause injury because of the excessive trauma that can occur from an extra tight muscle being overly stretched or wrenched if the runner trips or stumbles.

It is recommended that the woman do a few modified sit-ups to tighten the abdominal muscles. Sit-ups should be performed with knees flexed to take strain off the back muscles. They should be performed slowly; the number should be increased until 15 or 20 are done at one time. It is very important to stretch the hamstring muscles and Achilles tendons. For the hamstring muscle stretches, the woman should lie on her back, right knee flexed, foot on floor, and left leg straight. The left leg is slowly raised until it is perpendicular to the floor with the foot plantar extended. Repeat with the other leg and do five or six repetitions. To stretch the Achilles tendon the woman should face a wall, place her palms against it, and shuffle backward keeping the feet (especially the heels) flat on ground until strain is felt in the back of the legs. Hold the position for 30 seconds allowing the muscles to stretch. Repeat two or three times.

There are many other types of stretching exercises that can be performed and several good paperback books available on various stretching techniques. It is important to stretch slowly and not in a jerking motion. When a muscle is suddenly stretched it stimulates the myotatic reflex, which responds by suddenly shortening the muscle. Only when the muscle is stretched slowly and held in that position for a short time does it lengthen and remain that way.

Women who have chondromalacia patellae may find these stretching exercises painful. It is helpful to keep the affected knee slightly flexed when doing the stretching exercises and do extra quadriceps exercises on the affected knee to strengthen the muscles and tendons that support the kneecap. A common quadriceps exercise is to sit on a table and hang a weight over the toes and slowly straighten the leg. As one gains strength in the leg, increase the weight resistance. Repeat the exercises ten times.

It is necessary to begin the aerobic activity slowly. After a few minutes of being in motion, it becomes more natural to pick up the pace. Some people wait until they begin sweating, a sign that they are warmed up, before they increase the pace. While this may be an accurate sign for men, many women are slow to perspire and should increase their pace when they feel it is right for them.

When beginning an aerobic activity some women feel awkward because they are not used to doing the activity. The more one participates in the exercise the more efficient her style will become. It is a mistake to try to mimic someone else's actions. Fixx (1977) explains in *The Complete Runner* that every person's body is its own biochemical system with its own centers of gravity and articulation. The beginner should become familiar with the fundamentals of the aerobic activity but allow her own natural style to evolve. By following some guidelines, but not allowing the guidelines to dominate, exercise will be more enjoyable. Exercise should not be just for fitness. It is just as important to experience exercise as a special pleasurable happening for the mind and body. Fitness, style, and expertise will develop with time.

Pacing

Beginning participation in an aerobic activity should not cause strain. When a person begins to feel tired while cycling, running, etc., she should slow down and then pick up the pace again. Experts advise that one should be able to talk comfortably while exercising. Adaptation to the aerobic activity will occur over time, and eventually the person will be able to sustain a given pace for a longer time with the same effort.

Adaptation to exercise depends on the overload principle. By physically stressing the body to a certain limit, it is better able to endure stress. To achieve adequate use of the overload principle, an optimal heart rate needs to be sustained for a given time period. The minimal training heart rate can be estimated by taking the maximal heart rate of 220 (this can vary from person to person but is used as a constant) subtracting the person's chronologic age and taking 20% of the difference and subtracting that from the person's maximal heart rate.

Standard maximal heart rate	220
Minus age in years	35
Difference	185 (personal maximal heart rate)
Multiply by 20%	37.00
Subtract	37
from	185
Individual heart rate	148

It is important to keep the heart rate around that level. It can vary 10 beats higher or lower and still remain in the optimal training range. It is not beneficial to go above the maximal individual heart rate. Optimal training results are obtained when the heart rate is kept at the optimal training level rate. Faster training results are not obtained when the pulse rate is kept near the maximal rate. The aforementioned formula is an estimation and does not take individual differences into account. It is advisable to multiply the individual maximal heart rate by 0.30 instead of 0.20 if the woman is a smoker, more than 20 pounds overweight, or recuperating from surgery or a serious illness. A person may still find herself tiring in trying to maintain her optimal heart rate. In this case she should slow down a bit and aim for a lower optimal heart rate. Perceived exertion is a more accurate account of how much benefit is being obtained rather than trying to force oneself to fit a chart or general formula.

It is not necessary to check the pulse during every exercise period unless indicated by the health examina-

tion results. Otherwise, once a week is sufficient. Measuring the radial or carotid pulse by counting the beats accurately for six seconds and adding a zero is recommended. Pulse counting for a longer period does not ensure accuracy because the more physically fit a person becomes the faster the heart rate drops when exercise is stopped.

It is important to start out slowly and slow down the session when one becomes tired. As conditioning improves, exercise sessions lasting 15 to 20 minutes maintaining optimal pulse rate is needed to improve conditioning. The sessions should be done four or five times per week.

Cooling down

When the exercise session is over, it is important to take time for a cooling down period. Cycle, swim, or walk slowly for a few minutes. Stretching exercises are beneficial because the muscles are warm and supple at the end of an exercise session and stretch easily. Stretching also helps to eliminate metabolic wastes that have accumulated in the muscles as a result of the exercise.

Muscle soreness

Some degree of muscle sensation is unavoidable for the person who begins exercise. The feeling should be more of a tingling awareness and not pain. If one experiences muscle pain, the exercise is too strenuous. A long, hot bath and muscle massage do a lot to alleviate the discomfort. Continuing to exercise will actually make the muscles feel better since the improved circulation in the working muscles will enhance dissipation of metabolic wastes that are causing the soreness.

There are common injuries that result from certain types of aerobic activities. Running and jumping rope are more likely to result in leg and back discomfort. Knee discomforts account for about 25% of running injuries. The most common symptoms are parapatellar pain when running, walking, and extending the leg. Knee discomforts will decrease if the exercise sessions are shortened; increase the amount of quadriceps exercise and avoid running or jumping rope on a hard surface. If the woman is still troubled by knee pain, she may need to find a different type of shoe that alters foot support patterns and shifts the kneecap/femur contact area.

"Morton's toe" has recently been labeled a causative factor in heel, ankle, and knee discomforts. Morton's toe is a condition in which the first toe is shorter than the second. The first toe normally absorbs the greatest stress (two times more than the remaining four toes combined). With Morton's toe, the stress is displaced to the second toe and problems can ensue. The exact cause and effect relationship has not been discovered. Women with a Morton's toe may need a special type shoe or insert to correct the weight bearing.

Inflamed muscles and tendons on the anterior aspect of the lower leg accompanied by pain are commonly called shin splints. They range greatly in severity. Shin splints result from repeated jolts and by running or jumping too high on the toes. They are more common in women who elect to "run in place" because of the tendency to land on the ball of the foot and toes when performing this exercise.

For knee and shin discomforts it is recommended that the person continue to exercise unless the pain is worsened by the exercise. Frequent use of heat to the affected area between exercise periods is helpful. Following exercise, use of an ice pack for 10 minutes reduces the inflammation. For severe inflammatory response, aspirin, 600 mg three times a day (if not contraindicated), is frequently helpful.

Low back pain is a common complaint when exercise is begun. Back pain occurs especially in the multiparous woman who has never participated in physical activity, and in women with unequal leg lengths. Low back pain is frequently the result of poor abdominal muscle tone. Symptoms include an aching feeling in the lower back and radiating pain down the buttock and posterior leg. Bent-leg sit-ups and hamstring stretching exercises help to prevent lower back discomfort. Women who are troubled with chronic low back pain may find swimming to be a good aerobic activity (especially the side stroke) since there is less jarring of the back muscles.

Wearing apparel

Until recently women have had difficulty finding exercising clothes that were made specifically for women. Some women can wear men's shorts but others find that men's shorts are too big in the waist, too small in hips, and too narrow in the crotch. No special clothing is necessary. Whatever is worn should be easily washable, nonconstricting, and comfortable. Most beginners have a tendency to overdress because they do not realize the amount of heat their bodies will generate while exercising. Research shows that the amount of clothing needed to keep a resting person comfortably warm at 70° will keep a runner warm at −5° F (Fixx, 1976).

When exercising outside in the winter it is advisable to wear layers of clothing. An absorbent cotton T-shirt underneath a heavier sweatshirt or sweater is recommended. Wear just enough to remain pleasantly warm. Light cotton clothing is best for exercising in warm environments. Cotton is better than synthetic fabrics because it is more absorbent and allows for better air circulation. Properly fitting shoes are the most important equipment needed for any aerobic activity requiring leg

and foot work, especially running. Running causes extra pressure on lower leg muscles and tendons because of the heel-to-toe gait. As the heel contacts the surface the gastrocnemius and soleus muscles of the calf and the Achilles tendon are forcibly stretched. When weight is shifted forward to the sole of the foot, the gastrocnemius and Achilles are further stretched. Pushing off and getting ready to plant the opposite heel places extra stress on the anterior lower leg muscles. Running shoes are designed so that the heel is slightly raised, which allows for maximal cushioning on contact and prevents overstretching of lower leg muscles and tendons. They also have thin flexible soles that allow the foot to bend easily and facilitate pushing off. In the past women had difficulty purchasing running shoes because they were made only in men's sizes. Now companies are making running shoes in narrower widths which make them more acceptable for women.

Some women feel more comfortable exercising without a bra; however, many large-breasted women find participating in physical activity uncomfortable unless they are wearing a good supporting bra. A "Jogbra" is being developed that offers adequate support for both large- and small-breasted women and is comfortable. The Jogbra is made of soft, slightly stretchy fabric. It is made in a step-in design that holds the breasts close to the body. It has no metal hooks or strap holders, no traditional cups, and an "inside out" design so that seams and labels are outside and the smoothest part is toward the skin. This type of garment offers good support and greatly reduces the chance of nipple and skin chafing.

Developing the exercise habit

In developing the exercise habit it is important for the woman to assess her own life-style and the kinds of exercise facilities that are available in her community.

Many types of aerobic activities require a special setting or equipment such as a pool, bicycle, or handball court. Running and jumping rope are popular because they require minimal equipment and can be done anytime, anyplace. Women find difficulty in setting time aside for exercise because daily responsibilities usually do not stop with a 9-to-5 job. It is helpful for the woman to review her daily schedule and her own behavior. Some find it easier to exercise at night; others exercise in the morning. It is becoming popular to take time over the lunch hour to participate in exercise. It is hoped that places of employment will supply adequate locker rooms for women who are interested in exercise. Many companies already have such facilities for men. Once a time is set aside, avoid thinking of excuses for delaying exercise. It takes extra energy to develop the exercise habit, but the payoff is well worth it. Authorities recommend keeping a diary of a personal exercise routine that includes heart rate, weight, amount of exercise performed, and feelings toward the experience.

Women are more likely than men to be troubled with male hasslers, and they have a greater fear of mugging and body assault. According to Fixx (1977), the hasslers can be dealt with by ignoring them or "replying with oaths that would shock a stevedore." Fear of muggers and rapists is a real concern in some areas of the country. Exercising outside with a friend gives some added protection. Some women carry a stick, large hat pin, dog repellents, or a loud whistle to scare would-be attackers. Fixx believes that muggers are more likely to attack a woman carrying a purse or wearing jewelry than a woman running, but cases have been reported of women being assaulted while exercising. It is best to exercise in patrolled areas or where there are other people.

REFERENCES

Andersen, K. L., Rutenfranz, J., Masironi, R., and Seliger, V., editors: Habitual physical activity and health, Copenhagen, 1978, World Health Organization, Publication #6.

Astrand, P. O., Hallbaik, I., and Kilbom, A.: Reduction in maximal oxygen uptake with age, J. Applied Physiol. 35:649, 1973.

Astrand, P. O., and Rodahl, K.: Textbook of work physiology, New York, 1977, McGraw-Hill Book Co.

Barmeyer, J.: Physical activity and coronary collateral circulation, Adv. Cardiol., 18:104-112, 1976.

Barnard, R. J.: Long Term effects of exercise on cardiac function, Exer. Sports Sci. Rev. 3:113-133, 1975.

Beecher, H. K.: Surgery as placebo, a quantitative study of bias, J.A.M.A., 176:1102-1107, 1961.

Biles, F. R.: Self-concept change in college freshman women in a basic physical education course using two methods of instruction, Ph.D. thesis, Ohio State University, Columbus, 1978.

Borgman, F.: Exercise and health maintenance, J. Nurs. Educ., 16:6-10, 1977.

Brammell, H. L., and Niccoli, A.: A physiologic approach to cardiac rehabilitation, Nurs. Clin. North Am., 223-236, June, 1976.

Bruce, R. A.: Methods of exercise testing: step test, bicycle, treadmill, isometrics. In Amsterdam, E. and others, editors: Exercise in cardiovascular health and disease, New York, 1977, Yorke Medical Books.

Claremont, A. D.: Taking winter in stride requires proper attire, Physi. Sports Med., pp. 65-68, Dec. 1976.

Cureton, T. K.: Improvement of psychological states by means of exercise fitness programs, Assoc. Phys. Mental Rehab. 17:14-17, 1963.

Dale, E., Gerlach, D., and Wilhite, A.: Menstrual dysfunction in distance runners, Obstet. Gynecol. 54:47-53, 1979.

Daniels, J., Fitts, R., and Sheehan, G.: Conditioning for distance running, New York, 1978, John Wiley & Sons.

DeVries, H. A.: Immediate and long term effects of exercise upon resting muscle action potential level, J. Sports Med. 8:1-11, 1968.

Drinkwater, B. L.: Physiological responses of women to exercise, Exer. Sports Sci. Rev. 1:125-153, 1973.

Erdelye, G.: Gynecologic survey of female athletes, J. Sports Med. 2:174-176, 1962.

Erdelye, G.: Effects of exercise on the menstrual cycle, Phys. Sports Med. pp. 79-81, Mar. 1976.

Erkkola, R., and Rauramo, L.: Correlation of maternal physical fitness during pregnancy with maternal and fetal pH and lactic acid at delivery, Acta Obstet. Gynecol. Scand. 55:441-446, 1976.

Fixx, J.: The complete book of running, New York, 1977, Random House.

Garlick, M., and Bernauer, E.: Exercise during the menstrual cycle: variations in physiological baselines, Res. Q. Am. Assoc. Health Physical Ed. 39:533, 1968.

Gendel, E.: Pregnancy, fitness, and sports, J.A.M.A., 201:125-128, 1967.

Gendel, E.: Psychological factors and menstrual extraction, Phy. Sports Med., pp. 72-75, Mar. 1976.

Gendel, E.: Lack of fitness a source of chronic ills in women, Phys. Sports Med., pp. 85-95, Feb., 1978.

Gollnick, P. D., and others: Effect of training on enzyme activity and fiber composition of human skeletal muscle, J. Applied Physiol. 34:107-111, 1973.

Harris, D. V.: An investigation of psychological characteristics of university women with high and low fitness indices, Ph.D. thesis, University of Iowa, Iowa City, 1965.

Harris, D. V.: Involvement in sport: a somatopsychic rationale for physical activity, Philadelphia, 1973, Lea & Febiger.

Harris, G., and Frankel, L.: Fitness after fifty, New York, 1977, Plenum Press.

Haycock, C., and Gillet, J.: Susceptibility of women athletes to injury: myths vs. reality, J.A.M.A., 236:163-165, 1976.

Hellison, D. R.: The effect of physical conditioning on affective attitudes toward the self, the body and physical fitness, Ph.D. thesis, Ohio State University, Columbus, 1969.

Hitchcock, M.: The manipulative approach to management of primary dysmenorrhea, J. Am. Osteopath. Asso., 75:909-918, 1976.

Kiessling, K. H., and others: Mitochondrial volume in skeletal muscle from young and old physically untrained and trained healthy men, J. Clin. Sci., 44:547-554, 1973.

Lamaze, F.: Painless childbirth: psychoprophylactic method, Translated by Celestin, L. R., Chicago, 1956 (1970), Regnery.

Layman, E. M.: Psychological effects of physical activity. In Wilmore, J. E., editor: Exercise and sports science reviews, New York, 1974, Academic Press, Inc.

Morehouse, L. E., and Miller, A. T.: Physiology of exercise, St. Louis, 1976, The C. V. Mosby Co.

Morgan, T. E., and others: Effects of long term exercise on human muscle metochondria. In Pernon, B., and Saltin, B., editors: Muscle metabolism during exercise, New York, 1971, Plenum Press.

Nadel, E. R., editor: Problems of temperature regulation during exercise, New York, 1977, Academic Press, Inc.

Neill, W. A.: Coronary and systemic circulatory adaptations to exercise. In Amsterdam, E., and others, editors: Exercise in cardiovascular health and disease, New York, 1977, Yorke Medical Books.

Ogden, J. E.: Personality correlates of athletic participation among college women and men, Ph.D. thesis, University of Texas, Austin, 1977.

Penpargkul, S., and Scheuer, J.: The effect of physical training upon the mechanical and metabolic performance of the rat heart, J. Clin. Invest. 49:1859-1868, 1970.

Rushmer, R. F.: Cardiovascular dynamics, Philadelphia, 1976, W. B. Saunders Co.

Selye, H.: Implications of stress concept, N. Y. State J. Med. pp. 2141-2142, Oct. 1975.

Selye, H.: Stress in Health and Disease, Boston, 1976, Butterworth, Inc.

Selye, H.: Stress, Montreal, 1950, Acta, Inc.

Vincent, M.: Comparison of self-concepts of college women: athletes and physical education majors, Res. Quart. 47:218-225, 1976.

Wentz, A., and Jones, G.: Managing dysmenorrhea, Portgrad. Med. **60:**161-164, 1976.

Whitehouse, F.: Motivation for fitness. In Harris, G., and Frankel, L., editors: Fitness after fifty, New York, 1977, Plenum Press.

Wilmore, J. H.: Acute and chronic physiological response to exercise. In Amsterdam, E., and others, editors: Exercise in cardiovascular health and disease, New York, 1977, Yorke Medical Books.

Wilmore, J. H.: Individualized exercise prescription. In Amsterdam, E., and others, editors: Exercise in cardiovascular health and disease, New York, 1977, Yorke Medical Books.

Wynaham, C. H., Morrison, F. F., and Williams, C. G.: Heat reaction in male and female Caucasians, J. Applied Physiol. **20:**357, 1965.

Zaharieva, E.: Olympic participation by women: effects on pregnancy and childbirth, J.A.M.A., **221:**992-995, 1972.

Zaharieva, E.: Sports during pregnancy, other questions explored, Phys. Sports Med., pp. 82-85, Mar. 1976.

Zhanel, K.: Fencing in relation to menstrual cycle and gestation, J. Sports Med. **11:**120, 1971.

20

Women and the workplace

Nancy Fugate Woods
James S. Woods

During the last decade, women have been entering the labor force in increasing numbers. This trend has led to a renewed interest in the effects of employment outside the home on women's health and that of their offspring. Although some researchers claim that employment has positive effects on women's health (Nathanson, 1975), others are concerned about occupational exposure of women to physical, chemical, and other safety hazards in the workplace. Much of the concern in recent literature has focused on potential offspring rather than the health of the woman herself (Howell, 1972). The purposes of this chapter are to explore the wide range of women's work; to discuss the possible effects of women's roles on their health; to document known and suspected health hazards that are associated with occupations in which women are commonly employed; to document mutagenic and teratogenic agents found in occupational settings; and finally, to analyze the health hazards impinging on women whose work is in the home.*

WOMEN'S WORK

Throughout the history of the United States, women's work has made an important contribution to society. It was not until the mid-nineteenth century, however, that American women were employed outside their homes in large numbers. Rapid industrialization led to a desire for cheap labor, and both women and children were exploited in the textile mills. An abundance of occupational hazards led to an investigation of the status, experiences,

and difficulties of employed women in 1908. As a result protective legislation, restricting women to certain types of work, was enacted. World War I saw women entering a variety of male strongholds—munitions plants, smelters, and so on, at an accelerated pace. Unemployment was high for women and blacks during the Depression, but World War II prompted the return of women to the labor force. It was during this era that the United States Army sponsored a comprehensive investigation of the occupational health problems of women, *Women In Industry* (Baetjer, 1946). As early as 1946 Dr. Anna Baetjer warned of the effects of toxic substances—benzene, carbon monoxide, carbon disulfide, hydrocarbons, lead, mercury, and radiation—on pregnant women and their fetuses. She pointed out, however, that there was no proof that toxic substances had effects on nonpregnant women different from those on men. After World Ware II, many women left the labor force, and interest in special occupational health problems of women waned. The recent increase in the number of women employees has led to a resurgence of interest in the health effects of occupational exposure. Before considering the hazards of the workplace for women, it is important to examine the kinds of work most women do.

Distribution of women in the labor force

Today women comprise nearly 40% of the labor force in the United States. More than 40 million women were in the labor force in 1978, a figure representing 50% of all women 16 years of age and older (U.S. Department of Labor, 1978). Married women comprise about 60% of all women workers and over 40% of all married women are in the labor force. More than half of all female heads of families are employed.

Although there has been a tendency in past decades for women to leave the labor force while in their twenties (probably for marriage and childbearing), this is no longer the case. The United States Department of Labor

---

*In this chapter, the term "homemaker" will be used to denote those women whose work is the maintenance of the home environment and the care of children or other family members in the home. This is not to imply that women who are employed outside of the home do not engage in these same activities. Rather this term will be used in preference to "housewife," for women are not married to their houses. In addition, women who are not employed outside their homes will not be described as "not working," for anyone who is a homemaker is by definition, engaged in several kinds of work.

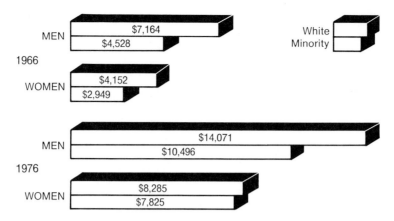

Fig. 20-1. Fully employed women continue to earn less than fully employed men of either white or minority races. (Prepared by the Women's Bureau, Office of the Secretary, United States Department of Labor, Published by the Bureau of the Census, U.S. Department of Commerce, Aug. 1978.)

Table 20-1. Total money earnings of civilian year-round, full-time workers, by occupation group and sex, 1974 (persons 14 years of age and over)*

Occupation group	Women	Men	Dollar gap	Women's earnings as a percent of men's	Percent men's earnings exceeded women's
TOTAL	$6,772	$11,835	$5,063	57.2	74.8
Professional, technical, and kindred workers	9,570	14,873	5,303	64.3	55.4
Managers and administrators	8,603	15,425	6,822	55.8	79.3
Sales workers, total	5,168	12,523	7,355	41.3	142.3
Retail trade	4,734	9,125	4,391	51.9	92.8
Other sales workers	8,452	13,983	5,531	60.4	65.4
Clerical workers	6,827	11,514	4,687	59.3	68.7
Craft and kindred workers	6,492	12,028	5,536	54.0	85.3
Operatives (including transport)	5,766	10,176	4,410	56.7	76.5
Service workers (except private household)	5,046	8,638	3,592	58.4	71.2
Farmers and farm managers	†	5,459	—	—	—
Farm laborers and supervisors	†	5,097	—	—	—
Nonfarm laborers	5,891	8,145	2,254	72.3	38.3
Private household workers	2,676	†	—	—	—

*From United States Department of Labor, Bureau of Labor Statistics: Current population reports, P-60, No. 101, Washington, D.C., U.S. Government Printing Office.
†Base less than 75,000.

indicates that the number of working women whose children are under 18 years of age has increased nine-fold since 1940; indeed more than one third of working women have children of preschool age. There appears to be a trend for women to be employed throughout their adult lives, with a diminishing proportion of women leaving the labor force for pregnancy and parenting. Such a trend raises new concerns for those clinicians caring for employed women.

Occupations of women

Despite their increasing representation among the employed, women still do not enjoy equal representation in all occupations. In general, women tend to be concentrated in low-paying jobs. Fig. 20-1 presents evidence that fully employed women earn less than fully employed men, even when race is taken into consideration. The earnings gap increased by a significant amount over the decades 1955 to 1975. In 1955, women's median earnings constituted 63.9% of men's; in 1974 women's median earnings were only 56.9% of men's. The gap persists even when occupational group is held constant (see Table 20-1). Educational level does not account for the earnings gap, since women's median income constitutes 52% to 65% of that for men when education is held constant.

Women also are restricted in the types of work they perform. Overrepresented as private household work-

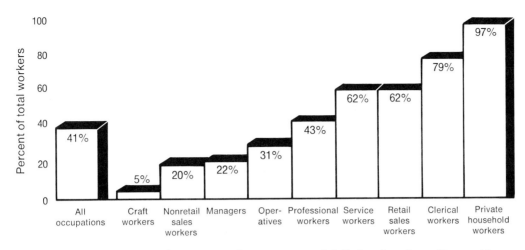

Fig. 20-2. Women are underrepresented as managers and skilled craft workers. (Prepared by the Women's Bureau, Office of the Secretary, from data published by the Bureau of Labor Statistics, U.S. Department of Labor, 1977.)

Table 20-2. Occupations of women: 1950, 1960, and 1970*

Occupational group	Women as percent of all persons in occupation		
	1950	1960	1970
TOTAL	28.1	32.8	38.0
Professional and technical workers	39.0	38.4	39.9
Managers and administrators, except farm	13.7	14.8	16.6
Sales workers	34.2	36.2	38.6
Clerical and kindred workers	61.9	67.9	73.6
Craftsmen	3.1	3.1	5.0
Operatives	27.4	28.7	31.5
Laborers, except farm	3.6	5.1	8.4
Farm workers	8.8	9.6	9.5

*From Women's Bureau, Employment Standards Administration, United States Department of Labor. Data reprinted from the Economic Report of the President, 1973.

Table 20-3. Women in the labor force, October 1978, (women 16 years of age and over)*

Occupations of employed women	All women	Women of minority races†
Number (in thousands)	40,049	5,069
Percent of women	100.0	100.0
Professional and technical workers	15.7	13.7
Managers and administrators (except farm)	5.8	2.9
Sales workers	6.6	3.1
Clerical workers	34.9	28.1
Craft and kindred workers	1.9	1.4
Operatives, except transport	11.2	15.3
Transport equipment operatives	0.8	0.7
Nonfarm laborers	1.2	1.4
Private household workers	2.8	7.6
Service workers (except private household)	17.6	25.1
Farmers and farm managers	0.4	0.1
Farm laborers and supervisors	1.0	0.7

*Data distributed by Women's Bureau, U. S. Department of Labor, December 1978.
†Includes all races other than white; Spanish-speaking persons are included in the white population.

ers, clerical workers, retail sales workers, and service workers, women are *under*represented as craft workers, nonretail sales workers, managers, operatives, and professional workers (see Fig. 20-2). Furthermore, one can readily discern from Table 20-2 that the biggest gains for women in the civilian labor force from 1950 to 1970 have been among clerical and kindred workers.

The percentage of all employed women and women of minority races for 1978 for each occupation is given in Table 20-3. Clerical work is the most common occupation for women. Minority women tend to be overrepresented as service workers or private household workers and are underrepresented as managers and administrators and sales workers.

Labor unions

Many labor unions have discriminated against women, with some barring women from membership as late as 1972. It is interesting to note that there are few women in leadership positions, even in the unions that represent a predominantly female work force. There are, however, several women's organizations and unions that are concerned about women workers' special interests. The United Auto Workers (UAW) and International

Union of Electricians (IUE) have active women's departments; the Oil, Chemical and Atomic Workers International (OCAW) has published a Handbook for OCAW Women that deals with legal rights of women in the workplace. The Coalition of Labor Union Women (CLUW), begun in 1974, is attempting to achieve affirmative action in work settings and is working for legislative action on women's issues, organizing more women, and encouraging women to participate more actively in their unions. Union WAGE (Women's Alliance to Gain Equality), begun in 1971, works for equal opportunity and equal pay, an end to male domination of unions, extension of protective legislation for all workers, and organization of unorganized workers (Hricko and Brunt, 1976).

Variables influencing the kinds of work available to women

The kinds of work currently available to women reflect beliefs about women's work capabilities, their roles as wives and mothers, their pregnancy potential, and the need for an expendable source of cheap labor. Stereotyping of women and men has led to labeling of certain jobs as "women's work" or "men's work." Hiring of only male workers for jobs that require lifting heavy objects was justified on the basis of variability in physical strength between the sexes. Having mostly female secretaries probably reflects the low pay associated with most clerical jobs, a factor that makes these jobs less attractive to men. Beliefs that women are "less stable" than men have been grounded in misconceptions about the effects of the menstrual cycle and pregnancy; yet they have probably served as effective deterrents in electing women to high government offices or corporate management.

The image of women as perpetually pregnant has no doubt limited their attractiveness to employers who provide extensive job training and therefore require a long-term commitment from their employees. Attitudes that women workers would regard their employment role as less important than their roles as wives and mothers have probably limited the recruitment and hiring of women for high-commitment positions. Having a potential source of cheap labor has been an attraction for many industries; keeping women in reserve as an exploitable source of labor has been fostered by employment policies that kept women out of high paying, long-term jobs.

Apprenticeships

Apprentice programs have recently become more accessible to women. New equal employment and equal pay legislation has facilitated the entry of women into some training programs. A recent California law re-

quired joint apprenticeship programs to establish goals for admitting women. In addition, the 31-year-old age limit for entry into apprenticeship programs may be eradicated as a result of a lawsuit. The rule has been effective at limiting possibilities for older women who return to the labor force after raising their children (Hricko, 1977).

"Protective" legislation

Although there are currently laws to prohibit sex discrimination in employment and pay, early legislation that was designed to protect women from hazards of the work environment may have served to bar women from certain occupations. Such legislation limited the amount of weight women were allowed to lift and the number of hours they could work. While these attempts to limit the exposure of women to hazardous conditions in the workplace probably were motivated by concern and compassion for deplorable working conditions, they were never applied to men. They thus became subverted as an instrument of discrimination.

Avoidance of success

A final variable influencing the distribution of women in various occupations has been studied only recently. Several researchers suggest that women have been socialized to avoid success.

Throughout history the notion persisted that femininity and individual achievements reflecting intellectual competence or leadership were desirable, but mutually exclusive, goals. Horner (1972) suggests that the motive to avoid success, an anxiety about achievement that grew out of the anticipation of negative consequences such as social rejection, is more prevalent among women. In a classic study she asked a group of college females to respond to the situation:

After first term finals, Anne finds herself at the top of her medical school class.

A group of college males were asked to respond to the same situation, but with respect to a male character. Whereas more than 90% of the male students described positive consequences for the character in the study, 65% of the females were disconcerted or confused by the sentence. Loss of femininity, personal or societal destruction, and social rejection were anticipated. It is interesting that since Horner's first study, the major difference in testing subsequent samples is that men express increasing concern about success. It is also interesting that in junior high school samples only 47% of the seventh graders demonstrate fear of success while fear of success imagery ranges from 60% to 88% in female college samples. The consequences of this fear are seen in women who disguise or apologize about their abilities and withdraw from the mainstream of achievement in the society. Horner cautions that this does not happen to women without a dear price: the individual experiences negative interpersonal and emotional consequences, and society loses a human and economic resource.

Myths about women in the workplace

Many beliefs about women workers are myths. Although the myth that a woman's place is in the home should have been dispelled by the influx of women into the labor force, it probably persists in some quarters and is expressed in subtle or more sophisticated form. Another myth is that women work only for extra money and therefore are not seriously committed to being employed. The statistics in Fig. 20-3 illustrate that most women work because of economic need. According to U.S. Department of Labor Statistics, only 20% of the women in the labor force in 1974 were married to husbands who earned $15,000 or more per year. Some contend that women are out of work because of illness more frequently than men are, which is expensive to industry, yet the recent absentee rates for illness are comparable for men and women; women miss an average 5.6 days per year and men 5.2. Another myth is that because women do not work as regularly or for as long as their male counterparts, their training is expensive and ultimately wasted. Current trends, however, suggest a decline in the proportion of women who leave the labor force. Even when women leave employment for childbearing and rearing, they still have 25 work years available to them (U.S. Department of Labor, 1974).

It is argued by some that married women take jobs away from men, yet most unemployed men lack the education or skills required for many of the jobs that women now fill. Furthermore, there would be a considerable number of unfilled positions since working women outnumber unemployed men. Others contend that women should not compete for "men's" jobs, yet tradition rather than the content of the job has been used to label jobs. Some suggest that women do not want job responsibility; yet women successfully perform professional and technical as well as managerial jobs. There have been contentions that the employment of women in supervisory positions would cause men to be unhappy, yet most of the men and women who have worked for women supervisors rate them positively. A final myth is that employment of mothers causes juvenile delinquency; recent studies suggest that maternal employment does not appear to be an important determinant (U.S. Department of Labor, 1974).

"Just a housewife"

The industrial production of goods and services caused work to be redefined in terms of its market value in trade. Because the work women performed in the home was not bartered or sold, it received no market value. It subsequently was not considered work. Even though some women perform private household work for pay they continue to be among the lowest paid workers. This seemingly reinforces the low value assigned to housework (Stellman, 1977).

Yet many household workers perform long hours, working at disagreeable and monotonous tasks. Despite the similarity of skills and working hours required for housework with those required in some industries, housework is not considered to have labor market value. There is little wonder that in a society where rewards for productivity and achievement are monetary ones, a woman whose work is the maintenance and care of the home may describe herself as "just a housewife."

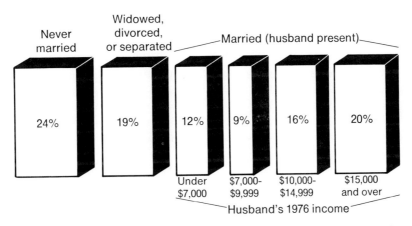

Fig. 20-3. Most women work because of economic need. (Prepared by the Women's Bureau, Office of the Secretary, from data published by the Bureau of Labor Statistics, U.S. Department of Labor.)

The value of women's work

The value of women's work is attested to by its contribution to the Gross National Product (GNP). Whereas job-related services contribute to the GNP, nonmarket work (housework) does not. Attempts to attach a dollar value to work in the home, however, are limited because there are few data about the monetary values of services performed and also because of the difficulty in assigning value to intangibles such as the continuous relationship with children. The fact that no monetary reward is provided for housework often leads women to forsake routine, repetitive tasks at home for routine, repetitive tasks in the labor force. Thus nonmarket activities are likely to become undervalued, with the growth of the national income confirming society's view that the contribution of women increases as they enter the labor force. If the nonmarket work of providing services in the home were rewarded in an economic sense, then perhaps fewer women would be drawn into the job market; women heads of household would have another option in addition to employment outside the home (Kreps, 1971). Of course, such a change in economic strategy could eliminate a large pool of cheap labor— women.

WOMEN'S ROLES, HEALTH, AND ILLNESS
Women's roles and their health

The literature dealing with women's roles and health-illness outcomes is primarily concerned with the comparison between women in traditional wife-mother roles and those who are employed outside the home. Many of the earlier studies in this area were predicated upon the assumption that employment of women would undermine the maternal-child bond, threaten the marriage, and probably would be hazardous to the woman's health. Studies in the literature since the feminist movement became popular in the United States sometimes reflect the assumption made by Nathanson (1975a) that work outside the home may be the single most important contribution to a woman's health.

Early studies focused on mental and physical health of the mother and the effects of woman's employment on marital happiness and roles.

Employment and health

Feld (1963) studied a probability sample of 2460 women in the United States. Of these, 438 were white, married, had children living at home, and were either employed full-time or were full-time homemakers. In 1957 this sample had been given several measures of distress, tapping such complaints as worry, unhappiness, projected unhappiness in the future, history of nervous breakdown, lack of uniqueness of self, lack of self-acceptance, shortcomings in the self, and lack of strong points in the self. Marital inadequacy, problems and unhappiness, negative orientation to children, problems in childbearing, feelings of inadequacy as a parent, anxiety, and physical ill health were also documented. The Health Opinion Survey was administered to the sample also.

Results indicated that the employed mothers were more accepting of themselves and demonstrated fewer physical symptoms of distress than the nonemployed mothers. The employed mothers were also less likely than homemakers to complain of pains and ailments in various parts of their bodies and of not feeling healthy enough to carry out the things they wanted to do. However, the employed mothers demonstrated doubts about their maternal adequacy more frequently than the homemakers. Even when education and family income were controlled, employed mothers reported more marital unhappiness than the control group of homemakers. However, it is impossible to determine whether marital unhappiness preceded or followed employment among the employed women.

Using the same 1957 data as Feld, Sharp and Nye (1963) found that among 1993 mothers living in three Washington towns, the employed mothers had no more psychosomatic symptoms than the nonemployed. Socioeconomic status and education did not influence the amount of anxiety the women experience. However, being employed in a blue collar occupation and having preschool children was associated with a high level of anxiety among these women.

Unemployment and depression

Of forty-six women seeking employment counseling services, eighteen were found to be very depressed as determined by several depression scales. Of these, seventeen who found work were significantly less depressed and pessimistic 4 months after seeking counseling. Although the women in this sample were self-selected, the results of the study shed some light on possible relationships between women's roles and their health. Many of the women who were most depressed anticipated relocating in the next 5 years. Frequent moves, usually as a result of the husband's career, were often cited as the reason they were unable to find satisfying employment. Other difficulties cited by the women included the stress of carrying out multiple roles and the problem of reconciling their own needs with those of their children and spouses (Weissman, 1973).

Employment and symptoms

Finseth and coworkers (1975) used data from 9847 enrollees of a New Haven Health Maintenance Organization (HMO) to show that employment status did not seem to affect disease prevalence patterns.

Pope and McCabe (1975) interviewed 2603 persons enrolled in the Kaiser Foundation Health Plan (1402 of these were women). Of the female respondents, 519 were not employed outside the home and 561 were. Employment and occupational status were used as independent variables. The dependent variables included: (1) general and physical health status; (2) mental and emotional health status; and (3) self-concept and personal sense of well-being. Respondents were queried with regard to a self-assessment of their health, a self-report of their utilization, an index of six symptoms selected because of their potential psychosomatic origin, and absenteeism from work for employed females. No index of social role incapacity was obtained for women not employed outside the home. As an index of mental health, the twenty-two item mental health scale from the Midtown Manhattan study was used. Medical records were searched to establish utilization, number of contacts for physical diseases, and number of new conditions treated during the 2-year study period. Medical record data were also obtained regarding diagnosis of mental illness and utilization for the same. Another symptom list was derived for psychosomatic complaints. Finally, the Bradburn and Caplowitz' "affect balance" and a worries scale were used as indices of well-being. Women were also queried directly about their happiness, self-acceptance, and life satisfaction.

The findings included the following:

1. There was no difference in health and well-being for employed vs unemployed women.
2. The homemakers had significantly more worries than employed women.
3. Blue-collar employed women had greater self-acceptance than either the white-collar employed women or homemakers.

Education, social class, and income were positively related to perceived health status and mental health status. These variables plus marital status were related to affect balance and life satisfaction. Employed women perceived their health as better, and reported better mental health and fewer worries than women who were not employed. However, all but the latter variable did not differ significantly across employment status when age, marital status, education, social class, and family income were controlled. Selection of healthier women into the work force was not considered as a variable.

The fourth study in this area sought to identify the effects of family contextual variables on whether and how women responded to their own illnesses. Context was defined in terms of structural variables, such as the number of role obligations a woman had, as well as by the woman's and her husband's attitudes toward illness and the medical care system. Data from 1214 women who had participated in the Baltimore household survey were used to test the hypotheses mentioned above. Women with the least demanding immediate family situation (no children) and whose broader social arenas were most demanding (poor nonwhites) and reported the most morbidity for the 2-week recall period (Rivkin, 1972).

In most studies, employed women tend to report fewer symptoms of ill health than do homemakers. One possible explanation for this phenomenon is termed the "healthy worker effect" (McMichael, 1976). Simply stated, this means that women with poor health get selected out of the labor force and therefore one would expect women who are employed to appear healthier than those who are not employed.

Women's roles and illness behavior

Empirical evidence regarding employment and illness behavior is equivocal. Finseth and coworkers (1975) demonstrated that women registered as female spouses stood out as high users of HMO services when compared to female participants (those in whose name the HMO policy was registered.) These latter women used the service much less frequently than female spouses, but more frequently than male participants. Further, female spouses made more visits to the HMO and received more prescription medications. Pope and McCabe (1975) also found that compared to homemakers, employed women reported fewer total physician office visits and fewer physician contacts for disease with a large emotional component.

Rivkin's findings (1972) demonstrate the reverse: employed women used health services for illness more than women who were not employed. Further, she documented that the presence of children seemed to influence nearly every relationship between independent variables and illness behavior. Among women with children, those women who were married, employed, who used fewer unprescribed drugs, and had positive attitudes toward medical care tended to use health services more than other women. Among women with children, disability days were strongly associated with nonemployed women with high anxiety, high use of nonprescribed drugs, and high skepticism of medicine. Among women with no children there were few significant relationships with utilization. However, those who were from the upper classes, had high anxiety, used many nonprescription drugs, and who had negative attitudes toward medical care tended to have the most disability days. Family structural variables other than economic class and presence of children did not greatly influence utilization patterns.

Mortality rates

In 1946 Baetjer wrote that "very few data are available to determine the influence of occupation on the mortality rates of women, or to predict whether the increasing employment of women will appreciably raise the death rate of this group." (p. 213) It is lamentable that Baetjer's description is still accurate.

To cope with this dilemma, Baetjer analyzed the mortality associated with occupations for men and extrapolated from these to predict expected trends for women as a result of their expected employment. Marital status, social class, and age appear to be codeterminants of mortality in the groups of women studied—marital status has a protective effect on mortality, as does social class.

A recent study of female production workers in the rubber industry reveals that there was an excess of deaths caused by cancer of the trachea, bronchus, and lung, and by myocardial infarctions. Both of these causes of death have been clearly associated with cigarette smoking, but smoking histories were not available for the women in the study. There was a deficit of breast cancer deaths in this same population. The investigators point out that because of the long latency period between exposure and some causes of death, it may be many years before we can fully evaluate the effects of occupational exposure in women who are now entering the labor force (Andjelkovic and Taulbee, 1976).

Another study of professionals of the Wisconsin work force for 1968 to 1972 reveals a reversal of the male/female death rate differentials (Ladbrook, 1976). A disproportionately high number of professional women suffered from deaths associated with behaviors such as smoking and driving after drinking. There was a higher incidence of suicide among professional women than men, as well as a higher incidence of cancer deaths. Cancer of the breast and genitourinary system were responsible for the cancer deaths. There was also a diminution of the traditional male excess of lung cancer deaths. This study implicates professional life-style variables in the reversal of the usual mortality differentials for men and women. Ladbrook suggests that several mechanisms may be involved:

1. Professional women take on more risk factors once characteristic of males, e.g. smoking, drunken driving.
2. The marriage opportunities for professional women are more limited than those for professional men, thus limiting a source of social support for women.
3. There are rich support facilities for professional men whereas some of these familial (or "wifely") supports are not present for professional women.
4. The division of labor in the professions may be disadvantageous to women.
5. Individual modes of adapting to stress may account for the differences in mortality trends.

Women who are employed may simply adhere to a set of norms different from those of women who are not employed. That is, it may be less acceptable for them to admit to illness. Increased socioeconomic resources available to families and involvement of the woman with other workers in a supportive network may offset some of the strains associated with employment.

Finally, the rewards inherent in the work the woman does, over and above the monetary rewards she accrues, may lead to increased self-esteem; on the other hand, if the woman perceives herself as a failure, she may develop illness, and perhaps leave the labor force because of her inability to remain healthy in this situation.

Role proliferation: a special hazard

A special hazard to employed women is role proliferation. Rather than encountering a transitional sequence from one role to another, women encounter an accumulation of roles as they enter the labor force. They take on a combination of disparate and dissociated roles, for example, employee and mother roles, both of which require deep commitment. Role expectations frequently compete because the demands are synchronous and continuous.

Boulding (1976) contends that a triple role for women of breeder-feeder-producer has existed from the days of the hunting and gathering societies to the age of highly industrialized societies. She points out that in nearly every type of human society, women have been responsible for the bearing of and caring for children (breeding) and the feeding of humans of all ages in addition to any other producing activities in which they engage. Data from recent studies in the Western world substantiate her claim, for even when both spouses are employed, the feeder and breeder roles still are considered to be "women's work."

Feelings associated with role proliferation may be frustration, inadequacy, or failure. Some persons might regard the pressures associated with role proliferation as the spice of life, whereas another might perceive them as overwhelming.

Johnson and Johnson (1976) suggest several mechanisms women might use to cope with role proliferation. These include:

1. Establishing a hierarchy of importance among roles
2. Insulation of some roles from observation
3. Receiving mutual support from peers
4. Compartmentalizing roles
5. Delegation of some roles
6. Elimination of some roles
7. Role bargaining

Establishing a hierarchy of importance presents difficulties for career-oriented women inasmuch as normative demands inherent in wife-mother roles are especially powerful and widely reinforced. Insulation or "privatization" of career and family roles may be difficult as women are "expected to move in a more intimate interpersonal environment which is particularistic, personalistic and responsive to emotional demands" (Johnson and Johnson, 1976, p. 38). Mutual support from status peers may be difficult to find for women in the traditionally male areas. Compartmentalization of roles is another way of dealing with strain. It requires suppressing concerns about one role while performing another. Delegation of some roles may be difficult, and elimination of some roles, whether that of spouse, mother, or employee may become necessary. Role bargaining may be used as a means of decreasing achievement expectations in some roles and assuming greater responsibility for roles more compatible with the woman's commitments.

Any combination of these mechanisms can be explored. For women who perform multiple roles and who have little reinforcement, mutual support from status peers might be recommended. This might involve entering a support network such as a consciousness-raising or homemakers' group, or perhaps initiating a support group of women with similar concerns. Women with many roles and poor evaluation of their role performance might also benefit from such groups as a source of feedback. Massive social change would be required to reform the stressful social arenas that limit women from racial minorities and lower social classes.

HEALTH HAZARDS OF THE WORK ENVIRONMENT

An analysis of health hazards of the work environment, with special reference to women, must consider: the types of populations of women who are at high risk of hazardous exposures; those physical, chemical, microbial, mechanical, temporal, and social stressors impinging on the woman; similar stressors impinging on the woman's offspring; and, finally, the hazardous exposure of a large population of women who are not protected by any occupational regulations—women whose work is at home.

Types of high-risk populations

Conibear (1977) suggests that two types of high-risk populations can be identified. The first is a "situational or environmental" high-risk population, which includes a population of workers who have been or are currently exposed to a hazard but exhibit no signs of negative health. In this instance, it is the environment that creates the risk rather than variables intrinsic to the population of workers. For example, we know that exposure to asbestos carries the risk of developing mesothelioma. The second type of high-risk population is the "intrinsic" high-risk population. Because of some variable in-

trinsic to the population, certain workers are more likely than others to experience negative health outcomes from their exposure. Because of genetic predisposition, personal habits, nutritional patterns, life-style, intercurrent disease processes, and age, certain groups of workers are at greater risk of harmful health effects than others. Conibear cites the examples of increased risk of ill health in persons with kidney disease who are exposed to lead or in heavy drinkers who are exposed to solvents. Smokers who are exposed to asbestos constitute another high-risk population.

A current problem facing women in the workplace is determining whether or not they constitute an intrinsic high-risk group because they are female. Some arguments about characteristics associated with being female have been used, in the past, to classify certain jobs as "women's work," or, conversely, to keep women out of these jobs. Some of the traits used to build the case for women as an intrinsic high-risk population include such contentions as:

1. Women's physical strength, dexterity, and stamina are inferior to those of men.
2. Women have a special susceptibility to certain toxic substances by virtue of supposed physiologic differences between the sexes.
3. Because they bear children, women should be concerned about genetic transmission of effects of hazardous exposure to future offspring (e.g., mutagenesis).
4. There are differences in women's responsibilities (e.g., caring for home and children in addition to keeping a job), and these must be considered in opening certain jobs to women.
5. Women become pregnant, and because of the danger of prenatal exposure of their offspring (teratogenesis), they must be regarded as a population with intrinsically high risk.

There appears to be little support for the first four of the five traits cited above. There is not much evidence to suggest that presumed sex differentials in physical strength should be used to assign jobs, inasmuch as some women are stronger than some men, and vice versa. Excluding childbearing, the biochemical and physiologic processes of men and women are more similar than different, thus it is unlikely that women can be presumed to be especially susceptible to certain substances, except insofar as they affect embryonic or fetal development. The third argument probably applies to men as well as women. Given that the worker has any reproductive ability, exposure to mutagenic agents would be hazardous to both men and women. Indeed, Conibear (1977) points out that men might be *more* susceptible to mutagenic agents because the process of spermatogenesis is so rapid. The fourth argument for women as an intrinsically high-risk population is also open to debate. As Conibear points out, certain aspects of men's life-styles, such as greater use of alcohol and higher incidence of smoking, could constitute a basis for men to be considered an intrinsic high-risk population.

The final situation, pregnancy, does merit special concern. Fetal exposure to toxic and stressful agents may be a special case inasmuch as exposures that are not thought to be hazardous to adult workers *may be* hazardous to the fetus. Thus action to limit hazardous exposure of the fetus is needed. This leads Conibear (1977) to conclude that fetuses must be considered an intrinsically high-risk population. This should not create a certain dilemma in the workplace, for a safe and healthful workplace is guaranteed to all workers by the Occupational Safety and Health Act, and Title VII of the Civil Rights Act prohibits exclusion of workers from certain jobs on the basis of sex. Conibear emphasizes the need for epidemiologic and toxicologic studies to determine mutagenic, teratogenic, and carcinogenic substances and the acceptable level of risk for these; education of workers, employers, and health personnel to the known hazards; and reduction or elimination of exposure to mutagens, teratogens, and carcinogens.

Exposure of the woman herself
Physical stressors

A number of physical stressors impinge on women in the workplace, including noise, heat, physical labor requirements, postural limitations, and ionizing radiation.

Noise. Noise is unwanted sound and can be stressful. While there is no single noise-induced disease except hearing loss, noise triggers physiologic changes in the endocrine, cardiovascular, and auditory systems. Noise also interferes with worker's ability to communicate.

The pituitary-adrenal axis has a very low threshold for stimulation by noise, estimated to be as low as 68 dB linear.* Activation of the pituitary-adrenal axis leads to increased secretion of ACTH and subsequent increase in adrenocortical activity. Thus noise can be considered a nonspecific stimulus capable of inducing ACTH release, and seems to cause a biphasic pattern of hormonal release.

In addition, noise appears to stimulate the adrenal medulla, resulting in increased urinary excretion of epinephrine and norepinephrine. The cardiovascular response to noise includes peripheral vasoconstriction. It is believed that vasoconstriction in the spiral vessels supplying the organ of Corti is the change probably re-

---

*Intensity of noise is measured in decibels (db) where db(A) represents the range perceived in the human ear. The frequency of the sound is described in Hertz. PNdb is the perceived noise level.

sponsible for hearing loss in humans. Animal studies demonstrate that exposure to noise produces decreased placental blood flow, increased incidence of abnormalities in fetal development, and smaller litters.

In human adults, 80 dB(A) seems to be the maximal sound intensity that is unable to induce sensorineural hearing loss, regardless of duration. This means that at levels above 80 dB(A), exposed persons risk hearing loss.

The intensity of exposure can be increased if the duration is lessened, thus minimizing risk. The National Institute for Occupational Safety and Health (1975) recommends the following exposure limitations:

dB(A)	Hours/day
90	8
92	6
95	4
97	3
100	2
102	1½
105	1
110	½
115	¼

It is recommended that exposure to 115 dB(A) be considered the maximum. Impulsive or impact noise should be limited to 140 dB(A). The human ear is much more sensitive to effects of high-frequency sound than to low-frequency sound. Thus loss from high-frequency sound results in a more profound loss of hearing acuity.

Stellman (1977) estimates that noise levels in secretarial areas caused by typing, accounting, and business machines might reach 63 dB(A), or a perceived level of 78 PNdB. Indeed, keypunch operators, laundry workers, and some hospital workers probably are exposed to noise levels greater than 85 dB(A).

Heat. Exposure to a hot environment not only produces discomfort but also threatens health. Physical exertion decreases tolerance for heat in the external environment. Exposure to heat interferes with body's ability to dissipate heat inasmuch as evaporation is slowed. Workers exposed to heat stress usually adapt to some degree; their cutaneous blood vessels dilate, and there is minimal effect on the vital organs. On the other hand, persons not accustomed to heat may experience compensatory vasoconstriction to kidney, liver, and digestive organs as the cutaneous vessels dilate. Persons not acclimatized to heat also perspire in only a few places, thus limiting the amount of heat loss. Very humid air, such as that found in laundries, slows the evaporation process. Persons exposed to heat on a continuous basis may perspire excessively, become dehydrated, and even experience shock. It appears that heat is tolerated better by younger persons than by older people and those with circulatory impairments. It is estimated that

4 to 6 days of work are necessary for acclimatization to heat to occur, and that when one is absent from the hot environment for 3 weeks, adaptation must begin anew. The health outcomes of chronic exposure to heat are not well documented (Stellman, 1977).

Physical exertion. The risk of injury and illness as a result of physical exertion is difficult to determine. Rather than adhering to general guidelines for the amount of exertion by workers, Chaffin (1976) recommends that personal strength testing be performed before an employee begins a job. The tests used must be repeatable, easily administered, safe, and measure the personal risk involved. Such a procedure as advocated by Chaffin would involve following people whose jobs are rated to have various lifting requirements to determine the incidence of illness and injury for each. Using the outcome of low back pain, there seemed to be little difference in the incidence rates between men and women. It is likely that strength might be a much more relevant criterion than sex, and that matching the job requirements with the person might protect men as well as women. Nurses and other health services workers are frequently exposed to heavy lifting (e.g., transferring and moving patients).

Postural requirements. The postures required to perform certain jobs frequently include sitting or standing. Sitting at a desk, keypunch machines, typewriter, or telephone switchboard may lead to impairment of circulation to the lower limbs resulting in pooling in legs and feet. Hemorrhoids and varicose veins may occur in women who must sit or stand for long periods of time without interruption or who use chairs that create pressure over the popliteal space.

Sitting posture is influenced by the type of chair, height of equipment, and type of activity performed. Chairs that do not provide back support require the person to contract muscles of the back resulting in perceived muscular tension and ache. Jobs requiring a great deal of concentration lead to muscle tightening, strain, and fatigue of the entire body. The optimal position when sitting in a chair is with the back supported and leaning slightly forward. Table or desk height must complement the design and height of the chair.

Standing also leads to stress on muscles in the back, legs, and feet as well as development of varicose veins. If the structural integrity of the vein has not been damaged, support stockings may improve the varicosities. On the other hand, the woman whose veins are damaged may anticipate swelling of the feet and legs, blistering, skin ulcers, and rashes.

Women whose work requires standing may require opportunities to sit down at regular intervals, and they should not wear constricting garments such as girdles. Writing can lead to overexertion of the muscles of the

hands, fingers, and wrists; writer's cramp occurs when the muscles are fatigued. In addition, typists may develop tenosynovitis of the wrists. These tendons become inflamed as a result of overexertion or stress (Stellman, 1977).

Ionizing and microwave radiation. Women are exposed to ionizing or microwave radiation in a variety of occupations. The increasing possibility of occupational exposure to radiation from various sources underscores the importance of understanding the nature of the effects of radiation on biologic tissues and the preventive measures necessary for avoiding excessive radiation exposure.

The principal hazard from ionizing radiation is the destruction of vital organs occurring when X-rays, gamma rays, or alpha or beta particles pass through biologic tissues exciting the atoms and changing them to electrically charged ions. The net result of this effect varies with the dose and type of radiation received, and may range from no noticeable change in organ function to genetic damage or cancer.

The principal occupations in which women may be exposed to ionizing radiation include dentistry, X-ray technology, radiology, nuclear medicine, nuclear power engineering, and laboratory work. In these occupations ionizing radiation may be encountered from X-ray generating machines or from chemical isotopes used in power generation, medical therapy, or for diagnostic or experimental analysis.

Acute exposure to sources of ionizing radiation is of clinical significance only when the dosage is sufficiently high to cause tissue destruction resulting in cell death and loss of vital organ function. Such exposure would be expected only in cases of accidental exposure to massive doses of radiation or ingestion of isotopes of high specific radioactivity. Symptoms of acute high dose radiation exposure range from burns to "radiation sickness," which is characterized by loss of hair, sore throat, diarrhea, purpura, and damage to rapidly proliferating tissues such as bone marrow. The actual extent of radiation poisoning from acute exposure episodes depends largely on the dose received and may range from relatively mild symptoms to death.

The more insidious form of occupational radiation poisoning comes from long-term exposure to low-level radiation sources such as might be encountered in occupations such as those mentioned above if proper protective measures are not practiced. Although little is currently known about the long-range effects of prolonged low-level radiation exposure in humans, animal studies suggest that exposure for long periods may produce tissue damage at the subcellular level leading to a variety of adverse health effects including cataracts and cancer. Since radiation exposure is cumulative with respect to changes induced in biologic tissues, the risk of adverse health effects increases with continuing exposure. For this reason, federal agencies have established maximum radiation exposure levels; once one has reached this maximum exposure level, no further exposure is permitted until an appropriate time interval has passed.

Protection from the adverse health effects of ionizing radiation is essential to women employed in occupations where exposure to radiation sources may occur. This includes the use of proper shielding for X-rays and wearing of protective clothing when working with radioactive chemicals. Many agencies require that long-sleeved protective uniforms or lab coats be worn in areas where radiation may be encountered. Lead-lined aprons and gloves and protective eyeglasses made with lead-impregnated glass are also recommended for close-up work involving radioactive substances. Personal radiation monitoring devices should always be worn by persons working in areas where sources of radiation are present. Such devices usually consist of badges of film impregnated with a radiation-sensitive chemical for monitoring individual cumulative radiation exposure. All radioactive chemicals should be appropriately labeled and kept in well-marked radiation storage or disposal areas. Unnecessary exposure to radiation sources should be avoided.

In contrast to ionizing radiation, microwaves are electromagnetic waves, having a frequency between 30 and 30,000 MHz. Microwaves are not ionizing and produce effects on biologic tissues primarily through the production of heat. The principal occupational sources of microwave radiation exposure to women are from microwave ovens used by commercial and institutional food processors, and from diathermy machines used by therapists. Although the biologic effects of microwave exposure have not been clearly established, it is now recognized that long-term exposure to microwaves may damage the eyes, possibly leading to the formation of cataracts. Other vague symptoms such as increased fatigue, dizziness, headaches, insomnia, and changes in light, sound, and olfactory sensitivity have been reported among workers exposed to continuous microwave radiation. A controversy currently exists with respect to other adverse effects of low-level microwave radiation, such as possible changes in the function of pacemakers and other metallic implants. The basis of these effects remains to be substantiated.

Chemical stressors

Women are exposed to numerous types of chemical stressors in the occupational environment. Many of these, such as anesthetic gases, organic solvents, and halogenated hydrocarbons, are directly utilized in the production and delivery of goods and services, so that exposure to them may be both intentional and to some extent unavoidable. For many years the adverse health effects resulting from exposure to such chemicals were considered primarily in terms of their acute health effects, such as headache or skin rash, and little thought was given to the possible long-range health hazards that those symptoms might portend. In recent years, however, the possibility of serious life-threatening effects resulting from prolonged exposure to chemicals in the work environment has been recognized, leading to both increased worker awareness of long-term occupational health hazards and legislative action oriented toward reduction of hazardous chemical exposure in the work environment. Some of the more commonly encountered occupational chemicals and their short- and long-term health effects are given in Table 20-4.

Among the most insidious adverse health outcomes now recognized as being associated with prolonged exposures to occupational chemicals are: (1) cancer, resulting from occupational exposure to arsenic, asbestos, halogenated hydrocarbons, and other organic substances; (2) chronic organ damage, associated with the use of metals and petroleum products; and (3) irreversible neurologic dysfunction, caused by exposure to lead, mercury, and other trace elements.

Cancer is of particular concern because of the growing numbers of chemicals identified as either carcinogenic or cocarcinogenic,* and because of the recognition of increasing numbers of nonoccupationally encountered chemicals that increase the risk of cancer in otherwise low-risk individuals. An excellent example of this situation is the greatly increased risk of lung cancer in asbestos workers who smoke cigarettes compared with those who do not smoke. Similarly, diet, medications, and other chemicals encountered both in and out of the work setting may substantially affect the risk of cancer produced by specific chemicals employed in the work setting.

Among the various classes of occupational chemicals, organic solvents and other petroleum products probably constitute the greatest long-term health risk to exposed workers. Solvents such as benzene, toluene, and xylene are encountered in a wide variety of work activities where women are employed, ranging from housekeeping and clerical work to jobs in heavy industry. Used primarily to dissolve grease, ink, paint, and other oil-based substances, organic solvents produce a spectrum of adverse health effects when they are ingested or absorbed through the skin in sufficient quantity. The immediate consequences from such exposure include dizziness, fatigue and headache, and , if high enough concen-

---

*A cocarcinogen is a substance that must be present in order for a second substance to be carcinogenic.

Table 20-4. Health effects of common occupational chemicals

Chemical (class)	Health hazard		Occupation
	Short-term	Long-term	
Asbestos	Respiratory system irritation	Mesothelioma, cancer of lung and pleura, chronic respiratory disease, asbestosis	Clerical workers, shipyard workers, beauticians, textile workers

Anesthetic gases
  Cyclopropane
  Divinyl ether
  Ethyl ether
  Trichloroethylene
  Ethyl chloride
  Vinyl ether
  Halothane
	Reflex depression, cardiovascular depression, respiratory depression, gastrointestinal depression, spontaneous abortions	Hepatotoxicity, birth defects	Operating room personnel, dental and medical assistants, veterinary personnel, laboratory workers

Halogenated hydrocarbons
  Trichloroethylene
  Bischloromethyl methyl ether
  Vinyl chloride
  Chloroprene
  Dichlorobromopropane
  Perchloroethylene (PERC)
  Carbon tetrachloride
  Chloroform
  Polyhalogenated biphenyls (PBBs, PCBs)
	Hepatotoxicity, headache, fatigue, nausea and vomiting, dizziness, narcosis, mucous membrane irritation	Liver necrosis, cancer of lung, liver, and skin	Laundry and drycleaning personnel, clerical workers, textile finishers, plastics manufacturers, beauticians, cosmetologists, hairdressers, electrical workers, agricultural workers, housekeeping

Organic solvents
  Benzene
  Toluene
  Xylene
  Triethanolamine
  Formaldehyde
  Dimethyl formamide
  Alcohol
  Acetone
  Diethylene dioxide (dioxane)
  Turpentine
	CNS depression, bone marrow suppression, liver toxicity, eye and skin irritation, depressed red and white blood cell count	Leukemia, dermatitis, allergies and sensitization, circulatory failure, respiratory arrest, liver and kidney damage	Rubber workers, laboratory workers, textile workers, beauticians, cosmetologists, petroleum manufacturers, dry cleaners and launderers, clerical workers, housekeepers, histology workers

Trace elements
  Lead
  Cadmium
  Mercury
  Arsenic
	Acute respiratory effects, bronchitis, coughing, chest pain, shortness of breath, porphyrinuria	Neurologic dysfunction, brain damage, cancer, liver and kidney damage, tremor, erethism	Chemical and pesticide workers, battery plant workers, dental assistants, welders, agricultural workers, paint manufacturers, electric workers, seed dressers

Acids and alkalis
  Hydrochloric acid
  Nitric acid
  Sulfuric acid
  Sodium hydroxide
  Bleaches
	Nose and upper respiratory tract irritation, skin irritation, tissue destruction in large doses	Allergies and sensitization	Laboratory workers, chemical workers, laundry personnel, housekeepers

Cotton dust	Chest tightness, shortness of breath, cough	Byssinosis, chronic bronchitis, emphysema	Textile and apparel workers, agricultural workers

trations are involved, narcosis. Skin rashes and dermatitis are also common among persons who permit regular contact of organic solvents with the skin. Of greater concern, however, are the long-range effects of these substances, which may not appear until many years after initial exposure to them has occurred. The major chronic toxic effects include anemia or leukopenia resulting from bone marrow damage, or thrombocytopenia caused by decreased production of platelets required for clotting. Benzene exposure is of special concern in this respect, having been linked to asplastic anemia resulting from destruction of marrow cells, and leukemia, a malignant disease of the reticuloendothelial system.

Chlorinated and other halogenated hydrocarbons are also recognized as producing a broad spectrum of long-range toxic effects in humans, including cancer. These substances, such as chloroform, carbon tetrachloride, and trichlorethylene (TCE), are found in many types of occupational activities in which women are engaged, including dry cleaning, textile finishing, and laboratory work. On a short-term basis these substances have a narcotic effect, producing dizziness, loss of coordination, and unconsciousness. Irritation of the skin, eyes, nose, and mouth are also common effects. If taken internally the chlorinated hydrocarbons are extremely toxic to the liver and kidneys, and prolonged exposure may cause cancer in various organ sites. Women working as cosmetologists, hairdressers, and beauticians are especially likely to experience long-term occupational exposure to organic solvents and halogenated hydrocarbons, since these agents are common ingredients in many hair sprays, hair dyes, wave solutions, and other cosmetic preparations.

Another class of chemicals found in many occupations where women are employed is the trace elements, including mercury, arsenic, and lead. These substances share as their principal long-range toxic effect brain damage and other types of neurologic dysfunction. Some of these elements may be carcinogenic as well. Dental assistants are at particularly high risk from mercury poisoning, which is routinely used in the preparation of amalgam for use in dental fillings. Many inorganic mercury compounds are used in the manufacture of drugs, dyes, explosives, and ink whereas organic mercury has been employed in the production of drugs and pesticides. Organic mercury, because of its ability to easily cross lipid membranes, is much more toxic to the nervous system than are inorganic forms, and during prolonged exposure may cause blindness and severe brain damage.

A second occupationally encountered trace element that has a high level of toxicity is arsenic. Women working in the manufacture of ceramics, paints, and arsenical pesticides, and in smelting and refining of copper and other metals are at particularly high risk to arsenic exposure. Ingestion of dusts and inhalation of fumes containing arsenic compounds are the most common routes of exposure, resulting in irritation of the conjunctiva, skin, and mucous membranes, and occasionally, perforation of the nasal septum. Chronic exposure may lead to liver damage, neurologic dysfunction, and cancer of the liver, lung, or other organ systems.

Lead poisoning may also occur in a variety of occupations in which women are employed. A partial list of occupations in which lead exposure may occur includes ceramics and glass makers, enamel workers, painters, and plumbers. The early signs of lead poisoning are nonspecific and are difficult to distinguish from symptoms of minor seasonal illnesses such as decreased physical stamina and appetite. As a cumulative poison, lead may cause neurologic damage, loss of kidney function, and damage to bloodforming organs after exposure for long periods.

A variety of inorganic acids and alkalis are utilized in many occupations populated by women. Laundry workers, chemical manufacturers, and laboratory workers in particular are inclined to be exposed to these substances. The principal immediate health effects resulting from exposure to acids and alkalis include skin irritation and possible burns of exposed tissues if direct contact with concentrated solutions occurs. Long-term use of acids and alkalis may lead to allergic sensitivities to other chemicals found both inside and out of the occupational setting.

Dusts and vapors resulting from the processing of natural products may also pose a serious health threat to persons exposed to them in the workplace. One of particular concern to women is cotton dust. Exposure may be high in agricultural, textile and apparel manufacturing industries. Short-term exposure to raw cotton dust causes shortness of breath, tightness of the chest, and cough, all of which are symptoms of the long-term health consequence, byssinosis. Also known as brown lung disease, byssinosis is thought to be caused by an allergic-like reaction to some substance in the dust. The long-range prognosis for byssinosis is very poor and can lead to the development of severe respiratory diseases including emphysema.

Microbial hazards. Women who work with sick persons are at special risk of infection. They are frequently exposed to infectious agents such as tuberculosis and hepatitis before the patient has even been diagnosed. Nurses and other health workers are directly exposed to patients' secretions, open wounds, and excretions. Health workers handle contaminated linens, syringes, and food trays, often without knowing they are contaminated. While most hospitals have infection control protocols, they do not always have procedures for routinely handling potentially infectious materials. A list of some of the infectious agents and preventive measures is given in Table 20-5.

Table 20-5. Partial list of commonly occurring infections and communicable diseases and preventive measures for hospital workers*

Infection	Preventive measures
Amebiasis	Preemployment screening recommended for food handlers
Bacterial enteric infection (*Shigella, Salmonella, E. coli*)	Avoid direct contact with feces, other gastrointestinal secretions
Bacterial meningitis	
H. influenza B	Isolation of patient
Meningococcus	Isolation of patient, if contact with patient intimate (e.g., resuscitation or handling secretions) prophylaxis with Minocycline or rifampin; otherwise employees treated only if febrile disease develops.
CNS viral infections (viral meningitis, encephalitis, meningoencephalitis)	Enteric isolation; regular handwashing (LCM and arboviruses not transmitted from human to human.
Chickenpox (varicella)	Isolation of patient until all vesicles are scabbed over.
Diphtheria	Initial immunization with adult Td antigen; booster DT for those previously immunized antitoxic serum (DIG); antibiotic for unimmunized contacts.
Hepatitis A	Immune serum globulin (5 ml IM) can be given to employees who experience puncture wounds from instruments contaminated with blood from patients who are suspected to have or recently had hepatitis.
Hepatitis B	Immune serum globulin not completely protective against Hepatitis B. Hepatitis B immune globulin given to workers with percutaneous exposures if the hepatitis B surface antigen status is positive. Preexposure prophylaxis may be considered for hemodialysis and may be considered for personnel.
Herpes progenitalis (genital herpes)	Avoid direct contact with lesions.
Herpes labialis (fever blisters)	Avoid direct contact with lesions.
Herpes zoster	Isolation of patient; avoid direct contact with lesions.
Influenza	Offer immunization, warning of possible complications.
Measles (rubeola)	Immunization; if doubtful, can give immune globulin to nonpregnant employees within 3 days of initial contact.
Measles (rubella)	If female is of childbearing age, rubella HAI done; if 1:16, and the woman is *not* pregnant, offer immunization.
Mumps	Immunization.
Pertussis (whooping cough)	Immunization; for unimmunized contacts, diphtheria antitoxic antiserum, therapeutic antibiotic.
Poliomyelitis	Immunization.
Rabies (hydrophobia)	Gloves to protect personnel.
Smallpox	Immunization.
Staphylococcal infections (dermatitis, enterocolitis, pneumonia, wounds, burns, skin infections)	Handwashing, barriers, and patient isolation.
Streptococcal infections (pharyngitis, pneumonia, scarlet fever)	Handwashing, barriers, and patient isolation.
Syphilis	Prophylactic antimicrobial therapy available for those who had needle or mucous membrane exposure to congenital or acute disease.
Tetanus	Booster can be given every 5-10 years.
Tuberculosis	Tuberculin test and chest films can identify those who may convert to candidates for prophylactic therapy.
Viral gastrointestinal infections	Limit direct contact with gastrointestinal secretions; fomites; handwashing; enteric isolation of patient.
Viral respiratory infection (influenza and adenoviruses)	Barrier precautions; use of gloves; regular handwashing.

*Data from: Wehrle, P.: Employee health service, Connor, J. D.: Epidemiology and control of common communicable disease; Deschairo, D.: Isolation; and Mosley, J.: Control and prevention of viral hepatitis. In Barrett-Connor, E. and others, editors: Epidemiology for the infection control nurse, St. Louis, 1978, The C. V. Mosby Co.

Temporal stressors. Women in the workplace are exposed to temporal stressors, including the effects of shift work, erratic working hours (such as those of airline stewardesses who suffer jet lag and waitresses who work split shifts) and the time stresses of assembly line work.

Many women are employed in settings that require shift work. For example, some hospital personnel not only are required to work during the times that most persons sleep, but also may rotate from one shift to another, sometimes working two or three different shifts in the course of a week. A recent NIOSH conference on shift work suggests that shift workers have (Akerstedt, 1976):

1. A variety of sleep problems, such as short sleep time, trouble falling asleep and staying asleep, and awakening without feeling rested. Effects of these problems are most likely to occur during the night work period and may be manifest as bad mood or restlessness.
2. Excess minor nervous disturbances.
3. Excess gastrointestinal problems.
4. No clear absence of mortality effects.

Yet a number of questions about shift work remain unanswered. Characteristics of work, task, and environment probably interact with one another to produce some short- and long-term effects in performance, accidents, illnesses, and occupational diseases (Akerstedt, 1976; Ayoub, 1976).

Wofford (1976) reports that the most outstanding effect of airline flying seems to be tiredness and hazardous fatigue. She points out that cumulative sleep deficits, time changes, and upset circadian rhythms (in addition to other stressors) contribute to this fatigue. Flight attendants experience cumulative sleep deficiency with 65% encountering problems staying asleep. Little is known about the effects of disrupted circadian rhythms subsequent to time changes except sleep deprivation and impaired performance. Some attendants report changes in the menstrual cycle, including altered length of the cycle, dysmenorrhea, and so on. The long-term effects of these changes has yet to be evaluated, although the average tenure of the flight attendant today is about 7 years.

A final temporal stressor is the pace required by some types of work, for example, assembly line or piece work. In situations where the pace is excessive, the worker may perceive tension; those exposed to a slow pace may feel boredom and monotony. Both can be stressful.

Safety hazards. Women in the workplace are exposed to a number of safety hazards including those accruing from industrial accidents and mechanical equipment. In hospitals and clinics, workers are exposed to puncture wounds and lacerations from needles and blades, and because there is a high-risk of infection in these settings, these wounds are particularly dangerous. Accidents also occur in offices where falls and disabling injuries result from lifting office equipment and working with office machines. Women who perform domestic work are exposed to safety hazards from equipment, especially electrical equipment. Laundry workers can be injured by machinery such as mangles; lacking protective guards and automatic shut-off devices, these pieces of equipment can produce serious injuries such as crushing of limbs, amputation, denuding, and removal of parts of the scalp (Stellman, 1977).

Social stressors. Women in the labor force are exposed to a number of social stressors, including those associated with traditional roles, nontraditional roles, child care, and pressures emanating from work at home. Women who are employed in jobs that are traditionally regarded as "women's work" are exposed to low economic incentives for their participation in the labor force, which reinforces the low value attached to their work. Often these women have great economic needs. Women who do "women's work" such as domestic tasks or who work in the service sector may be exposed to high risks. In hospitals or homes they may be allocated the least desirable jobs, such as cleaning, that expose them to microbial, physical, and chemical hazards. Often the traditional jobs allocated to women provide only limited satisfaction; they may be repetitive, monotonous, fast-paced, and offer little opportunity for advancement.

Women who perform nontraditional roles in the labor force also must deal with social stressors. Often there is a lack of female role models for women and, consequently, women do not have access to an example or have no one with whom to discuss or compare experiences. In many instances social networks that are important for occupational advancement are primarily male and perhaps closed to women entirely (e.g., men's clubs such as the Rotary club). Women in new roles may not have the same types of social support systems as do their male counterparts. It is less likely that the spouse of a woman professional would provide the same (wifely) social supports as would the spouse of her male counterpart. In addition, the woman in a nontraditional occupation may receive little support from women who are not employed or are employed in lower status positions since she may not have the opportunity for contact with these women.

Child care remains a barrier for women who are employed, regardless of the type of occupation in which they are involved. Worry about the welfare of their children is commonly cited by women in a wide range of occupations, some of which was induced by the belief that continual presence of a mother was essential for the child's normal development. Child care continues to be limited to specific (usually daytime and weekday) hours; it presents a considerable financial burden to some families; it may not be convenient to the workplace; and it is usually not supported or subsidized by employers or government. Furthermore, "flexitime," a system in which workers can perform their tasks on a flexible time schedule, has not been widely implemented in this country, and the sharing of an occupation by husband and wife—as is done in some European countries—is extremely rare.

A final stressor for many women is the lack of assistance they receive with their responsibilities at home. It is still customary for women to perform the homemaking functions in addition to their market work. There is not yet much sharing of the traditional homemaker's chores in families where both men and women have full-time employment.

Thus while these stressors need not serve as obstacles to women being employed, it is important that they are not dismissed altogether. Solutions such as better economic incentives for traditionally "female work"; the provisions of female role models and support networks for women in nontraditional roles; improvement of the availability, accessibility, and quality of child care resources; and a greater sharing of the nonmarket work—or even payment for housework—might significantly improve the health of women in the labor force.

Exposure of pregnant women and their offspring

It has been estimated that almost 1,000,000 babies born in 1970 were exposed to the occupational environs of their mothers—some safe and some unsafe (Hunt, 1975). The recent increase in the number of women in the labor force precipitated renewed interest in hazards to pregnant women and their offspring. Yet concern about exposure of pregnant women and their offspring was evident as early as a 1944 U.S. Department of Labor report entitled "The Industrial Nurse and the Woman Worker":

The problem appears to be of some moment to employers at this time for several reasons. The majority of working women are in the child-bearing years, and the inexperience of some employers with women workers causes them a bit of panic in the face of possibilities that they scarcely know how to handle. It is the usual practice in plants not to hire women who are known to be pregnant; and it is almost equally common to discharge them as soon as pregnancy is discovered. Such a policy, however, encourages women to conceal their pregnancy as long as possible. Under such circumstances a woman may continue to work at a job or in a place that offers considerable hazard to her health and safety. Moreover, the first three months of pregnancy, which are the most easily concealed, are also more precarious than the next three

months. At this early date, then, women particularly need protection; but unless there is a policy in the plant that will encourage them to report their condition, they cannot avail themselves of protection. The plant will profit from knowledge of the women's condition by assuring itself that women will be kept on suitable jobs and thus experienced workers will not be lost, and by being protected against the risk of accident among women doing heavy or hazardous work at a time when they are not fitted to do it.

The points to be considered for such a maternity policy are: The importance of judging each case individually; the time at which a woman should stop work before the birth of her child, and how soon afterward she may return to work; the types of jobs that should be avoided because of danger of physical strain or injury from toxic substances; the preservation of seniority rights, the opportunity to return to her job, the length of hours and rest periods, and other conditions of work.

It is unfortunate that the guidelines from this 1944 report have not been implemented well since the time of their writing. Instead, industry has tended to respond to reports of toxic substances and birth defects, still-births, and miscarriages by excluding *all* women of child-bearing age from such exposures. Although a prudent means of limiting legal liability, exclusion has the possible outcome of sex discrimination. Furthermore, such exclusionary practices ignore the harmful effects of the exposure on *male* reproductive systems. Yet the actual probability of harmful exposure may be relevant only during about a 6-day period when the fertilized ovum would be at risk, and men's semen would be continuously exposed. Few men or women have the luxury of choosing whether or not to be employed. Furthermore, the 1972 amendments to the 1964 Civil Rights Act ensure women benefits from health insurance plans for disability from pregnancy, miscarriage, abortion, childbirth, or recovery from these. Thus it is difficult to set limits of exposure for pregnant women without discriminating in employment on the basis of sex. How to handle this dilemma? Hunt (1978) recommends that attention be given to promoting a safe work environment for men and women rather than moving pregnant women out of the workplace.

Early studies (Stewart, 1955) showed that employment for women was associated with a high perinatal death rate and increased incidence of low birth weight and premature infants:

Occupation	Perinatal death rate	Low birth weight	Premature births (matched pairs) (n = 143)	(n = 152)
Housewives	2.8%	4.7%	2.1%	1.3%
Employed before 28 weeks	4.9%	8.4%	4.9%	—
Employed after 28 weeks	7.5%	11.1%	—	7.3%

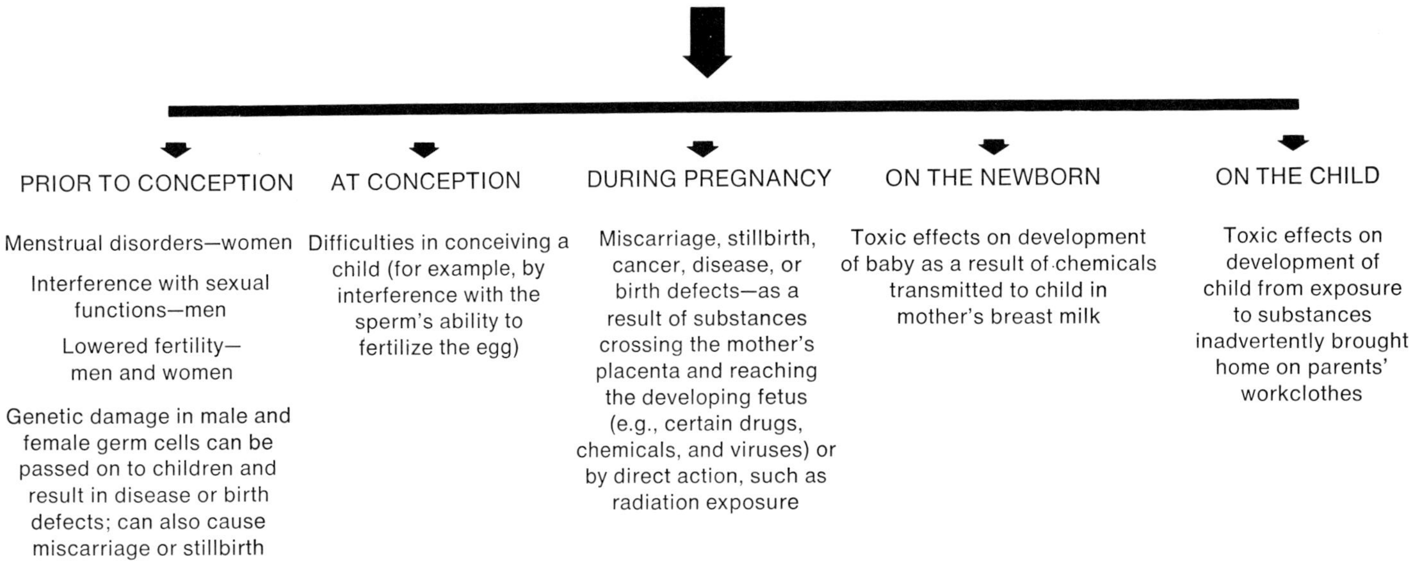

Fig. 20-4. Chronology of potential adverse effects of job exposures on reproduction or on the ability to have normal healthy children. (From Hricko, A.: Working for your life: a women's guide to job health hazards, Labor Occupational Health Program/Health Research Group, 1976.)

Yet Stewart commented that the occupations of the pregnant women were not exceptionally dangerous or exacting when compared to housework. McDonald (1958) demonstrated that a higher percentage of mothers of infants who had major congenital defects (e.g., anencephalus, hydrocephalus, congenital heart defects, hypospadias) were employed in heavy work, such as laundry work. There was, however, no effect on prenatal or neonatal death, and lifting and pulling were not associated with miscarriage. These early studies indicate the need for concern about the hazards of employment for pregnant women.

The potential points at which occupational exposures might have adverse effects on pregnancy outcome are given in Fig. 20-4. It can be seen that hazards may impinge on *both* men and women prior to the conception of their children.

Mutagenesis and teratogenesis

Mutagenesis is the process that occurs when chemicals, radiation, or biologic agents interact with living cells to cause a change in the genetic material of that cell. Such a change is called mutation, and the substance producing the change, a mutagen. Most mutations are harmful and often result in the death of the individual cell. Mutations may also cause abnormal cell division, which can result in cancer (unchecked somatic cell growth) or altered cell function. If a mutation occurs in a germ cell (sperm or egg) prior to conception, it may be incompatible with life, resulting in infertility or death of the fetus. Alternatively, mutations in the offspring may occur, manifested as mental retardation,

congenital defects, or, possibly, qualities superior to those of the parents. It is not known to what extent the rate of mutations in human cells may be increased by occupational or environmental exposure to chemical agents. However, 25% of the diseases in the United States are estimated to have some genetic origin, and 30% of spontaneous abortions are found to involve chromosomal aberrations that may be caused by chemical exposure.

Teratogenesis is the process that occurs when chemicals, radiation, or biologic agents alter fetal development during gestation to cause fetal death or abnormalities such as cleft palate or missing limbs. Exposure to the fetus generally occurs by way of the placenta to substances in the mother's blood, although direct exposure, such as to radiation, may also occur. The developing fetus is uniquely sensitive to chemicals that may be teratogenic even if not harmful to the mother. The first trimester (from 0 to 60 days after conception) is thought to be the period of greatest susceptibility to teratogenic insult. However, teratogenic effects of varying degrees of severity may occur throughout gestation.

Alterations in physiology during pregnancy

There are a number of alterations in a woman's physiology during pregnancy. During the *first trimester*, the kinds of symptoms women experience are highly variable. The most common ones are nausea, fatigue, tenderness and swelling of the breasts, and increased frequency of urination. There is an increase in maternal blood volume, with increased cardiac output, increase

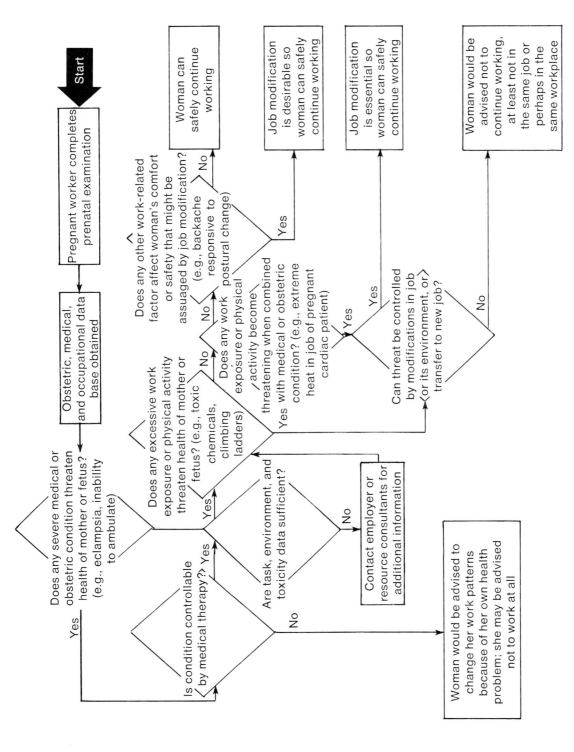

Fig. 20-5. Algorithm for decision-making about pregnant women and work guidelines on pregnancy and work. (Adapted from American College of Obstetricians and Gynecologists, Cincinnati, 1977, U.S. Department of Health, Education and Welfare, National Institute for Occupational Safety and Health.)

in ventilation rate, increase in glomerular filtration rate, and increase in renal plasma flow.

During the *second trimester*, there is a great increase in uterine size, which accentuates pelvic lordosis and thoracic kyphosis. The symphyseal and sacroiliac joints become increasingly mobile. Some women experience low back discomfort and stiffness. Others experience dizziness or syncope with prolonged standing or heat, attributable to decreased venous return and peripheral vasodilation.

During the *third trimester*, the uterus continues to enlarge rapidly. There is a tendency for women to have peripheral edema and decreased venous return from the legs because of pressure of the uterus on the pelvis veins. Many women experience fatigue, dyspnea, and insomnia, and general discomfort from the increase in body size; balance and equilibrium may be difficult to maintain in some activities. Myalgias and low back pain may result from the stretching of abdominal muscles and use of new muscles to maintain balance. Constipation, hemorrhoids, and varicosities may cause discomfort.

The general physical condition of the pregnant worker can also be affected by her age; weight and nutrition; use of cigarettes, alcohol, and drugs; and access to prenatal care. These factors should all be considered in the assessment of the woman's ability to work.

An adaptation of the approach to decision-making recommended by the American College of Obstetricians and Gynecologists (ACOG) is given in Fig. 20-5. While the ACOG algorithm emphasizes the safety of the unborn fetus and the mother, it is written in a way that suggests that physicians make the decision about the woman's ability to work. The algorithm has been adapted to reflect the philosophy that women can make their own decisions, and that medical workers can only advise. Furthermore, the algorithm as it was initially devised, places the cost of occupational exposure in pregnancy on the woman. Therefore, the outcomes have been rewritten in a way that suggests that the workplace and society bear some of the cost.

Chemical exposure

The hazards of chemical stressors encountered by women in the occupational environment may be complicated extensively when the potential effects on reproductive capacity, fetal development, and birth outcome are considered. This fact is particularly pertinent in light of the growing numbers of women remaining in the work force throughout their reproductive years and the proliferation of new chemicals, few of which have been thoroughly investigated with respect to their mutagenic or teratogenic potential.

Chemical effects on reproduction may best be considered in terms of the hazards they pose at specific stages of the reproductive process. Thus occupationally encountered chemicals may interfere with sexual functioning leading to decreased fertility or interest in sexual activity; or chemicals may induce genetic damage to egg or sperm cells leading to difficulties in conceiving a child or mutational changes manifested in the fetus at the time of conception. During pregnancy, chemicals may cause teratogenic effects in the developing fetus resulting in spontaneous abortion or in congenital defects. Following delivery, chemical damage to the offspring may still be induced if the occupationally exposed mother is breast-feeding or exposes the child to substances brought home on the work clothes.

Because the physiology of the woman is altered during pregnancy, there is an increased susceptibility to the toxic effects of many chemicals (both to herself and the fetus) that would not be expected in nonpregnant women. Of particular concern in this respect are the effects of nonoccupational chemical exposure from cigarette smoke, alcohol, and drugs taken before or during pregnancy, which can confound the health hazards associated with occupational chemical exposure manyfold. Examples of the principal classes of chemicals to which women are at risk during their reproductive years are given in Table 20-6.

Anesthetic gases are encountered by women who work in operating rooms, experimental laboratories, clinics, and dental offices. Unless carefully controlled, anesthetic gases routinely escape into the work environment causing continuous occupational exposure to those in the immediate surroundings. As general depressants of all physiologic activities, anesthetic gases may have pronounced depressant effects on reproductive function, ranging from ability to perform sexually to growth and delivery of the fetus. Halogenated hydrocarbon anesthetics, such as halothane, readily pass the placenta and may be highly toxic to the liver and other organ functions in the fetus.

Women working in occupations where exposure to anesthetic gases occurs have been shown to have up to three times a greater rate of spontaneous abortions (miscarriages) as nonexposed female medical workers, and their offspring have a two-fold higher risk of congenital birth defects as those who are not exposed. The risk of birth defects in children of wives of male anesthetists has also been shown to be 25% greater than those of unexposed men.

Trace metals are another class of chemicals that are particularly hazardous during pregnancy. The toxicity of these substances rests on the heightened sensitivity of the rapidly developing fetus to central nervous system damage owing to the immaturity of membrane barriers that partially protect the brain from such substances later in life. Lead is probably the most well-known cause of fetal damage from metals, causing increased

Table 20-6. Occupational chemicals affecting reproduction

Chemical (class)	Suspected effect on reproduction
Anesthetic gases	
Halogenated hydro-carbons	Reduced fertility, spontaneous abortion, mutagenesis, teratogenesis
Trace metals	
Lead	Reduced fertility, spontaneous abortion, teratogenesis, impaired neonatal develop-ment, neurologic damage
Mercury	
Cadmium	
Arsenic	
Organic solvents	
Benzene	Mental disturbances, fetal organ damage, mutagenesis, teratogenesis
Toluene	
Xylene	
Trichloroethylene	
Halogenated hydrocarbons	
Carbon tetrachloride	Reduced fertility, spontaneous abortion, mutagenesis, teratogenesis, impaired neonatal development
Chloroprene	
Dibromochloropropane	
Ethylene dibromide	
Polyhalogenated biphenyls (PCB, PBB)	
Tetrachloroethylene	
Trichloroethylene	
Dioxin (TCDD)	
Pesticides	
Chlorinated hydro-carbons: (chlordane, hepane, mirex)	Reduced fertility, spontaneous abortions
Miscellaneous agents	
Carbon disulfide	Increased menstrual flow, spontaneous abortions, fetal suffocation, fetal death, ner-vous system defects, cere-bral palsy
Carbon monoxide	

rates of miscarriages, stillbirths, and nervous system disorders in offspring of exposed women. Mercury is also known for its transplacental toxic effects, including severe mental retardation and neurologic dysfunction in children of women exposed to mercury during pregnancy. Severe cerebral palsy and damage to kidneys and other organs have also been observed in offspring of women exposed to mercury. Trace metals also interfere with the sexual function and behavior of adults when prolonged occupational exposure to these substances results in neurologic deterioration or chronic debilitating effects.

Perhaps the most hazardous class of chemical substances in terms of their adverse effects on the range of reproductive activity and function are the petroleum products, especially the organic solvents. Benezene, toluene, and xylene, for example, have been associated with menstrual disturbance, including more prolonged and intense uterine bleeding than normal. The ease with which these substances cross the placenta poses a particular hazard to the fetus in terms of damage to rapidly developing organ systems such as the liver and other hematopoietic tissues. The observations of chromosomal alterations in bone marrow cells of workers exposed to benezene raises the possibility of both mutagenic and teratogenic effects in women who are employed in jobs where routine exposure to benzene occurs.

Another class of petroleum products, the halogenated hydrocarbons, also rapidly cross the placenta and post a high hazard of fetotoxicity. Carbon tetrachloride, for example, is extremely hepatotoxic to both the mother and fetus and increases the risk of both fetal death and birth anomalies in animals. Trichloroethylene (TCE), a compound chemically similar to the carcinogen vinyl chloride, is widely used as an industrial solvent, and has been shown to be mutagenic in microbial and plant assay systems. A related chemical, chloroprene, is used extensively in the rubber industry, and has been shown to produce degenerative changes in wives of workers exposed occupationally to this substance.

Various other organic compounds to which women are exposed in the work setting may adversely affect reproduction in various ways. These include polychlorinated and polybrominated biphenyls (PCBs and PBBs), dioxin (TCDD), and various pesticides such as mirex and kepone. PCBs, for example, are known to be embryotoxic and produce chromosomal alterations in birds. Pregnant women who have ingested PCBs have produced offspring with decreased birth weight, jaundice, skin discoloration, and impaired postnatal development. TCDD, a contaminant of the once widely used herbicide 2,4,5-trichlorphenoxy acetic acid (2,4,5-T), is one of the most potent chemicals known in terms of its toxicity to various organ systems, as observed in experimental animal studies. The principal fetotoxic effects include internal hemorrhages in fetal rats, and increased frequency of cleft palate and kidney abnormalities in fetuses of mice. While teratogenic effects such as these have not been observed in offspring of humans exposed to TCDD, an increased incidence of miscarriages has been suggested from studies of women living in areas where exposure to this substance has occurred.

Several miscellaneous substances to which women receive substantial occupational exposure should be mentioned here. Carbon disulfide, used in the production of viscose rayon, has led to menstrual difficulties in some women, as well as increased spontaneous abortions and threatened abortions in pregnant workers. Carbon monoxide, a gas formed whenever incomplete combustion of any carbon-containing material occurs, greatly increases the risk of fetal death or nervous system defects, such as mental retardation or cerebral palsy in the offspring. Since carbon monoxide is one of the many hazardous substances contained in cigarette smoke, pregnant women who smoke cigarettes or who are employed in places where smoke from cigarettes or other sources is present suffer greatly increased risk of injury to their unborn children as well as to themselves in terms of chronic health problems.

Physical exposure

Noise. It is unfortunate that little is known about the effects of noise and vibration on pregnant women and their fetuses. Although sound can transmit to the fetus, no harmful effects have been documented to date. Neither vibration (frequencies less than 20 Hertz) over the entire body (referred to as infrasound) nor ultrasound seem to have demonstrable effects on the woman or fetus, but The American College of Obstetricians and Gynecologists recommends that each instance of vibratory exposure be evaluated individually (NIOSH, 1977; Hunt, 1975).

Heat. Although temperature regulation in women is altered, there has been no study of heat tolerance in the pregnant woman (Hunt, 1975). Pregnant women have some difficulty demonstrating reflex vasodilation in response to a heat stimulus late in pregnancy.

Physical labor. There has been one study of effects of maternal work on the fetal heart rate. The fetuses responded in three ways:

1. Some were not affected at all.
2. Some fetal heart rates increased gradually with a maximum occurring at the beginning of a steady state, and decreasing to the starting value toward the end of the maternal effort.
3. Some fetal heart rates accelerated with a maximum at the end of the effort and with a decrease below the starting rate at the restitution period.

The greater the reaction of the woman to work, the greater the reaction of her fetus. Pokorny and Rous (1967) suggest that the fetus of a woman who is physically fit would be advantaged when the mother exerted herself.

On the other hand, the change in fetal heart rate markedly increased during exertion of pregnant women with diabetes and toxemia. It is clear that more research is needed to determine whether or not exercise leads to hypoxia in the fetus by means of diverting blood supply from the fetus to the muscles being exercised.

Posture. Prolonged sitting or standing in the same position can lead to venous stasis in nonpregnant women, and this becomes pronounced in pregnant women during the later months of pregnancy. As the fetus grows, there is an increase in pressure over the blood vessels supplying the lower extremities. Thus stasis induced by postures with pressure over the popli-

teal space, poor sitting, or prolonged standing exacerbates the stasis produced by the growing fetus.

Ionizing and microwave radiation. Occupational exposure to ionizing radiation represents a particular health hazard with respect to reproductive function in women because of its ability to produce both mutagenic and teratogenic effects. In the former case, ionizing radiation may produce chromosomal alterations in germ cells so that conception is either impaired or results in a fetus in which mutagenic changes are manifested. Such mutations are often incompatible with life, and spontaneous abortion may occur during gestation. In contrast, if a child bearing those mutations survives, they may be passed on to future generations. Germ cell mutations from ionizing radiation are of greater potential concern to women than men, since a single exposure episode may place at risk the entire lifetime complement of germ cells with which a woman is born. In contrast, males continuously regenerate sperm cells such that a single point exposure episode to ionizing radiation of mutagenic strength is not necessarily of continuing concern with respect to ability to ever conceive normal offspring.

Exposure of women during pregnancy to ionizing radiation represents a risk of teratogenic effects to the fetus because of the enhanced rate of cellular proliferation of fetal tissues. If such effects are not lethal, children may be born bearing congenital anomalies such as anatomic defects, impaired growth, or mental retardation. Such children also have a greater chance of developing leukemia or other cancers later in life.

Microwave radiation is not ionizing to biologic tissues and therefore is not known to represent a hazard to germ cells or the developing fetus unless exposure is great enough to produce burns. Tissues such as the eyes and testicles are known to be most susceptible to injury from prolonged microwave exposure. However, the effects of microwaves on those tissues in the fetus are not known. The reduction in the numbers of maturing spermatocytes found in adult males exposed to microwaves has been found to be readily reversible.

Microbial hazards. Infection may have a number of adverse effects on the fetus. Perhaps the best known example is that associated with rubella. There is growing evidence that some viruses cause intrauterine death of the embryo whereas others produce selective kinds of damage. Table 20-7 shows the teratogenic effects of some viral and nonviral diseases on the fetus.

Social stressors. The pregnant worker is exposed to some social hazards, especially as her pregnancy progresses. Some employers and fellow workers may harass her about her continued employment. In the past pregnant women were expected to leave work when they began to "show." Taylor and Langer (1977) suggest that

Table 20-7. Teratogenic effects of viral and nonviral diseases*

Disease	Effects
Viral diseases	
Rubella	Abortion, developmental defects, fetal disease
Measles (rubeola)	Abortion, developmental defects, fetal disease, congenital disease
Mumps	Abortion, developmental defects, fetal disease, stillbirth, congenital diseases
Herpes zoster	Abortion, developmental defects
Herpes simplex	Abortion, developmental defects
Influenza	
Asian-D	Developmental defects
1918-A	Abortion
Lymphocytic choriomeningitis	Fetal disease
Hepatitis A	Abortion, stillbirth
Cytomegalic inclusion	Fetal disease
Anterior poliomyelitis	Abortion, developmental defects, fetal disease, stillbirth, congenital disease
Coxsackie	Abortion, developmental defects, fetal disease, stillbirths, congenital disease
Smallpox	Congenital disease
Chickenpox	Congenital disease
Nonviral diseases	
Typhus (rickettsia, typhoid bacillus)	Abortion, developmental defects, fetal disease
Tuberculosis (mycobacillus)	Possible abortion, developmental defects, fetal disease, congenital disease
Syphilis (spirochaeta)	Abortion, developmental defects, fetal disease, stillbirth, congenital disease
Toxoplasmosis (protozoa)	Possible abortion, developmental defects, fetal disease, stillbirth, congenital disease
Malaria (protozoa)	Possible abortion, developmental defects, fetal disease, stillbirth, congenital disease
Listeriosis (coccobacillus)	Possible abortion, developmental defects fetal disease, congenital disease
Brucellosis (coccobacillus)	Abortion, developmental defects
Cryptococcosis (fungus)	Possible abortion, fetal disease, congenital disease

*Adapted from Hunt, V.: Occupational health problems of pregnant women, pp. 48-48A.

because pregnancy is a novel stimulus, others respond to the pregnant woman with staring and avoidance, with men's reactions being more pronounced than women's. In Taylor and Langer's experiments other women liked the pregnant woman better when she was passive rather than assertive, but they also rejected her as a companion. These investigators propose that a cycle exists in which:

Clearly, the cycle could be interrupted if pregnancy were a less novel stimulus. This would be possible if more pregnant women continued activities they were involved in when they were not pregnant.

In addition to considering the stressors associated with pregnancy as a stigmatized state, researchers should consider the possible effects of other social variables. Both job satisfaction and economic need could be associated with employment status and pregnancy outcomes.

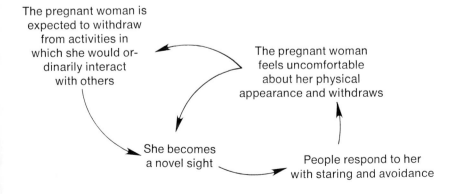

Time stressors. No research has been done to document effects of shift work and long working hours on pregnant women. There are, however, a number of instances in industry and the health professions in which pregnant women not only rotate from shift to shift, but also work more than 8 hours per day.

Safety hazards. Accidents and injuries from hazardous machinery or employment conditions have not been investigated specifically in relation to pregnant women. The fetus is well protected from physical trauma by the amniotic fluid. The change in the woman's center of gravity during late pregnancy might require additional alertness to prevent falls.

Recommendations for research

Hunt's report (1975) on occupational health problems of pregnant women concludes with several recommendations, among them the collection of birth certificate and census data to enable study of occupational effects on pregnancy outcomes. In addition, she recommended that data already collected as part of other epidemiologic studies which have information about occupational history of the mother and pregnancy outcome be analyzed. She also recommended that the pregnant worker be considered in all studies of occupational safety and health standards. Clinicians and epidemiologists should be cognizant of the importance of occupational history in studies involving reproduction and pregnancy outcome. Finally, Hunt recommends that health education programs be provided at all educational levels to promote understanding of the desirable conditions for a successful pregnancy.

Hazards of housework

Women whose work is at home lack visibility in the occupational health literature, probably a reflection of the low economic value attached to their services and their not being organized to barter for protection of their health as are those who perform market work. Yet those women constitute an immense segment of our society. Not only do the hazards associated with housework impinge on women whose work is only at home, but also affect women who are employed outside the home and perform household services in addition to their paid employment. Because little value has been attached to housework and nearly all women perform household services, special attention must be devoted to the attendant hazards of this work.

Social hazards

In 1971 Oakley conducted a study of the sociology of housework. Forty London homemakers (women, other than domestic servants, who were responsible for most of the household duties) were interviewed. Half of the women were working class and half middle class; social class was based on the husband's occupation.

Dissatisfaction with housework was evident, with 70% of the women expressing discontent. Monotony, fragmentation, and excessive pace were commonly experienced, but only monotony was a cause of dissatisfaction. While loneliness was a frequent complaint, autonomy was the most valued feature of being a homemaker. The woman's perception of her own low status was associated with her dissatisfaction with housework.

The most disliked aspect of being a homemaker was housework. Although there was considerable variability in the way women ranked the tasks associated with being homemaker, cooking, shopping, washing, cleaning, washing up, and ironing were most liked, in the order given. Although the women created their own standards and routines, they spent from 48 to 105 hours per week doing housework; the mean work week was 77 hours! The self-derived standards appeared to constitute a self-reward system for these women.

Incongruence between the status of jobs women had held in the past and their current status as a homemaker resulted in dissatisfaction. Furthermore, dissatisfaction with housework was greater among women who had been previously employed in jobs that gave them great satisfaction.

There was a difference between women's feeling about housework and their orientation to the homemaker role. High personal identification with the role of homemaker meant that housework was the woman's personal responsibility. Women with high identification also had highly specific standards and routines. The woman's mother served as an important role model in shaping identification with the domestic role, but the woman's responses included not only imitation but also rebellion. Beliefs in "natural" feminine domesticity were associated with the woman's identification with the homemaker role. Thus it was possible for women to dislike housework but have a positive orientation to being a homemaker and vice versa.

The women in Oakley's sample had predominantly negative attitudes toward women's liberation, expressing considerable anxiety about the meaning and consequences of changing sex roles. Their strong identification with more traditional definitions of womanhood might keep these women in a position of internalizing their own oppression. Furthermore, performance of the homemaker role has the capacity to insulate women from other women, thus preventing them from raising one another's awareness about the felt need to do housework and to compulsively adhere to standards. Although the medical literature deals with dissatisfaction among homemakers as a disease (e.g., "Housewife's Disease" in the Yearbook of Neurology, Psychiatry, and Neurosurgery, 1964-1965), Oakley would recommend a macrosocial solution to these women's dissatisfaction: deconditioning women who have acquiesced to their own subordination.

Physical hazards

Despite "women's work" being generally regarded as less strenuous or dangerous than work usually regarded as "men's work," women whose work is in the home are exposed to a number of physical hazards. In the following pages we will explore several physical stressors impinging on women who perform housework. A summary of these is given in Table 20-8.

Physical stress induced by standing can lead to stasis and ultimately varicosities. Pregnant women and women over 40 are at special risk for the development of varicosities. Lifting, bending, and carrying heavy household appliances, furniture, and children may result in back injuries. Kneeling to scrub floors can lead to knee injuries. Accidents resulting in cuts, burns, and falls can be responsible for injuries ranging from minor lacerations to extensive burns and severe head injuries. Noise associated with some household appliances may be severe enough to cause some hearing loss, particularly if the woman is continuously exposed (see Table 20-9). Fortunately, most of this equipment is not used continuously, but several appliances are likely to be used in one day, and women who are exposed to noise on the job as well as at home could be subjected to increased risk of hearing loss and the other health effects of noise mentioned earlier in this chapter (Stellman, 1976).

Table 20-8. Physical hazards associated with housework

Hazard	Examples	Possible health effects
Physical stress	Lifting, bending, standing; carrying household furnishing, groceries, children; kneeling to scrub floors	Back injuries, varicose veins, knee injuries
Accidents	Cuts and burns associated with food preparation; falls on wet floors or downstairs	Lacerations, possible amputations, infection, scarring, contusions, abrasions, fractures, head injuries
Noise	Household appliances such as blenders, vacuum cleaners	Hearing impairment
Thermal	Burns from cooking utensils, ovens	Infection, scarring
Electrical	Frayed electrical wires or defective appliances	Electrocution

Household chemical hazards

The modern home environment poses multiple chemical threats to every individual regardless of age. The cleaning cabinet, laundry room, garage, and bathroom medicine cabinet generally contain a variety of drugs and chemicals that pose potential toxic hazards. Accidental overdoses of therapeutic agents, as well as occupational and environmental exposure to various chemicals, may compound the possible hazards associated with exposure to chemicals found in the home.

Among the dangerous household chemicals in common usage in modern homes, petroleum products, carbon monoxide, pesticides, and drugs, including salicylates, barbiturates and tranquilizers, are considered to be the most troublesome. These agents account for 30% to 36% of nonfatal accidents and for nearly 40% of the fatalities. Of these carbon monoxide, salicylates, and petroleum products cause most toxic emergencies. Other household agents including cleaning preparations, cosmetics, and toilet articles account for the rest.

Household cleaning preparations. Thousands of incidents involving toxic ingestion of soap, detergents, bleaches, and cleaners are reported annually. The majority of cases involve children under 5 years of age. Accidents such as these are largely preventable by proper handling and storing of these products out of reach of children. Fortunately, severe toxic affects occur infrequently and fatalities are rare.

A list of toxic cleaning agents and some of their properties is given in Table 20-10. Soaps, which are salts of fatty acids, generally have low toxicity; when ingested in sufficient quantity, however, they may cause gastrointestinal irritation with vomiting and diarrhea. Detergents are also freely available in every home. These products contain a number of toxic substances, including surfactants and "builders," which are substances designed to reduce water hardness. The principal manifestation of poisoning from ingestion of detergents are

Table 20-9. Some typical noise levels in the home*

Source	Noise level (dB [A])†	Perceived noise level (PNdB)
Garbage disposal	81	93
Vacuum cleaner	74	87
Dishwasher	70	82
Stove/hood exhaust	75	88
Central-heating system	58	71
Food mixer	—	80

*Data from Stellman, J. M.: Women's work: women's health, myths and realities, New York, 1977, Pantheon Books.
†Recommended PNdB for the home is 53; noise above 80 dB can induce hearing loss.

Table 20-10. Toxic properties of household cleaning agents

Agent	Symptoms
Soaps	Gastrointestinal irritation and vomiting
Detergents	
Sufactants	
Cationic	Vomiting, collapse, coma, convulsions
Anionic	
Nonionic	
Builders	
Polyphosphates	Severe gastroenteritis, vomiting, diarrhea, esophageal stricture
Calcium precipitators	Corrosive burning of mucous membranes
Bleaching and bactericidal agents	Gastrointestinal irritation
Cleaning, polishing agents	Gastrointestinal irritation, vomiting

Table 20-11. Toxic properties of cosmetics and toilet articles

Agent	Toxic effect
Shampoos	Eye irritation (lysol shampoos), injury to internal organs (dry shampoos)
Hair coloring preparations	Skin irritation: inflammation of eyes and ears
Hair coloring agents	Asthma, vertigo, hypertension, gastritis, methemoglobinemia, tremors, convulsions, coma
Depilatories	Gastrointestinal and skin irritation, vomiting, possible convulsion and respiratory failure
Suntan preparations	Ethanol intoxication
Hair sprays	Thesaurosis (storage disease), ocular irriation, keratitis
Deodorants and antiperspirants	Relatively innocuous

vomiting, coma, and sometimes convulsions and esophageal stricture.

Bleaching agents (chlorine-releasing agents) or bacterial agents (mild concentrations of quaternary ammonium compounds) have been included in the formulation of a number of household detergent preparations. These additives are only moderately toxic. Furthermore, since the concentrations are low, they are not likely to influence the toxicity of the product significantly.

A large number of cleaning and polishing agents are available varying from relatively innocuous liquids and creams with mild inert abrasives to the very potent dip type cleansers. The latter contain strongly corrosive substances such as thiourea, sulfuric or phosphoric acid, or sodium hydroxide, ingestion of any of which requires emergency treatment.

Furniture polishes, metal cleaners, and abrasives usually contain petroleum distillates, mineral seed oil, cedar oils, industrial alcohols, silica, alkali, and other toxic ingredients. A number of potentially toxic products are commercially available for removing grease from ovens, grills, and stoves and for cleaning bathtubs, showers, and toilet bowls. Some of these preparations contain sodium hydroxide in concentrations up to 10%. If ingested, these caustic alkalis can cause severe damage to mucous membranes of the upper gastrointestinal and respiratory tracts.

Cosmetics and toilet articles. Throughout much of the world vast amounts of money are spent annually on the production and purchase of face powders, lipstick, cleansing creams, eye makeup, face lotions, shaving cream and depilatories, hair sprays, lotions, hand creams, perfumes, bath salts, and deodorants. While most products are safe when used as directed, some preparations can be strong sensitizers and contain chemicals that can be quite dangerous if ingested in large quantities or are otherwise misused. Allergenic or photosensitivity (increased sensitivity to sunlight) reactions, which can cause severe inflammation of the skin or mucous membranes, may occur in susceptible individuals. In general, however, most cosmetics have relatively low toxicity. It has been estimated that most preparations show an acute oral LD_{50}* in rats in excess of 10 Gm/kg. This means that a child weighing 10 kg would have to ingest 100 Gm or more before life is endangered. The toxic properties of some cosmetics and toilet articles are summarized in Table 20-11.

Petroleum products. Many types of materials found in the home for use in general housekeeping chores, home maintenance, and hobby activities contain potentially toxic petroleum products. General household solvents, including carbon tetrachloride, trichloroethylene, denatured alcohols, turpentine, kerosine, gasoline, paint thinners, and various aromatic hydrocarbons, have extremely toxic properties and should be handled with great care. Effects of overexposure to most of these agents range from vague symptoms such as headache or light headedness to serious internal injury, disability, or death. In contact with the skin, these substances remove skin oils and may cause dermatitis or sensitization. When taken internally they are severe depressants of the central nervous system and may cause toxic systemic effects including damage to blood and hematopoietic organs, liver, kidney, nervous, and other tissues as well. Many petroleum products can produce

*LD_{50} is the dose that will kill 50% of exposed animals.

cumulative systemic effects from repeated exposure. Some of the more widely utilized household agents are also frequently encountered outside the home in many occupations where women are employed. The potential toxic effects resulting from exposure to these substances were reviewed previously. Chemical pneumonia resulting from exposure to petroleum products is the most common cause of toxic emergencies and hospitalization in children.

Cements and glues. Plastic household cements are comprised primarily of volatile hydrocarbons, both aromatic and aliphatic, which include acetone, toluene, xylene, benzene, amyl acetate, butyl alcohol, isopropyl alcohol, and methyl cellosolve acetate. Carbon tetrachloride, chloroform, or ethylene dichloride may also be present. This latter group of solvents may have extensive toxicities involving the central nervous system, heart, gastrointestinal tract, liver, and kidneys. All of these solvents are central nervous system depressants; some can cause central nervous system stimulation as well.

In recent years there has been an outbreak of intentional inhalation of the vapors of plastic cements and glues by adolescents. The toxic effects of sniffing these vapors include a depressant action in the central nervous system resembling acute ethyl alcohol intoxication. While a few whiffs initially suffice, larger inhalations are soon needed to produce an intoxicating effect.

Acids and alkalis. A variety of corrosive substances are found in most households for use primarily as cleaning agents. These are principally solutions of inorganic (mineral) acids and alkalis, many of which may cause harmful burns on skin contact or destruction of internal tissues if swallowed or inhaled.

The most commonly encountered mineral acids include hydrochloric, nitric, phosphoric, and sulfuric acids. While somewhat less hazardous than the others, phosphoric acid may cause burns on contact with any part of the body and local injury if taken internally in concentrated solutions. Hydrochloric, nitric, and sulfuric acid solutions are extremely hazardous in concentrated form, producing tissue irritation and skin necrosis on contact. Inhalation of vapors or mists of mineral acids may result in edema and severe irritation of the upper respiratory tract. If acids are swallowed in aqueous solution, the stomach and esophagus can be badly burned as well as the upper part of the small intestine. The entire mucosa may eventually slough and disappear. Death from shock may occur. Coma and convulsions are sometimes the terminal events.

Some low molecular weight organic acids found in the home may also present a similar hazard. These include formic, acetic, lactic, and trichloracetic acids. These acids are strong irritants but are somewhat less corrosive than mineral acids. Acetic acid may cause esophageal stricture and, possibly, pyloric stenosis. Trichloracetic acid resembles acetic acid in its toxicity. Lactic acid is toxic even when diluted with milk and may produce both esophageal and gastric injury.

The strong corrosive alkalis include caustic soda, caustic potash, sodium and potassium hydroxides, carbonates, oxides, and peroxides and are known in general as "lyes." Lyes are commonly used around the home as cleaning agents and are present in many washing powders, drain-pipe cleaners, and paint removers. Most reported cases of poisoning have resulted from the careless practice of leaving lye solutions in familiar open containers within the reach of children.

The strong alkalis are remarkably corrosive and penetrating because of their solubilizing reactions with proteins and collagen, saponifying effects of lipids, and dehydrating action in tissue cells.

When ingested or exposed to skin and other tissues, these compounds combine with protein to form proteinates and with fats to form soap, which accounts for the deep caustic and penetrating burns they produce. Damage is related to the concentration of the alkali ingested.

Alcohols and glycols. Many alcohols and glycols are commonly found around the home and are used for a variety of purposes. Those principally found include ethyl, methyl, isopropyl, and amyl alcohols and ethylene, diethylene, hexylene, and propylene glycols.

Probably the most commonly utilized alcohol is ethanol (ethyl alcohol), available in the home in drug formulations, cosmetic preparations, rubbing alcohol, and intoxicating beverages. All preparations except the latter are commonly "denatured" by the addition of substances intended to induce vomiting (e.g., brucine) or to produce a bitter and objectional taste on consumption (e.g., diethyl phthalate).

If ingested within a short period, the fatal dose in an average adult is 1½ to 2 pints of 40% to 55% alcohol as whiskey or gin. Intoxication with alcohol may be stimulated by certain pathologic conditions such as hepatitis, diabetic acidosis, epilepsy, uremia, head injuries, and various CNS depressants (e.g., barbiturates) or stimulates (e.g., atropine). Hepatic toxicity is also likely when ethanol is consumed by persons undertaking chemotherapeutic drug regimens for cancer or other diseases.

Isopropyl alcohol is an isomer of propyl and a homologue of ethyl alcohol. Although similar to the latter in its properties when used for external purposes, it is more toxic than ethyl alcohol when ingested. It is an important industrial solvent and is also employed as an ingredient of various cosmetics and for medicinal preparations for external use, such as rubbing alcohol.

The toxic effects of isopropyl alcohol per se include

a wide variety of clinical manifestations, which are also common to ethanol intoxication, although to a greater degree. The central nervous system is especially vulnerable to the toxic effects of isopropyl alcohol, which may cause deep refractory narcosis and depressed respiration. Isopropyl alcohol is also more irritating to the gastrointestinal tract and more likely to produce nausea, vomiting, and abdominal pain than ethyl alcohol.

Methyl alcohol (methanol) is another common household solvent and is extremely toxic following either acute or chronic ingestion. Its toxicity is attributed to both the slow and incomplete oxidation of methyl alcohol in the tissues to formic acid (in contrast to ethyl alcohol, which is converted into carbon dioxide and water). Severe acidosis is produced by formic acid, and the pH of the urine may reach 5.0 as a result of the large amounts of formate excreted. As a powerful nerve poison, methyl alcohol attacks the central nervous system, especially the optic nerves, causing impairment of vision or blindness. Degenerative damage of the kidneys, liver, and heart may also occur. Symptoms of methyl alcohol poisoning may be delayed as long as 36 hours after ingestion and include sudden dimness of vision, coma, and respiratory failure. Dermatitis is a common local effect.

Amyl alcohol, also known as fusel oil, is about four times as toxic as ethyl alcohol and produces major, severe, and prolonged symptoms. The amount present in alcoholic beverages is very small and its consumption in liquor has not been demonstrated to produce toxic effects aside from those associated with "hangover." Poisoning from its use in industry is rare, although severe poisoning has resulted from oral ingestion. The symptoms associated with oral overdose of amyl alcohol include headache, vertigo, nausea and vomiting, diarrhea, stupor or delirium, and coma. Methemoglobinemia, methemoglobinuria, and glycouria have also been reported. In some cases recovery may be delayed or death may result.

Glycols are heavy liquid with a sweet, acid taste and are excellent solvents for many water-insoluble substances, including drugs. The principal glycol found around the home is ethylene glycol, which is used in a few cosmetic preparations. However, "permanent type" automobile antifreeze is the main source of poisonings.

The toxicity of glycols arises from their conversion in the body to glycolic and glyoxylic acids, which are then metabolized to oxalic acid. The latter damages the brain and causes impairment of renal function and anemia. Severe central nervous system depression may also occur and is similar to that produced by ethyl alcohol. The initial symptoms in severe poisoning are those of alcoholic intoxication including weakness, ataxia, stupor, prostration, cyanosis, anemia, unconsciousness, and convulsions. Death may occur early from respiratory failure or later from pulmonary edema or renal failure. Chronic poisoning from inhalation of glycols may produce any of the above symptoms in lesser degree.

Gases. A variety of gases (natural, manufactured, propane) are used in a number of household applications. While most of these are inert or of low toxicity when properly utilized, high concentrations encountered either intentionally or by accident may have serious toxic effects.

Natural gas consists chiefly of volatile hydrocarbons including methane (85%), ethane, and hydrogen. Inert and of low toxicity, natural gas contains no carbon monoxide unless it is contaminated. Carbon monoxide can be formed, however, whenever carbonaceous material is burned in insufficient oxygen.

Carbon monoxide (CO) is responsible for a greater number of severe chemical poisonings than any other single agent. The principal toxicity of carbon monoxide results from its formation of a reversible complex with hemoglobin, carboxyhemoglobin, thus depriving cells of necessary oxygen. Because the binding affinity of carbon monoxide with hemoglobin is over 200 times that of oxygen, a small concentration of CO in the inspired air can tie up a large proportion of hemoglobin in the blood. Exercise, fever, and anemia increase the hazard of collapse from CO, and young children are more susceptible than are adults.

The nature of toxic symptoms associated with CO poisoning are sometimes correlated with the blood level of carboxyhemoglobin. The control organs are those that are most susceptible to oxygen deprivations, notably the brain. Myocardial anoxia is also sometimes sufficient to precipitate untoward reactions. The characteristic cherry red color of the skin is caused by a low concentration of reduced hemoglobin and a high level of carboxyhemoglobin in the blood. Miscellaneous and atypical reactions accompanying CO poisoning include various skin lesions, sweating, and anginal pain. In severe CO poisoning death is usually the result of respiratory arrest from severe CNS depression.

Pesticides. Pesticides are also an important source of poisoning around the home. Warfarin, which causes dangerous problems only with repeated dosing, accounts for nearly 50% of the nonfatal rodenticide poisonings. Arsenic and anticholinesterases account for a large number of fatalities. Other toxic agents, such as strychnine, thallium, and squill are also implicated in pesticide poisonings around the home.

Probably the most important group of household pesticidal agents with respect to their overall toxicity are the synthetic organic insecticides including the chlorobenzene derivatives, indane derivatives, phosphate esters, and the carbamates. The best known of the chlorobenzene derivates is chlorophenothane (DDT). Since this chemical is fat soluble and is very stable after application, DDT and its metabolites accumulate and persist in body fat for long periods of time. The absorbed pesticide is partitioned between adipose tissue and blood and is partly converted to a much less toxic metabolite, DDE. Some DDT is converted directly to an acetate derivative, DDA, which is conjugated in the liver and is excreted in the bile and urine. A large portion of ingested DDT is never absorbed and is excreted in the feces.

Following ingestion of toxic doses of chlorobenzene derivatives, salivation, nausea, vomiting, and abdominal pain may occur. After absorption through the skin or by inhalation, symptoms may include irritation of the eyes, ears, nose and throat, blurring of vision, cough, pulmonary edema, and dermatitis. Chronic poisoning causes anorexia, loss of weight, liver and kidney damage, and emaciation. Disturbances of the central nervous system and skin irritation may also occur.

Another group of synthetic organic insecticides, the indane derivatives, includes chlordane, aldrin, and dieldrin. These compounds are fat-soluble chemicals that are used either singly or in mixtures for the control of flies, mosquitos, and field insects. Aldrin is the most toxic of these, being two to four times as toxic in animals as chlordane. The other derivatives have intermediate toxicity. Symptoms of poisoning in humans occur after ingestion or skin contamination with 15 to 50 mg/kg of body weight of these preparations. Acute poisoning from the ingestion, inhalation, or skin contamination is characterized by hyperexcitability, tremors, restlessness, ataxia, and tonic and clonic convulsions. Since liver function is impaired well below lethal levels, the toxicity of these derivatives is enhanced in people with previous liver damage.

Organophosphate esters, including parathion, malathion, and chlorthion, are also widely used for eradication of insect pests in and around the home. These agents are readily absorbed from the skin, lungs, and gastrointestinal tract. The hazard from respiratory exposure is estimated to be three times greater than that from oral exposure and ten times as great as that following dermal absorption.

Carbamates are used as broad-spectrum insecticides against a variety of insect pests. They are manufactured as flowable formulations, dusts, and wettable powders and are absorbed by all portals including the skin. Concentrates may produce skin irritation as well as systemic poisoning. Since these insecticides are cholineserase inhibitors, the symptoms are not unlike those that occur with the organophosphate esters.

A number of insecticidal agents are utilized for insect pest control as fumigants and repellants. These include a wide variety of chemical compounds that are highly toxic when ingested or inhaled. Those of major interest are cyanides; carbon tetrachlorides; naphthalene; paradichlorobenzene; methyl bromide, chloride, and iodide; dimethylphthalate; indalone; and diethyltoluamide. The least dangerous ones are those repellents intended for local application to the skin, including dimethylphthalate and indalone. The most toxic types are the soil fumigants such as the cyanides and the halogenated hydrocarbons.

Naphthalene and paradichlorobenzene are important because of their wide use in the home as moth repellents. The poisonous properties of naphthalene are not generally recognized, and it is often placed in locations easily accessible to children. Ingestion of naphthalene can result in severe toxicity including a rapidly progressive hemolytic anemia. The lethal dose of ingested naphthalene is approximately 2 Gm.

A number of household pesticidal agents are used specifically to kill, repel, and control rodents. Rodenticides may be comprised of a variety of organic and inorganic compounds as well as agents derived from botonical sources. The principal effectiveness of the inorganic preparations results from the toxic effects of metal salts they contain. The most important chemicals are salts of arsenic, fluoride, cyanide, thallium, selenium, and phosphorus. The toxicity of these agents is related to their ability to interrupt metabolic processes through inhibition of regulatory enzymes or other mechanisms. Thus severe systemic toxicity ranging from shock to death may result from ingestion of these substances. The principal organic rodenticidal agents include chemicals such as warfarin, an anticoagulant. Although dangerous to humans only with repeated dosing, warfarin, as mentioned before, accounts for nearly 50% of the nonfatal rodenticide poisonings around the home.

Fungicides are employed in the home to eradicate fungi and protect materials from rot and decay. These also include a large number of inorganic and organic compounds, some of which are highly toxic to humans. Among these are mercury compounds, pentachlorophenol, dithiocarbamates, and iodine. The toxic effects of these agents range from skin irritations to severe systemic poisoning including death.

Finally, a variety of pesticidal agents are used to control the growth of weeds. Some such "herbicides" are selectively toxic to certain types of weeds and grasses but not dangerous to animals or humans. Others are toxic with whatever they come in contact, including humans. The latter include sodium chlorate, potassium cyanate, arsenicals, caustic acids and alkalis, and petroleum distillates. Localized or systemic toxicity ranging in severity from skin irritation to death may occur following contact or ingestion of these agents.

Time stressors

Estimates of the amount of time devoted to housework are surprisingly high. Oakley's (1971) study reveals that, on the average, women spend about 77 hours per week doing household tasks. Indeed, these hours are comparable to those reported by women in Western countries from 1929 to the present (Oakley, 1974). Kreps (1971) estimates that married women typically perform 2053 hours of unpaid housework per year.

Changing levels of expectation contribute to the large amount of time devoted to housework. People in the Western world want more possessions, larger homes, and so on. The advertisements for household products and the portrayal of women as ideal mothers and wives help to increase women's expectations of themselves. Women have increasingly become passive consumers of goods and services rather than active producers of these. Thus the time allocated to housework can expand to fill the time available. Each new product can create a demand for its use, and pushed to the extreme, the commodity comes to dictate the household tasks rather than the essential tasks dictating the commodity.

The time allocated to housework is influenced by two factors: employment outside the home and childbearing. It is estimated that, on the average, women who are employed outside the home are engaged in work activities in both the place of employment and the home 80 hours per week. By contrast, their husbands average approximately 50 hours of work per week (Stellman, 1977). Furthermore, child care imposes constraints inasmuch as it is not a 9-to-5 occupation. At least for a brief period, one of the parents must provide continuous child care, and usually this is the woman. Thus women who are employed outside the home are often required to perform three roles: homemaker, parent, and employee.

One of the time stressors that Oakley's (1971) sample associated with housework was excessive pace. If women are fairly autonomous in the performance of their household tasks, why do they complain of excessive pace? One reason may be that increasing expectations for cleanliness and quality of family life must be contained within a finite period of time. Careful examination of women who have high identification with the homemaker role and high standards for work performance might reveal the same type of characteristics more commonly attributed to women in business, or the prototype for type A behavior—the American businessman!

Although it is tempting to assume that labor-saving devices have liberated women from the time devoted to housework, Vanek (1974) uses data from national surveys to illustrate that women who are not employed outside the home spend as much time in housework as their grandmothers did. Whereas nonemployed women spend 55 hours per week in housework, employed women spend only about 26 hours in similar pursuits. These differences do not appear to be attributable to nonemployed women having larger families, younger children, or less help with housework.* Rather it appears that since the value of housework is not clear, women who are not employed outside the home feel pressure to spend more hours in household chores than women who are employed; employed women may not perceive the same pressure.

REFERENCES

Akerstedt, T.: Shift work and health: interdisciplinary aspects. In Rentos, P. G., and Shepard, R. D., editors: Shift work and health: a symposium, Cincinnati, NIOSH USDHEW, July 1976.

American College of Gynecologists: Guidelines on pregnancy and work, Cincinnati, 1977, NIOSH, USDHEW.

Andjelkovic, D., and Taulbee, J.: Mortality of female industrial workers. Presented at APHA meeting, October 19, 1976.

Arena, J.: Poisoning: toxicology, symptoms, treatments, ed. 3, Springfield, Ill., 1974, Charles C Thomas, Publisher.

Ayoub, M. M.: Shift work and health: an erogonomic approach, In Rentos, P. G., and Shepard, R. D., editors: Shift work and health: a symposium, Cincinnati, 1977, NIOSH USDHEW.

Baetger, A. Women in industry, Philadelphia, 1946, W. B. Saunders Co.

Barrett-Connor, E., and others: Epidemiology for the infection control nurse, St. Louis, 1978, The C. V. Mosby Co.

Bernard, J.: Women, wives, mothers: values and options, Chicago, 1975, Aldine Publishing Co.

Boland, B. M., editors: Cancer and the worker, New York, 1977, New York Academy of Science.

Boulding, E.: Familial constraints on women's work roles, Signs J. Women Cult. Soc. 1(3, Part 2):95-117, Spring 1976.

Calabrese, E. J.: Pollutants and high risk groups, New York, 1978, John Wiley & Sons.

Casarett, L., and Doull, J., editors: Toxicology—the basic science of poisons, New York, 1975, The Macmillan Co., Inc.

Chaffin, D.: Hazards related to personal physical strengths. In Bingham, E., editor: Proceedings of the Conference on Women in the Workplace, Washington, D.C., 1977, Society for Occupational and Environmental Health.

Chemicals and Health, Report of the Panel on Chemicals and Health of the President's Science Advisory Committee, September 1973. Science and Technology Policy Office, National Science Foundation.

Coburn, D.: Job-worker incongruence: consequences for health, J. Health Social Behav., pp. 198-212, 1978.

Cole, S., and LeJeune, R.: Illness and the legitimization of failure, Am. Soc. Rev. 37:347-356, 1972.

Conibear, S.: Women as a high risk population. In Bingham, E., editor: Proceedings of Conference on Women and the Workplace, Washington, D.C., 1977, Society for Occupational and Environmental Health.

DeBruin, A.: Biochemical toxicology of environmental agents, Amsterdam, 1976, Elsevier/North Holland Biomedical Press.

Feld, S.: Feelings of adjustment. In Nye, F. I., and Hoffman, L. W.: The employed mother in America, Chicago, 1963, Rand McNally and Co., pp. 331-352.

Finseth, K., Dallal, G., Lynch, J. T., and Brynjes, S.: Health problems of employed women enrolled in an HMO, presented at APHA meeting, November 1975.

*It is interesting to note that husbands of employed women give no more help than those of nonemployed women.

Gleason, M., and others: Clinical toxicology of commercial products, Acute poisoning, ed. 3, Baltimore, 1969, The Williams & Wilkins Co.

Horner, M.: Toward an understanding of achievement-related conflicts in women, J. Soc. Issues 28(2):157-175, 1972.

Howell, M. C.: Employed mothers and their families: I, Pediatrics 52(2):252-263, 1973.

Howell, M. C.: Effects of maternal employment on the child, II, Pediatrics 52:327-343, 1973.

Hricko, A., and Brunt, M.: Working for your life: a women's guide to job health hazards, Labor Occupational Health Program, University of California, Berkeley, Health Research Group, 1976.

Human health and the environment; some research needs. Second Task Force Report. U.S. Department of Health Education and Welfare Publication, No. NIH 77-1277, 1977.

Hunt, Z.: Occupational health problems of pregnant women: a report and recommendations from the office of the Secretary of Health, Education and Welfare, Washington, D.C., 1975.

Hunt, Z.: The health of women at work, Evanston, Ill., 1977, Northwestern University, Program on Women.

Johnson, F., and Johnson, C.: Role strain in high-commitment career women, J. Am. Acad. Psychoanalysis 4(1):13-36, 1976.

Key, M. M., and others, editors: Occupational diseases. A guide to their recognition, 1977 (revised ed.), USDHEW: CDC/NIOSH.

Kreps, J.: Sex in the marketplace: American women at work, Baltimore, 1971, Johns Hopkins Press.

Kryter, C.: The effects of noise on man, New York, 1970, Academic Press.

Ladbrook, D.: Mortality of professional women. Presented at APHA meeting, October 20, 1976.

Levy, R.: Psychosomatic symptoms and women's protest: two types of reaction to structural strain in the family, J. Health Social Behav. 17:122-134, 1976.

Loomis, T.: Essentials of toxicology, ed. 2, Philadelphia, 1974, Lea & Feibiger.

Lopata, H.: Occupation housewife, New York, 1971, Oxford University Press.

McDonald, H. D.: Women at work: maternal health and congenital defect: a prospective investigation, N. Engl. J. Med. 258:767-773, 1958.

McLean, Alan, editor: Occupational stress, Springfield, Ill., 1972, Charles C Thomas, Publisher.

McMichael, A. J.: Standardized mortality ratios and the "healthy worker effect," J. Occupat. Med. 18:165-168, 1976.

McRee, D. E.: Environmental aspects of microwave radiation, Environ. Health Perspect. 2:41-54, 1972.

Nathanson, C. A.: Sex, illness and medical care, a review of data, theory, and method, Soc. Sci. Med. 2(1):13-25, 1977.

Nathanson, C. A.: Illness and the feminine role: a theoretical review, Soc. Sci. Med. 9:57-62, 1975.

National Clearing House for Poison Control Centers, 1972.

National Institute on Occupational and Safety Hazards: Guidelines on pregnancy and work, Cincinnati, NIOSH USDHEW, September 1977.

Nye, F. I., and Hoffman, L. W.: The employed mother in America, Chicago, 1963, Rand McNally and Co.

Oakley, A.: The sociology of housework, New York, 1974, Pantheon Books.

Oakley, A.: Woman's work: The housewife past and present, New York, 1974, Pantheon.

Pokorny, J., and Rous, J.: The effect of mother's work on fetal heart sounds, In Hroky, J., and Stembera, Z., editor: Proceedings of the International Symposium on Intrauterine Dangers of the Fetus, Amsterdam, 1967, Excerpta Medica.

Pope, C., and McCabe, M.: The employment status of women and their health and well-being, presented at APHA meeting, November 1975.

Rentos, P. G., and Shepard, R. D., editors: Shift work and health: A symposium, Cincinnati, July 1976, NIOSH USDHEW.

Rivkin, M. O.: Contextual effects of families on female responses to illness, unpublished Ph.D. dissertation, Johns Hopkins University, Baltimore, 1972.

Salmon, V., Mills, J. S., and Peterson, A.: Industrial noise control manual, Cincinnati, NIOSH, June 1975.

Sharp, L. J., and Nye, F. I.: Maternal mental health. In Nye, F. I., and Hoffman, L. W.: The employed mother in America, Chicago, 1963, Rand McNally and Co., pp. 309-319.

Stellman, J. M.: Women's work: women's health. Myths and realities, New York, 1977, Pantheon Books.

Stellman, J., and Daum, S.: Work is dangerous to your health, New York, Vintage Press.

Stewart, A.: A note on the obstetric effects of work during pregnancy, Br. J. Prevent. Soc. Med. 9:159-161, 1955.

Taylor, S. E., and Langer, E. J.: Pregnancy: a social stigma? Sex Roles 3(1):27-35, 1977.

U.S. Department of Labor, Women's Bureau: Women in the labor force—January 1976-1977, Washington, D.C., February 1978, U.S. Government Printing Office.

Vanek, J.: Time spent in housework, Sci. Am. 231:116-120, 1974.

Waldbott, G. L.: Health effect of environmental pollutants, ed. 2, St. Louis, 1978, The C. V. Mosby Co.

Weissman, M., and others: The educated housewife: mild depression and the search for work, Am. J. Orthopsychiatry 43:563-573, 1973.

Wofford, S.: Health problems in the airline industries. In Bingham, E., editor: Proceedings of the Conference on women in the workplace, Washington, D.C., 1976, Society for Occupational and Environmental Health.

Women's Bureau, Employment Standards Administration, United States Department of Labor: The myth and the reality, May 1974.

21

Nutrition

Catherine Ingram Fogel

"You are what you eat" is a widely accepted trusim that has particular significance for women. Nutritional status has a profound effect on the health of women. For example, there is growing evidence that nutritional interventions during pregnancy can have a significant effect on pregnancy outcomes. Ideas about what constitutes adequate dietary patterns during pregnancy are undergoing radical changes, while preconception nutritional status is now recognized as a crucial factor in the ability to conceive and bear healthy children.

The differing nutritional needs of women throughout the life cycle are beginning to be identified and the knowledge incorporated into health care teaching. Obesity may be the most common chronic illness in American women today. Furthermore, obesity has been implicated as a risk factor in the development of many chronic diseases to which women are increasingly prone. The youth-conscious culture of America encourages many women to use suspect dietary practices and reducing diets in order to remain slim and youthful-looking, even though these may jeopardize their nutritional status and health. Women continue to be the primary food buyers, food preparers, and transmitters of nutritional information to their families so that they have a direct impact on the health of others.

The role of nurses in teaching has long been recognized, particularly in the areas of nutritional needs, dietary patterns, and therapeutic diets. The purpose of this chapter is to increase the nurse's ability to provide comprehensive nutritional counseling to her clients by increasing her understanding of the factors that influence food patterns; identifying nutritional needs throughout the life cycle of women; and analyzing nutritional disorders common to women. Woven throughout are specific nursing assessment skills and management strategies appropriate to specific nutritional needs and problems.

FACTORS INFLUENCING FOOD PATTERNS

Food is a common denominator for everyone: it is essential not only for physiologic needs but also for so-cial and emotional needs. Even though food meets common needs for all of us, food patterns are infinitely complex and are influenced by many variables, including early experiences and social, economic, geographic, ethnic, religious, and environmental factors. All people must eat to survive; they must obtain enough food of acceptable quality to satisfy nutritional requirements; however, enormously different solutions are developed to meet this need. Cultural foodways—those behaviors that affect what people eat—show infinite variety. They determine what is and is not considered food, what are acceptable methods of preparing and combining foods, and what rules govern food distribution.

Food patterns are among the oldest and most entrenched aspects of any given culture; change is not easily accomplished and it can produce unexpected and unwelcome reactions. Foodways play an important part in cultural identity. Most people hold the view that other people's foodways are irrational and their own are natural and sensible. Health care practitioners tend to ascribe to this belief as well and to reject patterns of behavior different from their own; we may label food patterns that differ from ours as "bad" or "wrong." This ethnocentricity or cultural bias can severely hamper the effectiveness of our teaching. Unless cultural biases can be put aside and food patterns viewed as part of a greater cultural whole, client education will be severely hampered. The old adage, "start where the patient is," is never more true than when dealing with food and eating.

People usually do not automatically choose to eat what is best for them. They tend to eat what is available and may learn through trial and error what foods are better for their health than others. This approach is at best time consuming; it can be hazardous to health and may bring gross misconceptions about foods. The circumstances under which one eats are largely determined by one's culture. Every cultural group has customs dictating which foods should or should not be eaten. Although these belief systems are not grounded in scientific fact, they are usually rigidly held and highly resistant to change. There can be extreme emotional reactions to attempts to effect acceptance; for example, a Jewish woman once reported to me that the accidental eating of a shrimp caused her to be extremely nauseated. In developing countries, food taboos can accentuate malnutrition. Many food taboos are associated with women, particularly menstruating and pregnant women. In some cultures it is believed that if a menstruating woman touches particular foods or crops, they will spoil. In parts of the rural South, it is thought that a menstruating woman should not make pickles as they will not "pickle" correctly. Often pregnant women are encouraged to eat specific foods to ensure the infant's well being. The idea that a pregnant women must "eat for two" may have arisen from just such a myth. (Specific cultural variations in diet during pregnancy are discussed later in this chapter.)

The family probably has the greatest influence on the individual's diet patterns, and the woman in the family is particularly important. Usually, she purchases food and plans, prepares, and serves the meals. The values she holds about food will be transmitted through all of these acts. In turn her values are based on income, geographic region, level of education, knowledge of nutrition, and cultural belief system.

The mother not only determines which foods and how much of them reach the table; she also has a major influence on what emotional connotations are placed on food. The young child learns early that many emotions can be expressed through food. Further, food has been used as a means of communication since the beginning of history. Friends are honored with food. Food is often used as a reward, punishment, or means of bribery; children are rewarded with sweets or punished by being deprived of a favorite food. Adults often reward themselves with special food or an expensive meal after a difficult day or experience. A family may feel rewarded and loved when served their favorite foods or punished and unloved when meals include foods they dislike. Food is also a part of religious observances and festivals. Sympathy is expressed and solace given by foods. Food may be a weapon to express anger or an attention-getting device. The offer of security through food is universal. Security foods are those that give comfort during anxiety and serve as reassurance. They are usually foods that the individual has been given in infancy or childhood and are interpreted as evidence of love and acceptance. Bread and milk are examples of security foods.

It is essential for the nurse to understand the emotional meaning food has for the individual. Without this knowledge, attempts to modify food habits and effect changes in eating patterns are doomed to failure. For example, weight reduction diets should not be undertaken when an individual is experiencing a great deal of stress. Eating serves as a way of coping with life's stresses. It is more difficult to deny oneself food, which represents security, when one is already feeling insecure and anxious.

The nurse should be aware of the individual's typical meal patterns because eating has social values. To eat with someone implies that you are valued; eating alone may mean that you are not worthy of companionship. Eating together may also have status connotations. Throughout history one's seat at the table has indicated one's social position. Still today, in some homes, women must wait until the males of the family are fed before eating themselves; often the choicest morsels are reserved for men. In other situations, the children are fed separately from adults.

Social status or prestige may be expressed through serving foods that are expensive, difficult to obtain, distinctive in flavor, or time-consuming to prepare. Examples of such foods are caviar, lobster, filet mignon, crepes suzette, and champagne. Other foods are scorned as lacking status or being associated with the poor; fish, stews, and ground meats are examples. Some individuals derive satisfaction from being an epicurean or gourmet and view this as indicative of high status.

Often a good deal of ritual is associated with a specific meal. A certain food may be identified as basic to life and a meal not considered complete without it. Food preparation may be highly significant for some. Emphasis on all natural ingredients or "making it from scratch" can convey caring and concern for others' well being. Being a good cook can be a source of pride and identity, and any refusal to consume all food prepared a rejection to the cook. Remember the stereotype of the Jewish mother who says, "If you love me, you'll eat."

The mass media have a tremendous impact on food patterns. Manufacturers often create a desire for their products by appealing to the emotions. Food consumption is pictured in situations suggesting fun, social status, and group acceptance. Often the message is, "If you care about your family you will serve this food item." Foods may then be bought to meet an emotional need rather than for their nutritional value.

In almost all religions there are some regulations on the use of food. Certain foods are forbidden by religious proscription—for example, pork to Orthodox Jews or flesh foods to Seventh-Day Adventists. Certain foods may become associated with a specific religion; for example, bread and wine are symbols of Christianity, and maize is associated with the Indians of Mexico. Fasting is a component common to most religions. On days of fast either total abstinence from food or the substitution of one food for another may be practiced. A substitute food is likely to be associated with denying oneself and could not be chosen when seeking enjoyment. Perhaps the most well-known example is the traditional substitution of fish for meat on Fridays by American Catholics, a practice no longer used.

Often foods are categorized as suitable for a given age group or more suitable for one sex or another, and this can affect nutritional intakes. Peanut butter and jelly are foods for children while martinis, olives, and coffee are adult foods. Adolescents often adopt the current food fads and are inveterate junk food eaters. Heavy, starchy, filling foods such as meats, potatoes, and pie are thought to be preferred by men, while women supposedly prefer lighter foods such as salads, fruits, and vegetables. There are many myths or old wives' tales about the food preferences of men and women. It is a commonly held belief that women like sweet foods more than men do (Bender, 1976). There is little scientific evidence to support this belief; however, there are many nursery rhymes and sayings that emphasize it. For example, according to one nursery rhyme, women have a decided preference for strawberries, sugar, and cream; another states that women have a preference for hot cross buns, and a third says they prefer bread and honey. In contrast, men are pictured as preferring meat—the king who ate a blackbird pie and Jack Spratt who would eat only "lean." Finally, we have all been taught that little girls are made of "sugar and spice" while little boys come from more substantial matter. Bender says that it is uncertain whether any clear differences in food preferences exist between the sexes. The only firm conclusions that have been drawn from research are that women have a greater preference for fruit and a lesser preference for milk; they are less apt to eat a cooked breakfast; and they have a more adventurous palate than men.

The amount of information the individual has about nutrition will affect nutritional status. If one does not know what makes up an adequate diet or how to prepare it, the chances of obtaining a nutritionally healthy diet are poor. Often, misinformation or food myths contribute to the problem. A survey made by the FDA (1974) to determine what consumers know about nutrition found that food shoppers generally have a working knowledge of nutrition. The younger shoppers and those with a college education were likely to know most. According to the survey, educational efforts should be directed at the poor, the old, the less educated, and minorities. Interestingly, many people had accurate information about milk and meat products but they seemed to know very little about the value of vegetables. School was ranked as the most common source of information about nutrition, followed by magazines and newspapers, and then by "mother." American shoppers are primarily concerned about two things when they go to the grocery store: (1) providing nourishing meals at (2) reasonable prices. Many are concerned about being able to provide adequate diets in the face of constantly rising food prices.

Many myths abound about nutrition. Some of the most common are these:

1. Food prepared from "scratch" is more nutritious or better for you than convenience foods that are canned or frozen.
2. Snacks are not as nutritious as food eaten at regular meals.
3. If you eat a variety of foods you will be well nourished.
4. Vitamins that occur naturally in foods are better than those added to foods or vitamin supplements.
5. You should take supplemental vitamins.
6. Organically grown or unprocessed food is more healthful.
7. Your body will tell you what it needs, or if you eat what you want you will be well nourished.
8. If you weigh what you should, you are properly nourished.

Obviously, a person who believes all of these myths and bases food selection and diet on them will be at greater risk for dietary insufficiencies. The more accurate the knowledge one has, the more potential there is for selection of a diet that will meet nutritional needs. Knowledge does not ensure adequacy but it does increase the potential for it.

Income will have an important influence on a person's food habits. The less income available, the more limited are food choices: you buy what you can afford. The time available for food shopping and meal preparation will also influence the types of food one eats and the adequacy of the diet. People with little time are more apt to rely on "fast food" meals, convenience foods, or foods that take little preparation, such as sandwiches.

The nurse who wishes to change undesirable food patterns must first have an intimate knowledge of the client's belief system about food and present food habits. Prior to attempting any change she must identify all those factors that influence the client's particular food pathways; and she must evaluate the psychologic and social functions of the food problem. Proposed changes should be developed with all these specifics in mind; generalizing to a common diet will not be effective. In attempting to effect change, it is important to use the positive aspects of the client's present diet. Change is more likely to occur if some familiar aspects can be retained and if the client feels some of what she has been doing is good. It is important to set realistic goals that are determined by the client. Only if the client sees the necessity for change will change occur. All teaching should begin where the client is, both in terms of motivation and ability to understand. If dietary recommendations make use of known foods and food pathways, the likelihood that they will be followed is greatly increased. It is also important that follow-up be done by the same person, that constant encouragement be given, and that evaluation be done systematically and continually. When all of these principles are observed, the client is more likely to make permanent changes in her food patterns.

NUTRITION THROUGHOUT THE LIFE CYCLE

Traditionally, health care practitioners have addressed themselves to improving dietary habits of women during pregnancy and given little or no thought to nutritional status prior to or following pregnancy or to women who won't ever be pregnant. This shortsightedness ignores the impact that general health status can have on reproduction and fertility. It has been suggested that we are what we eat, and what we eat will tell us how well we reproduce. Frisch (1977) has found that onset and maintenance of regular menstrual functioning are dependent upon maintenance of a minimum body weight for height. There is, apparently, a critical amount of fat storage that is essential for regular menstrual activity. Loss of about one-third of body fat will result in amenorrhea. Excessive body fat also affects menstrual functioning; very obese women are often amenorrheic or have irregular cycles. It seems that too little or too much fat is associated with interruptions in reproductive ability (Frisch,

1977). In addition, food intake can directly affect fecundity, and therefore undernutrition or malnutrition may be a factor for some who are unable to conceive or reproduce.

Poor nutrition can shorten the length of a woman's reproductive lifespan and reduce its efficiency. The undernourished woman will experience menarche later and menopause earlier than a well-nourished woman will. She will have a higher frequency of irregular and anovulatory cycles and may stop menstruating completely if undernutrition is severe enough. When pregnant, she has a higher probability of miscarriage or stillbirth. After delivery, lactational amenorrhea may last longer and result in longer birth intervals than those of a well-nourished woman (see Fig. 21-1).

Given the influence that adverse nutritional states have on a woman's ability to conceive and bear healthy children, it is crucial that nursing practitioners make interconceptual nutritional teaching a part of established health care for women. Interconceptual care is defined as "specific maternal and child health practice that applies the principle of the periodic health examination throughout the entire cycle of human reproduction" (Gold, 1969, p. 27). It begins with birth and extends

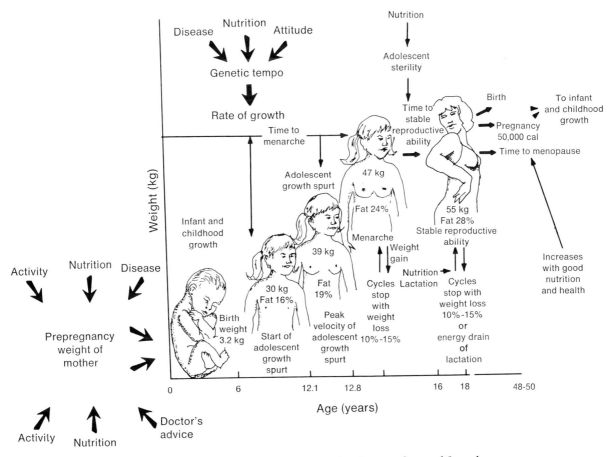

Fig. 21-1. Influence of nutrition on the female reproductive life cycle.

through infancy, childhood, adolescence, and young adulthood to conception, then resumes following delivery and continues until the next conception or menopause occurs. The long-term nutritional history of the mother is as important to fetal outcome as is diet during pregnancy. In order to ensure the best possible reproductive outcomes for both the mother and infant, it is essential that good dietary habits be formed early in life and practiced throughout life. Nursing interventions should be directed toward this end. It is a matter of keeping the long-range perspective (i.e., good general health status) always in mind while focusing on short-term specific goals, for example, diet during pregnancy.

Infancy and childhood

The nutritional needs of the infant and child do not differ according to sex. Both sexes need a diet that is nutritionally adequate in all respects to meet their continuing needs for physical growth and development. Nutritional status and food habits developed in infancy and childhood may have far-reaching effects on adult nutritional status and eating patterns. The girl who is overfed as an infant or young child may find she has a problem with obesity throughout her adult life. Malnutrition begun in the early years will affect reproductive ability and outcomes and general health as an adult. Learned behavior about food and eating will affect nutritional status throughout life.

Adolescence

With the onset of adolescence, special dietary considerations emerge. Adolescence is a unique period of change. Increased nutrients are needed to meet accelerated physical growth needs; and therefore increased amounts of food are needed. The adolescent's specific nutritional needs relate directly to the timing and extent of the pubertal growth spurt. The character and timing of physical growth and sexual maturation differ greatly from individual to individual; however, in general, linear growth is not complete in the adolescent female until 4 years after menarche.

The increased energy requirements needed during rapid growth periods are generally met without concentrated effort on the adolescent's part. Appetite usually increases and increased food intake is the normal response. One factor that can adversely affect this is the pressure many teenage girls feel to be "fashionably" thin. In an effort to achieve this, many girls severely limit their food consumption to levels far lower than are needed to meet normal growth demands. The long-term effects of caloric restriction by teenage girls are not presently known. It has been hypothesized that effects will be directly related to the time in the growth period when caloric restriction is imposed. If it occurs at the height of the rapid growth period, normal growth of the

skeletal system may be compromised and the long bones particularly affected; the dimensions of the pelvic girdle will also be adversely affected. Caloric restriction after the growth spurt will not be as devastating; however, nutritional status may be poor and tolerance to stress and disease lower (Worthington et al., 1977).

Protein deposition and nitrogen retention are greatest during the period of most active growth in adolescence and slow down as growth slows. Most studies indicate that protein intakes generally exceed recommended levels (see Table 21-1). Usually, protein makes up at least 10% of all calories consumed and frequently the proportion is higher (Committee on Maternal Nutrition, 1970). Most adolescent girls prefer protein foods with low caloric intake. Often diets are reasonably high in protein but low in calories so that some dietary protein is used for energy, leaving less for building body tissues. For this reason adolescent girls should be encouraged to plan diets that contain enough energy to allow for an adequate amount of protein for tissue synthesis.

Iron needs for the adolescent girl are large because of the iron necessary for enlarging muscle mass and blood volume. Extra iron is needed to maintain adequate iron stores. Additional stress is placed on the girl by body iron losses during menstruation. The recommended daily allowance for adolescent girls and women is at least 18 mg daily of iron; this amount will allow build-up of sufficient iron stores, though it may be difficult to obtain since dietary sources of iron are limited. Several studies* have noted that iron consumption is less than the recommended daily allowance; while the incidence of iron deficiency anemia is low, the problem of low iron stores is widespread.

Calcium absorption and retention increase prior to menarche and the growth spurt. This is necessary if adequate mineralization of the skeleton is to take place. Teenage diets frequently appear to be low in calcium (King et al., 1972; Osofsky et al., 1971). The restricted diets that many adolescent girls eat often contain inadequate amounts of vitamins and trace minerals, particularly vitamin A.

The emotional and psychologic growth that takes place during adolescence also influences nutritional status. As she seeks to establish her own identity, the adolescent tests, rejects, and/or accepts her parents' values and beliefs. Dietary habits may be challenged because parents advocate them. Often teenagers are told to eat something because it is good for them, whether they like it or not. Adolescents usually do not experience the nutritional disaster predicted by their parents if they practice poor food habits. As long as they feel well they are not

---

*Hueneman et al., 1968; King et al., 1972; Osofsky et al., 1971; Worthington et al., 1977.

Table 21-1. Recommended daily dietary allowances for women through the life cycle*

	Young teenager (11-14 yrs)	Adolescent (15-18 yrs)	Childbearing years (19-50 yrs)	Older women (51+ yrs)	Adult pregnancy increase	Teenage pregnancy increase	Lactating
Energy (calories)	−2400	2100	2000-2100	1800	+300	+300	+500
Protein (Gm)	44	48	46	46	+30	+30	+20
Calcium (Gm)	1.2	1.2	.8	.8	+0.4	+0.4	+1.2
Phosphorus (Gm)	1.2	1.2	.8	.8	+0.4	+0.4	+1.2
Iron (mg)	18	18	18	10	0e	0e	0e
Magnesium (mg)	300	300	300	300	+150	+150	+150
Iodine (μg)	115	115	100	80	+25	+25	+25
Zinc (mg)	15	15	15	15	+5	+5	+10
Vitamin A (IU)	4000	4000	4000	4000	+1000	+1000	+2000
Vitamin D (IU)	400	400	a	0	0	0	0
Vitamin E (IU)	12	12	12	12	+3	+3	+3
Vitamin C (ascorbic acid) (mg)	45	45	45	45	+15	+15	+15
Niacin (mg)	16	14	b	12	+2	+2	+4
Riboflavin (mg)	1.3	1.4	c	1.1	+0.3	+0.3	+0.5
Thiamine (mg)	1.2	1.1	d	1.0	+0.3	+0.3	+0.3
Folic acid (mg)	0.4	0.4	0.4	0.4	+0.4	+0.4	+0.4
Vitamin B_6 (mg)	1.6	2.0	2.0	2.0	+0.5	+0.5	+0.5
Vitamin B_{12} (μg)	3.0	3.0	3.0	3.0	+1	+1	+1

a. 400 IU required for ages 19-22 years; more recommended for ages 23-50; b. 14 mg recommended for ages 19-22 years; 13 mg for ages 23-50; c. 1.4 recommended for ages 10-22 years; 1.2 recommended for ages 23-50 years; d. 1.1 recommended for ages 19-22 years; 1.0 recom- mended for ages 23-50 years; e. Supplemental iron is recommended. *Adapted from Recommended daily dietary allowances, Washington, D.C., 1974, Food & Nutrition Board, National Academy of Sciences– National Research Council.

concerned about nutrients. Many adolescents have a sense of invulnerability about their bodies; they find it difficult to imagine long-term adverse effects.

Peers and peer activities are essential for adolescents. Often these activities revolve around fast-food places and result in the ingestion of empty calories, which replace balanced meals. Peer reinforcement of slimness as a valued objective can result in fad diets and severe caloric restrictions.

In a study done by Dwyer and associates (1967) 15% of 446 adolescent girls were obese but 60% were currently on or had been on reducing diets. Many of them were reducing for appearance rather than for health reasons. Nutritional knowledge was limited, even with respect to calories.

Food is only one component of an active life; what teenagers need and will eat is not always available at the times and places where they do eat. Irregular eating habits are characteristic of most adolescents. Teenagers tend to eat more than three times a day. Girls appear to eat more often than boys. The obese eat less frequently and tend to skip breakfast. Snacking is a normal pattern of teenagers and should be used in meal planning; as much as one fourth of all calories may come from snacks (Hampton, 1967).

Meal regularity is positively associated with socioeconomic status: blacks tend to eat all meals less frequently than whites. The most preferred meal is dinner and lunch is skipped most often. Obese teenagers tend to eat fewer dairy products, vegetables, and fruits. Sweets and desserts are consumed most by blacks. The teenagers most at risk nutritionally appear to be the obese and black females (Hueneman, 1968).

There is no magic formula for helping maturing teenage girls to adopt healthful dietary habits. Perhaps most crucial is development of a trusting relationship. Often the nurse must deal first with other health concerns before the girl is ready to consider her diet. Fortunately, there are some plus factors that provide hope for teenagers to be well fed: they get hungry, they like to eat, they value energy and want to be able to compete successfully. Many have established good food habits earlier in their lives.

Many adolescent girls have nutritional intakes that meet their needs, but knowledge of nutritional needs and the relationship of nutrition to health is poor. The diet of adolescent girls needs much improvement in order to maintain adequate nutritional status and prepare for possible pregnancy and lactation.

Childbearing years

The nutritional needs of pregnant and lactating women are many, complex, and individual. The nutritional demands of pregnancy and the nurse's role in assisting the client to meet these demands are discussed in detail later in this chapter. Nutritional needs of women who do not exercise their reproductive capabilities are similar to those women between pregnancies.

Middle age

The special needs of the woman in her reproductive years subside as reproductive capabilities and menstruation cease. Basal metabolic rates are lowered and activities are often lessened. Energy needs may decrease by 15%; there are no other significant decreases in estimated needs of other nutrients except iron. Reduction of caloric intake with increasing age requires care in food selection to make sure essential nutrients are not compromised. The woman needs to include higher proportions of foods of high nutrient density in order to maintain good nutritional status. It is important that women enter the middle and aging years in good physical condition to meet the possible stressors of endocrine changes at menopause and physiologic changes that occur with the aging process with its accompanying hazards of diabetes, cardiovascular disease, obesity, and osteoporosis.

Old age

Studies of the nutritional status of the older woman find that caloric intakes are often low: diets fail to meet nutrient standards for weight and age. Nutrients most limited are protein, iron, and vitamin A. Dietary intakes tend to decrease with age, income, and educational level. Black women have poorer diets than white women (Todhunter, 1977).

In addition to the changing nutritional needs of women as they move through the life cycle, there are special conditions and illnesses that have a profound effect on nutritional status and general health.

PREGNANCY
Nutritional influence on pregnancy

Without food, life cannot be sustained. Unless an adequate supply of food and essential nutrients is available, the human organism cannot grow and develop normally. Despite these obvious facts, the influence nutrition has on pregnancy and its outcome has not always been adequately recognized. Gossip, old wives' tales, and medical advice not founded in fact have frequently been the primary sources of dietary recommendations for pregnancy. Since time began, pregnancy has been shrouded in mystery. Because of this, the pregnant woman has suffered all types of deprivations and proscriptions aimed at shielding her from evils that might cause a miscarriage or birth of a child with a defect. In the absence of scientific fact, she has been the receipient of every fad and fallacy that man could conjure up.

Dietary advice has been based on beliefs that obvious physical properties of different foods could have specific effects on either the mother or child. Such beliefs often were influenced by the mysticism that surrounded the childbearing experience. For example, salty, sour, or acid foods might be forbidden for fear they would cause a child with a "sour" disposition. During the late nineteenth century, Prochownick, a German obstetrician, recommended semi-starvation in the form of a low-carbohydrate, high-protein, fluid-restricted diet. The justification for the diet was that women who followed this regime produced smaller infants and had less discomfort and difficulty in labor and delivery. Remnants of this type of diet during pregnancy persist today, even in the face of overwhelming evidence that the diet is harmful.

Another belief that persists is that the maternal organism is somehow mysteriously endowed with an innate ability to produce a viable offspring regardless of maternal health or nutritional status. It is assumed that the pregnant woman will instinctively eat to meet the health needs of herself and infant. Another old view that is still influencing nutritional advice is the conviction that as long as the mother takes plenty of vitamins, the fetus will get all the nourishment it needs, no matter what the mother's nutritional status is (Shank, 1970).

Today maternal nutrition is considered critically important to both mother and fetus. Maternal nutrition can and does interfere with the ability to conceive. It also seems reasonable to expect that it can cause spontaneous abortions, congenital defects, and low–birth weight infants. The risks for preterm and growth-retarded infants are so well documented that low birth weight in itself is considered an unfavorable outcome of pregnancy (see Chapter 10). It has been estimated that between 10% and 20% of all low–birth weight infants are the result of intrauterine growth retardation; i.e., the infant experienced malnutrition in utero. Fetal malnutrition is defined as a reduction in maternal supply or placental transport of nutrients so that fetal growth is significantly restricted. A number of factors influence fetal growth; maternal malnutrition is but one of these, however crucial.

The timing and duration of nutritional restriction are significant. During the embryonic stage of fetal development, cells differentiate into three germinal layers. Growth during this time occurs only by an increase in the number of cells. The fetal stage is the time of most rapid growth. During this time, growth is almost continuous and is accompanied by increase in cell size. Most organ cells continue to proliferate after birth. It is thought that growth in cell size begins at around 7 months' gestation and can continue for 3 years after birth. Given this sequence of growth, it is possible to suggest the effects malnutrition might have at different stages of gestation. During the embryonic phase, a severe limitation in nutrients could have teratogenic effects causing malformation or death. While malnutrition occurring after the third month of gestation would not have teratogenic effects, it could cause fetal growth retardation. During the last trimester, nutritional needs are at a peak as cells increase in both size and number. Poor nutrition in the latter stages of pregnancy affects fetal growth, while malnutrition in the early months affects embryonic development and survival.

In addition to the relationship between nutritional status and fetal outcomes of pregnancy, nutritional status has an effect on maternal well-being. Nurses need to know specific nutritional requirements of pregnancy so that they can advise clients to meet their nutritional needs. When pregnant, the woman has specific needs for calories, protein, fat, vitamins, and minerals; these are summarized in Table 21-1.

Nutritional requirements of pregnancy

Weight gain during pregnancy has been a subject of great controversy. Opinions on what constitutes optimal total weight gain vary greatly. It is difficult to obtain reliable average figures for normal weight gain during pregnancy under physiologic conditions because most physicians advise their clients to eat less than their appetites would dictate. One study (Higgins, 1972) analyzed weight gain of primigravidas who were not being advised to restrict food intake; the investigators found that total weight gain averaged 27.5 lbs, with an average rate of gain of 1.1 lbs per week in the second half of pregnancy. This amount of gain was found to be associated with the lowest overall incidence of pre-eclampsia, low birth weight, and perinatal mortality.

There is general agreement that the optimal weight gain in pregnancy follows a pattern, showing little gain in the first trimester, a rapid increase in the second, and some slowing in rate of increase in the third. This brings a gain of 1.5 to 3.0 lbs in the first trimester, approximately 14 lbs by the end of the second trimester, and approximately 24 lb by the end of the third trimester. Most of the weight gain associated with the products of conception takes place in the second half of pregnancy, while maternal stores are laid down very rapidly before midpregnancy, then slow down and appear to stop before term (see Table 21-2). About 8.8 lbs of weight gain are unexplained and water free. The only tissue that can be stored in such a quantity and under such conditions is fat. Such fat represents energy stores that would be enough to sustain fetal growth in the last trimester or to subsidize energy needed during lactation. This energy storage may serve no useful purpose for many women in the United States today and it can be the foundation for

Table 21-2. Average components of weight gain (in pounds) in each trimester of pregnancy*

Component	Trimester		
	First	Second	Third
Fetus	Negligible	2.2	7.5
Placenta	Negligible	0.7	1.3
Amniotic fluid	Negligible	0.9	2.2
Fetal subtotal		(3.7)	11.0
Increased uterine size	0.7	1.8	2.2
Increased breast size	0.2	0.7	1.1
Increases blood volume	0.7	2.9	3.3
Increased extracellular fluid	0	0	3.3
Maternal subtotal	(1.5)	(5.3)	11.0
TOTAL GAIN ACCOUNTED FOR	1.5	9.0	20.9

*Contrasting increased maternal and fetal weight shows the maternal component accounts for most of the gain in the first trimester, about 60% in the second trimester, and about 40% in the third. From Pitkin, R. M., and others: Maternal nutrition: A selective review of clinical topics, Obstet. Gynecol. **40**:777, 1972.

subsequent obesity. There is some evidence that progesterone may provide the stimulus for fat storage, possibly by acting centrally to reset a "lipostat" in the hypothalamus.

One of the most striking features of weight gain in pregnancy is its variability. Young women tend to gain slightly more weight than older women, primigravidas slightly more than older women, and thin women slightly more than fat women. Similarities in total weight gain may conceal large differences in the components of gain. Healthy, well-nourished women who begin pregnancy with a high weight-for-height gain relatively large amounts of water and relatively little "dry" weight, whereas women who are underweight for height gain more fat and less water.

Calories

Growth is a process that requires energy. Therefore, additional calories, above those required for maintenance, are needed during periods of growth. Table 21-1 gives the recommended dietary allowances for calories to provide optimal weight gain at various ages, to meet growth needs of the fetus, placenta, and associated maternal tissues, and to take care of the increased maternal basal metabolism. Caloric needs may often be partially offset by decreased activity. Calories are essential to protect protein. If caloric intake is not adequate for energy needs, protein will be used for energy and thus unavailable for growth. Furthermore, protein breakdown leads to acidosis.

Protein

Protein needs are increased in pregnancy. Protein is essential for synthesis of hemoglobin and provides the nitrogen and amino acids essential for forming body tissue. Protein intake should be increased from 46 gm to 86 gm per day in pregnancy for all females. The pregnant adolescent often needs even more protein to sustain her during a period of rapid growth for herself as well as her fetus. Efficiency of protein utilization decreases as protein intake is increased, the point of maximal usage is 92 gm per day, according to the Committee on Maternal Nutrition.

Dietary restrictions

Caloric restriction in pregnancy is a firmly rooted dictim not based on scientific fact. Earlier it was thought that dietary restrictions limiting caloric intake would help prevent toxemia and decrease the incidence of dystocia and other maternal complications. Numerous studies of experimental animals subjected to dietary restrictions during pregnancy have demonstrated profound negative effects on maternal physiologic adjustments and fetal growth and development (Pitkin et al., 1972). Larger maternal weight gain is generally associated with larger birth weight; however, this increase is not sufficient to cause mechanical difficulties during labor and delivery. Pitkin states that several recent studies fail to establish a relationship between excessive weight gain based on fat accumulation and toxemia of pregnancy. There appears to be little evidence that excessive weight gain in pregnancy predisposes to other obstetric complications such as abortion, dystoxia, and postpartum hemorrhage.

There appears to be a relationship between excessive weight gain in pregnancy and subsequent obesity. This is significant, given that obesity is a common, serious condition in American women. It is likely that some women become obese because excessive fat is laid down during pregnancy and is not lost between pregnancies; there is an additive effect in successive pregnancies. Gestational obesity often results from misguided eating habits, "eating for two," and cravings. For this reason it may be sensible to limit weight gain to some degree. However, severe caloric restrictions or fad diets are not indicated; rather, a diet soundly based on the basic food groups and relatively free of empty calories is needed. The Committee on Maternal Nutrition considers an average weight gain in pregnancy to be 24 lbs. At no time is severe limitation of weight gain considered justifiable because of the possibility of adverse effects on birth weight and neurologic development of the infant.

Problems associated with weight gain

The client who enters pregnancy significantly under- or overweight is at risk. Prepregnant weight and pregnancy weight gain exert independent and additive influences on birth weight. The importance of adequate nutrition before conception and during pregnancy has already been established. Deviations in weight gain are common problems in obstetric practice. Pitkin (1977) suggests the following definitions as guidelines:

Underweight—prepregnant weight is 10% or more below standard weight for height and age

Overweight—prepregnant weight of 20% or more above standard weight for height and age

Inadequate gain—less than 2.2 lbs per month in second and/or third trimester

Excessive gain—more than 7 lbs are gained in 1 month

The obese pregnant client is at increased risk for several complications. If a woman is obese the chance of her having hypertension of pregnancy is increased sevenfold. She is also at greater risk for diabetes during pregnancy. Obesity probably increases her chance of pyelonephritis and breech presentation. In the primigravida obesity appears to increase the risk of dystocia and cesarean section; these risks are not increased in the multigravida. Obesity seems to play a role in maternal mortality, possibly by a factor of six (Travers, 1976).

In the past caloric restriction has been advocated for the obese pregnant client in order to hold weight constant or even lose weight during pregnancy. The pregnant woman may see pregnancy as a time to get rid of excess pounds. This is no longer considered advisable in *any* circumstances.

Weight loss or no weight gain during pregnancy brings serious risks. Insufficient intake of nutrients at crucial developmental stages may result in infants with a defect or low birth weight. Marked caloric restriction, even if adequate protein is provided, may result in use of protein for energy, making it unavailable for tissue growth and repair and fetal needs. In addition, when maternal intake is severely restricted, maternal fat stores are catabolized to meet energy requirements, resulting in ketosis and ketonuria. Maternal ketonuria may be associated with neurologic damage to the fetus. Pregnancy should never be viewed as a convenient or easy time to correct maternal obesity.

The undernourished woman begins her pregnancy with inadequate stores to meet the increased nutritional demands. The additional metabolic needs of pregnancy, increased hormones, nausea, and vomiting in early pregnancy, and the psychologic adjustments to pregnancy may all compound the problem. The principal hazard is delivery of a low–birthweight infant. The underweight category includes those women who seem uninterested in food and those who do not understand the link between food and health. The underweight woman should be considered high risk and encouraged to gain as much as she can within reasonable limits (at least 25 to 30 lbs).

The client with inadequate caloric intake may also be deficient in other nutrients.

Sodium

The restriction of sodium in the pregnant woman's diet has been standard practice for decades. Recently, it has been recognized that the healthy pregnant woman retains salt normally and to restrict her salt intake may be dangerous. There is a positive sodium balance in normal pregnancy, resulting from significant changes in renal and hormonal function. The glomerular filtration rate increases by 50% in early pregnancy and remains elevated until late in the third trimester, filtering sodium into the renal tubules. At the same time progesterone exerts a salt-losing natriuretic action in the kidneys retarding absorption of filtered sodium through the renal tubules.

In the absence of some compensatory mechanism, severe electrolyte imbalance can occur. The renin-angiotensin-aldosterone system acts as a compensatory mechanism in normal pregnancy. Renin, a proteolytic enzyme of the kidneys acting on circulating plasma renin substrate, causes the release of angiotensin. Angiotensin, in turn, stimulates the adrenal cortex to secrete aldosterone, which counterbalances the salt-losing tendencies of progesterone. Urinary excretion of dietary sodium is decreased as a result of increased renin and aldosterone secretion.

Sodium is conserved to meet the additional amounts needed for expanded tissue and fluid compartments. Therefore, sodium retention is an expected component of normal pregnancy. To maintain fluid balance and osmotic integrity when sodium is retained, water must be retained as well. This retained water will contribute significantly to weight gain. Salt-restricted diets have been routinely prescribed to prevent or treat what is now thought to be a normal physiologic component of pregnancy. Restriction often resulted in sodium depletion. It appears that sodium restriction so severely stresses the physiologic mechanism of sodium conservation as to cause the system to breakdown; then blood volume cannot be expanded and hyponatremia develops in fluid and tissues (Pitkin, 1972; Oakes et al., 1975).

Iron and folic acid

Pregnancy imposes a severe burden on the maternal hematopoietic system. Normal hematopoiesis requires a nutritionally adequate diet. Hemoglobin is a complex molecule of protein and iron. To produce it there must be protein to provide essential amino acids and sufficient additional iron. Various vitamins and minerals, such as copper, zinc, folic acid, and vitamin B_{12} are needed to serve as cofactors in synthesis of heme and globin. The limiting factor in the synthesis of hemoglobin is usually the availability of iron.

The requirement for iron during pregnancy is slightly less than 1 gm; fetal needs are approximately 300 mg at term, and augmented maternal erythropoiesis requires about 500 mg. Dietary iron intake provides only slightly more than the amounts lost through stool, urine, and skin. The average healthy young American woman has approximately 300 mg of iron stores. A significant proportion of women enter pregnancy without any iron stores, usually because of menstrual blood loss or previous pregnancy.

Anemia is a relatively common complication of pregnancy because the small amounts of usable dietary iron ingested combined with low iron storage cannot meet the increased need for iron. Iron deficiency during pregnancy is easily prevented by giving iron supplements. It is recommended that all pregnant women receive ferrous iron in doses of 30 to 60 mg/day during the last two trimesters (Pitkin, 1972). Continuation of iron supplements following delivery is also recommended to replenish iron stores. It is theoretically possible that augmentation would pose a hazard by increasing total iron content within the body, which would then have to be excreted when blood volume returned to normally postpartally. Pitkin (1972) believes these concerns are groundless because of the documented blood loss during delivery; he says there is no evidence that oral iron supplements during pregnancy cause a harmful iron overload.

Folic acid requirements are increased during pregnancy because of augmented maternal erythropoiesis and fetal and placental growth. Folic acid is an essential coenzyme in purine and pyrimidine metabolism and in DNA synthesis. Megaloblastic anemia, the principal effect of folic acid deficiency, is not as common as iron deficiency anemia, but it does occur in high-risk clients such as those of low socioeconomic status and those with a multiple pregnancy or chronic hemolytic anemia.

The decision to use routine folate supplementation is controversial because it is questionable how many pregnant women actually have megaloblastic anemia, since the indices for diagnoses are unclear. Furthermore, it is unclear what beneficial effect, if any, this would have on the course and outcome of pregnancy. Pitkin and associates (1972) recommend that supplementation, while unnecessary as a routine, should be considered when dietary intake is low, or when the woman has chronic hemolytic anemia, a multiple pregnancy, or is on anticonvulsant drug therapy. Recommended supplementation is 200 to 400 μg/day.

Minerals

Increased calcium is needed during pregnancy for fetal bone development. Increases of up to 50% are recommended in pregnancy, and even more is needed during lactation. When calcium intake is inadequate, fetal needs will be met by demineralizing the maternal skeleton. Diet, the preferred source, can provide adequate amounts of calcium needed during pregnancy and lactation. For example, four glasses of milk or 1¼ oz of cheese will supply the needed daily requirement. Even though calcium is usually included in prenatal vitamin-mineral supplements, it is unnecessary in routine practice. Needs for phosphorus are met when calcium needs are met.

Iodine is an essential component of the thyroid hormones and is an essential nutrient for women. The need can easily be met by using iodized salt. Various other minerals, such as copper, zinc, and magnesium, have been found to be essential in trace amounts.

Vitamins

Two irrational beliefs tend to influence our use of vitamins. The first is that one is nutritionally safe if an adequate supply of vitamin is taken. The second is that if a little is good, more is even better. Vitamins are essential to good nutrition and health; however, this does not always mean that dietary intake needs to be supplemented. According to Pitkin and associates (1972) overt evidence of vitamin deficiency is rare in developed countries. This statement is probably accurate for middle and upper class women; however, this assumption should always be validated by a careful diet history and assessment, because many women of low socioeconomic status and women attempting to remain thin do not eat nutritionally adequate diets.

Given an adequate diet, vitamin supplements do not appear to have any beneficial effects, nor do they appear to have any harmful effects generally. A possible exception is vitamin D. There is some evidence to suggest a relationship between maternal hypervitaminosis D and subsequent development of severe infantile hypercalcemia with craniofacial abnormalities and supravalvular aortic and pulmonary stenosis (Pitkin et al., 1972). An additional potential danger in routine vitamin supplementation is a false sense of security about deficiencies of essential nutrients. Vitamins cannot make up for poor food habits. Vitamin supplements should not be routinely prescribed for healthy pregnant women consuming an adequate diet.

Vitamin A, a fat-soluble substance, is essential for the integrity of epithelial cells and for stimulating new cell growth. It also aids in maintaining resistance to infections. There is an increased need for vitamin A in pregnancy and lactation because these are times of rapid cell growth and relative vulnerability. Hypervitaminosis A can cause bone fragility, liver and spleen enlargement, and skin peeling. Excessive carotene, a form of vitamin A, can result in carotenemia causing yellow discoloration of the skin.

Vitamin D, another fat-soluble vitamin, is essential for maintenance of calcium absorption and utilization and skeletal integrity. Inadequate supplies can cause rickets; this is not usually a problem in the United States because food products such as milk and cereals are routinely fortified. Excessive amounts of vitamin D (1000 to 3000 IU/kg/day) are potentially dangerous to children and adults. Excessive doses mobilize calcium and phosphorus from the tissues, reversing the effect of normal doses. Nausea, anorexia, diuresis, and headaches can result from hypervitaminosis D.

Vitamin E, a third fat-soluble vitamin, is also essential for human growth and metabolism. The necessary requirements for vitamin E can easily be met with an adequate diet.

Vitamin C (ascorbic acid) is involved in tooth formation, bone development and repair, and wound healing. It is probably related to capillary integrity and synthesis of certain adrenal gland steroids. It is the least stable of the vitamins and poorly stored in the tissues. Although daily intake is essential, it is not difficult to meet this need, given an adequate diet that includes citrus fruits and juices daily. Smoking interferes with the absorption of vitamin C and it is suggested by some authorities that smokers double the recommended intake.

The need for the B complex vitamins—thiamine, riboflavin, niacin, B_6, and B_{12}—is slightly increased in pregnancy. Vitamin B_6 functions in carbohydrate, fat, and protein metaboiism; its major function is related to protein and amino acids. Vitamin B_{12} is essential for normal functioning of all cells, particularly bone marrow, nervous system, and gastrointestinal tract. Its most important function is metabolism of nucleic and folic acids, although B_{12} is also involved in protein, fat, and carbohydrate metabolism. Megaloblastic anemias can result from Vitamin B_{12} deficiencies. Vegetarian diets may often be low in vitamin B_{12} because the principal source of the vitamin is animal protein. Niacin is implicated in the development of pellagra. Thiamine deficiencies result in beriberi, while deficiencies in riboflavin cause irritation of the eye, tongue, and mouth.

Clinical applications for the nursing practitioner who is assisting the pregnant client to meet her nutritional needs are these:

1. The routine provision of vitamin-mineral supplements is no longer considered mandatory. It should not be considered a substitute for thorough nutritional counseling, or a solution to poor food habits. This provision is probably neither beneficial nor harmful unless hypervitaminosis results. The cost of the supplements relative to the cost of improving the woman's diet must be considered.

2. Daily iron supplementation of 30 to 60 mg is necessary during the second and third trimesters and

through lactation, or 2 to 3 months postpartum if not breast-feeding.

3. A daily supplement of 0.2 to 0.4 mg of folate should probably be recommended as prophylaxis against megaloblastic anemia of pregnancy.

4. Caloric intake should be increased by 10% (approximately 200 to 300 calories/day) over nonpregnant requirements for age. Daily protein intakes should equal at least 80 gm/day.

5. Total weight gain should be at least 24 to 27 lbs. This gain should follow a pattern of minimal gain in the first trimester and about 1 lb per week in the second half of pregnancy.

6. There is no scientific justification for routine restriction of weight gain to less than 24 to 27 lbs. Severe caloric restriction is harmful to both the fetus and the mother.

7. The routine restriction of sodium in the diet is of questionable value. It probably does not prevent toxemia and may have the adverse effect of decreasing the intake of essential nutrients because the diet is unpalatable or does not contain foods with high sodium content.

Specific dietary problems in pregnancy
Anemia

Anemia is the most common complication of pregnancy. Two types, iron deficiency and folate deficiency, are related to nutrition. The normal maternal physiologic adaptations to pregnancy cause a "physiologic" anemia when blood volume increases without a corresponding increase in total cell volume. Blood volume increases by about 50% in order to supply the increased circulatory needs to the fetus, placenta, and enlarged maternal structures. This increase begins in the third month of gestation, reaches a peak during the third trimester, and returns to normal by the third postpartal week. Red blood cell mass increases by 25%, starting at 6 months, peaking at term, and returning to normal by 6 weeks postpartum. It is evident that the increase in red blood cells does not compensate for the marked increase in plasma volume. Therefore, through dilution, a physiologic anemia results with decreasing hematocrit and hemoglobin values (Table 21-3).

As many as 56% of pregnant women are anemic (Worthington et al., 1977). For the majority of these women the anemia is nutritional in origin, with iron deficiency being the most common (approximately 77%) of the nonphysiologic anemias of pregnancy. Women often have low iron stores during the reproductive years because of menstruation; therefore, they are vulnerable to iron-deficiency anemia during pregnancy. The iron cost of pregnancy is high, and negative balances easily result. The increased demand for iron is the result of increased

Table 21-3. Hematocrit and hemoglobin values for women

	Hemoglobin (Gm/100 ml)	Hematocrit (packed cell vol %)
Pregnancy		
Normal	12.0	36 to 40
Borderline	9.5 to 11.9	30 to 35
Anemia	9.5	30 or below
Nonpregnant		38 to 44

need for hemoglobin synthesis and storage of iron in the fetal liver to meet the iron needs of infancy. At least 2 years of normal diet are needed to replace the iron lost during pregnancy.

A diagnosis of iron-deficiency anemia is made when the hematocrit is less than 33 or hemoglobin is less than 11. Iron preparations of up to 200 mg/day of iron are given. Iron-deficiency anemia can be prevented by a daily supplement of 30 to 60 mg of iron. The most commonly used preparation is ferrous sulfate. The inclusion of food sources rich in iron in the daily diet will also help prevent anemia. It is particularly important to institute these measures early for the woman who is at risk for iron deficiency—the woman who has a poor diet, has had frequent pregnancies, or a prior history of iron-deficiency anemia.

Folic acid deficiencies can produce megaloblastic anemia in pregnancy, most often in combination with iron deficiency. During pregnancy, folic acid absorption is somewhat decreased while there are increased maternal-fetal tissue synthesis needs. Dietary intake is frequently inadequate to meet the needs in pregnancy, particularly in low socioeconomic groups. Therefore, the National Research Council on Maternal Nutrition recommends supplemental sources 200 to 400 μg/day as well as assuring food sources in the diet.

Toxemia

Toxemia of pregnancy, a disease of the third trimester, is characterized by hypertension, albuminuria, and sudden excessive weight gain accompanied by edema. The cause of the disease is unknown and there are conflicting opinions on management. It seems increasingly evident, however, that nutritional factors play an important role. Standards of living and, therefore, quality of prenatal care and nutritional status appear related to the incidence of toxemia. The highest mortality rate occurs in the lowest income group. Factors associated with poverty that affect the outcome of pregnancy and appear related to development of toxemia are availability and quality of prenatal care, general poor health with chronic conditions, prevalence of poor nutrition resulting from a lifetime of poor food habits, ignorance of good health practices, emotional stress, and young age at first pregnancy.

The organ most affected by toxemia appears to be the liver. Multiple hemorrhagic changes occur, possibly caused by intense vasospasms of the hepatic arterioles. It is also thought that liver tissue changes may be the result of metabolic malfunction caused by malnutrition (Worthington et al., 1977). Renal tissue is also severely compromised. Pregnancy requires enormous physiologic and metabolic changes in the human organism. The liver, as the major metabolic organ of the body, must meet the increased functional demands; therefore, a healthy functioning liver is basic to a healthy pregnancy. In order to have a healthy liver, optimal nutritional input is essential. The role of nutrition is critical in the development and outcome of toxemia.

Protein is essential to provide the basic amino acid, necessary for growth in pregnancy. In addition, three functional roles of protein need to be considered in relation to toxemia:

1. Fluid and electrolyte balance. Albumin is of major importance in the maintenance of serum osmotic balance and, thereby, the capillary fluid shift mechanism. The liver is the sole source of albumin, which it constructs from amino acids derived in large part from dietary protein. Thus the two factors necessary for synthesis of albumin and normal operation of the capillary fluid shift mechanism and water exchange throughout the body are continuous optimal dietary sources of adequate protein and a healthy functioning liver.
2. Lipid transport. Protein is the major means of transporting lipids in the bloodstream. The transport vehicles, the lipoproteins, are formed mainly in the liver. When this process is interfered with by inadequate supply of protein or a malfunctioning liver, fat is not converted to lipoprotein transport and fatty deposits build up in the liver.
3. Tissue synthesis. Protein is the basic ingredient needed for building and maintaining protein. Therefore, the maintenance of a healthy functioning liver is dependent upon optimal protein supply and utilization.

These basic protein functions are related to the metabolic functioning of the liver and, therefore, to toxemia. It has been demonstrated that hypoalbuminemia and hypovolemia are characteristic of pre-eclampsia and eclampsia (Worthington et al., 1977).

A sufficient supply of nonprotein calories is essential to meet energy needs and protect protein sources. This assumes additional significance in relation to toxemia, in light of the widespread practice to restrict calories in an effort to control weight and thereby supposedly reduce the risks of toxemia. This practice is dangerous and unfounded in scientific fact. There is a greater incidence of toxemia in underweight women and in women who do not gain weight normally during pregnancy. Eastman (NRC, 1974) refutes the notion that excessive weight gain is correlated with increased incidence of toxemia. What is important is not the total amount of weight gain but rather the quality of the gain as measured by nutritional intake and pattern of weight gain.

Sodium has also been erroneously restricted in an effort to decrease edema and thereby toxemia. In pregnancy, when the total extracellular fluid is increased, the total amount of its major cation, sodium, must also be increased. In toxemia, sodium retention increases in direct relation to increased edema. Edema and sodium retention are decreased by re-establishing normal circulating blood volume through correcting hypoalbuminemia and thus getting better operation of the capillary fluid shift mechanism. Sodium retention only compounds the problem by stressing the renin-angiotensin-aldosterone system, causing exhaustion of the adrenal secretory cells. Another common practice, the use of diuretics to decrease edema, can further impair renin secretion and damage the structure and function of the adrenals. Pitkin and associates (1972) state that diuretics are of no value in preventing toxemia and in treatment are of limited value at best. At times their use can lead to extreme electrolyte imbalances. Routine sodium restriction and use of diuretics are potentially dangerous in normal pregnancy and in toxemia.

The best way to handle toxemia is to prevent it. The most effective way to prevent it is through good prenatal care, and a primary ingredient of good prenatal care is sound nutrition. Establishment and maintenance of a good nutritional status are basic to a healthy pregnancy with good maternal and fetal outcomes.

Diabetes

Pregnancy is a diabetogenic event. In order to care for the pregnant person with diabetes the nurse needs an understanding of the metabolic states of pregnancy and the way in which diabetes affects and alters these. In pregnancy, energy needs and fuel requirements to meet these needs are increased. Glucose is the primary fuel, particularly for the growing fetus. The fetal uptake rate of glucose is at least twice that of an adult. To meet fetal needs, glucose is transferred rapidly from the mother to the fetus through simple diffusion and active transport. While glucose crosses the placental barrier, insulin does not, and the fetus is dependent upon its own supply for development. Maternal fasting blood glucose levels drop as a result of rapid fetal uptake of glucose and glucose precursor amino acids. The drop in maternal blood levels decreases the fasting insulin levels, which leads to starvation ketosis. The net response of the mother to even brief fasting is hypoglycemia, hypoaminoacidemia, hypoinsulinemia, and finally hyperketonemia. The ketosis can be taken by the fetus as an alternative fuel source; however, this carries a risk of fetal brain damage. Changes in maternal fasting glucose levels result not only from fetal demands but also from increased secretion of placental hormones. Normal glucose tolerance is maintained, however, by increased maternal secretion of insulin.

The normal energy metabolism of pregnancy and the maternal-fetal relationship have certain implications for the person with diabetes. During the first half of pregnancy the increased transfer of maternal glucose to the fetus along with the often lowered food intake because of nausea and vomiting may result in reduced insulin requirements. The decreased availability of maternal circulatory blood glucose may create a decreased need for insulin. In the second half of pregnancy the diabetogenic effects of the placental hormones override the continuous fetal drain of glucose so that insulin requirements are increased by as much as 65% to 70%. At the same time that insulin efficiency is decreased, the tendency to ketoacidosis is increased because blood glucose levels do not increase markedly. The pregnant diabetic may have ketonuria reflecting starvation ketosis or diabetic ketosis. It is essential that the practitioner be able to differentiate between the two.

Diet is critical in the management of the pregnant woman who has diabetes. Energy input or calories must balance energy needs to reach and maintain ideal weight. During pregnancy, total energy needs are determined by maternal-fetal growth demands and overall increased metabolic needs. The National Research Council on Maternal Nutrition recommends that the diabetic pregnant woman consume from 2000 to 2400 calories daily. The proportions of nutrients used to meet caloric needs are important. Approximately 45% of total calories should be supplied by carbohydrates. It is best that the carbohydrates be in complex forms such as starches, vegetables, and fruits, which are slowly digested and absorbed. The pregnant diabetic should consume at least 100 to 120 gm of protein each day. This is greater than the general recommendation of 86 gm for pregnant women because of the importance of protein for diabetes control. Fat needs are not primary in pregnancy and should be kept at moderate levels of about 30% to 35% of total calories.

Regular distribution of the total diet throughout the day to balance insulin activity is important. A pattern of three meals a day with afternoon and evening snacks is advisable. Each meal and snack should include both protein and carbohydrate. The usual diabetic food exchange system can be used to make selections. For any diabetes except class A or gestational diabetes, insulin is needed throughout pregnancy. Insulin requirements usually drop in the first half of pregnancy but rise in the second half with dosage requirements increasing 70% to 100% above nonpregnant needs.

Starvation ketosis may occur more easily in pregnancy because of rapid fetal uptake of glucose, possibly compounded by nausea and vomiting or caloric restriction. In this condition, blood ketones may be elevated two to three times above normal but hyperglycemia is *not* present. Treatment consists of glucose solution and food rather than insulin. *Diabetic ketoacidosis* occurs in the presence of hyperglycemia. Treatment involves administration of rapid-acting regular insulin, hypotonic fluids, and potassium supplements.

Pica

Pica is the general term for the habit of eating nonfood substances. Varieties of pica found in the United States include clay, starch, chalk, and unusual quantities of ice. Pica is found in all ages and both sexes; however, the practice is most common in pregnant women. The underlying cause of pica is unknown. Pica is associated with a higher incidence of malnutrition. There is also a strong link between pica and iron deficiency; however, the exact relationship is not clear.

Pica is thought by some researchers to cause anemia by binding dietary iron, making it useless to the body. Clay with a high cation exchange capacity effectively blocks iron absorption. Magnesium oxide found in antacids used for pica prevents iron absorption. It has also been suggested that nonfood substances take the place of iron-containing foods, causing anemia. For example, laundry starch provides empty calories, thus decreasing hunger; but these are calories without iron. Other researchers believe that depleted iron stores lead to pica—that pica is a consequence, not a cause, of iron deficiency.

The reasons for pica have not been clearly identified. One important factor is culture and tradition. In a study in Alabama it was determined that women ate substances such as clay, cornstarch, flour, and baby powder because they believed these substances would relieve nausea, prevent vomiting, relieve dizziness, cure swelling, relieve headaches, and make sure the children were attractive.[38] Other women have reported a belief that clay contains substances that are beneficial for the child. Frustration of cravings are considered to be a delicacy. One of the author's clients once very carefully described when the "best" clay was found on the river bank and how to cook and clean it. Moore (1978) reports that women describe the best clay as being "good, gummy, crunchy, or bitter." Starch is described as "good, smooth, sweet, bitter, or thick" (p. 270). These women appeared to enjoy eating clay or starch.

Pica is potentially dangerous for both the woman and her baby. The ingestion of empty calories instead of foods containing essential nutrients can lead to malnourishment. Anemia is commonly associated with pica, as already noted. Intestinal and pyloric obstruction in the mother, prematurity, toxemia, and perinatal mortality have all been linked to pica during pregnancy (Luke, 1977b).

It is not easy to discourage ingestion of nonfood substances in those pregnant women who practice it. For the nurse, the most immediate need is to identify pica. Often direct questions about diet will uncover the fact. An open-ended question about cravings or eating unusual substances is most likely to detect pica. The nurse should determine how much is being eaten, why it is being eaten, and when the woman practices pica. With this information and a thorough dietary assessment, the nurse can begin nutrition education. She needs to provide the client with in-depth nutritional guidance, including explanations of the significance of good diet and the potential harm current eating practices may cause. Iron supplementation is essential.

Food taboos

Superstitions and taboos about food are as old as human life. Pregnancy seems to be a time of high concern about food taboos with strong connotation as to what is beneficial or harmful. When these taboos are grounded in ignorance, they can have a deleterious effect on the pregnant client's diet. Bartholomeu and Poston (1970) found many superstitions associated with protein and protein-rich foods. For example, milk would supposedly cause cancer if you were pregnant, while pork or fish would "rot" the uterus. Cheese was thought to cause "dry labor," as were peanuts. Green leafy vegetables were taboo because they would "mark the baby." From these examples it is easy to see why dietary inadequacies of protein, calcium, iron, and vitamins A and C might occur. While poor nutrition is most often the result of nutritional ignorance, specific food dislikes, inavailability, superstition, and bizarre food traditions can be significant.

Lactose intolerance

The majority of the world's population is unable to digest varying quantities of milk because of low levels of activity of the lactose enzyme. The mother who says she just cannot drink milk because it makes her sick may be lactose intolerant. In cultures that never kept dairy animals or included milk in the adult diet, the population has an almost 100% intolerance. There is also a very high percentage of intolerance (85% to 100%) in cultures that may have kept dairy animals but never include significant quantities of milk in the adult diet. Such populations include the Chinese, Thais, Filipinos, and most African blacks. The incidence of intolerance is low (15% to 25%) in the cultures of the Middle East, the herdsmen of eastern Africa, and most Europeans and their descendants. These cultures use lactose-rich foods in their diet. The intolerance is insignificant because the black populations of the United States were drawn primarily from the "high-intolerance" areas of Western Africa. Other ethnic groups, such as the Vietnamese, may also have problems.

Lactose is the enzyme responsible for the hydrolysis of lactose into glucose and galactose. If lactose is not broken down it enters the large intestine undigested where it pulls water from the surrounding tissue into the intestinal lumen. It is also fermented by bacteria present in the colon, producing organic acids, carbon dioxide, and hydrogen. These cause the symptoms of lactose intolerance—abdominal cramps, bloating, diarrhea, and flatulence (Luke, 1977a).

A quart of whole milk supplies 100% of recommended dietary allowances of vitamin D and calcium and 50% of the protein recommended during pregnancy. Milk is economical, convenient, and readily available in the United States. For these reasons it is always included in dietary recommendations for pregnancy. For lactose-intolerant women, it is not an option. Another problem facing these women is that lactose facilitates the body's use of minerals and protein and its absorption of calcium. The ingestion of milk by women with lactose intolerance produces harmful effects—calcium is lost through the feces and they develop a negative calcium balance. Pregnant women with lactose intolerance or low calcium intake appear to be more prone to skeletal demineralization and hyperparathyroidism secondary to nutritional factors; and their infants are more likely than other infants to have neonatal hypocalcemia (Luke, 1977a).

All pregnant women need to be counseled to include adequate calcium-rich foods in their diet. Women who cannot or will not drink milk should be advised of alternative foods. Cheese, which is an excellent source of calcium, has a very low lactose content. Many lactose-intolerant women find they experience fewer and less severe symptoms if dairy products are well chilled. The nurse might suggest ice cream as a substitute for milk. Of all the milk substitutes, cheese is the most valuable for its calcium, lactose, and protein content per ounce. It can be used in a variety of ways and should become a staple in the lactose-intolerant pregnant woman's diet. If the woman dislikes all cheeses, calcium supplements may be used as a last alternative. They supply calcium but do not contribute the other nutrients found in dietary sources.

Adolescent pregnancy

When pregnancy occurs in adolescence, there are potential physical and psychologic risks. Adolescence is a period of rapid growth and development that requires substantial nutritional intake. Increased amounts of food are needed, as well as specific nutrients related to pubertal growth spurts. Teenagers who become pregnant in the 4 years following menarche are at biologic risk because they are anatomically and physiologically immature. Pregnancy may occur before skeletal growth, most particularly of the pelvis, is completed. In addition, nutritional states at conception and during pregnancy determine in part the nutritional state and reproductive capability of the subsequent generation. These may be compromised in the adolescent who is pregnant.

Caloric needs are usually greater during pregnancy and during adolescence. Caloric requirements for the pregnant teenager may be as much as 400 calories/day greater than for the nonpregnant woman. This assumes additional significance in light of the teenager's widespread practice of dieting and the still-prevalent notions of weight control in pregnancy. Protein needs are also high for the pregnant teenager to meet both her own and her baby's growth needs. The need is intensified for the teenager who has a poor nutritional history. A protein intake of 92 gm/day is recommended. More calcium is needed to provide for fetal skeletal development and to prevent compromising the maternal skeleton by demineralization. Iron needs are at least 18 mg/day. Adequate nutritional intake of all other vitamins and minerals, as outlined in Table 21-1, is recommended.

Several studies have attempted to determine the nutritional status of pregnant adolescents in order to ascertain exactly what problems exist. McGanty et al. (1977) has found that intakes of calcium, iron, vitamin A, and niacin are low in the pregnant adolescent. Many adolescents enter pregnancy with unacceptable stores of iron, vitamins A and C, and riboflavin. Pica was present in 28% of the girls surveyed. Smith (1969) reports that only 30% of the girls he surveyed had diets rated as good. Milk and dairy products, fruits, and vegetables were consumed in low quantities, resulting in low dietary intakes of calcium, vitamin A, and vitamin C. Most had a fair intake of protein.

Teenagers consume more food during pregnancy than when they are not pregnant, according to a study done by King (1972), but he found that not one nutrient was adequately supplied. Protein intake was most nearly adequate, while calcium, iron, vitamin A, and energy sources were least adequate. Eighty-five percent had some nutritionally based problem such as inadequate weight gain, proteinuria, anemia, glycosuria, rapid weight gain and/or clinical edema. Osofsky and others (1971) corroborated other findings that teenage diets were inadequate in iron, calcium, and vitamin A; they also found poor protein intakes. Skipped meals and fad diets were common. In addition, Seiter and Fox (1973) found that although dietary supplements improved the diets of some pregnant girls, erratic use of the supplements was reported, and few girls appeared to take them throughout pregnancy.

Given the pregnant adolescent's increased nutritional needs to provide optimal growth conditions for herself and her offspring, and given the fact that adolescents frequently do not meet their needs for several essential nutrients, it is imperative that the nurse encourage positive nutritional patterns for the adolescent. This requires an individualized approach to the problem for each girl.

Nursing implications

Nutritional counseling is an integral component of comprehensive nursing care for the maternity client. Counseling begins with an in-depth assessment of maternal nutrition early in prenatal care and proceeds to individualized guidance based on the assessment. Three basic methods of assessment will provide the data necessary to determine nutritional needs. These are (1) a thorough history, (2) physical examination, and (3) laboratory tests. Primary factors to include in the basic history are age, marital status, previous obstetric history, and prior medical, social, personal, and nutritional histories. The nurse should be able to recognize factors that place the client at nutritional risk, collect a nutrition history, perform selected physical examination procedures, and interpret laboratory tests to assess nutritional adequacy.

Many factors may place the client at increased nutritional risk. These are summarized in Table 21-4. The presence of one or more of these indicates a need for a more intensive nutritional assessment than that provided by routine history, physical examination, and laboratory tests. The information gathered from carefully taken medical, obstetric, and personal histories is a good way to begin determining the client at nutritional risk.

The diet history is an indispensable component of nutritional assessment, yet it is rarely a routine component of clinical practice. This may result from lack of training and experience, time constraints, or lack of recognition of its value. A diet history need not be time-consuming, and it can be both informative for the practitioner and educational for the client. The process is begun by collecting some general data. The pregnant woman is first a person with specific attitudes towards food, emotional responses to food, cultural beliefs about food, and information about nutrition that must be explored. It is also important to know how she views health, being pregnant, and bearing a child. It is important to explore her

Table 21-4. Nutritional risk factors

Factor	Significance
Age	The adolescent whose reproductive biologic age (chronologic age minus menarche age) is less than 3 is at particular risk because of her own growth needs. Adolescent pregnancy may also be associated with emotional, financial, and educational risks. Advanced age may be associated with high parities. Age of menarche is significant in that it can be delayed by poor nutrition.
Reproductive performance	Short interconceptual periods are a risk factor, particularly when coupled with high parity. Past obstetric history of abortions, poor weight gain, anemia, generalized edema, stillbirth, toxemia, low birth weight infants, and premature labor are also factors.
Chronic systemic illness	Anemia, thyroid dysfunction, diabetes, chronic infection, malabsorption syndromes, and severe emotional/psychosocial problems constitute risk factors, as do drugs used to treat these illnesses that may interfere with nutrition.
Weight	Low pregnant weight or low weight (less than 85%) for height may indicate long-term nutritional inadequacy. Inadequate weight gain during pregnancy is a risk factor, as is obesity above 120% of standard weight for height.
Unusual nutritional patterns	Food fads and/or constant dieting can result in inadequate food intake. Pica is a special risk. Special dietary restrictions because of ethnic or cultural factors may also cause nutrition problems.
Substance abuse	Use of tobacco, drugs, or alcohol may decrease nutrition intake and directly affect fetal growth and development.
Economic deprivation	Inability to purchase adequate amounts of the required nutrients and chronic, low level nutritional inadequacy constitute risks.

Table 21-5. Symptoms of nutritional deficits

Deficit	Symptoms
Calories	Underweight, short stature, weight loss, lethargy, anemia, edema, acetone breath
Protein	As for calories, plus sizable nondependent edema
Iron/folate	Anemia, filiform papillary atrophy of tongue, glossitis
Iodine	Goiter
Vitamin A	Follicular hyperkeratosis of upper arms, growth failure, night blindness
Vitamin C	Swollen, red papillae of gums
Riboflavin	Photophobia, dermatitis

cial practices, food allergies or intolerance, and medication or supplements routinely taken must be ascertained.

Once the nurse has gathered the requisite background information, a specific diet history should be obtained. A technique suited to many types of clinical practice is the 24-hour recall. It is relatively accurate, simple, and brief, and does not require a lot of experience to use it. Fig. 21-2 is an example of a 24-hour recall diet history form. During the process of taking a diet history, much valuable information about the woman's level of nutritional knowledge and tips for counseling methods can be obtained. In addition to the types of food eaten, amounts and method of preparation should be recorded. At times it is useful to supplement the 24-hour recall with a 7-day list of foods eaten.

A thorough general physical examination is a standard component of prenatal care. Unfortunately, physical evidence of poor nutrition usually appears relatively late and is often nonspecific and subtle. The practitioner needs to be careful to distinguish between nutritionally significant findings and normal maternal physiologic changes of pregnancy (for example, dependent edema or gingival hyperplasia). Symptoms of specific nutrient deficiencies during pregnancy are given in Table 21-5.

Perhaps the single most significant physical finding indicating nutritional adequacy is weight—both prepregnant weight and gain during pregnancy. Clients who weigh less than 85% or more than 120% of the standard weight for height are judged nutritionally inadequate. In addition, poor weight gain during pregnancy or sudden, excessive bursts of weight gain can indicate nutritional problems. Obesity may indicate poor protein and iron intakes.

Intrauterine growth retardation or failure may indicate poor nutritional status. Significant negative discrepancy between gestational age and fundal height indicates intrauterine growth retardation. Dental caries and peri-

cultural beliefs about food, particularly in relation to appropriate foods during pregnancy. Determining her birthplace and early childhood home can help identify cultural food influences. The nurse needs to identify the value food holds for the client in terms of nutritional status, appetites, and emotional significance. Inquiry should be made as to the impact of economic factors on food selection, storage, and preparation. It is helpful to know how much control the pregnant woman has over food preparation and purchasing. The expectant mother's education and occupation should be noted. Any spe-

```
(Questions on this form can be adapted for use with any patient)

                   NUTRITIONAL HISTORY FORM

Name_____ Address_____

Race_____ Age_____ Height_____ Weight_____

Vitamin or mineral supplements taken_____

Salt intake: light, moderate, or heavy

                 Foods eaten in last 24 hours
```

Kind and amount of food and drink (List main foods in mixed dishes)	Number of servings				
	Milk	Meat	Veg/ fruits	Bread cereal	Misc. (list)
Morning					
Midmorning					
Noon					
Afternoon					
Evening					
Before bed					
Total servings eaten Recommended servings Comparison	___	___	___	___	___

What food and drink do you think people should have to keep healthy?

Fig. 21-2

odontitis may cause mechanical difficulties that interfere with eating.

More objective precise information about nutritional status can be obtained from laboratory assessments. Laboratory tests often reflect poor nutrition well before it is clinically evident. Interpretation may be difficult because established norms for pregnant women are not always available, and the relationship of certain nutrients to pregnant and pregnant status is not always clear. Table 21-6 summarizes those laboratory tests that appear to be most significant.

Once all baseline data from the physical, dietary, and general history and laboratory studies have been gathered, evaluation of the client's nutritional status may be done jointly by the nurse and client. The diet is analyzed to determine its adequacy to meet the increased nutritional needs of pregnancy. Using a food chart, the diet is analyzed for calories, protein, calcium, iron, and key vitamins and minerals. The diet is then compared with the recommended dietary allowances for pregnancy (see Table 21-1). These findings along with laboratory data and physical findings will identify the strengths and weaknesses of the expectant mother's diet and nutritional status. From this point, nutritional counseling may proceed.

Table 21-6. Laboratory assessment of nutritional status in pregnancy

Test	Rationale	Normal values	
		Nonpregnant	Pregnant
Hematocrit/hemoglobin	To determine presence or absence of anemia	>12/30	>11/33
Serum iron/iron-binding capacity	To detect iron-deficiency anemias	>50/250 to 400 μg per 100 ml	>40/300 to 450
Serum albumin	To detect protein deficiency	3.5-5 mg/100 ml	3-4.5 Gm
Fasting blood sugar	To detect gestational diabetes	70-100 mg/100 ml	65-100
Folic acid, serum	To determine folic acid deficiency/ megaloblastic anemia	5-21 mg/ml	3-15
Urinalysis for protein and glucose levels	Protein: detection of preeclampsia Glucose: screen for diabetes	0/0	0/0*

*Occasionally trace protein results may indicate contamination of specimen with vaginal secretion.

Table 21-7. Summary of available sources and amounts of recommended dietary allowances for pregnancy

Nutrient	Daily amount	Purpose	Food sources	Basic 4 food group
Protein	76 to 90 Gm	Rapid fetal tissue growth	Milk	1 qt daily
		Amniotic fluid	Cheese	2+ oz hard cheese or ½ cup cottage cheese
		Placenta growth and development	Eggs	2
		Maternal tissue growth; uterus, breasts	Meats	2 (¾ oz.) servings
		Increased maternal circulating blood volume:	Grains, breads, cereals	4-5 slices or servings whole grains and enriched
		Hemoglobin increase	Legumes, nuts	Occasionally as substitute for meat (6-8 oz) or in combination
		Plasma protein increase		
		Maternal storage reserves for labor, delivery, and lactation		
Calories	2400	Increased BMR, energy needs	Carbohydrates	Milk group
		Protein sparing	Fats	Bread group
			Proteins	Meat group
Calcium	1200 mg	Fetal skeleton formation	Dairy products	1 qt milk (as above)
		Fetal tooth bud formation	Grains, whole or enriched	4-5 slices or servings (as above)
		Increased maternal calcium metabolism	Green leafy vegetables	1 serving
Phosphorus	1200 mg	Fetal skeletal formation	Milk	1 qt
		Fetal tooth bud formation	Cheese	2 oz cheese
		Increased maternal phosphorus metabolism	Lean meats	2 (3-4 oz) serving
Iron	18 mg (30-60 mg supplement)	Increased maternal circulating blood volume, increased hemoglobin	Organ meats, especially liver	1-2 servings per week
			Egg yolk	2
		Fetal liver iron storage	Green leafy vegetables or dried fruits	1-2 servings
		High iron cost of pregnancy	Grains, enriched	4-5 slices or servings
Iodine	125 μg	Increased BMR—increased thyroxine production	Iodized salt	Daily in cooking and on foods
			Seafood	1-2 servings per week

Table 21-7. Summary of available sources and amounts of recommended dietary allowances for pregnancy—cont'd

Nutrient	Daily amount	Purpose	Food sources	Basic 4 food group
Magnesium	450 mg	Coenzyme in energy protein metabolism	Whole grains	
			Nuts	Occasionally as meat substitute
		Enzyme activator	Soybeans	
		Tissue growth, cell metabolism	Dried beans and peas	
			Cocoa	With milk
		Muscle action	Seafood	As part of daily meat allowance
Vitamin A	5000 IU	Essential for cell development, hence tissue growth	Butterfat (whole milk, cream, butter)	2 tbsp butter (or fortified margarine)
		Tooth bud formation (development of enamel-forming cells in gum tissue)	Liver	1-2 servings per week
			Egg yolk	2 servings per week
			Dark green or deep yellow vegetables or fruits	1-2 servings
			Fortified margarine	2 tbsp
Vitamin C	60 mg	Tissue formation and integrity	Citrus	1 or 2 servings
		Cement substance in connective and vascular tissues	Other fruits—papayas, strawberries, melons	Occasional serving to substitute for 1 citrus portion
		Increased iron absorption	Broccoli, potatoes, tomato, cabbage, green or chili peppers	1 serving as a substitute for 1 citrus occasionally
Folic acid	800 μg	Increased metabolic demand in pregnancy	Liver, dark green vegetables, dried beans, lentils, nuts, (peanuts, walnuts, filberts)	1 serving
		Prevention of megaloblastic anemia in high-risk patients		
		Increased heme production for hemoglobin		
		Production of cell nucleus material		
Vitamin D	400 IU	Bone growth	Fortified milk	1 qt
		Absorption of calcium and phosphorus, mineralization of bone tissue, tooth buds	Fortified margarine	
Vitamin E	15 IU	Tissue growth, cell wall integrity	Vegetable oils	
			Leafy vegetables	2-3 servings
		Red blood cell integrity	Cereals	
			Meat	3-4 servings
			Egg	2
			Milk	1 qt
Niacin	15 mg	Coenzyme in energy metabolism	Meat	2 servings
			Peanuts	Occasional substitute
		Coenzyme in protein metabolism	Beans and peas	Occasional substitute
			Enriched grains	4-5 servings a day
Riboflavin	1.5 mg	Coenzyme in energy metabolism and protein metabolism	Milk	1 qt
			Liver	2-3 times a week
			Enriched grains	4-5 servings
Thiamine	1.3	Coenzyme for energy metabolism	Pork, beef	2 servings
			Liver	2-3 times a week
			Whole or enriched grains	4-5 servings a day
			Legumes	Occasionally
Vitamin B₆	2.5	Coenzyme in protein metabolism	Wheat, corn	2 servings a day
			Liver	2-3 times a week
		Increased fetal growth requirement	Meat	2 servings a day
Vitamin B₁₂	4.0 μg	Coenzyme in protein metabolism, especially vital cell proteins such as nucleic acid	Milk	1 qt
			Egg	2
			Meat	2 servings
			Liver	2-3 servings per week
		Formation of red blood cells	Cheese	2 oz a day

In beginning nutritional counseling, the practitioner needs to recognize that nutrition may not be a top priority with the pregnant woman. She may not be aware of its significance to her own and her infant's well-being. She may have no concept of the relationship between health and food ingestion. Cultural beliefs may prevent proper nutrition in pregnancy. The woman may not have control of food preparation or food purchasing. There can be a sense of futility—a focusing on the present—that makes it difficult for the woman to plan for the future. She may be experiencing high stress levels with corresponding reactions that are not conducive to good nutrition; for example, some persons overeat in periods of stress, while others experience anorexia and do not eat at all. Any or all of these factors prevent adequate nutrition.

All of the knowledge nurses have about prenatal nutrition is useless unless it is used by the client. Many expectant mothers are interested and motivated to make the changes needed in their diets. For these women, providing information initially and following up at subsequent prenatal visits is all that is usually required. There is a second group—those women who are either not able, interested, or willing to change their diets—who may require the nurse's most creative intervention to motivate them to improve their diets.

Learning is more easily effected when the client is ready to learn, which includes possessing motivation to learn. Two principles of health behavior motivation help explain nutritional behavior: (1) a person's health behavior is a result of perceived health benefit or threat and belief about courses of action available; (2) individual's motives and beliefs about courses of action often conflict and the behavior seen is a resolution of these conflicts (Rosenstock, 1960). It is important for the practitioner to recognize that health behaviors often are based on feelings and beliefs and not necessarily on facts. Therefore, it is essential to assess the client's value system as well as to determine her knowledge level. When this is done, the nurse can give her facts to deal with her beliefs. Facts can fill gaps in information and correct misinformation. Success in altering nutritional behavior will be in direct proportion to how well the practitioner understands the client. Nutrition counseling should be adapted to the woman, not the reverse.

Nutrition counseling begins where the individual woman is and is tailored to meet her needs. The goals should be clearly identified, realistic, and challenging yet attainable. Nutritional instruction must be meaningful and not beyond the client's ability to comprehend. New material is built on what is already known so that it is readily associated. Using a variety of teaching aids increases the likelihood of understanding and remem-

Table 21-8. Basic daily meal plan during pregnancy

Meat	2-3 servings
Milk	4 cups
Grains	4-5 servings
Vitamin C–rich fruit and vegetables	1 serving
Vitamin A–rich fruit and vegetables	1 serving
Other fruit or vegetable	2 servings

bering. Material to take home, such as pamphlets, can be used for continued reference.

The "basic four," as described by the U.S. Department of Agriculture, is an excellent guide for well-balanced nutrition. It is a foundation on which nutritional counseling is built. From this foundation, the nursing practitioner can help the pregnant woman or couple convert recommended dietary allowances into specific amounts and types of food. Table 21-7 summarizes this information; Table 21-8 is an example of a basic meal plan during pregnancy.

Individual prenatal nutritional counseling should include reinforcement of good food habits as well as new information. The nurse can strengthen good habits by pointing out the relationship of positive food practices to nutritional needs in pregnancy, by reviewing the reasons for the increased nutritional needs, and by giving warm praise for good habits. Nutritional deficiencies can be corrected in a constructive manner by helping the client identify the difficulties herself and the reasons for them. This can be followed by exploring possible alternative solutions to the problem. The woman should participate in the determination of nutritional assets and the diagnosis of nutritional deficits. She devises her own plan of care, thus enhancing self-care activities and the possibility of effecting positive change.

Many expectant mothers have special nutritional needs during pregnancy because of individual cultural, economic, or physiologic specifics. There is no standard diet in the United States. During pregnancy, ethnic variations in diet can prevent optimal nutrition. The practitioner needs to be familiar with cultural variations in diet and potential problems.

The American Indian diet has many tribal variations and many have become Americanized. Because of poverty, the diet may be inadequate in all nutrients. Carbohydrate intake is often high, while protein sources, fruits, vegetables, and milk are severely limited. Alcoholism, obesity, dental caries, and iron-deficiency anemia have also been identified (Jensen, 1977).

Oriental customs vary from one nationality to another; in addition, traditional diet patterns have become Americanized. Milk is rarely used and thus calcium and vitamin D need to be supplemented. Rice is a basic sta-

Table 21-9. The menus below show the cultural variations possible when planning a nutritionally adequate prenatal diet. All meet the Recommended Dietary Allowances for calories, provide a minimum of 90grams of protein, and exceed the Recommended Dietary Allowances for vitamin A and C and calcium. Only the Black and Mexican dietary pattern meets the Recommended Dietary Allowances for iron, providing 21.9 mg and 23.1 mg. The Regular, American-Indian, and the Oriental pattern provide 15.3 mg, 15.8, and 15.3 respectively. The Lacto-Ovo plan provides only 12.0 mg.*

	Regular	Mexican	Black	Oriental	American Indian	Lacto-ovo
Breakfast						
2 energy foods	1 cup Cream of Wheat 1 tbsp. sugar	2 corn tortillas 2 tbsp jelly	1 cup grits 1 tbsp. sugar	1 cup rice 1 tsp. sugar (in tea)	1 cup corn mush 1 tbsp. sugar	1 cup brown rice 1 tbsp. honey
1 calcium/protein food	1 cup milk	½ cup evaporated milk in coffee	1 cup milk or 1½ oz cheese	1 cup milk or 1½ oz cheese	1 cup milk	1 cup milk
1 vitamin C food	1 cup orange juice	1 cup orange juice	1 cup orange juice	1 cup orange juice	1 cup orange juice	1 cup orange juice
Lunch:						
1 energy food	1 slice bread	1 tortilla	1 2" square corn bread	½ cup rice	1 slice Indian fried bread	1 slice whole wheat bread
2 protein foods	2-1 oz. slice cheese	1 cup beans	1 cup pork and beans	3½ oz. tofu 1 egg	1 cup pinto beans	1 cup lentils
1 calcium/protein food	1 cup milk	½ cup evaporated milk and chocolate	1 cup milk	1 cup milk	1 cup milk	1 cup milk
1 vitamin A food	½ cup spinach	½ cup spinach 1 green pepper	½ cup collard greens	3/5 bok choy	½ cup spinach	½ cup spinach
1 vitamin/mineral food	1 banana	1 banana	1 banana	1 banana	1 apple	1 banana
Dinner:						
1 energy food	1 small baked potato	½ cup Spanish rice	2 halves candied yams	½ cup rice	½ cup fried potatoes	1 small baked potato
3 protein foods	3 oz. beef roast	1 cup beans 1 cup caldo	3½ oz. fried pork chops	Okazu (stewing beef 3 oz. and ½ cup broccoli and 2 oz. tofu)	3½ oz. fish	3½ oz. cheese (Cheddar)
1 calcium/protein food	1 cup milk	½ cup evaporated milk and coffee	1 cup milk	1 cup milk	1 cup milk	1 cup milk
2 vitamin/mineral foods	1 stalk broccoli 1 cup fruited Jello	1 cup fruited Jello	1 cup peas 1 cup fruited Jello	1 cup fruited Jello	1 stalk broccoli 1 cup fruited Jello	1 stalk broccoli ½ cup fruited Jello
Snacks:						
1 calcium/protein food	1 cup custard	1 cup flan	1 cup custard	1 cup custard	1 cup custard	1 cup custard
1 vitamin/mineral food	1 pear	1 pear	1 pear	1 pear	1 pear	1 pear
1 energy food	2 oatmeal-raisin cookies	2 oatmeal-raisin cookies	2 oatmeal-raisin cookies	2 oatmeal-raisin cookies	2 oatmeal-raisin cookies	2 oatmeal-raisin cookies

*From Cross, A. T., and Walsh, H. E.: Prenatal diet counseling, Reprod. Med. 7(6): 1971.

ple and should always be enriched and not washed. Large assortments of fruits and vegetables are used. Meats and fish are used in small quantities. Often protein and calorie intake is inadequate. Northern Chinese may have more grease in their cooking, while the Japanese may have an excessive salt intake.

The Spanish-American or Mexican woman may limit her meat intake because of limited finances. She eats little milk and milk products. Lard and sugar are often used in excessive amounts. Few leafy green or yellow vegetables are used. Vegetables may be boiled excessively. Consumption of carbonated beverages and other empty calorie foods is high. This client should be encouraged to use corn tortillas rather than flour-based ones.

The black culture makes extensive use of frying and fats such as salt pork, lard, and fat back. Carbohydrate intake is often high. Vegetables are often cooked excessively. Intake of citrus fruits and enriched breads is often insufficient. Limited amounts of milk are drunk.

Table 21-9 demonstrates how cultural variations may be used to plan a nutritionally adequate diet.

Vegetarian diets are becoming increasingly numerous for a variety of socioeconomic, cultural, religious, and personal reasons. Limited intake of protein can create hazards for the fetus and mother. There are three basic types of vegetarians: (1) pure vegetarians, who exclude all animal foods; (2) lacto-vegetarians, who allow the inclusion of dairy products; and (3) lacto-ovo-vegetarians, who include eggs and dairy products in the diet. In all three diets meat and poultry are excluded while all types of fruits, vegetables, legumes, grains, and nuts are allowed. Obviously, the more limited the diet, the more hazardous it is.

Vegetarians can have nutritionally adequate diets when they consume wide varieties of grains, legumes, fruits, vegetables, nuts, seeds, milk and milk products, and eggs in the right combinations so protein can be utilized. There are health advantages to vegetarian diets. Obesity is unusual, highly processed foods are usually avoided, and blood cholesterol levels are frequently lower than with other diets. Potential problems in pregnancy result from inadequate intake protein and calories, vitamin B_{12}, vitamin D, riboflavin, calcium, and iron. If dairy products are eaten, vitamin B_{12}, vitamin D, riboflavin, and calcium needs will be met. It is possible to plan a vegetarian diet that is adequate for all nutrients. In order to ensure an adequate diet, the use of milk, milk products, and eggs should be encouraged. In planning the diet, the basic four are still used. Meat is replaced with a generous intake of legumes, nuts, and meat analogues made from wheat and soy products. The milk group is altered toward use of greater amounts of low-fat milk and milk products such as cheese and cot-

tage cheese. Intake should increase slightly—fruits and vegetables are used to make up the needed caloric intake so that amounts selected are important. Vegetarians who adhere to the strictest form of the diet must have calcium, vitamin B_{12}, and vitamin D supplements. Iodized salt should always be used and iron supplements prescribed.

The foods that pregnant women need most, those high in protein, vitamins, and minerals, are often the most expensive. Women with limited incomes and poor nutritional knowledge often eat foods that fill their stomach—usually foods high in carbohydrates. It is frequently a serious challenge to the practitioner to assist the low-income client to devise a nutritionally sound, inexpensive diet. Suggestions such as the following may be useful:

1. Use nonfat dry milk whenever possible
2. Cheese is a good value because there is no waste and much nutritive value per ounce
3. Fish is a relatively inexpensive food with a high-protein per-ounce and per-unit cost ratio
4. Meats should be compared on a cost per serving basis
5. Cooked cereals are less expensive and a better source of nutrition than cold cereals

In all cases of nutritional counseling it is mandatory that food plans be realistic. For most women minimal guidance and assistance will result in a diet sufficient to meet their needs. For those women with real dietary problems and/or substantial pregnancy risks, careful supportive counseling is essential. Some type of follow-up support and evaluation must be a part of the ongoing nursing care. In all cases, nutritional counseling will enhance the pregnancy outcome, and in some isntances it may determine the success of the outcome.

NUTRITIONAL DISEASES
Effect of oral contraceptives on nutritional status

In America at present, large numbers of women in their reproductive years take oral contraceptives for extended periods of time. Recently, health care professionals have begun to ask what effect oral contraceptives may have on nutritional status and, in particular, whether the effect is unfavorable.

Oral contraceptives typically consist of a synthetic estrogen and one of several synthetic progestins taken in combination form. A number of studies (Prasad, 1976) suggest that women taking oral contraceptives experience altered metabolic needs for several nutrients. These are summarized in Table 21-10. Many of these changes appear to be reversed when hormone use is discontinued.

These alterations take on added significance in the woman who is already undernourished, for she is more likely then other women to develop deficiencies more

Table 21-10. Effect of oral contraceptives on nutritional needs

Need increased	Need decreased
Vitamin B_6 (similar to amount needed in pregnancy)	Vitamin A
	Copper
Folic acid	Iron (due in part to decreased menstrual flow)
Vitamin B_{12}	
Vitamin C (estrogen appears to increase rate of ascorbic acid breakdown)	

quickly. Vitamin C is involved in iron absorption, capillary maintenance, and wound healing. Symptoms of vitamin C deficiency are bleeding gums, capillary fragility, bruising, and anemia. Vitamin B is involved in many phases of protein metabolism and carbohydrate and fat utilization; deficiency causes depression, mood change, and alterations in sleep patterns. When folic acid stores are deficient, anemia, diarrhea, intestinal malabsorption, and sprue may result.

Carbohydrate metabolism may be altered in users of oral contraceptives. Estrogen can cause increased insulin secretion, increased secretion of growth hormone, and an elevation of serum glucose levels. Results of the glucose tolerance test are abnormal in 10% to 11% of women who have taken oral contraceptives for a year (Belsey, 1977). This is usually reversed within 3 months of discontinuation. Certain women may be more prone to have abnormal results of the glucose tolerance test. These are women who have a family history of diabetes or history of previously abnormal test results, have delivered large babies, are obese, are older, or have high parity.

Oral contraceptives have an effect on protein metabolism similar to pregnancy. The concentration of blood coagulation factors increases. There is a clear relationship between oral contraceptives and thromboembolic disease (see Chapter 22). The interactions between oral contraceptives, nutritional state, and thromboembolic occurrences are not known; nor is the exact role nutrition might play in enhancing or preventing thromboembolic disease known. If the woman is in a poor nutritional state for protein, oral contraceptives will possibly have a further deleterious effect.

Oral contraceptives are associated with increased levels of triglycerides, cholesterol, phospholipids, and lecithin. Increased serum lipid levels are associated with an increased risk of vascular occlusive disease. There is a definite association between increased myocardial infarction and oral contraceptives, but it is not known whether this is the result of thromboembolic effects or altered lipid metabolism.

The World Health Organization suggests three questions that need to be explored for women with nutritional disorders who are taking oral contraceptives (Belsey, 1977):

1. Do oral contraceptives aggravate existing borderline deficiencies or chronic infections?
2. Are there effects of oral contraceptives that improve existing disease status?
3. Is the presence of nutritional deficiency or other disease associated with higher or lower risks of metabolic side effects?

The existing information about the effect of oral contraceptives on nutritional status suggests the need for a careful assessment of dietary patterns if malnourishment is suspected. All clients should be provided with dietary teaching to increase amounts of vitamin C, vitamin B_6, folic acid, and vitamin B_{12} in their diets. Women who are at risk for the problems associated with oral contraceptives, such as those with diabetes, hypertension, and obesity, as well as older women, should be carefully monitored. Counseling about alternative methods of contraception for women at risk should be provided.

The intrauterine device is associated with increased incidence of anemia because of hypermenstruation. Some recommend routine iron supplementation for all women with an IUD. Certainly, a hematocrit should be performed at 6 months following insertion and at yearly intervals thereafter.

Nutritional anemias

Approximately one-third to one-half of all American women of reproductive age are anemic, as compared to 10% of males and 13% of women over 40 years (Herbert, 1977). Up to 60% of all pregnant women are anemic. Menstrual loss of iron is the primary source of loss in nonpregnant women (about 20 mg iron per cycle). In women who experience menorrhagia, the loss may be as high as 80 mg iron per cycle. In pregnancy, the fetal need for iron combined with low prepregnant stores results in anemia. Absorption of iron from different food sources is highly variable, usually only about 10%. This is significant because the average American diet provides an iron intake from dietary sources that is borderline for adolescents and adult women in the reproductive years and that is definitely inadequate for pregnant women. Many women enter pregnancy with inadequate iron stores in the face of increased demands. The iron needs of pregnancy should be met by iron supplementation. Menorrhagia may also cause a need for iron supplementation.

Anorexia nervosa

Anorexia nervosa has been described as a disease of "the young, the rich and the beautiful" (Bruch, 1970).

Ninety percent of those suffering from anorexia are women, usually adolescent girls. It is rarely found in the lower socioeconomic classes and, in fact, according to Bruch, has never been described in an underdeveloped home. The girls are usually well-educated, intelligent adolescents who achieve well in school. Most of them have been raised in financially secure homes by parents who appear, at least initially, to have stable marriages. Family size is usually small, approximately 2.8 children per family. The parents are often older and the siblings are usually sisters (Bruch, 1970).

Anorexia nervosa is usually a disease of adolescence with age of onset often being around puberty or early teens. The age range of many girls with anorexia is between 15 and 20 years. Often these girls are considered plump or somewhat overweight prior to the onset of anorexia. In general, the incidence of anorexia in psychiatric hospitals or clinics is about one in 300 patients (Szyrynski, 1978). Bruch (1978) feels the incidence is increasing as a result of several factors:

1. The enormous value our culture places on thinness. The message often given is that one can only be loved and respected when one is slender.
2. The freedom to use one's talents and abilities, engendered by the women's liberation movement, is perceived not as an opportunity but as a demand.
3. Expectations of and demands on the modern teenager have been compared to those experienced by a 40-year-old executive prior to a heart attack.
4. The greater sexual freedom prevalent today may emphasize an expectation that the girl is not really ready for.

Mortality rates between 5% and 15% have been reported (Arcuni, 1977).

Anorexia nervosa was first described in the medical literature in 1689 by Morton and later in 1868 by Sir William Gull. While the condition has been recognized for hundreds of years, its cause and effective treatment are recent discoveries. Anorexia is a distinct illness whose outstanding feature is a relentless pursuit of thinness. The name itself is incorrect because appetite is not lost; hunger is not absent nor is there a lack of interest in food. Rather, it is a psychosomatic disorder characterized by an active refusal to accept food; a more correct term might be "psychogenic food refusal syndrome" (Szyrynski, 1973).

Three symptoms appear to be classic: (1) voluntary resistance to eating, (2) conspicuous weight loss in excess of 20% of the premorbid state, and (3) amenorrhea. In some cases amenorrhea initially brings the client into contact with the health care system. In appearance these girls resemble walking skeletons. They are hyperactive, restless, and involved in exhausting exercise. They experience constipation and often make excessive use of

laxatives and/or diuretics. Their bodies are often covered with lanugo. They may alternate between severe starvation and food binges followed by self-induced vomiting. They are irritable, exhibit excessively overcontrolled behavior, and are obsessed with exercise. Blood pressure is usually low, basal metabolism rates are below normal, protein-bound iodine values are at low normal, and follicle-stimulating hormone level is low. Frequently moderate anemia, hypoproteinemia, and nutritional edema are found (Szyrynski, 1978). Depression and suicidal intent may often be seen.

Bruch (1977, 1978) delineates three areas of disordered psychologic functioning that are characteristic of clients with anorexia nervosa. The first is a disturbance in body image and body concept of delusional proportions. The girls insist that their cachectic appearance is normal and that they are not too thin. The second characteristic is a misinterpretation of internal and external stimuli. Most prominent is the failure to interpret signals (hunger) indicating nutritional need. Awareness of hunger and appetite in the ordinary sense seems to be lacking. Anorectics train themselves to consider hunger as a pleasurable, desirable sensation. Another manifestation of the misinterpretation of stimuli is an inability to acknowledge fatigue. Their constant hyperactivity is not associated with a perception of fatigue. The absence of sexual feelings and failure of sexual functioning can also be considered a perceptive and conceptual deficiency. The third feature is a paralyzing sense of ineffectiveness. There is a tremendous feeling that they are helpless to change anything about their lives. This is often expressed as extreme negativism and stubborn defiance.

Most anorectic girls appear to experience an essential fear of sexuality. They are afraid of growth and maturity and have difficulty accepting their sexual identity. Fear of pregnancy is often present, and pregnancy is symbolized by food—getting fat. Fantasies are often formulated, such as oral impregnation (Dikowitz, 1976; Szyrynski, 1978).

Hostility is another important factor often seen in anorexia nervosa. An anorectic's basic delusion is not having an identity of her own. Anorexia occurs in families where the mother is dominant and the father is rather passive and ineffective. The mother may be overprotective and unable to see her daughter as a separate being. She may even specifically have told the child when she was hungry and when not. The most frequent conflict is an attempt to gain independence from the mother; in addition, there may be rebellion against identifying with a mother who is seen as fat or shapeless.

Hostility toward the mother may lead the girl to deny her femininity even more by denying the maternal model. There is a deeper anxiety of being forced to grow up, to become a woman. Some change or new demand occurs with which the girl does not feel prepared to cope and she begins dieting. Dieting is a means to undo the bodily changes of adolescence, to achieve control over the body again. Anorectics blame the body for their discomfort and try to solve their problems by changing the body through starvation and exhausting activities. There is a self-punishing element in the denial of comfort and pleasure. The illness is an effort to make time stand still; to avoid growing up with its attendant need for self-reliance, independence, and separate identity. Anorexia nervosa may be a wish to return to childhood size and functioning (Bruch, 1970).

Frequently, anorectics come from homes where great importance is attached to food. There may be excessive concern about proper nourishment, and a belief that a fit child equals a healthy child. Some parents with repressed hostility toward their children attempt to expiate it through excessive concern about their eating habits, while other parents may contribute to the development of anorexia by following food fads or being preoccupied with dieting. Their mothers are weight conscious themselves or preoccupied by dieting. Their fathers may criticize them for being plump or tease them about being overweight.

A typical triad in anorexia nervosa clients, particularly boys, has been identified. It includes great importance of food to the parents, resistance of the client to growing up sexually and otherwise, and regression to old patterns of adjustment with the revival of primitive conflicts.

The anorectic child is often described as ideal—bright, obedient, cooperative. Eating disturbances are rarely remembered. The negative and oppositional behavior usually seen between 24 and 36 months was absent. The anorectic is never allowed to express anger. Good behavior is expected always, and there is frequently much emphasis on academic achievement. The obligation to live up to this "specialness" is a tremendous burden. The anorectic is always trying to live up to expectations and always feels she is not good enough. She is overvalued by her parents and too much is expected in return.

Effective treatment for anorexia is crucial since it is literally a life-and-death situation. Treatment should be determined by the basic psychiatric psychodynamic clinical findings and the physical condition of the client when she is first seen. Treatment methods include psychotherapy, behavior modification, traditional physical support, and family therapy.

Numerous studies report high success rates for various treatment approaches; however, these results should be viewed with caution since they are often based on poor research methods. Garfinkel et al. (1977) report that most patients with anorexia improve regardless of the method of treatment, while some patients do poorly no matter what therapy is used. No one specific treatment has been shown to be superior in influencing outcome. The most sensible approach in the treatment of anorexia appears to be an eclectic one. Reversal of the starvation process is of paramount importance; the human organism must receive support or death will occur.

Treatment in most cases includes hospitalization to effect weight gain initially. Behavior modification techniques have been used with success in many cases. Behavior modification of anorexia requires total control of the client's environment and is done in the hospital. Here the client is deprived of the privileges or positive reinforcements of everyday life. Reinforcing activities such as watching TV, crafts, and reading are made contingent upon weight gain. The client is given meals at regular intervals and instructed to carefully monitor food intake and weight regularly.

Once the starvation process is halted and the client has gained weight, psychotherapy is often begun to work through the underlying intrapsychic conflicts. Many authors feel that treating the anorectic in terms of weight gain alone should be avoided. If she is not helped to deal with the stresses that necessitated the anorectic state in the first place, severe depression and possibly suicide may result. Bruch (1970) emphasizes that the psychotherapeutic approach should evoke awareness of feelings and thoughts, and impulse organization in the client herself rather than following the more traditional psychoanalytic approach.

Concurrent counseling for the parents or family therapy is as important as weight gain and individual psychotherapy. Without alterations of the family dynamics that created and perpetuated the situation, treatment and a positive prognosis for the anorectic client are more difficult.

No one specific therapy has a long-term high success rate for anorexia nervosa. A combination of treatments, which provide physiologic support with attendent weight gain, resolution of individual psychodynamic factors, and alterations in family patterns are needed to bring long-term positive results.

Obesity

The American woman is concerned about obesity and continually exposed to messages about the importance of remaining slim and youthful. She may avail herself of one or more of the approximately 17,000 weight reduction methods published to date and contribute to the $10 billion diet industry in the United States. Her concern about becoming overweight, however, stems more from a desire to remain attractive than from concern about health risks. At the same time there is a growing awareness on the part of health care practitioners that obesity is a major health problem in America. It is considered the number one nutritional problem, with far-reaching medical and psychologic consequences. Nurses have a responsibility to educate their clients about the risks inherent in being obese and to facilitate weight reduction and maintenance at optimal levels.

Several terms are used to designate an individual who is too fat. The *overweight* person is one whose weight is greater than normal when compared to standard weight tables. There is excess weight of all tissues in the body. *Obesity* refers to abnormal amounts of body fat. It is an accumulation of fat in excess of that needed for optimal health (Mayer, 1975). The terms are not the same but are often used synonymously. For all practical purposes the individual is obese if she is 15% to 20% overweight.

Obesity can be divided into two types on an anatomic basis: (1) *hypertrophic* obesity is characterized by a normal number of enlarged fat cells; (2) *hyperplastic* obesity is characterized by an increased number of enlarged fat cells. In infancy, and perhaps prenatally, adipose tissue grows mainly by an increase in the number of fat cells. At some point, probably early in life, the number of fat cells becomes fixed and from this point on, increases in adipose tissue occur only by an increase in the size of individual fat cells (Stunkard, 1975). It is thought that during periods of rapid growth, such as prenatally, during infancy, and during the adolescent growth spurt, fat cells can be laid down in increasing numbers. *Juvenile obesity* occurs when the individual gains most of her excess weight as a child. This type of obesity is characterized by both hypertrophic and hyperplastic fat cells. In adult-onset obesity, which accounts for 95% of all obesity in adults, the excess weight is gained as an adult. These people have the same number of fat cells as the nonobese but they are hyperplastic. Much adult obesity is characterized by the "creeping waistline" syndrome, in which some sort of weight equilibrium was maintained until approximately age 25 and then a yo-yo process of gaining weight, losing weight, and gaining weight began. Each time more weight is gained than is subsequently lost, and there is a gradual expansion of the waistline and accumulation of excess pounds.

Etiology

Obesity results when energy intake (calories) exceeds energy expenditure (activity), but to attribute obesity to overeating alone is to oversimplify. There is not one cause common to all fat people. There are definite medical causes for some obesity, for example, obesity caused by hypothalamic irregularities or endocrine disorders; by genetic diseases, or certain drugs. However, these represent only a small fraction of the total number of

obese people. Most cases of obesity are more probably caused by:

1. A gradual decrease in activity coupled with either an increase or no reduction in calories
2. Social and cultural patterns that encourage excessive food intake
3. Ignorance of food values and factors essential for weight control

Gluckman (1972) feels that psychologic factors are important in the development of obesity. Data indicate that in most types of human obesity, there is probably a relationship between psychosocial, biochemical, neurophysiologic, hereditary, and environmental factors. Psychotherapeutic data suggest that many obese patients did not experience an appropriate maternal response to their nutritive and nonnutritive needs during infancy and childhood.

There are two small subgroups of obese persons who are characterized by abnormal, stereotypic food intake patterns. The *night eater* is most often a woman with morning anorexia, evening hyperphagia, and insomnia, usually precipitated by stressful life situations. Once the syndrome is begun, it tends to recur daily until the stress is alleviated. The *binge eaters* suddenly and compulsively eats large amounts of food in very short periods of time, with subsequent feelings of anxiety and self-condemnation. This is also a reaction to stress. These obese individuals who later develop anorexia nervosa were usually binge eaters. Among women, adult obesity is often related to being a fat child. Travers (1976) estimates that 42% of adult obese women were obese as children. Pregnancy also can precipitate or compound obesity. As many as 30% become obese during pregnancy, often the result of misguided eating habits, compulsive eating, cravings, and the erroneous idea that the pregnant woman must "eat for two." At this point, a woman may join the "obesity cycle."

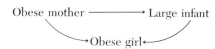

Epidemiology

Obesity is very common in women: 25% between the ages of 30 to 39 exceed their optimal weight by 20%; 40% of all women aged 40 to 49, and 46% of those 50 to 59 years are obese (Hashim, 1977). At least one in three women is obese, and if one considers those who are "only" overweight, then two out of three women are overweight. Obesity is more common in women than men and is more prevalent in black women than white women.

Certain social factors have been linked to obesity (Stunkard, 1975). There is a marked inverse relationship between socioeconomic status and prevalence of obesity (Gain et al., 1976). The prevalence in the lower socioeconomic class is six times that in the upper class. This relationship is usually stronger for women than for men (Oken et al., 1977). The longer a woman's family has been in the United States, the less likely she is to be obese. Religious affiliation is another social factor linked to obesity. The greatest prevalence of obesity is found among Jews, followed by Roman Catholics, and finally Protestants. It is apparent that in Western urban settings, social factors have more influence on women than on men: women in the United States have become slightly thinner during the last 20 years, while men have continued to become fatter.

Age appears to be a factor in obesity also. Obesity is not only more prevalent in poor girls but it is established earlier and increases at a more rapid rate than among upper-class girls (Gain et al., 1977). There are a growing number (15% to 30%) of children who are obese, and the earlier obesity develops, the more difficult it is to "cure."

Fatness and leanness appear to run in families. When parents are obese, the children also tend to be fat. Husbands and wives tend to reflect leanness or fatness (Gain, et al., 1977). This may be a reflection of attitudes toward food, eating, and exercise. The question of whether or not obesity has a genetic component is yet to be answered satisfactorily—genetics and environment are difficult to separate.

Obese people tend to select greater quantities and more servings of high-calorie, low-nutrient foods (Food Choices, 1974). Fullness of the stomach does not seem to affect the appetite of the obese as it does the nonobese. Taste does appear to affect amounts eaten, however. If the food is unpalatable, whatever the nutritional status, the obese do not eat it, while normal-weight subjects appear to adjust their intake to nutritional needs. The obese are less apt to organize their eating patterns around the time of day. They tend to eat fewer meals a day than the nonobese but to eat more rapidly and to consume more at any one meal (Crow, 1974).

Risks

Obesity is a serious health risk and is related to many chronic diseases. Mackenzie (1976) states that all medical risks, including risk of cancer and accidents, increase once one reaches the level of 30% overweight. Obesity makes breathing more difficult and increases the work of keeping the body oxygenated. Tolerance to any exercise is diminished as is tolerance of any respiratory infection. Very marked obesity can lead to a pickwickian syndrome (Mayer, 1975). Hypertension is more prevalent in the obese, and the obese hypertensive has a greater mortality and morbidity. In women, obesity is strongly associated with a higher risk of coronary heart disease (Gordon et al., 1977). Hirsutism and menstrual irregularities are far more common among obese women than other women (Mayer, 1975). Diabetes is also more common in obese women and responds dramatically to weight reduction (Gordon et al., 1977).

Serum cholesterol levels appear to be related to high calcium intake and respond positively to a negative caloric balance (Mann, 1974). There is a significant association between obesity and gallbladder disease, particularly in women. Obesity often leads to rashes, inflammation of furuncles because of excessive perspiration trapped in skin folds and constant friction. Complications of varicosities, such as ulceration are exacerbated by obesity; arthritis, low back pain, and foot problems are also exacerbated by excess weight. Surgery is technically more difficult to perform on the obese and postoperative complications are increased. Iron-deficiency anemia is more commonly found.

The obese experience many physical limitations because of the difficulty of moving large amounts of fat. They are accident prone and are more uncomfortable in warm weather because of the thermal insulation properties of fat. Obesity is an occupational hazard. The obese are less agile; obesity is a major health problem associated with unemployment (Roe and Eichwort, 1976). (The problems of obesity and pregnancy were discussed earlier in this chapter.) Sexual performance and libidinal desires do not appear to be affected by obesity; however, hyperobesity does constitute a major social obstacle that limits sexual experience (Wise and Gordon, 1977).

The psychologic consequences of obesity are likewise serious. The obese often exhibit traits similar to those subjected to intense prejudice: heightened sensitivity, obsessive concern with weight, passivity, withdrawal, and expectations of rejection. The "jolly fat man" is a myth with little basis in fact. The obese often suffer from distorted body image, alienation, and feelings of despondency, dependency, and manipulation (Bruch, 1978). Often the key behavioral reaction is hostility.

The obese do not like being fat and often describe themselves as unattractive and uncomfortable (Bruch, 1973). Fat people face stigma and social discrimination; the prevailing message in America today is that fat is ugly, weak, self-indulgent, immoral and unhealthy. The near hysteria many women feel about being plump is associated with the American beauty standard of thinness and the society's emphasis on the negative aspects of fatness. The obese are continually reminded of their inferior status when they buy clothes, watch television, or read magazines, and in the reactions of people they come in contact with. Overweight applicants are at a disadvantage in college admissions. It is more difficult to get a job; positions in which contact with the public is essential are often not open to the overweight (Dwyer and Mayer, 1970).

The practitioner needs to be sensitive to the negative self-concept obese women generally have. When this is kept firmly in mind, it is easier to cope with the hostile defensive front that the client may project. The obese are a minority with all the attendant effects of discrimination; the nurse who incorporates this knowledge into the plan of care and develops a relationship with her client will be more successful.

Treatment

Success rates for all types of treatments for obesity have not been good. From 60% to 75% of those who seriously try to lose weight have a fair degree of success, but only about 5% maintain weight loss. Most obese people do not seek treatment for obesity. Of those who do, most will not follow through; of those who do follow through, most will not lose weight; of those who lose weight, most will regain it. Many of those who do lose weight will pay an emotional price for it with symptoms such as nervousness, weakness, and irritability (Stunkard, 1975).

Any treatment for obesity should be based on a thorough assessment that includes: (1) a history of how weight was gained; (2) a complete diet history, (3) accurate determination of caloric intake and energy expenditures, and (4) family history. For optimal results, weight loss should approximate 1 to 2 lbs/week. This is achieved by reducing intake, increasing activity, or both. Reduction of caloric intake must result from a diet that is nutritionally adequate and of sufficient satiety. Increased activity is always desirable unless it is medically contraindicated. Psychologic support is essential and can be achieved through individual or group approach.

Success rates are highest when the obesity is of the adult-onset variety, when weight reduction is approached in gradual steps, and when group therapy is used. The individual who is reducing for the first time, who is emotionally mature, married, or of a higher socioeconomic group is also more apt to experience success.

Treatment modalities abound and all produce some weight loss. The key is to maintain weight loss. For too long a time, it was believed that just losing weight would somehow magically instill the will power necessary to keep weight off. It is now recognized that this belief is fallacious. Greater emphasis is now being placed on a gradual, practical transition from the weight loss phase to the weight maintenance phase. This text describes those aspects of therapy that the practitioner herself might use or would need information about in order to inform and refer clients.

Psychotherapy can function as an indirect treatment of obesity. It may be most helpful in the client whose disturbances in eating functions have been a problem throughout life. The therapist can assist the client with emotional conflicts associated with weight loss and body image changes. Attention can be given to those anxieties that continue to produce overeating or resistance to making major life-style changes for the sake of appearance or health. Psychotherapy should focus on increasing the client's awareness of self-initiated feelings, thoughts, and behaviors. Working with the family is also beneficial. Dietary change should be postponed until the client experiences some competence in some area of living and can recognize emotional problems as separate from nutritional needs (Bruch, 1973b).

Behavior modification methods have been used for control of obesity since 1967. They are based on a belief that obesity is a learned response and as such can be unlearned. Stunkard (1975) describes numerous studies demonstrating the ability of behavior modification to increase the effectiveness of treatment of obesity by a factor of two. The basic behavioral program consists of four parts:

1. Description of the behavior to be controlled: The client is asked to keep careful records of all the food she eats and the circumstances surrounding food consumption. This vastly increases the client's awareness of her eating patterns.
2. Control of the stimuli that precede eating: The client is asked to limit all stimuli that make her want to eat. The amount of high-calorie foods in the house is limited and low-calorie foods are substituted. The client is to eat only in the kitchen using only one type of silverware.
3. Development of techniques to control the act of eating: The speed of eating is decreased and awareness of food is enhanced while eating. Food is savored. For example, each mouthful is chewed a certain number of times and the act of swallowing is made conscious.
4. Modification of the consequences of eating: A system of formal rewards for changing behaviors and reducing pounds is used. The rewards are tangible, such as seeing a good movie or buying a new dress, and prompt.

These elements of the behavior modification approach to obesity control can be easily incorporated by the nursing practitioner.

The self-help group approach to weight loss also appears to be useful. This approach stresses the benefits of group support and peer pressure to achieve success.

Diet plans that are nutritionally sound are provided, and progress is monitored with weekly weighing and records kept of pounds lost. Stuart and Mitchell (1978) have reviewed several studies of self-help weight control groups and conclude that the "self-help group approach with the application of behavioral self-management techniques is the current treatment of choice for the mild to moderately overweight individual" (p. 702). The nurse should know where these resources are available and suggest them to appropriate clients. She should follow up with her client to determine whether the client followed through with the suggestion and whether or not she found it helpful.

A decreased caloric intake, coupled with increased activity, is basic to all successful weight reduction programs. The diet needs to be nutritionally adequate and to provide sufficient calories to permit physical activity. The dieter should take at least 300 calories at each of three to four meals, without snacking. Suggestions on how to prepare foods using low-calorie methods of cooking and seasoning should be given to the client. Menu plans and recipes should also be provided. The client should be encouraged to exercise sufficiently to increase the body's capacity to process oxygen while remaining relatively free of side effects. The exercise should be interesting, produce desirable fatigue, and last between 15 and 40 full minutes; it should be done three to four times a week.

Once weight loss is achieved, the most difficult task of maintaining the loss begins. The client is encouraged to weigh on the same scale at least every 10 days and to take corrective measures immediately if weight rises more than 2 to 4 pounds. The daily diet should be based on the basic four food groups and no foods should be prohibited. High-calorie foods should be eaten only on spe-cial occasions and in small quantities. Exercise should be continued on a regular basis.

Obesity is a major health problem that can be corrected with persistence and determination. The nurse can facilitate weight loss and maintenance of the loss by the development of a supportive long-term relationsip with the client.

Fad diets

Successful weight loss requires self-denial, often of foods viewed as highly desirable. Anyone who has ever tried to lose weight has wished for a painless, quick method. It is this wish that is the basis of the success of fad diets. They all promise a swift, easy, painless way to lose weight, and they often work, at least initially. Weight loss is achieved if the directions are followed. However, the loss is seldom permanent because the diets do not provide directions for maintaining weight loss through good eating habits. Weight is often regained once the individual returns to her traditional eating habits. These diets are often nutritionally inadequate and can be deleterious to health if used for long periods of time.

Table 21-11 provides a summary of several popular weight control programs. Knowledge of these and similar diets will assist the practitioner in assessing a client's nutritional status. The client's understanding of the inadequacy of fad diets should be enhanced. The axiom that the only effective way to take weight off and keep it off is to follow basic rules of sound nutrition should be stressed. The client with a weight problem must accept the fact that a change in food habits is essential for weight loss to occur and that this change must be lifelong. She must accept the fact that successful dieting requires motivation, discipline, and transitory discomfort.

Table 21-11. Analysis of common reducing diets*

Name of diet	Calories	Techniques employed	Comments
Dr. Atkins' Super Energy Diet. R. C. Atkins, Crown Publishers, New York, 1977.	2800	Unspecified energy level; unbalanced energy sources (very low carbohydrate); use of famous name and biochemical claims; vitamin-mineral supplements.	This is diet 1, the "super energy weight reducing diet." It is an extremely high in fat, low in carbohydrate. Portion sizes and types of foods are specified so that if the meal plan is followed, calorie counting is avoided. Levels of vitamin C are slightly low, but levels of other nutrients are those recommended. Vitamin and mineral supplements are suggested. The meal plan provides fewer servings of breads and cereals and fruits and vegetables than does the Basic Four plan, but more servings of the meat and dairy groups.

*From Dwyer, J.: Twelve popular diets—brief nutritional analysis, Psych. Clin. North Am. 1(3):623-627, 1978.

Table 21-11. Analysis of common reducing diets—cont'd

Name of diet	Calories	Techniques employed	Comments
You Can Be Fat Free Forever. Diet from book by the same name by L. M. Elting and S. Isenberg, St. Martin's Press, New York, 1974.	2000	Unspecified energy levels; special conditions for eating; monotony; unbalanced energy sources (low carbohydrate).	Incorporates a number of useful behavior modification techniques, exhortation and a diet plan low in carbohydrate. The dieter is allowed to eat unlimited amounts of foods high in protein from the meat group, but dairy products and breads and cereals (also high in protein) are absent from the plan. The diet is low in calcium.
Water Diet. As presented in "The Doctor's Quick Weight Loss Diet" by I. M. Stillman and S. S. Baker, Dell Publishing Co., New York, 1977.	2000	Unspecified energy level; unbalanced energy sources (very low carbohydrate); monotony; special conditions on eating (use of at least 8 glasses of water a day); famous name.	Also known as the Stillman diet, this diet works by specifying the types but not the amounts of foods which are permitted. Foods from the fruits and vegetable or bread and cereals groups are to be eschewed, while large numbers of servings from the dairy and meat groups are permitted. Many of the foods which are allowed are quite high in saturated fat. Vitamins A and C, thiamine, and iron are likely to be low. A large quantity of water and vitamin-mineral supplements are also suggested.
Dr. Solomon's Great New Health Diet. From "The Health Diet Book," by Neil Solomon, Good Housekeeping, April, 1978.	1400	Specified energy level (set or fixed menu); balanced energy sources; addition of special food (foods high in roughage); famous name.	Foods high in roughage, dietary fiber, and "natural" foods are given special emphasis. It is claimed that the bulk of the liberal amounts of fruits and vegetables which are provided furnishes the eater with a feeling of fullness or satisfaction, which has not been substantiated. In comparison to the basic four food groups, slightly less than the usual servings of dairy products are suggested, and more servings of fruits, vegetables, breads and cereals along with usual suggestions from the meat group. Iron content is slightly low.
The Fake Mayo Diet. In "A Mini-Dictionary of Diets," Epicure, Summer, 1973.	1400	Unspecified energy level (but diet consists only of a few foods); monotony; unbalanced energy sources; biochemical claims and hints of scientific breakthrough.	This is one version of a popular crash diet also called the Mayo Clinic diet, the Egg and Grapefruit diet, the Tomato Juice Diet. The diet is not approved by the Mayo Clinic. The unsubstantiated claim is made that there is a special enzyme in both tomato and grapefruit juice which dissolves fat and causes it to be burned off. While the diet does not limit pattern or amount of foods, so few foods are permitted that boredom soon sets in. Breads and cereals are not permitted and dairy products are also sharply restricted. Foods from the meat and fruits and vegetables groups are provided in larger amounts than usual. Calcium and iron are low.
Pritikin Diet. From "Live Longer Now: The First One Hundred Years of Your Life." N. Pritikin, Grosset and Dunlop, New York, 1974.	1400	Unspecified energy level; unbalanced energy sources (extremely low fat); special conditions on eating (portion size control); famous name; unsubstantiated scientific breakthrough; low sodium; prophylactic claims.	This diet is exceedingly low in fat (only about 10% of total calories). While the types of foods allowed meet the basic four guide, particular emphasis is given to large amounts of fruits and vegetables and breads and cereals. Some commonly eaten foods are forbidden: sugar, table fats, beef, oil, and dairy products unless they are made from skimmed milk. Slightly low in iron.

Table 21-11. Analysis of common reducing diets—cont'd

Name of diet	Calories	Techniques employed	Comments
The Ayds Plan Diet. From the diet instruction provided with Ayds Candy, produced by the Campana Corporation, Batavia, Illinois.	1200	Unspecified energy level (set menus); balanced energy sources; addition of special food (candy); use of rewards; unsubstantiated biochemical claim.	The diet itself is a good one, but the candies are not necessary. Each candy provides 25 calories, and 1 or 2 are suggested before each meal. All of the usual foods in the basic four are allowed but amounts are limited. Iron intake is likely to be slightly low.
"Our High Fiber Reducing Diet" Marilyn Mercer, McCall's Magazine, September, 1975. and **The Save Your Life Diet.** Theodore Isaac Rubin.	1200	Balanced energy sources; specified energy intakes; addition of special food (dietary fiber high foods); famous name.	These diets are quite similar in giving special attention to dietary fiber, which is claimed, by its bulking effect, to fill the dieter. This claim has not been demonstrated to date, but fiber-rich foods do improve laxation. Fewer servings of dairy and bread-cereal group foods are permitted than is suggested by the basic four pattern, and the fruits and vegetable group given special prominence. Calcium and iron may tend to be low.
The Doctor's Quick Teenage Diet. I. M. Stillman and S. S. Baker, Warner Books, New York, 1972.	1100	Unbalanced energy sources (low carbohydrate); increased physical activity via exercise; unsubstantiated scientific claims; famous name.	This diet *not* suitable for a growing adolescent! It is low not only in energy, but also in vitamin A, thiamine, iron, and calcium. The rapid weight loss promised in the first few days is due to its very low carbohydrate content, which encourages diuresis. Breads and cereals and fruits and vegetables are provided only in very small amounts, while much emphasis is given to meat group selections.
Carnation Slender Liquid Diet Formula	900	Specified energy level; balanced energy sources; formula diet; monotony; low sodium.	This formula diet differs from those which prescribe protein supplements in that it is not low in carbohydrate and does not induce ketosis. Since it is a liquid, monotony may set in if used exclusively. It is a milk-based product; thus the recommended dose is high in dairy products and lower in all the other food groups than the basic four pattern. It fulfills needs for all nutrients but is rather low in bulk.
Last Chance Refeeding Diet. From "The Last Chance Diet" by R. Linn, Bantam Books, New York, 1977.	500	Specified energy level; unbalanced energy sources (very low carbohydrate), special formula required as well as food, famous name, unsubstantiated claim for a scientific breakthrough.	This diet is that which follows the protein supplemented fast which Dr. Linn advocates. A high protein powder, called Pro-Linn, is suggested for the fast itself. Such fasts are dangerous in that they may induce ketosis but also hypokalemia and other complications when attempted by persons not under medical supervision. During the fast, vitamin and mineral supplements, potassium, and folic acid are also prescribed with at least two quarts of noncaloric fluids per day. Gradually food is introduced; this is called the refeeding phase and is detailed here. The ProLinn powder is still used twice a day. Danger of dehydration, hypokalemia, etc., if directions not followed. Intake of vitamin A, roboflavin, thiamine, iron, and calcium is inadequate.

Table 21-11. Analysis of common reducing diets—cont'd

Name of diet	Calories	Techniques employed	Comments
Fasting is A Way of Life. From the book of the same title by L. Cott, Bantam Books, New York, 1977.	500	Specified energy level (fast followed by formula); unbalanced energy sources (low carbohydrate).	*The type of fasting described in this diet is extremely dangerous and may result in serious problems if done without medical supervision.* This book suggests a total fast followed by a low calorie diet of liquid meals. The diet is very low in the meat group and breads and cereals compared to the basic four. It is lower than recommendations in protein, niacin, riboflavin, thiamine, calcium, and iron. The diet is ketogenic because of the low carbohydrate levels.

REFERENCES

Abramson, E.: A review of behavioral approaches to weight control, Behav. Res. Ther. 11(4):547-556, 1973.

Arcumi, A. J.: Anorexia nervosa: diagnosis and treatment, Female Patient, pp. 29-32, Aug. 1977.

Aubry, R.: The assessment of maternal nutrition, Clin. Perinatol. 2(2):207-219, 1975.

Bartholomeu, M. J., and Poston, F. E.: Effect of food taboos on prenatal nutrition, J. Nutr. Educ., pp. 15-17, Summer, 1970.

Belsey, M. A.: Hormonal contraception and nutrition. In Moghissi, K. S., and Evans, T. N., eds.: Nutritional impacts on women, New York, 1977, Harper & Row, Publishers.

Bender, A. E.: Food preferences of men and women, Proc. Nutr. Soc. 35:181-189, 1976.

Brasel, J. A.: Factors that affect nutritional requirements in adolescents, Curr. Concepts Nutr., Vol. 5, 1977.

Bruch, H.: The importance of overweight, New York, 1957, W. W. Norton Co.

Bruch, H.: Changed approaches to anorexia nervosa, Int. Psychiatr. Clin. 7:3-24, 1970a.

Bruch, H.: Psychotherapy in primary anorexia nervosa, Int. Psychiatr. Clin. 7:54-67, 1970b.

Bruch, H.: The psychological handicaps of the obese. In Obesity in perspective, NIH Conference Proceedings, DHEW Pub. no. 75-708, Washington, D.C., 1973a, U.S. Government Printing Office.

Bruch, H.: Eating disorders: obesity, anorexia nervosa, and the person within, New York, 1973b, Basic Books, Inc.

Bruch, H.: Psychological antecedants of anorexia nervosa. In Vigersky, R. A., editor: Anorexia nervosa, New York, 1977, Raun Press.

Bruch, H.: The golden cage, Boston, 1978, Harvard Press.

Cassel, J.: Social and cultural implications of food and food habits, Am. J. Public Health 47:732-740, 1957.

Chappelle, M. L.: The language of food, Am. J. Nurs. 72(7):1294-1295, 1972.

Clark, A., and Affonso, D.: Childbearing: a nursing perspective, ed. 2, New York, 1979, F. A. Davis.

Committee on Maternal Nutrition, Food and Nutrition Board, National Research Council: Maternal nutrition and the course of pregnancy, Washington, D.C., 1970, National Academy of Science.

Crisp, A. H., and others: The long-term prognosis in anorexia nervosa: some factors predictive of outcome. In Vigersky, R. A., editor: Anorexia nervosa, New York, 1977, Raven Press.

Cross, A. T., and Walsh, H. E.: Prenatal diet counseling, J. Reprod. Med. 7(6):265-274, 1971.

Crow, R.: Experimental studies of obesity, Nurs. Times, Jan. 24, 1974, pp. 103-105.

Dikowitz, S.: Anorexia nervosa, Mental Health Serv., p. 28, Oct. 1976.

Dunning, H. N.: What do consumers know about nutrition? FDA Consumer, DHEW Pub. no. 75-2005, June 1974.

Dwyer, J.: Twelve popular diets, Psych. Clin. North Am. 1(3):621-628, 1978.

Dwyer, J. T., Feldman, J. J., and Mayer, J.: The social psychology of dieting, J. Health Soc. Behav. 11:269-287, 1970.

Dwyer, J. T., and Mayer, J.: Potential dieters: who are they? J. Am. Diet. Assoc. 56:570-574, 1970.

Dwyer, J. T., and others: Adolescent dieters: who are they? Am. J. Clin. Nutr. 20(10):1045-1056, 1967.

Edwards, C. H., and others: Clay and corn starch eating in women, J. Am. Diet. Assoc. 35:810-815, 1959.

Fineberg, S. K.: Diet: the realities of obesity and fad diets, Nutr. Today, pp. 23-26, July/Aug. 1972.

Food and Drug Administration: What do consumers know about nutrition? DHEW Pub. no. 75-2017, Washington, D.C., 1974, U.S. Government Printing Office.

Frisch, R. E.: Nutrition, fatness and fertility: the effect of food intake on productive ability. In Mosley, W. H., editor: Nutrition and human reproduction, New York, 1977, Plenum Press.

Fusillo, A.: Food shoppers' beliefs: myths and realities, FDA Consumer, DHEW Pub. no. 75-2017, Oct. 1974.

Gain, S.: Trends in fatness and origins of obesity, Pediatrics 57(4):443-456, 1976.

Gain, S., and others: Levels of education, level of income and level of fatness in adults, Am. J. Clin. Nutr. 30:721-725, 1977.

Garfinkel, P. E.: The outcome of anorexia nervosa: significance of clinical features, body image and behavior modification. In Vigersky, R. A., editor: Anorexia nervosa, New York, 1977, Raven Press.

Gluckman, M. L.: Psychiatric observations on obesity, Adv. Psychosom. Med. 7:194-216, 1972.

Gold, E.: Interconceptual nutrition, J. Am. Diet. Assoc. 55:27-30, 1969.

Gordon, T., and others: Diabetes, blood lipids, and the role of obesity in coronary heart disease risk for women, Ann. In. Med. 87(4):393-397, 1977.

Greenwood, M. R. C., and Johnson, P.: Adipose tissue cellularity and its relationship to the development of obesity in females, Curr. Concepts Nutr. 5:119-135, 1977.

Haley, E. S.: Promoting adequate weight gain in pregnant women, Maternal Child Nurs., pp. 86-88, Mar./Apr. 1977.

Hampton, M. C., and others: Calorie and nutrient intakes of teen-agers, J. Am. Diet. Assoc. **50**:385, 1967.

Hashim, S. A.: Hunger and satiety in man. In Winick, M., editor: Nutritional disorders of American women, New York, 1977, John Wiley & Sons.

Herbert, V.: Anemias. In Winick, M., editor: Nutritional disorders of American women, New York, 1977, John Wiley & Sons.

Higgins, A. C., and others: Nutritional states and the outcome of pregnancy, Amsterdam, 1972, Excerpta Medica, pp. 1076-1077.

Hueneman, R. J., and others: Food and eating practices of teen agers, J. Am. Diet. Assoc. **53**:17-24, 1968.

Jacobson, H. N.: Weight and weight gain in pregnancy, Clin. Perinatol. **2**(2):233-241, 1975.

Jensen, M. D., Benson, R. C., and Boback, I. M.: Maternity care: the nurse and the family, St. Louis, 1977, The C. V. Mosby Co.

Johnson, B. S., and Ritchie, V.: Milieu management of the patient with anorexia nervosa. In Kneisl, C. R., and Wilson, H. S., editors: Current respective in psychiatric nursing: issues and trends, St. Louis, 1976, The C. V. Mosby Co.

King, J. C., and others: Assessment of nutritional state of teenage pregnant girls, Am. J. Clin. Nutr. **25**:916-925, 1972.

Kreutner, A., and others: Adolescent obstetrics and gynecology, Chicago, 1978, Year Book Medical Publisher, Inc.

Lakey, C.: Pica—a nutritional anthropology concern. In Bauwens, E. E., editor: The anthropology of health, St. Louis, 1978, The C. V. Mosby Co.

Leverton, R. M.: The paradox of teen age nutrition, J. Am. Diet. Assoc. **53**:13-16, 1968.

Lewis, C.: Family nutrition, Philadelphia, 1976, F. A. Davis Co.

Lorenberg, M. E.: The development of food patterns, J. Am. Diet. Assoc. **65**:263-268, 1974.

Luke, B.: Lactose intolerance during pregnancy, Maternal Child Nurs. pp. 92-96, Mar./Apr. 1977.

Luke, B.: Understanding pica in pregnant women, Maternal Child Nurs., pp. 97-100, Mar./April, 1977.

Mackenzie, M.: Obesity as failure in the American culture, Obesity/Bariat. Med. **5**(4):132-133, 1976.

Mahoney, M. J.: Behavior modification in the treatment of obesity, Psychiat. Clin. North Am. **1**(3):651-659, 1978.

Mann, G. V.: The influence of obesity on health, New Engl. J. Med. **291**(5):226-232, 1974; **291**(4):178-185, 1974.

Mayer, J.: Obesity, Prog. Food Nutr. Sci. **1**(2):115-122, 1975.

McGanty, W. J.: Nutrition in the adolescent. In Moghissi, K., and Evans, T. N., editors: Nutritional impact on women, New York, 1977, Harper & Row, Publishers.

McGanty, W. J., and others: Pregnancy in the adolescent, Am. J. Obstet. Gynecol. **103**(6):778-788, 1969.

Moore, M. L.: Realities in childbearing, Philadelphia, 1978, W. B. Saunders Co.

National Research Council, Committee on Maternal Nutrition: Maternal nutrition and the course of pregnancy, Washington, D.C., 1970, National Academy of Sciences.

Oates, G. K., and others: Diet in pregnancy: Meddling with the normal or preventing toxemia? Am. J. Nurs. **75**(7):1134-1136, 1975.

Oken, B., and others: Relation between socioeconomic status and obesity changes in 9046 women, Prevent. Med. **6**:447-453, 1977.

Osofsky, H. J., and others: Nutritional status of low income pregnant teenagers, J. Reprod. Med. **6**(1):52-56, 1971.

Pitkin, R. M.: Nutritional during pregnancy: the clinical approach. In Winick, M., editor: Nutritional disorders of American women, New York, 1977, John Wiley & Sons.

Pitkin, R. M., and others: Maternal nutrition: a selective review of clinical topics, Obestet. Gynecol. **40**(6):773-785, 1972.

Prasad, A.: Commentary: oral contraceptives and nutrition, J. Am. Diet. Assoc. **68**:419-420, 1976.

Prasad, A., and others: Effect of oral contraceptives on micronutrients and changes in face elements due to pregnancy. In Moghissi, K. S., and Evans, T. N., editors: Nutritional impacts on women, New York, 1977, Harper & Row, Publishers, pp. 160-188.

Pritchard, J. A., Whalley, P. J., and Scott, D. E.: The influence of maternal folate and iron deficiencies on intrauterine life, Am. J. Obstet. Gynecol. **104**(3):388-395, 1969.

Ritenbaugh, C.: Human food ways: a window on evolution. In Bauwens, E. E., editor: The Anthropology of Health, St. Louis, 1978, The C. V. Mosby Co.

Robinson, C. A.: Fundamentals of normal nutrition, ed. 3, New York, 1978, The Macmillan Co.

Roe, D., and Eickwort, K.: Relationship between obesity and associated health factors with unemployment among low income women, J.A.M.W.A. **31**(5):193-194, 1976.

Rosenstock, I. M.: What research in motivation suggests for public health, Am. J. Public Health **50**:295, 1960.

Rosman, B. L., and others: A family approach to anorexia nervosa: study, treatment and outcome. In Vigersky, R. A., editor: Anorexia Nervosa, New York, 1977, Raven Press.

Seiter, J. A., and Fox, A. M.: Adolescent pregnancy: association of dietary and obstetric factors, Home Econ. Res. J. **1**:188, 1973.

Shank, R. E.: Chink in our armor, Nutr. Today, pp. 2-11, Summer 1970.

Smith, F.: Dietary habits of girls pregnant at 16 and under, Pub. Health Rep. **84**:213, 1969.

Stein, J. S.: Weight control programs, Curr. Concepts Nutr. **5**:137-155, 1977.

Stevan, M. A.: What shoppers are concerned about, FDA Consumer, DHEW Pub. no. 75-2012, Sept. 1974.

Stuart, R. B., and Mitchell, C.: Self-help weight control groups, Psych. Clin. North Am. **1**(3):697-711, 1978.

Stunkard, A. J.: From explanation to action in psychosomatic medicine: the case of obesity, Psychosom. Med. **37**(3):195-236, 1975.

Stunkard, A. J.: Basic mechanisms which regulate body weight, Psychiat. Clin. North Am. **1**(3):461-472, 1977.

Szyrynski, V.: Anorexia nervosa and psychotherapy, Am. J. of Psychother. **27**(4):492-505, 1973.

Task Force of Nutrition: Assessment of maternal nutrition. Chicago, 1978, American College of Obstetrics and Gynecologists and The American Dietetic Association.

Toddhunter, E. N.: Nutrition in menopausal and postmenopausal women. In Moghissi, K. S., and Evans, T. N., editors: Nutritional impacts on women, New York, 1977, Harper & Row, Publishers.

Travers, C. K.: Obesity and pregnancy: a review, Obesity/Bariatr. Med. **5**(5):172-177, 1976.

Williams, E.: Vegetarian diets in pregnancy, Birth Family J. **3**(2):83-86, 1976.

Wise, T. N., and Gordon, J.: Sexual functioning in the hyperobese, Obesity/Bariat. Med. **6**(3):84-87, 1977.

Worthington, B. S., Vermeersch, J., and Williams, S. R.: Nutrition in pregnancy and lactation, St. Louis, 1977, The C. V. Mosby Co.

22

Fertility control

Catherine Ingram Fogel

Women need effective, safe, comfortable, inexpensive, reversible, and easily available methods of controlling their reproductive functions. Only when such methods exist will women be able to realize their highest potential, free from the notion of biologic destiny propounded by Freud. Women should be able to utilize the concept of fertility control in its fullest sense. It can be a method of postponing pregnancy, of spacing between pregnancies, or of avoiding pregnancy altogether. It should include using modern methods of conception control to establish adequate intervals between births to ensure that every pregnancy is a wanted pregnancy. When every child is a "wanted" child, high-level wellness and optimal health are more apt to be realized. Nurses who are involved in the health care of women have a responsibility to assist them with fertility control needs. This chapter is designed to enhance the nurse's ability to meet her responsibilities by providing requisite information in the following areas: the need for fertility control, risks and effectiveness of contraceptives, contraceptive methods, and contraceptive counseling and nursing management strategies.

NEED FOR FERTILITY CONTROL
Population growth

Excessive population growth and development of programs to solve the problems of overpopulation have become matters of world interest. Nurses traditionally have focused on the individual and family: the number and spacing of children born to specific parents have been more important than fertility and reproductive rates of the nation and the world. But these broader concerns affect us as individuals and as nurses. As individuals we are all a part of and affected by the problems that overpopulation can cause in the world. As nurses we will be affected by governmental attitudes in funding of population programs. In addition, our views of family planning, which can be influenced by our perception of the problems of overpopulation, will be reflected in the type of care we offer our clients.

Although at present birth rates in the United States are decreasing (Moore, 1978), there is still a potential for population problems. It is important to consider how the goals of our nation can be compromised by overpopulation. It is not enough to maintain the status quo: rather, we need to move ahead to reduce the numbers of underprivileged, decrease the amount of poverty and numbers of unemployed, make available to each child the best education he or she is able to use, provide for the aged, and make health care available to all.

Higher fertility rates among the underprivileged mean larger portions of the next generation growing under conditions of economic and cultural deprivation. Education level, which is a good measure of income or socioeconomic status, is closely correlated with fertility; the higher the education or income, the fewer the children. Research has documented that unwanted children constitute 35% to 45% of the U.S. population increase (Kintzel, 1977). This is far from the goal of making every pregnancy the result of an informed personal decision, with the outcome being a wanted child.

On a worldwide scale, the question of how many people the earth can sustain becomes even more imperative to answer. A second question is, sustain on what level? It is thought by some that possibly the world has already reached its capacity in terms of the number of people who can be fed using available resources (Moore, 1978). Who is to feed the poor of the world and how are the major concerns of this century that are yet to be answered. Starvation is not the only problem of unrestrained population growth. The quality of life and economic standards are both adversely affected. Poverty leads to high fertility, which in turn leads to worsened poverty. Another concern is the effect of high population density on the quality of life. When overcrowding occurs, high stress levels exist, which can be severely detrimental to life itself.

Family health

The individual and family may be adversely affected in many ways by overpopulation. The risk of stillbirth, while relatively high in first deliveries and lowest in second births, increases with each subsequent pregnancy and rises sharply after the fifth and sixth births. As the number of children in a family increases, so does the risk of infant and early childhood mortality—no matter what the social class. There is some thought that rates of specific diseases, such as respiratory infection and gastroenteritis, rise with larger family size. Data on this relationship are conflicting, most probably because of social class variation and use of the health care system (Moore, 1978; Siegel and Morris, 1975).

The risk of prematurity is greater when there is less than 12 months between pregnancies. Prematurity is a major cause of both neonatal death and infant morbidity. As family size increases, marital satisfaction decreases. Furthermore, large families have been correlated with diminished maternal care. (The effects of high parity on maternal health and infant well-being are discussed in Chapter 10, High-Risk Pregnancy.)

Social and cultural issues

Control of reproductive functioning through fertility control has a potentially revolutionary impact on women's relationships with men and their own self-concept. Basic to the notion of birth control are the concepts of freedom of choice and the individual's right to self-determination. Until the mid-nineteenth century, control of reproductive capabilities was not feasible. Women continually risked getting pregnant unless they abstained from heterosexual—usually marital—relations with the attendant social disapproval. It was only through pregnancy that women achieved their approved social roles. Motherhood was demanding, unpredictable, usually inevitable, and more or less continual through the reproductive years—a major portion of a woman's life span. It was the inescapable lot of women with all of its attendant demands, and it strongly influenced women's relationships with men, their position in society, and their self-concept. With the advent of reliable, available, and relatively safe birth control methods, women have begun to try to alter their role in society. The opportunity to play roles divorced from the biologic imperative of motherhood is a powerful force for fertility control.

Fertility control behaviors

The decision to use contraception or not is a complex one based on a multitude of interrelated factors. The conscious or unconscious decision-making process that leads to contraception is an expression of a woman's overall health behaviors and self-image. As defined by Sandelowski (1976), contraceptive behaviors are considered to be "repeated, haphazard, or one-time performance or non-performance of specific acts, which over a period of time may or may not result in interference of the biologic consequences of sexual relations—pregnan-

Table 22-1. Factors influencing family planning behaviors

Host (potential contraceptive user)
Perception of problem
Meaning of contraception
Motivation
Knowledge of choices
Ability to act
Environment
Social forces
Role
Health care delivery system
Significant others
Agent (method of contraception)
Effectiveness
Acceptability

cy." The factors that will influence the decision to use contraceptives or not can be considered by using Suchman's (1967) model as adapted by Sandelowski and further modified by the author. This model explores several aspects of the potential contraceptive user (host), environment, and agent (method of contraception) that influence a woman's decision to use or avoid contraception. The model is outlined in Table 22-1.

Host

The woman who is a potential user of contraceptives must first perceive some difficulty or problem that would result from a pregnancy. If she is going to use contraception successfully she must perceive the risk of pregnancy as one she does not wish to incur. Obviously, an unwanted pregnancy can create a variety of medical, emotional, social and financial problems. Any or all of these can be seen as serious enough to want to avoid pregnancy; however, it is also important to realize that the use of contraception may itself cause problems in one or more of these areas. Therefore, each woman has to choose between using nothing at all and risking pregnancy or using a birth control method. The decision will depend on which of the two choices is perceived as the least difficult or risky.

The woman who practices birth control has to accept personal responsibility for having intercourse, with the knowledge that pregnancy is a possible consequence of sexual activity. Inherent in this acceptance is an acknowledgement that sexual intercourse will occur or is wanted. Denial of her sexuality, belief that she is infertile, or belief that she is immune from conception because impregnation has not yet happened may cause the woman to decide contraception is not needed.

The woman must be willing to act and be accustomed to taking action, because action is necessary to avoid pregnancy. The individual must *do* something in order to interrupt the natural progression of events that follow sexual relations. Motivation to act is closely linked to a predisposition to action. The woman must feel she has some control over her own life, that she has free will, and that she can effect change in her life. Motivation involves a positive self-image and a view of oneself as a controlling being. Also related to motivation is perception of the threat of pregnancy; if this is perceived as real, then the woman will be more highly motivated to use contraception. Time perception likewise influences motivation: whether the woman is present- or future-oriented is important. If planning in the present for possible future consequences is not a part of her health behaviors, she will be less likely to use contraception. Present planning for future consequences is also affected by other conflicts occurring in her life at the time; if these appear more immediate and more deserving of attention than avoidance of something that might not occur at all, it is less likely that birth control will be practiced.

A woman's perception of the risk of pregnancy, her predisposition to act, and her motivation are all integrally related to the meaning that contraception and childbearing have for her, and the motivation for childbearing each woman experiences. Attitudes and behaviors concerning contraception must be considered within the woman's value system, as determined by her culture. A woman's health care values will also affect her behavior. The values that sex, marriage, reproduction, children, and family have for a woman profoundly influence her throughout the maturity cycle. Values will change as social, economic, and technologic conditions change.

The motivations for pregnancy are many and will be only briefly reviewed here. According to Moore (1976) childbearing may be viewed as:

1. A rite of passage. Pregnancy and delivery are seen as the transition in role status from childhood to adulthood. Pregnancy may be viewed as an affirmation of competency as an adult.
2. A way to save or maintain a relationship. One or both partners may believe that a child will save or stabilize a relationship or marriage. There is the hope, often unconscious or unexpressed, that a child will provide common experiences and a bond to share, or will force one or both to become more responsible.
3. A substitute for a relationship. The child may be viewed as a replacement for the love or relationship that is lacking with a partner.
4. A way to get needs met. For some women having a child is seen as a way of getting needs for love or dependency met. The baby is viewed as an object whom she can love and who will love in return.
5. A result of pressure to produce. Expectations of others, be they peers, parents, or social reference group, may exert sufficient pressure to ensure that pregnancy occurs. In other cases there may be pressure to produce an heir or a child of a specific sex.
6. Replacement of a loss. Pregnancy may occur after the loss of a significant other such as a child or parent.
7. Affirmation of masculinity or femininity.

In addition to these reasons why a woman might wish to have a child or become pregnant, there are other reasons, principally psychologic and interpersonal, that also operate consciously and unconsciously. Most women are ambivalent about pregnancy at some point in their reproductive lives (Sandberg and Jacobs, 1971). This ambivalence is exacerbated by conflicts between the values a woman holds and those she may be exposed to. Conflict about contraception needs to be considered because conscious and unconscious arguments for and against its use often exist simultaneously. Behavior does not always conform to apparently rational, voiced attitudes; it appears that, for some, psychologic conflicts are influential. These forces seem to be changeable in type and strength and vary with time, age, situation, and partner. Thus there is a necessity for repeated decision-making, which can lead to discontinuation of contraception. Sandberg and Jacobs have identified several psychologic forces that result in a woman not using contraception; in some cases pregnancy is an accidental aftermath, and in others pregnancy is the goal and lack of contraception is a necessary but incidental factor.

1. *Denial.* This can take three forms: (a) of the possibility of pregnancy, (b) that contraceptive measures work, or (c) of personal responsibility for contraception.
2. *Sacrifice.* Love may be equated with self-sacrifice and a willingness to take risks and pregnancy may be considered a sacrifice or demonstration of love—a gift that may or may not have been solicited.
3. *Guilt.* Some women feel greater guilt with the use of contraceptives than with their nonuse. Pregnancy may be considered the "normal" result of coitus and without pregnancy, intercourse is for "no purpose." Contraception is seen as a denial of God or nature.
4. *Shame.* Some women would be ashamed or embarrassed if others discovered they were using contraception.
5. *Coital gamesmanship.* Sexual intercourse can be used to achieve control of a relationship.
6. *Sexual identity conflicts.* In the majority of the world's cultures, a woman who feels herself to be fertile also feels more feminine, attractive, and desirable. A male may also view her this way if he

sees her as a prospect for demonstration of his virility through impregnation.

7. *Hostility.* At times pregnancy may be an immature revengeful act—a way of "getting even."

8. *Masochism.* Hostility is directed inward even though the individual "cuts off her nose to spite her face". A sense of worthlessness can be verified by allowing oneself to be used sexually.

9. *Eroticism.* Sexual pleasure is accentuated by or derived from the thrill of taking risks.

10. *Nihilism.* This is reflected in the abject apathy so often seen in association with poverty, and it influences all attitudes and actions. The woman is too apathetic to make plans and to carry them through. Pregnancy occurs simply because of inertia and ennui.

11. *Fear and anxiety.* There may be anxiety over potential side effects or fear of body damage. Anxiety can result from concern about control of sexual impulses. There are fears that contraceptions will lead to sexual loss of restraint or, conversely to loss of libido. There may also be concern about the effect of contraception on future reproductive capabilities.

12. *Opportunism.* There are some who will accept the possibility of pregnancy for the advantages to be gained from intercourse at a particular time.

The use of contraception may have other meanings and implications for a woman as well. She may desire to limit her fertility for any number of reasons related to personal convenience, economics, social values, and life-style. She may have a desire to achieve, to be in control. For some women control of reproductive functioning represents freedom of choice. Not only are unwanted pregnancies avoided, but other life-styles and options are opened up. Use of contraception may reflect a wish to have more time to devote to mothering and wifehood, to decrease economic burdens and achieve financial stability, to enhance upward socioeconomic mobility, or to pursue a career. All of these will influence whether or not a woman chooses to use contraceptives.

The woman (host) who is a potential user of contraceptives must be physically and psychologically ready to act and she must know how to act. If she has no knowledge of birth control or sex education available to her, she cannot avoid pregnancy. In order to use contraception a woman must know what is available. The individual must also believe in the action; the action must be reconciled with her personal, moral, and religious values, and she must believe that the action is worth it.

Environment

There are many influences from without that impinge on the woman who is making decisions about contraception. Social pressures may be perceived as forceful or weak. Sociocultural factors, such as current trends in family size, the size of her family of orientation, the importance that a particular cultural group places on children, and the stress placed on having a male child all influence a woman's decision. Occupational and economic realities also can play a major part in decision-making. One's religious beliefs will help determine how and what contraception is used. An individual's perception of the broader environmental issue of global overpopulation may also influence her. The role a woman sees for herself in society and her concept of self have been mentioned repeatedly; these are influences by her cultural reference group and will be an important consideration for the potential contraceptive user.

Information on birth control and sex is restricted in this country in part because of persistent Victorian attitudes, which hold that sex is sinful, shameful and something to be ignored. In many areas laws and policies continue to restrict the dissemination of needed information to the public. What often results is ignorance and misinformation. In the 1960s and 1970s the public moved towards advocacy of more open presentation of sexual facts; however, the old habits die hard and sex education for all is still more of a dream than a reality.

The women's movement has provided a stimulus to limit family size through birth control and move society toward acceptance of different roles for women. The feminist movement has brought into the open the notion that childlessness is acceptable and that a woman's lot in life is not just motherhood. As the challenges to the conventional norms about women's role in society continue and gather strength, fertility control will become more acceptable to women.

The health care system is a potent environmental force in the acceptance and use of contraception; unfortunately, it is not always a positive one. There is often an iatrogenic basis for nonuse of contraceptives. Negative attitudes and ambivalence on the part of health care personnel are often encountered by women seeking birth control. Overly enthusiastic authoritarianism, demeaning attitudes, apparent ignorance, oversight, or unconcern can all be equally damaging. Incomplete or inaccurate instruction can sabotage contraceptive practices. Equally detrimental are misconceptions transmitted by the health care worker that lead to rejection of contraception (Sanberg and Jacobs, 1971).

The Boston Women's Health Collective (1976) has made the statement that "our society is not working with us to ensure control of our bodies." Individuals and agencies other than the client often control the choice and acquisition of birth control methods. Much of the information available to women about birth control is published by drug companies that have vested interests. Often physicians do not have up-to-date information about birth control from unbiased sources, and what they do know they do not always communicate. Financially, birth control is expensive. Often the costs of office visits and prescriptions prevent women from receiving adequate birth control.

The significant others that a woman is involved with also influence her fertility control behavior. The partner's wishes and concerns have a lot to do with how effectively a woman uses birth control. If a man feels uncomfortable or threatened by a specific method, his partner is less apt to use it successfully. Most of today's methods are for women, and that responsibility is a burden for many unless it is shared. Total responsibility can create angry feelings, which can prevent adequate use. The partner's attitude is significant: two people prevent pregnancy far more effectively than one. Women often do not talk about birth control with their partners; they hesitate to inconvenience the man, fear to displease him, do not want to deny him. All of these lead to haphazard use of birth control (Boston Women's Health Collective, 1976).

Agent

The general characteristics of the method chosen need to be personally agreeable to the woman. Theoretically, the method can be capable of preventing pregnancy but individual use governs its real effectiveness, and this can decrease effectiveness considerably. The method should be at least minimally displeasurable. As little effort as possible should be involved in the use of the contraceptive. Often there is a balance between the types of effort needed for use; for example, remembering to take pills has to be balanced against repeated insertions or visits to a clinic. Previous experience, either personal or vicarious, influences acceptance and use of contraception, as does the way in which the method is introduced.

Obviously, decisions about fertility control are multifaceted and based on many factors including biopsychosocial and external factors, and the characteristic of the method chosen. The nurse who wishes to be influential in her client's health choices must be cognizant of all these factors.

CONTRACEPTION: RISK VS USE VS EFFECTIVENESS

When assisting a woman to select a satisfactory method of birth control, the factors of risk (mortality and morbidity), effectiveness of the method, and potential usage must all be considered.

One of the most common questions asked by contraceptive users concerns effectiveness. It is important to realize that two types of effectiveness rates are often quoted. The *theoretical effectiveness* of any method is the ideal—its effectiveness when used under ideal con-

ditions and without error—that is, when the method is completely understood and always used correctly. If a contraceptive measure is used in this way, any pregnancies that occur result from method failure or an imperfection in the contraceptive measure itself. The degree of success in the method used under ideal conditions is the maximal effectiveness of the method. In contrast, *use effectiveness* considers all users of a method, those who are careless and those who use the method without error. This measure of effectiveness takes into account the method's effectiveness in preventing pregnancy under actual conditions of use; that is, when some people use it correctly and others do not. Pregnancies resulting from incorrect or careless use of a method reflect *patient failure* as well as method failure (Martin, 1978; Hatcher et al., 1978).

Failure rates are most often expressed in pregnancies per 100 woman years, using the Pearl formula in which the number of pregnancies per woman years equals 1300 times the total number of failures per total number of cycles (Martin, 1978). Hatcher notes that reservations about using the Pearl index as a means of evaluating contraceptive effectiveness have resulted because the index is often incorrectly interpreted as the number of women out of a 100 who would become pregnant in 1 year. This occurs because the Pearl index replaces each woman who becomes pregnant with another. The 100 women per year do not remain constant. That is, as a woman becomes pregnant she is no longer counted in the sample but is replaced by another nonpregnant woman. For the purposes of this chapter the more conventional effectiveness measure—pregnancies per 100 woman years—will be used because this continues to be the way in which most effectiveness rates are computed. See Table 22-2 for a summary of method effectiveness.

When evaluating contraceptive methods or in choosing a method to use, a major factor to consider is the risk-benefit ratio. The risks most often considered are the medical ones, particularly mortality. These risks are compared with the risks associated with pregnancy and childbirth since unprotected intercourse will often result in pregnancy. It is commonly believed that pregnancy is more dangerous than contraceptive usage and that any contraception is safer than no contraception. Statements to that effect are found in standard obstetric-gynecologic textbooks, such as the Romney text (Romney et al., 1975). Tietze et al (1976) conclude that all the major reversible methods of fertility control—oral contraceptives, IUD, condom, diaphragm, and abortion, used alone or in combination—have lower maternal mortality rates than does pregnancy and childbirth when no fertility control measures are used. The one major exception the authors note is use of oral contraceptives after age 40 (see Table 22-3).

Blake (1977) points out that the view that young wom-

Table 22-2. Method effectiveness: theoretical and actual use rates (Number of pregnancies during the first year of use per 100 non-sterile women initiating method)*

Method	Used correctly and consistently (Theoretical effectiveness)	Average U.S. experience among 100 women who wanted no more children (Actual use effectiveness)
Abortion	0	0+
Abstinence	0	?
Hysterectomy	0.0001	0.0001
Tubal ligation	0.04	0.04
Vasectomy	0.15	0.15+
Oral contraceptive (combined)	0.34	4[a]-10[b]
I.M. long-acting progestin	0.25	5-10
Condom + spermicidal agent	Less than 1[c]	5
Low dose oral progestin	1-1.5	5-10[b]
IUD	1-3	5[a]
Condom	3	10[a]
Diaphragm (with spermicide)	3	17[a]
Spermicidal Foam	3	22[a]
Coitus Interruptus	9	20-25
Rhythm (Calendar)	13	21[a]
Lactation for 12 months	25	40[d]
Chance (sexually active)	90[e]	90[e]
Douche	?	40[a]

*From Hatcher, R. A., and others: Contraceptive technology 1978-1979, ed. 9, New York, 1978, Irvington Publishers, Inc.

[a]Ryder, Norman B., "Contraceptive Failure in the United States, "*Family Planning Perspectives* 5:133-142, 1973.

[b]Oral contraceptive failure rates may be far higher than this, if one considers women who become pregnant after discontinuing oral contraceptives, but prior to initiating another method. Oral contraceptive discontinuation rates as high as 50-60% in the first year of use are not uncommon in family planning programs.

[c]Data are normally presented as Pearl indices. For conversion to the form used here, the Pearl index was divided by 1300 to give the average monthly failure rate n. The proportion of women who would fail within one year is then $1 - (1 - n)$.

[d]Most women supplement breast feedings, significantly decreasing the contraceptive effectiveness of lactation. In Rwanda 50% of non-lactating women were found to conceive by just over 4 months postpartum. It might be noted that in this community sexual intercourse is culturally permitted from about 5 days postpartum on (Bonte, M., and van Balen, H., *J. BioSoc. Sci* 1:97, 1969).

[e]This figure is higher in younger couples having intercourse frequently, lower in women over 35 having intercourse infrequently. For example, MacLeod found that within 6 months 94.6% of wives of men under 25 having intercourse four or more times per week conceived. Only 16.0% of wives of men 35 and over having intercourse less than twice a week conceived (MacLeod, *Fertility and Sterility* 4:10-33, 1953).

Table 22-3. Continuing pregnancy rates and deaths due to contraceptive methods or pregnancies per 100,000 fertile women per year having regular intercourse*

Method	Continuing pregnancies	Death due to continuing pregnancies	Deaths due to birth control	Total deaths
No contraception	80,000	16	0	16
Rhythm	25,000	5	0	5
Early abortion	0	0	2.6-4	2.6-4
Diaphragm	12,000	2	0	2
IUD	3,000	1	1	2
Oral contraceptive	500	0	3	3

*From Martin, L.: Health care of women, New York, 1978, J. B. Lippincott Co.

en enjoy relative immunity from health risk from oral contraception appears to be based on the computations used by Tietze when he compared morbidity risks of contraception, pregnancy, and abortion. According to his calculations, the dangers of oral contraceptives in younger age groups appear slight in comparison to the higher mortality associated with childbirth- or abortion-related mortality. It should be noted, however, that these pregnancy- and abortion-related risks assume that the average woman will experience 13.4 pregnancies (no birth control used) and 28.9 abortions (only birth control method used) in her lifetime. Such average rates of pregnancy and abortion are not the norm in large populations that use no contraception; therefore, the associated mortality risks are inflated. In addition, when other methods are available, the relative risks of oral contraceptives for young women should become more of a focus of concern. It should be noted that risks to life are influenced by the individual's health status. There are many conditions that make pregnancy and childbearing more hazardous for a specific woman. These same conditions can also increase the slight mortality risks associated with first trimester abortions. In addition, mortality rates will be higher for those users of a specific contraceptive measure who have health factors that would contraindicate this usage.

It is important to realize that while mortality is the most serious consequence, it is only one possible adverse result of childbearing or fertility regulation. Moreover, it is a very rare one. There are numerous other possible side effects that are less serious but occur far more frequently and have the potential for causing adverse health consequences to both women and their offspring. Furthermore, it should be understood that the idea that any contraception is better than no contraception is now beginning to be qualified by exceptions, and,

Table 22-4. Contraceptive methods: factors affecting usage*

	Foam	Condom	Oral contraceptives	IUD	Early abortion	Diaphragm
Cost	$25/yr.	$25/yr.	$60/yr.	$60/yr.	$150 each	$60/yr.
Effectiveness (theoretical)	97%	97%	99.66%	97-99%	100%	97%
Morbidity						
Major	a	a	1%	1%	1%	a
Minor			40%	40%	8%	
Mortality (per 100,000 users/yr.)	a	a	0.3-3	1.5	1.9	a
Reversibility	100%	100%	100%	+100%	0	100%
Skill required[b]	1	1	1	2	⅔	2
Anesthesia type	0	0	0	0/local	Local	0
Time away from work	0	0	Office visit	Office visit	½ day	Office visit
Hospital or office time	0	0	5-15 min.	5-15 min.	10-15 min.	15 min.
Recovery time	0	0	0	0	1 hour	0
Facility	Across the counter		Office	Office	Office/outpatient	Office/across the counter

*From Hatcher, R. A., and others: Contraceptive technology 1978-1979, ed. 9, New York, 1978, John Wiley & Sons.
[a]Related to pregnancy only.

[b]On scale of 1 to 5: 1-lay, 2-short course, 3-medical, 4-surgical/gyn; 5-surgical/endoscopy.

as research continues, the list of exceptions will probably grow.

The ideal contraceptive is one that is 100% effective, 100% safe (with no side effects), simple to use, easy to understand, cheap, completely reversible, not connected with the act of intercourse, able to be widely distributed, and easily available (Martin, 1978). None of the currently available methods meet all these criteria. Therefore, decisions are made on the basis of the individual's understanding of the following: health, effectiveness, convenience, moral and ethical beliefs, lifestyle, cost, and reversibility (see Table 22-4 for a review of these factors).

Consumers should be informed to the greatest extent possible about all of the advantages and disadvantages of each available method and combination of methods, so that they can make informed choices. The issue of informed consent is critical in contraceptive counseling because most methods are requested by healthy women in the absence of illness (the traditional medical reasons for treatment). There are potentially serious dangers, and often the risk to a particular woman cannot be fully determined in advance. Certain characteristics that can be identified by history or physical examination may contraindicate the use of a given method. Even with a negative history and physical examination, complications occur and it is the patient's right to know about these risks.

The question of how much to tell a client, particularly about side effects and complications, is an issue that continues to be discussed. It has been said that telling a client about a specific problem will be suggestive and may even create the problem. Even though this may be so, it is not an adequate reason for not discussing complications. Legally and morally, the health care professional has the responsibility to provide adequate information to help the client make an informed decision, and the client has a right to this information. The client who has a thorough understanding of the method she chooses and its potential problems will be more apt to use it effectively. The U.S. Department of Health, Education and Welfare guidelines for informed consent to voluntary sterilization can be adapted for use as a model:

Informed consent is the voluntary, knowing assent from the individual to whom a contraceptive is to be provided after she has been given:
1. A fair explanation of the proposed method
2. A description of attendant discomforts and risks including all major (life-threatening) and common minor risks
3. A description of the benefits to be expected
4. An explanation of alternative methods and effectiveness rates
5. An offer to answer any questions about the method
6. Instruction that the individual is free to withdraw consent to the method at any time without affecting future care or loss of benefits
7. A written consent document detailing the basic elements of informed consent and the information provided. This should be signed by the patient, by a witness of the patients' choice, and by the person obtaining consent.

An important part of a woman's choice of contraceptive measure is the information she receives about each method. It has been found that the biases held by family planning professionals and personnel clearly affect the information given about contraceptive effectiveness. Trussel (1976) found that the theoretical effectiveness rates are given for those methods that family planners feel are best, while use effectiveness or lower rates are given for the other methods. In this study the responses were biased in favor of oral contraceptives and the IUD, which tended to drive clients away from other safe, effective methods of birth control such as foam, condoms, and diaphragms. Clients should be given both rates so that they will have complete information to make a decision.

Oral contraceptives

Oral contraceptives were first proposed in the 1930s after a breakthrough in knowledge of the menstrual cycle made it possible to understand the mechanism of fertilization. Once the basic hormonal interrelationships were identified, attempts to alter these patterns so as to control fertility were begun. Progesterone was isolated in 1934 from a Mexican Yone and in 1937 it was demonstrated that progesterone could inhibit ovulation. By the late 1950s, oral contraceptives had been used in Puerto Rico and found to be very effective. They have been widely available since the 1960s, and since the late 1960s it has been clear that the most serious side effects and many of the minor side effects are estrogen related. Since that time many attempts have been made to decrease the amount of estrogen used and to deliver progestins alone (Hatcher, 1978).

At present between 80 million and 100 million women in the world (10 million to 15 million women in the United States alone) are using oral contraceptives to prevent pregnancy. Oral contraceptives are among the most widely used medications in the world—and one of the most casually taken and supervised in actual practice (Martin, 1978). They were first approved for sale in America by the FDA on the basis of studies of 132 women who had taken oral contraceptives for 12 or more months and 718 who had taken them less than 1 year (Corea, 1977). Since then extensive studies have documented the enormously important fact that oral contraceptives affect virtually every organ system. There is steadily accumulating evidence of widespread effects on physiology, complex endocrine alterations, long-term side effects, and significant dangers to life and health. In the face of this mounting evidence, it is essential that the nurse understand mechanisms of action, potential complications and side effects, contraindication to usage, and management so that she may effectively counsel her clients.

Effectiveness

The theoretical effectiveness of the combined drugs is almost 100%, with a reported failure rate of 0.1 pregnancies per 100 woman years (Hatcher, 1978). The Royal College of General Practitioners (1974) reports a failure rate for combined pills of 0.34. Pills containing only progestin have a failure rate of 2.5. Use effectiveness is considerably lower, however, and is related to forgetting or skipping pills, or discontinuing them without beginning an alternate method of contraception. Hatcher (1978) points to a mean failure rate of ten pregnancies per 100 woman years of use (the range is 2 to 16 pregnancies). Oral contraceptive users experience a high attrition rate; only 40% to 75% of the women who begin taking oral contraceptives continue taking them for 1 year. Because of this high attrition rate, it is advisable to instruct every woman receiving oral contraceptives about an alternative birth control method to use if she discontinues the pill.

Among the major reasons for discontinuing the pill are intercurrent morbidity (33.6%), anxiety about side effects (15.5%), and actual side effects (7.1%) (Hatcher, 1978). The risks of taking oral contraceptives become greater the longer the client takes them, both in actual terms and in the perception of clients. It is often stated that despite all of its adverse effects, both potential and proved, oral contraceptives are safer than pregnancy. This argument becomes increasingly less convincing as we consider some of the facts:

1. The statement assumes that women who do not take oral contraceptives become pregnant. There are other safer contraceptives that many women who choose not to use the pill may use rather than become pregnant.
2. The risk of pregnancy is not the same for all women. Most maternal mortality results from poor or nonexistant prenatal care or prior poor health of the woman.
3. The cumulative absolute risk for oral contraceptive usage may be much higher when we consider the broadening range of diseases with relatively higher risks for users. We cannot continue to include major diseases for which the relative risk is two to eight times greater among pill users and not begin to incur absolute effects.
4. The longer oral contraceptives are in usage the more is learned about potential damaging side effects and risks to the users. As yet we have little knowledge about long-term (20 years) impairment to women; however, it seems reasonable to assume that there will be deleterious side effects based on the past record.

For all of these reasons nurses need to continue to question absolute statements of safety and to be increasingly more aware of the risk-benefit ratio for women when considering oral contraceptives.

Mechanism of action

Oral contraceptives prevent pregnancy through four mechanisms of action: (1) prevention of ovulation, (2) alteration in tubal transportation, (3) endometrium changes, and (4) alterations in cervical mucus. Most combination pills which include both estrogen and progestins prevent ovulation by suppressing the midcycle luteinizing hormone peak and depressing follicle-stimulating hormone. This is accomplished through the effect of estrogen on the hypothalamus, which then suppresses pituitary function. Ovulation is not always suppressed by lower doses of estrogen (50 μg or less) or progestin alone. Estrogen accelerates movement of the fertilized ovum through the tubes while progestins seem to slow transportation. After ovulation high doses of estrogens have an antiprogesterone effect on the uterus, causing an alteration in the normal secretory development of the endometrium, resulting in areas of marked edema alternating with areas of dense cellularity. There is also a reduction in carbonic anhydrase, which may result in a decrease in pH, thus making implantation or survival of the zygote impossible. Progestins cause a regression of the proliferative endometrium, and rapid progression through the progestational phase, resulting in an exhausted, atrophic endometrium. Estrogens favorably affect cervical mucus, thus facilitating capacitation of sperm, releasing it from the effects of seminal fluid. However, progestins produce scanty, cellular mucus with increased viscosity that is resistant to sperm penetration and does not allow the capacitation process to take place (Hatcher, 1978).

Types of oral contraceptives

The oral contraceptives available are constantly changing. Although there are more than twenty brand names available, only six different progestational agents and two different estrogens are used. In most cases, the dosage of either the progestogen or the estrogen or both is different. In some, however, only the trade name varies, contributing to the confusion. The oral contraceptives currently available are in combined form or progestin only (mini-pills). The vast majority of combination pills have 2.5 mg or less of progestogen combined with 20 to 100 μg of estrogen. At one time sequential pills, which provided a higher dose of estrogen alone for 14 to 15 days and then a progestogen was added for the last weeks of the cycle, were available. These were thought to have one of four advantages: high estrogen effect, low progestational effects, low androgenic effect, or reduced suppression of the hypothalamus-pituitary-ovarian axis. However, their effectiveness rate was lower and complication rates higher than for combined pills. They have been banned by the Food and Drug Administration because studies suggested an increased risk of endometrial cancer.

In addition to the combination pill, a low dose progestin without estrogen is available, which is taken without interruption. These mini-pills have significant advantages over combined pills in that they are easier to take (one every day); are safer (less serious complications); produce less nausea, weight gain, premenstrual tensions, headaches, leg pain, and depression (more common side effects of estrogen); and they have less effect on lactation. They have a lower theoretical effectiveness rate and are associated with spotting and irregular menses in some women.

Systemic effects

It is now universally acknowledged that oral contraceptives with their powerful synthetic hormones affect almost all body systems, creating many metabolic and endocrine changes. The following is a synthesis of known physiologic alterations.

Reproductive system. Most women who take the combination form of oral contraceptive (containing both estrogen and progestin) experience some changes in their menstrual cycle. Often these are viewed as positive changes, both physically and emotionally. The menstrual cycle becomes regular and shorter. For many, oral contraceptives reduce or completely relieve spastic dysmenorrhea and premenstrual tension syndrome. Often endometriosis and menorrhagia are relieved by the combination drug. A woman's bleeding pattern for a specific estrogen-progestin combination is usually established in the first 6 months of use; however, there may be a gradual decrease in flow for a year or so. Hypomenorrhea is becoming a concern for an increasing number of women. Some women believe that a certain amount of bleeding is essential to good health; others become fearful of pregnancy when the flow is scant or absent. Hypomenorrhea is fairly common in women who are taking potent antiestrogenic progestins, while a gradual reduction in flow is common with lower dosage estrogen pills. Hypomenorrhea does not appear to have any harmful effects and can be corrected by switching to an oral contraceptive containing a higher level of estrogen or a less antiestrogenic progestin (Huxall, 1977).

Breakthrough bleeding, spotting, and amenorrhea all occur in women who are on oral contraceptives. Breakthrough bleeding can occur during the first few cycles of use while the endometrium is accommodating to the additional hormones introduced by combined oral contraceptives. At first there is insufficient estrogen to maintain endometrial growth, with resulting degeneration of blood vessels and adjacent stroma causing staining or bleeding. This gradually decreases and usually disappears following the third or fourth cycle. If it does not disappear, then recommended therapy is to increase the dosage of estrogen. The most common type of breakthrough bleeding begins early in the cycle before taking the fourteenth pill and is usually continuous. Menses is often scant. Early breakthrough bleeding is related to an imbalance in estrogen and progestin. Changing to a pill with either increased progestational and androgenic potency or estrogen potency will usually correct early breakthrough bleeding.

A second type of breakthrough bleeding occurs late in the cycle; it is almost always the result of insufficient progestational potency and may be analogous to the bleeding in corpus luteal insufficiency. It may be associated with heavy menses and dysmenorrhea. This type of bleeding may improve spontaneously after three or four cycles; also, changing to a higher progestational potency will correct late breakthrough bleeding. If breakthrough bleeding persists or recurs after estrogen is increased, then appropriate diagnostic measures (endometrial biopsy or curettage) should be done to detect disease.

Commissioner Kennedy in the *Federal Register* of January, 1978, recommends that nonfunctional causes should be considered in all cases of breakthrough bleeding. According to Kennedy, for any undiagnosed persistent or recurrent abnormal vaginal bleeding, adequate diagnostic measures should be employed to rule out pregnancy or malignancy. If pathology is ruled out, time or changing to another type of oral contraceptive may correct the problem. However, changing to an oral contraceptive containing a higher estrogen content, while potentially useful in minimizing menstrual irregularities, should be done only if necessary because of the increased risk of thromboembolic disease. It should also be noted that alterations in menstrual patterns are likely to occur in women who are taking the mini-pill or compounds containing only progestin. The amount and duration of flow, length of cycle, spotting, breakthrough bleeding, and amenorrhea can be quite variable.

Most women quickly resume their previous menstrual cycle patterns after they stop taking oral contraceptives. In a group of 211 women, Taylor et al. (1977) found that after the first cycle, cycle length and regularity were comparable to previous norms in most cases. A few women develop true secondary amenorrhea; usually these are women who experienced irregular or anovulatory cycles before they started using oral contraceptives.

Women with previous histories of very irregular cycles as well as sexually immature, young teenagers should not be given oral contraceptives to "regulate" their periods. These women may have hypothalamic-pituitary-ovarian dysfunction or immature development of the pathways of the hypothalamic-pituitary-ovarian axis and oral contraceptives will suppress these conditions rather than correct them. The amenorrhea is a result of the suppressive effect of oral contraceptives on the secretion of gonadotropin. In women whose pituitary-ovarian axis is already compromised, oral contraceptives are at least partially responsible for subsequent amenorrhea and possible sterility (Martin, 1978; Romney et al., 1975). Women with cycles of 60 to 90 days or more should not use oral contraceptives. These women are more likely to have hypothalamic-pituitary dysfunction which can be easily aggravated by oral contraceptives, especially in prolonged use (Kistner, 1976).

Tatum and Schmidt (1977) have found that in progestin-only oral contraceptive failures the chance of an extrauterine pregnancy appears to be significantly greater than would be expected in the normal, unprotected population. This is probably related to the progestin's effect on deceleration in ovum transport. The ovaries under the influence of oral contraceptives appear inactive. There is some early follicular development that is soon arrested (Romney et al., 1975).

Kistner (1976) raises the possibility that pelvic inflammatory disease (PID) among oral contraceptive users is related to the increased freedom for sexual activity associated with the method. However, he acknowledges that the precise incidence of PID in oral contraceptive users is not known. Oral contraceptives have been implicated in the marked increase in vaginal infections, particularly monilia *(Candida albicans)*. Cervical erosion is also diagnosed more often among pill users than among users of other methods such as the IUD and diaphragm (Family Planning Digest, 1976). Women using the pill are less likely to develop certain types of ovarian cysts.

Thyroid. Women taking oral contraceptives often have abnormal laboratory values for thyroid functioning. Estrogen causes an increase in thyroxin-binding globulin with a subsequent increase in protein-bound iodine and T_4, and a decrease in T_3 intake. Thyroid function does not appear to be altered, however, because basal metabolism rates, cholesterol, and free thyroxin levels remain normal. There is no evidence that oral contraceptives cause either hypo- or hyperthyroidism and the abnormal test results disappear 2 to 4 months after pills are discontinued (Romney et al., 1975).

Skin. Chloasma is reported in 29% of oral contraceptive users. Unfortunately, unlike chloasma of pregnancy, that caused by oral contraceptives does not entirely disappear after use is discontinued. It is more likely to appear in women who had chloasma during pregnancy or who have had prolonged exposure to sunlight. Acne may be improved in women who take estrogen-dominant pills since estrogen causes a decrease in subaceous gland activity (Romney et al., 1975). Conversely, some women will have a flare-up of acne or develop hirsutism when taking progestin-dominant pills. Women who have a history of acne or excess body hair should not be placed on androgenic oral contraceptives. Scalp hair loss is not commonly experienced while taking oral contraceptives but may occur while a woman is on the pill or soon after discontinuation (Dernison, 1976).

Weight gain. Weight gain is probably the most common reason that women discontinue taking oral contraceptives. Some 40% to 50% of women who take oral contraceptives report a 3 to 5 lb weight gain, usually most severe in the first 3 months and less pronounced after a year. Lecoq et al. (1967), in a study using two different combination drugs and a constant caloric intake, report a consistent increase in lean body mass without weight gain, as well as a positive nitrogen balance indicative of accumulated body protein. Most often weight gain is associated with increased appetite resulting from the progestational and anabolic properties of progestin. Estrogen can stimulate a particular type of weight gain in some women. Estrogen is responsible for an increase in subcutaneous fat distribution, especially over the thighs, hips, and in the breasts. In addition, cyclic weight gain from fluid retention is often caused by estrogen (Waller, 1975).

Carbohydrate metabolism. According to Romney et al. (1975) studies of the effect of oral contraceptives on carbohydrate metabolism are conflicting. It may be that estrogen affects carbohydrate metabolism, but the effect depends on the type of estrogen, the dosage involved, and the client's carbohydrate status. Obesity or a history suggestive of diabetes places a woman at greater risk for abnormal carbohydrate metabolism. It appears that progestins have no adverse effect on carbohydrate metabolism and may improve glucose tolerance. Women taking oral contraceptives have a three-fold increase in human growth hormone (HGH) resulting in a compensatory increase in insulin caused by the anti-insulin effect of HGH. At the same time blood sugar levels are increased. These factors interact to produce abnormal glucose tolerance test results in most women. Clients with normal beta cell function will respond to the estrogen in oral contraceptives with an elevated HGH level and a compensatory increase in plasma insulin, allowing them to maintain normal glucose tolerance. Patients with impaired functioning will have altered glucose tolerance. There appears to be no contraindication to the use of oral contraceptives in insulin-dependent diabetics because they have very little, if any, endogenous insulin. However, medical control of diabetes may be more difficult, as it is in pregnancy. The women at risk are those potential diabetics whose compensatory production of insulin is reduced. Studies of short-term users point to prompt reversal of cell changes once oral contraceptives are discontinued; long-term effects are not yet known.

Lipids. Increased plasma triglyceride and phospholipid levels have been found in oral contraceptive users. This is a dose-dependent estrogen effect, not related to progestin. The mechanism is unclear but may be related to increased hepatic production. At this time the long-term effects of lipid increases are not known, but they may be associated with circulatory disorders and acute vascular accidents (Martin, 1978).

Hypertension. An increase in blood pressure has been reported in women taking oral contraceptives. There appears to be a direct relationship between the estrogen component and hypertension. Estrogen appears to cause increases in the concentration of angiotensenogin and plasma renin activity (Waller, 1975). It is also possible that the direct action of estrogen on the juxtaglomerular cells causes a blunting of the normal feedback control (Martin, 1978). Romney et al. (1975) state that the incidence is from 15% to 18% of women taking oral contraceptives. Oral contraceptive users are six times as likely as nonusers to develop hypertension.

Increases in systolic and diastolic pressure occur in both normotensive and hypertensive women as early as 1 to 3 weeks after beginning oral contraceptives. Usually, blood pressure will return to premedication levels within 1 to 3 months of discontinuation of the pill. In the first year of use, the prevalence of hypertension in women using oral contraceptives may be no higher than in a comparable group of nonusers; however, the prevalence among users increases with longer exposures, and by the fifth year of use it is 2.5 to 3 times greater than the prevalence reported in the first year. Age is closely correlated with the development of hypertension. Women who have experienced hypertension in pregnancy may be more likely to develop blood pressure elevation while on oral contraceptives.

Thromboembolitic effects. As stated in the *Federal Register* (1978), "An increased risk of thromboembolic and thrombotic disease associated with the use of oral contraceptives is well established." There is an increased risk of fatal and nonfatal venous thromboembolism and stroke, both hemorrhagic and thrombotic. Women who use oral contraceptives are four to eleven times more apt to develop these diseases without other evident cause. Several factors are apt to be implicated in this thrombogenic potential, including production of vascular lesions, venous stasis, and alterations in the blood. Women taking oral contraceptives also have more rapid fibrin formation and increased clot firmness (Fisch and Freedman, 1975). Vessey (1973) states that the risk of thrombotic stroke is related to estrogen content of oral contraceptives and low-dose preparations should be used whenever possible. British investigators have concluded that the risk for thromboembolism is directly related to the dosages of estrogen used in oral contraceptives (Martin, 1978). Preparations containing 100 μg or more of estrogen show more association with an increased risk of thromboembolism than those containing from 50 to 80 μg of estrogen. Further analysis suggests that quantity of estrogen may not be the sole factor involved (Federal Register, 1978).

Blood alterations begin within a few days of pill usage and disappear within 2 months of discontinuation. Estrogen has been implicated in clotting problems; it causes increases in blood factors VII, IX, and X and platelet counts (Martin, 1978). Progesterone antagonizes the estrogenic effect by causing an increase in the rate of fibrinolysin; however, progesterone may also increase the likelihood of thrombophlebitis by causing venous relaxation and therefore dilation of veins and venous stasis. In a study by Jick and associates (1967) the risk of thromboembolism was found to be three times greater in women with blood types A, B, or AB. A history of varicosities or other circulatory disorders increases the risk of thromboembolism.

Users of oral contraceptives are exposed to seven to eight times greater risk from thromboembolic disease than are nonusers. Inman and Vessey (1968) have found the risk of hospital admission for venous thromboembolism to be about nine times greater in women who used oral contraceptives than in those who did not. They calculate that one in every 2,000 women using oral contraceptives is admitted to the hospital with "idiopathic" venous thromboembolism, in contrast to one in every 20,000 women not using them. They also conclude that oral contraceptives can be a cause of cerebral vascular insufficiency.

An increased risk of myocardial infarction among users of oral contraceptives has been reported (Federal Register, 1978; Mann and Inman, 1975;). The greater the number of associated risk factors for coronary artery disease, such as cigarette smoking, hypertension, obesity, diabetes, and history of pre-eclampsia, the greater the risk of developing myocardial infarction whether or not the client is using oral contraceptives. However, oral contraceptives have been found to be a clear additional risk factor.

The risk of fatal heart attack is greatly multiplied in the woman who smokes and takes oral contraceptives. Oral contraceptive users who do not smoke are twice as likely to have a fatal heart attack as nonusers who do not smoke. For women who smoke and take oral contraceptives the risk is five times that of users who do not smoke, and ten to twelve times the risk for nonusers who do not smoke. The amount of smoking is an important factor. Age is also closely related to the risk factor of smoking (Federal Register, 1978). Jain (1977) found the risk of death from oral contraceptive use in women aged 15 to 29 years to be lower than the corresponding risk from childbearing, for nonsmokers as well as smokers. He further states that for 15 to 29 year-old-women who are heavy smokers oral contraceptives may be more hazardous than any other method of fertility regulation, al-

though less hazardous than using no contraceptive method. For nonsmokers over age 30 the risk of death from oral contraceptive use is substantially lower than risk of death from childbearing. However, for pill users between the ages of 30 and 39 years who smoke, the risk is slightly higher than when no fertility control method is used. For the woman over age 40 who smokes and takes oral contraceptives the risk of death is substantially higher—up to four times greater than that associated with absence of fertility control. While there are other factors associated with risk of myocardial infarction, smoking is the greatest risk factor. Increased age also appears to have a synergistic effect, increasing the risk involved. So great is the risk that the FDA now requires the following statement to be placed on all oral contraceptive "patient package inserts":

Cigarette smoking increases the risk of serious adverse effects on the heart and blood vessels from oral contraceptive use. This risk increases with age and with heavy smoking (15 or more cigarettes per day) and is quite marked in women over 35 years of age. *Women who use oral contraceptives should not smoke.* (italics added.)

A four-to six-fold increase in the risk of postoperative thromboembolic complications has been reported in oral contraceptive users. When possible, these should be discontinued at least 4 weeks prior to any surgery associated with an increased risk of thromboembolism or extended immobilization (Federal Register, 1978).

A recent analysis by Tietze (1979) of United States mortality statistics for men and women during the years 1950 through 1976 casts serious doubts on the applicability in the United States of British findings that women who use oral contraceptives are four times more likely to die of cardiovascular disease than are nonusers. Analysis shows that deaths among women of reproductive age from cardiovascular disease have dropped much more steeply than have death rates for men. This decrease has occurred in face of an increase in women who smoke and who are exposed to the stress of the workplace, both of which are believed to be associated with cardiovascular disease. Tietze points out that this analysis does not disprove that a relationship exists between cardiovascular disease and oral contraceptive use but it does suggest that caution be exercised in accepting levels of relative risk of death.

Cancer. The exact relationship between oral contraceptives and cancer will probably not be clearly determined for several more years. It is known that the pill causes benign cervical polypoid hyperplasia, but there is no evidence that this condition progresses to malignancy (Martin, 1978). Studies have reported an increased risk of endometreal carcinoma in postmenopausal women associated with prolonged use of exogenous estrogen. Silverberg and Makowski (1975), reported on endometrial adenocarcinoma in women under 40 on oral contraceptives. Among those women who had no predisposing risk factors, such as irregular bleeding prior to onset of taking oral contraceptives or polycystic ovaries, nearly all cases occurred in women who used sequential oral contraceptives. This type of oral contraceptive has since been withdrawn from the market. There is no reported evidence of an increased risk of endometrial cancer in users of combination or progestogen-only oral contraceptives.

The lower incidence of benign breast tumors in users of oral contraceptives has been well documented. This protective effect appears related to progestin dose and duration of use (Population Reports, 1975, 1975; Federal Register, 1978). At present no causal relationship has been established between breast cancer and oral contraceptives. Certain types of breast cancer are estrogen-dependent and grow more rapidly in a hyperestrogenic state (for example, pregnancy). Concern has been expressed that oral contraceptives, which also create a hyperestrogenic state, might initiate or promote the development of breast cancer. Several studies have found no increased incidence of breast cancer in women taking oral contraceptives or estrogens (Federal Register, 1978). Fasal and Paffenbarger (1975) did find, however, that while there was no overall increased risk of breast cancer in women taking oral contraceptives, there was an increased risk for women on oral contraceptives who had documented benign breast disease. As noted before, studies in the United States and Great Britain have consistently demonstrated that women taking oral contraceptives have a lower incidence of benign breast tumors than nonusers (Population Reports, 1975, 1977; Federal Register, 1978).

According to the *Federal Register*, there is at present no confirmed evidence in human subjects of an increased risk of cancer associated with oral contraceptives. Nevertheless, close clinical monitoring of all women on oral contraceptives is essential. All cases of undiagnosed, persistent, or recurrent abnormal vaginal bleeding should be promptly examined to rule out malignancy. In our opinion those women who have a familial history of breast cancer or who have breast nodules, fibrocystic disease, or abnormal mammograms should not be placed on oral contraceptives.

Liver. Oral contraceptives cause an alteration in liver function that is apparently related to estrogen rather than progestin; it is dose related and easily reversible when the woman stops taking the drug. It appears that oral contraceptives alter hepatic cell permeability rather than being hepatotoxic (Romney et al., 1975). Benign hepatic adenomas have been found to be associated with oral contraceptive usage. These tumors appear to be re-

lated to prolonged usage (incidence increases after 4 years), type of estrogen, and potency (Martin, 1978). This appears to be a rare complication, one for which there is no obvious method of prevention or early detection. It does seem feasible to regularly examine the abdomen of women taking oral contraceptives. Health care practitioners should be aware of the possibility of hepatic adenomas in any young woman and should regard abdominal pain, particularly hepatomegaly, as suspicious. Ruptured hepatic adenoma should be considered in the differential diagnosis of acute abdominal disease in women who are taking oral contraceptives or hormonal replacement therapy (Kent et al., 1977; Waschek and Helling, 1970).

Gallbladder. There is an increased risk of gallbladder disease in users of oral contraceptives. Apparently the risk is related to prolonged use (Federal Register, 1978).

Eyes. Some women develop mild corneal swelling as a result of fluid retention from estrogen effect. They may find contact lenses fail to fit properly. The swelling is usually worse in the first three months of usage, after which it may improve (Martin, 1978). Neuro-ocular lesions, such as optic neuritis and retinal thrombosis, have been reported to be associated with oral contraceptives (Federal Register, 1978).

Urinary tract. Users of oral contraceptives have been noted to have an increased incidence of urinary tract infections, probably related to ureteral dilation from hormonal influences and asymptomatic bacteruria (Martin, 1978). A greater incidence of vaginitis from *Candida albicans* (monilia) and *Trichomonas vaginalis* has been reported and may be associated with urethral irritation and reports of burning upon urination.

Lactation. Low-dose estrogen oral contraceptives will cause a significant decrease in milk supply. Small amounts of exogenous hormones are excreted in the milk during lactation (Martin, 1978). What effect this may have on the breast-fed infant is undetermined at this time.

Genetic effects

The use of estrogenic and progestational hormonal agents in early pregnancy may seriously damage the fetus. An increased risk of congenital anomalies, including heart and limb defects, has been reported with the use of sex hormones, including oral contraceptives, in pregnancy. Data suggest that the risk of limb defects is somewhat less than one in 1,000 births (Federal Register, 1978).

There is no evidence to definitely link an increase in fetal abnormalities to use of oral contraception prior to conception. An increased number of early spontaneous abortions has been linked to oral contraceptive usage, as has an increased incidence of triploidy among abortuses from women who conceived soon after stopping the pill (Martin, 1978).

Psychological effects

Kane (1976) states that from 10% to 40% of oral contraceptive users may suffer mild to moderate depression syndromes resulting from a variety of mechanisms, such as alterations in folate, pyridoxine, and vitamin B_{12} metabolism. Interactive effects may result such as impaired coping mechanisms and psychologic defenses caused by altered central nervous system functions. The effect of oral contraception on libido is extremely variable according to reports by individual women. Certainly, it is possible that the hormones could alter physiology enough to affect sexual desire and functioning. However, multiple factors are usually operant, and it is difficult to say with certainty that oral contraceptives are always a factor. Mood, sexual interest, and enjoyment appear to be affected both positively and negatively in different women.

Side effects

The side effects that occur while taking oral contraceptives are the same as those symptoms that occur during natural periods of hormone excess or deficiency. The symptoms of hormonal excess are similar to the common symptoms and physiologic changes of pregnancy and can be caused by estrogen or progesterone. One of the most confusing aspects of these side effects is that their occurrence is so variable. Some women experience them more often than others and with some drugs more often than with others. Furthermore, the same contraceptive can cause symptoms of hormonal excess in one woman and symptoms of deficiency in another because women differ in the amount of estrogen and progesterone that their bodies produce and metabolize. Most of the minor side effects can be classified in two ways: (1) by the hormone they are related to (estrogen and progesterone) and (2) by amount (excess or deficit). See Table 22-5 for a summary of the hormonal etiology of side effects and Table 22-6 for a time framework of side effects.

Symptoms of estrogen excess can be divided into three types. The first includes those symptoms caused by estrogenic effect on blood vessels, such as vascular headache, and changes in serum proteins caused by estrogenic effect on liver enzymes. The second group of symptoms result from the estrogenic effect on the reproductive system and include increased uterine fibroid growth, cervical exotrophia, mucorrhea, cystic breast changes, and hypermenorrhea. The third group consists of those symptoms related to estrogenic effect on sodium and fluid retention, such as nausea, dizziness, leg cramps, bloating, visual changes, and nonvascular headache. These are the same as the premenstrual syndrome

and are related to progesterone withdrawal followed by rebound sodium and fluid retention. While the symptoms of fluid retention tend to improve in 3 months (just as in pregnancy) because of a readjustment in the ho-

Table 22-5. Side effects of oral contraceptives

Estrogen excess*
Vascular system and liver enzyme effects
1. Vascular headache
2. Hypertension
3. Thromboembolic disease
4. Increase in serum proteins and lipids
5. Telangiectasia
Reproductive system effects
1. Mucorrhea
2. Uterine enlargement
3. Fibroid growth
4. Cervical extrophy
5. Cystic breast changes
6. Increase in breast size (ductal and fatty tissue)
7. Hypermenorrhea, menorrhagia, dysmenorrhea
Fluid retention effects
1. Nausea and vomiting
2. Epigastric distress
3. Dizziness, Syncope
4. Edema, leg cramps
5. Irritability
6. Bloating, cyclic weight gain
7. Visual changes
8. Nonvascular headaches
Estrogen deficiency†
1. Spotting and bleeding (day 1-14)
2. Decreased flow (hypomenorrhea)
3. No withdrawal period
4. Pelvic relaxation
5. Nervousness
6. Vascular symptoms
7. Atrophic vaginitis

Progestin excess‡
Progestational effects
1. Tiredness
2. Feeling weak
3. Depression
4. Breast tenderness
5. Increase in breast tissue (alveolar)
6. Decreased libido
7. Dilated leg veins
8. Pelvic congestion syndrome
9. Decreased days of flow
10. Moniliasis
11. Anovulation following discontinuation
12. Noncyclic weight gain
13. Increased appetite
Androgenic and anabolic effects
1. Increased libido
2. Oily skin and scalp
3. Acne
4. Hirsutism
5. Rash
6. Pruritus
7. Cholestatic jaundice
Progestin deficiency§
1. Late spotting or breakthrough bleeding (day 15 to 21)
2. Heavy flow and clots
3. Dysmenorrhea
4. Delayed withdrawal bleeding

*Symptoms tend to decrease in severity in a few months' time.
†Symptoms get worse with time and may not appear until months or years of use.
‡Symptoms get worse with time.
§Symptoms may improve in 3 to 4 months' time.

Table 22-6. Side effects of oral contraceptives; a time framework*

Worse in first 3 months	Over time: steady-constant	Worse over time	Worse post-discontinuation

1. Nausea plus dizziness
2. Thrombophlebitis (venous) Leg veins
   [a] Pulmonary emboli
   [a] Pelvic vein thrombosis
   [a] Retinal vein thrombosis
3. Cyclic weight gain edema
4. Breast fullness, tenderness
5. Breakthrough bleeding
6. [a] Elevated serum lipid levels even to the extent of pancreatitis
7. [a] Abnormal glucose tolerance test
8. Contact lenses fail to fit because of fluid retention
9. Abdominal cramping
10. Suppression of lactation
11. Failure to understand correct use of oral contraceptives; pregnancy
	1. Headaches during 3 weeks that Pills are being taken
	2. [a] Arterial thromboembolic events, blurred, vision, stroke
	3. Anxiety, fatigue, depression
	4. Thyroid function studies Elevated PBI Depressed T3 resin uptake
	5. Susceptibility to amenorrhea post-Pill discontinuation
	6. Change in cervical secretions—mucorrhea
	7. Decrease in libido
	8. Autophonia, chronic dilatation of Eustachian tubes rather than cyclic opening and closing
	9. Acne
		1. Headaches during week Pills are not taken
		2. Weight gain
		3. Monilial vaginitis
		4. Periodic missed menses while on oral contraceptives
		5. [a] Chloasma
		6. [a] Myocardial infarction
		7. Spider angiomata
		8. Growth of myoma
		9. Predisposition to gallbladder disease
		10. Hirsutism
		11. Decreased menstrual flow
		12. Small uterus, pelvic relaxation, cystocele, rectocele, atropic vaginitis
		13. Cystic breast changes
		14. Photodermatitis—sunlight sensitivity with hypopigmentation
		15. One form of hair loss—alopecia
		16. Hypertension
		17. Focal hyperplasia of liver and hepatic adenomas
			1. [b] Infertility, amenorrhea, hypothalamic and endometrial suppression, and miscalculation of the expected date of confinement
			2. One form of acne
			3. Hair loss—alopecia

*From Hatcher, R. A., and others: Contraceptive technology, 1978-1979, ed. 9, New York, 1978, John Wiley & Sons.
[a] May be irreversible or produce permanent damage.

[b] N.B. To avoid this complication in many patients, advise women desiring to become pregnant to discontinue Pills 3-6 months prior to desired pregnancy.

meostatic mechanisms, the other symptoms related to estrogen excess remained the same or worsen.

Symptoms of estrogen deficiency are similar to those associated with the childbearing years. The most common is breakthrough bleeding and spotting caused by lack of stimulation of the endometrium, often accompanied by scant flow or amenorrhea. Often these symptoms do not appear until the drug has been taken for months or years; usually they then become progressively worse.

Symptoms of progestin excess can be related either to the progestational effects or the androgenic activity by the progestin. Progestin-related symptoms are like those that may be seen in the second and third trimester of pregnancy (fatigue, increased breast size, depression, decreased libido, and weight gain associated with an increased appetite). Smooth muscle relaxation, a progesterone effect, can cause decreased dysmenorrhea and venous dilation leading to varicosities. The androgenic symptoms of progestins and similar to those found in Stein-Leventhal syndrome (for example, acne, oily

scalp, hirsutism, rash, pruritus, cholestatic jaundice, and increased libido). Monilia vaginitis may result from either progestin excess or estrogen deficiency. Symptoms of progestin excess are seldom serious but have a high nuisance effect, causing women to stop taking oral contraceptives.

Progestin deficiency results in heavy menstrual flow associated with clots and longer intervals between when the last pill was taken and menses begins. Dysmenorrhea is experienced more often. Breakthrough bleeding after the fourteenth day is also associated with progestin deficiency.

Some side effects are difficult to attribute to any specific steroid component of oral contraceptives. For example, headache can be caused either by excess estrogen or excess progestin, depending on when in the cycle it occurs.

Management

A woman should not be placed on oral contraceptives hastily or without adequate assessment. A woman who receives a prescription for oral contraceptives has begun long-term use of an extremely potent medication with widespread multiple effects on most body systems. The principles of informed consent must be followed and careful follow-up planned for. The decision to place a woman on oral contraceptives should be preceded by thorough history taking and physical examination to identify any contraindications to taking them, as well as any history or physical condition that would indicate that one type is better than another. The initial history-taking should include the following:

1. Family history, specifically of diabetes, cancer, thromboembolism, and cardiac disorders
2. Personal medical history including diabetes; cancer; thyroid, liver, kidney, cardiac, and thromboembolic history; hospitalization and surgeries; and allergies. For each of these, dates, location, or type of condition and treatment should be noted.
3. Detailed menstrual history to detect irregularities, dysmenorrhea, onset of menarche, and disruption of the period.
4. Previous obstetric history, if any, including number of pregnancies, deliveries, abortions
5. Contraceptive history including current knowledge level, method preferred by woman and partner, method currently being used and woman's satisfaction with it and its usefulness
6. History of smoking
7. Subjective data on headaches, vision, edema, or anything else the woman wishes to report

The client's history may uncover medical conditions indicating that the risk of taking oral contraceptives is too high for the client. Adverse behavior patterns that would affect the client's ability to take the pill may also be noted.

A complete physical examination must be done to discover at the outset any conditions that would contraindicate usage of oral contraceptives. This also provides baseline data for future follow-up. Special attention should be given to:

1. Blood pressure and weight
2. Visual disturbances
3. Breast masses
4. Alopecia
5. Thyroid enlargement
6. Abdomen (gallbladder tenderness, liver size and consistency)
7. Pelvic (uterine size, cervicitis or erosion, ovarian tenderness or enlargement, vaginal discharge, bladder tenderness)
8. Extremities (peripheral circulation, bruising, varicosities, edema)

Laboratory diagnostic tests that should be done are Pap smear, cervical culture for gonorrhea, urinalysis for glucose and protein, hemoglobin and hematocrit, blood test for syphilis, and possibly a prothrombin time (Cowart and Newton, 1976).

Specific contraindications* to the use of oral contraceptives have been identified and include the following:

Absolute contraindications
  Thromboembolic disorder (or history thereof)
  Cerebrovascular accident (or history thereof)
  Impaired liver function
  Coronary artery disease (or history thereof)
  Hepatic adenoma (or history thereof)
  Malignancy of breast or reproductive system (or history thereof)
  Pregnancy (known or suspected)
  Smoking
  Undiagnosed abnormal vaginal bleeding
Strong relative contraindications
  Termination of term pregnancy within past 10 to 14 days
  Severe vascular or migraine headaches
  Hypertension
  Diabetes, prediabetes, or strong family history of diabetes
  Gallbladder disease, including cholecystectomy (or history thereof)
  Previous cholestasis during pregnancy
  Mononucleosis, acute phase
  Sickle cell disease or sickle C trait
  Elective surgery planned in next 4 weeks (e.g., hysterectomy, exploratory laparotomy, or elective orthopedic procedures)
  Long-leg casts or major injury to lower leg
  Over age 35 to 40 (risk is even greater if obese, hypertensive, heavy smoker, diabetic, or if patient has high cholesterol levels)
  Fibrocystic breast disease and breast fibroadenomas
  History suggestive of infertility and anovulation
  Lactation
  Conditions that prevent patient from following instructions
  Depression
  Varicose veins
  Cardiac or renal disease
  Uterine fibroids
  History of hepatitis
Possible contraindications
  Chloasma or has had chloasma during pregnancy
  Asthma
  Epilepsy
  Acne

Once the decision has been made that oral contraception is the desired means of birth control and contraindications have been eliminated, a specific drug must be prescribed. The risk of the client developing

---

*This list is adapted from Hatcher (1978) but reflects our analysis of the seriousness of potential side effects.

major or minor side effects should be minimized. Cost is also an important factor (Hatcher, 1978). The recommendation to use a specific drug should be based on the following assumptions:

1. At this time, it is difficult to predict which women will develop serious complications.
2. The estrogen component causes most of the major complications and most of the minor side effects responsible for discontinuation.
3. Some minor side effects are caused by progestin and result in discontinuation.

Selection of the appropriate drug for the individual woman can be extremely difficult given the large number available from which to choose. There are two forms of estrogen used—ethinyl estradiol and mestranol. Both are similar in estrogenic potency and contraceptive effectiveness; it is thought that ethinyl estradiol may be somewhat more potent. At present six progestogens are used; all of them are 19-nortestosterone derivatives. The biologic properties vary, such as anabolic effects, antiestrogenic components, conversion to estrogen, progestational potency, and androgenic potential. When these hormones are combined into various oral contraceptives, the complexity of action and interaction is enormous. Because individual women differ in the amount of estrogen and progesterone they need for balance and a given oral contraceptive when combined with their own physiology may create an excess or deficit in hormonal needs, it can be useful to assess the drugs on a scale of estrogen dominance to balanced to progestogen dominance. This will facilitate initial selection or changing of drugs because of the development of side effects (Martin, 1978).

It is usually best to begin with a pill containing 50 μg or less of estrogen in order to minimize thromboembolic risks. Over 90% of women can take oral contraceptives with 50 μg of estrogen or less. If side effects are reported, they need to be evaluated as to possible cause; for example, estrogen excess or deficiency, or androgen excess, or progestin deficiency (see Table 21-5). Most women should be encouraged to stay on the initially chosen drug for two or three cycles since many minor side effects will disappear after this time. Most women take combination oral contraceptives and usually one can be found that is compatible with individual needs.

Dosage modification related to side effects can be summarized as follows:

1. *Spotting, early or late:* Taking the contraceptive at exactly the same time of day can sometimes control spotting. Spotting is a potential problem in all 50 μg pills; at times it is necessary to switch to a type with a higher estrogen content. Those containing only 20 to 30 μg estrogen are associated with a higher incidence of breakthrough bleeding and/or spotting.
2. *Nausea:* The amount of estrogen should be decreased.
3. *Weight gain associated with increased appetite:* A low-androgen drug or one low in anabolic effects is effective.
4. *Weight gain caused by fluid retention.* This is associated with estrogenic excess and is best ameliorated by oral contraceptives containing 0 to 50 μg of estrogen.
5. *Hypertension:* It is best to use 0 to 50 μg of estrogen, and after a trial of 3 to 6 months on a combined form and antihypertensive therapy, to switch to a mini-pill. The combined drug should not be continued indefinitely with a client experiencing continued elevated diastolic blood pressure. If the diastolic pressure exceeds 100 mm Hg on two subsequent visits, estrogen-containing contraceptives should not be used.
6. *Oily skin, acne:* A low-progestin, low-androgen drug preferably with 50 μg of estrogen, should be used. Any oral contraceptive can cause acne to worsen but those highest in androgens are especially troublesome.
7. *Hirsutism:* A low-androgen type should be used.
8. *Depression:* Depression can be caused by high estrogen levels resulting in fluid retention; by high progestin levels; or by very low estrogen levels. It is often difficult to decide what dosage alteration to make. Furthermore, depression can become more severe or improve while oral contraceptives are being used. Each user must be questioned carefully (Hatcher, 1978).

Client education

Given the wide variety of oral contraceptives with different packaging and schedules, the numerous misconceptions and fears about them, and the various troublesome side effects and potential serious complications that occur, client teaching is of prime importance. Details as to how to take oral contraceptives, side effects, symptoms of serious dangers, and follow-up care should always be discussed. Instructions should include the following:

1. The first pack is started on the fifth day of the next menstrual cycle or 4 weeks postpartum. One pill should be taken every day until the pack is finished. If the 21-day variety is used there will be one week when no pills are taken and then the new pack is begun on the same day of the week as when originally begun. If the 28-day variety is used, the woman will always take a pill, beginning a new

pack as soon as she finishes the last one. The 28-day type has seven inert pills, usually containing iron, so that the pill-taking habit is not interrupted.

2. A second method of birth control should be used for the first month oral contraceptives are used because full protection is often not achieved for the first month. Foam and condom is a good alternative.

3. The pill should be taken at the same time each day. This ensures a constant drug blood level and better protection. If the pill is associated with a specific daily routine such as brushing the teeth, it is easier to remember.

4. If *one* pill is missed, it should be taken as soon as the woman realizes she has forgotten it. The next day's pill should be taken at the regular time. It is unlikely that pregnancy will occur. If *two* pills are missed, both pills should be taken the next day. Some spotting may occur and another contraceptive should be used during the rest of the cycle. If *three* or *more* pills are missed, the woman should take no more pills in that pack and use another method of contraception immediately. Spotting or bleeding will probably occur. A new pack should be started one week after the old pack was discontinued even if bleeding is still present. An alternative method of birth control should be used for the entire time the woman is not taking the pill and for the first 2 weeks of the new pack.

5. If one or more pills is missed and the woman's period is skipped, she may be pregnant and should seek health care. If no pills are missed and a period is skipped, it is unlikely that pregnancy has occurred. If two periods are missed, even if no pills were skipped, pregnancy should be suspected and checked for.

6. If a woman wishes to discontinue taking oral contraceptives, it is best to stop at the end of a pack to avoid irregular bleeding. Another method of birth control should be used immediately if pregnancy is to be avoided (Martin, 1978).

7. If the woman is seen by a physician for other reasons, she should always inform him or her that she is using oral contraceptives.

All women using oral contraceptives should be informed of their side effects and possible consequences. Approximately 40% of users will experience side effects of one kind or another. When discussing these with the couple or woman, adequate time should be given for the client to ask questions and voice concerns. These should be discussed in detail. Instructions related to side effects and potential serious complications should include the following:

1. The woman should be informed of those symptoms that may cause serious trouble. These are (Hatcher, 1978):

Symptom	Possible problem
Abdominal pain (severe)	Gallbladder disease, hepatic adenoma, blood clot
Chest pain (severe) or shortness of breath	Pulmonary embolism or myocardial infarction
Headache (severe)	Stroke or hypertension
Eye problems: blurred vision, flashing lights, blindness	Stroke or hypertension
Severe leg pain (calf or thigh)	Thrombophlebitis

If she experiences any of these she should contact her physician at once. The symptoms should not be ignored nor should the woman wait to see if they will go away.

2. If the woman is concerned about any minor symptoms she should call for information or an appointment. If symptoms persist for more than three cycles they should be re-evaluated.

3. The benefits of taking oral contraceptives should be carefully weighed against the hazards. At present, the long-term effects are not completely known even when there are no specific contraindications for taking oral contraceptives. Weighing the risk-benefit ratio is even more important for the woman who may have relative contraindication or risks in taking oral contraceptives.

Follow-up is essential. The woman should be evaluated after two cycles have been completed. If there are no apparent problems or significant side effects, the woman should be seen at least yearly; if problems arise, she should contact a health care provider sooner. On each visit the following should be done (Martin, 1978):

1. Check weight, blood pressure, and urinalysis (Pap smear, hematocrit, gonorrhea culture and serologic test for syphilis yearly).

2. Question client specifically about headaches, blurred vision, leg pain, chest pain, abdominal pain, bleeding or spotting, or any other symptoms she may bring up.

3. Review pill-taking procedures to be sure they are being taken correctly.

4. Ascertain if the woman is satisfied with oral contraceptives; offer alternatives if appropriate.

5. Review the symptoms of serious complications and what to do should they occur.

As women are becoming more informed, there is a growing trend toward conservatism in the use of oral contraceptives. It is an essential responsibility of the nurse to assist clients in making an informed decision regarding whether or not to use oral contraceptives.

Other hormonal methods
"Morning after" pill

Diethylstilbestrol (DES) is the most common postcoital contraceptive agent used today in the United States. It was approved by the FDA in 1975 as an emergency measure only. Its mechanism of action is the same as that of the estrogen described earlier in the section on oral contraceptives. Hatcher (1978) states that "DES is probably an effective postcoital contraceptive." However, failures do occur because (1) implantation is already established, (2) too long a time has elapsed between unprotected intercourse and treatment, (3) dosage is inadequate, (4) regurgitation of DES has occurred, or (5) the drug itself has failed. To be effective it must be taken within 72 hours of midcycle, unprotected intercourse; the dosage must be high (50 mg diethylstilbestrol; 3 to 5 mg ethinyl estradiol; or 25 mg conjugated estrogen), and it must continue for 5 to 6 days (Martin, 1978).

Side effects include nausea and vomiting, headache, menstrual irregularities, and breast tenderness. DES is contraindicated in the presence of established pregnancy, tumors of the breast or reproductive organs, and conditions contraindicating high estrogen in oral contraceptives. There is the possibility of thromboembolic complications. Finally, there is a relationship between DES and subsequent development of reproductive tract cancer in users and their offspring exposed in utero (Hatcher, 1978). This fact and the questionable efficacy of DES as a postcoital method of contraception raise serious questions as to whether this method is a realistic method of birth control.

Long-lasting progesterone injections

Depo-Provera is given in 150 mg doses every 3 months to prevent pregnancy. It is used in many countries but was rejected by the FDA in April, 1978, for use as a long-acting contraceptive in the United States.

Intrauterine contraceptive devices (IUD)

Intrauterine contraceptive devices have been used for thousands of years for fertility control as well as for a variety of gynecologic disorders. IUDs were mentioned in the writings of Hippocrates. During the nineteenth century intracervical devices were used to correct uterine displacements and for contraception. These early models fell into disrepute because they were associated with pelvic inflammatory disease, which was difficult to treat and often fatal. In 1930 Grafenberg published his report of over 2000 insertions of IUDs for contraceptive purposes. These were made initially of silkworm gut and later of silver wire. The pregnancy rate was reported as 1.6%. After a brief period of popularity, the Grafenberg ring was condemned, apparently because of the occurrence of occasional intrauterine infections. Oppenheimer, in 1959, reported on over 20 years of successful use with 1500 women and no serious complications. These results, along with those of a similar study in Japan, led to a resurgence of interest in IUDs, and a variety of devices were developed. At present, the search for the "ideal" IUD goes on. Currently, 15 million women in the world are using IUDs (Hatcher, 1978; Kintzel, 1977).

Effectiveness

The theoretical effectiveness of intrauterine devices is between 95% and 99%. The differences in effectiveness of various IUDs is attributed to factors such as size, shape, and presence of copper or progesterone. Use effectiveness is close to theoretical effectiveness—about 90% to 94%—because clients can make relatively few errors using an IUD. Use effectiveness is determined by administrative, client, and medical variables such as ease of insertion, clinician experience, likelihood of expulsion, likelihood that expulsion will be detected, and client's ease of access to medical services (Hatcher, 1978).

Mechanisms of action

The exact mechanisms of action are not known; however, it appears that inflammatory and immune reactions are involved. It has been postulated that the IUD has an inflammatory effect on the endometrium with an attraction of macrophages to the surface of the IUD. This may cause lysis of the blastocyst or phagocytosis of spermatozoa. The IUD may make the endometrium unfavorable for implantation or it may effect a mechanical dislodgement after implantation. The increased immunoglobulin G and M levels present in women with IUDs lend support to the idea that the IUD has an immunologic antifertility mechanism. Copper, which is added to certain IUDs increases the effectiveness as it interferes with sperm migration and implantation. Copper may also inhibit carbonic anhydrase and alkaline phosphate activity and interfere with the estrogen uptake of uterine mucosa or with the cellular uptake of DNA in the endometrium (Martin, 1978). It is also thought that IUDs may cause increased local production of prostaglandins, which inhibit implantation (Hatcher, 1978).

Types of IUDs

There are a number of types of intrauterine devices and their advantages and disadvantages vary. Figure 22-1 illustrates the most common. The Lippes Loop is the most popular IUD used today (Hatcher, 1978). The Copper-7 has copper wrapped around it, while the Pro-

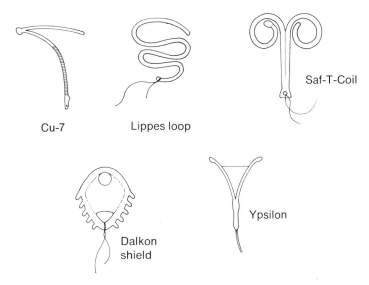

Fig. 22-1. Types of intrauterine devices.

Table 22-7. Intrauterine devices

Device	Advantages	Disadvantages	Present status
Lippes Loop	Proved relatively safe. Easy to insert and remove. Comes in four sizes.	Expulsion or bleeding sufficient to require removal in approximately 25% of cases.	In use
Saf-T Coil	Proved relatively safe. Two sizes (small size designed for nulliparous women).	Expulsion or bleeding sufficient to cause removal in approximately 27% of cases.	In use
Cu-7	Smallest diameter of inserter. Easy to insert. Well tolerated by nulliparous women. Less bleeding.	Small amounts of copper released systemically—effect not clear. Less effective after 2 years; should be removed.	In use
Cu-T	Similar to Cu-7 but slightly larger.	Similar to Cu-7.	
Progestasert	Increased effectiveness. Beneficial to use with client who has history of painful or heavy menses.	Slightly larger, more difficult to insert. Long-term effect of released hormonal agent not known. Needs to be replaced periodically.	In use

gestasert has progesterone deposited in it. See Table 22-7 for a comparison of the types.

Advantages and disadvantages

The primary advantage of the IUD is that once it is inserted, it does not require any continuing action, motivation, or equipment on the part of the woman in order to be effective. The IUD is particularly advantageous for the woman who has trouble following directions or remembering to use a contraceptive. The woman does not need to be involved with the IUD, although it is recommended that she check the strings to make sure it remains in place. The IUD has none of the systemic metabolic effects associated with oral contraceptives, and there is no delay in return of fertility once this method is discontinued. IUDs are highly effective, ranking just below combination oral contraceptives. The risk of mortality appears to be lower than that associated with oral contraceptive use and it does not increase with age.

Tietze et al. (1976) state that the risk of mortality is constant at about 1.2 per 100,000 IUD users.

Disadvantages are related to the necessity that a skilled professional insert the device, the discomfort associated with insertion, the potential for increased menstrual flow and dysmenorrhea, and potential complications. While mortality rates are lower, morbidity rates are generally higher with IUD use than with oral contraceptive use. Almost twice as many women (two per 1000 IUD users vs one per 1000 oral contraceptive users) are hospitalized for treatment of a method-related condition (Tryer, 1977).

Complications and side effects

Bleeding. The most frequent side effect of IUDs is an alteration in uterine bleeding patterns. Menorrhagia usually results from IUD use; this, along with the occurrence of intermenstrual bleeding and spotting, is the major reason for discontinuation of use. The primary cause of IUD bleeding is damage to the endometrium by abrasion and/or pressure necrosis from the IUD foreign body. It also appears that increased vascularity and congestion of the endometrium occur, resulting in interstitial edema and bleeding. Bleeding may also be a consequence of an antifertility agent such as copper introduced in or on the IUD. Other theories include changes in coagulation patterns and specific changes in the fibrinolytic activities of the endometrium.

Although the specific etiology of IUD-related bleeding is not completely understood, reduction of the physical trauma caused by an IUD is essential to prevent the bleeding. The IUD should be of a shape and size to fit the uterine cavity easily in its smallest dimensions. Usually, total blood loss in an IUD user is demonstrably above normal levels during the menstrual cycle. Bleeding is serious enough to require hospitalization in 1% of IUD users. Normal blood loss during the menstrual period is 35 ml; it is more than double this in a woman using the Lippes Loop or Saf-T-Coil. Blood loss is less (50 ml or less) with medicated devices because these are usually smaller and cause less distortion of the uterine cavity. The problems of blood loss acquires additional significance with the increasing prevalence of nutritional deficiencies (Tatum, 1977; Connell, 1977; Tryer, 1977).

Pain. Pain is commonly associated with IUD insertion and use and is a major reason for discontinuation of the method. Insertion in the nulliparous woman is usually painful; insertion pain in any woman can vary from slight cramping to severe pain, and it is occasionally associated with serious vasovagal responses such as bradycardia, syncope, and nausea. Paracervical block and the administration of atropine will help reduce these responses.

The cramping experienced in the uterus and the discomfort in the lower abdomen and back are the result of increased contractions of the uterus in its efforts to rid itself of a foreign body. Pain is more common during the first 3 months after insertion and usually decreases after that. Dysmenorrhea can be initiated or aggravated by the IUD; however, studies have shown that dysmenorrhea is decreased by the use of the Progestasert device (Fryer, 1977). Severity of pain is an indication of the degree of distension of the uterine cavity and myometrium caused by the IUD; pain can be kept to a minimum by using an IUD that causes the least amount of distortion. Usually the discomfort can be alleviated by nonnarcotic analgesics (Tatum, 1977; Romney et al., 1975).

Perforation. One of the problems inherent in all IUDs is the risk of perforation. It may occur at the time of insertion or at any time thereafter; it is most common at the time of insertion. The risk varies with the size, shape, and consistency of the device; the technique of insertion; the status and configuration of the uterus; and, most importantly, the expertise of the clinician. Most perforations are asymptomatic and may never be detected. Perforation is more likely to occur when (1) the IUD is inserted by the push-out rather than the withdrawal technique; (2) the IUD is forced through the cervical canal without an insertion tube; or (3) the IUD is inserted less than 12 weeks postpartum.

Perforation should be suspected when an intrauterine pregnancy occurs, when the tail of the IUD cannot be visualized in the cervical os, or when sharp pain occurs with insertion. If perforation is suspected, pregnancy must first be ruled out. If the woman is not pregnant, then the IUD should be located by X-ray or ultrasonography. Sources differ as to management. Connell (1977) recommends that all devices be removed because of the risk of intestional strangulation and obstruction. Tatum and Schmidt (1977), on the other hand, say that this is not necessary in all cases, though they do recommend it for "psychological manifestations" or when it is a medicated device, a closed type IUD, or an IUD with a complex, multifilamental tail. Removal should be effected by the simpliest method possible.

Pregnancy. An unplanned pregnancy occurring with an IUD in utero is a potentially serious problem. If the woman wishes to terminate the pregnancy it should be done as soon as possible; if she wishes to carry the pregnancy, she should be informed of the complications that might develop. If the IUD is left in utero, approximately 50% of the pregnancies will terminate by spontaneous abortion; if the IUD is removed, the rate of spontaneous abortion decreases to 30% (Tatum, 1977). There is also the possibility of midtrimester septic abortion associated with leaving an IUD in place during pregnancy. According to Cates et al. (1976) risk of death from spontaneous abortion is over fifty times greater for women who continue these pregnancies with a device left in place than for those who do not. Therefore, it is essential that IUDs be removed, if possible, as soon as pregnancy is confirmed, regardless of whether or not the woman wishes to continue her pregnancy (Connell, 1977; Tatum, 1977).

Pregnancies that occur in women wearing an IUD are more likely to be extrauterine than when no contraceptive is used. It appears that IUDs are a causal factor in ectopic pregnancy and, further, that this is more likely to occur when the IUD has been used for a prolonged period. There does not appear to be any difference in this regard between medicated and nonmedicated IUDs. Any woman who has had an ectopic pregnancy is not a candidate for the use of an IUD (Tatum, 1977).

Infection. Infection is the most serious complication of IUD use and the major cause of mortality associated with IUDs. Anytime an IUD is placed in the uterus, bacteria are simultaneously introduced into the endometrial cavity from the vagina and external cervical os. The initial invasion rapidly clears up and the uterus sterilizes itself within 30 days after insertion (Tatum and Schmidt, 1977). According to Tyrer (1977), studies indicate that the approximate risk of pelvic infection is three to five times higher for IUD users than for nonusers. Pelvic infections that occur shortly after insertion are probably caused by the IUD; those occurring later are more apt to be coincidental. Early reports suggested that the majority of infections were gonorrheal in origin; however, it has now been demonstrated that a variety of organisms are responsible for IUD-related infections (Connell, 1977).

IUD infections can present several different clinical pictures. Severe pelvic infection manifests itself with acute pelvic pain, bleeding, and general sepsis with high fever. This type of infection should be treated immediately with a broad-spectrum antibiotic effective against gonorrhea and other organisms. The IUD is left in place, but if there is no improvement in 24 hours, it is removed. The second type of infection is mild, smoldering, and at times almost asymptomatic. This type of infection produces progressive endometritis, usually noted 6 to 12 months after insertion. The woman frequently complains of vaginal spotting or bleeding and foul-smelling vaginal discharge. Adnexal and parametrial tenderness, at times with a distinct mass, can be noted. The IUD should be removed, cultures taken, and antibiotic therapy begun (Connell, 1977). Over time there is an increased incidence of endometritis in symptomatic women with IUDs in place, as well as some chronic endometritis associated with IUDs (Martin, 1978). Problems of sepsis and infection if pregnancy occurs are associated with all types of IUDs; every woman should be informed of these potentially serious risks.

Management

It is essential that a careful gynecologic history be taken and a thorough pelvic examination be performed to determine whether an IUD is suitable for the woman. For example, a woman with very heavy menses or severe dysmenorrhea or uterine abnormalities would not be a good candidate for an IUD. Contraindications to IUD insertion are (Hatcher, 1978; Martin, 1978; ACOG, 1976):

Absolute
Pelvic infection, acute or chronic
Pelvic inflammatory disease, acute or chronic
Septic abortion
Postpartal endometritis
Pregnancy
Cervical or uterine malignancy
Abnormal Pap smears
Uterine abnormalities
History of ectopic pregnancy

Relative
Hypermenorrhea
Dysmenorrhea
Acute cervicitis
Valvular heart disease
Endometriosis
Anemia
Uterus less than 6 cm
Marked antiflexion or retroflexion
Abnormal uterine bleeding
No previous pregnancies

The choice of IUD must be individualized for each client. Questions that should be asked in determining which IUD to select include the following:

1. Is the woman using the IUD for termination of childbearing or for spacing? If the IUD is to be used for permanent prevention of pregnancy, one that need not be removed or replaced at set intervals should be used. If the IUD is to be used for spacing, any IUD is acceptable.
2. Has she ever been pregnant? If the woman is nulliparous, then a small IUD should be inserted with the use of a paracervical block during insertion. Following abortion, a small or medium IUD should be used; following an uncomplicated full-term delivery, almost any IUD is acceptable; following a full-term cesarean delivery, an IUD that uses a withdrawal insertion technique rather than expulsion should be chosen.
3. Is there a history of painful or heavy menstruation? If dysmenorrhea is present, a Progestasert might be used. It is important not to insert an IUD that is too large. If heavy bleeding is a problem, the Progestasert-T should be considered or possibly a copper-containing device.
4. How large is the uterus? If the uterus is less than 4.5 cm, no IUD is likely to be well tolerated. A uterus that is 4.5 to 6.5 cm may tolerate an IUD with a vertical length of less than 3.0 cm. If the uterus is 6.5 to 9.9 cm, most IUDs will be acceptable. A uterus of 10.0 cm or more needs a large IUD and a back-up method of contraception.
5. What other medical, social, or personal factors might indicate or contraindicate use of a specific IUD? For example, allergy to copper would contraindicate the use of copper-containing devices. The client who is using an IUD after midcycle unprotected intercourse should use a copper IUD. The woman who has a history of IUD expulsion may need a different size or a more rigid IUD. Also, the Progestasert has been used successfully following multiple expulsions of other IUDs. For the woman who may have difficulty returning for periodic examinations, an IUD that must be re-

placed at certain intervals should not be used. If a client specifically requests a certain IUD, try to meet this request. *Never* use an IUD the client objects to (Hatcher, 1977).

Many practitioners prefer inserting an IUD during menses or shortly thereafter because the cervix is slightly softer and dilated at that time. The risk of pregnancy is also minimized. However, many others do not limit IUD insertion to this time. Some think that a woman may be more susceptible to the development of infection from IUD insertion during menses. Many women experience pain and faintness upon insertion, a vasovagal response that usually disappears in a few minutes. A paracervical block is recommended to prevent pain. This is particularly helpful for the woman who has never been pregnant.

Client education

It is essential that the woman selecting an IUD as a method of birth control know the relative effectiveness of the method as well as its advantages and disadvantages. She should be informed of potential major and minor side effects. All of this information should be given the client so that she can make an informed decision as to whether or not she prefers to use an IUD.

Before insertion of the IUD the woman should be told that she may experience some pain or nausea right after insertion; she may want someone to accompany her in the event she needs to be driven home.

After insertion the following points need to be clearly made to the client:

1. It is normal to experience some spotting and cramping and these should gradually decrease. Irregular spotting may be experienced for the first 2 to 3 months. The menstrual period may be longer and heavier than usual.
2. It is essential to periodically check the IUD strings to be sure the IUD is still in place. The woman should be able to feel the strings before she leaves the office after insertion. Expulsion is most likely right after insertion or during menstruation. The strings should be checked frequently during the first several months and following menses thereafter. If at any time the string cannot be felt, the woman should come in to be examined and use another method of birth control.
3. Another method of birth control, such as foam or condoms, should be used the first 2 months to prevent pregnancy. An alternate method should be kept in reserve in case of expulsion. Some women also choose to use a second method at midcycle for extra protection.
4. The Copper-7 and Copper-T must be replaced every 2 to 3 years and the Progestasert every year.

All others may remain in place longer if no problems develop.

5. Nuisance side effects of the IUD most commonly reported are dysmenorrhea, spotting, and heavy menstrual flow. If these become intolerable, the IUD can always be removed. Increased menstrual bleeding can be serious if the woman is anemic. A hematocrit should be done yearly.
6. If at any time the woman experiences fever, pelvic pain or tenderness, severe cramping, or unusual vaginal bleeding, she should contact a health care provider. These can be signs of life-threatening infections, which should be treated at once.
7. If a period is missed or pregnancy is suspected, a health care provider should be contacted at once. If the woman is pregnant, the IUD should be removed.
8. A woman should never attempt to remove her IUD herself, nor should she allow her partner to attempt it.
9. Follow-up care is essential. The IUD should be checked yearly, and a Pap smear and breast examination done; a gonorrhea culture is also recommended. The woman's hematocrit should always be checked.

In teaching the woman who is using an IUD as a method of birth control, emphasis should be placed on the danger signals of IUD use: abdominal pain, bleeding, chills, fever, purulent vaginal discharge, and early signs of pregnancy.

Spermicidal agents

Spermicidal agents such as vaginal foams, jellies, or creams are introduced into the vagina immediately prior to intercourse and act as a chemical barrier at the cervical os. They consist of two components: an inert base, which holds the spermicidal agent in the vagina against the cervix, and a spermicidal chemical. The aerosol foams expand at once to cover all vaginal folds, leaving a lasting invisible coating. Cream spreads more evenly than jelly but jelly has greater lubricating ability. Creams and jellies spread more slowly over the vaginal surface than do foams, often taking up to several minutes. When the spermicidal preparations mix with semen, they release an immobilizing spermicide that inhibits the sperm's movement through the cervical os into the uterus. Since the semen and spermicidal chemicals neutralize each other, a separate application is necessary for each act of intercourse.

Hatcher (1978) states that creams and jellies should not be recommended for use without a diaphragm. Other authorities are not so specific in their recommendations. The theoretical failure rate for foam is three pregnancies per 100 women per year, while the actual use rate is twenty-two pregnancies per 100 women per year. High failure rates reflect both the inherent likelihood of failure of the method and carelessness of the users. The foam user can make many mistakes: using too little, not realizing the foam bottle is empty, not shaking the foam bottle vigorously enough, not interrupting intercourse to insert the foam, and douching too soon after intercourse. Effectiveness rates become much higher when foam is used with condoms and is used correctly and consistently (Hatcher, 1977).

There are some real advantages to the spermicidal preparations. They are available without a prescription, they are relatively simple to use, and they have almost no side effects except an occasional allergic reaction to the chemicals. They are particularly useful as an interim measure until more effective contraception can be started. They are often recommended for use following delivery until the postpartum check-up and for the first month after oral contraceptives are begun or an IUD is inserted. Spermicidal agents can be used if a woman chooses to stop oral contraceptives for a few cycles or or change IUDs. Foam slightly increases the chances of contracting gonorrhea or trichomoniasis.

There are also very real disadvantages to the use of spermicidal preparations. They are closely associated with the act of intercourse; they must be inserted a few minutes before penetration, and no longer than 30 minutes should elapse between insertion and intercourse. Some women or couples find spermicidal agents esthetically displeasing; they may also cause excessive lubrication, feel unpleasant to touch, taste bad, or create oral anesthesia. They may also feel "drippy" or "messy." The primary disadvantage is their low effectiveness rate when used alone; they must be used correctly every time, and still the effectiveness is not nearly that of other contraceptive methods such as oral contraceptives or IUD.

Client education

It is essential to give the woman careful instructions concerning use. The preparation should be inserted into the vagina within 30 minutes of coitus. The applicator

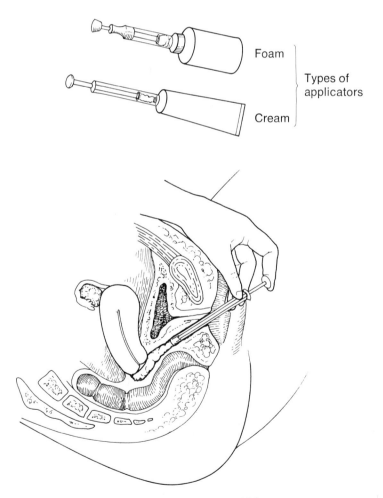

Fig. 22-2. Inserting a spermicidal agent.

should be filled according to the manufacturer's instructions. It should be inserted with the woman lying on her back. The applicator is inserted as far as possible into the vagina and then withdrawn slightly (about ½ inch) before depressing the plunger. This pushes the spermicide to the cervical os (see Fig. 22-2). Often two full applicators can be used for additional protection. The spermicide should always be inserted before any penile-vaginal contact is made. The movement of the penis distributes the spermicide throughout the vagina and over the cervix. If the woman gets out of bed before intercourse, she should insert another application of spermicide. For every sex act, a separate application should be made. It takes approximately 6 to 8 hours for the immobilization and killing of the sperm to be accomplished; the woman should not douche during this time. All of these points should be a part of client instruction in the use of spermicidal agents as a method of birth control. Other points the practitioner should make are these: (1) if one brand of foam seems to irritate the woman or her partner, try another brand; (2) since foam has an unpleasant taste, insert it after oral-genital contact; (3) keep a spare container since it is often difficult to tell when the foam is about to run out; (4) be sure that the woman knows what she is buying and using since products are often unclearly labeled and their effectiveness varies greatly; and (5) always shake the can well because spermicide tends to settle to the bottom and the more bubbles the foam has, the better it blocks the sperm.

Encare oval

The Encare Oval is the most recently introduced contraceptive in the United States. The contraceptive action is two-fold: it is a spermicidal agent and its effervescent action in the presence of moisture and warmth forms a thick barrier that occludes the cervical os.

When the Encare Oval was first released, effectiveness rates implied by promotional literature were "a pregnancy rate of one per 100 woman years." Recently, concern has been expressed over these effectiveness rates; the FDA has raised serious questions as to the reliability of the studies upon which the claims of "99% efficacy" are based. The FDA (1978) states that it considers "recent labeling and advertising claims of 99% efficacy for Encare Ovals to be unsupported and therefore to present a possible health problem." At this point the safest approach is to consider the Encare Oval to be similar to foam in its effectiveness.

The Oval has real advantages in that it is small and convenient, it is available without prescription, is apparently safe without serious complications, has a pleasant odor, uses no hormones, provides a premeasured dose of the contraceptive agent, and may slightly decrease the spread of sexually transmitted disease.

There are also definite disadvantages. Heat will cause it to soften in the package (though placing it in cold water will correct this). It has an unpleasant taste, thus hampering free oral-genital expression. There is the possibility of allergic or chemical irritation. It creates a small amount of heat as it effervesces, which could be viewed as either unpleasant or pleasant. If the woman has minimal vaginal lubrication it can feel gritty. There may be a slight vaginal discharge. It takes 10 minutes to dissolve and may not completely dissolve in some women in this amount of time. It is "messy" for some women, causing postcoital discharge. Some women find it difficult to open the wrapper.

Mechanical barriers
Diaphragm

A diaphragm is a dome-shaped cup made of latex rubber with a flexible metal rim (Fig. 22-3). It is available in sizes of 50 to 110 mm rim diameter and four basic rim types: flat spring, coil spring, arc spring, and the rigid bow-bend shape. Three types are used most frequently. The arcing spring diaphragm with a firm rigid rim is used with women who have poor mucle tone and relaxed pelvic organs. The softer more flexible coil spring is used by women with good pelvic musculation or by those who find the firm arc spring uncomfortable. Less frequently, the flat spring is used when the coil spring is appropriate but the rim is too thick and therefore does not fit snugly.

The well-fitted diaphragm is positioned as follows: The front rim fits snugly with just a little give behind the pubic bone. The side rims extend outward, comfortably distending the vaginal walls without bending upward or downward. The back rim rises behind and beneath the cervix with the cup extending lengthwise in the vagina to cover the cervix completely. During intercourse, the diaphragm should fit snugly against the vaginal roof and cover the cervical os completely.

The contraceptive effect of the diaphragm comes from two sources: (1) the barrier mechanism it provides by covering the cervix and decreasing the contact of the cervix and semen, and (2) its ability to hold a spermicidal agent against the cervix.

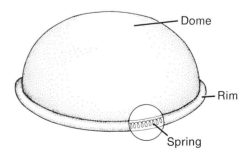

Fig. 22-3. Diaphragm.

According to Hatcher (1978) the theoretical failure rate is two pregnancies per 100 women per year. Lane (1970) reports an overall use failure rate of two pregnancies per 100 users; therefore, the theoretical failure rate is a conservative estimate. Hatcher cites a use effectiveness rate of seventeen pregnancies per 100 woman years of use. When used correctly and conscientiously the diaphragm can be a highly successful method of birth control; the client's success with the use of the diaphragm depends greatly on how well she is prepared by the practitioner. Nurses can and should assume much of this role.

To be effective the diaphragm must be used. The essential factor in effective use of a diaphragm is motivation. The diaphragm works best when the wearer is highly motivated to prevent pregnancy, uses the method consistently, and cares for the diaphragm correctly. It requires a certain level of sophistication on the part of the woman using it—a knowledge of reproduction and some degree of comfort with her body.

There has been a recent resurgence of interest in the diaphragm, which is seen as a highly effective alternative to other birth control methods that may hold significant risks of side effects. Bradbury (1975) identifies several reasons for this awakened interest: the diaphragm's unquestioned safety; the increasing accessibility, availability, and acceptance of early abortion as a back-up method; the increasing awareness of women to their own bodies and sexual responses; and a steady increase in the number of women using tampons for menstrual protection.

Other reasons why women may wish to use the diaphragm include uneasiness about real or imagined side effects of other methods, distaste for the artificiality of some methods, and growing concern about the interference with normal bodily processes inherent in methods such as oral contraceptives or IUDs. For other women there is the satisfaction of feeling in control of one's body. Diaphragms are seen as reliable interim methods; and they can also be used as a hygienic measure during menstruation. The diaphragm is inexpensive, it does not necessarily interfere with sexual pleasure, and fertility is resumed as soon as the device is discontinued.

Yet with all of these advantages, only about 10% of women practicing contraception are using the diaphragm (Kilby-Kelberg, 1975). Many women view the diaphragm as inconvenient. For others it is uncomfortable and difficult to insert or remove. Sometimes the partner complains that he can feel it. Other women are influenced by the negative opinions of health care practitioners who create a climate of mistrust and/or distrust because of negative bias. Many of these disadvantages, as well as actual failures resulting in the "dia-

phragm baby syndrome," can be successfully overcome by a careful, thoughtful, skilled clinician.

There are almost no *health* contraindications for diaphragm use except for the possibility of individual sensitivity to latex rubber or to the spermicidal agent (which can be cured by switching to another agent). *Anatomic contraindications* are more numerous; for example, damaged pelvic floor or relaxation of the pelvic musculature; anatomically short vagina, prolapsed uterus, severe cystocele or rectocele, or abnormally small cervix will all prevent satisfactory fitting. There are also women with anatomic conditions that prevent reaching into the vagina, such as short fingers, excessive abdominal fat or an extremely long vagina, which would prevent proper insertion (Bradbury, 1975).

There are many psychologic, social, or educational contraindications to diaphragm use. The woman who has an aversion to touching her genitalia will have difficulty using the diaphragm correctly. Seaman (1972) has suggested that our culture's masturbation taboos explain why some women are uncomfortable inserting their fingers into their vagina. Since the diaphragm requires some degree of practice and experimentation, it may not be emotionally comfortable for all women. Insertion of the diaphragm in advance may disturb the traditional stereotype that the man should initiate sex; when the diaphragm is inserted during foreplay, it may be perceived as ruining spontaneity. Rainwater (1960) found that lower socioeconomic class individuals had many criticisms, doubts, and confusions about using the diaphragm. They found it difficult to understand how it worked since the concept of fertilization was not clearly understood. Its effectiveness in relation to the condom was doubted because it cannot be seen or felt.

Others are not candidates for diaphragm use because there is a lack of motivation for protection or a disgust with the whole idea. Still others lack the privacy necessary for insertion, removal, and cleaning of the diaphragm and for keeping the diaphragm and spermicidal agent out of reach of others. Finally, the partner can exert pressure against using the diaphragm.

Once contraindications to diaphragm usage have been considered for each client, and those women who would not be successful candidates for this method of birth control are advised to use other methods, there are three areas of critical importance as identified by Bradburg (1975) to be implemented for successful use of the diaphragm. All are within the parameter of the nurse clinician. They are technique, teaching, and time.

It is essential that the practitioner be skilled in assessing the woman's pelvic structures for suitability and type of diaphragm. She must be skilled in determining what type and size of diaphragm will be best. She must also understand female sexual response and how this affects diaphragm use. She must be patient, gentle, matter-of-fact, and sensitive. The practitioner must be able to give encouragement, present a positive attitude as well as practical, commonsense approaches to using a diaphragm.

Client teaching is critical; it is crucial that the woman thoroughly understand use of the diaphragm and be successful with insertion and removal before she leaves the office. Teaching is not just didactic explanation and a pamphlet or list of instructions. It is demonstration and return demonstration with success. All of this takes time—up to 45 minutes to do an adequate job of fitting and teaching. It is imperative that adequate time be allowed for this. Clients have individualized needs that cannot be fitted into a neat little package to be handled quickly. If these general principles are met, the failure rate can be significantly reduced.

Client use and education. Diaphragms are sized according to their diameter, and range from 50 to 110 mm. They are available in 5 mm progressions. The majority of women need a 70- to 80-mm size. A woman's height or weight has no bearing on what size diaphragm she will need. Nor does the number of children she has had; however, usually a parous woman will need a larger size than will a nullipara. Correct fit depends on each woman's particular pelvic structure. When fitting a woman for a diaphragm it is important to realize that tenseness during the pelvic examination and fitting can result in giving her a diaphragm that is too small for her under more relaxed conditions. The excitement phase of the sexual response cycle in the woman causes the upper two-thirds of the vaginal barrel to expand; thus a diaphragm that fits in the sexually unstimulated state may slip during sexual excitement, allowing penile penetration above the rim of the diaphragm. For these reasons the diaphragm size prescribed should be the very largest that is comfortable.

There are other factors that can cause slippage or incorrect positioning of the diaphragm. If excessive lubrication is present, particularly around the rim, it can cause the rim to slip from its normal midline position. In the female superior position during intercourse, the penis can penetrate between the rim in front and the upper roof of the vaginal wall. The woman should check penile placement carefully to prevent this. During multiple mountings, it is difficult to maintain diaphragm placement that will provide adequate cervical protection, no matter what position is used. During multiple orgasms the diaphragm will frequently move from behind the pelvic bone with repeated penile thrusting.

There is a greater risk of reintroducing the penis between the upper vaginal wall and the rim of the diaphragm with increased sexual excitement in either partner (Bradbury, 1975). The nurse must be able to discuss these factors comfortably and matter-of-factly with the client so that she will be aware of the relationship of sexual response and practices to diaphragm placement or displacement.

It is crucial to remember that successful continued use of the diaphragm depends in large measure on the amount of success or frustration the woman experiences as she first learns to use the diaphragm. Enough time for adequate teaching is essential at the initial visit. The following format designed by Bradbury (1975) is excellent for ensuring that the goal of successful use is met.

1. Initial interview: The woman's history is taken. Her attitudes toward sexuality, touching her genitalia, using tampons, and contraception should be assessed. It is important to know if abortion would be acceptable "backup" if pregnancy should occur. If pregnancy would be a "disaster" and abortion not an alternative, another method of birth control should be recommended. The woman should know that the diaphragm is not foolproof and that pregnancy might occur.

2. Preliminary teaching should include demonstration of the diaphragm with a model of female pelvic anatomy. Then the woman is able to visualize her anatomy and how the diaphragm works, and imagine what a diaphragm feels like. She is able to visualize insertion and removal, demystifying the procedures.

3. Examination and fitting are done next. First a thorough physical examination including breasts, abdominal palpation, speculation, and bimanual examination is done. Pap smear and gonorrheal culture should be taken. Once a determination is made that the woman's pelvic structure is favorable for diaphragm fitting and use, she is raised to a semi-sitting position, which is similar to the position she will use for self-insertion. She is helped to feel as comfortable and relaxed as possible. It is essential that the practitioner be positive, encouraging, matter-of-fact, gentle, and understanding in this awkward and potentially embarrassing situation. As the practitioner begins to fit the woman she demonstrates (a) how to apply the spermicidal agent (about 1 tsp in the cup of the diaphragm, which is spread around the inner side aspect of rim); (b) how the diaphragm should be held for insertion, pressing the rims together tightly; and (3) insertion. The nurse demonstrates how to find the vagina with one hand while holding the diaphragm with the other and inserting the protruding end of the diaphragm with a slightly upward movement momentarily and then back and down toward the rear, using both hands to push in one continuous motion. Once the proper size is ascertained, the woman bears down and the diaphragm is removed. It is essential that the diaphragm size selected be the very largest size that can be tolerated. A diaphragm is too large if it protrudes from the vagina when the woman bears down or fits so snugly against the pubic bone that it causes nagging pain in the low back or groin after being in place awhile.

4. Once proper fit is achieved, the woman should go

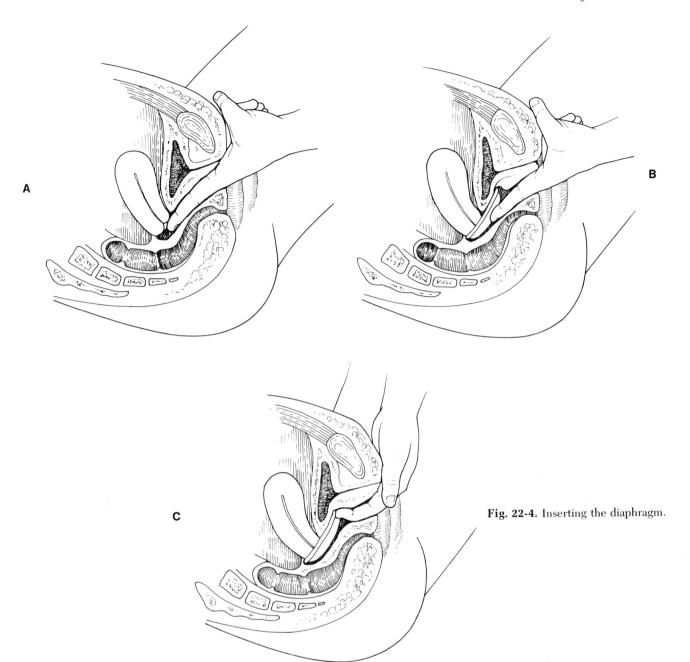

A

B

C

Fig. 22-4. Inserting the diaphragm.

through all the steps of insertion and removal herself. The practitioner should remain with her the entire time to encourage, answer questions, and assist whenever needed. At least two or three practice sessions should be done before the woman leaves the clinic.

5. Another teaching session should follow the examination and fitting. This should include details about use and care of the diaphragm, how to check to see if it is in proper place (see Fig. 22-4), what type to get, and where to get the diaphragm, and spermicidal agents and how much they cost. This is also the time to provide the client with some tips and practical points about using a diaphragm, such as:

a. Always empty the bladder and bowel before inserting the diaphragm.

b. The diaphragm can be inserted at any time; insertion does not have to be related to the time of coitus.

c. If intercourse does not occur in 4 hours, or if it is repeated, more spermicidal agent should be applied to the outer aspect of the diaphragm dome with the fingers or an applicator. The diaphragm should not be removed.

d. Diaphragm insertion or application of a spermicidal agent can be incorporated into sexual foreplay.

e. If the diaphragm fits correctly and is in place, neither partner should feel it.

f. It should not protrude into the vagina or dislodge in most coital positions although some caution should be used with the female-astride position.

g. A spermicidal agent must always be used with a diaphragm. It should be spread liberally over the inside cup and lightly on the rim so that there is direct contact with the cervix during intercourse. Additional jelly or cream should not be added right after insertion because it can cause slippage. It is also messy.

h. Spermicidal cream is better than jelly since it distributes more immediately and more evenly about the cervix and vagina. Jelly is more viscous and therefore takes longer to spread evenly (Masters and Johnson, 1966).

i. A diaphragm should always be left in place 6 to 8 hours after sexual intercourse and it can be left in place indefinitely. Any normal activities can be carried out without removing the diaphragm—voiding, defecating, bathing. Position of the diaphragm should be checked after defecation.

j. Douching is not recommended. It should only be done after removal of the diaphragm and only with warm water.

k. The diaphragm should be cleaned with warm water and mild soap, dried thoroughly, and powdered with cornstarch before it is put away. The diaphragm should be carefully inspected for holes, tears, or scratches before and after every use.

l. With careful use, a diaphragm can last 3 years.

m. Never use the diaphragm with any lubricant other than a spermicidal agent and *never* use it *without* a spermicidal agent.

6. Follow-up consists of two parts. First the woman should wear her diaphragm for at least 8 hours every day for a week to determine how comfortable it is. She can have intercourse but another method of contraception should be used also. She should return to the practitioner with the diaphragm in place so that the nurse can see how well it is working and answer any questions. Again, emphasis should be placed on the fact that a diaphragm is an excellent method of birth control if it is used.

Long-range follow-up consists of yearly visits for diaphragm assessment. The woman should bring the diaphragm with her when she comes for the annual check-up. If the woman loses or gains 15 lbs or more, has pelvic surgery, becomes pregnant, has an abortion or loses or damages her diaphragm, she should return immediately for a new diaphragm.

Cervical cap

Recently another type of mechanical barrier device for women has been rediscovered in the United States—the cervical cap, a thimble-shaped object that fits snugly over the cervix. First described in 1838 by a German gynecologist, the cervical cap has been used in England and other parts of Europe for the past 50 to 100 years (Whartman, 1976). In the United States it and the diaphragm were used prior to the advent of oral contraceptives and IUD in the 1950s and 1960s (Boston Women's Health Collective, 1980). Until recently the cervical cap was seldom mentioned in medical literature, although the reasons for this are difficult to ascertain. It is thought that some physicians did not recommend the cap to clients because they believed the method was too complicated for the average woman (Whartman, 1976).

The cervical cap, most often made of thick rubber or plastic, fits over the cervix and blocks only the cervix. The cap is usually about 1.5 inches long and encompasses almost the entire cervix. It is widest at its opening and has a thick semirigid rim. The rubber cervical cap comes in sizes according to the width of its opening.

The cap, with or without spermicide, provides an effective mechanical block against sperm. If the cap is to be left in place for longer than 24 hours, application of spermicidal jelly or cream will enhance its effectiveness. Population Reports (Whartman, 1976) states the cervical cap has an effectiveness rate similar to that of the diaphragm. Because a properly fitted cap attaches by suction deep in the vaginal canal, it is less likely than the diaphragm to be displaced during the excitement phase of intercourse. Unfortunately there have been no recent thorough studies of the cap. Tietze et al. (1955) performed the last major study in 1953 and found that for each 100 women using the cervical cap, 7.6 will become pregnant. His study included women who used poor technique, used the cap sporadically, or omitted it completely.

The cervical cap has several advantages: (1) because it is a barrier method there are no known side effects; (2) when used properly, it is an effective contraceptive method; (3) use can be dissociated from sexual activity because it can be inserted long before intercourse takes place; (4) cost is low; and (5) use of a cervical cap can provide information about one's own vagina and cervix.

Disadvantages are few: (1) some women may find self-insertion and removal to be somewhat difficult because the cap must cover the cervix, which is deep in the vagina; and (2) some women notice a malodor if the cup is left in place for a long time. Some health care providers have raised the concern that continued contact of the cervix with the cap might cause erosion or irritation. It is unlikely that either condition would occur if the device is properly fitted (Whartman, 1976).

Contraindications to the use of the cervical cap are (Whartman, 1976): (1) cervical erosion, lacerations, or cervicitis; (2) cervical malformation, including extremely long or short cervix; (3) inflammation of adnexa; and (4) inability of women to insert, place, or remove cap correctly.

The cervical cap must be fitted by a health care professional. Correct size is essential for successful use. During her fitting, the woman is taught how to insert and remove her cap in much the same manner as described for diaphragm fitting. Recommended instructions for use are similar to those for diaphragm usage: application of a spermicide to the inside bottom of cap, insertion of the cap prior to sexual activity, and allowing the cap to remain in place at least 8 hours after intercourse. Nursing interventions described for the diaphragm are equally applicable to the client using a cervical cap.

At present the FDA has not approved the cervical cap for use in the United States except for a few research projects. Interest in the cervical cap is growing, particularly among women dissatisfied with alternative methods of contraception. It is anticipated that as interest and enthusiasm grow and more research is done, pressure upon the FDA to release the cervical cap for widespread use will increase.

Condom

Since ancient times, the condom or a sheath over the penis has been used for decoration or as a protection against disease or to prevent pregnancy. The present day condom is a rubber or processed collagenous tissue sheath that fits over the erect penis to contain the ejaculate and thus acts as a mechanical barrier to prevent sperm from entering the cervix.

Used consistently and correctly, the theoretical failure rate is three pregnancies per 100 woman years. Actual use failure rate is much higher, however—often as high as fifteen to twenty pregnancies per 100 woman years. If spermicidal foam is used with the condom, the effectiveness rate approaches that of oral contraceptives (Hatcher, 1978).

The advantages of the condom are its availability without prescription, its ease of use, absence of side effects, and low cost. A primary advantage lies in its ability to prevent transmission of sexual disease. The disadvantages usually expressed are decreased sensation on the part of the male (which could be partially taken care of by using the thinner condoms) and the necessity of interrupting foreplay to put the condom on. This can be overcome by incorporating it into foreplay.

If the condom is to be effective it must be used correctly every time. It can only be used once and should not be more than 2 years old. Heat will cause deterioration. It must be applied before there is any penile-vaginal contact and about ½ inch of space should be left at the tip (or a nipple condom used) for the ejaculate. This will help prevent tearing or overflow. Lubricated condoms or a water-soluble lubricant will also decrease the potential for tearing. Once ejaculation has occurred the partially erect penis should be withdrawn from the vagi-

na while holding the condom rim tightly around the penis to prevent leakage. For each act of intercourse a new condom should be used. If the condom tears or falls off, contraceptive foam or jelly should be used at once.

Natural fertility control methods

The concept of natural fertility control and those birth control methods utilizing this concept are becoming increasingly popular. As more and more women express a desire for birth control that does not have damaging side effects, does not interrupt normal bodily functions, involves no external or internal devices, involves her sexual partner in the responsibility, and is effective, more attention is focused on natural methods. The Federal Health Revenue Sharing and Health Services Bill passed in late 1975 requires family planning agencies receiving federal funding to provide information and counseling on natural family planning methods. Many individuals are opposed to the introduction of artificial devices or drugs into their body. Others have religious beliefs that prohibit the use of artificial contraceptives.

Natural birth control methods are a realistic alternative for certain women—those who are able to carefully observe their bodies during the different phases of the menstrual cycle, who are willing to not be completely spontaneous in their sexual activities, who have a cooperative partner, who are highly motivated to prevent pregnancy, and who are able to learn the necessary concepts.

All methods of natural family planning require periodic abstinence from sexual intercourse and depend on the observation and recording of events in the menstrual cycle. All methods are based on the assumption that the woman will be able to recognize body signs indicating whether she is in a fertile (unsafe) or unfertile (safe) period in her menstrual cycle. Four recognized methods of natural family planning are currently used: basal body temperature (BBT), calendar rhythm, ovulation, and sympto-thermal. All are based on the fact that hormonal fluctuations in the menstrual cycle produce physical signs that can be detected and used for fertility awareness. In addition to these contraceptive uses, natural fertility control methods have the potential for teaching women a great deal about their bodies.

The reproductive functions of a woman's body are controlled by gonadotropic hormones, which fluctuate on a delicate, negative feedback system (see Chapter 5). During the menstrual cycle numerous changes take place in the cervix and cervical mucus. Approximately 100 mucus-secretory crypts are present in the normal woman during her reproductive years. These produce several types of mucus, two of which are significant in natural family planning: type E, which predominates at ovulation, and type G during the luteal phase of the menstrual

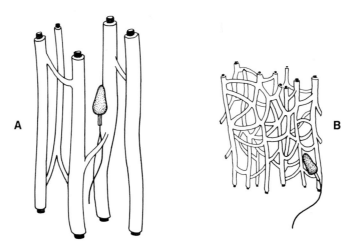

Fig. 22-5. Sperm passage through cervical mucus. **A,** Type E mucus; **B,** type G mucus.

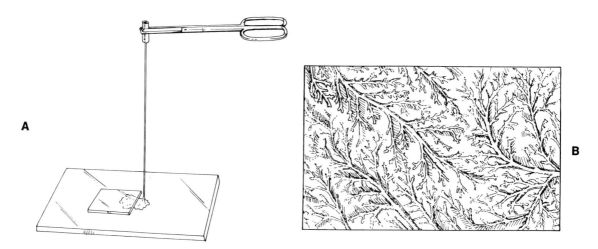

Fig. 22-6. Fern patterns.

Estrogens   Estrogens Progesterone   Progesterone Estrogens

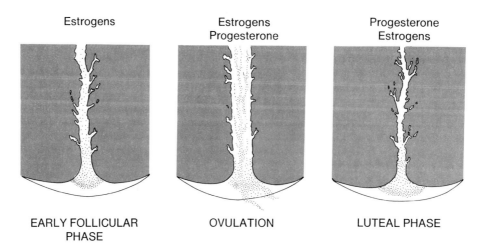

EARLY FOLLICULAR PHASE   OVULATION   LUTEAL PHASE

Fig. 22-7. Sperm migration through the cervical canal.

cycle. Type E allows increased permeability of the mucus to sperm and facilitates the upward passage by use of mucin fibers. These fibers lie parallel to each other and to the cervical canal, thus providing easy access through the cervix for the sperm. Type G mucus, which is thick and sticky, is present during the luteal phase of the menstrual cycle, when taking oral contraceptives, or during pregnancy. The mucin fibers prevent upward migration of the sperm by cross-linking the cervical canal and forming a net that traps the sperm (Fig. 22-5). Cervical mucus changes throughout the menstrual cycle because of the effect of estrogen and progesterone. At the time of ovulation, the cervical mucus increases in amount and becomes clearer and more stretchable. In addition, near ovulation, sodium chloride can be identified in the mucous through the appearance of a fern pattern when the mucus is dried on a glass slide (Fig. 22-6). These characteristics result from the effect of estrogen on the mucus crypts. Progesterone causes the viscid, tacky, cellular mucus of the luteal phase.

Spinnbarkeit is the term used for the characteristic stretchability of cervical mucus. During the ovulatory phase of the cycle this becomes more pronounced. Under the influence of estrogen at the time of ovulation, the cervix becomes softer, more open, and rises in the vagina. During the follicular phase, the cervical os is narrower, while in the luteal phase the cervix is closed, firm, and lower in the vagina (Fig. 22-7).

Each woman's basal body temperature reflects changes in her menstrual cycle. These sequential variations in temperature occur because of fluctuations in estrogen and progesterone. Basal body temperatures are generally lower in the follicular phase than in the luteal phase of the menstrual cycle.

Rhythm or calendar method

This method enables the woman to predict or calculate her "unsafe days," or fertile period, for each menstrual cycle. The calculations are based on three assumptions: (1) ovulation occurs on day 14 ± 2 before the onset of the next menses; (2) sperm are viable for only 2 to 3 days; and (3) the ovum survives for 24 hours. A woman wishing to use the rhythm method must keep a menstrual calendar. To begin, she records the length of her menstrual cycles for the preceding 8 months. She then determines the earliest day she is likely to be fertile by subtracting 18 days from the length of her shortest cycle. The latest day of potential fertility is obtained by subtracting 11 days from the length of her longest cycle. These two numbers represent the beginning and end of her fertile period. For example, if a woman's shortest cycle was 26 days, she would subtract 18 from 26 and find that on the eighth day she must begin to abstain from sexual intercourse or use another method of birth

control. If her longest cycle was 35 days, she would determine that the twenty-fourth day (35 − 11) was the day upon which the period of abstinence might safely be ended.

The effectiveness of this method increases if the woman's cycle is regular. If cycle variability is only 1 to 2 days, for example, from 27 to 29 days, the period of abstinence is much shorter, from the day 9 to the day 10, thus enhancing the couple's ability to abstain and decreasing the possibility of failure. The rhythm method is less likely to be successful for young, postpartum, postabortion, or premenopausal women, whose cycles are often irregular. If these women choose to use this method, they should combine it with one of the other natural family planning methods.

Basal body temperature method

This method can reliably determine the end of the fertile interval. The basal body temperature (BBT) is the lowest temperature reached by the body of a healthy person in waking hours. Recording BBT will not allow prediction of ovulation, but rather the beginning of the safe luteal phase. This method depends on a single variable, ovulation, rather than a number of variables such as the calendar method does. The BBT method is based on the fact that the basal body temperature drops prior to ovulation and then, under the influence of progesterone, rises in 1 to 3 days after ovulation and remains slightly elevated throughout the remainder of the cycle. The time in which the drop occurs is short and temperature rise is considered to be the best indicator that ovulation has taken place. Because of ovum and sperm survival, conception can occur for up to 72 hours after the rise in temperature; therefore, a woman using the BBT method must refrain from intercourse until her temperature has been elevated for at least 3 days. Since occasionally a woman may ovulate as early as day 7 of the cycle, anyone using the BBT method alone should avoid unprotected intercourse from day 7 until the third day after temperature elevation (Hatcher, 1978). Every woman using the BBT method must keep a chart of her basal body temperature patterns. Fig. 22-8 illustrates a model pattern. In this chart there are two so-called safe or nonfertile periods. The strict BBT method restricts intercourse to the second safe period only—from day 3 after the thermal rise to the onset of menses. The failure rate for the strict method is 0.8%, which is comparable to the rate for oral contraceptives. There is 3.1% failure rate for the BBT method when both safe periods are used (Deibel, 1978).

The woman who wishes to practice the BBT method of birth control must take her temperature the first thing in the morning upon waking, after at least 2 to 3 hours of sleep (length of recommended sleep time varies; some

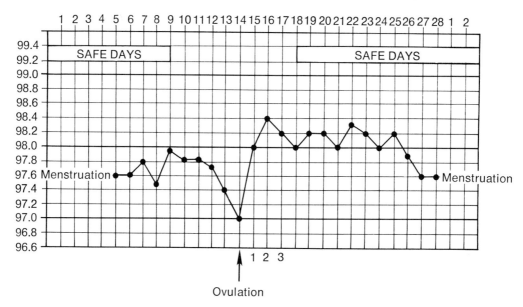

Fig. 22-8. Model basal body temperature pattern.

sources recommend as much as 5 to 6 hours) (Britt, 1977). The same site should be used every time; though no one site is preferable to others for convenience, oral is most often suggested. There is some controversy about whether the woman must take her temperature before any activity takes place or whether she may move around in bed or go to the bathroom. Common sense should be the guide here: if a woman is comfortable she is more apt to follow the routine, and routine is essential to assure accuracy. After obtaining her temperature, the woman records it on a graph and notes any circumstances that might have caused a temperature variation, such as sleeplessness, illness, emotional upsets, medications, intercourse, or an electric blanket. The woman should keep a chart for 1 month while refraining from intercourse, and then return to her clinician for interpretation and to answer any questions. After the couple or woman feels comfortable and competent with the system, she needs only to take her temperature from day 7 until her temperature has remained elevated for 3 days (Britt, 1977; Deibel, 1978; Hatcher, 1978). Many couples choose to practice a form of birth control that is a combination of the calendar rhythm method and the BBT method. The rate of effectiveness is greater than that for either of the two when practiced alone.

Ovulation method

This method was first developed by Drs. John and Evelyn Billings of Australia and is based on the fact that fertilization is impossible without favorable cervical mucus. It is also predicated on the belief that a woman can learn to assess and identify the changes that occur in her cervical mucus throughout the menstrual cycle. She can therefore identify her safe and unsafe days.

In the ovulation method, there are four identifiable phases of the menstrual cycle: menstruation, early safe days, unsafe days, and late safe days. The primary signs that the woman notices are variations in feelings of wetness or dryness around the vagina and changes in the physical properties of the mucus. The woman should assess feelings of wetness or dryness daily, preferably in the evening when she has had a full day of impressions. After menstruation there are usually a few dry days, which are safe for intercourse. As ovulation approaches, there is an increased sensation of wetness. At first the mucus appears cloudy and feels sticky; as ovulation comes closer, the mucus gradually becomes clear, slippery, and stretches without breaking—the Spinnbarkeit phenomenon. The mucus is very thin, clear, smooth, and slippery, similar to egg white (see Fig. 5-22).

The day on which the woman notices the greatest sensation of wetness, the longest stretch in mucus, and the highest degree of smoothness is called the "peak symptom day." It corresponds to the peak in estrogen levels immediately prior to ovulation (Britt, 1977). Ovulation follows the peak symptom; however, because mucus can prolong the life of sperm, conception can result from intercourse on any wet day prior to ovulation. The mucus becomes opaque or sticky again after ovulation and the woman will again experience a sensation of dryness, although there may be some opaque nonsticky mucus present. In order for this method to work, there can be no penis-vaginal contact on wet days; only during the dry days is intercourse safe.

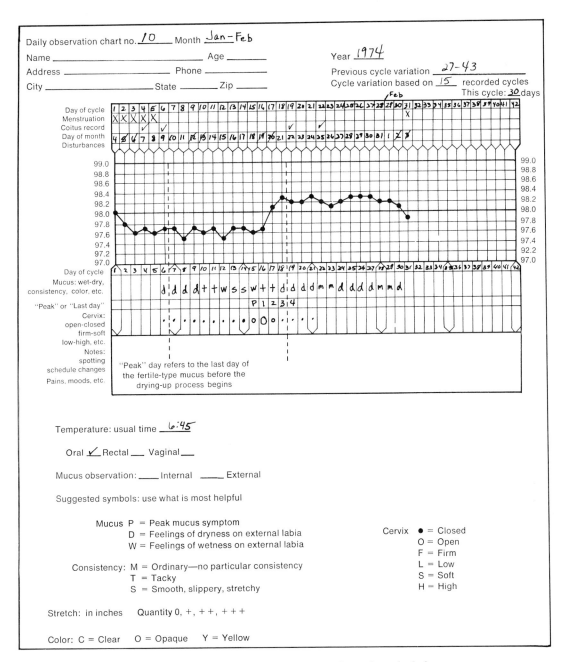

Fig. 22-9. Example of completed sympto-thermal method chart.

Billings (1975) recommends that the method be communicated from woman to woman. It is thought that a woman feels more comfortable asking questions of another woman, and that as a woman gains experience and confidence using the method, she can offer useful tips to another woman.

A woman using the ovulation method should keep a record that involves color-coded stamps. Red stamps denote menstruation and green stamps stand for the dry days. These are considered to be the safe days and

stamps. White stamps with an outline of a baby on them indicate fertility, or unsafe days, while light green stamps with an outline of a baby indicate the unsafe days following ovulation. An X is placed on the white stamp that corresponds to the peak symptom day (Billings, 1975).

With this method there is an emphasis on the couple's relationship, although the woman makes the observations and does the recording. She is expected to assess her feelings of wetness and dryness every day as well as the consistency of her mucus even during menstruation. Abstinence from intercourse is necessary during the menstrual and proliferative phases of the cycle so that the woman can identify fertile mucus. There is some question about using this method when vaginitis or cervicitis is present. Billings does not feel that this need be a concern because a woman can learn to identify abnormal discharge. He does suggest the use of BBT as an additional temporary aid in such situations. A woman may also recognize and use other bodily symptoms, such as mittelschmerz, as further indicators of impending ovulation.

The ovulation method can be successfully used by women who have irregular cycles because it depends on the presence of mucus, and ovulation is always accompanied by cervical mucus changes. This method is useful for the lactating and premenopausal woman.

The efficacy of the method has been rated very high by the proponents—often as high as 98% reliable. Hatcher (1978) reports a pregnancy rate of 2% to 3%. Deibel (1978) states that an African study had only one failure in 200 woman years and cites a personal interview with Sister Magdalino of the Philippines who claims 100% effectiveness in 4329 couples.

Sympto-thermal method

This method is really a combination of methods that involves both partners in the responsibility for prevention of conception. It is based on determination of basal body temperature, observation of cervical mucus changes, and recognition of secondary symptoms. The woman identifies the signs and symptoms while the partner keeps the records. Together the couple interprets the records to determine safe and unsafe periods. They use a special chart such as the one in Fig. 22-9. The chart records days of cycle, coitus, days of month, disturbances in routine, temperature, mucus, peak day, cervical changes, and any special notes. Once a chart is completed, it is interpreted by the couple to determine phases of the cycle. Users of the sympto-thermal method divide the cycle into the relatively infertile phase, the fertile phase, and the infertile phase, which are roughly the same as the menstrual, secretory, and proliferative phases of the woman's menstrual cycle. With this method, secondary symptoms noted may include increased libido, spotting or breakthrough bleeding, mittelschmertz, fullness or tenderness in the pelvic area, vulvular swelling, or bearing-down pains. The woman or her partner periodically checks her cervix to determine changes. Prior to ovulation, the cervix dilates slightly, becomes softer, rises in the vagina, increases mucus production, and feels more slippery. The couple learns to identify all of the signs and symptoms that are indicative of ovulation (Britt, 1977).

As with the other methods, abstinence is necessary during the fertile or unsafe days. Many who use this method report improvement in their marriage relationship (Britt, 1977; Moore, 1978). Efficacy rates for this method are not known but are believed to be similar to those of the other natural family planning methods.

Advantages and disadvantages of natural fertility control

For the woman and perhaps the couple, these methods offer added insights into the functioning of the female body. These methods can enhance self-esteem and appreciation of one's own body. They can be practiced by the woman alone, allowing her a sense of control over her own body. They can also enhance communication between the couple. They can facilitate the development of alternative methods of sexual expression and enhance expression of intimacy in ways other than penile-vaginal intercourse. They do not require the introduction of foreign materials into the woman's body nor do they use any external devices.

A disadvantage is related to the high degree of motivation and understanding needed in order to practice them successfully. In addition, either partner can experience feelings of frustration because of long periods of abstinence. Finally, the effectiveness rates vary greatly and these methods are not for everyone.

Sterilization

Permanent resolution of the need for contraception is becoming more and more popular in the United States. Hatcher (1978) states that for married couples over age 30, sterilization is now the most commonly used method of birth control. Over 9.5 million adults in the United States today have opted for this method of birth control. Sterilization is being used not only by couples who have completed their families but also by single people or couples who have decided not to have children.

In the last few years there have been many changes in the laws and regulations governing sterilization procedures. Hatcher (1978) identifies several critical needs that every practitioner who does birth control counseling should be aware of:

1. From a practical and legal standpoint, it is essential to conform strictly to the guidelines for informed choice and consent as set down by HEW.
2. Partner consent is not a legal requirement.
3. To be eligible for federal funds for sterilization procedures, the woman must be at least 21 years of age and legally competent.
4. HEW and some state regulations require waiting periods of varying lengths between counseling and performing the procedures.

Factors that most influence client satisfaction with

sterilization as a method of birth control are related to the maturity, motivation, understanding, and adjustment of the woman (and her partner). If at all possible both partners should be involved in the decision-making process and should agree. Common concerns often expressed are fear of pain with the procedure, complications or side effects, effect on physiology, and effect on sexual functioning. Counseling must deal with these concerns while also providing accurate information and allowing couples to explore their feelings about ending reproductive functioning. Informal consent is essential; to ensure this Hatcher (1978) recommends the use of the following guidelines:

Benefits: Permanent, effective; repeated decisions or cost not necessary.

Risks: Surgery has attendant morbidity and mortality; expensive in the short-run; not 100% effective

Alternatives: All options of reversible contraception; exploration of possibility of partner sterilization

Inquiries: Client should be encouraged to ask questions; clear up misinformation and myths

Decision to change: Woman should feel she can fully decide not to be sterilized if she wishes without punitive repercussions.

Explanation: All aspects of procedure and side effects in detail. Clearly emphasize the permanence of the procedure and give accurate estimates of possibility of reversal. Any psychologic and/or physiologic effects on hormones, weight, menses, and sexual response should be described. Cost, availability, and accessibility of procedure should be explained.

Documentation: Any written instruction; written risks, and written, signed, witnessed consent form.

When individuals are correctly informed and counseled and choose freely from healthy motivation, sterilization for the woman should not adversely affect sexual functioning, physiology, or self-concept.

The various sterilization procedures and their physiologic and psychologic ramifications are discussed in Chapter 15, Reproductive Surgery.

INEFFECTIVE METHODS AND NONMETHODS
Withdrawal or coitus interruptus

This is one of the most ancient contraceptive techniques known and worldwide it continues to be one of the most commonly practiced. The man and woman who choose to use this method have intercourse anyway they wish until the point of ejaculatory inevitability is reached. At this point the male withdraws his penis from the vagina and ejaculates away from her external genitalia, theoretically preventing conception. Withdrawal as a contraceptive measure has real advantages in that it involves no artificial devices or chemicals and is available at all times at no cost. There is one major disadvan-

tage, however; its failure rate is quite high—a theoretical effectiveness rate of 15 pregnancies per 100 women per year and 25 pregnancies per 100 women per year among actual users.

Failure occurs for several reasons, one of which is a built-in source of error. Pre-ejaculatory fluid, which usually escapes before the penis is withdrawn, contains sperm capable of impregnation. This method also requires considerable self-control on the part of the male, which is not always possible.

Withdrawal can contribute to the development of sexual dysfunction as the couple become focused on the timing and success of withdrawal. There is the potential for the man to develop premature ejaculation while the woman can experience orgasmic dysfunction or unrelieved build up of pelvic myotonia and congestion. Closeness between the couple can be hampered severely. Many couples who use this method are able to develop their own patterns and alternative methods of sexual pleasuring that are highly enjoyable to both and enable both to experience orgasmic responses. But for the majority of couples the method is probably unsatisfactory; it is a primitive, male-oriented method.

Abstinence

Some authorities list abstinence as a method of birth control. It is the most effective method known and has been used for centuries. For it to be legitimately considered as a form of birth control, however, there needs to be a potential for sexual activity to occur. Many couples use periodic abstinence as a method of birth control; it is part of the framework of the natural family planning methods. There are no physical side effects so long as prolonged sexual arousal is followed by orgasm to relieve pelvic congestion. Psychologic side effects depend on the reasons why the choice was made and the motivations surrounding it.

Douching

Many women believe that sperm can be "washed away" by douching. This is an "old wives' tale"; douching can, in fact, facilitate the movement of sperm up the cervical canal.

Avoidance of orgasm

Avoidance of orgasm is another of the old wives' tales still believed by some women. Orgasm or the lack thereof has no effect one way or the other on fertility.

Lactation

On a worldwide basis, lactation probably prevents more births than any other form of contraception (Hatcher, 1978). Lactation prevents pregnancy by suppressing the return of ovulation after childbirth. Ovarian functioning is suppressed but not completely depressed by lactation. Deibel (1978) states that the suckling stimulus rather than lactation acts on the pituitary. In order to use lactation as a method of birth control, total or complete breast-feeding must be practiced. To be successful, the mother must never leave her infant, particularly for the first 12 to 15 months. He should even sleep with her. The baby is allowed to remain at the breast after nutritionally satisfied; only the breast is available for comfort and nourishment. In addition, the woman must wait 6 months before giving the infant solids and then use finger foods. The baby should be at least 9 months old before being given other liquid unless he expresses strong desire for a cup (Deibel, 1978). If this regimen is followed, success rates close to 95% can be expected according to Kippley (1974). This strict regimen is not possible for most women; in these cases, use effectiveness rates are closer to 40 pregnancies per 100 women per year, while the theoretical effectiveness rate is about 15 pregnancies.

CONTRACEPTIVE COUNSELING

It is the goal of nursing to promote high-level wellness to the degree possible for each client. For this reason, responsibility for facilitating the process of responsible fertility control by women and their partners lies within nursing's role. Fertility control involves the total relationship between a man and a woman, including health, fertility, and socioeconomics; and it is essential for the development and maintenance of a sound family relationship and individual well-being.

The critical factor in assisting individuals or couples in the use of contraception is helping them to find a method that they will use. Whether a particular method will be used or not outweighs the given method's reliability. The desired outcome is that the woman selects a method she understands and is comfortable with and that is compatible with her individual health problems, physical status, and life-style. Taylor (1976) proposes using a decision-making model as a teaching strategy to actively promote contraceptive problem-solving and provide information about birth control and sexuality. This model is based on the assumption that the process of deciding will provide an outcome that is satisfying and acceptable to the individual.

To clarify the application, consider how a woman might reasonably choose a method of birth control. First she makes a tentative decision to avoid pregnancy and focuses on a particular method of birth control. Then alternatives to the initial decision are considered—pregnancy, abstinence, or another method of contraception. If conflicts arise as the woman considers the possible consequences of or barriers to her initial decision, she re-evaluates the alternatives in light of their implications. She may decide to modify or abandon the initial decision. The first stage is to make a commitment to a specific course of action. This type of decision-making process allows the woman to organize information and arrive at conclusions appropriate for her own value system.

The role of the nurse in this process is that of facilitator rather than decision-maker. The nurse provides information and asks questions that will help the client identify her own feelings and concerns. Nondirective questioning can help the client discover what specific obstacles are preventing contraception and what motivating factors leading to contraception are present. Such an approach will strengthen the individual's self-awareness, self-understanding and self-control. This approach is predicated on the assumption that knowledge is not enough; rather, motivation to use contraception stems not only from the rational level but also from the belief system—attitudes, values, norms, roles, and relationships.

An essential part of any contraceptive counseling is the history-taking and physical examination. Family history of diabetes, heart disease, hypertension, bleeding or clotting disorders, kidney or liver disease, migraine headache, seizure disorders, anemia, tuberculosis, stroke, cancer, or mental problems should be obtained. This information will provide baseline data on diseases the client may be at risk for; it also is essential for determining the suitability of oral contraceptives. The woman's past medical history should be taken next. She should be asked whether or not she has experienced any of the above problems, and about previous hospitalizations, operations, or other major illnesses. A detailed menstrual and obstetric history is essential; any complications or abnormalities should be carefully described (see Chapter 6 for information on how to obtain these histories). Any allergies should be recorded, as well as medications the woman is currently taking. It is important to discuss her previous use of and experience with contraceptives; this will provide valuable clues as to appropriate selection. Key questions to ask while obtaining the history are these:

1. When did menarche occur? Are menses irregular? Either late menarche or irregular menses could indicate anovulatory cycles, in which case oral contraceptives should not be used.
2. Does she experience heavy periods with clotting and cramping? This will be exaggerated by the IUD; oral contraceptives can bring improvement. Before an oral contraceptive is prescribed, however, extremely heavy flow should be investigated as to cause.
3. Does she have a history of pelvic inflammatory disease? An IUD would be contraindicated.

4. Is there a history of severe migraine, cerebral arterial insufficiency, cardiovascular disease, liver disease, severe diabetes, genital or breast cancer, thromboembolytic problems, hypertension, or family history of cardiovascular accidents? If any are present, oral contraceptives are contraindicated.

5. What contraceptives has she used before? Were they effective? If not, why not? The answers to these questions will give some idea of the client's level of knowledge and understanding.

6. What does she see as the most important reasons for contraceptive use? Answers will give clues as to whether expectations are realistic or not. Misconceptions can come to light and be cleared up. Goals and priorities can be identified. Prevention of pregnancy as a goal will dictate use of a highly effective method, while a desire to delay or space children might call for a method with a somewhat greater pregnancy risk but no systemic or local alterations (Martin, 1978).

Hatcher (1978) has developed a series of questions that will help to identify factors that might lower the use effectiveness of a given method. A yes answer indicates these factors.

Am I afraid of using this method of birth control?
Would I really rather not use this method?
Will I have trouble remembering to use this method?
Have I ever become pregnant while using this method?
Are there reasons why I will be unable to use this method as prescribed?
Do I still have unanswered questions about this method?
Has my mother, father, sister, brother, or a close friend strongly discouraged me from using this method?
Will this method make my periods longer or more painful?
Will prolonged use of this method cost me more than I can afford?
Is this method known to have serious complications?
Am I opposed to this method because of my religious beliefs?
Have I already experienced complications from this method?
Has a nurse or doctor already told me not to use this method?
Is my partner opposed to my using this method?
Am I using this method without my partner's knowledge?
Will the use of this method embarrass me?
Will the use of this method embarrass my partner?
Will my partner or I enjoy intercourse less because of this method?
Will this method interrupt the act of intercourse?

After the initial history-taking and counseling session, a physical examination should be done. A breast and pelvic examination with Pap smear is the absolute minimum required. It is preferable that a thorough screening physical be done, particularly if the woman plans to use oral contraceptives or an IUD. The following should be included (Martin, 1978):

Eyes: Check for condition of retina, condition of veins and arteries, and signs of glaucoma.

Ear, nose, throat: General screening.

Thyroid: Examine for nodules, diffuse enlargement. Oral contraceptives alter thyroid function tests.

Chest: Examine lung fields; heart and great vessel murmurs, bruits, or abnormal lung sounds should be investigated.

Breasts: Check for masses, nodules, nipple discharge. Positive findings contraindicate oral contraceptives until consultation.

Abdomen: Examine for masses, bruits, or heptosplenomegaly. Positive findings require consultation.

Extremities: Varicosities are a contraindication for oral contraceptives. Absent or weak peripheral pulses indicate possible circulatory or arteriosclerotic problems, which should be investigated. Oral contraceptives should not be prescribed.

Pelvic examination: Pelvic relaxation with prolapse, cystocele, or rectocele, or anatomic anomalies such as a small cervix or short anterior vaginal wall contraindicate use of a diaphragm. Endocrine problems can be indicated by presence of an infantile cervix or uterus, in which case an IUD or oral contraceptives should not be prescribed. PID or extensive cervicitis rules out the use of oral contraceptives; IUDs are difficult to insert when fibroids are present. In such cases foam, condom, or diaphragm would be the method of choice. If ovarian or tubal masses are found, no contraceptives should be begun until the condition is diagnosed and treated. Severe retroversion or anteversion of the uterus contraindicates the use of the IUD. If vaginitis is present, it should be treated.

Weight: Obesity is considered to be a contraindication to oral contraceptives because of the effect on carbohydrate and lipid metabolism. Obesity also increases the risk factor for other potential serious complications, such as thromboembolic or coronary happenings. It is difficult to fit the obese woman with a diaphragm or to insert an IUD. Until weight is lost, foam with condoms is the contraceptive of choice.

Age: Serious consideration should be given to the advisability of prescribing oral contraceptives for the very young whose endocrine system is immature or the woman over age 35, because of the greater risks they carry.

Hypertension: Even marginal elevations constitute contraindications for the use of oral contraceptives.

Laboratory tests: Pap smear, gonorrhea culture on sexually active women, urinalysis, complete blood count, and serologic test for syphilis should be done. If there is a question as to liver function, liver enzyme studies should be determined; impaired liver function is an absolute contraindication to oral contraceptives.

Motivation for contraception differs from person to person. Furthermore, some clients are highly motivated and desire only specific information; others may have fears and misconceptions. Still others we seek out because we think they need contraceptive advice. The common denominator in counseling these disparate women is determining what factors will motivate them to use contraception successfully. It is also crucial that we recognize when a client does not wish to practice birth control. The woman or couple must decide what method, if any, is desired and feel free to reject any method. In most cases the client's wishes can determine the method she uses; there may be some clients, however, for whom specific methods will be contraindicated and the reasons should be made clear to them. Once a method is chosen, the woman must be carefully and thoroughly informed as to the most effective use of the contraceptive chosen. She needs plenty of time to practice and describe to the nurse how she will use the method. Practical matters such as cost and where to get supplies should be dealt with.

A final consideration in contraceptive counseling is informed consent. This is particularly crucial because fertility control methods are usually initiated at the request of the client without traditional medical indications for treatment. The HEW guidelines for nontherapeutic sterilization provide a definition of informed consent, and a way to ensure that each client is protected when receiving contraceptive counseling. HEW defines informed consent as "the voluntary knowing assent from the individual [for] whom any [contraception] is [provided] after she has been given (as evidenced by a document executed by such individuals):

1. A fair explanation of the proposed method
2. A description of attendant side effects, major risks, common minor risks, and common discomforts
3. A description of the benefit to be expected
4. An explanation of appropriate alternative methods of fertility control and the effect and impact of the proposed method, including the effectiveness rate and the fact that nothing is 100% effective
5. An offer to answer any questions
6. An instruction that the individual is free to withhold her consent to the treatment at any time prior to use of the method with prejudicing her future care and without loss of other programs or project benefits to which the patient might otherwise be entitled.
7. The documentation referred to in this section should be provided by one of the following methods:
   a. Provision of a written consent document describing all of the basic points of informed consent as detailed in 1 through 6 above.
   b. Provision of a short-form written consent document stating that the basic elements of informed consent have been presented orally to the client. This must be supplemented by a written summary of the oral presentation. The written summary is signed by the person obtaining consent and the witness. The witness is to be chosen by the client.
   c. Each consent document must display the following, printed prominently at the top:

NOTICE: Your decision at any time not to use contraception will not result in the withdrawal or withholding of any benefits provided by programs or projects.*

REFERENCES

Ambsni, L., and others: Are hormonal contraceptives teratogenic?, Fertil. Steril. **28**(8):791-797, 1977.

American College of Obstetricians and Gynecologists: The intrauterine device, ACOG technical bulletin, No. 40, Chicago, June 1976.

Billings, J. J.: Natural family planning, ed. 3 (American), Collegeville, Minn., The Liturgical Press, 1975.

Blake, J.: The pill and the rising cost of fertility control, Soc. Biol. **24**(4):267-280, Winter 1977.

Boston Women's Health Collective: Our bodies, our selves, ed. 2, New York, 1976, Simon & Schuster.

Bradbury, B. A.: Preventing the diaphragm baby syndrome: a matter of technique, teaching and time, J. Obstet. Gynecol. **4**(2):24-32, 1975.

Brillman, J.: The cervical cap, reprint, Boston Women's Health Book Collective, 1980.

Britt, S. S.: Fertility awareness: four methods of national family planning, J. Obstet. Gynecol. Nurs. **6**(2):9-18, 1977.

Cates, W., and others: The intrauterine devices and deaths from spontaneous abortion, N. Engl. J. Med. **295**:1155-1159, 1976.

Connell, E. B.: Side effects of intrauterine devices, Int. J. Gynecol. Obstet. **15**:153-156, 1977.

Corea, G.: The hidden malpractice, New York, 1977, Wm. C. Morrow & Co.

Cowart, M., and Newton, D. W.: Oral contraceptives: how best to explain their effects to patients, Nursing '76 **6**:44-48, 1976.

Deeker, E. L.: Side effects of the pill: trivial or serious? Nurs. Update, pp. 5-9, Mar. 1976.

Deibel, P.: Natural family planning: different methods, Mat. Child Nurs., pp. 171-177, May/June 1978.

Dernison, C. F.: One look at the risk of the pill, Nurs. Update, pp. 3-4, Mar. 1976.

Family Planning Digest: Family Plan. Perspect. **8**(5):241-245, 1976.

Fasal, E., and Paffenberger, R. S.: Oral contraceptives as related to cancer and benign lesions of the breast, J. Natl. Cancer Inst. **55**:767-773, 1975.

Federal Register: Oral contraceptives. Fed. Reg. Part II. Jan. 31, 1978.

Fisch, J. R., and Freedman, S. H.: Oral contraceptives and ABO blood group and in vitro fibrin formation, Obstet. Gynecol. **46**:473-479, 1975.

Fischman, S. H.: Change strategies and their application to family planning programs, Am. J. Nurs. **73**(10):1771-1774, 1973.

Gordon, L.: The politics of birth control, 1920-1940: the impact of professionals, Int. J. Health Serv. **5**(2):253-277, 1975.

Greene, G. R., and Sartwell, P. E.: Oral contraceptive use in patients with thromboembolism following surgery, trauma or infection, Am. J. Public Health **62**(5):680-685, 1972.

Hatcher, R. A., and others: Contraceptive technology, 1978-1979, ed. 9, New York, 1978, John Wiley & Sons.

---

*Adapted for use with contraceptive counseling from HEW Guidelines.

Huxall, L.: Today's pill and the individual woman, Mat. Child. Nurs., pp. 359-363, Nov./Dec. 1977.

Inmann, W. H. W., and Vessey, M. P.: Investigation of deaths from pulmonary, coronary and cerebral thrombosis and embolism in women of childbearing age, Br. Med. J., pp. 193-199, Apr. 1968.

Jain, A. K.: Cigarette smoking, use of oral contraceptives with myocardial infarction, Am. J. Obstet. Gynecol. **126**(3):301-307, 1976.

Jain, A. K.: Mortality risk associated with the use of oral contraceptives, Studies Fam. Plan. **8**(3):50-54, 1977.

Jick, H., and others: Venous thromboembolic disease and ABO blood type: a comparative study, Lancet, pp. 539-542, Mar. 8, 1967.

Kane, F. J.: Evaluation of emotional reactions to oral contraceptive use, Am. J. Obstet. Gynecol. **126**(8):968-971, 1976.

Kapor-Stanulovie, N., and Snowden, R.: In defense of a psychological approach to studying fertility regulating behaviors, IPPF Med. Bull. **10**(5):1-2, 1976.

Kent, D. R., and others: Liver tumors and oral contraceptives, Int. J. Gynecol. Obstet. **15**:137-142, 1977.

Kilby-Kelberg, S.: Why some won't try the diaphragm method; why others try and fail, J. Obstet. Gynecol. Nurs. **4**(2):24-25, 1975.

Kintzel, K. C.: Advanced concepts in clinical Nursing, Philadelphia, 1977, J. B. Lippincott Co.

Kippley, S.: Breastfeeding and natural child spacing, the ecology of natural mothering, rev. ed., New York, 1974, Harper & Row, Publishers.

Kistner, R. W.: DC's & IUD's: a challenge to modern gyn care, RN pp. 55-62, Sept. 1976.

Klaus, H.: The ovulation method, Nurs. Digest, pp. 13-14, Mar./Apr. 1975.

Lane, Mary E., and others: Emotional aspects of contraception, Bull. Nurse-Midwives **15**(1):16-25, 1970.

Lecocq, F. R., and others: Metabolic balance studies with norethynodrel and chlormadinone acetate, Am. J. Obstet. Gynecol. **99**:374, 1967.

Mann, J. I., and Inman, W. H.: Oral contraceptives and death from myocardial infarction, Brit. Med. J. **2**:245-248, 1975.

Martin, L. L.: Health care of women, Philadelphia, 1978, J. B. Lippincott Co.

Moore, M. L.: Realities in childbearing, Philadelphia, 1978, W. B. Saunders Co.

Muller, C.: Fertility control and the quality of human life, Am. J. Public Health **63**(6):519-523, 1973.

Population Reports: Oral contraceptives, Series A, #2, Mar. 1975.

Population Reports: Oral contraceptives, Series A, #4, May 1977.

Rainwater, L.: And the poor get children, Chicago, 1960, Quadrangle Books, 1960.

Report of the Royal College of General Practitioners: Oral contraceptives and health, London, 1974, Pittman Medical.

Romney, S., and others: Gynecology and obstetrics. In Romney, S., and others, editors: The health care of women, New York, 1975, McGraw-Hill Book Co.

Sandberg, E., and Jacobs, R.: Psychology of the misuse and rejection of contraception, Am. J. Obstet. Gynecol. **110**(2):237-241, 1971.

Sandelowski, M.: An epidemiologic view of family planning, J. Obstet. Gynecol. Nurs. **5**(2):35-37, 1976.

Seaman, B.: Free and female, Greenwich, Conn., 1972, Faucet Crest.

Seaman, B., and Seaman, G.: Women and the crisis in sex hormones, New York, 1977, Rawson Associates Publishers, Inc. (Bantam paperback, 1978.)

Selstad, G. M., and others: Predicting contraceptive use in post abortion patients, Am. J. Public Health **65**(7):708-713, 1975.

Siegel, E., and Morris, N.: Family planning: its health rationale, Nurs. Digest, pp. 55-57, May/June 1975.

Silverberg, S. G., and Makowski, E. L.: Endometrial carcinoma in young women taking oral contraceptives, Obstet. Gynecol. **46**:503-506, 1975.

Suchman, E.: Preventative health behavior: a model for research on community health campaigns, J. Health Soc. Behav., pp. 197-209, Sept. 1967.

Tanis, J. L.: Recognizing the reasons for contraceptive non-use and abuse, Am. J. Mat. Child Nurs. pp. 364-369, Nov./Dec. 1977.

Tatum, H. J.: Clinical aspects of intrauterine contraception: circumspection 1976, Fertil. Steril. **28**(1):3-28, 1977.

Tatum, H. J., and Schmidt, F. H.: Contraceptive and sterilization practices and extrauterine pregnancy: a realistic perspective, Fertil. Steril. **28**(4):407-421, 1977.

Taylor, D.: A new way to teach teens about contraceptives, Am. J. Matern. Child Nurs. pp. 378-383, Nov./Dec. 1976.

Taylor, R. N., and others: Changes in menstrual cycle length and regularity after using oral contraceptives, J. Gynecol. Obstet. **15**:55-59, 1977.

Tietze, C.: The pill and mortality from cardiovascular disease:another look, Fam. Plan. Perspect. **11**(12):80-89, 1979.

Tietze, C., Bongaarts, J., and Schearer, B.: Mortality associated with the control of fertility, Fam. Plan. Perspect. **8**(1):6-14, 1976.

Tietze, C., and others: The effectiveness of the cervical cap as a contraceptive method, Am. J. OB/GYN **66**:904-908, 1955.

Timby, B. K.: Ovulation method of birth control, Am. J. Nurs. **72**(6):928-929, 1976.

Trussell, T. J., Faden, R., and Hatcher, R. A.: Efficacy information in contraceptive counseling: those little white lies, Am. J. Pub. Health **66**:761-767, 1976.

Tryer, L.: The benefits and risks of IUD use, Int. J. Gynecol. Obstet. **15**:150-152, 1977.

Vessey, M.: Oral contraceptives and stroke, New Engl. J. Med. **17**:906-907, 1973.

Waller, D.: Oral contraceptives. Unpublished paper, Feb. 8, 1975.

Waschek, J., and Helling, D. L.: Oral contraceptive associated liver tumors, Drug Intell. Clin. Pharm. **12**:523-527, 1970.

Weidenbach, E.: The nurses' role in family planning, Nurs. Clin. North Am. **3**(2):355-365, 1968.

Weir, R. J.: Blood pressure in women taking oral contraceptives, Am. Heart J. **92**(1):119-120, 1976.

Werley, H., and others: Professionals and birth control: student and faculty attitudes, Fam. Plan. Perspect. **5**(1):42-49, Winter 1973.

Whartman, J.: The cervical cap, Population Reports, Series H, #4, Washington, D.C., 1976, George Washington University Medical Center.

23

Abortion

Catherine Ingram Fogel

Women have long considered abortion to be a solution to unwanted pregnancy and a way to control fertility. In the United States today, induced abortion constitutes a significant portion of women's health care (Martin, 1978). Abortion is a complex emotional, social, political, and legal issue about which most practitioners feel strongly. Because of the influence values and attitudes about abortion have on health care delivery, the topic needs to be examined by nurses who care for women during their reproductive years. There is a need for prepared nursing practitioners who are able to care for clients seeking induced abortion. The purpose of this chapter is to meet this need by:

1. Examining the factors influencing a woman's decision to abort
2. Determining the scope of the issue
3. Exploring the historical determinants of abortion
4. Discussing legal considerations
5. Describing available abortion methods
6. Identifying the risks and complications of abortion

Nursing responsibilities, appropriate interventions, and counseling techniques are also discussed.

FACTORS INFLUENCING THE DECISION TO ABORT

It is important to know what factors influence the decision-making process for the woman. What makes her decide to terminate or carry the pregnancy? According to a study done by Steinhoff (1973), four areas need to be explored: (1) the relationship between the woman and the father of the pregnancy, (2) in what context the decision-making took place, (3) the woman's goals in life for herself, and (4) the woman's self-concept and her view of self regarding her sexual activity. Clark and Affonso (1976) state that decision-making and the behavior of pregnant women may take place in three time frames: (1) preconception (was anything being done to prevent conception if a child was not wanted?), (2) after pregnancy was a reality, and (3) postpregnancy (how will she prevent another pregnancy?).

As discussed in Chapters 11 and 12, preconceptual decision-making appears to be irrational. The woman may be unable to view herself as sexually active and therefore will not use contraception. A woman may feel pressured into sexual activity by her partner. Some authorities suggest that there may be a predisposition to risk an unwanted pregnancy through ineffective use of contraception when the woman, married or single, has a history of role redefinition in the family of origin. The components of role redefinition are: (1) the daughter assumes some of the mother's role as wife or homemaker, (2) the daughter and mother are alienated, and (3) there is intimacy between father and daughter that excludes the mother. Often women who risk unwanted pregnancy feel they have poor support systems from other women and that their significant relationships have been with men. Finally, they state they dislike sex and sexual relations.

Decisions to abort a fetus are more apt to be based on objective factors and are related to the woman's perception of her ability to care for a child, quality of the relationship with her partner, and her own personal goals. Comparatively, very few women seek abortion for medical reasons alone. Reasons given are more apt to be: (1) reluctance to interrupt career plans, (2) lack of money, (3) fear of a loss of personal freedom, (4) uncertainty about the relationship with the male involved, (5) single status, (6) have enough children, (7) need for child spacing, and (8) do not want children.

Swigar et al. (1976) studied abortion applicant "dropouts" to determine what factors influenced these women to carry a pregnancy to term. Women who were experiencing extreme conflict about the unwanted pregnancy and who believed that abortion was morally wrong were most likely to carry the pregnancy to term. Women whose partners desired a baby also more often elected to remain pregnant. Partners who strongly objected to abortion had a definite influence. A third factor in deciding not to have an abortion was fear of the procedure. Many women hold misconceptions and myths about what the procedure involves, so much so that their fear prevents them from obtaining an abortion. Women who found that marriage was possible often decided not to have an abortion. It appears that conceiving was a way of inducing a boyfriend to marry and that abortion was a way out for the woman if marriage plans fell through or did not materialize. At times a woman, usually an adolescent, conceives out of rebellion against her family. In these instances abortion would just continue the problem in the woman's mind, not solve it. Finally, for some women abortion is equated with loss of a part of self and therefore is intolerable.

HISTORY OF ABORTION

Abortion as a solution to unwanted pregnancy is as old as recorded time. Ever since the connection between intercourse and pregnancy was made, women have been trying to find effective methods of abortion. Francke (1978) describes such techniques as swallowing fourteen live tadpoles 3 days after a missed period or drinking quicksilver in oil in hopes of stimulating a period. Egyptian women, in 1500 B.C., douched with honey and salt or inserted plugs made of crocodile dung and paste. In slightly more modern times Russian women have attempted abortion by squatting over a pot of boiling onions, and women belonging to certain Indian tribes climbed up and down palm trees hitting their stomach against the tree trunk.

Even today women continue to use their own home remedies—brews of castor oil, turpentine, or special herbs such as horseradish or mustard—as abortifacients. More dangerous potions such as lye or ammonia have also been used in a desperate attempt to get rid of an unwanted fetus. Sometimes these work by injuring the woman's body so severely that she spontaneously aborts. Other women have attempted to abort themselves with coat hangers or knitting needles, the most common result being uterine perforation, hemorrhage, infection, frequently permanent sterilization, and sometimes death. At present women no longer have to resort to these dangerous, barbaric practices, or at least most women do not. For the moment, at least, abortion is available to most; the future is more uncertain.

The morality of abortion has varied according to the period and culture; even within the same religious framework, views have changed. For example, it is only within the past 100 years that abortion became illegal in the United States or was decreed a mortal sin by the Roman Catholic Church. Under English common law, abortion was not even included in the criminal code although it was against Church laws (Romney et al., 1975). Until about 100 years ago, abortion under certain circumstances was acceptable and condoned by both Church and state.

For centuries the Catholic Church accepted abortion in a woman before quickening occurred. It was at time of quickening that the "animate soul" was believed to enter the fetus changing it from "inanimate soul" to person. Quickening is usually experienced between the sixteenth and twentieth weeks of pregnancy; however, the Catholic Church defined quickening as being 40 days' gestation. This was based on Aristotle's belief that males quickened at about 40 days while females took 80 days to acquire a soul. Hippocrates was not quite as sexist, for he thought a fetus became a male at 30 days and a female at 42 days. It is not recorded how a woman was supposed to find out what sex she was carrying, and so the compromise date of 40 days was adopted by the Church (Francke, 1978).

Unfortunately, the Church became increasingly more uncomfortable with its arbitrary stand on abortion as medical knowledge grew and it became more embarrassing to pinpoint just when body and soul began. In 1869 Pope Pius IX banned abortion altogether. Abortion became a sin and grounds for excommunicating, and was considered homicide. Apart from religious values, social reasons also made abortion unacceptable. European wars had depleted the Catholic numbers, which was of concern to the Church hierarchy. Also, abortion was becoming more popular and used more frequently in Europe and America. According to the 1869 law, the mother was not subject to excommunication but was considered an innocent party until 1917 when the word "mother" was added to the list of sinners who participated in abortion.

At about the same time that religious views were undergoing drastic changes, abortion was being questioned by the medical establishment, legislators, and industrialists. Until the nineteenth century under American and English common law abortion was legal unless the woman died. Only then was a crime committed and it was not the woman but the abortionist who had committed it. Abortion, though risky and painful, was widely sought and its popularity was its undoing. There was an upsurge in puritanism, and abortion became one of its targets. Martin Luther's words were widely accepted: "If a woman grows weary and at last dies from childbearing, it matters not"; and "Let her only die from bearing, she's in there to do it." The decimation of the population resulting from European Civil Wars was another factor in increasing resistance to abortion, which was then a primary method of birth control. In addition, the antiabortion movement gained impetus from business and farming factions whose economic future depended on more workers. Women were thought of as assets as breeders. Both white and black women were expected to be good breeders—good workers were hard to find!

The medical establishment of the time (predominantly

male) also played its part in the antiabortion movement. As health standards were raised, death or injury from abortion became less and less tolerable. Surgery still entailed a high risk in the nineteenth century and many physicians felt the ends did not justify the means in abortion. The movement of the times was away from midwives to male physicians who were less sympathetic to the wishes of women who wanted to terminate unwanted pregnancies. By 1880 almost every state had a law restricting abortion to life-threatening situations only. At this point abortion on demand went underground and stayed there until the early 1970s when a few states passed less restrictive laws. In 1973 the Supreme Court returned the right of controlling reproduction to the women who were actually doing the reproducing.

There is approximately one abortion performed for every three live births in the United States today (U.S. National Center for Health Statistics, 1977). This means that approximately 1,100,000 abortions are performed annually in the United States. Approximately one-third of women receiving abortions are teenagers, one-third 20 to 24 years old, and one-third is over 25 years. More pregnant adolescents below the age of 15 have an abortion than deliver a live birth. The same trend also holds true for women over age 40. Of the women experiencing legal abortions 67% are white and 33% are nonwhite. Although white women account for the majority of abortions being done today, nonwhites have higher abortion rates than whites.

Twenty-seven percent of the women who had abortions in 1975 were married; therefore, the vast majority of women choosing therapeutic abortion are nonmarried. Not only are most women receiving abortions not married but also the majority have no living children at the time of the procedure. It should be noted that there is a bimodal distribution when one looks at abortion ratios to live births in that the highest rates occur in the nulliparous women and then again in the grand multipara.

Suction curettage or D & E is the most common (77%) type of abortion method used, followed by sharp curettage (D & C, 12%), intrauterine instillations (8%), and hysterotomy/hysterectomy (0.6%). Eighty-four percent of all abortions are performed before the thirteenth week of pregnancy, which correlates closely with the type of method used. There is an ever-increasing trend toward performance of abortion in the first trimester. Furthermore, the percentage of women having an abortion at 8 weeks' gestation or less is also increasing. Over 10% of all women who have abortions have had a previous one. Several important trends emerge from all these figures that are significant for nurses in anticipatory counseling and planning nursing care for clients.

It is obvious that abortions are now an accepted part of American society; the number of abortions performed annually continues to rise. Accessibility of services has improved since 1973 and until recently limited financial resources were not an insurmountable barrier.

LEGAL CONSIDERATIONS

Existing antiabortion laws began to be challenged beginning in the early 1960s, and a few state legislatures passed less restrictive laws permitting abortions under specific conditions (when there was a threat to the life and physical or mental health of the mother, when there was a high risk of physical or mental defect in the fetus, or if pregnancy was the result of rape or incest). The various legal challenges were successful, and the Supreme Court decisions, *Roe v Wade* and *Doe v Bolton*, were handed down in January, 1973. These cases held that during the first 3 months of pregnancy, women have the right to obtain abortions without interference from the state. After the first trimester of pregnancy, the state can impose regulations safeguarding maternal health. Later, when the fetus has become "viable," the state may regulate abortions to protect the life of the fetus and may even prohibit abortions except when necessary to preserve the life or health of the mother. Viability was defined by the court as the time when the fetus is "potentially able to live outside the mother's womb albeit with artificial aid."

In the summer of 1976, the Court again addressed the issue of abortion. In a series of cases, the rights of adult women were expanded and some of these rights were extended to minors. In the case *Planned Parenthood v Dunforth* the Court ruled that the state cannot impose the requirement of consent by a third party on a woman's right to consent. That veto power cannot be exercised by spouse, parent, or guardian. In another ruling the court held that health care workers can provide family planning services to minors who receive AFDC and Medicaid funds.

The legal status of abortion is presently under strong attack. Antiabortionist groups are lobbying strongly for a Constitutional Amendment prohibiting all abortions.

ABORTION METHODS

The goal of any abortion method is to remove all products of conception, which include the placenta or chorionic villi, fetal parts, and some of the decidual tissue. Before the abortion is performed the health care worker should obtain a thorough medical history from the client. Included in this history are:

1. Date of last menstrual period, when coitus occurred, and method of contraception if any
2. Previous obstetric history including details of all prior pregnancies and reproductive surgeries
3. Past contraceptive use and plans for future contraception (reasons for failure and expectations of birth control methods should be explored)

4. Known allergies to anesthetics, analgesics, antibiotics or other drugs
5. Current drug usage
6. Past medical/surgical history by systems to identify acute or chronic illness that might influence performance of the abortion procedure. (For example, an outpatient abortion is not indicated for a woman suffering from cardiac, pulmonary, hematologic, or metabolic diseases. Physical conditions such as anemia, sickle-cell disease, liver, kidney, or heart diseases, diabetes, and epilepsy should be identified (Moore, 1978). While the history is being taken, the nurse should be alert to signs of undue anxiety or ambivalence that could indicate a need for further counseling.

Following the history, a brief physical examination including vital signs, heart, lungs, breasts, and abdomen and a thorough pelvic examination should be done. The pelvic examination should determine uterine size and estimated length of gestation; position of uterus (whether anteflexed or retroflexed), and any abnormalities such as fibroids. In addition, the client's hematocrit or hemoglobin should be checked so that if the woman is severely anemic (<30%) blood can be available. Rh determination should be done so that RhoGam can be given if the client is Rh negative. A Pap smear should be taken and a gonorrhea screening culture should be done to decrease the risk of postoperative infection by preprocedure treatment (Hatcher, 1978). The abortion methods used currently in the United States are:

Early abortion:
Menstrual extraction
Vacuum or suction curettage
Dilatation and curettage (D & C)
Second trimester:
Dilation and evacuation (D & E)
Intrauterine instillation of drug
Hysterotomy/hysterectomy

The length of pregnancy (week of gestation) and the woman's condition usually determines the appropriate type of abortion procedure. Fig. 23-1 gives a summary of assessment and decision-making in an abortion flowchart.

Early abortions
Menstrual extraction or regulation (ME)

Menstrual extraction is a procedure in which a flexible polyethylene catheter is inserted through the cervix into the uterus. Suction is applied through a syringe or pump, and the endometrium and contents of the uterus are aspirated. Cervical dilation is rarely necessary; however, paracervical blocks are frequently used. This procedure is usually performed within 6 weeks of the last menstrual period; however, it may be performed until 8 weeks after the last period. The procedure is performed on an outpatient basis. After the client receives adequate postoperative and contraceptive counseling and cramps have subsided, she can return home or to work with no physical or sexual restrictions.

The two risks associated with menstrual extraction are continuation of the pregnancy and complications. Over 99% of abortion clients undergo this procedure. It is important that only physicians experienced in the use of the technique perform it because the failure rates become much higher (as great as 10%) when performed by inexperienced practitioners (Brenner, 1977). The incidence of complications and risks such as uterine injury and bleeding are low when compared to other abortion methods. The risks become greater when the client is nulliparous and more than 6 weeks amenorrheic (Brenner and Edelman, 1977). It is essential that all clients experiencing menstrual extraction receive adequate contraceptive counseling and that a variety of contraceptive choices be made available.

A major problem with ME is that not all women who request the procedure are pregnant. Better patient selection would minimize the number of nonpregnant patients being exposed to the risks, inconvenience, and discomforts of the procedure. The proportion of women who are pregnant increases with length of amenorrhea; however, if the abortion is delayed until after 40 days of amenorrhea, when at least 75% of the women are pregnant, the complication rate increases threefold. What is needed is a universally available, sensitive, specific early pregnancy test that would enhance the selection process so that no nonpregnant clients would undergo ME. Some feminist groups advocate use of this technique by women in their own homes. It is not yet clear whether there might be a danger in repeated MEs in the same woman. Most authorities agree it should not be used as a substitute for contraception.

Vacuum curettage

Vacuum curettage is a widely used technique in which complete emptying of the uterus is accomplished in a short time period through small cervical dilations and under paracervical block. It can be done through 12 weeks' gestation. The cervix is gradually dilated mechanically, although often laminaria are inserted 6 to 24 hours prior to the procedure. Laminaria are small sticks of dried seaweed that expand slowly as they absorb moisture. They are placed in the cervical canal so that they dilate both the internal and external ossa. It is relatively painless and very effective. It has the drawback of requiring an extra visit to the physician and may possibly increase the occurrence of endometritis. Following the insertion of a vacuum curette, the products of conception are evacuated (Fig. 23-2).

Bleeding after the procedure is usually about the same as a heavy menstrual period; cramps are rarely severe.

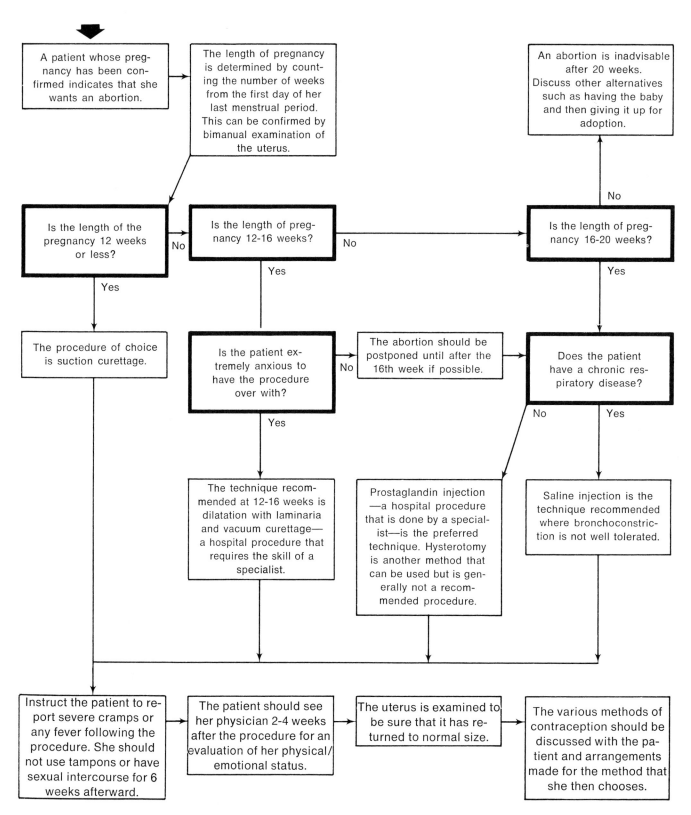

Fig. 23-1. Summary of decision-making process in therapeutic abortion (From Jensen, M., Benson, R. C., and Bobak, I. M.: Maternity care: the nurse and the family, St. Louis, 1977, The C. V. Mosby Co.)

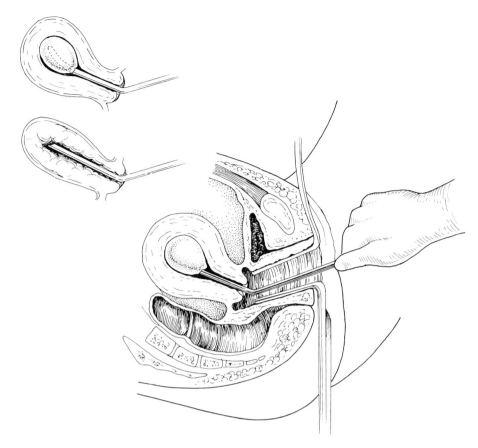

Fig. 23-2. Vacuum curettage abortion method.

The most common complications are infection, uterine perforation, and/or excessive bleeding caused by incomplete evacuation or retained placental fragments.

In a study done by Wolff (1977) the incidence of complications was found to be 1.54%; the earlier in pregnancy the procedure is performed the less likely it is that major complications will occur. Jensen and associates (1977) report that infection such as endometritis or salpingitis occurs in about 8% of all patients, and approximately 2% must have subsequent dilation and curettage for excessive bleeding. Several studies have documented that this procedure can be performed safely in an outpatient setting provided there is appropriate back-up available.

Dilation and curettage

The traditional D & C uses a sharp metal curette instead of vacuum curettage. This procedure necessitates more cervical dilation and is more painful than the suction curettage. It requires general anesthesia, causes increased blood loss, and may result in less complete uterine evacuation. It is used primarily when the other procedures are not available.

Dilation and evacuation (D & E)

The D & E is an extension of the traditional D & C and the vacuum curettage. It is particularly useful for the woman who is 13 to 16 weeks pregnant. The cervix needs to be more fully dilated, usually with the assistance of laminaria, and the products of conception are larger, requiring evacuation through a crushing instrument followed by vacuum curettage. After a paracervical block or general anesthesia is administered, the uterus is entered through the dilated cervix and the products of conception are removed. Often a vacuum instrument is used in the final curettage.

Late abortions

Second trimester abortions include instillation of drugs into the uterus, hysterotomy/hysterectomy, and D & E.

Instillation of drugs

Prostaglandins. Prostaglandins are fatty acids that occur normally in many human tissues. They are widely used to induce labor and, thereby, abortion in second-trimester pregnancies. The client is admitted to the hospital and an amniocentesis is performed (see Chapter 10). Approximately 8 ml of PGF is inserted into the amniotic sac. Prostaglandins induce abortion by stimulating contractions of the uterine smooth muscle. In most cases, expulsion of the uterine contents occurs within 24 hours. Because these substances stimulate smooth muscle of the gastrointestinal tract as well as the uterus, nausea, vomiting, abdominal cramps and diarrhea are common side effects. These can be controlled by Demeral and Compazine. This method should not be used for women who have asthma, epilepsy, hypertension, or glaucoma because it occasionally causes bronchospasms, convulsions, or transient blood pressure elevations. Hatcher (1978) states that prostaglandins have the following disadvantages: possible need for a second intraamniotic injection, high incidence of gastrointestinal symptoms, associated cervical lacerations, high cost of medication, and the potential for delivery of a live fetus.

Hypertonic saline. Saline has been used for many years as an abortifacient by intrauterine instillation through amniocentesis. Approximately 200 ml of amniotic fluid is withdrawn and a similar amount of 20% sodium chloride solution is injected. Uterine contractions usually begin within 8 to 40 hours. In many cases oxytocin augmentation is necessary to effect abortion in a reasonable time period. The advantages of this method are that it is relatively inexpensive, readily available, and feticidal. Complications of second trimester hypertonic saline abortion are: (1) postinjection infection (10%), (2) incomplete placental separation (15%), (3) excessive bleeding with transfusion (2%), (4) failure to abort (19%), and (5) rarely, consumption coagulopathy, disseminated intravascular clotting, or hypernatremia. The major danger to the woman is the risk that the hypertonic sodium chloride will enter her circulation causing neurologic or cardiopulmonary damage or death from acute hypernatremia. It is also possible to cause myometrial necrosis if the solution is extravasated (Hatcher, 1978; Jensen et al., 1977; Moore, 1978).

Hysterotomy/hysterectomy

Occasionally, urea or hypertonic glucose is used as an intra-amniotic abortifacient. Hysterotomy or hysterectomy are also still used occasionally. The overall morbidity and mortality rates of these procedures limit their use however.

RISKS AND COMPLICATIONS

Safety of the abortion procedure is often related to early diagnosis of pregnancy, prompt referral, and early intervention. Clients are less likely to experience complications if (Hatcher, 1970):

1. The abortion is performed early in pregnancy
2. The client is in good health
3. The practitioner is experienced
4. There are no abnormalities of the uterus
5. Local anesthesia is used
6. The client understands the danger symptoms and her care
7. Twenty-four-hour follow-up care is available
8. The evacuated contents of the uterus are carefully inspected to detect any ectopic or molar pregnancy
9. Rh-negative women receive RhoGam
10. There are no pre-existent infections such as gonorrhea
11. Client is not ambivalent about abortion

Mortality

The risk of dying from abortion is really very slight. According to Cates et al. (1977), there is less risk of dying from legal abortion than from any other commonly performed surgical procedure or from carrying a pregnancy to term. The death to case rate for legal abortions was 3.1/100,000 abortions in 1974. The risk of mortality increases with length of gestation of pregnancy and is also clearly related to the type of procedure used. This is understandable because length of pregnancy usually dictates choice of the procedure.

Analysis of data from the Center for Disease Control for the years 1972 through 1975 shows that deaths increase at higher gestational ages and that the risk of death from abortion is highest with hysterotomy and lowest with suction curettage. Second trimester instillation procedures are associated with higher rates of mortality than first trimester curettage procedures (Cates et al., 1977). Hemorrhage, infection, and saline-associated causes account for over 80% of the deaths directly related to abortion, while anesthesia-associated events and vascular accidents account for the majority of deaths indirectly related to abortion. Hatcher (1978) states that many of the deaths, including those related to anesthesia, hemorrhage, or infection, can be prevented, and implies that this can be accomplished through a knowledge of the possible causes of death, which will assist in counseling and evaluating clients for specific procedures. It appears that the key to the reduction of abortion-related mortality is the performance of the least traumatic procedure at the earliest time possible in the pregnancy.

Morbidity

The most common postabortion complications are infections, retained products of conception, continued pregnancy, cervical or uterine trauma, and bleeding. Infection can be minimized by proper preabortion screening and treatment (particularly for gonorrhea), by treatment for severe cervicitis, and by making sure all products of conception are removed during the procedure. Many physicians recommend and use prophylactic antibiotics. The symptoms of infection are cramping, fever, foul discharge, and pelvic discomfort. All clients should be instructed to contact the practitioner immediately if any of these appear. Infection, if prolonged, can become pelvic inflammatory disease (PID) and cause subsequent infertility.

The second most common problem is excessive bleeding either from retained products of conception, cervical lacerations, or inability of the uterus to contract properly. The client needs to be instructed concerning what to expect in terms of bleeding. Bleeding should not be more excessive than a heavy menstrual flow; it should not last over 7 days or return in less than 4 weeks. If abnormal bleeding occurs, the client should contact her physician. If hemorrhage occurs, a D & C and/or uterine contracting agents (oxytocin or ergotrate), and/or uterine massage may be used.

Grimes and associates (1977) found that in abortions performed on women after 13 or more weeks' gestation, D & E was significantly safer than abortion by prostaglandins or saline, and abortion by saline safer than that by prostaglandins. Moreover, second trimester D & E was believed to be both safe and practical. It is a direct and rapid procedure that can be performed on an outpatient basis. Although prostaglandins accelerate the time required for abortion, morbidity is also significantly increased. In comparing clients who underwent saline abortion with those who had prostaglandin abortion, the latter had significantly higher rates of infection, hemorrhage, and retained tissue. There were also higher rates of convulsions reported, as well as higher rates of operative treatments for complications. In fact, the higher rehospitalization rates may offset the principal advantage of prostaglandin abortion—fast induction to abort tissues. Fever, endometritis, hemorrhage, retained products of conception, and urinary tract infections were more frequent among saline-treated women, while cervical injury and uterine perforation were more frequent among D & E clients. Even with these complications, D & E appears to be both safe and practical. It precludes the uncertainty of a prolonged labor and the systemic effects of the instillation methods. It also spares the client the potential psychologic trauma associated with an uncomfortable labor and the possible dilemma of a surviving fetus.

In 0.1% to 0.3% of cases the attempt to terminate the pregnancy will be unsuccessful. There should be careful evaluation of the products of conception done by a pathologist. Furthermore, a pregnancy test should be made on the follow-up postabortion visit. If the pregnancy has not been terminated, an ectopic pregnancy should be considered. However, continued pregnancy is usually the result of inadequate uterine curettage in an early pregnancy (Hatcher, 1978). Smith and associates (1970) have documented that complication rates can be reduced by at least 30% if the abortion procedure with the least risk of complications at each length of gestation is selected.

There is much concern about the long-term effects of induced abortions. While mortality rates and the number of immediate complications are low, the long-term effects may be more severe than those for other means of fertility regulation, particularly for women who choose abortion as a means of postponing initial childbearing or of spacing children. Although no causal link has yet been established between abortions and such complications as secondary infertility, ectopic pregnancy, etc., Hogue (1977) has found significant associations in several studies. The following complications appear to be significantly associated with a history of induced abortion; bleeding during pregnancy, prolonged third stage of labor, premature delivery, and low birth weight. Harlap and Davies (1975) found that mothers with a history of one or more induced abortions were more likely to report bleeding during the first 3 months of a present pregnancy. They were subsequently less likely to have a normal delivery and more of them needed assistance in the third stage of labor. In births following induced abortions, the relative risk of early neonatal death was doubled and later neonatal deaths were increased three to four times. There was a significant increase in the frequency of low birth weight infants and increases in major and minor congenital malformations. A study by Pantelakis (1973) confirms these findings. He found the percentage of stillbirths and premature births among women who had had a previous abortion, induced or spontaneous, to be double that of a control group.

PSYCHOLOGIC EFFECTS OF ABORTION

There is probably no psychologically painless way to cope with an unwanted pregnancy, whether it is voluntarily interrupted or carried to term. While an abortion may evoke feelings of guilt, regret, or loss, such alternatives as forced marriage, becoming a single parent, giving up a child for adoption, or adding an unwanted child to a family may also carry its burden of psychologic problems for the woman, the child, and the family.

For many years it was assumed that there were severe negative psychologic or psychiatric sequelae for all clients undergoing abortion. Much of the extensive psychiatric material or alleged psychologic trauma consists of impressionistic case reports (David, 1972, 1974). The majority of these reports are unsubstantiated by reputable research designs and were reported before abortion became legalized. It is important to dispel these myths of permanent severe postabortion psychologic damage by what is now known based on solid fact and reputable studies. It is also important to keep in mind that studies of psychologic sequelae prior to the 1973 Supreme Court decision may be biased inasmuch as the women who sought abortion often was compelled to do so in violation of the law.

Although it is possible that an individual woman would experience none of the feelings commonly associated with abortion, it is reasonable to assume that most women will. Therefore, nurses need to watch for these and recognize when the expression of feelings is within the realm of normal or when additional counseling is needed. Anger, guilt, fear, and sadness are common emotions expressed by women prior to and following abortion. The anger may be at herself or at her partner. Some degree of guilt is not unusual; for most women some ambivalence and sadness may also be present. There may be concern over religious standards, which produce guilt, or over social mores, which also evoke guilt feelings or shame. Fear may also be present—of procedures, of pain, of aftereffects, or that someone will find out about the abortion. The degree to which these emotions result from living in a culture that for so long has considered abortion a sin is not clear.

Relief that the abortion is over, gratitude that abortion is possible, and new self-understanding may also occur. Both positive and negative feelings can be present in the same woman. It is not known how long these feelings will last; for some women they are immediate and transient and for others they are likely to persist for a long time.

The American literature suggests that an immediate negative response to abortion is not uncommon among women experiencing a therapeutic abortion and that short-term guilt and unhappiness may be a part of the normal response (Donovan et al., 1975; Friedman et al., 1974). The proportion of women with serious psychiatric complications is probably less than 10%. It is important to remember that abortion is a double challenge to the woman—both a termination of a pregnancy and a surgical procedure that causes a complex of feelings related to invasion of the body. In the study done by Donovan et al. (1975) the comments of the women were quite varied, sometimes indicating conflict, guilt, and sadness as well as relief. Those expressing negative feelings did not see themselves as emotionally disabled, nor did they appear to be psychiatrically ill to the researchers. This study suggests that women who have made relatively conflict-free decisions feel relieved after an abortion. Women who saw the fetus as a baby—who appeared emotionally attached to the fetus, who were in the second trimester, who were being aborted for medical reasons but wanted the pregnancy, or who mourned its loss—felt guilty or sad in the postabortion period. It

also seems that a woman's style of coping with abortion is consistent with her general coping style. All of these points are valuable to the nurse in planning relevant care for clients. Several factors have predictive value in determining postabortion difficulties: (1) pre-existing severe psychiatric illness, (2) failure of the family to support the decision, (3) abortion for medical indications, (4) severe ambivalence, and (5) coercion by family or physician.

Infrequently, psychiatric symptoms appear following an abortion. They may range from sexual dysfunction to psychiatric decompensation. Often they are a continuation of a pre-existing illness but occasionally they are not. The symptoms need to be differentiated from the mild transient negative emotional responses of guilt, sadness, and regret, which are part of the normal responses to abortion but which may be increased by cultural attitudes.

The Donovan study (1975) suggests that several aspects of the woman's decision-making process are crucial. The vulnerable woman who is coerced or accepts abortion reluctantly in light of a strong wish to have a child is more likely to experience difficulty later than the vulnerable woman whose decision is made with little ambivalence on the basis of pressing reality. An inability or reluctance to make a decision with resulting continued ambivalence can trigger severe symptomatic responses in the postabortion period.

Belsey et al. (1977) also found that although a small number of women actually develop emotional disturbance following abortion, the dominant factor is the degree of adjustment existing before pregnancy. Those most likely to be disturbed were those with a history of psychosocial instability, poor or no family ties, poor work patterns, and those who had commonly failed to use contraception, suggesting possible ambivalence. Neswander (1974) found that those women who had doubts most frequently were those having an abortion for medical reasons such as rubella; although these clients were generally satisfied with the abortion, they suffered the greatest doubts about the decision. Walter (1970) states that legal abortions can be performed without fear of severe psychic trauma to the woman. The reaction of the woman appears to be determined by her previous psychologic set. Legal abortion leaves its mark just as does every other important event in a person's life. It is an unnatural way of solving conflict involved in an unwanted pregnancy. In women who are psychologically vulnerable, an unwanted pregnancy involves extra stress whatever decision is made.

In summary, for the healthy woman with an adequate support system who is able to make the decision to have an abortion with relatively little conflict, abortion will not result in psychologic trauma and is most often truly therapeutic. These women, who constitute about 90% of all women having abortions, experience some transient guilt, grief, or regret. However these feelings will be resolved relatively quickly and easily. It is the other 10% of women having abortions, who can often be recognized by the high degree of ambivalence and difficulty with decision-making, who will experience severe postabortion emotional symptoms and who most need our best, most highly skilled nursing care.

NURSING CARE FOR WOMEN WHO ELECT ABORTION

The nurse has a unique contribution to make in the total care of women experiencing abortion. The combination of health knowledge, social awareness, and feminine understanding that the nurse brings to her clients provides the uniqueness that enhances the client care. Abortion counseling from beginning to end is an appropriate role function for nursing and is multifaceted. Ideally, preabortion counseling should help the client gain insight into her feelings about pregnancy and abortion in order to cope better with the abortion procedure and to complete the experience with a minimum of painful emotional after-effects. Gedan (1972) suggests that factors indicating the need for preabortion counseling are:

1. Abortion is a significant event in the life of the woman and will affect her. The meaning the prospective abortion has to the woman and the way she copes with her reaction to it will determine the effect the procedure has on her.
2. It is a life crisis. There are many problems that prompt a woman to seek an abortion. The feelings about these problems need to be consciously explored; if repressed, they may reappear later as emotional difficulties.
3. Many patients have fears and misconceptions about abortion procedures. Important in the preabortion care is the ventilation of these fears and clarification of them.
4. Unconscious motivations are often the reasons why unwanted pregnancies occur. The exploration of these will assist the client in understanding the needs that influenced her becoming pregnant.
5. Most women have feelings about being pregnant and about terminating their pregnancy. Counseling that explores these normal emotional reactions can help relieve and/or prevent guilt, anxiety, and depression.

The importance and significance of preabortion counseling as a positive factor in successful resolution of a life crisis for the woman is clearly documented. Davila (1972) found that counseling just prior to, during, and following induced abortion can help prevent future unwanted pregnancies through contraceptive use. The counseling procedure will bring the woman through the crisis with minimal trauma and help her gain an understanding of how this happened in the first place and therefore lead to action that will prevent future unwanted pregnancies.

Bracken et al. (1973) examined what type of abortion counseling was most effective. It was generally found that women who experience individual counseling responded most favorably to the counseling process itself. However, these same women had a worse reaction to all aspects of the abortion procedure when compared with women who had group counseling. A significant difference was found when the variable of age was examined. While all women still preferred individual counseling, it was the younger woman (below 20 years) who reacted most negatively to abortion following individual counseling. Older women (21 years and over) had the most positive reaction to the abortion if they were counseled individually.

Abortion counseling should have the following aspects: (1) allow the woman to work through her feelings about the pregnancy to reach the best decision for herself, (2) help her cope with the stress, ambivalence, and guilt she feels, (3) assist her to understand the psychologic reasons why contraception was not used, (4) help her to thoroughly understand the abortion procedure, and (5) assist her to potentially explore her relationship with her family and significant others (Nadelson, 1974).

Prior to any induced abortion, every woman should be counseled in such a way that she: (1) understands the meaning of abortion and is sure that this is what she wants, (2) does not feel she has been coerced by others (partner, parents, friends, counselor), (3) has considered her own value system, (4) has considered alternatives to abortion, and (5) is knowledgeable about effective contraception (Moore, 1978).

Assessment of the woman's feelings

Verbalizing how she feels about the pregnancy is essential to helping the woman eliminate the need to repeat the experience in the future. Accepting the responsibility for the pregnancy and for having the abortion must ultimately be faced by the woman. In assessing the woman's feelings the following questions should be answered:

1. Have all possible alternatives been considered objectively with the advantages and disadvantages of each weighed?
2. Is this solely her decision?
3. What is the relationship with the partner involved? Does he know of the pregnancy and the plan to terminate it? Does he agree? Will he help financially? If she has not told him, why not? What type of role does she expect him to play in her future?

4. How does she feel about being pregnant? Does she understand it? How does she picture pregnancy at this stage—as a blob of cells or a fully formed baby? How does she conceive of abortion? Does she consider it murder? How is she going to feel about herself in the future? Will she regret not having the baby?

5. Is she thinking realistically? Has she gone through the decision-making process or is this an impulsive act? Is she thinking of her future or only the present? Are her responses consistent or contradictory? Is her behavior appropriate?

6. What support systems are available and will they continue to be available to her?

In addition, the nursing assessment should include answers to the following (Clark and Affonso, 1976):

1. Where and at what age did she receive information about sex, pregnancy, and contraception?

2. What is the woman's pattern of sexual behavior?

3. What does she know about birth control? How does she use it?

4. What is the duration of the pregnancy? When was decision to have the abortion made?

5. What does she think about abortion and people who have abortions (values)? What does she feel about having an abortion (the reality of the decision)?

The second phase of abortion counseling is information-giving and education. Information about the following must be imparted before the woman can decide on an alternative:

1. Anatomy and physiology of reproduction and pregnancy. Assess the woman's knowledge, review what she does not know, and encourage questions.

2. Procedure and common after-effects of a therapeutic abortion. Assess what she knows and explain procedures. Go over each procedure step by step using diagrams and models. Give the client all information available, including side effects.

3. Information about contraception, assessing the woman's level of previous knowledge, and building upon it to correct misinformation.

Once the woman has decided definitely on abortion, the nurse can give her all the relevant information about where to go and how to make the arrangements for the abortion. Her financial situation, scheduling, wish for privacy, and particular fears all need to be considered in referring her to the best possible resource.

The woman undergoing therapeutic abortion needs considerable support during this stressful situation. Often the nurse is able to provide some of this support; in addition, the woman should be urged to utilize as fully as possible her usual support systems—family, friends, partner.

Guilt is a feeling often expressed to the nurse. Abortion may be the only rational alternative for the woman but she may still feel she is a "bad" person. The nurse can encourage her to verbalize her feelings, thereby helping her to reduce the anxiety generated by guilt. Ambivalence may also need to be explored. The woman may feel a sense of pride in the ability to conceive, and she may wish the baby. She may even have fantasies about the developing fetus. Again, there is the reality of not being able to have the child. The woman needs to express these feelings to a nonjudgmental person.

The woman will experience grief and sadness after the abortion and the nurse can help her begin the grieving process. Denial of feelings about being pregnant may be expressed. This defense mechanism takes energy and may leave the client vulnerable to anxiety and panic. The nurse can confront the woman with her denial and help her to accept reality by verbalizing and validating it. Anger, disappointment, and sadness may all surface when denial is given up and the feelings are expressed. The nurse can support the expression of these feelings (Clark and Affonso, 1977).

Providing information

The woman needs detailed information about the technique to be used. This will help to decrease fear of the hospital or clinic and the abortion procedure itself as well as correct misapprehensions. Some women have very unrealistic ideas about how simple the procedure is and they experience great anxiety when faced with reality; this is particularly true with second trimester procedures. Since the woman's anxiety level is often quite high, the information should be available in written form.

The abortion client has a low tolerance level for frustration. Once she has made the decision to abort, she wants it over immediately. Bureaucratic red tape, rules, and regulations represent frustrating barriers. Acknowledging the client's frustration and explaining why these regulations are necessary can help. Reasonable explanations can enable the client to accept rules that would otherwise seem unnecessarily restrictive. There are some clients who will display open hostility. As an authority figure, the nurse may represent an identifiable barrier and for this reason be the target of hostility or anger.

The nurse is one to whom the client can communicate both positive and negative feelings resulting from projection, displacement, fear, and justified anger at the health care delivery system. In an atmosphere of safety and acceptance, the client can feel free to express anger and frustration. Anxiety will often be such that the client's perceptual field and attention span are limited. The presence of a caring person can be very important.

Whenever a client puts into words negative feelings she is experiencing she takes the risk of rejection. By being accepting and nonjudgmental, the nurse can encourage the continued expression of feeling and emotions, be they rational or irrational.

Nursing care
First trimester abortions

Safety and comfort for the woman experiencing a therapeutic or induced abortion are paramount. For those women undergoing first trimester abortion the risks are minimal (as previously indicated) and most women will experience only mild cramping and minimal bleeding. The client is usually sent home in an hour or two with specific postabortion instructions.

Second trimester abortion

For the woman who is experiencing second trimester abortion safety and comfort become more crucial issues since the risks are greater and she is experiencing labor and delivery. During the abortion procedure the nurse is involved in monitoring vital signs to detect quickly hemorrhage or infection, monitoring intake and output, and encouraging fluid intake to maintain proper hydration. Many patients will be receiving intravenous fluids concurrently with oral intake of fluids. It is essential that nursing interventions be directed toward the prevention of infection and hemorrhage. Careful perineal hygiene is essential in preventing infection. Frequent, accurate monitoring of the progression of labor will assist the nurse to correctly identify when abortion and therefore increased potential for hemorrhage are likely to occur.

In essence, the client experiencing an instillation abortion is undergoing labor and delivery and careful monitoring of contractions is necessary. The nurse should use all of the customary nursing interventions for a laboring woman specific to the prevention of infection and hemorrhage. Once the client has aborted the fetus, the nurse should carefully clamp the cord and remove the fetus. It is then crucial to watch for the expulsion of the placenta and to monitor the amount of bleeding. Often oxytocin or other synthetic oxytocic drugs is administered intravenously or intramuscularly to aid in the contraction of the uterus and to prevent excessive bleeding.

Comfort measures are important nursing interventions for the woman who is experiencing an abortion in the second trimester. The uterus contracts, the cervix dilates, and pain is experienced. In many cases the pain threshold is lowered because of anxiety and pain may be perceived as very intense. It has been documented (Anderson et al., 1976) that a modified form of the Lamaze method of psychoprophylaxis will benefit the abortion client. Education and concentrated relaxation and breathing exercises produce a more controlled, positive experience for the client. It is thought that psychoprophylaxis emphasizing breathing and relaxation techniques may even decrease the need for analgesia during the abortion process. Physical discomfort can also be reduced by keeping the client clean and dry and providing medication for pain and nausea as needed.

One of the most important ways of providing comfort for the client is through psychologic support. The presence of a caring person who provides an opportunity for expression of feelings and an explanation of progress may be the most important variable in making the client comfortable. The importance of the nurse's use of self to provide support in a crisis situation cannot be overemphasized nor should it be underestimated. The client can receive the most meticulous physical care possible and still experience nontherapeutic nursing care if the element of care and giving of self is not present.

Postabortion care

There are specific objectives for care of the client following an abortion that the nurse needs to observe. To diminish the risk of Rh immunization in Rh-negative women RhoGam is administered. The patient should understand specific and general hygiene measures as well as signs of possible complications. Finally, all clients experiencing abortion must be offered contraceptive advice (Clancy, 1973).

It is extremely important that clients receive proper instruction following an induced abortion. It often is the nurse's responsibility to do this or to reinforce the information given by others. The client should be told which symptoms indicate serious complications; this information should also be given to them in writing.

Postabortion nursing care includes assessment of the physical, emotional, and contraception needs of the client. In follow-up contacts the nurse needs to assess the client's physical status beginning with the woman's general health status. At this time the nurse can give the client the opportunity to become an active participant in her own health care by encouraging her to evaluate her own status.

Because of the increased risk of uterine infection, cervical laceration, and pelvic inflammatory disease, any evidence of infection should be noted—vaginal discharge, unusual temperature elevation, pain, or bleeding. Any difficulties with menses—dysmenorrhea, amenorrhea, irregularity, increased flow—should be noted. Finally, the woman should be given the opportunity to verbalize any problems she may have even if they are not necessarily related to the abortion. It is a popular misconception that all postabortion women experience depression, guilt, anxiety, and a negative self-

---

Discharge instructions*

You may eat or drink what you wish and resume normal activities. Strenuous activities should be avoided for the next few days. It is best to be guided by how you feel. Do whatever seems comfortable to you. Follow the instructions given you and be sure to contact the physician if a problem or question arises.

What to expect. The amount of bleeding and cramps women experience varies considerably but most experience cramps and bleeding during the first 2 weeks following the abortion. Spotting may occur for up to 4 weeks after the abortion. The next normal menstrual period should begin in 4 to 6 weeks. Because it is possible to become pregnant before menstrual periods resume you should begin using a method of birth control before your first period occurs.

Dos and Don'ts

To protect yourself from infection:

1. Use sanitary pads only; no tampons for the first week.
2. Avoid intercourse for 1 week.
3. Do not douche for 1 week.
4. Take your temperature twice a day at the same time for 1 week. Notify the physician if it is 100° f or more.
5. If Tylenol or aspirin are used for pain, take your temperature before you take the medication.
6. Return for postabortion check-up in 2 weeks.

Notify the physician at once if:

1. Temperature is 100° F or more prior to return appointment.
2. Severe pain or pain unlike menstrual cramps occurs.
3. Bleeding for 2 consecutive days is heavier than heaviest day of normal period.
4. Heavy bleeding continues longer than 2 weeks.
5. The first menstrual period does not begin in 8 weeks.

*Based on Hatcher, R. A., and others: Contraceptive technology 1978-1979, ed. 9, New York, 1978, John Wiley & Sons.

---

concept; however, they may have some transient feelings of guilt, regret, or remorse. The postabortion client may feel ambivalent and will profit from skilled counseling that will permit her to discuss her conflicting feelings and identify and resolve them.

The nurse cannot remove all negative feelings for the patient or pretend that things are as they were before the abortion. What she can do is to help the woman to see the positive aspects of the experience, focus on her positive feelings, and move toward a more positive concept of herself. It is essential that the nurse be aware and nonjudgmental in listening and assisting the client to clarify her feelings.

An essential part of the postabortion counseling process is anticipatory guidance for the future in learning how to avoid pregnancy until it is desired. This involves teaching contraceptive control and sex education as appropriate and indicated. This aspect of preventing unwanted pregnancy is discussed in Chapter 22.

NURSES' ATTITUDES TOWARD ABORTION

Nurses have long been aware that their own attitudes influence the kind of care they are able to give and the patient's response to that care. Harper et al. (1972) found that in hospitals where staff members view abortion less favorably, abortion patients perceive the nursing care as less satisfactory. Because nurses have attitudes toward abortion, they must decide whether or not they can care for abortion clients safely, compassionately, and nonjudgmentally. It is possible that nurses will have moral and ethical conflicts while working with women who have abortions. Some of the issues involved are:

1. Nurses are educated to preserve life; abortion may be perceived as the destruction of life.
2. Nurses are often educated to influence or control others to achieve health; abortion clients are controlling their own life by deciding to terminate the pregnancy.
3. Identification with the woman may cause conflict between two value systems: society's value system against unconventional sexual behavior and nursing norms that state nurses are nonjudgmental.
4. The traditional image of the nurse being subservient to the male physician conflicts with the feminist view of woman having control over their own body.
5. Nursing education does little to help students work through their values about sexuality and sexual behavior. There is almost no opportunity for clarification of values.

If the nurse has not dealt with these conflicts and reached effective resolution and awareness of her feelings, she should not be doing abortion counseling. The nurse needs to understand how her early cultural conditioning and values influence her beliefs and actions. No nurse who has conflicting or negative feeling about abortion should be caring for abortion clients. It can only be detrimental to both. The attitude of the nurse toward the client is of paramount importance. It must be nonjudgmental, caring, attentive, warm, and supportive. As David Mace (1972) so accurately states, "If you find a wise counselor—one who knows the subject really well, but is also a patient listener; one who will encourage and help to think the issue through, to come to terms with conflicting emotions, and arrive at a decision that can be lived with—if you can find such a counselor, beat a path to her door and count yourself fortunate."

REFERENCES

Anderson, C., and others: Psychoprophylaxis in midtrimester abortions, JOGN Nurs., pp. 29-33, Nov./Dec. 1976.

Belsey, E. M., and others: Predictive factors in emotional response to abortion, Soc. Sci. Med. 11:71-82, 1977.

Bracken, M. B., and others: Abortion counseling: an experimental study of three techniques, Am. J. Obstet. Gynecol. 117(1):10-20, 1973.

Brenner, W., and Edelman, D.: Menstrual regulation: risks and abuses, Int. J. Gynecol. Obstet. 15:177-183, 1977.

Butts, R. Y., and Sproakowski, M. J.: Unwed pregnancy decisions, J. Sex Res. 10(2):110-117, 1974.

Cates, W., and others: Abortion as a treatment for unwanted pregnancy: the number two sexually transmitted condition, Adv. Plan. Parent. 10(3):115-121.

Cates, W., and others: The risk of dying from legal abortion in the United States, 1972-1975, Int. J. Gynecol. Obstet. 15:172-176, 1977.

Clancy, B.: The nurse and the abortion patient, Nurs. Clin. North Am. Vol. 8, No. 3, Sept. 1973.

Clark, A. L., and Affonso, D.: Childbearing: a nursing perspective. Philadelphia, 1976, F. A. Davis Co.

Cornish, J.: Women's experiences with abortion. In McNall, L. K., and Galeener, J. T., editors: Current practices in obstetrical and gynecological nursing, Vol. 1, St. Louis, 1976, The C. V. Mosby Co.

David, H. P.: Abortion in psychological perspectives, Am. J. Orthopsych. 42(1):61-68, 1972.

David, H. P.: Abortion research: international experience, Lexington, Mass., 1974, Lexington Books.

Davila, B., and others: Abortion counseling and behavioral change, Fam. Plan. Perspect. 8(2):23-27, 1972.

Denes, M.: In necessity and sorrow, New York, 1976, Basic Books, Inc.

Donovan, C. M., and others: Preabortion psychiatric illness, Nurs. Dig. pp. 12-16, Sept./Oct. 1975.

Fatal ectopic pregnancy after sterilization or abortion, Morbidity and Mortality Weekly Report, p. 75, March 4, 1977. New York, California.

Francke, L. B.: The ambivalence of abortion, New York, 1978, Random House.

Friedman, C. M., and others: The decision-making process and the outcome of therapeutic abortion, Am. J. Psych. 131(12):1332-1337, 1974.

Fussell, J., and Hatcher, R.: Women in need, New York, 1970, Macmillan Co.

Gedan, S.: Pre-abortion emotional counseling, ANA Clinical Session 1972, New York, 1972, Appleton-Century-Crofts.

Goldman, A.: Learning abortion care, Nurs. Outlook, pp. 300-352, May 1971.

Greene, J., and Hendershot, G.: Abortion attitudes among nurses and social workers, Am. J. Public Health 64(5):438-441, 1974.

Grimes, D. A., and others: Methods of midtrimester abortion: which is safest? Int. J. Gynecol. Obstet. 15:184-188, 1977.

Harlap, S., and Mectrail, D. A.: Late sequelae of individual abortion: complications and outcome of pregnancy and labor, Am. J. of Epidemiol. 122(3):217-224, 1975.

Harper, M. W., and others: Abortion—do attitudes of nursing personnel affect the patients' perception of care? Nurs. Res. 21(4):327-331, 1972.

Hatcher, R. A., and others: Contraceptive technology, 1978-1979, ed. 9 (rev.), New York, 1978, John Wiley & Sons.

Hodgson, J., and Portmann, K.: Complications of 10,453 consecutive first trimester abortions: a prospective study, Am. J. Obstet. Gynecol. 120(6):802-807, 1974.

Hoffman, H.: Psychological aspects of legal abortion and contraception, J. Sex Res. 4(1):7-15, 1968.

Hogue, C. J. R.: An evaluation of studies concerning reproductive after first trimester induced abortion, Int. J. Gynecol. Obstet., No. 15, pp. 167-171, 1977.

Institute of Medicine: Legalized abortion and the public health, Washington, D.C., 1975, National Academy of Sciences.

Jensen, M., Benson, R. C., and Botish, I. M.: Maternity Care, St. Louis, 1977, The C. V. Mosby Co.

Keller, C., and Copeland, P.: Counseling the abortion patient is more than talk, Am. J. Nurs. 72:102, 1972.

Kimball, C. P.: Some observations regarding unwanted pregnancies and therapeutic abortion, Obstet. Gynecol. 35(2):293-296, 1970.

Lanaham, C.: Anxieties and focus of patients seeking abortion. In McNall, L. F., and Galeener, J. T., editors: Current practice in obstetrics and gynecologic nursing, vol. 1, St. Louis, 1976, The C. V. Mosby Co.

Mace, D. R.: Abortion: the agonizing decisions, New York, 1972, Abington Press.

Margolis, A. J., and others: Therapeutic abortion follow-up study, Am. J. Obstet. Gynecol., pp. 243-249, May 15, 1977.

Martin, L.: Health care of women, Philadelphia, 1978, J. B. Lippincott Co.

Monsour, K., and Stweart, B.: Abortion and sexual behavior in college women, Am. J. Orthopsych. 43(5):804-814, Oct. 1973.

Moore, M. L.: Realities in childbearing, Philadelphia, 1978, W. B. Saunders Co.

Nadelson, C.: Abortion counseling: focus on adolescent pregnancy, Pediatrics 54(6):765-769, 1974.

Neswander, K., and Patterson, R.: Psychologic reaction to therapeutic abortion, Obstet. Gynecol. 29(5):702-706, 1967.

Osofsky, H. J., and Osofsky, J. D.: The abortion experience: psychological and medical impact, New York, 1973, Harper & Row, Publishers.

Osofsky, J. D., and others: Psychological effects of abortion: with emphasis upon immediate reactions and follow-up. In Osofsky, H. J., and Osofsky, J. D.: The abortion experience: psychological and medical impact, New York, 1973, Harper & Row, Publishers, pp. 188-205.

Pantelakis, S.: Influence of indirect and spontaneous abortions on the outcomes of subsequent pregnancies, Am. J. Obstet. Gynecol. 116(6):799-805, 1973.

Romney, S. L., and others: Gynecology and obstetrics, New York, 1975, McGraw-Hill Book Co.

Schonberg, L.: Complications of outpatient abortion, Adv. Plan. Parent. 10(1):45-48, 1975.

Smith, R., and others: The potential reduction and medical complications from induced abortion, Int. J. Gynecol. Obstet. **15**:337-346, 1978.

Steinhoff, P.: Background characteristics of abortion patients. In Osofsky, H. J., and Osofsky, J. D.: The abortion experience: psychological and medical impact, New York, 1973, Harper & Row, Publishers.

Swigar, M. E., and others: Interview follow-up of abortion applicant proponents, Soc. Psychiatry **11**(3):135-143, 1976.

U.S. National Center for Health Statistics: Vital statistics of the United States, 1977, Annual, Washington, D.C., 1977, U.S. Government Printing Office.

Vincent, C.: Unmarried mothers, New York, 1961, The Free Press.

Walter, G.: Psychologic and emotional consequences of elective abortion, Obstet. Gynecol. **36**(3):482-491, 1970.

Wolff, G. J. L., and others: Elective abortion—complications seen in a free-standing clinic, Obstet. Gynecol. **49**(3):351-357, 1977.

Zimmerman, M. K.: Passage through abortion, New York, 1977, Proege Publishers.

24

Alternatives in childbirth

Nancy Fugate Woods

Pregnant women confront a number of decision points during their pregnancies. Many of these decision points occur very early in the pregnancy; such is the case for women who choose abortion as an alternative to childbirth. Other decision points may go unnoticed, as in the case when health practitioners have not offered options to the woman or have not fully informed the woman of the degree of freedom she has in her birthing process.

Many decision points occur during stressful periods or in contexts in which decision-making is difficult, if not impossible. Yet some of these decision points might be anticipated and possible alternatives explored by women and health workers alike. The purpose of this chapter is to explore the existing alternatives to the usual approaches to in-hospital birth in the Western world. The justification for new alternatives will be emphasized, since current practice is already addressed in most standard obstetric texts. What follows is not a mandate for changes in practice. Instead, alternatives that could be valuable to women with few or no risk factors for obstetric complications will be presented. Because research on alternatives has not yet been fully explored, this chapter will therefore simply outline some of the issues that might be considered.

Preparation for childbirth affords the woman and her family an opportunity for consciousness-raising about birthing, for information about alternatives in the birthing experience, and for skills to facilitate a comfortable and safe birth. The birthing experience also affords the woman a number of options. Finally, the immediate parenting experience invites the woman to choose from several alternatives including those related to breast-feeding, infant nurturing, and family functioning. Each of these aspects of the birthing experience will be explored in an attempt to illustrate alternatives to current practice.

PREPARATION FOR CHILDBIRTH
Rights of the client

The Pregnant Patients' Bill of Rights (see box) as endorsed by the International Childbirth Education Association (ICEA) and the National Association of Parents and Professionals for Safe Alternatives in Childbirth (NAPSAC), contains guidelines for caring for the pregnant woman. Ideally, these rights would be communicated to the pregnant woman early in her preparation for childbirth. Each of the sixteen specific rights could be addressed as issues for discussion in the context of childbirth preparation classes. The pregnant client should have the right to participate in decisions that affect her well-being or that of her unborn child. In emergency situations, decision-making may be delegated to health professionals, but even in these instances the woman may be able to participate in decision-making, if only in a limited fashion.

Informed consent vs ignorance

Many of the issues to be addressed in preparation for birthing relate to iatrogenic hazards from drugs and procedures. Most relate to the woman's right to be an informed rather than an ignorant participant in the birthing process. In addition to rights to information about the birthing process, the woman should be given information about *who* is providing her care and who actually attended the delivery. Not only is the woman's right to have a support person with her acknowledged, so also is her right to nurture and feed her infant according to its needs rather than the hospital's needs. Finally, the woman should be assured access to information about her infant's health status and to pertinent medical records.

Many of the alternatives that women confront prior to childbirth have been identified earlier. There are a few, however, that deserve special attention, such as breast-feeding and the method of preparing for childbirth.

Breast-feeding

Breast-feeding is discussed in detail in Chapter 25. What is important to consider here is that many women are indirectly discouraged from breast-feeding by lack of information; others are directly discouraged by some

The Pregnant Patient's Bill of Rights

1. The Pregnant Patient has the right, prior to the administration of any drug or procedure, to be informed by the health professional caring for her of any potential direct or indirect effects, risks or hazards to herself or her unborn or newborn infant which may result from the use of a drug or procedure prescribed for or administered to her during pregnancy, labor, birth or lactation.

2. The Pregnant Patient has the right, prior to the proposed therapy, to be informed, not only of the benefits, risks and hazards of the proposed therapy but also of known alternative therapy, such as available childbirth education classes which could help to prepare the Pregnant Patient physically and mentally to cope with the discomfort or stress of pregnancy and the experience of childbirth, thereby reducing or eliminating her need for drugs and obstetric intervention. She should be offered such information early in her pregnancy in order that she may make a reasoned decision.

3. The Pregnant Patient has the right, prior to the administration of any drug, to be informed by the health professional who is prescribing or administering the drug to her that any drug which she receives during pregnancy, labor and birth, no matter how or when the drug is taken or administered, may adversely affect her unborn baby, directly or indirectly, and that there is no drug or chemical which has been proven safe for the unborn child.

4. The Pregnant Patient has the right if Cesarean section is anticipated, to be informed prior to the administration of any drug, and preferably prior to her hospitalization, that minimizing her and, in turn, her baby's intake of nonessential pre-operative medicine will benefit her baby.

5. The Pregnant Patient has the right, prior to the administration of a drug or procedure, to be informed of the areas of uncertainty if there is NO properly controlled follow-up research which has established the safety of the drug or procedure with regard to its direct and/or indirect effects on the physiological, mental and neurological development of the child exposed, via the mother, to the drug or procedure during pregnancy, labor, birth or lactation—(this would apply to virtually all drugs and the vast majority of obstetric procedures).

6. The Pregnant Patient has the right, prior to the administration of any drug, to be informed of the brand name and generic name of the drug in order that she may advise the health professional of any past adverse reaction to the drug.

7. The Pregnant Patient has the right to determine for herself, without pressure from her attendant, whether she will accept the risks inherent in the proposed therapy or refuse a drug or procedure.

8. The Pregnant Patient has the right to know the name and qualifications of the individual administering a medication or procedure to her during labor or birth.

9. The Pregnant Patient has the right to be informed, prior to the administration of any procedure, whether that procedure is being administered to her for her or her baby's benefit (medically indicated) or as an elective procedure (for convenience, teaching purposes or research).

10. The Pregnant Patient has the right to be accompanied during the stress of labor and birth by someone she cares for, and to whom she looks for emotional comfort and encouragement.

11. The Pregnant Patient has the right after appropriate medical consultation to choose a position for labor and for birth which is least stressful to her baby and to herself.

12. The Obstetric Patient has the right to have her baby cared for at her bedside if her baby is normal, and to feed her baby according to her baby's needs rather than according to the hospital regimen.

13. The Obstetric Patient has the right to be informed in writing of the name of the person who actually delivered her baby and the professional qualifications of that person. This information should also be on the birth certificate.

14. The Obstetric Patient has the right to be informed if there is any known or indicated aspect of her or her baby's care or condition which may cause her or her baby later difficulty or problems.

15. The Obstetric Patient has the right to have her and her baby's hospital medical records complete, accurate and legible and to have their records, including Nurses' Notes, retained by the hospital until the child reaches at least the age of majority, or, alternatively, to have the records offered to her before they are destroyed.

16. The Obstetric Patient, both during and after her hospital stay, has the right to have access to her complete hospital medical records, including Nurses' Notes, and to receive a copy upon payment of a reasonable fee and without incurring the expense of retaining an attorney.

It is the obstetric patient and her baby, not the health professional, who must sustain any trauma or injury resulting from the use of a drug or obstetric procedure. The observation of the rights listed above will not only permit the obstetric patient to participate in the decisions involving her and her baby's health care, but will help to protect the health professional and the hospital against litigation arising from resentment or misunderstanding on the part of the mother.

*From Haire, D. B.: The pregnant patient's bill of rights, J. Nurse-Midwifery **20**:29, Winter 1975.

health professionals and the culture that has defined a woman's breasts as sexual organs to the exclusion of their nurturant capacity. Women cannot freely choose to breast- or bottle-feed their infants unless they have adequate information about both alternatives. Therefore, it is important that childbirth preparation programs include accurate information on both options. Equally unfortunate as not giving information about breast-feedi. is the situation in which the woman is coerced into breast-feeding by overzealous health professionals. What is needed is a balanced perspective that allows women to choose freely without coercion. This choice must always be made prior to birthing, especially for breast-feeding mothers (see Chapter 25).

Childbirth preparation

A second issue that deserves special attention is the method of preparing for childbirth. Over the last decade there has been a proliferation of methods ranging from the general informational classes held by hospitals to specific techniques of psychoprophylaxis (such as Lamaze) and, more currently, biofeedback.

The current practice of childbirth preparation originated in the 1940s with Grantly Dick-Read's work that emphasized teaching women to relax, breathe correctly, understand labor, and develop muscle control. Soviet physicians at the same time were experimenting with pavlovian conditioning to help women cope with the pain of childbirth. In the 1950s Lamaze introduced the psychoprophylactic methods used in Russia to women in France, emphasizing the woman's participation in each stage of labor and the use of conditioned response and focal distraction to cope with the discomforts of labor. Sheila Kitzinger's (1978) psychosexual methods stress both physical and psychic education for childbirth. Bradley (1965) emphasizes the importance of nutritional considerations in prenatal care, early (first trimester) prenatal classes, husband-coached participation, total avoidance of medications during the childbirth process, and home delivery.

The approaches available to women for childbirth preparation are variations on one or several earlier methods. It is often difficult for women to make informed decisions about which approach is best for them because comparable information on each method is difficult to obtain. Women are frequently channeled into a method by the health professional or hospital, or there may be only one option in some locales. Respecting the individuality of each pregnant woman warrants an exploration of available methods in one's locale and provision of comparable information on each to the woman. A checklist for assessing each available option in a given area is given in Table 24-1.

Table 24-1. Checklist for childbirth preparation methods

	Option 1	Option 2
Name of class/method		
Instructor and qualifications		
Fee		
Meeting times, places, frequency with which classes are offered		
At what point in pregnancy do women enroll?		
Are significant others invited? Spouses only?		
What points of information are shared in the classes?		
Topics to be discussed:		
1. Nutrition		
2. Medications		
3. Common discomforts and relief measures		
4. Contraception		
5. Sexuality		
6. What to expect in labor and delivery		
7. Parenting		
8. Feeding choices		
9. Myths and misconceptions		
What skills are taught (e.g. pain control, relaxation, breast-feeding techniques)?		
What assumptions or philosophies guide the classes?		
Is the instructor available for support during the actual birthing experience or afterward?		
Are both hospital and home delivery addressed?		

The place of birth

The place of birth is an issue currently drawing much attention from women and health professionals alike. Whether a woman should give birth at home or in the hospital was a moot point when hospitals were not available and during the 1950s and 1960s when it was assumed that a laboring woman's place was in the hospital. The influences of the populist health movement, increasing skepticism of medicine, and the feminist movement have encouraged many women to give birth at home. The current controversy often involves whether or not the woman has a right to have an unattended home birth, whether nurse midwives may legally attend home births without being accused of "practicing medicine," and whether or not the home is sufficiently safe for both the mother and infant, particularly when the birth is attended by a lay midwife (albeit one who has been prepared for her responsibilities).

Mehl (1978) has done extensive research on the outcome of home delivery in the United States. In a series of studies, some with comparison hospitalized groups of women comparable to those choosing home delivery, he has demonstrated that significantly more procedures were used in conjunction with hospital deliveries than home deliveries, more cesarean sections were done in the hospital delivery groups, and the hospital groups had significantly more intrauterine fetal distress, elevated blood pressure during labor, meconium staining, and shoulder dystocia. The home delivery groups had more second stage dystocia, bleeding during labor, and occiput posterior deliveries. The hospitalized women had more postpartum hemorrhage. Infants born in the hospital had more birth injuries and neonatal infections, babies received more oxygen and had more respiratory distress of 12 or more hours, and more total noncongenital neonatal complications. The newborns who were delivered in the hospital had lower 1 and 5 minute Apgar scores and required more resuscitation. About 10% of the mothers and/or infants from home births required hospitalization. Indeed, the home delivery population seemed to fare as well and, in many instances, better than the women who delivered in the hospital. Mehl concluded that for women who have few risk factors for complications of pregnancy, home delivery is an alternative to be pursued.

Studies in Great Britain (Tew, 1978) suggest that there is no evidence in favor of all women delivering in hospitals. Statistics from National Health Services Hospitals failed to show that an increasing rate of hospitalization for birth decreased perinatal mortality. Yet in many western European countries there is a movement to have all women deliver in the hospital.

The origins of the problems women encounter in hospital vs home delivery are eloquently described by Haire (1972), Arms (1975), Kloosterman (1978), Richards (1978), Ettner (1977), and Lomas (1978), among others. (Many of these will be discussed in a later section.) Consideration of such problems is becoming more common among women as they choose a place of birth.

An important related issue is the degree of freedom women have in choosing a source of childbirth care. Many women have no alternative (or are aware of none) but the obstetrician. Yet in many localities, nurse-midwifery is common, especially in countries such as Great Britain. In some areas health professionals have helped lay midwives prepare themselves to assist women who deliver at home (Fremont Birth Collective, 1977).

Some investigators have attended to the psychologic needs and experiences of women as well as their physical safety when evaluating the alternatives for delivery. It has been suggested that the psychologic outcome of birth influences the process of parental-infant attachment (Peterson and Mehl, 1977) and that separation from the infant necessitated by anesthetized birth or some hospital births may impair bonding.

Kitzinger (1978) describes the experiences of women who gave birth at home. She found that women preferred home births for several reasons:

Hospital routines and atmospheres are impersonal
Home provides safety from interventionist obstetrics
Infant care in hospitals interferes with bonding
The birth could be shared with children at home
Continuity of care was available in the personal relationship with the midwife
Husbands could fully participate
Breast-feeding was more easily established at home
Delivery could be as easy as possible

Seiden (1978) delineates five approaches that are necessary to provide women good systems of childbirth care that foster maternal joy and mastery. These include health professionals having a clear idea of when the illness model applies, being committed to providing adequate emergency obstetric care, restoring the mother's choice and control in normal deliveries, intruding only when absolutely necessary in hospital deliveries, and providing lifelong childbirth education in natural contexts (e.g., schools).

Many hospitals have attempted to provide family-centered maternity care, alternatives for birthing women, and relaxed visitation restrictions. This effort might afford women a greater chance of humane treatment as well as the emergency services a hospital can offer. There is, however, the danger that being in a hospital elicits a definition of birthing as an illness to be treated.

BIRTHING

During the course of labor and delivery, several additional decision points arise. This is usually a time during which women are stressed and in pain. Being carefully informed, however, allows women in these circumstances to be actively involved in decision-making. Issues that arise include:

Awaiting the natural onset of labor vs induction
Providing basic self-hygiene vs pubic shave and enema preparation
Taking food and fluids vs fasting
Using psychoprophylaxis vs medication
Having family members or significant others as attendants vs only professionals
Being ambulatory vs bedridden during labor
Delivery in a squatting or sitting position vs lithotomy position
Having auscultation vs fetal monitoring

First stage

Elective induction of labor carries several hazards, some of which are summarized in Table 24-2. In addition, it is important to note that fetal and maternal deaths have occurred in conjunction with induction. The contractions stimulated by oxytocin are difficult even for women who are well-prepared to tolerate (Hack et al., 1976; Haire, 1972; Maisels et al., 1977). Although some of these complications (e.g. prematurity) are preventable with fetal diagnostic procedures, these procedures are not with hazard. For example, amniocentesis is not a benign procedure. Needle puncture may occur to the fetus (Broome et al., 1976) and the mother's anxiety level may be high (Robinson et al., 1975).

The necessity of the *pubic shave* has not been found to give women an advantage in the prevention of infection, but it does give them a definite postpartum itch. Women may have their pubic hair clipped or simply left as is. *Enemas* seem to intensify contractions during the latter part of the first stage and are very painful during transition. A woman can use a small enema during the early first stage or allow the natural diarrhea often accompanying labor to empty the bowel.

The need for *nutrients and fluid* during labor seems clear as the woman is *working;* she will be hypoglycemic and dehydrated if forced to fast. Light fluid and food intake does not seem to have negative effects on the woman, and if anesthesia is necessary, stomach contents can be aspirated.

The *alternatives to pain medication* during labor include the relaxation skills and psychoprophylaxis taught in childbirth classes. Emotional support from significant others or a health professional can help the woman cope with pain. Nearly all obstetric medications cross the placenta and many interfere with the woman's ability to push. There is evidence that women who have had Lamaze preparation have significant benefits in many re-

spects when compared with their counterparts. Hughey et al. (1978) report one fourth the number of cesarean sections, one fifth the amount of fetal distress, and one third the number of postpartum infections in Lamaze births. Felton and Segelman (1978) found that Lamaze-prepared women were more likely to view themselves as being origins of control vs others controlling them. There is evidence that biofeedback (electromyogram or galvanic skin response) has been effective in decreasing the need for obstetric medications and has decreased the length of labor (Biofeedback Training for Childbirth, 1975).

Having supportive people present in the birth environment, including children, can lessen the sense of isolation the woman feels. Providing support to her may alleviate the stress of labor and decrease her anxiety, which in turn can facilitate labor.

Allowing women to remain *ambulatory* and to deliver in a semi-sitting or lateral position, on an obstetric stool or by squatting facilitates delivery. Caldeyro-Barcia (1978) found that while maternal position had no effect on time of rupture of membranes or on fetal head molding, labor was 25% to 36% shorter in women who were upright. Ninety-five percent of the women preferred the upright position. Ambulation during labor significantly decreased duration of labor, need for analgesia, and incidence of fetal heart abnormalities. Furthermore, Apgar scores were better for ambulatory women and there was less need for oxytocin among the ambulatory groups (Flynn et al., 1978).

A final concern is about *routine fetal monitoring vs auscultation*. While the use of fetal monitoring has been thought to decrease the chance of death in the fetus and to assist in prognosis of neonatal respiratory problems (Hon et al., 1975), it is not without hazard. A careful analysis shows that fetal monitoring does have a significant influence on neonatal death rates, but the effects of monitoring decrease as the inherent risk of the baby declines. While 109 lives could be saved of 1000 high-risk babies monitored, in the lower risk groups, the absolute benefit would be negligible (Neutra et al., 1978).

The increasing incidence of cesarean sections has been attributed, at least in part, to use of fetal monitoring vs auscultation. It seems important to establish clear guidelines for interpretation of the fetal data as a means of preventing nonessential cesarean births. Although not yet specifically documented, it appears that fetal monitoring carries an increased risk for maternal and fetal infection because of the increased number of vaginal examinations needed and the fetal electrodes. In addition, the forced immobilization required of the woman who is receiving fetal monitoring may lead to the development of complications.

Table 24-2. Hazards of elective induction

To the mother	To the infant	To both
Intrapartum infection	Prematurity	Tumultuous labor
Injury from amniotomy	Prolapsed umbilicus	Uterine spasm
Amniotic fluid emboli	Injury from amniotomy	Placental separation
Afibrinoginemia	Displacement of presenting part from amniotomy	
Lacerations of cervix and vagina	Trauma	
Postpartum hemorrhage	Anoxia	
Water intoxication	Intracranial hemorrhage	
Uterine rupture		

Second stage

During the second stage of labor, another set of issues emerges:

Risking tears vs having an episiotomy

Birthing in bed vs moving to a labor room

Delivering slowly in a vertical position or having fundal pressure or forceps used and delivering in a horizontal position

Having family members, friends, or siblings present vs delivery alone

The "routine" *episiotomy* has become increasingly unpopular among women with no documented advantage to mother or fetus. Instead, episiotomies can interfere with sexual pleasure and may create problems in relation to further tearing and repair. Alternatives to the episiotomy include avoidance of the lithotomy position or pudental blocks, using perineal support, and antepartal and postpartal exercise of the perineal (especially pubococcygeus) muscles. Perineal massage also discourages tears.

Birthing in the labor bed rather than moving to a delivery table has several advantages. First, it does not intrude or disrupt the woman's labor. Second, it does not place the woman and fetus in a pathologically oriented environment. To cope with emergencies, portable or permanent equipment, such as oxygen, can be available in the labor room.

Delivering naturally without anesthesia and in an upright position decreases the need for routine use of fundal pressure or forceps for delivery following a prolonged second stage. Each of these procedures carries risks for both the fetus and mother. Prolonged bearing down (more than 5 seconds) may lead to late deceleration of the fetal heart, marked falls in maternal systolic and diastolic blood pressure with resultant delayed recovery of the fetal heart rate, and fetal hypoxia and acidosis in some cases (Calderyo-Barcia, 1979). An extended second stage of labor frequently results in an exhausted woman who is unable to push effectively. Fundal pressure or forceps may then be used to accomplish delivery. An episiotomy is routinely done in these instances. Vaginal lacerations and extension of episiotomy into the rectum are common.

Having a *supportive network* of family, friends, and siblings at the birth instead of delivering alone can be helpful to women who perceive this as desirable. While most women now find the presence of a spouse desirable, fewer desire having the siblings present. There appears to be positive effects to having siblings at birth, and it is recommended that someone be present to care for them who is not also caring for the mother (Anderson et al., 1978).

Third stage

During the *third stage of labor*, alternatives to common practices include those related to expulsion of the placenta and clamping of the umbilical cord. Putting traction on the cord, manipulating the fundus, manually removing the placenta, or using uterine stimulants can be hazardous to the woman. When the mother is unmedicated and in a semi-sitting position for birth, and when the placenta has been allowed to transfuse to the infant, such procedures are less likely to be necessary. Allowing the umbilical cord to remain intact until it ceases to pulsate can be accomplished with ease when the woman delivers in a vertical position or when there is simply a space below the level of the placenta to put the infant until the cord stops pulsating.

Concerns about hospital deliveries

Much of the concern about hospital delivery involves weighing the safety of the mother and infant against the hazards of being in a hospital. Many of the procedures used in conjunction with traditional hospital deliveries possess inherent value, particularly for high-risk clients. There can be no debating the value of life-saving measures judiciously applied. There are, however, certain risks inherent in the routine application of many of these measures, and that is the basis for concern with the hazards of hospital delivery. Haire (1972) points out quite clearly that a single medical intervention often sets off a domino effect, inasmuch as it necessitates subsequent interventions. An illustration of the problem is given in Fig. 24-1.

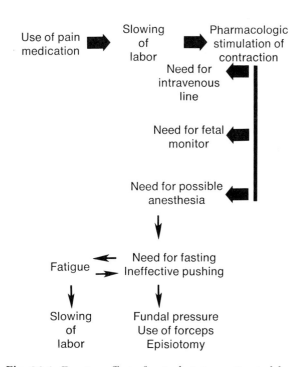

Fig. 24-1. Domino effect of a single intervention in labor.

EARLY PARENTING EXPERIENCE

During the early parenting experience, several alternatives may be offered to the woman and her family. These options relate to separation vs integration of the family members and the practices regarding breast-feeding.

Separation

Separation of mother, infant, father, significant others, and siblings is fostered by "routine" obstetric care. Klaus et al. (1972) have documented the importance of mother-infant togetherness during the first day following birth. Similar effects may obtain for father-infant attachment (McDonald, 1978). Putting the baby in the nursery conveys that the mother's care would not be adequate and probably inhibits her natural approach to caring. Rooming-in and allowing the infant to remain with the mother and significant others offers women a chance to establish early bonds with their infants. Restricting father and sibling visits is probably not necessary if appro-priate precautions are taken for infections and communicable diseases. Mothers should be permitted to regulate visitors in an effort to conserve energy.

Breast-feeding

Breast-feeding is discussed in Chapter 25. Briefly, there are three aspects that merit attention. First, infants can be safely nursed immediately after delivery, barring any complications. There is no need to delay the feeding if there is someone present who can intervene if the infant has a tracheoesophageal fistula. The literature supports several benefits of early breast-feeding. Glucose water is often offered first to breast-fed infants, and formula is often given to infants in the nursery. Neither of these practices is necessary since colostrum offers fluid and nutrients and does not pose allergy problems. Restriction of breast-fed infants to nursery schedules decreases suckling stimulation and thereby milk production; limits the antibodies the infant would get from colostrum; increases breast engorgement; and interferes with milk letdown. Keeping the infant with the mother allows for nursing on demand.

SUMMARY

This chapter was based on the premise that birthing women have a number of options regarding their experience. An attempt has been made to briefly address the decision points that occur before, during, and shortly after birth (Table 24-3). It is important to extend alternatives such as these to women who have few risk factors for complications for mother or fetus.

Table 24-3. Summary of alternatives in childbearing

Preparation for childbirth
Informed consent vs ignorance
Breast-feeding vs bottle-feeding
Childbirth preparation, alternative methods
Home vs hospital birth
Choice of facility (e.g., birthing room) vs usual labor and delivery setup
Choice of attendants (lay midwife vs nurse midwife vs obstetrician vs family vs team)

Birthing
First stage
Natural onset of labor vs induction
Self-hygiene vs pubic shave and enema
Food and fluid vs fasting
Psychoprophylaxis vs pain medication
Family, significant others in attendance vs health professionals only
Ambulatory vs bedridden labor
Auscultation vs fetal monitor
Second stage
Tears vs episiotomy
Birthing in bed vs delivery room
Delivering in vertical vs horizontal position, with risk of fundal pressure and forceps
Supportive others in attendance vs alone
Third stage
Allowing placental transfusion and natural delivery vs maneuvers to deliver placenta and early clamping of cord

Early parenting
Family separation vs integration
Breast-feeding:
On demand vs schedule
Immediate vs delayed
Spontaneous vs supplemented

REFERENCES

Anderson, S.: Siblings at childbirth. Presented at American Public Health Association Meeting, 1978.

Arms, S.: Immaculate deception, Boston, 1975, Houghton Mifflin Co.

Boston Women's Health Book Collective: Our bodies, ourselves, a book by and for women, New York, 1976, ed. 2. revised, Simon and Schuster.

Boston Women's Health Collective: Post-partum blues: as natural as childbirth, MS, Vol. 4, No. 9, Mar. 1976.

Bradley, R. A.: Husband-coached childbirth, New York, 1965, Harper & Row, Publishers.

Broome, D., Wilson, N., and others: Needle puncture of the fetus: a complication of second-trimester amniocentesis, Am. J. Obstet. Gynecol. **126**(2):247-252, 1976.

Caldeyro-Barcia, R.: Some consequences of obstetrical interference, Birth Family J., Vol. 2, No. 2, Spring 1975.

Caldeyro-Barcia, R. A.: The influence of maternal position on time of spontaneous rupture of the membrane, progress of labor, and fetal head compression, Birth Family J. **6**(1):7-15, Spring, 1979.

Caldeyro-Barcia, R. A.: The influence of maternal bearing down efforts during second stage on fetal well being, Birth Family J. **6**(1):17-21, Spring 1979.

Cetrulo, C., and Freeman, R.: Problems and risks of fetal monitoring. In Aladjem, S., editor: Risks in the practice of modern obstetrics, St. Louis, 1975, The C. V. Mosby Co.

Ettner, F.: Hospital technology breeds pathology, Women Health **2**(2):17-22, 1977.

Felton, G., and Segelman, F.: Lamaze childbirth training and changes in belief about personal control, Birth Family J. 5(3):141-150, Fall, 1978.

Flynn, A. M., Kelly, J., Hollins, G., and Lynch, P. F.: Ambulation in labor, Brit. Med. J. 2:591-593, 1978.

Fremont Birth Collective: Lay midwifery: still an "illegal" profession, Women Health 2(3):19-27, 1977.

Hack, M., and others: Neonatal respiratory distress following elective delivery: a preventable disease? Am. J. Obstet. Gynecol. 126(1):43-47, 1976.

Haire, D.: The cultural warping of childbirth, Int. Childb. Educ. Assoc., 1972.

Haire, D. B.: Pregnant patient's bill of rights, J. Nurse-Midwifery 20: 29, Winter 1975.

Hon, E. H., Zannine, D., and Quelligan, E. J.: The neonatal value of fetal monitoring, Am. J. Obstet. Gynecol. 122(4):508-517, 1975.

Howell, M. C.: What medical schools teach about women, N. Engl. J. Med. 291(6):304-307, 1974.

Hughey, M., McEelin, T., and Young, T.: Maternal and fetal outcome of Lamaze-prepared patients, Obstet. Gynecol. 51(6):643-647, 1978.

Kitzinger, S., and Davis, J. A.: The place of birth, New York, 1978, Oxford University Press.

Klaus, M., and Kennell, J.: Maternal-infant bonding: the impact of early separation or loss on family development, St. Louis, 1976, The C. V. Mosby Co.

Klaus, M., and others: Maternal attachment: importance of the first postpartum days, New Engl. J. Med. 286(9):460-463, 1972.

Kloosterman, G. J.: The Dutch system of home births. In Kitzinger, S., and Davis, J. A.: The place of birth, New York, 1978, Oxford University Press.

Kramer, R.: Giving birth: childbearing in America today, Chicago, 1978, Contemporary Books, Inc.

Leboyer, F.: Birth without violence, New York, 1975, Alfred A. Knopf, Inc.

Maisels, M. J., Rees, J., Marks, K., and Frideman, Z.: Elective delivery of the term fetus: an obstetrical hazard, J.A.M.A. 238(19):2036-2039, 1977.

Marieskind, H. I.: Restructuring Ob-Gyn, Soc. Policy 7(2):48-49, 1975 (special issue on Women and Health).

Marieskind, H. I.: Helping oneself to health, Soc. Policy 7(2):63-66, 1976 (special self-help issue).

Marieskind, H. I.: An evaluation of caesarean section in the United States, Final report submitted to Department of Health, Education, and Welfare, June 1979.

McDonald, D.: Paternal behavior at first contact with the newborn in a birth environment without intrusions, Birth Family J. 5(3):123-132, 1978.

Mehl, L. E.: The outcome of home delivery research in the United States. In Kitzinger, S., and Davis, J., editors: The place of birth, New York, 1978, Oxford University Press.

Neutra, R., and others: Effect of fetal monitoring on neonatal death rates, N. Engl. J. Med. 299(7):324-326, 1978.

Peterson, G., and Mehl, L.: Parental child psychology—delivery alternatives, Women Health 2(2):3-16, 1977.

Rich, A.: Of woman born, New York, 1976, W. W. Norton Co., Inc.

Richards, M. P. M.: A place of safety? An examination of the risks of hospital delivery. In Kitzinger, S., and Davis, J. A., editors: The place of birth, New York, 1978, Oxford University Press.

Robinson, J., Tennes, K., and Robinson, A.: Amniocentesis: its impact on mothers and infants: a one year follow-up study, Clin. Genet. 8: 97-106, 1975.

Seaman, B.: Pelvic autonomy: four proposals, Soc. Policy 7(2):48-49, 1975 (special issue on women and health).

Seiden, A.: The sense of mastery in the childbirth experience. In Notman, M., and Jadelson, C.: The woman patient, New York, 1978, Plenum Press.

Shaw, N.: Forced labor, New York, 1975, Pergamon Press.

Stewart, D., and Stewart, L., editors: Safe alternatives in childbirth, Chapel Hill, 1976, NAPSAC, Inc.

Tew, M.: The case against hospital deliveries: the statistical evidence. In Kitzinger, S., and Davies, J. A.: The place of birth, New York, 1978, Oxford University Press.

Waldbaum, D.: First time expectant fathers: the effect of childbirth classes on their fears and anxieties, ICEA Sharing 4(1):17-18, 1976.

Ward, C., and Ward, F.: The home birth book, Washington, D.C., 1976, Inscape.

Wertz, R. W., and Wertz, D. C.: Lying-in: a history of childbirth in America, New York, 1977, The Free Press.

25

Lactation

Gretchen Kramer Dery

Lactation, breast-feeding, nursing, and suckling are terms that are frequently used interchangeably. The nonspecificity of the terms has led to a lack of clarity in the literature and a lack of precision in studies of various components of the lactation process. Avery (1977) has initiated a beginning attempt to more clearly define the terms used when speaking about or studying the process. *Lactation* has been defined as an all-encompassing term that describes the process of milk secretion from its onset to its cessation. *Breast-feeding* is the maternal activity of supplying a child's sole or major nutritional needs by feeding milk from the woman's breast. *Nursing* is the maternal activity of giving a child the breast for suckling when breast milk is not the sole source of nutrition; in this case suckling also provides security, comfort, and affection. *Suckling* is the child's physical activity of drawing milk from the breast. Suckling may be done by the child for both nutritive or nonnutritive purposes. *Nursling* refers to the suckling child. Further clarification of terms is still needed, but an attempt will be made to use the terms as defined throughout this chapter.

Lactation is a complex phenomenon affected by multiple variables. A woman has the potential to exert a great deal of control over the variables influencing her lactation. It is the purpose of this chapter to give health care providers data that will allow them to facilitate and support a woman's decision to lactate, breast-feed, and nurse her child and to assist her to increase her awareness of options in directing the process.*

STYLES OF LACTATION

Two styles of lactation are frequently described in the literature. One style is called *primolactic*, a process in which the infant is allowed frequent and unre-

stricted access to the woman's breast, and food introduction and weaning occur gradually based upon the woman's observations of her child's readiness (Avery, 1977). The following is a narrative description of how such a process might proceed.

The woman, alert after she has given birth, puts the infant to breast immediately. The infant, in the quiet, alert phase that occurs for the first few hours after birth, uses his fully developed rooting and sucking reflexes to grasp hold of his mother's nipple. The child's suckling stimulates oxytocin, which consequently initiates the milk-ejection reflex. Oxytocin also stimulates the woman's uterus to contract vigorously, facilitating a return of the organ to the nonpregnant state. Mother, child, and significant others stay close together after the birth. Close skin and eye contact seem to facilitate a bonding between the mother and newborn. The infant is put to breast whenever he indicates discomfort. The suckling soothes him, and he may stay at the breast for up to an hour at a time. Frequent suckling stimulates the production of milk, and large quantities of milk appear within 24 hours of birth.

Woman and child sleep within touching distance and during the daylight hours, the child is generally in the woman's arms. The breast is offered on demand, and the infant seldom fusses. The woman has a strong attachment to the infant, sensing his needs and responding spontaneously. This behavior is enhanced by the influence of prolactin, which promotes maternal nurturing behavior. The woman needs the child close to her to empty her breasts, which become uncomfortable if overfilled. Each suckling causes the uterus to contract further. Breast-feeding is a sensual experience and is very pleasurable for the woman.

As the infant reaches approximately 6 months of age, he begins to indicate a readiness to try family foods. As nourishment begins to come from sources other than his mother's breast, her milk supply will gradually diminish. From 9 to 15 months after birth, lactation will decrease to the point that ovulation and menstruation will occur. At some period within the following years, the infant will gradually diminish suckling until he no longer wishes to suckle at all.

A second style of lactation, *mimelactic*, is a process in which the child is allowed access to the breast in a restricted or limited fashion. Supplemental formula

---

*Bottle-feeding will not be the focus of this chapter; however, this is in no way to suggest that the woman who chooses to bottle-feed does not need education and support.

and solids are introduced very early, and feeding is regulated by medical instruction or social custom rather than by the infant's readiness. Termination of suckling generally occurs at 3 to 6 months, if not before, and weaning is generally the result of an inadequate milk supply, the child's rejection of the breast, or maternal desire (Avery, 1977; Newton, 1971). A narrative description of how this style might proceed follows.

The woman, who had been medicated during labor and delivery, is too frightened and exhausted to see her baby for several hours after delivery. The infant, also sedated from the maternal drugs, has an impaired suckling reflex. She is placed in a central nursery and brought to her mother during the daytime hours on a strict schedule. Suckling time is severely limited, lactation is delayed, and ultimately the woman's breasts become engorged. The baby, still sleepy, has an even more difficult time nursing from the engorged breast. Glucose water and supplemental formula are given because she is not getting sufficient milk at her mother's breast, and the problem is compounded. If these problems are overcome, the woman may continue to lactate, and possibly supplement breast milk with formula. Cereal and other solids will be given when the infant is a few weeks old to help her sleep through the night and/or be quiet during the day. Night nursing will be infrequent, especially since the baby sleeps away from the woman in her own room. Daytime nursing is scheduled and suckling time limited. Pacifiers are used frequently, which also decreases suckling time at the breast. Weaning occurs within a few months, if not earlier.

These two descriptions represent extreme opposites in lactation styles. The second style probably comes closer to most women's experiences in the United States, but there are a growing number of women who are choosing a more primolactic style. There are many variations and possibilities of these two basic styles. To assist the woman achieve the style of lactation she desires, the nurse needs an understanding of the physiologic process and some data about the known advantages of human milk as an optimal nutritional source.

PHYSIOLOGIC PROCESS OF LACTATION

The physiologic aspects of the lactational process can be divided into three major phases: mammogenesis (mammary growth), lactogenesis (initiation of milk secretion), and galactopoiesis (maintenance of established milk secretion) (Schams, 1976).

Mammary growth

Growth occurs in the mammary organs during puberty and pregnancy (see Chapter 5). Glandular aveolar tissue increases, and it is this tissue that causes increased breast size during pregnancy. Although secretory tissue is generally fully developed by the sixteenth week of pregnancy, there is no milk secretion until after birth (Newton, 1962). During pregnancy placental tissues se-

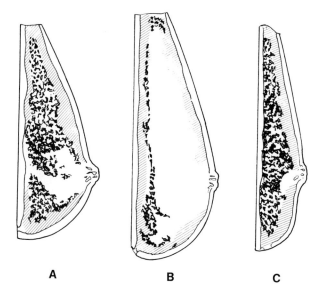

Fig. 25-1. Breast size is not a reliable indicator of potential milk secretion. This illustration depicts three types of breast tissue: Black = alveolar secretory tissue, white = fibrous tissue, cross-hatching = fatty tissue. Breast **A** is moderate in size with some fatty tissue and normal amounts of secretory tissue. Breast **B** is a larger breast, with large amounts of fatty tissue but minimal secretory tissue. Breast **C** is a smaller breast but with little fatty tissue and normal amounts of secretory tissue.

crete estrogens and progesterone in large amounts. The exact mechanism by which these hormones cause the mammary gland to grow is unclear (Schams, 1976); other steroids are also involved.

Breast size is not an accurate predictor of successful lactation (Fig. 25-1). Size is related to the amount of fatty tissue present and does not predict functional capacity. Breast size varies with age, heredity, pregnancy-lactation history, and support given to the breasts.

During pregnancy there is a significant increase in ducts and alveoli, and this growth is fostered by increased blood levels of estrogen (MacKeith and Wood, 1977). Nipple length and protractility also increase. Late in pregnancy the lobuloalveolar system reaches maximal development and is thought to be sensitized to the forthcoming effects of prolactin. Colostrum, a bright yellowish viscous fluid, is secreted in small amounts during the third trimester.

Milk secretion

During the last 3 to 5 weeks of pregnancy blood concentration of estrogens gradually increases. There is a further rapid increase during the final 2 weeks of pregnancy followed by a swift decline after birth (Schams, 1976). Increased serum levels of prolactin are seen in pregnant women at about the eighth week of gestation.

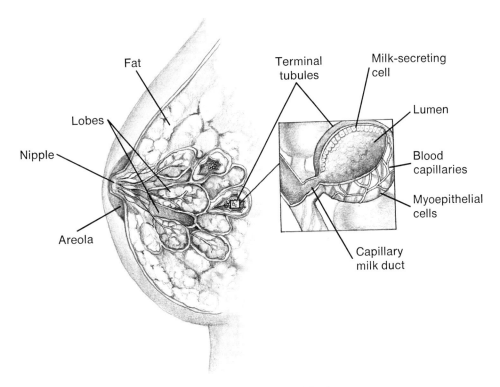

Fat

Lobes

Nipple

Areola

Terminal tubules

Milk-secreting cell

Lumen

Blood capillaries

Myoepithelial cells

Capillary milk duct

Fig. 25-2. Lactation system of the breast.

Prolactin reaches a peak level at birth. A woman who chooses not to lactate will return to a prepregnancy prolactin level within 2 to 3 weeks after birth, whereas a woman who lactates will continue to have increased prolactin levels (Schams, 1976). The fall in estrogens and rise in prolactin are thought to play a significant part in the initiation of milk secretion (MacKeith and Wood, 1977). Colostrum, which is the precursor to and chemically different from milk, is secreted from 24 to 96 hours after birth (Newton and Newton, 1962).

Milk is generally described as "coming in" suddenly. The sudden "coming in" sensation, described by many women in our culture, may be the result of overfullness of breasts that have been insufficiently suckled (Newton, 1962). Women who feed their infants in a primolactic style generally cannot describe a precise time when they feel their milk "coming in." During lactation, the milk is continuously secreted into the lumens of the alveoli. Prolactin is considered to be the chief lactogenic hormone for initiating and maintaining milk secretion.

There are three maternal reflexes involved in lactation. One is the *prolactin reflex*. Prolactin, produced by the anterior pituitary, is stimulated by the child's suckling. The released prolactin enters the bloodstream and is thought to act directly on the alveoli. The prolactin secreted, and thus the amount of milk produced, is directly related to the frequency, length, and intensity with which the child suckles the breast.

The second maternal reflex crucial to successful lactation is described as the *let-down reflex* (originally a dairy term) or the *drought* (an English term). Suckling is also considered crucial to the functioning of this maternal reflex, and this is confirmed by the fact that suckling alone can initiate milk production and flow. The let-down reflex is initiated by the child's stimulation of the richly innervated skin of the nipple. This causes transmission of impulses along the sensory nerve paths to the hypothalamus and down to the posterior pituitary, which then releases oxytocin into the bloodstream. The bloodstream carries the oxytocin to the breast. The network of smooth muscle (myoepithelium) around each alveoli contracts and squeezes the milk down the ducts and into the milk pools beneath the areola (MacKeith and Wood, 1977) (Fig. 25-2).

Newton and Newton (1962) attempted to identify signs and symptoms of an effective versus a noneffective let-down reflex. When they compared fifty-three women who were successfully breast-feeding with fifty women who were unsuccessful with breast-feeding, they found that those women defined as successful had a significantly higher incidence of the following four signs: milk dripping from the breasts before the infant was put to breast; milk dripping during a feeding from the opposite breast; uterine cramps (after-pains) during suckling; and cessation of nipple discomfort as the nursling obtained milk.

Women have described the let-down as a tingling or

prickly sensation, and one woman referred to it as a sensation "somewhere between a sneeze and an orgasm" (MacKeith and Wood, 1977). A newly lactating woman may not experience let-down immediately, and it may take several minutes of suckling to produce it (Newton and Newton, 1962). Sometimes when it occurs there may be spraying of the milk from the nipples (MacKeith and Wood, 1977). In women of other cultures or women who are breast-feeding their second or later child, the let-down can be very strong and controlled even from the first feeding. When the milk lets down and the milk sinuses fill and stand out in visible ridges under the areola, no leaking or dripping occurs (Newton and Newton, 1962).

The let-down reflex differs from the other reflexes in its susceptibility to psychoenvironmental stimuli. Newton and Newton (1948) demonstrated that the let-down reflex can be inhibited by severe cold, emotional conflict, or pain experienced by the mother. Emotional disturbance of a nursing woman decreased the mean amount of milk that could be obtained, from 168 to 99 Gm. Newton also demonstrated that the let-down reflex can be artificially induced by injection or intranasal spray of synthetic oxytocin. Disturbing a breast-feeding woman and administering oxytocin intravenously resulted in a mean volume of milk of 153 Gm.

Thus, distress can inhibit the let-down reflex. A woman who is anxious, uncertain, or tired also experiences stress, which can inhibit her let-down reflex. This usually results in a dissatisfied infant, who has received only minimal amounts of milk from the milk pools. The stressed woman is then additionally stressed by her unhappy child, her breasts become engorged and painful, and a vicious cycle begins.

The infant's sucking reflex is crucial to an adequate let-down reflex, because vigorous nipple stimulation promotes a good release of oxytocin from the posterior pituitary and hence a strong reflex flow. Also, as noted, suckling is essential for the milk secreting phase via oxytocin's action in the anterior pituitary to release prolactin. Thus, the milk-secreting phase and the milk-ejection phase are integrally interrelated (MacKeith and Wood, 1977) (Fig. 25-3).

The third maternal reflex necessary for lactation is the *nipple erection reflex.* This reflex is stimulated by the child's mouth on the nipple, which leads to nipple erection, making the nipple more proctractile and easier for the child to grasp (Jelliffe and Jelliffe, 1978). This is also generally a pleasurable sensation for women (see Chapter 5).

Maintenance of established lactation

This phase of lactation, while under complex hormonal control, is for all practical purposes primarily re-

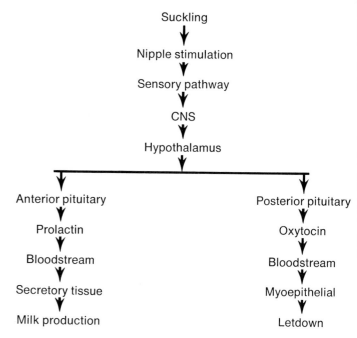

Fig. 25-3. Interrelation of milk secretion and milk ejection.

lated to continuing secretion of milk and based upon adequate production of prolactin, adequate maternal nutrition, and adequate suckling.

Prolonged lactation frequently delays the return of ovulation, and therefore delays the possibility of pregnancy. The exact mechanism is unknown, but it is thought to be related to the suppressive effect of prolactin and other hormones secreted in response to suckling. The woman who does not choose to lactate will generally have a return of her menses about 2 months after the birth. Lactating women seem to have a variable degree of amenorrhea, but it generally lasts substantially longer than 2 months. Breast-feeding practices and the woman's nutritional status appear to affect the duration of ovulation suppression (Knodel, 1977).

Menstruation, when it recurs, does not influence milk production to any significant degree. Increased irritability has been noted in some children during their mother's periods but it is thought that this might be in response to premenstrual tension in the woman being communicated to the child, versus a change in milk composition (MacKeith and Wood, 1977).

CHARACTERISTICS AND QUALITIES OF BREAST MILK

Breast milk is a highly complex and unique preparation, and is species specific (Consumer Reports, 1977; Jelliffe and Jelliffe, 1971). Many of the properties of human milk have been identified and studied. Comparisons are continually made between breast milk, cow's milk, and formulas, which are generally modified cow's milk and frequently referred to as "humanized." Until recently, it was widely accepted that formulas and breast milk were essentially similar both biochemically and nutritionally. As Jelliffe and Jelliffe (1976) note, however, the constituents of human milk and cow's milk are dissimilar in almost all respects excepting water and lactose content.

Composition

Protein. Breast milk contains less protein than cow's milk formulas, and high protein intake in early childhood can result in metabolic imbalances. The main protein in cow's milk is casein, which when acidified, precipitates and forms curds. The supernatant fluid remaining after curd formation is called whey. Cow's milk forms tough curds, which are difficult for human infants to digest. Breast milk contains lactalbumin as its chief protein, which forms soft, flocculent curds. These curds are rapidly and easily digested by the infant (Consumer Reports, 1977; Wing, 1977).

Amino acids. Taurine and cystine, amino acids, are present in high concentrations in breast milk and in very low concentrations in cow's milk and cow's milk formulas. Taurine functions in bile acid conjugation and may also have a role in the facilitation of nerve impulses. Cystine is involved in brain physiology (Jelliffe and Jelliffe, 1971; Wing, 1977).

Nucleotides. Breast milk and cow's milk both contain a large variety of nucleotides, which are required for protein synthesis. However, mature cow's milk contains only a small total amount of nucleotides, primarily orotic acid. Mature human milk contains a variety of nucleotides but no orotic acid (Gyorgy, 1971).

Lipids. Breast milk contains a higher content of linoleic acid (Gyorgy, 1971), the only dietary fatty acid considered essential for the child. Cow's milk and breast milk both contain much more cholesterol than formulas (Consumer Reports, 1977). The effect of the infant's diet on subsequent serum cholesterol levels is unclear (Wing, 1977).

Breast milk and cow's milk contain lipase, an enzyme that breaks down triglycerides to free fatty acids and glycerol. Human milk, but not cow's milk, contains additional lipase in the skim milk fraction, which is more active than that found in the cream fraction liberating more free fatty acids (Wing, 1977). Free fatty acids are the most important energy source for nurslings (Gyorgy, 1971).

The fat content of human milk is greater in hind milk, which is the milk released at the latter part of the feeding. This has been suggested to act as an appetite control mechanism for nurslings (Hall, 1978) in that the fore

milk would be more like a "drink" and the hind milk more like "food." Formulas, being of similar consistency throughout, would not provide this mechanism.

Minerals. The adequacy of iron content in breast milk is a highly controversial topic. Neither breast milk nor cow's milk contains large amounts of iron (Consumer Reports, 1977). Formulas are generally fortified with iron supplements, and supplements are also available for use by breast-fed children. Such supplemental iron has been, and still is, advocated for the breast-fed infant. However, recent studies show that the absorption of dietary iron depends greatly upon the food within which it is contained. An average of 49% of the iron present in breast milk is absorbed compared with 4% of iron absorbed from formulas. Studies suggest that if breast milk is ingested exclusively for the first year, iron intake may be adequate (Wing, 1977). Further study in this area is needed before conclusive recommendations are warranted.

Human milk contains less zinc than cow's milk (Wing, 1977) but absorption of the human variety is more effective because of differences in binding (Jelliffe and Jelliffe, 1971). Breast milk has a more favorable calcium-to-phosphorus ratio when compared to formulas (Consumer Reports, 1977) and cow's milk, where the ratio is considerably higher (Wing, 1977).

Because of the low protein and mineral content of breast milk, it is thought to provide less of a solute load for the infant's immature kidneys to excrete (Consumer Reports, 1977). The greater solute load in formula-fed children requires a larger obligatory water loss than for the breast-fed child, resulting in thirst. This thirst should be quenched with water to avoid dehydration. Breast milk, being a low solute food, provides both food and water. Supplemental water is not needed by the totally breast-fed child except in circumstances of excess water loss (Wing, 1977).

Calcium content in the breast milk of well-nourished women varies. While there might be indications that inadequately nourished women have normal to low calcium content in their breast milk (Jelliffe, 1976), for the most part this mineral is not thought to be affected by inadequate maternal nutrition. Iron, copper, and fluoride content of breast milk appear to be unaltered by maternal supplementation.

Variations in fluid intake within a wide range appear to have no physiologic effect on the volume of milk secreted, even though there is a prevalent belief that increasing maternal fluid intake will help assure copious volumes of milk. It cannot be denied that increasing fluid intake may have a confidence-building effect, and thus possibly enhance the let-down reflex. Prolactin has been demonstrated to have antidiuretic properties, and this may explain why the variations in fluid intake do not alter the volume produced (Jelliffe and Jelliffe, 1978), since the woman's body retains the needed fluids to produce the milk.

Vitamins. Formulas are vitamin fortified and contain at least the minimum FDA requirements. The vitamin content of breast milk varies with the woman's nutritional intake, and an adequate maternal diet will provide acceptable vitamin levels of all but vitamin D.

The level of vitamin D has been thought to be inadequate (Consumer Reports, 1977), but it has usually been assayed in the lipid portion of milk. A recent report indicates a previously unrecognized concentration of a water-soluble form of vitamin D in the aqueous fraction of human milk. Thus human milk contains greater quantities of vitamin D than previously supposed. It remains to be shown whether the nursling can utilize the vitamin D in the aqueous portion (Wing, 1977).

Colostrum is particularly rich in vitamin E, and is an important source of this vitamin for newborns. Vitamin K, normally produced by the intestinal flora, is unavailable to all newborns because the intestinal tract is sterile. Beginning with the second week of life, the supply of vitamin K produced by the fully developed intestinal flora will correct the physiologic deficit. Administering vitamin K to the pregnant/nursing mother or the newborn can prevent the possibility of transient hemorrhagic disease (Gyorgy, 1971).

Electrolytes and pH. Sodium and potassium concentrations in cow's milk are three times the concentrations in breast milk. Some cow's milk formulas have ranges of sodium and potassium that fall between the breast and cow's milk level, and some are made more like breast milk (Wing, 1977).

The pH of breast milk (7.0) is generally higher than that of cow's milk formulas, and there have been correlations between the pH of cow's milk and formula and acidosis in the child (Wing, 1977).

Sugar. Breast milk and formulas have the same carbohydrate, lactose, in similar amounts (Consumer Reports, 1977). Cow's milk has a lower concentration of lactose (Wing, 1977).

Fluoride. The fluoride content of human milk is thought to be low, even when present in optimal amounts in the water supply. Cow's milk contains almost twice the fluoride of breast milk (Wing, 1977). There is disagreement as to whether a nursling should be given additional fluoride (Filer, 1977), but there appears to be some benefits to the child (Thompson, 1978).

Protection against infection

The newborn's immune mechanisms are immature and immunologic defenses are weak (Grams, 1978). Breast-feeding is a hygienic, gradual method of protecting the infant until immunologic independence is reached (Gerrard, 1974). In Third World countries breast-feeding significantly affects both morbidity and mortality, but in the United States it is thought to have no more than a marginal effect on infection rates (Wing, 1977). However, current work has shown some important protective effects even in industrialized, sanitized circumstances (Jelliffe and Jelliffe, 1977b).

All classes of immunoglobulins, which form antibodies, are found in high levels in colostrum and in somewhat lower levels in breast milk (Mata and Wyatt, 1971). It is generally believed that immunoglobulins act locally on the child's intestine, providing a protective action for the intestinal mucosa against bacterial invasion. Recent evidence suggests that a small proportion of the immunoglobulins present in colostrum are absorbed and may play a role in systemic resistance to infection.

Antibodies to a variety of microorganisms have been demonstrated in human milk, including *Clostridium tetani* (tetanus), *Bordetella pertussis* (whooping cough), *Diplococcus pneumoniae* (pneumonia), staphylolysin and streptolysin (lytic enzymes produced by staphylococci and streptococci), *Corynebacterium diphtheriae* (diphtheria), enteropathogenic *E. Coli*, salmonellae and shigellae, and polio, Coxsackie, ECHO and influenza viruses (Wing, 1977).

In addition to immunoglobulins, breast milk contains other protective substances. One of these is an antistaphylococcal factor, which is thought to protect against staphylococcal infections. Lysozyme, an enzyme, is thought to contribute to the development and maintenance of the nursling's specific intestinal flora. The C-3 component of complement found in colostrum is active in the lysis of certain antibody-bound bacteria (Mata and Wyatt, 1971). Lactoferrin, found in higher concentrations in breast milk than any other biologic substance, possesses antimicrobial properties. Unsaturated vitamin B_{12}–binding protein is thought to compete for vitamin B_{12} with certain bacteria which take up this vitamin in the intestines. A nonspecific antiviral substance has also been discovered in the cream fraction of breast milk (Wing, 1977).

Colostrum and milk contain live white cells with immunologic capacity (Mata and Wyatt, 1971). These cells act by synthesizing immunoglobulins and/or by phagocytosis (Wing, 1977) to provide protection against certain bacteria and viruses (Consumer Reports, 1977).

The different composition of material entering the colon of the breast-fed versus the bottle-fed child reflects specific components of breast milk and results in differences in stool composition and intestinal flora. Nurslings have stools with a higher water content, less buffering capacity, a lower pH, a lower content of amino acids, and a higher content of reducing sugars. The low pH, lack of buffering activity, and the high sugar content in the colon are all favorable to the growth of the *Lactobacillus bifidus*. This organism dominates the nursling's intestinal flora. While *Lactobacillus bifidus* is present in the gastrointestinal tract throughout the life cycle, it outnumbers all other bacteria only in the nursling. Lactobacilli produce acetic and lactic acids in large quantities and this produces the low pH of the nursling's feces. The acidity of the feces interferes with intestinal colonization by enteric pathogenic bacteria (Wing, 1977), making the nursling less susceptible to intestinal infections than bottle-fed infants.

Protection against allergies

Even in the United States breast milk is superior to cow's milk for the prevention of allergic diseases (Wing, 1977). Since newborns cannot effectively break down proteins into amino acids or block partially digested or undigested protein from being absorbed through the digestive tract, these proteins can trigger an allergic response. Breast milk is thought to coat the intestinal tract and prevent such proteins from passing through. In addition, breast milk itself is nonallergenic (Consumer Reports, 1977).

Allergies to cow's milk occur in approximately 7% of bottle-fed children, and can cause such problems as recurrent rhinorrhea and bronchitis, colic, spells of diarrhea and vomiting (Gerrard, 1978), asthma, and eczema. Intestinal blood loss is commonly seen in formula-fed infants (Wing, 1977).

Although foods eaten by the lactating woman readily enter her breast milk and can precipitate an allergic reaction, this can easily be treated by removing the offending item from the woman's diet. If the specific food substance is unknown, common offenders such as dairy products, citrus fruits, or eggs can be eliminated on a trial-and-error basis (Gerrard, 1978).

Economics and convenience

When cost is considered a factor, the minimum cost of artificial feeding will almost always exceed minimum food costs to support lactation (Consumer Reports, 1977; McKigney, 1971). Breast milk also represents the original ready-to-serve 24-hour convenience food—precooked, preheated, prepackaged, and available in individual servings.

PREPARATION FOR LACTATION

Many techniques have been recommended to women to prepare their breasts for and avoid problems during lactation. Few of these techniques have been subjected to a critical analysis of their effectiveness and possible negative side effects. Some appear to be natural and reasonable, some have been used by large numbers of women who report success with their use, and some have

been proved detrimental. Long lists of things a woman "must" do to prepare her breasts can minimize the naturalness of the lactation process and make it appear very time-consuming and complicated.

Dress and hygiene

American women appear to be at risk for problems with nipple soreness during lactation. This is frequently presented as being especially true of blonde and redheaded women, presumably because they have fair skin (Pryor, 1973). Brown and Hurlock's (1975) study of fifty-eight lactating women was not able to substantiate that blondes and redheads had more nipple damage. Atkinson's (1979) study of seventeen primigravida women demonstrated that fair-skinned women reported more nipple soreness than olive complected women. Some women will choose not to prepare their breasts prenatally and nonetheless encounter no difficulties during lactation (La Leche, 1963).

Several aspects of our culture, such as the wearing of bras and the practice of frequently bathing with soap, may be operant in fostering susceptibility to nipple problems since women from cultures that do not espouse these practices have minimal problems. Bras protect the nipple and areola from air, sunshine, and the gentle friction of clothing. Assuming that the bra-wearing factor is inherent in problem development, there are several possible alternatives available. First, it is always possible, especially for women with small breasts, to refrain from wearing a bra for part or most of the time. If the woman has large breasts and would prefer to wear a bra, the area of the bra around the nipple and areola can be cut out or the nursing bra flap opened. Either of these options will let air reach the nipples and areola and also provide gentle stimulation to them from outside clothing (Pryor, 1973).

The largest sweat glands in the body are found at the nipple. Sebum, which is secreted from the sebaceous glands on the areola, has known bactericidal properties. During pregnancy the secretion of sebum increases, and the sweat glands in the areola hypertrophy. This increase in sweat and sebum is thought to make the nipple more supple (Newton, 1952). Colostrum secreted during pregnancy is also known to have lysozyme activity and provide bactericidal properties. Colostrum possesses an emollient quality and may be beneficial if not removed from the nipple. Therefore, it is frequently recommended that women refrain from using any potentially harmful cleansing agents on their nipples, such as soaps, alcohol, and perfumed creams.

Newton, (1952) notes that soap, the most frequently used cleansing agent, removes by mechanical action the dead horny cells and other materials derived from cellular disintegration. These materials, if not removed, will provide a protective covering for the skin. Alkaline watery solutions, such as soap, swell the outer epidermal layer. The swelling is followed by drying, loosening, and scaling of cells. Repeated applications of soap have a cumulative effect. Soap alkalinizes the skin, and it takes normal skin some time to recover its normal acidity after this alkalinization. Bacterial flora increase in alkalinized skin. Soap also removes the sebum. One possible reason that soap's harmful effects are seldom noted in our culture is that the skin is usually protected from hard usage. This is not the situation during lactation.

If the pregnant woman washes her nipples with soap, it is likely that she is counteracting her body's own natural attempts to prepare them for suckling. Plain water is recommended for adequate nipple hygiene. If a woman feels she must use soap, she can be encouraged to use it sparingly and rinse her breasts well (La Leche, 1963).

Ultraviolet lights

Assuming that ultraviolet light is partially responsible for making women in tropical cultures less at risk for sore nipples, two interventions can be recommended as potentially decreasing this risk for American women.

Exposing the breasts to sun (Eiger and Olds, 1972; Rees, 1976) is one option and can easily be done if a woman has access to a private outdoor place. It can also be done indoors directly in the sunlight shining in through a window (Rees, 1976). Exposure should be limited to 5 minutes the first day, and then can be increased by increments of 5 minutes up to a half hour per day. The time can be decreased to the previous day's time if any redness is noted (Eiger and Olds, 1972).

It is thought that a similar effect can be obtained from exposure to the artificial ultraviolet light in a sunlamp. *Extreme care* is needed by women choosing this alternative. Rees (1976) and Eiger and Olds (1972) recommend keeping the sunlamp 4 feet away from the body. Their recommended exposure schedule is given in Table 25-1. If at any time during the process any redness is noted, the previous day's schedule should be resumed and maintained for several days. Then the time can be increased by 30-second intervals. If longer periods are not tolerated, the woman should maintain the schedule that is nonirritating for her. Safety factors inherent in this method include: (1) using a watch or clock for timing, (2) covering one's eyes to protect them from damaging rays, and (3) using care in touching the bulb, since it becomes very hot during use. It is not necessary to buy an expensive sunlamp; ultraviolet bulbs that fit into any lamp fixture are available. Ultraviolet lights can also be used after birth for nipple soreness.

Ointments

Many women wish to use creams, ointments, or lotions on their nipples prenatally. Some health care pro-

Table 25-1. Recommended exposure schedule

Day	Exposure time
1	30 seconds
2	1 minute
3	1 minute
4	2 minutes
5	2 minutes
6+	3 minutes

viders feel a need to recommend them. Little conclusive evidence is available related to the value of these practices. Rees (1976) recommends avoiding the use of creams, ointments, or lotions that have perfumes or petroleum derivatives. Petrolatum, once widely used, inhibits the insensible evaporation of sweat from the skin. This leads to swelling and maceration of the horny layer; microorganisms may flourish under such conditions. Petrolatum also defats the skin (Newton, 1952); also, perfumes can act as chemical irritants.

Pure lanolin is frequently recommended and at least one study has demonstrated that while not particularly helpful, except perhaps psychologically, it was not harmful (Newton, 1952). Lanolin forms a protective coat that is resistant to penetration, yet it is miscible with water and allows normal evaporation from the skin. Since lanolin is a sheep's-wool product, this product is contraindicated for women allergic to wool (La Leche, 1974c). Pure lanolin is thick, sticky, and not perfumed, which may make it acceptable for use by the pregnant woman. Almost any druggist will provide some from their stock supply if asked.

Another commonly recommended ointment is A & D ointment. Newton (1952) has demonstrated that while it did not appear to help, it did not seem to contribute to nipple soreness or damage in lactating women.

Another frequently recommended cream for nipple preparation is Masse cream. Brown and Hurlock (1975) conducted a study in which nineteen women treated one breast during pregnancy by the application of this cream, and left the other breast untreated. No significant difference in objective or subjective measures of nipple pain and damage during lactation was noted.

Before a woman uses any lubricant on her breasts or nipples she can test its effect on her skin by rubbing a small amount on the soft skin in the bend of her elbow. It can then be observed several times over a 24-hour period for redness, irritation, or tenderness. If any reaction occurs, she can refrain from using that product on her breasts or nipples (Rees, 1976).

Nipple conditioning

Another recommended, though unproved, suggestion for pregnant women is some form of regular nipple conditioning, usually beginning some time during the last

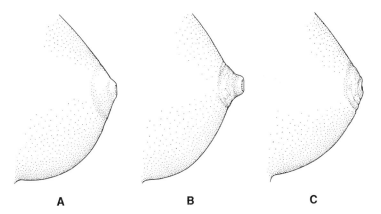

A   **B**   **C**

Fig. 25-4. A, Normal unstimulated nipple. Pseudoretracted nipple has similar appearance when in unstimulated state. **B,** Stimulated normal nipple showing protractibility. **C,** Appearance of stimulated pseudoretracted nipple, with nipple folding inward. True inverted nipples have their appearance before stimulation.

several weeks or 2 to 3 months of pregnancy. Two frequently suggested conditioning methods are nipple rolling and rubbing the nipples briskly with a terrycloth towel or washcloth after bathing.* Nipple rolling is accomplished by taking the nipple between the thumb and forefinger and pulling it out firmly, but not to the point of pain. Then the nipple is rolled between the thumb and forefinger for a minute or two. Some authorities recommend the application of a cream or ointment before this exercise (La Leche, 1963), while others recommend it after completion of the routine (Eiger and Olds, 1978). Others disagree with the practices altogether, believing they may be a source of irritation (Rees, 1976). One retrospective study concluded that nipple rolling during pregnancy did not prevent sore nipples (Whitley, 1978). Another study of nineteen women who used the nipple rolling technique on one breast and used the other breast as a control demonstrated no significant difference in objective or subjective measures of nipple pain and damage during early lactation between the treated and untreated breasts (Brown and Hurlock, 1975). However, less nipple pain was reported by seventeen women who used nipple rolling and nipple rubbing with a terrycloth towel from the thirty-fourth week of pregnancy until childbirth (Atkinson, 1979).

Assessing nipple protractility

It is important that the woman who wishes to lactate and breast-feed assess whether or not she has good nipple protractility. If she does, no further problem exists for her in this area. If she does not, she may have difficulty breast-feeding (as well as have nipples that are less sexually responsive). Checking for nipple protractility should be a normal part of prenatal care but frequently is not (Applebaum, 1975). Many physicians, aware that flat and inverted nipples naturally become increasingly protractile as pregnancy advances, do not systematically check women for this condition. Applebaum (1975) states that one third of mothers examined may have nipple retraction on stimulation.

There are variable degrees of nonprotractile nipples, sometimes classified as pseudoinverted nipples and true inverted nipples (Fig. 25-4). Pseudoinverted nipples can be demonstrated by grasping the areola with the thumb and forefinger just behind the base of the nipple (as in manual expression) and compressing it. The nipple, which may appear full-sized and normal, will fold back into the breast upon stimulation (Applebaum, 1975). This results from the nipple being anchored, rather than loosely attached, to the underlying structures. These adhesions at the nipple base can be broken by continual suckling after birth, but may interfere with the initiation of the lactation process.

Successful lactation and breast-feeding are partially dependent upon the infant's ability to mechanically stretch the nipple back to the hard palate of the mouth, allowing the let-down reflex to be properly stimulated (Applebaum, 1975).* Hoffman (1953) has recommended exercises for pseudoinverted nipples to help break the adhesions beneath the nipple, giving them increased protractility and subsequently allowing the infant an easier grasp. This exercise is performed by placing the thumbs or forefingers opposite each other on the areola close to the inverted nipples. The fingers or thumbs are

---

*La Leche, 1963; Eiger and Olds, 1972; Olson, 1978; Gerard, 1970.

*See also: Good news for "innies," up front facts, Keep. Abreast. J. 1: 46-57, 1976.

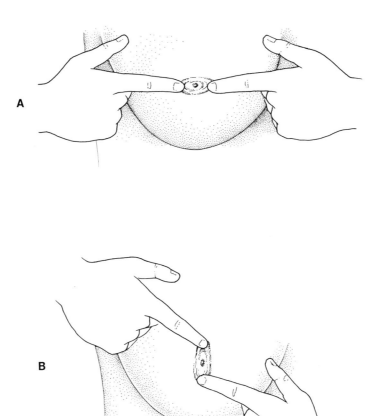

Fig. 25-5. Hoffman's technique for increasing nipple protractility. This method can be done with forefingers or thumbs. Place fingers (or thumbs) on opposite side of the areola **(A)** at its edge. Press inward toward chest wall and stretch in a horizontal direction. Then place fingers (or thumbs) at top and bottom areolar edge **(B)** and, again pressing inward toward chest wall, stretch in a vertical direction.

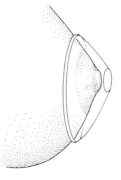

Fig. 25-6. Breast shields to be used primarily for inverted nipples, but also helpful if a woman's breasts are engorged.

then pressed in firmly and gradually pushed away from the areola (Fig. 25-5). Hoffman recommends this procedure be done four or five times a day prenatally.

A woman with true inverted nipples can wear a special shield (Fig. 25-6) for several months during the latter part of pregnancy to correct the inversion. These shields, which are placed over the nipple and areola, are worn under the bra and are painless. They exert an even, gentle pressure around the areola, which gradually forces the nipples through the central opening of the shield (Applebaum, 1976). (These shields should not be confused with nipple shields, which look like rubber nipples and are placed over real nipples while nursing.) A breast shield has two sections. The bottom section has a hole that fits over the breast; the top section fits over the bot-

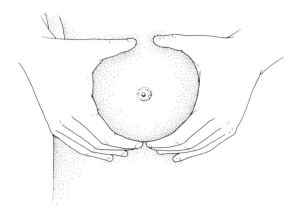

Fig. 25-7. Breast massage. The breast is encircled with thumbs and fingers. Gentle traction is exerted while moving hands from chest wall toward the nipple.

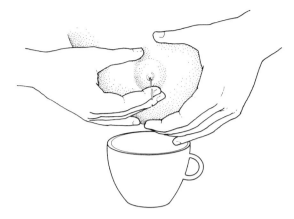

Fig. 25-8. Manual expression. While supporting the breast with one hand, place the thumb and forefinger of the other hand on the edge of the areolar area and push inward and back toward the chest wall.

tom, holding the bra away from the nipple, and after birth will catch any leakage. They are used prenatally and postnatally between feedings but never while the child is nursing. These shields can also be used by any woman who would like to improve the appearance and/or sexual responsiveness of inverted nipples.*

Manual expression and breast massage

Manual expression and breast massage are two other techniques that women are encouraged to practice during the last weeks of pregnancy. Applebaum (1975) suggests that prenatal manual expression will condition the woman's neurohormonal reflexes and thus enhance milk production and milk let-down after childbirth. Manual expression is also believed to open the milk ducts (La Leche, 1974c).

Breast massage has the effect of mechanically pressing milk from the alveoli through the ducts and locally stimulating myoepithelial cells, enhancing milk ejection. Dilation of the lactiferous ducts and sinuses has also been attributed to this technique, thus supposedly allowing for increased volume capacity of the breast. These practices are said to be helpful in reducing postpartum engorgement (La Leche, 1974c).

There is limited evidence available that disputes these claims. Whitley (1978), in a retrospective study of thirty-four lactating mothers, reported little differences in the incidence of engorgement, whether or not mothers practiced both techniques. Brown and Hurlock (1975) demonstrated that breasts prepared prenatally by expression of colostrum did not differ significantly on measures of objective or subjective damage or pain from breasts receiving no such preparation. In addition, weight gain,

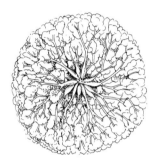

Fig. 25-9. Milk ducts radiating from the nipple.

used as an indicator of increased milk flow, was not significantly different in infants who suckled breasts prepared prenatally by the expressing of colostrum.

There appears to be little disagreement, however, that breast massage, and particularly manual expression, are valuable skills for the lactating woman to possess. Perhaps the technique is best learned at a time that allows practice and skill development in a relaxed environment. It is very difficult to learn these skills in a stressful situation, such as when postpartum engorgement occurs or during forced separation from the child.

The techniques are not complicated, but as previously stated, they do require practice. Breast massage is done by encircling the breast at the chest wall with the fingers and thumbs of both hands (Fig. 25-7). The hands are then gently moved toward the nipple, exerting gentle traction as they move. A cream may be used to prevent irritation caused by friction (Applebaum, 1975).

Manual expression usually follows breast massage, or it can be done alone. The woman grasps the breast at the end of the areola, with the thumb positioned above

---

* If not available locally, they can be obtained from La Leche League International, 9616 Minneapolis Avenue, Franklin Park, Illinois 60131.

and the fingers positioned beneath (Fig. 25-8). She then pushes her thumb and forefinger together, pushing in and back toward the chest wall. Then the areola is released and the process is repeated at another area. The finger and thumb should not be moved out toward the nipple (La Leche, 1974c) and the nipple is not pulled or squeezed at any time during manual expression (Rees, 1976). Since the milk ducts radiate out from the nipple in a manner similar to hands on a clock, (Fig. 25-9), this can be a useful analogy to help the woman visualize how to compress all the ducts. The woman can switch from one breast to another every few minutes. The first few times she performs this technique prenatally, she may not obtain any colostrum; however, after a few times, she will obtain a drop or two (La Leche, 1974c). Applebaum (1975) and La Leche League (1974c) recommend performing manual expression once or twice a day.

Additional research is needed in the area of techniques for prenatal preparation to avoid nipple pain and damage during the initiation of breast-feeding. Sore and damaged nipples can be a significant deterrent to the establishment and continuation of lactation.

SOCIOCULTURAL INFLUENCES
Barriers to lactation

Negative values about lactation are deeply rooted in our culture (Brack, 1975). Our society nurtures feelings of shame, guilt, and disgust about lactation. The frequency and duration of breast-feeding in America has fallen markedly during this century, although there appears to be a current trend to return to breast-feeding among women in the United States.

As previously noted, successful lactation depends upon two maternal reflexes, the let-down reflex and prolactin reflex. Since the first is inhibited by anxiety and the second is related to sufficient suckling stimulus, both are influenced by cultural attitudes and opportunities (Jelliffe, 1976). Successful lactation in this country is the rare exception, whereas failure has become the norm of expected behavior (Auerbach, 1976b).

Jelliffe (1976) describes a phenomenon called "linear Westernism," or those cultural changes resulting from scientific discoveries and ways of thought that occurred with the industrial revolution. This movement values the manufactured, the technologic, the mathematical, the provable, and the new—not the natural and traditional. The health care professions, especially organized medicine, have used the linear approach as a basis for its practice. Since anything manufactured is automatically regarded as better, the scientific approach has become the basis for infant feeding practices. Formulas are derived to provide the necessary nutrients that can be measured and administered at precise intervals.

Industry. The commercial baby food industry's interests in discouraging breast-feeding cannot be ignored.

The formula companies have a strong monetary interest in seeing that breast-feeding is deprecated. The "supplementary" bottles or "just-in-case" free samples undermine the lactating woman's confidence in her ability to feed her infant. Advertising is totally weighted in favor of bottle-feeding, and anyone looking at any media would think that there was no such thing as breast-feeding. Television and magazine ads encourage women to do what is "best" for their children, and what is "best" always involves purchasing their products. The baby food industry also has a strong interest in the encouragement of early introduction of solids. In a technical/commercial society, the influence of these groups upon women cannot be discounted (Brack, 1975; Jelliffe, 1976).

Sexual role of breast. In our society the breast is viewed almost exclusively as an object of eroticism rather than as a means of nurturing (Jelliffe, 1976). The result of this attitude is exemplified by the arrest of three women for indecent exposure while nursing their children in a park (Brack, 1975). (This and other similar incidents also reflect some of the cultural attitudes toward sexuality.)

Myths. The "super-mom" myth in the United States can negatively influence the lactating woman (Hall, 1978). This myth holds that the woman, shortly after childbirth, assumes a multitude of previous roles and tasks, simultaneously with the new demands placed upon her by the child. Thus she showers her partner and children with love and affection, is an immaculate housekeeper, chauffeurs the children, assumes her civic responsibilities, and returns to work. Attempts to make this myth a reality will lead to failure of lactation for most women. Reorganization of priorities, modification and sharing of tasks, and making choices are all part of changes necessary to accommodate to a new infant, and are crucial to successful breast-feeding.

Dress. Dress and clothing styles are another culturally influenced factor that can raise subtle barriers to breast-feeding. Western dress and clothing styles make breast-child contact difficult. (Fig. 25-10). Unobtrusive nursing can be accomplished, however. Two-piece outfits lend themselves most readily to easy nursing, especially if the top is loose-fitting. With a blouse or sweater pulled up on one side, the child covers any bare midriff and the garment covers the breast. Nursing nightgowns are available in department stores, but there are few daytime or evening clothes made specifically for nursing women. Women who do not choose to wear a bra will have easier access to their breasts. However, some women feel more comfortable wearing a bra, especially if breast size has increased during lactation. It is important for women to select a bra with a flap that can be easily manipulated (essentially with one hand) to avoid making daytime feedings a struggle.

Sleeping patterns. For more than 100 years Western

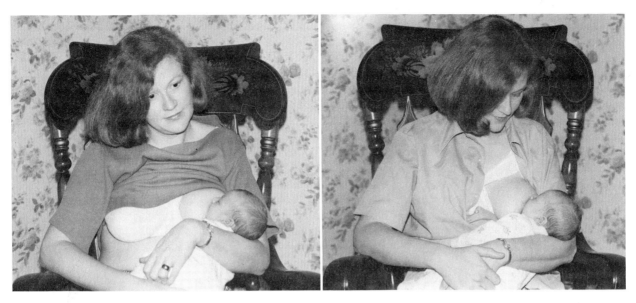

Fig. 25-10. Dress styles may be inhibiting to nursing. Loose overblouses or sweaters arc ideal for ease of nursing.

countries have strongly advocated the social custom of separate sleeping patterns. The advocacy is so strong that parents feel guilty when taking their children to bed with them. However, some parents do sleep with their children, and for a variety of reasons (Thevenin, 1976). The simplest and most convenient way for a woman to breast-feed an infant at night is with the child in bed lying next to her. It means that the woman can meet her child's needs with minimal interruptions of her sleep. Niles Newton notes that authorities who point to the psychologic harmfulness of sleeping with a child are either males or other people who have not had personal experience breast-feeding and caring for a child continuously throughout the night (Thevenin, 1976). One study involving 177 lactating women whose infants were between 1 and 2 months old were requested to complete a questionnaire related to four aspects of maternal behavior. These women were compared to nonlactating women, and the only measure of maternal behavior that they differed on was their willingness to share their bed with their infants (Newton, 1968).

Women are supposedly making choices about their decision to lactate. However, the previously mentioned sociocultural factors affect the lactation experience. A minority of women choose to breast-feed, and many of those have their efforts end in untimely weaning. Cole (1977) reports that of a sample of 332 middle class women in the Boston area, 57% intended to breast-feed, 42% to bottle-feed, and 1% were undecided. Yet 42% of those choosing to breast-feed ended up with early weaning (less than 1 month). The impact of overt and subtle sociocultural factors upon women desirous of breast-feeding cannot be dcnied.

Other variables have been associated with success or failure of women in breast-feeding, such as maternal age, parity, and educational level. One 1976 study of 102 nursing mothers reports that the older woman is more likely to initiate breast-feeding and to continue beyond the national United States norm of 12 weeks, usually weaning at 5 months. Younger women are more likely to bottle-feed, or if they do begin nursing, they are more likely to wean between 2 and 4 months. Previous breast-feeding experience of any length seems to be conducive to longer breast-feeding with subsequent children. There was a tendency for mothers to nurse their second child longer than they did the first child. One third of the women with a high school education or less chose not to breast-feed, compared to 16% of women with more education choosing not to breast-feed. When measured by years of formal schooling, women with the highest educational attainment were more likely than others to be nursing 6 months after childbirth (Auerbach, 1976a).

Anticipated feeding choice was significantly related to educational level, with more educated women selecting breast-feeding as their choice. Perhaps age, experience, and knowledge allow a woman to overcome the cultural norms and to successfully breast-feed despite a nonsupportive cultural milieu.

Support systems
Health care system

Many women decide how they wish to feed their children before they become pregnant; few appear to wait until the child's birth to decide. Guthrie and Guthrie (1979), in a study of fifty-five breast-feeding women, found that eighteen of the women decided to breast-feed prior to pregnancy, fourteen at the time of pregnancy, fifteen before the second trimester, four at a previous child's birth, and only four at the time of this child's birth. Information regarding alternatives must be given by providers as early as possible. An ideal method is to integrate information about lactation and breast-feeding as a part of all young children's education about their bodies. However, even if this is done it will take years to make an impact on childbearing women. Presently, it appears that early pregnancy is a good time to raise the question of feeding methods.

It is important for health care providers to be aware of what options a woman has selected for her birth experience, since the childbirth and immediate postpartum environment can be very influential in the establishment or defeat of a positive breast-feeding experience. Frequently, the activities of the health care providers reflect a negative attitude toward breast-feeding. Certain of these activities can negatively affect a woman's lactation and lead to untimely weaning. Breast-feeding is too often made a much more difficult experience than it needs to be (Newton and Newton, 1962).

Practices that can negatively influence the lactation experience can occur during labor. Barbiturate drugs, administered to a woman during labor, have been demonstrated to have an adverse affect on the child's suckling reflexes for a period of 4 to 5 days after birth (Haire, 1972). "Routine" episiotomies, common in the United States, can lead to or add to general discomfort after childbirth. One study demonstrated that the more "problems" that a woman experienced, the less likely she was to continue breast-feeding (Evans, 1969).

During hospital births, separation of the mother and child after birth and delay of the first breast-feeding remain common practice. The delay often involves a period up to 24 hours. Eppink (1969), in a study of thirty newborns, concluded that adjustment to breast-feeding was easier and more spontaneous when feeding was initiated early. Reasons frequently given for delaying the first feeding are excessive mucus and the possibility of a tracheoesophageal fistula. Since mucus does not generally interfere with nursing (Eppink, 1969) and the presence of tracheoesophageal fistula is rare (Applebaum,

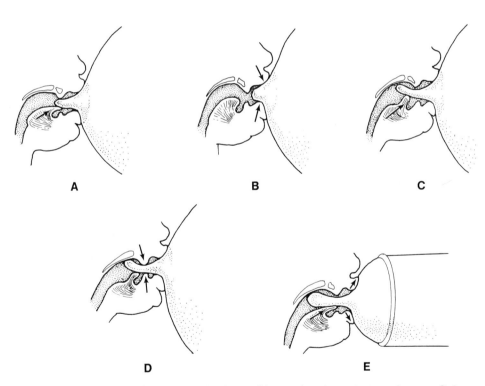

Fig. 25-11. Different mechanisms involved in suckling and sucking. **A,** Lips clamp in C shape at nipple-areolar junction, and cheek muscles are contracted. **B,** Tongue thrusts forward to grasp nipple and areola. **C,** Nipple is moved toward hard palate by backward pull of tongue, and areola is pulled into the mouth. **D,** Gums compress areola, with resultant milk flow against the hard palate. Milk flows from high pressure area in breast to negative pressure area in back of throat. **E,** Rubber nipple strikes soft palate. Tongue moves forward against the gum to control the flow. Lips form an O shape and cheek muscles are relaxed.

1970), perhaps a more supportive and sound approach would be to provide close surveillance during feeding periods rather than to delay feedings (Newton and Newton, 1948; 1962). Since evidence exists that (1) undrugged infants have strong sucking reflexes at birth, (2) early suckling is related to less engorgement and earlier appearance of milk, and (3) early breast-feeding leads to easier breast-feeding, it is time that specific alternatives developed for infants who may be at risk are used for those infants *only*. Practices needed to provide safe care for those women or infants at risk should not be indiscriminately applied to the care delivered to the majority.

Another common practice is the feeding of water and/or formula to newborns. When infants are bottle-fed formula or glucose water for any reason, stimulation to the breasts via suckling is reduced (Newton and Newton, 1962). There is no evidence to negate the safety of colostrum as the child's first food, but glucose water is still commonly recommended in its place. This is based on the assumptions that it "might" be aspirated and would be "safer" than colostrum. No data exists to support this contention.

Infants who are bottle-fed develop a measurably weaker sucking reflex by age 4 days. This again leads to less suckling stimulus for the breast. Feeding by a spoon (Newton and Newton, 1962) or an eyedropper (Eppink, 1969) can be a successful alternative when a *specific* problem necessitates this approach. Differences in suckling and sucking are considerable (Fig. 25-11). During breast-feeding, the child draws the mother's nipple into the mouth against the hard palate. The suction serves only to keep the nipple in place. The movement of the tongue in a posterior manner and subsequent squeezing of the end of the breast, areola, and nipple against the hard palate is the main element in suckling. When compared with bottle-feeding, there is more effort, especially jaw motion, involved in obtaining milk from the breast. Tongue movement and breathing patterns are also different (Jelliffe and Jelliffe, 1978).

Widely spaced feedings, such as every 4 hours, are based on experiences with cow's milk formulas and the convenience of schedules when infants are housed in a central nursery. This regimen restricts suckling stimulation of the breast, which leads to the vicious cycle of overdistention, poor let-down, pain, difficult nursing, and lactation failure. In the beginning it deprives the infant of colostrum and subsequently of adequate milk intake. It can lead to fluid and electrolyte imbalance in the child, or the need for supplemental feedings (Haire, 1972).

For the woman who has selected a hospital birth, it is essential that she be informed of the hospital's routine practices, and the effect, positive or negative, they may have on establishment of lactation. The care provided in many institutions is fragmented and invasive, and is not family oriented. A woman may find that the obstetrician has responsibility for caring for her breasts, whereas the pediatrician assumes total responsibility for directing her provision of infant nutrition. Frequently the nursing care is also divided according to the medical model; obstetric nurses care for the woman, while newborn nursery nurses care for the infant. Where these organizational patterns exists, the setting is ripe for conflicting advice, lack of support, and omissions of certain aspects of care. Many institutional practices were not derived for the convenience or support of an individual mother and her child, and such practices can frequently be based on assumptions that are irrelevant or obstructive to the woman who wishes to breast-feed.

Another indirect result of childbirth practices is that the model for lactating women is not set by other childbearing women, but by physicians (the vast majority of whom are men). In interviews with forty first-time breast-feeding women, it was found that 30% of the women had never seen a woman nurse her child (Hall, 1978). Obstetricians and nurses have considerable control over the situation in which breast-feeding is initiated, but as a rule they have limited understanding of the process and few solutions to common problems encountered by women during this period. Some may lack the desire to take the necessary time and effort to problem-solve with women (Brack, 1975).

In addition to being separated from other breast-feeding mothers, women are also often separated from or have limited access to their family or significant others during the immediate postpartum period. The rationale provided for restricted visitation is usually prevention of infections, yet there is evidence that the major sources of contaminants to newborns are nursery and hospital personnel (Haire, 1972).

Rooming-in arrangements can facilitate the lactation process. Cole (1977) found that two thirds of the 151 women who were still breast-feeding at 3 months had chosen rooming-in, whereas more than half of the group who were no longer breast-feeding their infants had utilized a central nursery. In many hospitals rooming-in is permitted only if there is a private room available, if the woman can pay, and only if the woman keeps her child with her all the time. As one nurse states, "It seems more like punishment rather than a pleasant learning opportunity" (Lawson, 1976).

The woman who knows what facilities are available in the hospital she has selected before delivery has a better chance of establishing, through negotiation or demand, the situation that is best for her and her child, within the constraint of the setting. It is unfortunate that many hospitals still fail to provide an environment conductive to breast-feeding; too many maintain practices that can hinder and discourage, if not defeat, a mother who wants to breast-feed her baby.

The woman who is planning on breast-feeding her child needs, from the moment of birth, special health care for herself and her infant. However, there appears to be a lack of understanding or a misunderstanding of the significance this experience can have for a woman and her child (Rees, 1976). As one physician has stated, "The degree of concern of the medical profession might be described as inversely proportional to the dimension of the problem." This physician questions whether the (primarily male) physicians' response would be the same in an analogous situation: "Would anybody suggest, seriously, that males abstain from intercourse, bind themselves, take drugs to relieve congestion, or be mechanically relieved routinely, and that it would be as good?" (Brack, 1975).

Nurses, who have a variety of potential roles in supporting the breast-feeding woman, also may reflect cultural bias against breast-feeding. There is limited information in many maternity nursing texts about breast-feeding and nursing (Estok, 1973), and information that is not possessed cannot be transmitted to consumers for their use.

Estok (1973), in a study of twenty-nine maternity nurses, reported the general inability of the nurses to identify common problems mothers have with breast-feeding after discharge from the hospital. Those nurses who definitely favored breast-feeding were more able to identify the specified problems, but overall twenty-five of the twenty-nine nurses identified no more than two of the seven given problems. Lawson (1976), in a survey of forty women who had given birth in a hospital, found that nineteen of the women perceived the nurses as helpful, whereas twenty-one women had negative feelings about the nursing staff.

Hall (1978) studied forty-nine first-time lactating women. These women were divided into two experimental groups and one control group. The control group received routine hospital care, the second group received routine hospital care plus teaching, and the third group received routine hospital care plus teaching and nursing support. All women in the study had expressed a desire to nurse until at least 6 weeks postpartum. Approximately half of the control group and the teaching group were still nursing at 6 weeks, whereas 80% of the group that received teaching plus support were still nursing. All the women in the teaching and support group and half of those in the teaching only group listed the researcher as the most helpful person in the hospital. Seventy percent of these women expressed disappointment in the hospital nurses, feeling they could have offered more help, especially during the first

breast-feeding experience. Whitley (1978), in a follow-up survey of thirty-four breast-feeding women, identified the physicians and nurses as the most frequently consulted resources. However, 67% of these women felt that the advice given by the nurses was inadequate.

In a study of 1124 women, Ladas (1970) demonstrated that individual support for the nursing woman from persons she perceives as significant (i.e., husband, mother, friends) was highly related to the successful outcome of breast-feeding. Other variables highly related to positive outcomes were group support and information. Information combined with support related more highly to outcome than either information or support alone. Conflict in individual support was not significantly related to outcome; that is, the breast-feeding behavior of a woman was not significantly affected if she belonged to a group that opposed breast-feeding, as long as she also belonged to one that favored breast-feeding. Causes of early weaning included maternal problems (not enough milk, sore nipples, or breast abscess) and what the women perceived as interventions by the physicians and/or hospital (medications given to end milk secretion, medications given that were transmitted in unsafe amounts in breast milk, supplementary bottles given in the nursery, baby too tired from crying to suck). Lack of information was significantly related to untimely weaning regardless of reason given for the weaning.

Evans and associates (1969) studied the needs of fifty-two breast-feeding women for a 6-month period. Approximately 40% of the women in the study were successful at breast-feeding and approximately 60% were unsuccessful. Discomforts expressed by all women were categorized into expected versus unexpected discomforts and then were correlated with successful or unsuccessful breast-feeding. Expected discomforts were identified as episiotomy, sore nipples, engorgement, leaking, let-down, and after-pains. Unexpected discomforts were cracked nipples, infected breasts, retention catheters, and hemorrhoids. Among successful women approximately 90% of the discomforts were expected; among unsuccessful women approximately 75% were expected. Discomforts did not appear to be as influential in discouraging breast-feeding women if they were anticipated.

Eighty-seven women completed questionnaires in one retrospective study (Brack, 1975). Fifty-eight of these women had attempted breast-feeding. Women who breast-fed all children or breast-fed later ones successfully (approximately 55%) were categorized as a "nursing" population. Those who did not breast-feed or breast-fed with little success were categorized as "nonnursing." Data from this study suggest that support from the physician, nurses, experienced women, and the woman's husband is related to successful breast-feeding, as is the opportunity for observing other women breast-feeding.

Physicians' attitudes also appear to have a strong influence on supporting or discouraging a woman's attempts at maintaining lactation (Newton, 1968). Halpen and associates (1972) in a study of 1753 children seen by eleven pediatricians in the Dallas, Texas area reported that an increased number of women breast-fed their children when the pediatrician felt positive toward breast-feeding.

Many obstetricians are either neutral or negative about breast-feeding (Countryman, 1973). They appear to be predisposed to ask the woman what she plans to do with regard to feeding her infant without providing data about the present level of knowledge of advantages and disadvantages of each method (Weichert, 1975). Physicians are regarded as "experts" on infant feeding although their education equips them to handle illness and pathology and rarely to deal with issues of breast-feeding unless the woman experiences complications such as mastitis (Brack, 1975). Male physicians have a tendency to formulate their attitudes toward breast-feeding as a result of their wives' experiences (Auerbach, 1976b). In a 1976 study of forty women who breast-fed for 1 or more months, thirty of the women reported that their obstetricians were not supportive or helpful, while ten perceived them as supportive (Lawson, 1976). Cole (1977) asked 151 breast-feeding women to select sources of "very helpful information about breast-feeding" from a checklist of fourteen possible sources. Only one third of the new mothers indicated that helpful information was supplied by the hospital nurses. However, of this third of the population, 79% were still breast-feeding at the time of the survey, 3 months after childbirth. The pediatrician's role was also described in relation to the discontinuation of breast-feeding. The third most common reason for ending breast-feeding was the "baby's doctor told me to stop." Thus it appears that health care personnel can provide support and facilitate a woman's lactation; specific interventions need further study.

Fathers

Supportive partners appear to be a significant factor for women who wish to breast-feed (Brack, 1975). There is general acceptance of the assumption that a supportive father can greatly influence a woman's success, and can just as significantly undermine her efforts. Bishop and Bishop (1978) list fifteen different ways a father can support a woman's attempt to breast-feed, and fathers can and have found breast-feeding a warm and enriching experience.

One distressing comment frequently made, however, is that an important disadvantage to breast-feeding is that the father cannot do it (Friedman, 1978)! It would seem unnecessary for women who want to breast-feed to deny themselves this opportunity because their partner cannot replicate the specific behavior. If this argument were carried to the extreme, a woman would also choose not to bear and give birth to a child in the first place, since her partner cannot replicate this behavior either.

Group support systems

The largest well-organized group support system available to both lactating women and health care providers is La Leche League International. This organization was founded in 1956 by a small group of women in Illinois, based on the assumption that women in the United States needed a formal organization to provide them with support and information (Knafl, 1976). The organization has a medical board of consultants, which approves the League's printed medical resources (La Leche, 1976). The League has a distinctive approach to lactation: it supports a more primolactic style, including early and demand feeding, exclusive feeding with breast milk for 4 to 6 months, and a longer duration of nursing with gradual, cooperative weaning (Meara, 1976).

Knafl (1976) found that women managed their lactation experiences in a very different manner after joining the League. Compared to the women's previous experiences breast-feeding, there was a 43% increase in demand feeding, a 93% increase in maintaining breast-feeding for 4 months or longer without solids or supplement, an 85% increase in gradual weaning, an 81% increase in duration of nursing past 9 months, and a 40% increase in early initial breast-feeding. Women who are League members attest to the difference this organization makes in assisting them to have a satisfying and successful experience (Knafl, 1976).

One problem often encountered that can be mitigated is a conflicting perspective on lactation between the League and health care providers. In interviews with nineteen obstetric nurses, Knafl (1951) documented a very common phenomenon of extremely negative attitudes toward La Leche League. Twelve of the eighteen nurses categorized La Leche League women as fanatics. They believed that the League overemphasized the importance of breast-feeding and that this was harmful. They had conflicting views with every aspect of lactation promoted by the League.

The League has a well-defined approach to lactation and a very strong underlying philosophy about which roles are the most important and desirable roles for women. There is, obviously, more than one approach to the management of lactation and there are many varied philosophies concerning women's options. While each woman's beliefs and values may not reflect those of the League, it remains the largest and most effective group support system available to a woman who desires to maintain lactation. Their vast knowledge and ready support are available to any woman who wishes them.

THE LACTATION EXPERIENCE

An interactional mode of describing the process of lactation has been advocated by Avery (1977). She depicts five phases of lactation, biekostal, oscular, nostalgic, and weaning. During each of the phases, women have needs, problems, and concerns that can be anticipated by informed health care providers.

Phases of lactation

Lactory phase

The lactory phase of breast-feeding is the period when all of the infant's nutritional needs are provided by breast milk. This can incorporate up to the first 6 months of a child's life. The woman has many varied needs during this phase. She needs a knowledge base of the anatomy and physiology of lactation. She needs to be aware of her increased nutritional needs, and she needs to be aware of the previously discussed cultural beliefs and values that may affect her "beginning" phase. She will need to know what type of support or opposition she can expect from the significant persons in her life and from health care providers. She will need to know how to handle or seek support to manage any problems that may arise with lactation. These needs are addressed throughout this chapter.

Biekostal phase

The term "biekostal" is derived from "bie kost," which is a noun used to refer to foods other than milk. The biekostal nutritional phase of nursing is the phase when foods other than breast milk are introduced, but breast milk is still a major source of nutrition. Suckling is beginning to serve nonnutritive, socializing functions (Avery, 1977).

There is no need for the woman to add any food to the breast-fed infant's diet for about the first 6 months (La Leche, 1963). There is no evidence that early feeding of solids is necessary or helpful, and it may lead to problems. A child full with solids nurses less well at the breast, which can lead to interference with established lactation. The child who is fed solids at an early age is ingesting a nutritional substance inferior to breast milk.

At some period around 6 months of age the infant may show an increased demand for breast-feeding and this demand continues despite more frequent nursings. This probably indicates a readiness for solids. Increased demands before age 6 months may result from other causes (i.e., a cold, increased tension in the mother, and so on) (La Leche, 1963).

An infant who has been suckling fed exclusively finds the first few attempts at spoon feeding a bit awkward, since spoon-feeding requires mouth and tongue actions different from suckling. A demitasse or small, long-handled feeding spoon is useful. At 6 months many infants can sit if well supported in a highchair, but a child seat or the mother's lap can be used.

It is easier to breast-feed the child prior to attempting spoon feedings. This accomplishes a dual purpose: it keeps the woman's milk supply up, and it makes the baby more malleable and cooperative in trying a new experience. Ravenous hunger interferes with the infant's ability to try something new.

Some women skip much of the spoon-feeding and move directly to finger foods for their babies. Since hand-to-mouth coordination has usually developed by this time, most babies are automatically putting everything in their mouths. Early finger foods should be hypoallergenic. Pieces of banana, pared apples, and pears are good beginners. Later, cubes of Cheddar or Swiss cheese, slices of cooked carrots, cooked peas and green beans, crusts of whole wheat bread, pieces of cooked hamburger, and pieces of cooked flaked fish make excellent finger foods (Eiger and Olds, 1972).

Commercially prepared baby foods are not necessary, are costly, and have a high water content. They often contain ingredients not needed by a child such as salt, sugar, and starchy thickener. Baby foods are easily prepared in a blender or inexpensive small food grinder. However, an assessment should be made of the woman's situation. If she hates to cook and no one else in the home likes this task either, it may be much more appropriate to use commercially prepared foods. When using food from jars, the woman should hear a "pop" when she opens the jar. The contents should be discarded if no "pop" is heard, because it may indicate that the seal has been broken. Also, unless the baby can consume the entire contents of the jar, the food should be transferred to another dish for feeding, since saliva transported back to the jar from the spoon will cause spoilage.

New foods should be introduced one at a time to allow identification of problem foods. A week between each new addition is a conservative recommendation (La Leche, 1963).

One problem women may experience during this phase is biting. This generally coincides with the onset of teething and can be very painful for the mother. The baby who is suckling properly cannot bite, and thus the biting generally occurs at the end of feedings (Eiger and Olds, 1972). Many women have found that saying "no" firmly and removing the infant from the breast and ending that feeding will rapidly eliminate the biting.

Oscular phase

During the oscular behavioral phase breast milk assumes a minor role in nutrition and suckling occurs primarily as a means of mother/infant interaction. The term "oscular" is recommended to replace "toddler nursing" due to the lack of specificity of that term. It is during the end of this phase and the entire next phase when strong cultural taboos affect the nursing woman. Many arguments, none of which has been substantiated, begin to be presented to women during this phase to encourage them to cease and desist nursing. The woman is accused of prolonging the nursing situation either for her own emotional and sexual needs or because this is her last child. She may be accused of using nursing in place of giving the child other forms of attention, or of making her child too dependent upon her (Avery, 1977). (These arguments have also been forcefully and equally applied against women who lactate past 3 months, 6 months, 9 months, 1 year, or 2 years of age.) The acceptable age limit for allowing children to suckle is highly dependent upon the cultural attitudes and beliefs of the person presenting the argument (Avery, 1977). A frequently offered comment to women who are in this phase of lactation is that the practice is "obscene."

One result of all the negative stereotypes that accompany nursing a baby at this phase is a phenomenon labeled "subrosa" or "closet nursing," i.e. the nursing behaviors are carefully shielded from outsiders. Women have been coerced into keeping some aspects of their nursing experience from physicians, nurses, family, friends, society in general, and even disapproving partners. Closet nursing presents one solution to the problem lactating women have when trying to meet their own and their child's needs, as well as outwardly comply with expected standards of behavior (Avery, 1977).

Avery (1977) conducted a pilot survey on weaning by surveying two groups of women who appeared to demonstrate different styles of lactation. The forty-five women in one group were participants at a La Leche League International convention, and were thought to be practicing a primolactic style of lactation. Sixty percent of the women in this group kept some aspect of their lactation secret. Reasons for secrecy included fear of lack of understanding, fear of isolation, fear of loss of self-esteem, and fear of punishment. Of all the children in this group, 64% were nursed over 1 year, 36% over 2 years, 18% over 3 years, and 10% over 4 years. The thirty-four women in the second group were receiving well-child or minor outpatient treatment in a medical clinic, and were thought to be practicing a more mimelactic style of lactation. Of these thirty-four women, only 6% kept any aspect of their lactation secret. Forty-four percent of the children were weaned before age 3 months, and most of these weanings occurred during the first month. Three children in this group were nursed longer than 1 year, two for 18 months, and one for 22 months. Avery proposed that because these women were practicing the more culturally accepted mimelactic lactation style they had little need to hide their nursing behaviors.

Nostalgic phase

During the nostalgic phase, the child is aware that suckling will soon end. This is a time of decision-making for the child regarding ending or continuing suckling (Avery, 1977). This phase includes nursing a preschool or older child. All the arguments and criticisms directed toward women in the oscular phase increase exponentially in the nostalgic phase. One of the more positive aspects of this phase is that the child is verbally interactive, and as weaning approaches, verbal communication can smoothe the way for both the mother and her child (Kadushin, 1977).

Weaning

Weaning is the end of the process of lactation—the end of suckling. As defined here, it specifically refers to the change in state of being nursed to no longer being nursed; the age or date when suckling ceases. Weaning can be of two general types, behavioral or "environmental." One behavioral type of weaning is "mother-led weaning," in which suckling ends as a result of the mother's desire to do so. "Child-led weaning," is the end of suckling as a result of the child's desire.

Weaning can be gradual or abrupt. In nearly all instances of mother- or child-led weaning, it is best done gradually. Sometimes in environmental weaning, abruptness is essential, but even here some adjustments can usually provide for some gradualness in the process. Despite recommendations to the contrary, there is no known "right" age to wean a child. Raphael (1973) notes that the time for weaning in Western societies coincides with attitudes of when a child is no longer a "baby," and the child begins to look unattractive to adults suckling at the breast.

Environmental weaning. Environmental, or untimely, weaning occurs when suckling is stopped because of factors that are out of the control of either the child or the mother, and before either is ready for the experience to end. This can occur because of serious illness of the mother or other emergency situations (Eiger and Olds, 1972). There is little scientific study about the impact of untimely weaning or its effects on the woman and her child, but there is some beginning interest in considering the area (Amsel, 1977). Individual women have reported that untimely weaning can be experienced very much as a loss, with resultant grief and grieving before resolution (Dascalos, 1977).

Abrupt weaning. Abrupt weaning has been described as "cold turkey." This type of weaning is undesirable. In addition to the possible impact of abrupt weaning on the emotional state of the mother and child, it induces a considerable amount of biophysical distress in the woman who has successfully established lactation. Breasts become engorged and more susceptible to mastitis and abscess formation. If abrupt weaning is unavoidable, the woman can obtain some relief from manual expression and application of compresses; hormonal preparations to decrease milk secretion may be indicated.

Mother-led weaning. The primary initiating factor in mother-led weaning is a need on the woman's part to terminate lactation. If a woman begins to perceive breast-feeding as a burden, begins to feel restricted by the process, or experiences some other negative feelings about situation, perhaps it is time for her to consider weaning. No matter what the child's age, if the mother is resentful about nursing the situation is certainly less than ideal. Mother-led weaning can be done gradually. Usually the first feeding to eliminate is the one in which the child has the least interest. A bottle or cup can be substituted, depending upon the child's age and interests. After 2 or more weeks, the next feeding can be eliminated in the same manner, until the woman is no longer nursing (Eiger and Olds, 1972; La Leche, 1963). Flexibility is a key concept, and special needs may temporarily interfere with the scheduled plan. It is important that feedings are not omitted during times of upheaval or stress (Parsons, 1978).

Child-led weaning. Child-led weaning refers to weaning that is done because of the child's desire to do so. As the child moves more and more to solid foods, she or he may lose interest in one feeding or another. The mother, responsive to the child's communication, just skips that nursing. She does not refuse the breast; she just does not offer it at that time unless the child changes her or his mind or the breasts are uncomfortably full. This process is very gradually repeated, taking cues from the child (La Leche, 1963). Some women wean so gradually that one day they realize that they have not nursed for a week or more—and for all intents and purposes their child is weaned.

Nutritional needs of lactating women

One crucial area of concern to the lactating woman is nutrition. Studies of the nutritional needs of lactating women and the effects of maternal nutrition on milk supply and quality have been addressed, but results have been fraught with methodologic difficulties. The standards recommended for dietary allowances for lactating women (National Academy of Sciences, 1974) are based on ideals, and are not directly transferrable to an individual woman's situation (E. Jelliffe, 1976). Studies of breast milk supply are difficult because there is no mechanism for gathering breast milk that is equivalent to the normal method (i.e., the child's suckling). Alternate techniques, whether by machine or manual expression, cannot be directly equated with the suckling process. In addition, environmental and psychosocial stress are known to inhibit the let-down reflex, and research designs to measure quantities of breast milk produced fre-

quently introduce stress of both types. Results of analyses of quality of breast milk are known to be influenced by the analytic technique used. It is also impossible to obtain a "representative" sample of human milk, because of diurnal variations in volume and composition, variations that occur during a single feeding, and seasonal variations in human breast milk (Jelliffe and Jelliffe, 1978).

The physiologic effects of lactation upon the woman will be partially dependent upon her nutritional state. Lactation requires even more energy than pregnancy, and in well-nourished women fat is stored during pregnancy to provide some of the energy needed for milk production. The well-nourished woman produces approximately 700 to 800 ml of breast milk per day (Wray, 1978). The energy obtained from maternal fat stores can subsidize lactation production energy requirements for 3 to 4 months (Jelliffe and Jelliffe, 1978). When the woman continues lactation past the time when the fat storage provides her with supplemental energy for the process, she will need to increase her calorie intake by 200 to 300 calories per day. A woman who gives birth to twins will deplete her reserve stores more rapidly, and when they are gone her daily supplemental energy needs will double (Worthington et al., 1977).

Lactating women need to take additional food to meet their energy requirements. According to our present knowledge, specific nutrients are needed by the lactating woman for the first 3 to 4 months (see Chapter 21). Specific nutritional components of breast milk have been studied, and some conclusions relating to the woman's intake of these have been reached. Caloric needs of the lactating woman include those she would normally need, plus those needed for the process of milk production and those needed in the milk itself. Present recommended allowances for the lactating woman is an additional 500 calories per day above the normal recommended intake. This recommendation is based upon the assumption that a fat store of 0.3 to 0.5 kg is present in the well-nourished woman who has given birth and which subsidizes lactation energy needs at a rate of 300 calories per day. The caloric content of breast milk itself is derived primarily from fat, lactose, and possibly protein. There is a good deal of variation in the calorie content of breast milk in well-nourished lactating women (Jelliffe and Jelliffe, 1978).

The protein needs of lactating women are currently recommended to be 20 Gm per day over the normal recommended intake (RDA, 1974). The protein content of breast milk does not appear to be appreciably affected by deficits in the woman's diet.

Fat, the main source of calories for the child in breast milk, also contains the fat-soluble vitamins, especially vitamin A. Fats are the source of fatty acids needed for central nervous system development. In well-nourished women the fat composition of milk resembles the fatty acid composition of the diet. Inadequately nourished women produce breast milk in which the fats in the milk resemble the same composition as human fat, mobilized from maternal stores. Fat content also appears to vary in the same woman, being higher in the morning and lower in the evening (Jelliffe and Jelliffe, 1978). The main influence on the fatty acid composition of the breast milk is carbohydrate intake (E. Jelliffe, 1976).

Lactose content is generally constant in the well-nourished lactating woman's breast milk, and does not appear to alter significantly with inadequate nutritional intake.

There is an additional recommended daily intake of several vitamins for lactating women, including vitamins A, B_{12}, C, thiamine, and riboflavin. Dietary inadequacy of these particular vitamins is reflected in breast milk, and supplementing the woman's diet will subsequently increase the amounts seen in breast milk (E. Jelliffe, 1976; Jelliffe and Jelliffe, 1978).

Lactation induces metabolism of body fats, even if the woman's food intake exceeds what is recommended for lactation (Appel and King, 1979). Lactation can thus be considered to have a slimming effect after childbirth in the well-nourished woman (Jelliffe and Jelliffe, 1978). The lactating woman should be aware that dieting during lactation may affect the quantity of her milk and the duration of lactation. The usual slow and desirable rate of weight loss after childbirth does not coincide with popular ideals of immediate return to prepregnancy body weight. The tremendous pressure in this culture to be thin may be counterproductive to the woman's desire to lactate.

Inadequate nutrition can affect three parameters of lactation: the quality of milk produced, the quantity of milk produced, and the duration of milk production. The quality of breast milk is the least sensitive of these factors to inadequate maternal nutrition, but is affected in serious cases of inadequate nutrition (Wray, 1978). Other influential factors affecting the quality of breast milk produced by the inadequately nourished woman are her previous nutritional status and the severity and length of her dietary inadequacies (Jelliffe and Jelliffe, 1978). Except in severe cases, maternal tissue depletion will provide the energy needed for lactation (Appel and King, 1979). The quantity of breast milk production is more sensitive to inadequate maternal nutrition, as is the duration of lactation (Wray, 1978). There is evidence that supplementing a nutritionally inadequate diet can improve both the quality and quantity of breast milk produced (E. Jelliffe, 1976).

Skill needs—the art of breast-feeding

The woman who is lactating for the first time will need to develop some basic breast-feeding skills. One of the most elementary things she must discover are positions that allow her and the child comfortable breast-feeding periods. Pillows are invaluable in this exploratory process. When sitting, whether in a chair or bed, the child can be placed on a pillow in the woman's lap (Fig. 25-12).

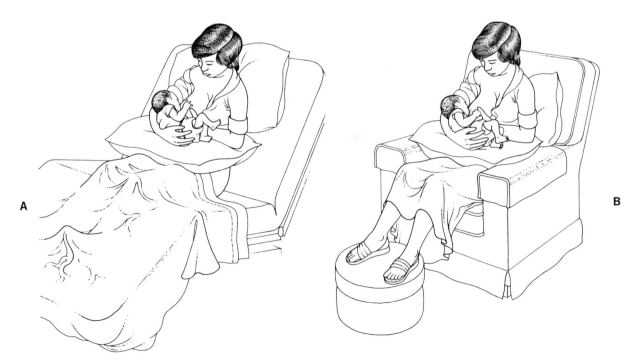

Fig. 25-12. A, Nursing in sitting position. **B,** Modified sitting position.

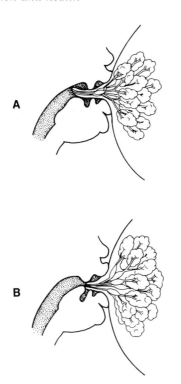

Fig. 25-13. A, Proper grasp of areola and nipple, **B,** Improper grasp of nipple.

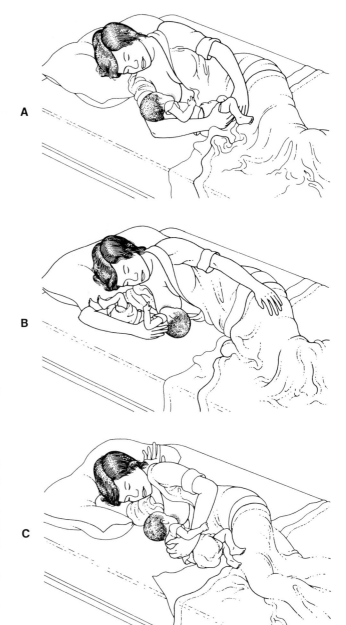

Fig. 25-14. Side-lying positions for breast feeding. **A,** Usual side-lying position. **B,** Alternate side-lying position. **C,** Nursing from both breasts while in one side-lying position by rolling body to one side.

This avoids having the woman slump over to reach the infant or strain her back, and also facilitates the infant's grasping the areola rather than the nipple (Fig. 25-13). The woman can experiment with several side-lying positions (Fig. 25-14), and some will need to be tried several times before the woman can assess her comfort with them.

Techniques for assisting the infant to properly grasp the breast need to be shared with the woman. The rooting reflex can be put to good advantage in the breast-feeding situation if the woman is aware of its presence. She should lightly touch the corner of the baby's mouth with her nipple, which will cause the infant to automatically move toward the nipple. Then the woman can gently bring the infant closer, and allow her or him to grasp the areolar area of the nipple. The nurse should be cautioned not to attempt to open the infant's mouth by putting pressure on both cheeks. If both sides of the face are simultaneously touched, the infant may become confused and frantic. The baby's head should never be pushed onto the breast, since this may cause obstruction of the nostrils by the mother's breast, and the baby may panic (Eiger and Olds, 1972). If the infant grasps only the nipple, the mother should be assisted to break the suction by inserting her finger at the corner of the baby's mouth (Fig. 25-15). The suction should always be broken before removing the child from the breast for any

reason, since this will avoid undue trauma and decrease nipple soreness (Applebaum, 1975).

In the early lactory phase, or when the woman has large or overfilled breasts, it is very helpful to compress the breast by placing the nipple and areola between the second and third forefingers (or thumb and forefinger) and compressing the breast toward the chest wall (Fig. 25-16). This facilitates proper grasp for the infant by projecting the nipple. It also helps maintain an airspace (Applebaum, 1975). Expressing some milk manually can also help this situation.

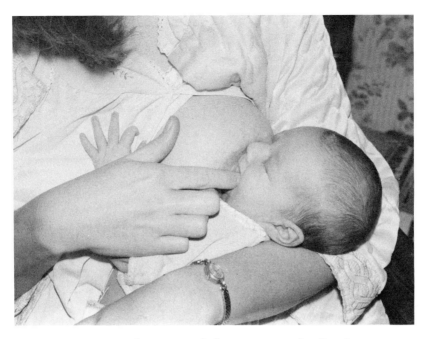

Fig. 25-15. Breaking suction before removing infant from breast.

Frequency and duration of feedings

The issue of frequency and duration of feedings seems to provoke myriad rules and regulations, each one differing from the other, and all without much substantive data to back up the arguments. Generally, breast milk is very easily digested by newborns, and most newborns indicate a need for feeding every 2 to 3 hours around the clock. There may be a longer stretch between feedings, but not always. A woman who chooses to practice a primolactic style of lactation may wish to satisfy not only her child's nutritional needs, but also the suckling needs. If such is her choice, then her infant may spend a good part of any 24 hours at her breast. If a woman does not wish to do this, she should remember the general 2- to 3-hour digestion period, and plan accordingly. A breast-fed infant *cannot* function on the popular 4-hour schedule. This schedule was initiated to meet the needs of formula-fed infants and is based on an entirely different situation.

Duration of feedings is a much discussed issue in our schedule-oriented culture. *After* the let-down (and this sometimes takes several minutes of suckling at first) most children can empty a breast in 10 minutes (La Leche, 1963; Pryor, 1973). Knowing this, the woman can adjust the suckling time to meet her and her child's individual needs.

"Feeding styles" of infants

It helps women to know that infants have very individual personalities and very different eating styles. Barnes (1953) delightfully categorizes some eating styles: "Bar-

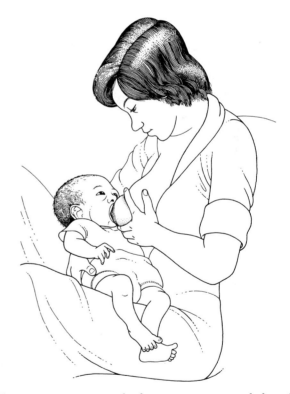

Fig. 25-16. Positioning the breast to prevent occluding the child's nostrils.

racudas" nurse vigorously and energetically when put to the breast. "Procrastinators" do not indulge themselves until the fourth or fifth postpartum day. They demonstrate no particular interest or ability in suckling during the first few days, but once they begin, they generally do well. Prodding and pushing are ineffectual! "Gourmets" or "mouthers" are infants who characteristically mouth the nipple, taste a bit, smack their lips, and generally approach the whole business with great delicacy. Once they indulge, however, they do quite well. They refuse to be rushed! "Resters" will suckle and rest, suckle and rest, suckle and rest. Breast-feeding these infants takes a good deal of time. They, also, refuse to be rushed.

Some mention needs to be given to the stoic child—the one who seldom indicates a need for feeding. If newborns are not eating approximately eight to ten times in 24 hours, the mother may have to periodically breast-feed her infant without waiting for his cry.

All children do not fall into these groups, and many combine characteristics of several styles. The woman can identify her baby's feeding style and try to meet his or her special needs. Some modifications may need to be made if the child's style and the woman's needs are highly incompatible. A child who wishes to suckle with no pattern and at frequent intervals may drive a highly organized woman to the brink, whereas other women may enjoy this type of interaction. Based upon a 2- to 3-hour recurring need to be fed, some scheduling can be introduced into the process if a woman feels the need for it.

Stools

The bowel movements of the breast-fed infant are usually quite different from those of formula-fed infants, and the lactating woman needs a reference point before her child's birth to avoid unnecessary concern. The newborn's first stools are dark green and are called meconium stools. These stools have been formed from cast-off cells from the liver, pancreas, and gallbladder (Eiger and Olds, 1972). Once the meconium stools have been passed, the stools range from a golden-yellow to a yellow-green or brownish color. The odor is mild and not unpleasant. The consistency is generally loose, and totally breast-fed children do not suffer from constipation. The amount and frequency of stools are not only highly variable among children, but also within the same child. At first it is not uncommon to have a bowel movement with every diaper change; later the child may not have a stool for as long as a week and still be perfectly normal. Many times the bowel movement on the diaper is only a stain (La Leche, 1963). Most women will not be aware of these patterns if this is the first child they have breast-fed, and may interpret these normal stools as abnormal. This is because most women learn what the usual pattern is for formula-fed children, which is not the same as that for breast-fed infants.

Indicators of sufficient infant nutrition

In our culture there seems to be a need to objectively measure everything. This leaves the breast-feeding woman at some disadvantage, since she cannot measure in ounces how much her child has consumed. However, the woman can be fairly objective in assessing the adequacy of her child's intake if she is giving only breast milk. The nurse should encourage her to simply be aware of the number of times per day the infant's diaper is wet, the concentration of the urine, and the number of bowel movements the child has. This will give her a good rough estimate of her child's intake. Six or more wet diapers a day with pale yellow urine and regular bowel movements (several small or infrequent larger ones) indicate sufficient intake (Eiger and Olds, 1972).

Weight gain is another indicator of sufficient intake. The average breast-fed infant gains from 4 to 6 oz a week during the first month, and from 6 to 8 oz a week during the next 3 months. However, this is highly variable (Eiger and Olds, 1972).

All children, especially during the first few months, experience growth spurts. At these times they have increased needs for breast milk, and generally let it be known. Increasing suckling over a 48 hour period will increase the supply enough to meet their increased needs (La Leche, 1963).

Woman's need for rest

One of the greatest foes of the woman who wants to breast-feed, especially in the early lactory phase, is fatigue. Regardless of what the woman's previous life-style and work roles were, she is now going to have to recuperate from childbearing, establish some style of parental role with her child, readjust her roles with other family members, and establish lactation. All this cannot be done without some modification of her previous life-style and schedule. Each woman must decide what her priorities are to be, but if breast-feeding is to be one of them, she needs to be aware of how easily fatigue can undermine her goals. Each woman will have varying needs for rest, but all will have increased needs at this time (Eiger and Olds, 1972; La Leche, 1963; Pryor, 1973). Raphael (1973) speaks of *doulas*, persons who surround, interact with, and aid a woman at any time within the perinatal period. Thus a doula can help protect a woman from many pressures and disturbances that may interfere with lactation. Almost anyone who is supportive and motivated can act in the doula role, allowing the woman a protected period in which to establish lactation.

SPECIAL PROBLEMS

Many women find themselves confronted with special problems during lactation. The following section describes some of these problems with suggestions for alleviating them.

After-pains

Women experience after-pains during the first few days of the lactory phase when the child is suckling. These pains can vary in intensity, but generally are stronger after a woman's second birth and with subsequent births. The pains may feel similar to menstrual cramps or mild labor contractions. The woman should be told about the pains before they occur so that she will realize they are normal. The nurse should explain that they are a sign that the uterus is contracting well and that the let-down reflex is functioning. Temporary use of analgesics can be helpful.

Leaking breasts

Leaking milk can be a bothersome problem to some women during the lactory phase. Some women never experience it, but others do and in varying degrees. It is very common to leak from one nipple while the child is suckling at the other. This usually presents no problem at home; a clean cloth can catch the drops. Some women leak quite a bit at night and will wake up drenched. This may be eliminated by more frequent nightfeedings; some women simply sleep over an absorbant towel. When a woman is away from home or fully clothed, leaking may be a problem. However clean handkerchiefs folded in squares or clean, cut diapers make excellent absorbant pads when tucked inside the bra. There are also commercial nursing pads available. The woman should not use anything with a plastic liner, since plastic frequently leads to retention of moisture and sore nipples. Many women experience the let-down reflex when thinking about their child or when hearing a baby cry. When the woman does not wish leaking to occur, she can press her palms or forearms against her nipples, and in a minute or two the let-down sensation will disappear and no more milk will drip from the breasts.

Engorgement

Engorgement can be an extremely painful, frustrating, and potentially defeating condition for the lactating woman. It is also thought to be a predisposing factor in nipple fissures and breast abscesses. Newton and Newton (1951), in a study of forty-seven women, demonstrated that breast engorgement was directly related to milk retention. Such milk retention (which in our culture generally occurs on days 3 to 5 of the puerperium), if unrelieved, can lead to secondary vascular and lymphatic stasis. The milk retention, in turn, is thought to occur because of a failure of the milk let-down reflex, primarily caused by restrictions on suckling from shortly after birth onward (Newton and Newton, 1951, 1962; Applebaum, 1975).

Engorgement should be treated as soon as it is observed, since severe engorgement is very difficult to treat rapidly or adequately. The woman who has breast engorgement should nurse more frequently and for longer periods. As milk residual is removed, the myoepithelial cells contract against decreased resistance of interconnective tissue, creating a stronger let-down. Blood supply to myoepithelial tissue improves with the decompression phenomenon. An increasingly efficient let-down reflex leads to a still further decrease in milk residual and milk tension, until milk tension normalizes as engorgement subsides (Applebaum, 1970).

Engorgement causes the nipple areolar junction, which normally is concave, to become convex. This results in the infant grasping the inverted nipple, causing nipple soreness and damage, and is very frustrating to the infant (Fig. 25-17).

To alleviate this situation the mother can manually express a small amount of milk with her thumb and forefinger (see Fig. 25-8). Manual expression can soften the areola, allowing the nipple to return to a more natural concave configuration, which the child can then get into his mouth so that the milk can be obtained (Applebaum, 1975). Ice applied to the nipples can help make them erect and can be soothing (Countryman, 1977). After nursing, the woman can also do breast massage and manual expression to remove any remaining milk from her breasts if she still feels engorged or if the child is suckling poorly. Electric breast pumps are useful for women

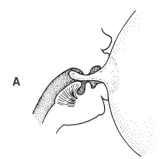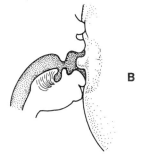

Fig. 25-17. A, Normal breast with child's lips around areola. **B,** Engorged breast with convex nipple-areolar junction. Child grasps nipple, causing increased nipple pain and damage.

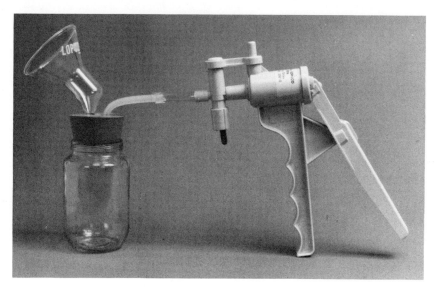

Fig. 25-18. The Loyd-B-Pump.

whose milk tension is elevated to a point that manual expression and massage are too painful to perform, but they are expensive and frequently are available only in the hospital. Local chapters of the La Leche League will often have a breast pump available for loan, but these may not always be available for an individual woman when she needs it. Most hand pumps can cause breast and nipple damage as a result of strong pressure and should be avoided (Applebaum, 1970; Grassley and Davis, 1978). One acceptable and reasonably accessible hand pump (Fig. 25-18) is called the Loyd-B-Pump.* Another slightly less expensive hand pump, called a Breast Milking Feeding Unit,† has also been successfully used by lactating women. Electric or manual breast pumps of acceptable design that do not induce nipple pain or damage and work effectively may be used by women in a variety of situations.

The application of heat using warm, wet towels, or taking warm showers is purported to facilitate relief of engorgement through vasodilation (Eiger and Olds, 1972; Grassley and Davis, 1978). However, there is disagreement on this particular treatment for engorgement; some believe that the vasodilation adds to the swelling. The alternate recommendation is cold packs, which is believed to reduce swelling and has the additional advantage of numbing nipples so that they are less sensitive during the first part of suckling (Eiger and Olds,

1972; Newton and Newton, 1972; Rees, 1976). Analgesics can also provide relief (Eiger and Olds, 1972; Newton and Newton, 1972).

Rubber nipple shields, which look like large formula bottle nipples, are frequently suggested for women with sore nipples. They are supposed to fit over the woman's nipples. They are contraindicated because they do not promote nipple extension and may be very irritating (Applebaum, 1975; Countryman, 1977). A glass shield is available that can be used but should be limited to as short a period as possible. It should be lubricated with water before placing it over the nipple. When the mother's nipple is drawn out, the shield is removed and the mother's own nipple substituted (Countryman, 1977). Even the use of these glass shields is controversial, because the milk is drawn out by suction alone, and they can interfere with adequate production (Pryor, 1973). The Woolwich Shield, previously discussed in relation to inverted nipples, can also be useful for the woman whose nipples are made concave by engorgement. When worn between feedings they can make it easier for the child to grasp the nipple by promoting the convex shape (La Leche, 1963; Countryman, 1973). Milk may drip into the shield if used in this manner, and women must be cautioned not to save this milk for feeding the infant because the milk remains at a warm temperature, which provides bacteria with optimal conditions for growth.

A supportive bra increases comfort for some women during engorgement, but care must be taken that it is not tight or further complications may occur from compression (Eiger and Olds, 1972).

---

*Available from Lopuco Ltd., 1615 Old Annapolis Rd., Woodbine, MD 21797.

†Available from Happy Baby Family Products, 1252 S. La Cienga, Los Angeles, CA 90035.

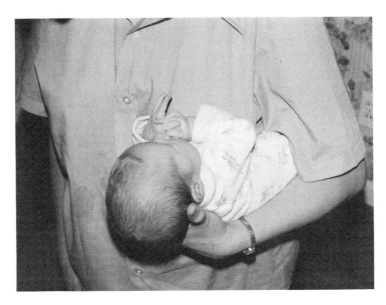

Fig. 25-19. Football hold.

Clogged ducts and breast abscesses

Clogged ducts, sometimes called "caked" breasts, can occur any time during lactation but are most likely to occur from 1 to 2 weeks after childbirth (Eiger and Olds, 1972). In this condition there is a localized area of inflammation caused by blockage of one or two of the milk ducts. The milk is unable to pass through them, resulting in stasis (Applebaum, 1975). It is not an infection, since at this point there usually are no microorganisms present (La Leche, 1963). Fever may or may not be present. The lactating woman may notice a small lump on the breast that is reddened and painful to the touch (Eiger and Olds, 1972). Any early localized soreness should cue the woman to seek professional help (Applebaum, 1975).

The precipitating causes of clogged ducts are factors that would increase milk tension. These include such things as wearing a tight bra, infrequent suckling, dried nipple secretions, sleeping in a prone position, or any factors that interfere with the let-down reflex (Pryor, 1973). The treatment for a clogged duct includes an increase in the frequency of suckling on the affected breast; twice the normal frequency has been recommended (Applebaum, 1975). The affected breast should be offered to the infant first to allow for more complete emptying (Eiger and Olds, 1972). Every conceivable position including cross-nursing and football hold (Fig. 25-19) should be used to facilitate better emptying of the ducts (Brown and Hurlock, 1975). After breast-feeding gentle breast massage and manual expression help to remove any remaining milk from the breasts (Applebaum, 1975; Eiger and Olds, 1972). When dried secretions are caked over the nipples, gentle removal with cotton saturated in clean water is indicated (Eiger and Olds, 1972). Lying prone with hot, wet compresses is thought to increase lymphatic drainage and decrease nipple edema if present. A warm washcloth, covered with plastic wrap, is an easy way to provide heat to the site of inflammation. A heating pad may be used on top of the plastic wrap to provide even warmth, but a heavy hot water bottle may impede drainage and should be avoided (Applebaum, 1970, 1975). Analgesics are indicated if the woman is uncomfortable, since such discomfort can diminish the let-down reflex, further complicating the problem. Rest is indicated, and the woman should go to bed if possible (Eiger and Olds, 1972; La Leche, 1963; Newton and Newton, 1962). Antibiotics are indicated if there are signs of chills, malaise, or an elevated temperature. When the above regimen is adhered to, mastitis and subsequent breast abscess can usually be avoided (Applebaum, 1970, 1975).

Mastitis and a localized breast abscess may follow an untreated clogged duct. Headache, painful engorgement, a breast that is hot and tender upon palpation, erythema, fever, and general aches and malaise frequently accompany this condition. Usually it is unilateral. The organism involved is usually *Staphylococcus*, which comes from the mother's skin or the baby's nasopharynx (Newton and Newton, 1962). A breast abscess is a localized complication during or following mastitis and is caused by localized accumulation of pus. It is treated with antibiotics and may require surgical drainage, which can be done on an outpatient basis. During the recuperative period breast-feeding can proceed on the nonaffected breast normally. The antibiotic selected needs to be one that is safe for the child. The milk on the affected side should be removed by manual expression or with a breast pump. This milk will need to be discarded. When healing is completed, breast-feeding can be resumed on the affected side (Eiger and Olds, 1972; La Leche, 1963).

"Losing" the milk

Most women in this country experience some degree of engorgement after childbirth. Their breasts may feel large, swollen, and lumpy. At some time during the first several weeks of the lactory period, engorgement no longer occurs and the breasts appear much softer and smaller. Many women have thought that this indicated their milk had "dried up," and subsequently have discontinued breast-feeding. What it does indicate is an adjustment to the lactation process. A woman needs to be aware of this phenomenon before it occurs to avoid an untimely end to breast-feeding.

"Nursing strikes"

Another problem that may occur at odd times, but generally between 4 and 10 months, is rejection of the breast. Babies sometimes suckle momentarily, pull away from the breast, arch their backs, and cry. If the woman tries to offer the breast, the infant refuses. Unless the woman wants to wean at this point, this is not the time to introduce bottles. If the child is taking solids, the woman can temporarily increase these portions. Fluids can be offered from a cup, or if the infant is too young, from a spoon or eyedropper. Trying to breast-feed the child when she or he is very sleepy also seems to work. Changing the positions generally used or changing routines has been used successfully in this situation. Because the infant cannot be forced to suckle, it is useless to recommend that the mother try force-feeding. Manual expression or an acceptable breast pump can be used temporarily.

Nursing strikes are thought to occur from a variety of different causes. Teething, extreme hunger, a strange new taste in the milk, increased tension in the lactating woman, infant's colds, and thrush have all been known to precipitate "strikes" (Eiger and Olds, 1972). If none of the above situations are identifiable, and yet the woman's child continues "on strike" for over a week, the child may be signalling to the woman that she/he is ready for weaning. More often, the "strike" ends in a few days.

Jaundice

There are many causes of jaundice in the newborn, and it should never be assumed that jaundice is benign until it is demonstrated to be so (Guthrie, 1978). In general, in the healthy term infant, blood bilirubin lev-

els below 20 mg/100 ml (1 decaliter) of blood are considered safe, although some recommend lower "safe" levels in healthy children (Tan, 1976). If the infant is sick or premature, the level of bilirubin considered safe is lower. When levels in excess of 20 mg/100 ml of blood exist in a term infant, it begins to be deposited in the brain resulting in progressive damage and even death. It is generally unnecessary to discontinue breast-feeding in the jaundiced child, since most neonatal jaundice is unrelated to the mode of feeding (Guthrie, 1978).

In 1963, a rare condition, "breast milk jaundice," was described (Arias et al., 1963). This type of jaundice occurs in approximately 1% of breast-fed children. It is considered to be another type of physiologic or idiopathic jaundice, and is thought to be caused by interference with or depression of glucuronyl transferase activity in the infant's liver, especially the hormone pregnandiol. This jaundice usually occurs after the mature milk comes in, and the main characteristic is its persistence, sometimes remaining 6 weeks or longer. Recently, the construct of "breast milk jaundice" has been disputed by a study that noted breast milk and pregnandiol had effects different from those noted in 1963 (Drew, 1978). Thus much remains to be learned about this type of jaundice.

One study of 1107 consecutively born children was done to determine if breast-feeding increased the level of jaundice. The investigators found that there was a higher level of jaundice after 72 hours of age in those children who were solely breast-fed when compared to artificially fed infants receiving combined breast and artificial feedings. However, the jaundice only rarely required active therapy (phototherapy and exchange transfusions). Of 13,102 other consecutively born children, 6.7% had serum bilirubin determinations because of clinical indications. In only one child was the jaundice proved to be caused by breast milk (Drew, 1978). In breast milk jaundice, serum bilirubin levels seldom exceed 15 to 20 mg/100 ml blood. Guthrie (1978) recommends a treatment regimen for true breast milk jaundice that is similar to the treatment of physiologic jaundice. Phototherapy is begun when the bilirubin exceeds 17 to 19 mg/100 ml. If the bilirubin exceeds 20 to 22 mg/100 ml, an exchange transfusion is indicated (Drew, 1978). Discontinuation of breast-feeding for 3 or 4 days results in rapid reduction of jaundice, and resumption rarely results in the jaundice becoming severe again (La Leche, 1971). Another recommended approach when bilirubin levels are high in a child over 1 week of age is discontinuation of breast-feeding for 12 to 24 hours once per week, which results in bilirubin drops of 5 to 10 mg/100 ml. After the interruption and drop in bilirubin level, it usually takes from 3 to 5 days to return to its previous level (Drew, 1978).

The concentration of serum bilirubin in infants with breast milk jaundice usually does not rise to levels that result in neurotoxicity (Johnson, 1975). When this does occur, proper medical management can make discontinuation of breast-feeding unnecessary. Women whose infants have this syndrome should not be discouraged from breast-feeding. A motivated mother and a sympathetic health care provider can maintain breast-feeding if they wish to try (Drew, 1978).

Certain drugs also may be potential causes of jaundice, and may reach the child by (1) direct administration after birth, (2) crossing of the placental barrier in utero, or (3) breast milk (Drew, 1978). Great discretion is necessary in this area until further knowledge is available.

Thrush

Thrush is a fungal infection that the infant can contract if the mother has an untreated vaginal monilial *(Candida albicans)* infection at the time she gives birth. Thrush in the newborn causes white, milky spots on the gums, cheeks, and tongue. It can also cause raw, red buttocks. Thrush can be subsequently transmitted to the woman's nipples by direct contact. In the lactating woman it can cause sore nipples or sharp, shooting breast pains, especially at the initiation of a feeding period (Newton and Newton, 1951).

One recommended treatment is washing the nipples after each nursing in a solution of 1 teaspoon of bicarbonate of soda mixed in a glass of sterile water, followed by gentle drying and the application of a mild cream (Eiger and Olds, 1972). The bicarbonate can also be made into a paste and put directly on the nipples (Newton and Newton, 1951). Refraining from wearing a bra or wearing a tea strainer in the bra keeps the air circulating to the nipples and has provided relief for some women. Bras are sometimes thought to be a source of reinfection, and it is recommended that they be changed daily (Newton and Newton, 1951). This condition can also be treated in both the infant and mother with prescription antifungal agents. Fungal infections can be very frustrating since they can persist for several months.

Environmental contamination of breast milk

Health care providers and lactating women need to be aware and informed of the potential contaminants of human milk. Contamination can be a problem for an individual woman in selected circumstances, such as when she requires a particular medication, or it can affect many women located in the same geographic area because of environmental pollutants. Arena (1970) categorizes contaminants as medicinal toxicants, social toxicants, and ecologic toxicants.

Several factors influence the passage of chemicals from the woman's plasma to her breast milk. The chemical's solubility, protein-binding capacity, and degree of ionization all influence transmission. Another factor affecting chemical passage is the composition of the milk (Rothermel and Faber, 1975). During the colostrum phase, the mammary gland is thought to be more permeable to a number of solutes, but little attention has been directed toward study of colostrum contaminants (Arena, 1970). The variability of fat content in breast milk— higher concentrations in the morning and during the latter part of a single feeding—will also affect the excretion of chemicals. Chemicals that are more fat soluble will more easily diffuse into breast milk as the fat content rises. The pH of breast milk is approximately 7.0 and the pH of a woman's plasma is approximately 7.4 (Savage, 1977). Thus the more acidic breast milk provides a better medium for diffusion of basic chemicals. Diffusion of basic chemicals can cause concentration of those chemicals in the woman's breast milk that are several times higher than the plasma concentration of such chemicals (Rothermel and Faber, 1975); this can be extremely dangerous to the infant.

Medicinal toxicants. Many drugs prescribed for the lactating woman are thought to be clinically insignificant and pose no hazard to the suckling child. In many instances less than 1% of the ingested dose is excreted in the breast milk, and the child may not absorb all this. However, some drugs must be completely avoided in the lactating woman; and others, when prescribed, must be followed with close supervision. It would be ideal if lactating women were to take no drugs, but in cases of necessity it is frequently possible to select medications that have not as yet been demonstrated to be potentially harmful to the nursling. If a potentially harmful drug is essential but only for a short term, the woman can pump her breasts and discard the milk during the treatment. Suckling can be resumed after the drug has been discontinued (Applebaum, 1977).

Social toxicants. Certain common social habits involving chemical intake also can affect the nursling. Alcohol in moderate amounts (1 to 2 oz per day) has not been demonstrated to be harmful to the nursing child (La Leche, 1974b; Savage, 1977). Cigarette smoking in the lactating woman can be problematic. Smoking may reduce the woman's milk volume, and the infants of women who smoke are smaller at birth than the infants of nonsmoking women. Nicotine is a toxic drug, and once in the bloodstream, it acts rapidly. Nicotine is fat soluble but gastrointestinal absorption of it is slow, and few severe nicotine toxic reactions are seen in infants whose mothers are very heavy smokers. Women who smoke heavily need to be aware of the possible hazards to their infants from heavy use of this drug (Arena, 1970).

The long-range effects of marijuana smoking on the

child have not been documented. However, the most active component of marijuana is fat soluble, and is likely to appear in breast milk (Arena, 1970).

Oral contraceptives appear to be contraindicated for lactating women. These drugs are known to inhibit lactation, but the exact effect depends upon how early after childbirth the drug is administered, how large the dose is, and what type of agents are involved (Grams, 1978). The effect of these hormone preparations on the developing endocrine system of the infant is unknown (Arena, 1970). Women should be informed of the above considerations and may wish to consider alternate forms of birth control during lactation.

Ecologic toxicants. All of us are exposed to a variety of environmental toxicants.

DDT. DDT was first reported in human milk in 1950, and has apparently been declining since that time, although breast milk contains more DDT than does cow's milk. The average daily intake of breast-fed children in the United States is only slightly, if any, greater than the conservative permissible rate set by the World Health Organization and the Food and Agricultural Organization after years of study (Arena, 1970).

PCBs and PBBs. PCBs (polychlorinated biphenyls), another environmental contaminant, are nonbiodegradable, fat soluble, and are principally excreted through the fat in breast milk. They have been used as heat-transfer agents in electrical systems, and have been discharged in large quantities into waterways as industrial wastes. Three routes of PCB intake are: ingestion, respiration, and absorption through skin and mucous membrane. Exposure occurs directly through contact with the chemicals or indirectly through eating fish obtained from contaminated waters. No damage to breast-fed children at the present PCB levels in human milk in the United States has been documented (Doucette, 1978).

PBBs (polybrominated biphenyls), another environmental contaminant, are also nonbiodegradable, fat soluble, and excreted through fat in breast milk. PBB contamination of human milk is not as widespread as PCB contamination. There is only one known incident where PBBs were included in animal feeds, and this was not discovered until a year after the accident. Studies of this situation revealed no immediate effects on nurslings whose mothers were exposed, but long-term effects are presently unknown (Johnson, 1975).

Lead. Lead has been widely found in human breast milk. Analysis of the other common milks fed to children, such as evaporated, evaporated skimmed concentrated formula, nonfat dry, and homogenized cow's milk, has demonstrated that all contain more lead than does breast milk. Maximal safe intake of lead has yet to be established (Johnson, 1975).

The "chemicalization" of modern living is an impor-

tant area for general caution, and more research is needed on the excretion of chemical toxicants in human colostrum and milk. Some toxicants are unavoidable, either therapeutically or as a part of mass production of food, but particular consideration needs to be given to minimizing the intakes of pregnant and lactating women, in view of the possible susceptibility of the child (Jelliffe and Jelliffe, 1978).

Special situations

Certain special situations that occur with the lactating woman need discussion. These situations generally require increased knowledge and perhaps support from health care providers for the woman to maintain lactation; anticipatory guidance appears to be crucial in these circumstances.

Employed women

Saloman and associates (1977) note that the question of the compatibility of a woman's economic productivity and her ability to humanely rear her children has been asked only since the Industrial Revolution and the resultant creation of special work places. The contemporary trend toward increasing employment and an increasing trend toward breast-feeding could be viewed as conflicting.

The woman who chooses to breast-feed is still in the minority, and the woman who works outside the home and chooses to breast-feed her child is even more rare. There is little data to support the contention that increasing numbers of women working outside the home are the same women choosing to breast-feed, but there is some indication that such might be the case.

In one study of 102 nursing mothers, 60% of the women planned to work outside the home. Currently, women with more years of formal schooling are likely to nurse longer than women with less education, and yet these women are probably the ones who feel that an outside career is important and would most likely return to work (Auerbach, 1976a). The assumption that employed women either do not want to or cannot lactate and breast-feed denies them choices. Many employed women have undoubtedly not attempted breast-feeding or have weaned their children before returning to work because of assumptions that breast-feeding and employment are incompatible.

It *is* possible for employed women to breast-feed their children, and key words to success in this endeavor are flexibility, determination, and a good beginning. Breast-feeding provides the employed woman's child with all the usual advantages, and in some ways provides additional advantages for the woman. Successful breast-feeding by the employed woman appears to be related to how well lactation has been established (Salomon et al.,

1977). All previously discussed factors, such as strong support from significant others, education, an early and more primolactic style of nursing, provision for rest and relaxation, and social support are all crucial. Several of the above points need special emphasis for the employed woman. The woman needs to be aware that some of the character traits that are desirable in the employment environment (i.e., high degree of motivation, independence, and assertiveness) can also ensure a successful lactation experience. However, breast-feeding is not a totally predictable process and does not lend itself to a high degree of organization and control as do some jobs. Nursing is a sensual, emotional, enjoyable experience and, especially in the early lactory phase, needs to be responsive to the child's needs—which are highly unpredictable.

One area that may need reinterpretation is independence. The lactating woman who is planning to return to her employment is even more "at risk" for trying to fulfill the super-mom myth previously mentioned. If the woman interprets independence as a total refusal for support, it seems likely that she will fail in her breast-feeding endeavors. She needs to accept support, both physical (as in allowing a rearrangement of responsibilities such as housework, shopping, cooking, and so on) and psychosocial (as in seeking and accepting information and emotional support from employed women who have successfully nursed their infants).

Although the La Leche League attempts to support all women who wish to breast-feed their children, the League's underlying philosophy strongly supports full-time mothering. Depending upon the leader's individual tolerance, some employed women have been able to find considerable support from this group. However, since working outside the home is seen as a less optimal choice, those who do so may feel some criticism directed toward them. This especially holds true for women who work primarily for nonfinancial reasons (Cahill, 1976). It is necessary for employed women to find support groups because they can be doubly criticized—on the one hand as a mother because they choose to work, and on the other hand as a worker because of their particular commitment to breast-feeding their child. Since disapproval is stressful, it can inhibit a woman's let-down reflex and thus interfere with her breast-feeding goals. The employed woman should contact the local La Leche League groups to see if they will provide her criticism-free support; they can also provide her with a knowledge base. It is their common practice to place a woman who is desirous of remaining employed while breast-feeding in contact with another woman who has or is successfully combining the two endeavors. And it is always possible for the woman to organize her own support group comprised of employed breast-feeding women in her area.

The lactating woman (as well as any woman who has given birth) should be encouraged to take at least a flexible 6-week leave from her job. This will allow time for establishment of the lactation process based on the woman's and infant's style and needs. Women who are unable to do this should not be discouraged from attempting to combine breast-feeding and employment. There are no studies concerning whether or not these women can be successful, but many women have established and maintained lactation in the total absence of suckling from their ill or premature infants, and it seems reasonable to assume that an employed woman could do the same.

If the employed woman can negotiate a 6-week leave, she can also use this time to finalize arrangements for her child's care during her absences. If the woman works in her home, or if a nursery is available at her place of employment, her needs will be similar to many women who work at home without reimbursement. However, few women in the United States have these options available to them.

If the woman has a substitute care-giver who can bring the infant during coffee breaks and lunch hour, her problems are minimized. There is no certainty that the child will choose to suckle at these specified times, but women have used this arrangement with good overall success. Hiring a caretaker who is willing to bring the child to the mother several times a day is generally an expensive proposition, and prohibitive for large numbers of women.

If a child-care center is available within minutes of the employment setting, this may allow minimally for lunch time feeding and, if close enough, for one or two "feeding breaks." Still another option is taking the child to the place of employment. This is usually a rare option, since most workplaces are too rigid to deal with this situation. However, during the early months, it has been a viable option for some women in certain types of employment.

For the large majority of employed women, however, the only choice is some type of substitute feeding. This can be carried out in two different ways. One is by substituting the "away" feedings with formula. Another is to feed the infant breast milk that has been obtained by manual expression or breast pump and then refrigerated or frozen.

If the woman chooses to use her own milk, she will have better results if she does some planning ahead and begins collecting her milk prior to returning to work. This will serve two purposes. It will help the woman become skillful at manual expression or using a breast pump and also provide a cache of milk in the freezer—a great psychologic boon during the adjustment period of returning to work.

The procedure for storing breast milk is not complicated. Breast milk can be preserved for 24 to 48 hours if kept refrigerated (Brown and Hurlock, 1975; Eiger and Olds, 1972). Milk kept longer than this needs to be quick-frozen and used within 2 weeks if in a standard refrigerator freezer (La Leche, 1963; Jelliffe and Jelliffe, 1977b). If stored in a separate freezer that maintains a temperature of 0°F (−18°C) milk can be kept for over 2 years (Eiger and Olds, 1972; Jelliffe and Jelliffe, 1977b). Breast milk freezes in layers but will mix again when thawed (Pryor, 1973). It should be thawed under cold running water, since boiling water can cause the milk to curdle. Sterilization of the collection equipment is recommended for infants less than 1 month of age. A dishwasher that heats the water to 180° can be used, or items can be boiled for 5 minutes (Eiger and Olds, 1972). Containers should be dated before storing.

Generally, the optimal time for beginning regular manual expression or pumping is before or during the first morning feeding, since breasts tend to be fullest at this time. Manual expression is much easier to do when the baby has initiated the let-down reflex on the opposite breast. When the mother first begins this routine, the infant may not get quite enough milk at this feeding because of the amount of milk expressed and saved. This is problematic only for a day or two, and soon the breasts will adapt to the increased demand (Brown and Hurlock, 1975).

Before returning to work it is wise to have a few practice runs. This allows the woman an opportunity to see how she and her baby will react. The first separation can be for a limited time, and the woman can check to see how her child is doing. Children who refuse a bottle from the nursing mother will sometimes accept one from an alternate care-giver without difficulty. Almost *all* breast-feeding children will drink from a bottle when hungry. Babies 6 months or older may prefer to wait long hours rather than drink from a bottle. This situation can be managed by giving solids (usually begun at this time) with high fluid content and using a spoon for fluid or trying a small glass or cup.

It is very important that the person(s) providing care in the woman's absence be supportive of her endeavors. It is not impossible to work around a nonsupportive person, but it certainly does add unnecessary stress to the lactating woman.

When she returns to her employment, the woman may find the following schedule or some modification helpful. Begin each day with manual expression (to be frozen or saved for mid-day feeding) and a relaxed feeding period. Assuming access to the child during the day is not an option, the woman can manually express her milk or use a breast pump at those times she would normally nurse her child or at those times when she has access to some semblance of privacy. She does not have to

isolate herself from other women, and she can also provide for her own nourishment at these times. The expressed milk can be refrigerated and saved for the next day. It is helpful if a routine time and place can be set to do this since this may help condition the let-down reflex to stimuli other than the child.

The return home in the evening is a critical period. This is usually a time of activity and stress for most families. The woman will have to make arrangements to decrease demands for the first half hour to one hour of her return, because this is an essential feeding session. Endless options to achieve this can be explored. If her child is cared for in a private home, she may find that relaxing and breast-feeding the child as soon as she arrives is helpful, especially since there are unlikely to be any demands upon the lactating woman in this setting and it provides an opportunity to talk with care-giver and learn about the child's day. If the care-giver is in the home, it may be possible to have her remain for a half hour or so until the woman has been able to sit down, relax, and breast-feed her child. The woman must negotiate and delegate responsibilities during this period, and her partner and older children can be encouraged to participate in the routine tasks to facilitate this breast-feeding session.

This feeding tends to be the most difficult; it takes planning, especially if there are other children in the home. During the remainder of the evening and night, the woman can move to a more primolactic style, suckling on demand or a semidemand schedule. Almost all infants will continue night time feedings until at least age 3 months, and this is an invaluable aid in maintaining the milk supply. In this situation it is crucial that breast-feeding be made as easy as possible, because the employed woman will not be able to nap during the day to make up for nighttime awakenings. The easiest and simplest method is to take the child to bed with her. Then she can breast-feed in an unrestricted fashion throughout the night. Even women who are very light sleepers can accustom themselves to this routine, experiencing minimal disturbance of rest. Partners may have their rest patterns disturbed by the nursling's presence. If this occurs, keeping the nursling in a basket/box/crib within arm's reach of the bed may be an acceptable compromise. Keeping the child in a separate room makes nursing difficult under any circumstances, and in this case can be the precipitating factor that leads to exhaustion and untimely weaning.

Several warning signals indicating excessive stress need to be recognized by employed women. Thoughts of "it's too much trouble," obsessive concern about manual expression and milk supply, or a significant reduction in milk supply are indications of approaching untimely weaning. If the time needed to pump or express breast

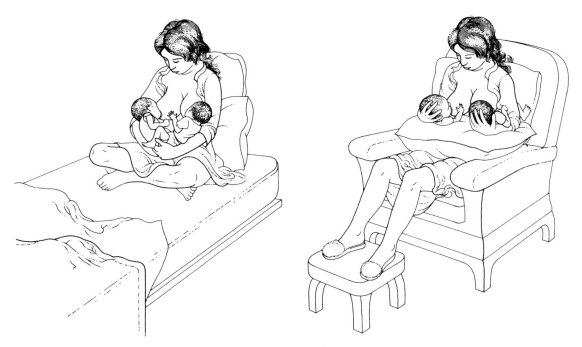

Fig. 25-20. Nursing of twins.

milk for the infant becomes burdensome, formula can be substituted for one or all "away" feedings rather than relinquishing breast-feeding. One recommended procedure when a woman has reached her limit is to take a day of leave, go to bed with the child, and force fluids (Salomon et al., 1977). Other situations need to be individually evaluated, and with help from supportive health care providers modifications can be made that will help the woman to achieve her goals.

One note of caution is necessary: breast-feeding a child while working for a 40 or more hours/week is an undertaking that requires high motivation and commitment. It is not a course to be recommended casually for all. Lactation must assume a high place in the woman's priorities, and if she has responsibility to other children and adults at home, it will require cooperation and support from them. Some women find that despite the organizational effort required, breast-feeding is still easy and satisfying. For others, this is not the case, and the nurse should take care not to make the woman feel guilty if she finds the process unacceptable and decides not to breast-feed. In addition, many modifications of the above recommendations can be made. Any amount of breast-feeding a woman chooses to engage in with her child is valuable, and if the woman has a joyful and satisfying nursing relationship with her child, by whatever description, she has achieved success.

Tandem nursing

Tandem nursing refers to the practice of breast-feeding nursing siblings of different ages. This would include nursing a child throughout a subsequent pregnancy and also nursing a child who stops nursing during the pregnancy but begins again after the sibling's birth (Avery, 1977). Advice on this issue is variable, with some discouraging the practice (Eiger and Olds, 1972) and others saying it depends upon the woman's feelings and desires. Lactation and pregnancy are both demanding, and if a woman chooses to tandem nurse she will need to be very much in tune to her body's needs for increased nutrition and rest. The milk supply generally tends to diminish as the pregnancy progresses, and some children wean themselves gradually during this period (Pryor, 1973).

Breast-feeding more than one

Breast-feeding twins (or even triplets) is possible and has been done. Since twins may have a lower birth weight than single-birth infants, they may benefit from certain protective advantages of breast-feeding. Nursing twins can be done separately, simultaneously, or in some combination (La Leche, 1963; Eiger and Olds, 1972; Pryor, 1973). When breast-feeding simultaneously, the woman needs to find a position comfortable for her and the infants. (Some ideas are depicted in Fig. 25-20.) Advice differs on whether to feed each child at its "own" breast or to alternate. There is no conclusive evidence of which is better.

If each twin has its own breast, each breast adjusts to that particular infant's supply needs. If the two children consume extremely different quantities of milk, the woman may notice some size difference in the breasts, but if she is not concerned about being a bit lopsided, this is not a problem. A woman breast-feeding twins has increased needs for rest and nutrition.

Relactation/induced lactation

Relactation is the physiologic process whereby human lactation is initiated at a time that is not related to the initial postpartum production of milk (Brown, 1977). Relactation can be initiated in a variety of circumstances for differing reasons. A woman who has experienced untimely weaning may wish to resume her nursing relationship with her child. Relactation has also been accomplished in adoptive mothers (Avery, 1973). Brown (1977) states three conditions essential for relactation: an adequately nourished woman interested in nursing, a child with a good sucking reflex, and a support system.

REFERENCES

Amsel, P.: The need to wean—as much for mother as for baby, Keep. Abreast J. **2**:188-196, 1977.

Appel, J., and King, J.: Energy needs during pregnancy and lactation, Fam. Community Health **1**:7-18, 1979.

Applebaum, R. M.: The modern management of successful breastfeeding, Pediatr. Clin. North Am. **17**:203-225, 1970.

Applebaum, R. M.: The obstetrician's approach to the breasts and breastfeeding, J. Reprod. Med. **14**:98-116, 1975.

Applebaum, R. M.: Breastfeeding and drugs in human milk, Keep. Abreast J. **2**:292-293, 1977.

Arena, J.: Contamination of the ideal food, Nutr. Today **5**:2-8, 1970.

Arias, I., and others: Neonatal unconjugated hyperbilirubinemia associated with breastfeeding and a factor in milk that inhibits glucuronide formation in vitro, Am. Soc. Clin. Invest. **42**:913, 1963.

Atkinson, L.: Prenatal nipple conditioning for breast-feeding, Nurs. Res. **28**:267-271, 1979.

Auerbach, K.: To breastfeed or not to breastfeed, Keep. Abreast J. **1**:316-323, 1976a.

Auerbach, K.: Where have all the nursing mothers gone? Keep. Abreast J. **1**:223-228, 1976b.

Auerbach, K.: A study of timing of first solid foods: comparison of breast and bottlefeeding mothers, Birth Fam. J. **5**:27-31, 1978.

Avery, J.: Closet nursing: symptom of intolerance or forerunner of social change? Keep. Abreast J. **2**:212-227, 1977.

Avery, J.: Induced lactation: a guide for counseling and management. Available from J. J. Avery, Inc., P.O. Box 6459, Cherry Creek Station Department, K. A., Denver, CO 80206.

Barnes, G., and others: Management of breastfeeding, J.A.M.A. **151**:192-199, 1953.

Bishop, W., and Bishop, P.: Father-assisted breastfeeding, Pediatr. Nurs. **4**:39-40, 1978.

Brack, D.: Social forces, feminism, and breastfeeding, Nurs. Outlook **23**:556-561, 1975.

Brown, M., and Hurlock, J.: Preparation of the breast for breastfeeding, Nurs. Res. **24**:448-451, 1975.

Brown, R.: Relactation: an overview, Pediatrics **60**:116-120, 1977.

Cahill, M.: Breastfeeding and working? Franklin Park, Ill., 1976, La Leche League International, Inc.

Coffin, L.: The doctor's role in breastfeeding and child nutrition, Keep. Abreast J. **3**:38-41, 1978.

Cole, J.: Breastfeeding in the Boston suburbs in relation to personal social factors, Clin. Pediatr. **16**:352-356, 1977.

Committee on Nutrition, American Academy of Pediatrics: Breastfeeding: a commentary in celebration of the international year of the child, 1979, Pediatrics **62**:591-601, 1979.

Countryman, B.: Hospital care of the breastfed newborn, Am. J. Nurs. **71**:2365-2367, 1971.

Countryman, B.: Breast care in the early puerperium, J. Obstet. Gynecol. **2**:36-40, 1973.

Countryman, B.: How the maternity nurse can help the breastfeeding mother (#118), Franklin Park, Ill., 1977, La Leche League International, Inc.

Dascalos, J.: Abrupt weaning: one mother's story, Keep. Abreast J. **2**:197-207, 1977.

Doucette, J.: Is breastfeeding still safe for babies? Matern. Child Nurs. J. **3**:345-346, 1978.

Drew, J. H.: Breastfeeding and jaundice, Keep. Abreast J. **3**:53-57, 1978.

Eiger, M., and Olds, S.: The complete book of breastfeeding, New York, 1972, Workman Publishing Co., Inc.

Eppink, H.: An experiment to determine a basis for nursing decisions in regard to time of initiation of breastfeeding, Nurs. Res. **18**:292-299, 1969.

Estok, P.: What do nurses know about breastfeeding problems? J. Obstet. Gynecol. Nurs. **2**:36-39, 1973.

Evans, R., Thigpen, L., and Hamrick, M.: Exploration of factors involved in maternal physiological adaptation to breastfeeding, Nurs. Res. **18**:28-33, 1969.

Filer, S.: Relationship of nutrition to lactation and newborn development. In Moghissi, K., and Evans, T., editors: Nutritional impacts on women, New York, 1977, Harper & Row, Publishers, Inc.

Friedman, E.: Physiological aspects of pregnancy. In Notman, M., and Nadelson, C., editors: The woman patient: medical and psychological interfaces, New York, 1978, Plenum Press.

Gerard, A.: Please breastfeed your baby, New York, 1970, New American Library, Inc.

Gerrard, J.: Breastfeeding: second thoughts, Pediatrics **54**:757-764, 1974.

Gerrard, J., and K.-T. Tan, L.: Hazards of formula feeding, Keep. Abreast J. **30**:20-25, 1978.

Good news for "innies," up front facts, Keep. Abreast J. **1**:46-57, 1976.

Grams, K.: Breastfeeding: a means of imparting immunity? Matern. Child Nurs. J. **3**:340-344, 1978.

Grassley, J., and Davis, F.: Common concerns of mothers who breastfeed, Am. J. Matern. Child Nurs. **3**:347-351, 1978.

Guthrie, H., and Guthrie, G.: The resurgence of natural childfeeding: a study of 129 middle class mothers in a college community, Clin. Pediatr. **5**:481-484, 1979.

Guthrie, R. A.: Breast milk and infant nutrition, Keep. Abreast J. **3**:34-37, 1978.

Guthrie, R. A.: Breast milk and jaundice, Keep. Abreast. J. **3**:49-52, 1978.

Gyorgy, P.: The uniqueness of human milk: biochemical aspects, Am. J. Clin. Nutri. **24**:1013-1021, 1971.

Haire, D. B.: The cultural warping of childbirth, Seattle, 1972, International Childbirth Education Association.

Hall, B.: Changing composition of human milk and early development of an appetite control, Lancet **1**:779-781, 1975.

Hall, J.: Influencing breastfeeding success, J. Obstet. Gynecol. Nurs. **7**:28-32, 1978.

Halpen, S., and others: Factors influencing breastfeeding: notes on observations in Dallas, Texas, South. Med. J. **65**:100-102, 1972.

Henderson, K., and Newton, L.: Helping nursing mothers maintain lactation while separated from their infants, Am. J. Matern. Child Nurs. **3**:352-356, 1978.

Hervada, A., and others: Drugs in breast milk, Perinatal Care **2**:19-25, 1978.

Hoffman, J.: A suggested treatment for inverted nipples, Am. J. Obstet. Gynecol. **66**:346-348, 1953.

Is breastfeeding best for babies? Consumer Reports **42**:152-157, 1977.

Jellife, D.: Community and sociopolitical considerations of breastfeeding. In Breastfeeding and the mother, Ciba Foundation Symposium 45, New York, 1976, Elsevier, North-Holland, Inc.

Jelliffe, D., and Jelliffe, E. F. P.: The uniqueness of human milk: an overview, Am. J. Clin. Nutr. **24**:1013-1021, 1971.

Jelliffe, D., and Jelliffe, E. F. P.: Alleged inadequacies of human milk, Clin. Pediatr. **16**:1104-1114, 1977a.

Jelliffe, D., and Jelliffe, E. F. P.: Current concepts in nutrition: breast is best: modern meanings, N. Engl. J. Med. **297**:912-915, 1977b.

Jelliffe, D., and Jelliffe, E. F. P.: Human milk in the modern world, New York, 1978, Oxford University Press.

Jelliffe, E. F. P.: Maternal nutrition and lactation. In Breastfeeding and the mother, Ciba Foundation Symposium 45, New York, 1976, Elsevier, North-Holland, Inc.

Johnson, J.: Neonatal nonhemolytic jaundice, New Engl. J. Med. **292**: 194-197, 1975.

Kadushin, A.: Breastfeeding and weaning a pre-school child, Keep. Abreast J. **2**:208-211, 1977.

Klaus, M., and others: Maternal attachment, New Engl. J. Med. **286**: 460-463, 1972.

Knafl, K.: Conflicting perspective on breastfeeding, Am. J. Nurs. **74**: 1848-1851, 1974.

Knafl, K.: Negotiating hospital care: La League members and hospital personnel, J. Obstet. Gynecol. Nurs. **5**:47-51, 1976.

Knodel, J.: Breastfeeding and population growth, Science **198**:1111-1115, 1977.

La Leche League International, Inc.: The womanly art of breastfeeding, Franklin Park, Ill., 1963, Interstate Printers and Publishers, Inc.

La Leche League International, Inc.: Breastfeeding and jaundice (#10) Franklin Park, Ill., 1971, The League.

La Leche League International, Inc.: Does your baby need a pacifier (#110), Franklin Park, Ill., 1974a, The League.

La Leche League International, Inc.: Inverted nipples (#108), Franklin Park, Ill., 1974b, The League.

La Leche League International, Inc.: Nipple care (#103), Franklin Park, Ill., 1974c, The League.

La Leche League International, Inc.: Losing your milk? (#83), Franklin Park, Ill., 1975, The League.

La Leche League International, Inc.: Why nurse your baby (#101), Franklin Park, Ill., 1977, The League.

Ladas, A.: How to help mothers breastfeed: deductions from a survey, Clin. Pediatr. **9**:702-705, 1970.

Lawson, B.: Perceptions of degrees of support for the breastfeeding mother, Birth Fam. J. **3**:67-72, 1976.

MacKeith, R., and Wood, C.: Infant feeding and feeding difficulties, New York, 1977, Churchill Livingston.

Magnus, P.: Impediments to human lactation, Keep. Abreast J. **3**:133-137, 1978.

Mata, L., and Wyatt, R.: The uniqueness of human milk: host resistance to infection, Am. J. Clin. Nutr. **24**:976-986, 1971.

McKigney, J.: The uniqueness of human milk: economic aspects, Am. J. Clin. Nutr. **24**:1005-1012, 1971.

Meara, H.: A key to successful breastfeeding in a nonsupportive culture, J. Nurse-Midwif. **21**:20-26, 1976.

Mohrer, J.: Breast and bottlefeeding in an inner city community: an assessment of perceptions and practices, Med. Anthropol. **3**:125-145, 1979.

Newton, M., and Newton, N.: The let-down reflex in human lactation, J. Pediatr. **33**:698-704, 1948.

Newton, M., and Newton, N.: Post-partum engorgement of the breast, Am. J. Obstet. Gynecol. **61**:664-667, 1951.

Newton, M., and Newton, N.: The normal course and management of lactation, Clin. Obstet. Gynecol. **5**:44-63, 1962.

Newton, N.: Nipple pain and nipple damage, J. Pediatr. **41**:411-423, 1952.

Newton, N.: Breastfeeding (Reprint #130), Franklin Park, Ill., 1968, La Leche League International, Inc.

Newton, N.: Psychologic differences between breast and bottlefeeding, Am. J. Clin. Nutr. **24**:993-1004, 1971.

Nicholas, M.: Effective help for the nursing mother, J. Obstet. Gynecol. Nurs. **7**:22-30, 1978.

Olson, J.: Breastfeeding: common problems and practical answers, Pediatr. Nurs. **4**:32-35, 1978.

Parsons, L.: Weaning from the breast: for a happy ending to a satisfying experience, J. Obstet. Gynecol. Nurs. **7**:12-15, 1978.

Peterson, J., and Bock, W.: Educating nursing mothers, Perinatal Care, Inc. **2**:44-47, 1978.

Pryor, K.: Nursing your baby, New York, 1973, Harper & Row Publishers, Inc.

Raphael, D.: The tender gift: breastfeeding, Englewood Cliffs, N.J., 1973, Prentice-Hall, Inc.

Ratner, H.: The new breastfeeding crisis: failure to thrive, La Leche League News **21**:21, 1979.

Reader's response: Fathers' talk about weaning, Keep. Abreast J. **2**: 235-236, 1977; **2**:230-234, 1977.

Recommended dietary allowances, Washington, D.C., National Academy of Sciences, National Research Council, 1974.

Rees, D.: Dialogue, Keep. Abreast J. **1**:137-144, 1976.

Rees, D.: Sore nipples are a pain! Keep. Abreast J. **1**:125-135, 1976.

Rothermel, P., and Faber, M.: Drugs in breastmilk—a consumer's guide, Birth Fam. J. **2**:76-88, 1975.

Salomon, M., Schauf, V., and Seiden, A.: Breastfeeding, natural mothering, and working outside the home. In Stewart, L., and Stewart, D., editors: Twenty-first Century Obstetrics Now, vol. 2, Chapel Hill, N.C., 1977, National Association of Parents and Professionals for Safe Alternatives in Childbirth, Inc.

Savage, R.: Drugs and breastmilk, J. Human Nutr. **31**:459-464, 1977.

Schams, D.: Hormonal control of lactation. In Breastfeeding and the mother, Ciba Foundation Symposium 45, 1976, New York, Elsevier, North-Holland, Inc.

Sims, S.: Dietary status of lactating women, J. Am. Diet. Assoc. **73**: 139-146, 1978.

Tan, L.K.-T.: Phototherapy for neonatal hyperbilirubinemia in "healthy" and "ill" infants, Pediatrics **57**:836-838, 1976.

Thevenin, T.: The family bed, P.O. Box 16004, Minneapolis, MN, 1976.

Thompson, A., Hytten, A., and Black, A.: Lactation and reproduction, Bull. W.H.O. **52**:337-349, 1975.

Thompson, R.: Breast milk and dental caries: the question of fluoride, Keep. Abreast J. **3**:108-113, 1978.

Weichert, C.: Breastfeeding: first thoughts, Pediatrics **56**:987-990, 1975.

White, M., and Thornton, M.: Together and nursing from birth (#20), Franklin Park, Ill., 1978, La Leche League International, Inc.

Whitley, N.: Preparation for breastfeeding: a one year follow-up of thirty-four nursing mothers, J. Obstet. Gynecol. Nurs. **7**:44-48, 1978.

Wing, J.: Human versus cow's milk in infant nutrition and health: update 1977, Curr. Probl. Pediatr. **8**:3-50, 1977.

Worthington, B., Vermeersch, J., and Williams, S. R.: Nutrition in pregnancy and lactation, St. Louis, 1977, The C. V. Mosby Co.

Wray, J.: Maternal nutrition, breastfeeding, and infant survival. In Mosley, W., editor: Nutrition and human reproduction, New York, 1978, Plenum Press.

26

Mental health

Anne Fishel

The mental health of women is profoundly affected by the social, economic, and psychologic consequences of inequality in our society today, for inequality increases women's vulnerability to stress and the potential for mental disorders. According to the President's Commission Report, (vol. III, 1978): "Despite the 1974 amendments to the Civil Rights Act of 1964 prohibiting discrimination on the basis of sex, discrimination against women continues in all the major institutions in this society." (p. 1027) The current status of women is summarized in the Commission report as follows (vol. III, 1978):

1. *Salary:* More than half of all women are now employed outside of the home but they are clustered in the lowest paying occupations and at the bottom of the achievement ladder. One woman in four compared to one man in 18 lives on an annual income of less than $4,000.
2. *Dual roles:* Whether or not a woman is employed outside the home, housework remains largely "women's work." Thus many American women have two full workdays in every 24 hours.
3. *Politics:* Only about 3.5% of the House, and 2% of the Senate of the United States and about 9% of the state legislators are women. This greatly reduces the political capacity of women to improve their status.
4. *Business:* It is still unusual to see women in the bastions of financial power and in high corporate echelons.
5. *Law:* In many states when a woman marries, she trades the rights of a person for the duties of a wife. A husband who deserts his wife and takes a temporary job in another state can seriously affect his wife's credit rating, right to vote, serve on juries, run for office, and so on. (Tavris and Offin, 1977). The legal system provides little economic support for divorced mothers. Fewer than 21% of divorced mothers regularly collect child support.

6. *Physical abuse:* According to the FBI, wife abuse occurs three times as often as rape (about 1.5 million times a year). Half of all American marriages may involve some physical abuse of the wife (Tavris and Offin). Sexual favors by women are exchanged for enough money from men to buy groceries for children. Women with large numbers of children, no education, and no job skills are trapped.

The mental health problems of women may be summarized as follows (President's Commission, vol. III, 1978):

- 175 women to every 100 men are admitted to hospitals for the treatment of depression.
- More women than men in the general population report that they experience symptoms of depression.
- 238 women to every 100 men are treated for depression in outpatient services.
- The highest rate for treatment in public facilities is for nonwhite women and among women between the ages of 25 and 44 years who are separated or divorced.
- Among married women in the general population symptoms of depression are more common among women whose children are living with them.
- Older women whose children have left home and women who never married show fewer symptoms of depression.
- Twice as many women as men use the two most popular minor tranquilizers, Valium and Librium.
- Fifty percent more women report having used barbiturates for medical purposes than men.
- Estimates of the proportion of alcoholic women in the population ranges from 20% to 50%.

This chapter discusses in detail the incidence and prevalence of mental illness among women and identifies women who are at high risk; presents facts essential to clarifying values about women and establishing a new psychology for women; discusses intervention strategies designed to improve the status of women in our society; and provides information and treatment strategies for such syndromes as depression, anxiety, and substance abuse.

INCIDENCE AND PREVALENCE OF MENTAL ILLNESS AMONG WOMEN

Women in the Western world live longer than men and have lower mortality rates for most causes of death. There is evidence that these differences are the result of women's constitutionally greater resistance to infection and degenerative diseases (Nathanson, 1975). However, women report more physical and mental illness than men and utilize health services at substantially higher rates (Mechanic, 1976). (One exception is the dormitory counseling system, which reports equal utilization by male and female students.) Levine (1974) reports that diagnoses that are not by definition sex-linked are overwhelmingly more often applied to females; schizophrenia, affective disorders, and psychoneurosis have become feminine disorders. Even situational personality disorders and psychophysiologic disorders occur preponderantly among women.

A psychiatric diagnosis depends not only on the patient's presenting symptoms but also on the psychiatrist's psychosocial biases. A study by Cohen (1978) of 267 cases from major psychiatric hospitals revealed a 12% (and statistically significant) discrepancy between the official discharge diagnosis and the residents' training report diagnosis. The discharge diagnosis, which was less severe and less socially stigmatizing than the earlier diagnosis, was said to be a "protective" diagnosis. Men were more protected than women, black men were more protected than black women, unskilled laborers and those on the lower end of the socioeconomic scale were more protected than professionals, and housewives were the least protected of any group. Protecting unskilled laborers over professionals initially appears at odds with other data citing psychosis as more prevalent in lower socioeconomic groups. Cohen offered an interesting explanation for this: there was greater protection for employed patients as a whole. The unskilled laborers and the greatest representation in the protected sample because they were seen as most vulnerable (it is harder to get a job if unskilled and crazy). The professionals, supervisors, and executives tended to receive less protection because they were perceived as more autonomous or powerful, and therefore needed less protection. The fact that women as a group received less protection could also be explained by the fact that they are unemployed. This study raises questions, however, about the validity of statistics taken from psychiatric hospitals.

Women tend to stay longer in psychiatric hospitals. Doherty (1978) found that female patients were rated by staff as becoming significantly healthier over time as compared to men. However, for female patients, staff ratings of severity of illness were *not* significantly related to type of referral recommendation (discharge or further hospitalization). In contrast, ratings for male patients were highly related to the type of recommendation made. In other words, women who were referred for further hospitalization received ratings similar to ratings received by males and females for whom discharge was recommended. Females referred for further hospitalization were single, unemployed, and younger than the discharged females; however, neither marital nor employ-

Table 26-1. Five leading diagnoses for admissions to outpatient clinics by race, sex, and rates per 100,000 population (May 1975)*

Whites	No.	Blacks	No.
Males		Males	
Adjustment reaction and behavior disorders of childhood	94.6	Adjustment reaction and behavior disorders of childhood	95.2
Adjustment reaction-adult	81.4	Schizophrenia	87.2
Personality disorders	73.0	Adjustment reaction-adult	65.5
Schizophrenia	64.6	Alcohol disorders	55.4
Depressive disorders	54.6	Drug disorders	54.0
Females		Females	
Depressive disorders	112.0	Schizophrenia	145.2
Adjustment reaction-adult	102.2	Adjustment reaction-adult	133.3
Neuroses	74.7	Depressive disorders	128.6
Personality disorders	67.1	Adjustment reaction and behavior disorders of childhood	61.2
Schizophrenia	60.9	Neuroses	58.2

*From President's Commission on Mental Health: Mental health of women, Task Panel Reports vol. III, Washington, D.C., 1978, U.S. Government Printing Office, p. 1047.

ment status was related to type of referral received by male patients.

Women considerably outnumber men in psychiatric outpatient therapy—60% to 75% women—and at least one study (Gordon et al., 1976) has shown an increase in the number of black women seeking help from outpatient psychiatric clinics. Yet Levine (1974) points out that from birth on, male children show a much greater prevalence of physical and emotional disorders than do female peers. Morbidity and mortality statistics for almost any disorder of childhood (cerebral palsy, congenital defects, childhood psychosis, behavior disorders, learning problems, hyperactivity) are overwhelmingly male dominated. After age 18, all anxiety-related symptoms are much higher in women than in men. The data in Table 26-1 from the President's Commission on Mental Health (vol. III, p. 1047) show the higher prevalence of psychiatric problems in male children. So why does the trend reverse in adults?

Psychiatric disorders rank third among conditions women present to general practitioners and seventh among conditions men present (Shepherd, 1964). In 1967, family doctors in the United Kingdom were consulted 20 million times for psychoneurotic disorders; 15 million of those visits were by women (Brandon, 1972). More recently, Weissman (1977), a psychiatrist, posed as a general practitioner and noted that of 152 women seen, sixty-six (or 43%) had symptoms of psychiatric disorder. Of the sixty-six, thirty-one were depressed and nineteen were anxious.

WHY HIGHER RATES OF MENTAL ILLNESS FOR WOMEN?

Many people have attempted to explain the existence of higher rates of mental illness among women. Mechanic (1976) speculates that most data collection tools are sex-linked and most frequently measure behaviors evidenced in females, such as neurosis. Behavior such as aggressiveness, violence, smoking, and alcohol and drug abuse—which are found more frequently among men— are less frequently measured. Women may also perceive more symptoms than men because of their interest in and knowledge about health. Mechanic also speculates that physicians are more likely to label a questionable symptom as psychogenic (instead of organic) if the patient is a woman, and especially if she also reports anxiety. Therefore, presenting problems of women get classified more often as psychologic. This is sex-role stereotyping.

However, this notion is challenged by McCranie and associates (1978), who designed a clinical simulation experiment in which general practitioners were asked to make clinical judgments about either a male or female patient having identical presenting symptoms (the symp-

toms could be either psychogenic or organic). It was hypothesized that if sex-role stereotyping were operating, the symptoms reported by the women would be more likely than those reported by men to be diagnosed and treated as reflective of psychogenic illness. The findings were negative; the physicians viewed patients' symptoms from an organic perspective regardless of sex. Since this was a recent report, one might think that perhaps physicians are changing, or that these were younger, less rigid doctors. (Mean age for the sample was, in fact, 51 years.) A caution about this study, however, is that sex-role stereotyping is activated by visual and auditory cues, which were not included in the written data collection tool.

Horwitz (1977) thinks women enter psychiatric treatment more frequently because they are more likely than men to recognize their problems and the need to discuss them. Women are taught that it is all right to seek help. Men, however, are more likely to be coerced into care or committed, and thus fewer are seen in organized mental health care centers. Other explanations given for the higher rates of mental illness among women are as follows (Levine, 1974):

1. Adult women are inherently emotionally weaker.
2. Statistics are unreliable.
3. Women have more time and freedom to indulge themselves in visits to a therapist.
4. Women are more open and emotionally honest, more expressive of their feelings than are men.
5. Physicians and therapists prefer female patients. Ninety percent of practicing psychiatrists in North America are male (two-thirds of clinical psychologists are male). Therapists are strong male authority figures who can be leaned on, but who also control and oppress women. Women continue in therapy because they think they cannot function on their own. Therapists do not get rich by curing people.
6. Society exacts a higher emotional price for women than for men by imposing rigid stereotyped sex roles on women; women pay the price for role rigidity (Davis, 1975).

Levine observed, "A woman 'on the couch' cannot win. If she acts according to society's and psychiatry's dictates, she feels like a fool, if she acts differently, she is labeled psychopathological" (p. 327). Phyllis Chesler (1973) notes that women have not been nurtured too well and take vacations in mental hospitals. Civilization, not people, is crazy. Most "crazy" people are just unhappily acting out their roles or rebelling against them.

A caution about interpreting the statistics is also issued by Maracek (1977b). Most data concern only those who have entered psychiatric hospitals for treatment, and many people seek treatment from outpatient clinics, private practitioners, family physicians, counselors, and friends. Thus statistics reporting hospital populations underestimate the total number of people with psychologic disorders. Also, the decision of whether or not to seek treatment is made on subjective and highly personal grounds. For instance, women may find it easier to share emotional concerns and thus be more inclined than men to seek psychotherapy. When all is said and done, "Women have been increasing their use of psychiatric facilities much more rapidly than men. It would be difficult to argue that attitudes and knowledge about psychiatry are changing faster in women than men. Instead, it is more plausible to argue that a rising amount of stress and conflict in women's lives is responsible." (Maracek, 1977a, p. 27).

Are there data to dispute the popular myth that women are inherently emotionally weaker than men? Earlier in this chapter reference was made to the higher prevalence of behavior disorders in males up until the age of 18. In addition, it may be helpful to look at sex differences/similarities and how menstruation affects mood. Garai (1970b) studied 280 elderly people (over age 60 years) in a resident community and found data to support his notion that women have greater investment in intimacy while men are more invested in achievement strivings. He found that: (1) women are more aware than men of the problems created by loss of a close confidant, (2) women are more likely to seek close relationships after a loss of intimacy, and (3) women have greater sensitivity to close relationships. Garai attributes the increased longevity of women to these assets. Perhaps the notion that women are emotionally weaker should be revised to say that women are emotionally (or interpersonally) more sensitive than men.

Other authors have noted that the male's activity level is higher (Goy, 1970; Money and Ehrhardt, 1972) and the female's tolerance for stress is greater (Lane, 1969; Teitelbaum, 1971). The most extensive review of sex differences published is in Maccoby and Jacklin's *The Psychology of Sex Differences* (1974). They reviewed over 2000 articles and books and concluded that many common assumptions about sex differences, including some that Garai maintains, are completely unfounded and are simply myths posing as facts. They also found that males and females do differ in interesting ways. (See Chapter 6 for detailed discussion.)

It seems safe to conclude, as Seiden (1976a) did, that girls have greater verbal ability after age 11, and boys have greater visual-spatial and mathematical ability beginning at age 12 or 13 and increasing through high school. It is not true that girls are *inherently* more socially oriented than boys, more suggestible, more auditory, less visual, less analytic, better at rote learning, or lower in self-esteem and achievement motivation, all of which

clearly indicates that most sex and social roles are learned.

Because of the cyclicity of female hormonal production, some traits may be exaggerated in a rhythmic way. An increase in drive and in the sense of competition and well-being occurs at ovulation (Money and Ehrhardt, 1972; Bardwick, 1974; Udry and Morris, 1968). Bardwick asked college girls to "tell me about an event in your life," and scored it using an anxiety scale for key words. Anxiety was significantly higher at premenstruation than at ovulation, and self-esteem and self-confidence were higher at ovulation. Women on combination oral contraceptives, however, had no significant mood fluctuations during the cycle. For these women both anxiety and hostility remained at the same high level throughout the month—as high as women not taking oral contraceptives experienced at menstruation. One criticism of Bardwick's study is that the girls knew it was related to the menstrual cycle and this could have influenced their responses (Tavris and Offin, 1977). Paige (1971) has suggested that the anxiety associated with menstruation may be related to the amount of flow—the more mess, unpredictable flow, and fuss, the more anxiety. Monthly mood changes (assuming they occur) have not been found to be great enough to affect a woman's ability to think and work (Tavris and Offin, 1977). "Well then, if menstruation doesn't make women dumber, perhaps it makes them dangerous . . . Half of the women who commit suicide, half of those who commit crimes, and almost half of those admitted to hospitals for psychiatric reasons are either menstruating or about to . . . Being arrested, having an accident, or entering a hospital are all highly stressful events, and great stress itself can bring on an early menstrual period . . . and because crime, accident, and suicide rates (though not suicide attempts) are much higher for males than for females, researchers might do better to study men at all weeks of the month than to worry about women during this one critical week." (Tavris and Offin, 1977). Some are suggesting that men also have rhythmic cycles due to testosterone production, although little research has been done on that. The "biorhythym" theories are another explanation for mood variations in both men and women.

Women at high risk

Guttentag and associates (1976) describe the high-risk female as being separated or divorced, nonwhite, poorly educated, and of low social status, who is coping with the combined stress of raising young children and being the breadwinner on a low income.

Social class

Of twenty studies reviewed, Dohrenwend (1965) found that in all but one, the highest rate of judged psychopathology occurred in the lowest socioeconomic status group. Social class is not simply a personal attribute, but a set of social conditions within which behavior occurs. More lower class individuals respond to stress with coping behaviors that stylistically mirror symptoms of psychoses than do upper class persons, whose response styles more closely approximate neurotic characteristics (Liem and Liem, 1978).

Women are overrepresented in the lower socioeconomic class. From the Department of Labor (1977) come the following data: Eighty-nine percent of women earn less than $9,000 a year, whereas only 49% of men earn less than $9,000 a year. Sexual discrimination within occupations is least obvious in professional groups (female median income as percentage of male is 67.5) and most obvious (40.3%) in the sales area. The female median percentage income of the male is about 55% for all levels of schooling until the number of years in school (beyond high school) reaches more than five. With more than five years of school beyond high school females make $11,000 a year and males make $16,900 yearly for a 65.4% of female to male income (no. 46, p. 3).

Among the fully employed who earned less than $3,500 in 1967, 45% were white women (10.6% were black females, 33.5% were white males, and 9.7%, black males). White women were only about 30% of the work force yet they were close to half of the fully employed working poor. Poor women have the highest incidence of mental illness (no. 46, pp. 20-21).

It is easy to see that social and economic discrimination can make women's lives more difficult. But what evidence is there that discrimination and lower status increase women's risk of psychologic disorders? Dohrenwend (1971) interviewed people from various social classes about recent life stresses and psychologic symptoms they were experiencing. She found that women reported significantly more life stress during the year preceding the interview than did men. Also, for women, psychologic symptoms were strongly associated with events that they could not control. Maracek (1977) notes that:

like other low-status groups, women face more stressful life events than their high-status counterparts. Second, these stressful life events produce symptoms of psychological stress; thus, women have more symptoms than men. However, when the contribution played by life events is held constant, both sexes have comparable rates of psychological symptoms. The third point is that women are not "weaker," less able to cope, or more reactive to external stresses than men (p. 271).

The President's Commission on Mental Health states:

Women who describe themselves in the socioeconomic status of working class represent a sizable portion of the female population who are most comfortable in the traditional societal roles as homemakers, wives and mothers . . . and have clung most tenaciously to traditional values and life styles. . . . These are the women who usually will not seek professional counseling . . . the problems faced by many working-class women at home and in the community have resulted in increasing social, psychological, and financial stresses (vol. III, p. 1033).

Race

Nonwhites show more utilization of state and county psychiatric facilities than do whites (Guttentag et al., 1976). They also make up a larger percentage of the lower socioeconomic class which is at highest risk for mental illness.

The inequalities that are barriers to full participation of women in American Society are multiplied for particular groups of economically and socially disadvantaged women. The Asian-American, Black, American Indian, and Hispanic women suffers discrimination because of her sex, because of her race and/or ethnic background, and because of physical and material oppression. . . . Psychologically, socially and economically the older minority woman faces the greatest risk in our society (President's Commission, vol. III, pp. 1032, 1033).

The women's movement has been viewed by some minority women with skepticism because black females are already in a better position than black men (Hare and Hare, 1972). They often have to marry into a lower socioeconomic class level. On college campuses today, the black female students greatly outnumber the black male students and competition for the small pool of affecting the social system educated males is readily visible. The self-esteem of black women will suffer if they continue to be unable to find suitable mates. If black women get better jobs as a result of women's liberation, then the difficulties of black's male-female relationships are further stressed.

Marital status

Gove (1972) examined data on mortality, suicide, and mental illness by marital status and sex, and found that married women generally had noticeably higher rates of mental illness than married men. He concluded that marriage had a protective effect on men but was detrimental for women. He cites the disadvantages of marriage for the woman as: (1) role restriction (men have both career and family with two sources of gratification), and (2) housekeeping (low prestige and time for brooding). Ramsey (1974) adds that the woman is exposed to a uniformly uninteresting environment, and her reaction time, sensory acuity, power of abstract reasoning, verbal ability, space visualization, and internal motivation to move, to daydream, or to think are all decreased. Gove compared single, widowed, and divorced females and males and found the overall incidence of mental illness among women was lower than among their male counterparts. These findings tend to support Gove's view that marriage has a detrimental effect on women.

Nathanson (1975) points out, however, that "happily" married women report less illness than single women (single includes divorced and widowed). Rivkin (1972) has also found lower reported morbidity among married women than among the single, widowed, or divorced. Age may also play a role in this difference. Renne (1971) found that divorced people in their early fifties, particularly women, were "consistently healthier, happier and less isolated than the unhappily married." One must be very cautious about interpreting findings about "single" women, since statistics on this segment of the population are confusing (President's Commission, vol. III). "Single" sometimes means "never married," but it may also include widowed, separated, and divorced people. Also, childrearing may or may not be a part of the "single" role. If "single" is considered to include all those women who are currently unmarried, the category comprises about one third of adult women in this country.

Children

Among unmarried women, those with children are more likely to use health care services than those without children. Working women with children have a higher utilization of services, fewer disability days, and higher anxiety than those without children (Nathanson, 1975). These findings are consistent with Rivkin's (1972) hypothesis that women with dense role responsibilities (children and no spouse or children and working) tend to get into the medical care system more often. Women with preschool children and employed women report less morbidity than their counterparts with older or no children, or who are housewives (Nathanson, 1975). Gove (1977) concludes that having children in the household generally contributes to poor mental health.

"Trapped young mother" syndrome. In a survey of the quality of American life (Seiden, 1976b), 89% of the young married child-free women reported life satisfaction, as compared to 65% of married women with young children. Though the 89% reporting life satisfaction appears very high, the actual number of young, married, child-free women is quite small in our society. One of five babies is born to an adolescent and many other women have their first child within the first 2 years of marriage. Indications of psychologic stress were greatest for both men and women during the early parental life stage. In striking contrast to the traditional belief that women require marriage and children for psychologic fulfillment, the child-raising period is equated with less life satisfaction, more stress, and more overt mental illness than other periods (Seiden, 1976b).

"Single parent" syndrome. The divorce rate in the United States is the world's highest and children are spending increasing amounts of time with an overburdened single parent (Seiden, 1976b). In 1970, over one fourth of American children under the age of 18 (and over one half of black children) were not currently living with both natural parents. More than one sixth of all children in America now live in single-parent families (usually headed by the mother) (President's Commission, vol. III). By the time they reach age 18, 35% to 45% of American children will have spent an average of 5 years in a single-parent home. Seiden reports that children are more vulnerable in single-parent homes than with happily married parents; however, the presence of any other adult in the single-parent home can reduce the child's vulnerability.

Divorced female parents report themselves as significantly less satisfied than their divorced male counterparts. The female single parents have a severe economic and emotional burden in childrearing. In 1975 only 14% received alimony; 44% received child support but less than half of these (21%) collected child support regularly. Even then it was usually inadequate (Seiden, 1976b). In 1975, 44% of the female-headed families with children had incomes below the poverty level. Low levels of child support and public assistance, and the continuing effects of sexism in hiring women and in wages paid to women contribute to this economic deprivation (President's Commission, vol. III). Loneliness and isolation also represent serious problems for single parents.

Employment

Employment has perhaps the most clearly positive effects on women's health of any variable investigated to date. Nathanson (1975) summarizes several studies that show when age, gynecologic illness, and occupational injuries are controlled for, employed women have lower sickness rates than housewives. Working women report less anxiety and many fewer physical symptoms than do housewives. Stevens (1978) considers homemaking an "occupational hazard." In spite of the adverse working conditions of women (low wages, household and child-care responsibilities in addition to job, low status jobs, and so on), employment has a healthy effect on women's mental status.

Warren (1976) reports that, in a study of 766 unemployed men and women, 9.3% of men as opposed to 33% of women reported symptoms of stress when they had lost their jobs. Employed women, many of whom ran households in addition to their jobs, were better off emotionally than the unemployed woman.

According to Gove and Geerken (1977), married women tend to be in poorer mental health than married men because of the roles they typically occupy. Since married women who are employed typically face much greater time and energy demands than their unemployed counterparts, an overload of actual tasks is not the prime cause of poorer mental health among women. Instead, it is the *kind* of demands found in the home and associated with children that produce the feeling of "incessant demands," not simply the *number* of tasks that must be performed. Employed married men are in the best mental health; unemployed married women are in the worst mental health, and employed married women are in between. Employed mothers were found by Feld (1963) to have more positive attitudes toward their children and to describe parenthood as less restricting, burdensome, and demanding than did unemployed mothers. Oakley (1975) found that women who devote themselves exclusively to their families experience the highest degree of dissatisfaction with their lives.

Eisenberg (1975) notes that increasing numbers of women are entering the labor force in response to the pressures of an inflationary economy, higher education costs for their children, opportunities for personal fulfillment, and a growing market for service occupations. Married mothers nevertheless continue to carry 70% to 80% of child-care and household duties even when both parents work.

Though women are returning to full-time employment, in actuality there is little shift in household or child-care responsibilities. A married mother who works has two jobs, a married father has one (Tavris and Offin, 1977):

Working wives have about ten fewer hours of free time each week than either housewives or employed men. Working wives use weekends to catch up on the cleaning and shopping. Working husbands use weekends to do odd chores, and then catch up on their rest, watch TV or play sports. As the family grows larger, the husband's participation decreases. He does less childcare, housework and cooking. The wife's housework time, however, increases between 5 and 10 percent with each child, whether she works [outside the home] or not (p. 231).

Employment outside the home is enhancing the mental health of women—or is it that the healthier women are employed outside the home? One wonders; however, what will be the impact of the loss of personal or fun time on the overall health of women in the future? Is the stress of being a full-time parent so great that the triple load of part-time parent, manager of household, and full-time employee is still less stressful? The United States is not the only country with a Catch-22 for women. In the Soviet Union, the domestic side of life is still regarded by both sexes as the woman's responsibility, regardless of her employment status. In China, 90% of the women work outside the home and there is a fairly extensive network of child daycare centers, but women continue to have responsibility for managing the house (Tavris and Offin, 1977).

In addition to the prediction of overload, many wom-

en are hesitant to engage in full-time employment because of the perceived negative impact on their young children. Group daycare for children has been discouraged based on at least two assumptions: (1) children would have more respiratory illnesses and (2) separation from the mother would cause irreparable harm to psychosocial development. The latter assumption in particular has kept women out of the job market for years and certainly has had an impact on the economic plight of women today. Few people dare postulate that perhaps the greatest danger to the mother and child occurs when they are isolated alone in a house. In fact, one could argue that group daycare is more similar to the way children were reared during past years when extended families and neighborhoods were closer and the number of children per family averaged six to ten. Since respiratory infections are the most common acute illnesses of young children, their nature and occurrence serve as useful indicators of environmental influences on health (Strangert, 1976). In comparing home care with family daycare (average of four children) and group daycare, the only daycare group with a higher incidence of illness was those children under age 2 years. When this group is controlled for socioeconomic class, the difference is apparent only in the upper socioeconomic class homes where there are no other children (Luda et al., 1972; Strangert, 1976).

There are no data to substantiate the myth that separation from the working mother causes harm to the child. Intellectual, social, and emotional development appears to be the same if not more advanced in group daycare children. There is, in fact, a significantly higher score on intellectual development of lower socioeconomic children who are in group daycare than in those who are not (Caldwell, 1972; Pines, 1971; Tavris and Offin, 1977).

Seiden (1976b) observes that children of employed mothers do best overall if the mother is doing what she prefers. Hoffman and associates (1974) found that maternal employment does not foster deprivation of the child and may, in fact, lead to greater marital harmony. Employment increases the power of the mother in the family, and working mothers are reported to be in better physical health and have greater self-confidence than mothers who are not employed. Mason and associates (1976) looked at changes in attitudes over a 10-year period beginning in 1964 and found a sharp decline in the proportion of women believing that maternal employment is harmful to their children's well-being. Birdbaum (1975), who compared housewives, married professionals, and single professionals, found that homemakers have the lowest self-esteem and feel the worst about their competence. The only thing missing for professional women is enough time to do all they want to do.

Impact of role conflict on the married career woman

Powell and Reznifoff (1976) suggest that no matter how desirable the changes presently occurring in role expectations for women, the process of change is, in itself, a painful and stressful experience. In a study of 136 graduates out of college 10 years and 132 out of college 25 years, neither employment status nor achievement motivation was significantly related to symptoms of mental illness. However, women with contemporary sex-role orientations exhibited significantly higher symptom scores. The class out of college 10 years had significantly more members with high need for achievement, contemporary sex-role orientation, advanced degrees with higher incomes, and higher symptom scores. The stresses may come from establishing oneself at a high professional level while simultaneously dealing with the responsibilities of young children in a society that still assigns this role primarily to women. Women making over $20,000, with or without children, exhibited significantly lower symptom scores than other employed women, suggesting that at this income level women are better able to make satisfactory arrangements for household help, in addition to enjoying the rewards of meaningful work.

Johnson and Johnson (1976), exploring the role strain in high-commitment, career, married women found that these women have role overload because of their commitment to two jobs, the domestic and occupational. In most instances, the woman's career is secondary to marriage and motherhood. The double-bind for women is obvious. If career investment is lowered, one faces diminished achievement and failure in competition with male colleagues. But if one lowers the commitment to mothering, that violates the most cherished social norms and can lead to social condemnation and reactive states of anxiety and guilt. With successful career women, the husband's support is the crucial ingredient. The typical husband, however, is reading the newspaper while his career wife is preparing dinner, and after dinner she bathes and beds the children, folds the laundry, makes out the grocery list, and writes a committee report—while he watches TV. The question in such homes is not who shall make the beds, but why aren't the beds made, or why haven't you, wife, made the beds? The options for the career married woman appear clear: she can eliminate some roles by changing her value system or hiring domestic help and/or she can bargain for role changes with family and employer.

The role strain is obvious among women physicians, who have a suicide rate that is twice as high as among women in the general population and a divorce rate that is higher than that among male doctors (Goldstein, 1975). Female physicians who had not pursued careers were found to have higher scores on depression, anxiety, and anger than either male or female practicing physicians; 46% of the practicing female physicians assumed responsibility for household planning, shopping, preparing and serving food, chauffering, child-care, and care of ill family members.

Alexandra Symonds (1976, 1978), who has written extensively on the difficulties experienced by women who move into careers, has observed that women have to make a character change from a predominantly compliant, dependent personality to a more expansive one, and this causes symptoms, anxieties, marital stress, and profound turmoil. Symonds argues that women already have the intelligence and skills for the careers they are now entering, but it will be some time before they develop the character patterns necessary to sustain the anxiety they are now experiencing. For example, women are poorly prepared for the competitive demands of our culture. Situations that men take for granted come as a complete surprise to women who are new in the field. When confronted with situations calling for aggressive protection of their rights, women often respond in inappropriate or ineffectual ways and feel puzzled and angry at the results. Anger may be expressed as tears; a woman may find she can fight only on the basis of weakness. Career women, says Symonds, experience symptoms as a result of "unresolved dependency needs," which may show up as a facade of self-sufficiency (in their tough and controlling manners) or may be evidenced by much turmoil in relationships with men. According to Symonds (1978), the largest group of career women:

> have achieved success in their work and have satisfactory personal lives but—owing to their underlying depression and conflicts regarding dependency—do not ever seem to be fulfilled. . . . These women work twice as hard as others because they work at their jobs and take care of their families as well. They are usually nurturing individuals who choose the helping professions (like nursing), with the compulsive need to be super-mom and super-wife. . . . [Besides doing extra work] they are constantly taking care of others. They give to others, often compulsively, but find it hard to allow others to give to them. This lack of nurturing takes its toll, and they often go into therapy because of depression (p. 203).

Fodor (1974) reports that women who are rated competent and who achieve in adult roles are said to have received more "maternal rejection" (defined as absence of mother love) as well as discipline that was more similar to what boys received. The fathers took an active role in the raising of their daughters and rewarded their independence and competence.

The elderly

Currently there are 23 million people over age 65 in the United States (11% of the total population). By the year 2000, the elderly will number 30 million and be 15% of the population (President's Commission, vol. II). Twenty-five percent of all suicides occur in the elderly.

Stresses affecting the elderly include social role changes, personal losses leading to bereavement, retirement from jobs, drop in income, economic worries, isolation, fear of crime, and concerns about health prospects (President's Commission, vol. II). An estimated 15% to 25% of the older persons have significant mental health problems. Three quarters of the elderly are living at home and of the remaining 25%, 20% are in community based care facilities while only 5% (largely females over 80 years) are in nursing homes.

In a small sample of black elderly persons, Faulkner and associates (1975) found that mobility was a critical variable in perceived happiness. Those who were not too happy were living with others and had restricted mobility. Those describing themselves as very happy were mobile.

Larson (1978) found a significant relationship between health and reported well-being in the elderly, but found that poor health had a greater impact on the well-being of the lower social classes. Other environmental features such as availability of transportation and social activities were significantly related to well-being.

Because of the tendency of women in this country to marry older men, and the likelihood that women will live 7 to 8 years longer than men of the same age, the average woman can expect to spend the last 10 years of her life as a widow. Within the population of elderly women, widowed women are particularly at risk. Twenty percent of American women are widows by age 60, 50% by age 65, and 67% by age 75 (President's Commission, vol. III). The most important unmet needs of elderly women are transportation, physical assistance, social affiliation, medical care, legal assistance, and financial assistance (Guttman et al., 1977). Many of the problems of the elderly women would be alleviated if more financial assistance were available. Specific means of assistance, says Guttman, include granting special reduced interest loans to improve the buildings in which older people live, subsidizing rent, building collective housing projects with services on the ground floor (such as canteens, hot meal services, recreational activities, hairdressing, and so on), providing protective dwellings for those who need some help and care, providing free or inexpensive domestic help, free home nursing care, day hospital care with transportation, and short educational courses on a wide variety of topics.

Toffler (1971) suggests engaging the elderly to help provide child care. Certainly, some involvement in community services could be rewarding for them as well as helpful to the community. Only a small percentage of elderly women are incapable of being productive citizens. The elderly are an untapped resource pool ready to be mobilized. Some of the "free" services mentioned earlier could be earned by providing community services, so that the community at large, elderly women, and taxpayers would all benefit.

WOMEN'S ATTITUDES TOWARD THEIR ROLE

When Cohen and Burdsal (1978) examined the role attitudes of 139 married women in Kansas, their most significant finding was that a satisfying relationship with her husband predicted a satisfied woman and vice versa. They also found that women with two or more children felt their husbands did not understand them; housewives who felt intellectually equal to their husbands felt that men use women as cheap labor. The higher the income of the woman's family, the more likely she was to consider childbearing a joint responsibility. Women who had helpful fathers expected help from their mates, and women who had working mothers felt good about working themselves.

R. Levy (1976) found that married women who were experiencing structural role strain in their marriages reacted in basically two ways: psychosomatic symptoms or political/social protest. Psychosomatic symptoms appeared more often in women who held traditional values and also were functioning in traditional roles. Women who protested manifested minimal psychosomatic symptoms.

Mason and associates (1976) examined changes in women's sex-role attitudes from 1964 to 1974 using data from five different sample surveys. They concluded that there has been considerable movement toward more egalitarian role definitions with change occurring equally among higher and lower class women. Educational attainment and employment were the most important variables for predicting women's attitudes (the well-educated and those with recent work experience had less traditional attitudes).

Dellas and Gaier (1975) discuss choices now available to the adolescent girl and list the role behaviors for (1) the traditional woman whose commitment is to the family, (2) the achievement model woman whose commitment is to a career, and (3) the bimodal sexual identity woman whose commitment to family coexists with allegiance to career. They subscribe to the belief that contemporary society affords the young girl an opportunity for alternative life-styles and roles. If this choice really exists, say Dellas and Gaier, then someone should tell the adolescent boys. In 1975, the same year that Dellas and Gaier published their article, Joesting reported that girls are changing but boys are not. The ninth grade girls in a Southern junior high school viewed their roles in an egalitarian manner and rejected traditional roles while their male peers maintained traditional views about women's roles:

- Girls did not think men are better leaders
- Boys did think men are better leaders
- Girls did not think husbands should make major decisions
- Boys did think husbands should make major decisions
- 49% of boys but 70% of girls thought women should be able to become lawyers

Joesting (1975) notes that the discrepancy in role perception could increase the anxiety of adolescent girls and contribute to increasing suicidal attempts, pregnancies, and other emotional disturbances.

Sex-role stereotyping

Sex-role stereotyping refers to "highly consensual norms and beliefs about the differing characteristics of men and women." (Broverman, et al., 1970, p. 4). Rigid sex-role stereotyping limits women's freedom to choose the life-styles most suited to their needs and abilities (Maracek and Kravetz, 1977). Confining women to stereotypic roles leads to depression, guilt, apathy, and other self-defeating behaviors. In addition, according to Maracek and Kravetz, social penalties are handed out to women such as divorcees, single women, married career women or child-free women, who do not elect to follow the stereotypic role.

A second damaging aspect of the traditional view of women is its devaluation of the female. People are generally taught to view the characteristics, activities, and achievements of men as superior to and more worthwhile than those of women. A third source of damage noted by Maracek (1977) is institutional sexism in the forms of legal, educational, economic, and political discrimination. "Thus, the social conditions arising from traditional cultural conceptions of women have had a detrimental effect on women's psychological health and personal growth" (p. 323).

The notion of sex-role stereotyping was highlighted almost 10 years ago by the classic Broverman studies. They sent out questionnaires consisting of 122 bipolar items to actively functioning clinicians with one of three sets of instructions: describe the healthy, mature, socially competent (a) adult, sex unspecified, (b) male, or (c) female. They found that clinical judgments about the characteristics of healthy individuals differed as a function of the sex of the person judged; these differences paralleled stereotypic sex-role differences. Moreover, behaviors and characteristics judged healthy for an adult (sex unspecified, reflecting an ideal standard of health) resembled behaviors judged healthy for men but differed from behavior judged healthy of females.

In other words, the mental health clinicians conceptu-

alized the ideal healthy adult and the ideal healthy male similarly. In contrast, the ideal healthy female was seen as significantly less healthy than the ideal healthy adult. Ideal women were viewed as: "more submissive, less aggressive, less competitive, more excitable in minor crises, having their feelings hurt, being more emotional, and more concerned about their appearance." Broverman notes that, "this is a most unusual way of describing any mature, healthy person."

Several researchers have re-examined the concept of a dual standard of mental health as found by Broverman. Instead of asking the practitioners their attitudes about women, Miller (1976) looked at the clients' charts from three mental health centers in southeastern United States. He found that attitudes toward women differed among professionals but seemed of little importance in terms of differential treatment excepting that women (more often than men) were perceived as needing to focus on family relationships and were more often seen in family therapy. Women received problem-oriented therapy while men received supportive therapy. Miller was *not* able to prove that women (in relation to men) were judged more disturbed, received more medication, were seen for shorter periods of time, or had less favorable prognoses.

Aslin (1973) used Broverman's sex-role stereotyping questionnaire and, using a similar design, collected data from 130 community mental health center (MHC) therapists (seventy-five women and fifty-five men) and eighty-two "feminist" therapists. Each of the subjects was given one of four possible instructions: Think of a normal adult, female, wife, or mother, and then indicate which of the following characteristics is mature, healthy, and socially competent. The clinical judgments of female MHC therapists and feminist therapists were similar on all scales. The clinical judgments of female and male MHC therapists were similar for adult and wife, but differed significantly on female and mother. The judgments of male MHC therapists and feminists therapists also differed significantly for both female and mother.

The male MHC therapists judged female, wife, and mother similarly but judged all of them as different from adult. The male MHC therapists (but not the female MHC or feminist therapists) responded to adult as more stereotypically male than female, wife, or mother.

Finally, Aslin found that therapists who described themselves as attempting to counter societal restrictions on women and as helping clients free themselves from stereotypes judged mentally healthy adults differently from therapists who described themselves as uninvolved in social change.

Two studies reported in recent literature on sex-role stereotyping in psychiatric nurses appear to arrive at contradictory results. Both researchers used the Broverman 82-item revised, short form of the sex-role questionnaire. Kjervik and Palta (1978) found that a healthy woman was rated closer to a healthy adult than was a healthy male. The descriptions of the healthy adult contained both the valued masculine and feminine traits, so that healthy females were found to possess valued masculine traits (such as achievement) without losing feminine valued characteristics (such as nurturance).

In contrast, Moscato (1978) concluded that psychiatric nurses held sex-role stereotypes with the traits for a healthy adult mirroring the stereotypical masculine sex-role characteristics. The nurses perceived themselves to be more closely associated with feminine, rather than with masculine, stereotypic sex-role behaviors.

Kjervik and Palta (1978) found that nurses who had longer experience as therapists and were older and still practicing viewed males and females as more alike. Moscato found no evidence that age or type of employment contributed to the nurses' stereotyping sex-role behaviors.

Bem (1975) has developed a tool designed to measure androgyny—the extent to which a person believes he or she possesses desirable attributes of both sexes. From testing of college students at Stanford University, Bem found about half to be traditionally feminine or masculine. Fifteen percent were cross sex-typed (scoring higher on traits associated with the opposite sex) and 35% were androgynous—scoring about the same on masculine and feminine qualities. Bem found that androgynous people were more flexible and this enhanced their mental health because they could adapt behavior depending on the situation—for instance, being nurturing with a baby and competitive in a job situation. Suter and Domino (1975) similarly found that highly creative women possessed a broader, less stereotyped sex-role identity.

Sources of sex-role stereotyping: the psychology of submission

Until recently feminine passivity was thought to be determined by an inadequacy of biologic origin, which also predicted many other inferior consequences.* Freud's psychology of women portrays them as inferior and incomplete males suffering from lack of a penis. Only lately through the research of Masters and Johnson (1966) has the myth that the clitoris is an inferior sexual organ been dispelled.

Karen Horney's (1945, 1950) theory of the learned dependent role of women is very relevant in a discussion of psychology of women. She states that females have been pressured from early childhood into the de-

---

*Miller, 1973; Rawlings and Carter, 1977; Carter, 1971; Mamalis, 1976.

pendent, submissive role in life and generally have accepted it. Girls are not encouraged to separate and develop in an autonomous manner as boys are. To the contrary, girls are encouraged to maintain their dependent relationships with parents and family and after marriage to transfer them to husband and children. Women are required not only to renounce their own achievements and need to succeed, but also to do it without feeling that they are sacrificing anything. To be lovely and non-aggressive, a female spends a lifetime keeping down resentful impulses. Healthy self-assertion is sacrificed since it may be mistaken for hostility. Women give up initiative and aspirations at a cost of becoming excessively dependent with a deep sense of insecurity and uncertainty about their abilities and worth (Symonds, 1976).

Traditional attitudes toward women, implying that they need special care and protection, that they are relatively frail, and that they are not as capable in "worldly" activities as men, have had specific harmful effects on women's emotional growth and development and on their concept of self (Symonds, 1974). Pressures of society have restricted women to developing about one third of their potential. Horney recognizes that from birth all humans have needs and potentialities in three main areas: dependency, detachment, and expansiveness. Humans need to develop all three. When the individual gets messages from the family or the culture that certain expressions are taboo, then the individual develops excessively in one direction and anxiously tries to repress the other needs. (For example, the dependent person must not acknowledge needs for separateness.) While few individuals ever achieve their full potential, women as a group have been encouraged to express *only* their dependency needs and have been actively discouraged and at times ridiculed for trying to meet needs of detachment or expansiveness. As Symonds (1974) states "As a result, the dependent personality is called feminine, as though it were biologically predetermined." The dependent person is considered the normal woman. "Women from early childhood equate self-fulfillment with being loved, finding a man, having a family. Men also need to have a woman and perhaps a family, but once this is settled, it becomes a background for growth and fulfillment in other areas" (Symonds, 1974, p. 180).

Society's tools to ensure sex-role stereotyping

Little girls are surrounded by sensory data that tell them being female is less desirable than being male as in the following examples.

Childrens books. A NOW task force (Women on Words and Images, WWI) conducted a survey of 134 elementary school readers published before 1972, from fourteen different publishers. They generally found that boys were shown doing brave, adventurous, even superhuman feats while girls most often were behind something, watching. Any random sample of children's books in a public library today will reveal stories and pictures about little white boys exploring and conquering their world. Girls and black children are written about infrequently and when they are, the girls are in passive or helpful roles. In a recent update using books published after 1972, the WWI found a 2:1 ratio for male to female biographies (much improved) but the ratio of boy-centered to girl-centered stories had worsened (from 5:2 to 7:2) (Tavris and Offin, 1977). WWI found 147 occupations represented for boys and only 26 for girls.

Television. Television (in 96% of homes) is the major medium of mass communication to the American family, with consequent implications for family mental health. Television delivers an average of 23.5 hours of "lessons" a week for the American child (President's Commission, vol. IV). Through television, the child learns about people and what kind of behavior is appropriate for them. Three fourths of all leading characters on prime-time network TV are male (Tavris and Offin). Wonder Woman, who was almost the only female among a large number of male "super friends" has recently left that role on TV. Even the women who are competent at jobs somehow end up needing a male to get them out of trouble. In a small survey of prime-time daytime and evening TV programs, it was found that the daytime soap operas were much more likely to stereotype the females in a feminine sex type than were the late evening programs (Whittenberg and Stoy, 1978). This tends to reinforce the feminine stereotype for housewives and young children.

Teachers. One recent study of teachers and children in fifteen nursery school classrooms supports the position that adults do treat boys and girls differently, but in subtle ways. "Even people who talk equality sometimes remain unconsciously traditional" (Tavris and Offin, 1977, p. 174). Serbin and O'Leary (1975) found that all fifteen of the teachers paid more attention to the boys. Boys got more rewards for academic work, they got more help than girls did when they asked for it, and they helped to problem solve.

Professional journals. A content analysis performed on 500 drug advertisements drawn from seven years of the *Medical Journal of Australia* and *Australina Family Medicine* revealed significant differences between ads for mood modifying drugs and ads for other categories of drugs (Darroch, 1975). For mood modifying drugs, pictures were more often of females than males, thus reinforcing the physician's expectation that the patient needing it will be female.

Benedek (1976) reports that of thirty-seven psychiatric and related professional journals, little effort is being made to increase the representation of women on editorial boards or in authorship of journals.

The sources of sex-role stereotyping are everywhere. The fact that "he" and "mankind" usually refer to both sexes is an everpresent subliminal reminder that it is a man's world. Recently, a patient was talking in a team meeting about a visit from a lawyer. The psychiatrist inquired about what he said. After the patient left the room, the group learned (from a female physician) that the lawyer was a woman. Men and women have lived with sexism so long that it is now a part of us and few are aware of how often it negatively affects our behavior and the self-esteem of women.

Psychologic consequences of stereotyping

O'Connell (1976) examined the differences in personal sense of identity in married women pursuing three different life-styles: (1) traditional (full-time housewives/mothers), (2) neotraditional (returned to paid employment after a period of childrearing), and (3) nontraditional (combining career with marriage and childbearing). O'Connell found that the traditional and neotraditional women did not perceive their self-identity as strong or related to their own personal development until after their last child was in school. These mothers with preschool children had a self-identity based on their husband and children's identities and were therefore vulnerable for quite a few years because of their dependency on the reflections of others for their sense of identity. In contrast, the nontraditional women experienced their identity as comparatively strong and personal at *all* stages of the life cycle. The appearance of children did not interfere with personal identity development, which grew stronger with each life stage. Beginning in adolescence, the traditional and neotraditional (but not the nontraditional) women underwent a "moratorium" in personal identity synthesis, which lasted until childbearing duties diminished. Women who chose a traditional or neotraditional role sacrificed identity development for a number of years.

Abernethy (1976) hypothesizes that a woman's internalization of a negative evaluation of female capacities promotes her withdrawal from competition. This could be a factor in explaining why school performance for girls begins to deteriorate in high school at the time of career choices. Girls perform as well as or better than boys until adolescence.

In a 3-year study of forty conflicted and twenty-five nonconflicted marriages, Alsbrook (1976) notes that the conflicted marriages are always composed of a superordinate and subordinate dyad—each struggling for control. From their subordinate position, women see themselves less positively than they see their husbands.

Even smoking behavior appears to be related to the

socialization process. Fear of weight gain (and unattractiveness) keeps women from stopping smoking (Dicken, 1978). The differential socialization of males and females with respect to independence and achievement may give males more confidence in their ability to affect important outcomes such as health, and leave females more inclined to attribute outcomes to external factors. Current trends show a decrease in male initiation of smoking and an increase in cessation. Females are unchanged on both. The females in Dicken's study reported taking things as they come, but the males were more apt to try to prepare for something that might happen in the future. The women were more likely than men to report using cigarettes to deal with emotional upset. Professional women were the only group who had higher smoking rates than comparable groups of males. Because of this, Dicken suggests that women may be using smoking to attain greater identification with a masculine mode of relating to the world—to achieve liberation from their stereotyped weak and subordinate role.

Levine (1974) suggests that to succeed and achieve are inconsistent with femininity in our culture. It is immensely important to the developing female to "be loved." Women tend to view their self-esteem in terms of "affiliation achievement." A highschool girl needs to be popular—which generally means being attractive and passive. Achievement is important for boys. But then when girls lose their attractiveness, they do not have anything else to bolster their self-esteem.

Horner (1972) began writing in the early 1970s about a "fear of success" in women. She found that college students, both male and female, perceived unpleasant consequences such as social alienation and ostracism when a girl was a high achiever. When she applied the test to black students, she got the reverse results. Fear of success was evident in the following:

White men	10%
White women	64%
Black men	67%
Black women	29%

For most black men and white women, attainment of success and/or leadership is seen as an unexpected event, making them the object of competitive assault or social rejection. Horner states that fear of success is learned early in life along with sex-role identity; it comes from parental attitudes and male peers. This fear of success bodes loss not only for the individual people but also for society.

Konstam and Gilbert (1972) reject Horner's ideas on fear of success and say the central dynamic is the negative reaction by one or both parents to the child's movement toward competence. The parents fear that the child will surpass their own level of competence. Konstam and Gilbert found that individuals who scored high on "fear of success" were less sure of their abilities and needed others to affirm their worthwhileness.

Other studies based on Horner's work show that men often fear success as greatly as women do. But the sexes do regard the consequences of achievement differently. Women associate success with social rejection; men question the value of success (Tavris and Offin, 1977). "Researchers still disagree about whether fear of success has actually kept anyone from succeeding in a career. But even if worry about being different does not actually block achievement, it may cause women to feel ambivalent and guilty about their accomplishments and create considerable personal anguish" (Tavris and Offin, 1977, p. 194).

Tavris and Offin also summarized evidence about the effect of stereotyping on self-esteem:

1. Females envy males more than males envy females. Among kindergartners, twenty-eight of twenty-nine boys would not want to switch sexes but six of the thirty girls were ready to change.
2. Many women devalue other women's intellectual competence. Two thirds of the kindergartners of each sex thought their own sex was smarter, but over half of the girls reported their fathers as smarter than their mothers.
3. Females have less self-confidence than males. Women will choose situations involving luck more often than situations involving skill because they are insecure about their skills.

A group of women was asked to judge the merits of an article. Half of the manuscripts carried a male author's name and half a female author's name. The marks were higher at a statistically significant level for the article allegedly written by a male.

Women perceive themselves as powerless but reality does not confirm this. Beck and Greenberg (1974) report on an experiment done by Olson in which young couples expecting a baby were asked questions such as: "Which one of you would decide whether to buy insurance for the baby?" or "Which one would decide the husband's part in diapering?" Olson also set up situations in which the couple had to arrive at a decision while he watched. He found that husbands perceived themselves as having more power than they actually had in the laboratory "reality" and wives perceived themselves as having less. Whereas 73% of the husbands overestimated their power in decision making, 70% of the wives underestimated theirs. It would seem from this research that women perceive their inadequacies as much greater than reality affirms. A perception of helplessness, however, will prevent women from acting on their own behalf.

INTERVENTION STRATEGIES TO ELIMINATE SEX-ROLE STEREOTYPING

There is little question that the price society pays for maintaining sex role stereotyping is very high. According to the President's Commission (1978):

. . . intervention in the social system has potential for effecting a far greater change than does individual or group psychotherapy. For example, implementation of affirmative action plans and a reduction in the extent to which jobs are segregated by sex would raise the earning potential of millions of women. The resultant increase in income would reduce the impact of life stress and raise the self-concept of women on a scale not possible through remedial psychotherapies. The development of a network of day-care systems in the community would free more welfare mothers to work and would relieve the stress of many mothers already working. Appointment of a representative number of women to policymaking positions in Federal, State, and local agencies would permit the concerns of women to be expressed in the decisions that impact on the lives of all American women. A change in the stereotyped portrayal of housewives thrilled with the sight of their detergent white laundry would influence the image of women to television viewers of both sexes and all ages. Legal enforcement of court-mandated child support payments would raise the living standard of millions of American women and children. Federal laws covering the kidnapping of children by the noncustodial parent would eliminate crisis situations for many parents and children. Such interventions in the social system are preventive measures and ultimately will reduce the need and the cost of remedial services (vol. III, p. 1065).

The data clearly indicate that even though work serves as a protection for women, the triple responsibility of work, childrearing, and household management places women under stress.

Strategies for social change

A renowned psychiatrist has written that mental health professionals should be involved in social change instead of just helping people to adjust to and maintain a status quo society (Hallbeck, 1978). The President's Commission on Mental Health (vol. III) made twenty-nine recommendations to change the social status of women and thereby lessen their need for mental health services. Those recommendations are summarized and discussed below.

1. Federal training funds should be given only to programs that demonstrate a commitment to nonsexist education. High priority should be given to programs devoted to training new or established mental health professionals in the psychology of women.
2. The Department of HUD should encourage states to develop supportive facilities for displaced homemakers, battered women, teenage runaways, the aged, and women offenders. The Secretary of HEW should estab-

lish under medicaid a class of intermediate care facilities that specifically recognize the needs of such women clients.
   a. A network of shelters for women should be established throughout the country. Emergency shelters offering protective care, medical, legal, and social services for women should be established in every metropolitan area.
   b. A broad, national campaign should be undertaken to educate the public of the existence of destitute and battered women. Community members should be encouraged to initiate shelter services on their own.
   c. Available government funding should be directed toward community-initiated programs demonstrating expertise in the delivery of services for the special needs of women (including battered, runaway, ex-offender, and destitute women).
3. Advocates who are experts on women's mental health needs should be included in any interagency group within the federal government that is coordinating community-based care for the mentally disabled.
4. The Departments of HEW and Justice should evaluate deinstitutionalism in terms of its effect on the family as well as the patients, especially women. The Departments of HEW, Labor, and Justice should cooperate in developing programs for institutionalized women that will give priority fostering integration back into the community.
5. The Department of HEW should give priority to training minority mental health personnel, minority researchers, and persons serving bicultural and bilingual groups.
6. The National Council on Health Planning and Development should include a person with expertise in special mental health needs of women and women should be represented in proportion to their numbers in the population.
7. The Secretary of HEW should analyze the impact on women of mental health coverage in private health insurance as well as national health insurance proposals including mental health benefits.
8. All restrictions on federal funding for abortion should be eliminated.
9. Legislation concerned with domestic violence should receive priority attention and such legislation should emphasize service delivery.
10. Research recommendations:
   a. New money should be earmarked for research that serves the needs of women. Emphasis should be placed on understudied stages such as early adolescence, young adults, women in midlife, and the elderly.
   b. Epidemiologic research should be undertaken that will profile the status of women as clients as well as providers in the mental health delivery system.
   c. Every agency within the Executive Branch of government should establish administrative positions

with responsibility for reviewing policies, regulations, and programmatic decisions for potential impact on the lives of women.

d. Adequate representation of women should be achieved and maintained on all NIH (National Institutes of Health) and ADAMHA (Alcohol, Drug Abuse, and Mental Health Administration) committees that review research on women's health, physiology, and reproductive systems.

e. A critical mass of women should be appointed to policymaking positions within ADAMHA agencies. Ongoing inservice training programs should be provided for staff of ADAMHA.

f. Funded training and service programs should be set up for up-to-date information on the status of women, sex-role assumptions, and the psychology of women as well as current perspectives on psychotherapy for women. Greater coordination of research efforts between the three ADAMHA agencies, NIMH (National Institute on Mental Health), NIDA (National Institute on Drug Abuse), NIDAA (National Institute on Drug Abuse and Alcoholism), should be fostered to reduce duplication of effort in research concerning women and promote a systematic approach to this research. The gap between research findings and training and service to women should be filled through regular publication of research results and dissemination to practitioners and trainers.

g. A task force should be appointed for ADAMHA with representation of staff and outside consultants to plan for the needs of women in the 1980s.

h. An interagency task force should be established between NIDA and FDA (Food and Drug Administration) to examine policies concerning drug testing and research with female subjects, including those within the childbearing ages.

11. The President and the Congress should endorse passage of the Equal Rights Amendment. This constitutional commitment to the eradication of the inequality between the sexes that is so devastating to this nation's mental health is a basic foundation for the strategies that are proposed.

12. The Congress and Executive Branch should endorse the National Plan of Action (of the International Women's Year, National Women's Conference) and request that the President give implementation of the plan highest priority as a strategy for prevention of the mental health problems of women.

Six recommendations proposed by the National Women's Conference are in relation to child care:

1. The federal government should assume a major role in directing and providing comprehensive, voluntary, flexible hour, bias-free, nonsexist, quality child-care and developmental programs, including child-care facilities for federal employees, and should request and support adequate legislation and funding for these programs.

2. Federally funded child-care and developmental programs should have low-cost, ability-to-pay fee schedules that make these services accessible to all who need them, regardless of income, and should provide for parent participation in their operation.

3. Legislation should make special provision for child-care facilities for rural and migrant worker families.

4. Labor and management should be encouraged to negotiate child-care programs in their collective bargaining agreements.

5. Education for parenthood programs should be improved and expanded by local and state school boards, with technical assistance and experimental programs provided by the federal government.

6. City, county and/or state networks should be established to provide parents with hotline consumer information on child care, referrals, and follow-up evaluations of all listed care-givers (President's Commission, vol. III, 1978, p. 1085).

The above recommendations refer to actions that can be initiated at the federal level to start a process of social change that will eventually affect the mental health of all people and especially women. Other strategies of a more specific nature are discussed here and in the clinical syndrome sections to follow.

Other strategies to improve the mental health of women
Work incentive programs (WIN)

These programs are funded by federal and state money with the purpose of helping people receiving welfare through Aid to Families of Dependent Children (AFDC) to achieve financial independence by offering them opportunities to acquire education and work skills for jobs. Data presented earlier in this chapter indicate that work has a positive effect on the mental health of women. In addition, some of the noneconomic benefits of participation in WIN programs were found to be (Department of Labor, p. 47):

• Working women reported increased self-esteem
• They reported fewer physical illnesses
• The women were interested in additional training
• The working mothers had a more effective home life and self-concept than nonworking mothers.

Work incentive programs are especially designed for poor, single parents with few job skills who are at the highest risk for mental illness. The 3-week program includes time to plan how to adjust their life-styles to the demands of the working world, to develop habits and methods of coming to work each day, and to make arrangements about family. They learn about birth control, budgeting, and inexpensive but proper nutrition (Messer and Lebrer, 1976). They were tested and trained for local job openings. In the first 2 years of WIN programs, 75% of the white women and 26% of the black women were able to get off welfare and feel better about themselves as a result of the program (Department of Labor, 1977).

Child care

One of the major reasons that the work incentive programs were only marginally successful was because the women could not earn enough money to cover the costs of child care (Department of Labor, 1977). They had more expendable income from welfare payments than from paid employment minus costs for child care. Social innovations in child care (such as mentioned above) are considered necessary if optimal conditions for child and family development are to be provided. The most necessary condition for successful child care and family adjustment in a home where both parents work is considered to be redistribution of household workload among husband, wife, and other members of the family. The notion of equalizing child care and housework tasks in the two-parent home is a good one but it appears to be unrealistic for the present, and many working mothers are single parents.

Reproductive freedom

Women must have control over their bodies. Availability of low cost contraceptives and abortions is a necessity if women are to take responsibility for themselves. The old cliché, "Keep her barefoot and pregnant," is not acceptable to women.

Division of household responsibilities

An equal division of child-care responsibilities for both parents along with an equal division of the low-status household tasks would improve women's lot. Delaying marriage (and especially childbearing) until the woman has her own occupational identity could be helpful. School systems need to be more sensitive to the problems of working mothers and provide scheduled activities for after school hours until the usual workday ends. Far too many children are staying at home unsupervised because schools close so early in the afternoon. Two-career families need a reliable social support system close by so that grandparents and friends can help with child care during high stress times. Because female roles are changing, this may have a positive impact on general mental health since both men and women will profit from the increased flexibility in gender role specifications (Abernethy, 1976).

Neighborhood helping networks

Professionals cannot and do not provide help for most individuals. Eighty percent of the problem with which people must cope are solved through help from the person's social network (President's Commission, vol. III).

The natural helping network includes spouses, neighbors, coworkers, friends, and acquaintances from church and civic groups. The self-help groups discussed in the section on depression are also examples of the social system taking over to reduce isolation and stressful life situations. These resources can and do provide major preventive and crisis help for women. Every new mother, for example, needs another mother with whom she can discuss the many concerns of parenting. Further development of community network systems should be encouraged.

Recent research suggests that those who have social supports are protected in crisis from a wide variety of pathologic states, both mental and physical. It is thought that these supports buffer the individual from the potentially negative effects of undergoing crises and changes and can facilitate coping and adaptation (Cassel, 1974; Kaplan et al., 1977). This concept is so important in promoting mental health that an entire section of the President's Commission on Mental Health is devoted to exploring ways to expand the community support systems model.

Leisure

McDowell (1976), discussing the theoretical constructs concerning leisure and mental health, mentions that the leisure experience and positive mental health are so closely related that one may consider them synonymous. From research data, however, it is not possible to draw conclusions about the relationship between leisure and mental health. Some recent evidence suggests the beneficial effects of exercising, such as jogging, on psychologic states. Certainly much more research needs to be done. Meanwhile, counseling people to participate in leisure experiences is assumed to be a helpful strategy.

Self-help groups

Part of the feminist therapy effort has been to promote alternatives to therapy, such as consciousness-raising groups and self-help counseling. Self-help groups are not only effective, their cost is minimal. Self-help groups, as opposed to therapeutic groups and group psychotherapy, for the most part, are organized and operated by group members themselves (Marram, 1978). Their purpose is to solve the problems of members as defined by members. They are groups of, for, and by the clients. When and if professionals participate in group meetings, they do so by invitation and are placed in an ancillary role. The most common denominator is that the person who has already lived through an experience is critical in helping others (Gartner, 1977). Not only does the person know what the experience is like, but also she has learned how to play the required new role (e.g., alcoholic who has stopped drinking, mother who returns to work). Often self-help groups become social advocacy groups.

The processes involved in self-help groups are: social affiliation, indoctrination in self-control, modeling of methods of coping with stress, and provision of an agenda of actions to change the social environment. The cognitive processes identified by Levy (1976) involve the following actions:

1. Remove mystification by providing a rational for problems
2. Give information and advice
3. Expand perceptions of problems and actions to cope with problems
4. Provide support for change
5. Decrease social isolation
6. Develop a new subculture for identification

The power of the self-help group, according to Riessman (1976), is that it enables members to feel and use their own strengths to control their own lives. Analysis of the effectiveness of self-help groups reveals the use of persons as helpers who have experienced and coped with the crises being experienced by the person seeking help. The rationale for effectiveness is similar to the idea proposed by Jerome Frank (1972) that psychotherapy works because it restores morale. The factors that facilitate progress in self-help groups are also quite similar to factors noted in Yalom's (1970) description of traditional group psychotherapy.

To date, not a single adequate study of the effectiveness of self-help groups exists (Lieberman and Bond, 1976). One way to measure effectiveness is by looking at membership figures. In the first 8½ years of its existence more than 3 million people attended one or more sessions of Weight Watchers (Bumbalo, 1973). For groups providing direct services to ex-patients and families, the average growth rate over three decades has been a consistent 3%. Within Alcoholics Anonymous, 60% of its members maintain sobriety for a year and 40% for 2 to 20 years (Riessman, 1976).

Members of self-help groups are more often members of voluntary community organizations, so that the self-help group may be a way to create new primary social groups. Perhaps everyone ought to be in mutual help or peer groups for "hearing and sharing of one another's burdens—way of life" (Gartner, 1976). In a study of twenty-two TOPS (Take Off Pounds Sensibly) groups in Philadelphia, Stunkard (1972) reports an impressive weight loss among those who remained in the group. These groups were compared with each other and with fourteen groups of obese patients being treated by various medical means. The most effective TOPS chapters were better than the most effective medically treated group. The average result for TOPS groups was similar to the average achieved by medical treatment. Most women report a much more positive self-image after successfully completing a weight reduction program.

The major focus in fifty self-help groups in the Boston area was as follows:

1. Twenty-nine were for therapy or anxiety reduction
2. Six were education/vocation groups, which taught coping skills
3. Fifteen were preventive—clients were not identified as having problems but were seeking support

At least thirty-nine of these groups believed in a societal basis for personal problems of women and were actively involved in social reform. Forty-one of the fifty had professional consultants. Upper class women were found in ten groups, middle class women in thirty (in seventeen of these they were the primary type of client), and lower class women in nineteen (in half of these as the primary type). Twelve groups served some women on welfare. The low-income woman with middle class values (students, widows, divorcees) was found as the primary type. Most were in their twenties, were white, and educated. These self-help groups are still largely inaccessible to poor black women (Barrett, 1976; Women and MH Project, 1976; Lieberman and Borman, 1976).

In a survey of 1700 women in consciousness-raising groups (99% white, high income, and well educated), 80% said they were "very effective" (Lieberman and Bond, 1976). The common bond experienced by 95% of the women was "sexual discrimination."

Feminist therapy

Contemporary views on the psychology of women need to be built into the core curricula and inservice education programs for mental health professionals. Women in therapy frequently comment that their therapists: (1) foster traditional sex roles; (2) have biases and expectations that devalue women; (3) use traditional psychoanalytic concepts in a sexist way; and (4) respond to women as sex objects. Levine, (1974) reviewed a psychiatrist, current literature and found overwhelming evidence that the psychiatric theory and practice are sexist in orientation, perpetuate and encourage inequalities between the sexes, and are based upon unsubstantiated and even incorrect premises about women. The preponderance of men in the top ranks of the health care industry has no doubt contributed to this. Medical knowledge and scientific definitions of women are determined by men, and legislation dealing with women's health needs is created by men (Marieskind, 1975).

Rice and Rice (1973) suggest that therapists need to be open to healthy redefinition of female sexuality and role behaviors in accordance with contemporary knowledge. Women's generalized feelings of hostility toward men is most appropriately expressed, accepted, and worked through, not just labeled transference. Many mental health professionals label role unhappiness as psychopathologic, yet society rewards those in achievement roles and assigns no value to parenting and no professional status to the important and difficult job of child-care workers.

Feminist therapy is counseling that meets the special needs of women. The major difference between feminist therapists and other therapists lies in the depth of their commitment to equality between the sexes, freedom from sex-role stereotypes, and the right to self-actualization. Phyllis Chesler (1973) has been one of the most vocal advocates of seeking out female clinicians who understand women's problems and the broad social conditions that have produced them.

Rice and Rice (1973) emphasize the active role of the feminist therapist and suggest that just sitting silently fosters regression, dependency, and superiority of the therapist. It reinforces the neurotic behavior patterns that distress many women, namely the passive infantile mode, reluctance to act, and preference for the "irrational" approach. Even the "client-centered approach" can fail women who come to therapy goalless, indecisive, and lacking identity, inspiration, or simply the information needed to search out new personal modes or solutions.

A woman therapist is veiwed by Golden and Golden (1976) as essential in sex therapy for women. She teaches the female client about her body and sexual responses while also providing a role model of a sexual and competent, knowledgeable woman.

Rawlings and Carter (1977) provide a summary of psychotherapeutic techniques that are compatible with feminist therapy:*

Cognitive level

The purpose of these techniques is to raise consciousness regarding sex-role socialization and to modify belief systems that prevent women from breaking out of traditional patterns.
Bibliotherapy
Cognitive reprogramming
Consciousness-raising groups
Rational emotive therapy
Sex-role analysis
Sex-role scripting (from transactional analysis)
Women's studies

Emotional level

The purpose of these techniques is to remove emotional blocks (guilt, anxiety, anger, fear) that prevent women from modifying traditional sex-role behaviors.

---

*From Rawlings, E., and Carter, D.: Psychotherapy for women, 1977. Courtesy of Charles C Thomas, Publisher, Springfield, Ill.

Bioenergetics
Creative fantasy
Gestalt exercises
Implosion
Psychodrama
Role play
Systematic desensitization

Behavioral level

The purpose of these techniques is to master skills for being more effective and competent in one's environment and to develop responsibility for overcoming feelings of helplessness and passivity.
Assertion training
Behavioral rehearsal (role play)
Contracts and homework assignments
Social and political action

Interpersonal level

The purpose of these techniques is to improve interpersonal communication and interpersonal skills.
Communications training
Egalitarian relationship counseling (for couples)
Transactional analysis

Physical level

The purpose of these techniques is to aid women to regain and improve physical power and strength, to overcome feelings of helplessness and passivity, and to increase positive body image.
Bioenergetics
Dancing
Karate
Physical fitness
Sports

Measures toward psychologic equality

All of society needs to become more aware of how sexism is manifested so that the treatment of women—and especially little girls—as inferior people will be stopped. Women's civic groups can be instrumental in making informal community investigation of discrimination that exists in TV, the school system, industry, local newspapers, radio stations, and children's books.

MENTAL HEALTH PROBLEMS
Depression
Incidence and prevalence

As noted earlier (see Table 26-1), depression is the most prevalent diagnosis among white women and the third leading diagnosis among black women admitted to outpatient psychiatric clinics. For every 100 men who are hospitalized for depression 175 women are hospitalized, and 238 women for every 100 men are treated as outpatients for depression (President's Commission, vol. III). Weissman (1977) reports a 2 : ratio of females to males who are treated for depression in every country except for some developing countries and India (where the ratio is reversed for "treated" depression). Community surveys, which include both treated and untreated cases of depression, show remarkable consistency. The prevalence rate ranges between 16% and 20%. The rates are highest for women, nonwhites, the separated and divorced, the poor, and the less educated (President's Commission, vol. III). Persons with these symptoms tend to seek general medical help, not psychiatric help, and usually receive psychotropic drugs for relief.

In one longitudinal study conducted in New Haven, Connecticut (Weissman et al., 1977b) only 18% of people suffering with depressive symptoms saw a mental health professional, and 4% were hospitalized. This points to the necessity for nonpsychiatric health professionals, and especially nurses, to become more involved in the recognition and treatment of depressive symptoms.

Although depressive symptoms are quite prevalent, current rates for clinical depressive syndrome are considerably lower (6.9% of the population, 8% for women and 4% for men) (President's Commission, vol. II). Lifetime rates of depression suggest that lower and upper class persons have the same rates of occurrence but lower class persons have a longer duration of illness. This may be a reflection of inadequate treatment. Major depressions can be prevented by early intervention when depressive symptoms are less severe. According to Spitzer (President's Commission, vol. II), only 35% of persons currently suffering from a major depression are receiving any general medical treatment and only 30% received psychiatric or mental health treatment in the year before the disabling episode. Psychiatric hospitalization is rare.

There are growing indications that the rates of previous suicidal attempts, mental hospital commitments, and depression among women sentenced to state prisons are significantly higher than rates among men prisoners. In one recent study of women offenders seeking medical treatment, 33% sought treatment for "anxiety and depression" and 28% for headaches, while the remainder sought treatment primarily for gynecologic problems (President's Commission, vol. III).

There are a few exceptions to the rule that depression is more prevalent in women than in men. Widowed and never married persons have equal rates of depression. Married unemployed men are more depressed than married unemployed women. Women working at professional or managerial level jobs have low levels of depression (President's Commission, vol. III). The incidence of depression by age does not necessarily support the theory of the "empty nest syndrome": there is no relationship between menopause and depression or between children leaving home and depression except in those women whose lives have been devoted to raising children. The data suggest that depression scores of parents increase with a decrease in age of the youngest child at home (Guttentag et al., 1976).

Kinds of depression

Mild depression or depressive symptoms. DeRosis and Pellegrino (1976) pose the following questions to enable women to recognize depressive symptoms:

1. Are you tired even when you've had enough sleep? Do you have difficulty getting yourself going in the morning? Do you accomplish less than you like?
2. Are you restless?
3. Have you lost interest in things? In your family? In your work? In your friends? In your sex life?
4. Are you unable to make decisions?
5. Are you continually angry and resentful?
6. Do you have bouts of anxiety? Do you often have feelings of dread, as if something terrible is going to happen?
7. Are you a chronic complainer?
8. Are you self-destructive?
9. Are you critical of yourself? Do you often feel inferior or inadequate?
10. Do you spend a great deal of time daydreaming?
11. Do you have 'up' weeks and 'down' weeks?

More severe depression or clinical depression. This syndrome can be identified by a few more questions posed by DeRosis and Pellegrino (1976)*:

1. Do you cry often? Do you cry more than you used to?
2. Have your sleeping habits changed? Doet it take you longer to fall asleep? Do you wake up several hours earlier than you want to?
3. Do you sleep more than you used to?
4. Does the thought of food make you almost sick? Have you lost weight recently without consciously dieting?
5. Do you feel full of guilt?
6. Do you often have nightmares?
7. Do you think about ending your life?
8. Do you feel 'unreal' as if you're in a fog?
9. Do you find you can't concentrate and that you go over and over certain thoughts?

Bipolar disorder. This includes both periods of depression and elation (or mania) and is the most serious and socially disruptive form of depression. It carries a significant risk of death by suicide. Its prevalence in the population is low (0.3% to 1.2%), and it occurs about equally in men and women. It appears to be more common in the upper social classes (President's Commission, vol. II).

Endogenous versus exogenous depression. Endoge-

---

*Excerpted with permission of Macmillan Publishing Co., Inc. from The book of hope, by Helen DeRosis and Victoria Pellegrino. Copyright © 1976 by Helen DeRosis and Victoria Pellegrino.

nous depressions are considered to have primarily a biologic origin and to be relatively uninfluenced by environmental or psychologic factors. Psychotic depressions, like the bipolar disorder described above, are usually put into this category. Exogenous depressions are considered to be reactive since they involve coping strategies employed in reaction to some stress. (Wilson and Kneisl, 1979).

Psychotic versus neurotic depression. Medical model terminology uses "psychotic" or "neurotic" to differentiate between the intensity of depression—whether it is mild or severe. *Psychotic* depression usually is associated with rather severe ego impairment (such as delusions, impaired judgment) and regression (inability to get out of bed or care for self). *Neurotic* depression indicates difficulty concentrating, much expressed guilt, and ruminating over the past (especially perceived losses and failures).

Nursing implications

The terminology for discussing depression is inconsistent, presenting problems for researchers and clinicians alike. Some familiarity with the various terms is necessary for nurses. An ability to assess whether a client is experiencing mild depressive symptoms or a more severe major clinical depression is essential. The generalist-prepared nurse should be held accountable in providing care for mildly depressed women, but a mental health specialist (nursing or other) and/or hospitalization may be necessary for the seriously depressed client. Knowing when to refer depressed clients to secondary care personnel is a critical nursing judgment. Knowing which community resources treat depressed women and their treatment philosophy is essential information for the nurse. For instance, if a facility is known to be heavily committed to women's issues with psychosocial treatment plans, then one would refer clients who are dealing with environmental stresses or role conflict issues (variously called exogenous, mild, or neurotic depression). If a serious bipolar depression, psychotic depression, or endogenous depression is suspected, then referral to a physician or health facility for physical and psychologic assessment should be considered first.

Clients who have received treatment for depression are often referred to nurses for follow-up. Making sure that medicine is taken is much more important with psychotic, bipolar, or endogenous depressions, for example, than with most other kinds. Also, nurses can determine which women have been placed unnecessarily on medications if they are aware of environmental stresses that may have precipitated the woman's depression. Nurses should use caution in interpreting research findings because there are many different kinds and degrees of depression. What works with one client may not be efficacious with another and vice versa. Another caution is

that we see and hear so much about depression that we tend to accept it as a fact of life just as clients often "accept" their own depression.

Although nurses do not usually refer clients directly for hospitalization, criteria used in referring depressed women for psychiatric hospital admission are: (1) an unexplained weight loss of more than 15 lbs over a 3- to 4-month period of time; (2) the person is dangerous to herself and others (suicidal or homocidal); (3) the person is unable to handle the activities of daily living; and (4) she is unable to sleep more than 3 to 4 hours a night for 5 to 7 days.

Anxiety vs depression —comparison of symptoms

Weissman (1975) compared a group of clinically depressed, outpatient clients receiving psychiatric care and a group of unhappy women not in treatment but attending a career guidance center. He found thier "moods" to be similar. The women in treatment, however, came in with somatic complaints and somatic anxiety as well as "depression."

Crary and Crary (1973) differentiate between symptoms of depression and anxiety as follows:

	Depression	*Anxiety*
Psychomotor activity	Slowed down movements and speech	Normal or speeded up
Speech pattern	Reluctant to discuss symptoms or emotional difficulties	Discusses easily and rapidly
Interests	Greatly decreased	Retains interests in some things
Enjoyment	Difficulty enjoying anything	Can enjoy some activities
Mood variation	Feels worse in morning or after sleep	Feels worse in evening; feels better after sleep
Weight	Weight loss and appetite loss	No weight loss, may eat constantly
GI system	Constipation	Diarrhea
Medication	Helped by antidepressants and worsened by tranquilizers	Helped by tranquilizers and worsened by antidepressants

Etiology

Though genetic and biochemical factors are obviously related to depression, the preponderance of depression in women suggests that psychosocial factors are responsible. Weissman (1977a) delineates three of these psychosocial factors as social status, learned helplessness, and marriage. With legal and economic discrimination, women are not able to take care of themselves; they have to depend on men. This dependency on others leads to low self-esteem and depression. Women also learn "helplessness" as a response pattern to stress. Women call their husbands (or fathers or lovers) when faced with a problem. Women develop limited response repertoires because they have learned that being dependent on men is the approved "feminine" behavior.

The higher incidence of depression in married women is well documented. Working class married women with young children at home are five times more likely to become depressed than middle class women. Lower class couples are also more likely to adhere to rigid patterns of sex-role behavior within their marriage. Brown and associates (1975) found that among working class women, the most important factor is preventing depression in the face of life stress was support from the significant men in their lives.

Dependence on men to make them feel good about themselves increases women's vulnerability. Part of the low self-esteem of women results from the fact that society does not value their accomplishments. These values are internalized by women, decreasing their self-esteem. Weissman (1973) has speculated that depression may occur not when things are at their worst but when there is a possibility of improvement; a discrepancy is then perceived between rising aspirations and the likelihood of fulfilling these wishes.

Mostow and Newberry (1975) hypothesize that the confinement of the role of housewife, the increasing automation of household chores, and the declining status of motherhood contribute to low self-esteem and feelings of worthlessness associated with depression. In a study of forty-two women patients aged 25 to 60 years and matched for age and marital status, he compared "workers" and "housewives." The workers were most impaired at the beginning of treatment but recovered faster than the housewives. Workers felt more competent in their work, less bored in free time and more at ease in social situations. Lower class women work out of economic necessity rather than for purposes of fulfillment. They usually are underpaid in relation to men, have full homemaking responsibilities in addition to work, suffer from the overall inadequacy of child-care facilities and have ambivalence about leaving children. Many wish they had the financial wherewithal to be full-time homemakers. Yet, in spite of the low potential for gratification in jobs held, the depressed workers in Mostow and Newberry's study were more interested in their work and felt more competent than housewives felt about housework. Thus, work appears to serve as a protection and diversion in depressed women regardless of social class.

Some researchers concerned with primary prevention see childhood experience as the major cause for depression. Jacobson and associates (1975) hypothesize that

childhood deprivation, defined as the lack, loss, or absence of an emotionally sustaining relationship prior to adolescence, is associated with the occurrence of adult depression. In comparing 347 depressed hospitalized women and 114 depressed outpatient women with 198 normal women (all white), Jacobson and associates (1973) reported that no significant relationship was found between overt childhood loss events (death of a parent or separation from biologic parents) and adult depression. Significant differences between the childhood experiences of the depressed patient group and normal women were that the normal subjects reported less separation of parents, less parental illness, less rejection and overprotection, and more affection in their childhood than did the patient group.

When actively depressed women were compared to their normal neighbors who had never had a depressive episode, it was found that depressed women's impairments reached into all aspects of their lives, but most specifically their relationships with their children were markedly disturbed (Endicott and Spitzer, 1977). During the height of illness, the depressed women had difficulty communicating with their children, expressed loss of affection, and considerable anger. Conflicts with adolescent children were especially serious.

Weissman (1972) compared the maternal role performance of depressed women with normal controls and found that depressed women were significantly more impaired mothers. They showed diminished emotional involvement, impaired communication, disaffection, increased hostility, and resentment. The depressed mothers of infants were inadequate in caring for their children (as evidenced by being overly concerned or directly hostile). Mothers of school-age children were irritable, uninvolved, and intolerant of children's noise and activity. The most severe problems occurred with adolescents who reacted to the mother's hostility and withdrawal with serious deviant behavior. Weissman concluded that early and intensive treatment of the depressed mother serves as major preventive work for the entire family. In conclusion, there is evidence that depressed women come from families in which they, as children, were deprived of adequate parenting. The helpless, dependent mother and the powerful, abusive father can set the stage for another generation of emotionally disturbed and probably depressed women.

Health improvement strategies

The general strategies related previously to improve the psychosociocultural and economic status of women in society today will have the greater impact on the mental health of women and especially on depression in women. Other strategies, especially for depressed women, are discussed here.

Self-help. Regular exercise appears to be particularly helpful for depression. In fact, some claim it is more effective than psychotherapy. Women generally get less exercise than men; perhaps this is another factor contributing to the higher incidence of depression in women.

Keeping up a daily routine is important. Women should get up at a regular time, plan events for the day and follow through with scheduled activities. Especially for the homemaker, it is important to finish jobs started. Sitting around waiting for the "mood to hit" is not successful. Going ahead with an activity will spark interest to continue.

Saving time for oneself is critically important. This means getting out of the house or away from the job by oneself or with a friend (not with children) to do something fun or relaxing.

Seeing family and friends is helpful but visits should be short and should not be in the woman's home, but someplace else.

Some people find it helpful to write about their experiences (and some even submit their story for publication). Everyone needs someone to trust and with whom to talk, someone to share innermost concerns, angers, fears, and disappointments. Talking helps to decrease depression.

De Rosis and Pellegrino (1976) give several suggestions for full-time mothers.

1. Arrange at least half a day or evening each week for yourself. This activity could be planned, as in taking a course or attending a club meeting, or unplanned, as in sitting quietly in a beautiful place.
2. Arrange a baby-sitting co-op with other parents.
3. Join a self-help group to discuss common problems and how to solve them.
4. Don't give up personal interests. Maintain a subscription to your favorite professional journal or magazine.
5. Plan one day a month to be out alone with your significant male person.
6. Get information on free or low cost entertainment, especially the kind offering free child care.
7. Do volunteer work.
8. Deepen friendships with other women and do things together on a regular basis such as bread making, shopping.
9. Find one or two couples compatible with you and your significant other person and plan monthly activities together.
10. Remember that vacations are for mom too.
11. Exchange weekend babysitting with acquaintances.

Self-help groups appear to be particularly helpful for persons experiencing grief reactions, such as widows or parents of babies who were victims of the sudden infant death syndrome. The Harvard Medical School hired "widow confidants" who had coped successfully with widowhood and matched them with new widows (Silverman, 1975). The service has continued to grow, pointing to its usefulness, even though research data are not available to prove its value. Barrett (1975) reports on a study in which seventy urban widows responded to a news release and were divided into three groups for a 7-week period or placed on a control waiting list group. The three experimental groups were: (1) self-help group, (2) confidant group, and (3) consciousness-raising group. There were minimal differences among the three experimental groups, but a significant difference was demonstrated between the experimental and control groups in their responses to a questionnaire measuring stress index. The experimental group was lower on the stress index and therefore were predicted to have better future health. Other self-help groups for widows have stressed coping skills, such as auto mechanics, how to travel alone, single parent concerns, and how to get a job, in addition to providing support for loneliness—the major identified problem (Miles and Hays, 1975). After the formal sessions end many groups continue on their own, which indicates their effectiveness.

Assertiveness training. The effectiveness of assertiveness training is well documented.* Clinical problems of women which Jakubowski (1977) thinks can be appropriately treated by assertion training include neurotic or exogenous depression. Summarizing Seligman's theories about women's depression and assertion, Jakubowski notes that these theories help to explain why women are more likely than men to become depressed. Because they are socialized into a dependent role, women depend on others to take care of them and consequently do not learn a wide repertoire of coping skills. When a woman's failure to act assertively makes her feel powerless and subsequently depressed, assertion training can be a useful treatment for the depression. Women who know they can assertively handle a situation feel in control of themselves (less helpless); therefore, assertion training is preventive of depression.

Assertiveness training is a behavior therapy procedure (Wolpe, 1958) aimed at reducing maladaptive anxiety that prevents a person from expressing herself directly, honestly, and spontaneously (Butler, 1976). Assertiveness training involves replacing irrational belief systems with belief systems that support individual rights, the internalization of truthful statements, and the practice of assertive responses. To accomplish these ends, Jakubowski (1977) outlines a four-phase training program.

---

*Butler, 1976; Percell et al., 1974; Tregeman and Kassinone, 1977; Galassi and Galassi, 1977; Jakubowski, 1977; Rimm, 1967.

1. Helping clients to distinguish among assertive, aggressive, and nonassertive behavior and motivating clients to become more assertive
2. Helping clients to identify and accept their interpersonal rights and to develop a belief system that will support their assertive behavior
3. Reducing or removing psychologic obstacles that prevent women from acquiring or using their assertiveness skills
4. Developing assertion skills through active practice methods, such as behavior rehearsal and modeling

Other models for assertiveness training are described in the literature (Bloom et al., 1975; Alberti and Emmons, 1974; Galassi and Galassi, 1977). Many schools of nursing offer assertiveness training courses through their continuing education programs. Every nurse should have beginning familiarity with this intervention strategy. It is widely applicable both in professional practice and in working with depressed women.

Psychotherapeutic medications. The most important clinical consideration in the use of medications for treatment of depression is that antidepressant drugs are not effective in all states in which a depressed mood prevails (Wilson and Kneisl, 1979).

In general, persons for whom antidepressants are indicated suffer from endogenous depression: a severely depressed mood with substantial feelings of guilt and unworthiness; motor retardation or agitation; and the vegetative signs—anhedonia, early morning awakening, anorexia and weight loss, constipation, and loss of libido. In fact, the vegetative signs are the features that most reliably predict response to drug therapy. A significant, and commonly overlooked, clinical consideration is that antidepressants have a delayed reaction onset. Thus, a client will not show lessening of depressed mood until a week to ten days following the institution of an adequate dose of tricyclics, for example. (p. 597)

There are three classes of antidepressant drugs, the tricyclics, the monoamineoxidase (MAO) inhibitors, and the stimulants. Since stimulants have no proved role in treatment, they will not be considered here. An overview of types of depression and types of treatment is presented in Table 26-2.

Halleck (1978a), summarizing recent research on comparative treatments for depression, notes that the more serious depressions, pharmacotherapy with tricyclics or MAO inhibitors has proved superior to psychotherapy or no treatment (Klein and Daves, 1969). One study suggests that family therapy might be as useful as pharmacotherapy, but the patients in this study were not severely depressed (Friedman, 1975). Minor depressions in younger people are probably not drug responsive.

Halleck also points out that studies of combined antidepressant therapy and psychotherapy with severely depressed patients suggest there is some advantage to combined treatment, particularly if outcome criteria are not restricted to symptom removal and include changes in social functioning (Kleiman, 1975). Drugs can reduce the acute symptoms of depression, improving mood and sleep, and restoring appetite and energy so that the patient can begin to engage in therapy aimed at social adaptation or change. Hollister (1978) thinks that the antidepressant drugs are probably underused and given in inadequate dosages.

Depressions associated with psychotic behavior are sometimes treated with antipsychotic drugs in addition to antidepressants (Halleck, 1978a). Retarded depressions respond well to tricyclics but this is not the case with agitated depression. It is generally agreed that when treated actively, even an acute, serious, depressive episode carries a good prognosis; the chance of recovery is excellent, and social function between episodes will be unimpaired (President's Commission, vol. II). However, data on the long-term course of depression suggest that depression is less benign than commonly believed (Weissman et al., 1976). Only 30% of the depressive women followed over a 10-year period of time remained completely asymptomatic; 10% reported mild recurring symptoms, including disturbances of mood, sleep, and appetite.

If drugs are used in grief reactions, antianxiety agents should be used, not antidepressants (Prange, 1975). If anxiety and depression are balanced, Prange recommends using both tricyclic and phenothiazine drugs.

Tricyclics. Tricyclic antidepressants have three main pharmacologic effects. The action considered most pertinent to relief of depression is blocking the reuptake of amine neurotransmitters (or norepinephrine) released into the synaptic cleft. There is also a sedative effect and

Table 26-2. Types of depression and types of appropriate treatment

Types of depression	Type of treatment				
	Tricyclics	**MAO**	**ECT**	**Lithium**	**Psychotherapy**
Grief reactions	—	—	—	—	Maybe
Exogenous depression	—	—	—	—	Yes
Endogenous—severe or psychotic	Maybe	Maybe	Yes	—	Yes
Bipolar	—	—	—	Yes	Maybe

Table 26-3. Dosage guide for antidepressants*

Drug	Total daily dosage (divided into 2-4 doses)	
	Outpatient range (mg)	Hospital range (mg)
Tricyclic derivatives		
Amitriptyline (Elavil)	50-150	75-300
Desipramine (Norpramin)	75-150	75-300
Imipramine (Tofranil)	50-150	75-300
Nortriptyline (Aventyl)	20-100	40-100
Protriptyline (Vivactyl)	10-40	15-60
Hydrazide MAO inhibitors		
Isocarboxazid (Marplan)	10-30	10-50
Nialamide (Niamid)	25-75	100-450
Phenezine (Nardil)	15-30	15-75
Nonhydrazide MAO inhibitors		
Tranylcypromine (Parnate)	20-30	20-30

*Adapted from Hollister, L.: Clinical use of psychotherapeutic drugs, Springfield, Ill., 1978, Charles C Thomas, Publisher.

a potent central- and peripherally-acting anticholinergic effect. This latter action contributes to the most bothersome side effects of these drugs (Hollister, 1978). The tricyclics are clearly the most effective class of antidepressants and have the least risk of side effects (Cole and Davis, 1975). Of the tricyclics, imipramine (Tofranil) and amitriptyline (Elavil) are the most frequently used because of their effectiveness. A large number of clients receiving amitriptyline maintenance were found to have experienced no deaths, cardiac arrhythymias, or liver, CNS, or blood reactions (Dimascio et al., 1975). Serious depressions that are not complicated by major sleep disturbances are usually treated with imipramine (Halleck, 1978a). Men usually respond better than women to imipramine. With neurotic depression and some anxiety, imipramine is the drug of choice (Prange, 1975). Amitriptyline has a mild sedative effect and is frequently used when the client is troubled with sleeplessness. Doxepin (Sinequan) is alleged to have fewer anticholinergic side effects than either imipramine or amitriptyline

Table 26-4. Antidepressants—tricyclics: general characteristics*

Precautions	Contraindications	Drug interactions	Effects on clinical tests
Use very cautiously in patients with: Urinary retention Narrow angle glaucoma Increased ocular pressure Convulsive disorders (may need increased anticonvulsants) Cardiovascular disorders Thyroid disease Benign prostatic hypertrophy Quiescent schizophrenia Organic brain syndrome Warn patient about driving vehicles or operating dangerous machinery Safe use during pregnancy not yet established Seriously depressed patients may be suicide risks Use caution in children under 12 Withdraw gradually if patient has been on more than 150 mg/day for more than 2 mo	MAO inhibitors: stop tricyclic a minimum of 14 days before beginning a MAO inhibitor Acute myocardial infarction Hypersensitivity *Do not* give barbiturates if MAO inhibitor and tricyclic are combined accidentally, as they will further depress respiration	Alcohol potentiates tricyclics Anticholinergic drugs: effect increased Anticonvulsants: increase CNS depression, but may need to increase to control seizures Antiparkinsonian agents: potentiates anticholinergic properties; at tonic levels may produce syndrome of agitation, convulsion, hyperpyrexia Estrogen: interaction reported in several cases Guanethidine (Ismelin): inhibits Ismelin (except Sinequan under 150 mg/day) Hypnotics and some tranquilizers: may affect tricyclic serum level (benzodiazepines do not) MAO inhibitor: may potentiate both (see contraindications) Minor tranquilizers: additive effect Phenothiazines: sedative effects additive (caution, but not contraindicated) Reserpine: inhibited Sympathomimetic amines (epinephrine, norepinephrine, amphetamines, many over-the-counter cold, cough, and sinus remedies): effects increased Veratrum alkaloids: effect decreased	(false increase or decrease) Alkaline phosphatase— may be ↑ Bilirubin—↑ BSP retention—↑ Cholesterol—may be ↓ FBS—may be ↓ or ↑ Transaminase—↑

*From Cain, R., and Cain, N.: A compendium of psychiatric drugs, Part I, Drug Therapy, January 1975.

Table 26-5. Antidepressants—tricyclics: side effects*

Serious adverse effects (rare) and treatment

Agranulocytosis (most frequently occurs between the 2nd and 8th weeks)	Stop medication; isolate from sources of infection; give antibiotics; hospitalize.
Cholestatic jaundice	Stop medication; bed rest; high protein/high carbohydrate diet.
Leukocytosis	
Leukopenia	
Loeffler's syndrome	Require immediate medical evaluation.
Eosinophilia	
Purpura	
Paralytic ileus	Stop medication; hospitalize.

Other adverse effects

Adverse effects	Treatment	Adverse effects	Treatment
Allergic		*CNS*	
Rash, itching (rare)	Stop medication; use antihistamine	Drowsiness† (except Vivactil)	Give single daily dose at bedtime
Photosensitivity	Wear protective clothes or use sunscreen (e.g., Pabafilm)	Jitteriness†	Decrease dosage or switch to another drug
		Seizures	
		Twitching	
Autonomic nervous system		Dysarthria	
Flushing	Needs no treatment	Paresthesia	
Dry mouth†	Rinse mouth frequently; if severe might try neostigmine 7.5-15 mg PO or pilocarpine nitrate 2.5 mg PO qid	Palsies	
		Ataxia	
		Sudden falls	
		Muscle tremor	Use muscle relaxant
		Weakness	Reassurance
Blurred vision†	If severe and cannot decrease dosage, might try 1% pilocarpine nitrate eyedrops	Fatigue	
		Headache	
		Insomnia	Give single daily dose in a.m.
Diaphoresis	Reassurance	Induced mania	Stop medication; treat as for any acute manic or schizophrenic state
Constipation†	Milk of magnesia	Activation of schizophrenia	
Urinary retention or frequency	Reassure; decrease dose	Visual hallucinations	
Aggravation of glaucoma	Concurrent tonometry, local cholinergics, and consultation	Delusions	
		Anger	If severe, stop and/or change medication
		Agitation	
		Vertigo	
Cardiovascular		*Gastrointestinal*	
Hypertension		Nausea†	Stop medication, or symptomatic treatment
Postural hypotension	Reassurance; avoid sudden changes in position; use surgical elastic hose if necessary	Vomiting	
Dizziness		Heartburn†	Take after meals
Tachycardia		Anorexia	Stop medication, or frequent small feedings
Palpitations			
Arrhythmias	Evaluate cardiac status	*Miscellaneous*	
Ankle edema		Peripheral neuropathy	Advisability of continuing medication must be weighed against the severity of sumptoms
Flattened T wave on EKG	Frequently benign but follow	Impotence	
		Galactorrhea	
Congestive heart failure, particularly over age 60	Stop medication; give digitalis; diuretics	Tinnitus	
		Bad taste in mouth	
		Weight gain	
		Weight loss	
		Orbital edema	
		Endocrine changes (estrogen effects)	

*From Cain, R., and Cain, N.: A compendium of psychiatric drugs, Part I, Drug Therapy, January 1975.
†Common side effects.

and is often used with elderly clients (Halleck, 1978?). When medicating the elderly, the entire dosage should not be given at bedtime as recommended for younger people. Amitriptyline may be more effective in the aged than imipramine (Prange, 1975).

MAO inhibitors. The MAO inhibitors are believed to increase the concentration of monoamines in the brain by slowing their rate of destruction (Halleck, 1978a). Because MAO inhibitors have not shown a superior efficacy over the tricyclics and because they have more serious side effects, they are used infrequently, and usually only when the tricyclics have failed (Halleck, 1978a; Prange, 1975). The most serious side effect of MAO inhibitors is the so-called hypertensive crisis that occurs when certain foods or other drugs are combined with MAO inhibitors. Usually, this complication is heralded by extreme headaches, but the client may also experience palpitations, nausea, vomiting, flushing of the face, photophobia, and sometimes cardiac and pulmonary complications. Blood pressure can rise to very high levels, followed by stroke or death. To prevent the hypertensive crisis, food and drug restrictions must be strictly adhered to (Table 26-6). Nurses must be keenly aware of the risks of the MAO inhibitor drugs and able to inform clients about necessary food and medication restrictions. According to Appleton and Davis (1973), phenelzine (Nardil) and tranylcypromine (Parnate) are the most effective of the MAO inhibitors.

Electroconvulsive therapy (ECT). Electroconvulsive therapy is generally used for depression only after pharmacotherapy has failed. Electroconvulsive treatment is clearly superior to no treatment or to psychotherapy in relieving the symptoms of severe depression (Detre and Jarecki, 1971). Some studies indicate the ECT may be superior to pharmacotherapy in treating the most severe depressions (Davis, 1975).

Avery and Winokeu (1976) found that an ECT-treated group had slightly lower mortality rates than a group receiving therapeutic levels of antidepressants. The ECT treated group had significantly lower mortality rates than a group receiving nontherapeutic levels of antidepressants, a group receiving placebo ECT treatment, and a

Table 26-6. Antidepressants—MAO inhibitors: general characteristics*

Precautions	Contraindications	Drug interactions
Warn patient to:	Tricyclic drugs	Alcohol: inhibits MAO inhibitor (possible hypertensive crisis if beverage contains tyramine)
Report headaches or unusual symptoms immediately	Stop MAO inhibitor minimum 14 days before beginning tricyclic	
Avoid self-medication (including over-the-counter drugs such as cold and sinus drugs, analgesics)	Amphetamines	Amphetamine: potentiates amphetamine, risk of hypertensive crisis
	Sympathomimetic amines	Anesthetics: increase CNS depression
Avoid tyramine-containing foods, such as cheese, wine (especially sherry and Chianti), beer, pickled herring, yeast extracts, chicken liver, cream, chocolate, fava beans, brood beans, snails, soy sauce, meat tenderizers, raisins, bananas	Hypertension	Anticholinergics: effect increased
	Cardiovascular disease	Antiparkinsonian agents: potentiated
	Headaches	Barbiturates: potentiated
	Pheochromocytoma	Chloral hydrate: potentiated
	Liver or advanced renal disease	Cocaine: potentiated or hypertensive crisis
	Quiescent schizophrenia	Curare: effect increased
Avoid excess amount of caffeine, chocolate, sour cream, yogurt, sauerkraut	*Avoid combination with:*	Foods with tyramine (see list under precautions): hypertensive crisis
Also avoid: Marmite, Bovril, yogurt, beestings	Dopa, amphetamines, hypoglycemics, alcohol, narcotics, diuretics, levodopa, meperidine, methyldopa, barbiturates, antiparkinsonian agents, insulin, guanethidine, sympathomimetic amines, reserpine, anticholinergics, antihypertensives, antihistaminics, hypnotics, other MAO inhibitors, anesthetics, phenothiazines, tryptophane	Insulin, oral: hypoglycemia; potentiated
Use analgesics in lower doses if needed		Meperidine: hypotension potentiated; may inhibit MAO inhibitor
Taper off when stopping		Methyldopa (Aldomet): hypertension, extation
Safe use in pregnancy not yet established		Minor tranquilizers: potentiated
		Other MAO inhibitors: additive
		Phenothiazines: potentiated; may inhibit MAO inhibitor
		Reserpine: excitation
		Sympathomimetic: potentiated; extreme hypertension
		Thiazide diuretics: hypotension; potentiate MAO inhibitor
		Tricyclic antidepressants: potentiate both

*Adapted from Cain, R., and Cain, N.: A compendium of psychiatric drugs. Part I, Drug Therapy, January 1975.

group receiving placebo drugs. The lower rate for the ECT group were explained as follows: (1) untreated depressed patients are usually malnourished and agitated and more susceptible to physical illness; (2) the risk of cardiotoxicity is a factor with the tricyclic antidepressant drugs; and (3) suicidal and drug therapy clients have a long recovery time and the drugs themselves can be fatal if ingested in a suicide attempt.

Avery and Winokin concluded that ECT is the preferred treatment for clients with severe, unipolar, psychotic depressions that also manifest high suicidal potential.

Lithium. In dealing with bipolar affective disorders, lithium carbonate is superior to psychotherapy or no treatment. There is some evidence that once the acute phase of the illness has subsided and the client is maintained on lithium, there is a higher remission rate if it is combined with psychotherapy (Benson, 1975). The efficacy of lithium in the treatment of mania ranges from 60% to 100% (Gershan, 1975). Because of its toxic effects, many physicians currently are advising to delay starting lithium (even with hypomania) until the second or third episode. With depressive recurrences, the best method is not clear. Gershan advises using lithium and an antidepressant or increasing the lithium dosage at the time of appearance of depressive symptomatology.

Nurses need to know that lithium is potentially very toxic, causing death if lithium blood levels get too high. Clients receiving lithium need to have lithium levels checked at weekly intervals during the final 4 weeks of treatment and every 4 to 6 weeks thereafter (Hollister, 1978). The lithium blood level should be maintained between 0.7 and 1.2 mEq/liter.

Significant side effects are usually correlated with blood levels of lithium about 1.5 mEq/liter. Common side effects include tremor, nausea, thirst, and polyuria. Severe lithium poisoning is a potential medical emergency. Early stages include vomiting and diarrhea, lethargy, and muscle twitching (Wilson and Kneisl, 1979). This can proceed to unconsciousness and cardiac arrest.

Psychotherapy/counseling. When psychotherapy was offered to a sample of working class depressed women, the focus was supportive and aimed at helping clients cope with life circumstances rather than resolving intrapsychic conflicts or enduring personality patterns (Weissman et al., 1973). The content themes discussed (listed in order of frequency discussed and time spent on topic) were: physical symptoms, mental symptoms, current treatment, practical problems, family of origin, spouse, sex, children, interpersonal relationships, and early experiences. Therapists may underestimate the benefit to the client derived from being able to share ev-

Table 26-7. Antidepressants-MAO inhibitors: side effects*

Serious adverse effects

Severe headaches (may be first sign of pending hypertensive crisis)	Stop medication.
Hypertensive crisis	Prevent by giving detailed list of things to avoid; no specific antidote; to lower blood pressure give Regitine (phentolamine) 5 mg IV if available; if not, Thorazine 50-100 mg IM may be used as emergency measure.
CVA Hepatocellular, toxic jaundice Leukopenia Anemia Shocklike coma Edema of glottis	Stop medication.

Other side effects

Autonomic nervous system: Perspiration, dry mouth,† blurred vision, delayed micturition, orthostatic hypotension, constipation,† epigastric distress, delayed ejaculation, impotence, paroxysmal hypertension

Cardiovascular: Hypotension, hypertension, tachycardia, palpitations, peripheral edema; may mask angina by suppressing pain

CNS: Insomnia,† drowsiness, overstimulation,† tremor, hyperreflexia, seizures, hypomania, mania, fatigue, dizziness,† weakness, headache, vertigo, ataxia, twitching, schizophrenic psychotic symptoms (anxiety, agitation, hallucinations), peripheral neuropathy, acute confusion with disorientation, mental clouding, and illusions

Gastrointestinal: Nausea, diarrhea, anorexia, abdominal pain, constipation

Miscellaneous: Rashes, hyperpyrexia, photosensitivity

*From Cain, R., and Cain, N.: A compendium of psychiatric drugs. Part I, Drug Therapy, January 1975.
†Most common.

eryday problems with a nonjudgmental, sympathetic listener. In a comparison of "completers" of treatment and "relapsers" (Jacobson et al., 1977), a significant difference was noted in the focus of sessions. Prolonged discussion of mental symptoms and the overt expression of negative affect, especially anxiety, were observed to be significant components of the therapy of the relapse group, while discussion of children was a dominant aspect of the therapy with the completers. The completers discussed their mental symptoms in the context of what could be done to alleviate them. Completers engaged in dynamic discussion of their life situations, including concerns about participation in major roles such as childrearing. This study should cause all of us to reconsider the indications for encouraging a depressed patient to express negative feelings.

Helping people to express anger outwardly and constructively is a major goal of therapy with depressed people. Bernadez-Bonesatti (1978) reports that repressed anger is not only responsible for depression but is central to the understanding of women's difficulties for depression but is central to the understanding of women's difficulties in creative and active pursuits. The cultural bias against expression of anger in women only allows women to express anger in defense of others, especially those more helpless than themselves. Infantile notions about women's omnipotence and devastating power are shared unconsciously by both men and women. All appear to be afraid of a woman's anger. The impulse to compete and the feelings of rivalry are so feared by many women that in order to avoid them, they do not enter competitive fields. Anger gets expressed by tears. The energy women spend in suppression, inhibition, and displacement of anger must be liberated if it is to be transformed into creative pursuits and social change (Bernardez-Bonesatti, 1978).

Cognitive therapy is very helpful with depressed women and can be practiced by generalist-prepared nurses (Beck and Greenberg, 1974). This therapy is based on the maladaptive cognitions theory; that is, people (especially women) behave on the basis of misconceptions and unrealistic thought patterns. The counselor allies herself with the client against the depressive symptoms that afflict the client. Beck and Greenberg note four approaches, described below:

1. The counselor helps the client learn to recognize idiosyncratic thoughts that may temper the depressed mood. The client must learn to distance herself emotionally from her thoughts, (that is, to view them objectively) with the critical perspective that will enable her to judge whether they are realistic or justified. A homemaker who sought help because of global feelings of depression, apathy, and inertia was instructed to pay close attention to her thoughts from the time she woke in the morning and throughout the day. After a day or so, she realized that when she began her household chores she would think, "I'm an incompetent housekeeper, I'll never be able to get this done." This is an example of reacting to a single, isolated failure by overgeneralization. The homemaker in the example was directed to look objectively at what exactly she was a failure at (she did not wash husband's favorite shirt by the time he wanted it) and recognize that one mistake does not constitute total failure. Another woman assumed that her friends no longer cared about her because no one telephoned for a day or two. She was helped to weigh the evidence on which her spontaneous conclusions were based, and to consider alternative explanations. (Actually, of her two best friends, Mary was sick and Joan was out of town.) Another client was overly absorbed in the negative aspect of her life. When she was required to write down and report back positive experiences, she recognized her selective attention to the negative.

2. The counselor calls attention to the client's stereotyped themes that influence her thinking. The automatic thoughts that constitute the woman's immediate reaction to an event may be a cognitive shorthand for elaborate ideas, deeply rooted in past experiences but no longer relevant. A woman who reported that she made a "fool of herself" in a job interview recognized that this assessment reflected not her actual performance but her tendency to see herself as a subject of humiliation. In reviewing her actual behavior, the counselor was able to shed doubt on the client's perception. In continuing to evaluate new experiences, the woman not only got a more realistic perspective on herself but she also learned new skills to cope with confirmed areas of difficulty.

3. The counselor observes that the client holds certain misconceptions, prejudices, and even superstitions, which need to be exposed and evaluated. One female nursing faculty member experienced intense depression when her manuscripts were not accepted for publication. She was helped to see that she held a set of interlocking premises, such as, "If I don't publish and become famous, my work and life are meaningless." The faculty member was helped to discover other areas of her academic role as well as her family that were rich sources of gratification. Subjecting her basic premises to a process of validation helped her to stop worrying about recognition and to get more enjoyment out of her work. Meanwhile, she worked with an editor and got published.

Sometimes the idiosyncratic cognitions take a pictorial rather than a verbal form. A woman who felt depressed following a dinner party told the counselor that she had a spontaneous fantasy during the evening in which her husband left the party with another woman. This woman felt inferior and believed her husband would leave her. With help she was able to recognize that she was, in fact, unusually accomplished and attractive, and her husband was exceptionally devoted; with this recognition, her depression lifted.

Clients can also learn to substitute pleasant fantasies for unpleasant ones. One woman who was depressed because her child required a minor operation was somewhat relieved when she pictured him in a year, playful and happy and without disability.

4. The counselor, in addition to these intellectual methods for changing the depressed cognitions, can use behavioral techniques, such as the graded task assignment. A depressed homemaker, for instance, may be given a series of tasks starting with simple jobs at which she has a good chance of succeeding, and progressing to more complicated tasks. At first she may only be asked to make the beds, then cook breakfast, etc. When she has clearly succeeded at a task, however simple, her lethargy decreases and she is motivated to try more.

Suicidal behavior

Suicidal thoughts and/or attempts are one of the most serious symptoms and require immediate assessment and intervention. Hospitalization may be indicated to provide a safe environment for the person. All depressed clients are potentially suicidal and deserve the nurse's attention. Suicide now ranks eleventh among the leading causes of death in the United States, with a mortality rate of 12.1 per 100,000 (and many are not reported because of the social stigma attached to death by suicide). Between 1963–1964 and 1973–1974, suicide rates among white women in the United States increased in every age group except the elderly. The rise in rates was most marked at ages 15 to 24 (up by 50%) and ages 25 to 34 (up by 20%) (Metropolitan Life, 1976). Despite the increase for women, suicides for white males continued to be higher (three men for each woman). Suicide attempts, however, occur at a rate of four women to each man (Garai, 1970a). Snyder (1977) notes that the increasing rate of suicidal behavior in women is a result of sociocultural factors. He cites the increased employment of women as occurring at the same rate as increased suicidal behavior in women and concludes that the most important need is for a new set of sociocultural values that allow membership in the labor force as an accepted female role.

Clinical and socioeconomic characteristics of 368 patients attending the British Royal Infirmary Accident and Emergency Department following a nonfatal act of deliberate self-harm were as follows (Morgan et al., 1975):
- There were twice as many women as men.
- Two thirds of the patients were in the 15 to 35 age group.
- Ninety-five percent had taken a drug overdose (tranquilizers, antidepressants, hypnotics, or analgesics).
- Seventy-eight percent of the drugs had been prescribed by a physician.
- Fifty percent of the patients mentioned interpersonal conflict as a major precipitating factor in the episode.
- There was a greater than average incidence of unemployment, overcrowded living conditions, and divorce.

Assessing suicide risk is oftentimes a responsibility of the nurse. "Understanding what a self-destructive person is trying to communicate is basic to helping the individual find alternatives to suicide. Assessment of suicide risk is a difficult task. It is made possible by recognition of signs that predict the likelihood of suicide for particular individuals. Assessment of suicide risk is an important basis for appropriate response to self-destructive people." (Hoff, 1978, p. 130) Inaccurate lethality assessment can cause problems ranging from too little attention for long range high risk persons to unnecessary hospitalization for low, immediate risk persons. However, important as is the task of assessing suicide risk according to research-based criteria, one should remember that it is nevertheless impossible to predict suicide in any absolute sense (Hoff, 1978, p. 118).

Lee Ann Hoff (1978, pp. 118-126) has summarized a number of predictive signs from the works of Brown and Sheran, Breed, Beck, Resnik, Lettieri, Farberow, Bush, Jacobs, Neuringer, Dublin, Hendin, Maris, Durkheim, Shneidman, and Alvarez. These include the following:

1. *Suicide plan.* The patient is considered high risk if she articulates an actual plan. High lethal methods include guns, jumping, hanging, drowning, carbon monoxide poisoning, barbiturates, lithium sleeping pills (especially Doriden), antidepressants, high doses of aspirin, car crashes, and exposure to extreme cold. Patients should be asked: "Has life become so hopeless that you've thought about killing yourself?" "What are you thinking of doing?" A specific plan with available means places one at great risk.

2. *History of suicide attempts.* Suicide risk is increased if the person has made several previous high lethal attempts and if the person has a negative perception of a counseling experience.

3. *Resources and communication with significant others.* Rigidity in problem solving is a higher suicidal risk because the person has fewer personal resources and perceives only one course of action or solution to a problem: suicide. Also, people who feel ignored or cut off from significant people are at greater risk than those with a good support system.

Research evidence (e.g., Brown and Sheran, 1972)

suggests that the nurse consider not only individual signs but the complex patterning of signs. Thus, Hoff (1978, p. 122) notes that if a person "a) has a history of high lethal attempts; b) has a specific, high lethal plan for suicide with available means; c) lacks both personality and social resources, his or her immediate and long range risk for probable suicide is very high regardless of other factors. The risk increases, however, if other factors are also present." These are as follows:

4. *Age, sex, race.* Suicide risk is increased for men, elderly whites, and separated, widowed, or divorced persons. The rate is increasing for adolescents, black and white women, and black men. Among young urban black persons between 20 and 35 years of age, the rate is twice that of white people the same age.
5. *Recent loss.* "Personal loss or threat of loss of a spouse, parent, status, money, or job increases a person's suicide risk. This is a very significant factor among adolescents."
6. *Physical illness.* Three out of four suicide victims have been under medical care or have visited their physician within 4 to 6 months of their death. The possibility of suicide is even greater if a person receives a diagnosis that affects her image of self or demands a major switch in life-style; for example, breast cancer, limb amputation, cancer of a sex organ.
7. *Drinking and drug abuse.* "Drinking increases impulsive behavior and loss of control and therefore increases suicide risk, especially if the person has a high lethal means available. . . . Half of the adolescents who die by suicide were involved in drug or alcohol abuse before their death."
8. *Isolation.* If a person is isolated both emotionally and physically, risk of suicide is greater than if she lives with close significant others.
9. *Unexplained change in behaviors.* Changes in behavior such as drinking by a previously sober person or withdrawal by a previously social person are important signs of impending suicide.
10. *Depression.* A large number of people who commit suicide (approximately 70%) have been diagnosed as depressed; however, the majority of depressed people do not commit suicide.
11. *Social factors.* Social problems such as family disorganization or broken home, and a record of delinquency and truancy increase a person's risk of suicide.
12. *Mental illness.* If a person hears voices directing her to commit suicide, the risk of suicide is obviously higher.

Even with these signs, the nurse is often in a position of trying to predict what the combination of signs say about the actual suicide risk now and in the future. She has to make a decision about whether to work with the person herself, utilize family and community resources, refer for mental health counseling, hospitalize immediately, recommend long-term hospitalization, etc. Effective assessment of lethality provides a scientific basis for nursing care plans, increases the appropriate use of hospitalization and other resources, and decreases the worker's anxiety (Hoff, 1978, p. 117).

Crisis intervention is frequently utilized by nurses to help suicidal people. Several techniques discussed by Hoff (1978, pp. 135-136) are particularly important for a person in a suicidal crisis:

1. Relieve isolation. If there is no friend or supportive relative with whom the person can stay temporarily, she may need to be hospitalized to provide safety.
2. Remove lethal weapons.
3. Encourage alternate expression of anger. Suicide is often a way of expressing anger at a significant other. Dumping the anger with the nurse may be adequate to temporarily prevent the act.
4. Avoid a final decision of suicide during the crisis.
5. Reestablish social ties. Referral to self-help groups may be life-saving.
6. Relieve extreme anxiety and sleep loss by medication. Life always seems more bleak at 4:00 AM, and a good night's sleep can temporarily reduce the suicide risk and put the person in a better frame of mind for problem solving.

If medication is needed, never give the person more than a 1- to 3-day supply and never without a specific return appointment. Unfortunately, the hopelessness and helplessness experienced by the client is contagious and the nurse may begin to feel very helpless in her role also. The nurse's helplessness in turn causes her to flee the client or make a hasty referral leaving the person even more desparate. It is critically important for nurses to handle their feelings while working with depressed, suicidal clients. For a fuller discussion of assessment and intervention techniques on behalf of suicidal women, the reader is referred to Chapters 5 and 6 of *People in Crisis* (Hoff, 1978).

Anxiety

Moulton (1977) notes that while the new feminism has opened up new paths for both sexes and loosened up sex-role stereotypes, it has also created new anxieties and problems in work and in sexual and family settings. She believes that rapid cultural change disturbs the established psychologic equilibrium, and both men and women experience personal anxieties and role strain. Equilibrium can be achieved only after the effects of change have been dealt with individually and socially.

Anxiety is a common experience for most women and occurs in the absence of defensive mechanisms. When defense mechanisms are used to control anxiety, the result is neurotic disorders such as phobia, obsessive-compulsive reaction, or conversion reactions. When neurotic disorders occur, anxiety is no longer experienced because it is being controlled by the defense mechanisms. Anxiety, or a fear of the unknown, is keenly felt by many women who are entering new life experiences with psychologic patterns that were developed for a totally different emotional climate. Women are poorly prepared for the competitive demands of our culture, and experience severe anxiety when faced with them (Symonds, 1976).

The subjective experiences described by persons suffering from anxiety reactions are described below. These have been adapted from the descriptions by Wilson and Kneisl (1979).

1. *Physiologic*
   Increased heart rate
   Elevated blood pressure
   Tightness in chest
   Difficulty breathing
   Sweaty palms
   Trembling, tics, or twitching
   Tightness of neck or back muscles
   Headache*
   Urinary frequency
   Diarrhea
   Nausea and/or vomiting
   Sleep disturbance
   Anorexia
   Sneezing
   Constant state of fatigue
   Accident proneness
   Susceptibility to minor illness
   Slumped posture
2. *Emotional*
   Irritability
   Angry outbursts
   Feeling of worthlessness
   Depression
   Suspiciousness
   Jealousy
   Restlessness
   Anxiousness
   Withdrawal
   Diminished initiative
   Tendency to cry
   Sobbing without tears
   Reduced personal involvement with others
   Tendency to blame others
   Critical of self and others
   Self-depression
   Lack of interest

3. *Intellectual*
   Forgetfulness
   Preoccupation
   Rumination
   Mathematical and grammatical errors
   Errors in judging distance
   Blocking
   Diminished fantasy life
   Lack of concentration
   Lack of attention to details
   Past-oriented rather than present- or future-oriented
   Lack of awareness of external stimuli
   Reduced creativity
   Diminished productivity
   Reduced interest

With the physiologic symptoms listed above, it is easy to understand why women go to their family physicians for help with what they perceive as physical problems. At least 50% of visits to the general practitioner are for psychologic problems (Weissman, 1977).

Anxiety attacks

Acute episodes may last from a few minutes to an hour and are terrifying. The woman usually experiences palpitations, rapid pulse, nausea, diarrhea, dyspnea, and a feeling of suffocation. The person often has a sense of impending death. In addition, there may be severe chest pain and an EKG is sometimes necessary to rule out heart attack. After the possibility of physical disorder is ruled out, measures can be taken to reduce the anxiety (Wilson and Kneisl, 1979):

*Nursing strategies**	*Rationale**
1. Stay physically with the client.	Being left alone may further aggravate feelings of panic.
2. Maintain a calm, serene manner.	Anxiety is easily communicated from staff to client.
3. Use short, simple sentences and a firm, authoritative voice. Make decisions for the client.	Convey sense of ability to provide external controls.
4. Encourage client to move to a smaller physical environment, such as her room, to minimize the stimuli. Decrease other stimuli such as noise and light. Speak softly, lower the lighting and do not touch the client.	The client is already overwhelmed by stimuli.
5. It is sometimes useful to focus the client's diffuse energy on	Physical exercise can sometimes drain off

---

*In a non-clinical sample of 451 women aged 15 or 44 years, 23% had headaches with two or more of the migraine characteristics (Markush).

*Adapted in part from Wilson, H., and Kneisl, C.: Psychiatric nursing, Palo Alto, 1979, Addison-Wesley Publishing Co., p. 300.

some physically tiring task such as moving furniture or scrubbing the floor.

6. It may be wise to recommend that an antianxiety medication be ordered for the client.

high levels of anxiety.

Certain somatic interventions are highly specific and effective in relieving anxiety attacks.

With mild or moderate degrees of anxiety the nurse can capitalize on the motivation triggered by anxiety and engage the client in problem solving to change her life situation. It is helpful to discuss one situation in the light of the specific precipitating factors. The nurse's thoughts should be focused on what the client expected to happen and what happened instead. Anxiety occurs when one's needs (or expectations) are not met. After helping the client clarify what needs were not met, it is necessary to think of ways she can express her needs more clearly to others or change the nature of her needs if they are unreasonable. Women often expect men to meet all of their needs. Not only is that unrealistic but often men are not aware of what the woman needs because she has not been able to express herself. As women get clearer about what they need from people, and as they experience some success in expressing their needs, anxiety can be prevented. Assertiveness training, mentioned previously, can help to reduce anxiety.

Antianxiety medications

Antianxiety drugs are minor tranquilizers. The two classes most frequently used are the glycerol derivates and the benzodiazepines. Meprobamate (Equinil, Miltown) is the most commonly used glycerol derivative, but tybamate (Tybatran) is occasionally used (Halleck, 1978a). Of the benzodiazepines, those prescribed most often are diazepam (Valium), chlordiazepoxide (Librium), and flurazepam (Dalmane). Their use is so widespread that Valium and Librium have become the two most frequently prescribed drugs of any type in the United States today. Dalmane is a better choice for sleep disturbances, since it is metabolized rapidly and does not interfere with dreaming (REM) sleep (Halleck, 1978a). Meprobamate was found to be significantly more effective than a placebo in some of the double-blind studies, and most comparisons showed tybamate to be significantly more effective than a placebo. Librium, Valium, and Serax have all been found to be better than a placebo in almost all of the studies done. Chlorazepate (Tranxene) is a newer minor tranquilizer found to be at least as effective as Valium and definitely superior to a placebo (Cole and Davis, 1975).

Since all antianxiety drugs have sedative effects, they potentiate the effect of alcohol and other psychotropic

drugs, and clients must be warned against their combined use. The major problem in using antianxiety drugs is that they are habituating (Halleck, 1978). These drugs make people feel good, and clients are not only willing but eager to take them. Addiction can be an especially serious problem with meprobamate; withdrawal from this agent can produce some of the same complications (such as seizure disorders) that are seen with barbiturate withdrawal. Since most clinicians believe that anxiety attacks are best understood and modified by examining the client's past learning experiences and current environmental interactions, the only rational use of an antianxiety drug is as an agent for temporary relief of symptoms—much as aspirin is used for a headache (Halleck, 1978a). Clients should be informed that antianxiety drugs are highly habituating and they should be responsible for using them judiciously.

Both the site and mechanism of action of the benzodiazepines are unclear at the present time (Hollister, 1978). See Table 26-7 for adverse effects of antidepressants.

Jeffrey Gray (1978) has concluded from extensive research on antianxiety drugs that these drugs reduce the capacity to react to changes in the environment; they inhibit the development of persistence in the face of unpredictable adversity. Gray states: "Since unpredictable adversity is one of the most predictable ingredients of life, this effect may make the price of the antianxiety drugs too high."

Pearlin and Schooler (1978) studied the structure of coping and conclude that individuals' coping interventions are most effective when dealing with problems within the close interpersonal role areas of marriage and childrearing, and least effective when dealing with the more impersonal problems found in one's occupation. The effective coping modes are unequally distributed in society; men, the educated, and the affluent make

Table 26-8. Dosage guide for antianxiety drugs*

	Dosage (mg)
Glycerols	
Meprobamate (Miltown, Equanil)	800-3200
Tybamate (Tybatran)	600-1200
Benzodiazepines	
Chlordiazepoxide hydrochloride (Librium)	15-100
Chlorazepate dipotassium (Tranxene)	15-60
Diazepam (Valium)	5-20
Oxazepam (Serax)	30-120
Flurazepam (Dalmane)	15-30

*Adapted in part from Hollister, L.: Clinical use of psychotherapeutic drugs, Springfield, Ill., 1978, Charles C Thomas, Publisher, p. 35.

Table 26-9. Minor tranquilizers—benzodiazepines and glycerols*

Adverse effects	Treatment
CNS: Drowsiness,† ataxia,† confusion,† slurred speech,† headache,† lethargy,† giddiness,† muscular incoordination, tremor, somnolence, dysarthria	Begin with initial low dose and increase over 3-4 days
Autonomic nervous system: Dizziness,† vertigo,† impaired visual accommodation,† salivation changes, incontinence, urinary retention, blurred vision	Reassurance or decrease dose, if severe
Cardiovascular: Hypertension, hypotension, syncope, hypotensive crisis rare, anaphylaxis	Begin with low dose initially and increase gradually
Behavioral: Euphoria, fatigue, weakness, depression, psychic dependency	Reassurance or decrease dose
Hematologic: Agranulocytosis, leukopenia, anemia, thrombocytopenic purpura	Stop medication
Hepatic: Jaundice, hepatic dysfunction	Stop medication
Gastrointestinal: Nausea, vomiting, constipation	Decrease dose
Dermatologic: Rash, urticaria, stomatitis, exfoliative dermatitis, Stevens-Johnson syndrome, erythema multiforme	Decrease dose / Stop medication
Endocrinologic: Menstrual irregularities, altered libido	Reassurance or stop medication
Paradoxical reaction: Acute excited states, anxiety, hallucinations, increased muscle spasticity, insomnia, rage, convulsions, sleep disturbances, stimulation	Stop medication
Miscellaneous: Chills, fever, paresthesias, edema, angioneurotic edema	Stop medication

*From Cain, R., and Cain, N.: A compendium of psychiatric drugs, Part I, Drug Therapy, January 1975.
†Most frequent side effects.

greater use of the efficacious mechanisms. Women were found to use "selective ignoring"—casting about for some positive attribute or circumstance within a troublesome situation—significantly more than men, and this was, in fact, the most common coping mechanism of women. In selective ignoring, once a positive circumstance is found, the person is aided in ignoring the negative aspects by anchoring her attention to what she considers more worthwhile and rewarding aspects. Selective ignoring of actually exacerbates stress in the marital and parenting areas. Pearlin and Schooler question whether the greater inclination of women to psychologic disturbance is a consequence not only of their having to bear more severe hardships, but also of their being socialized in a way that less adequately equips them with effective coping patterns. Their study implies that counseling anxious women should emphasize learning about more efficacious coping behaviors. In marriage, the most effective coping response is "self-reliance" rather than "advice seeking." In parenting, the most effective coping styles include "positive comparisons" and "self-reliance" as opposed to "advice seeking."

Phobias

Phobia refers to the occurrence of fear and anxiety in the presence of essentially harmless objects or situations. Phobia symptoms, particularly agoraphobia in women, and their associated syndrome—extreme helplessness and dependency—appear related to sex-role conflict. Stereotypically, women are viewed as emotional, submissive, passive, home-oriented, and showing a strong need for security and dependency. Under the realistic stresses of adult life and marriage, these stereotypically helpless women become anxious, wish to flee, and dream of being more independent or of rescue or escape. For some, the emotional stress is too great and phobia provides another solution (Fodor, 1974). They become more and more dependent on those around them and avoid autonomy, initiative, and assertiveness.

The most common severely disabling phobia is agoraphobia (Fodor, 1974). On the average, 84% of agoraphobics are female and 89% are married. Their personalities are typically dependent, anxious, and shy. The main fears are of (1) going out of the house—on the street, to movies, shop, etc.; (2) closed spaces—such as elevators; (3) travel—trains, buses, subway, shops, planes; and (4) bridges or tunnels (Fodor, 1974). Agoraphobia is characterized primarily by an inability to leave a safe place, usually home; some women are completely unable to leave the house; groceries must be ordered by phone, neighbors must be cajoled into chauffeuring children around, and trips out to dinner with the family or evenings at the movies are impossible. For the phobic woman, even the thought of going somewhere alone brings on a flood of anxiety. Many women, for instance, do not drive an automobile, which prevents them from facing many situations alone.

There are approximately 16 million Americans suffering from phobias that are debilitating enough to interfere with their functioning (President's Commission, vol. IV).

In about 1 million, phobias are severely disabling (they cannot work or manage common household tasks). There is a large percentage of people who avoid the very basics of health care, such as periodic injection, visits to the dentist, and other medical situations, because of irrational fears. Phobic relatives are a significant component of the overall problem of compliance with health care recommendations.

Theoretically, phobia involves a pattern of avoidance, particularly of activities that involve independent, self-assertive handling of the difficult, fear-arousing situations (Fodor, 1974). There appear to be at least two aspects of this avoidance reaction. One is a tendency to avoid assertion, especially of angry feelings, and the other is to avoid learning how to cope with and master feared situations that hinder the development of competence.

Symonds (1974) describes phobias in women as their "declaration of dependence." These women use the marriage relationship to get themselves taken care of. Young women who were independent, self-sufficient, and capable somehow change after marriage and develop phobias as a way of retreating from life.

Treatment

Desensitization is the technique deemed most effective with phobias (70% effective in mildly to moderately phobic women). It is a relaxation procedure that enables the client to learn alternative compatible responses to conditioned anxiety-producing stimuli. The client is asked first to imagine the feared situation in its least fearful design; then she builds up to talking about the most feared situation. The next step is to confront the less fearful situation with the therapist, then with friends, then alone in a series of slowly progressive steps. Relaxation tapes may be used and the therapist is very liberal with praise about the client's increasing autonomy. The client may be asked also to record phobic occurrences during the week, what was done to overcome fears, and what set them off (Fodor, 1974). Sometimes "flooding" is more effective with agoraphobia. Flooding involves prolonged exposure to the feared situation so that the client can "learn" that horrible imagined consequences do not come to pass (President's Commission, vol. IV).

Minor tranquilizers may be used at first, but they are not effective treatment. Group therapy is helpful, especially assertiveness training. A female therapist who is comfortable with her own identity is most helpful in enabling these women who have avoided being independent to see how such a woman can be happy and competent and "feminine" (Fodor, 1974). Family therapy is often effective, especially with male-female cotherapists. As the woman learns to be more independent, the man learns to feel comfortable with the role change. Often the husband has unwittingly reinforced the wife's dependence because of his fears that she will leave if she becomes autonomous. The greatest impact on phobias will occur, however, when society not only approves but requires adult role competence of both sexes instead of reinforcing sex-role stereotypes that force women into dependent roles.

SUBSTANCE ABUSE
Alcoholism

Alcoholism is a generic term referring to the chronic or repetitive use of alcoholic beverages to the extent that this interferes with one's economic, social, physical, or mental functioning. What all alcoholics have in common is drinking and damage (Whitehead and Ferrence, 1976). Female alcoholics are different from male alcoholics. James (1975) analyzed the responses of twenty-nine female alcoholics to a drinking history and symptoms questionnaire and compared them with the Jellinek alcoholism symptomology and phaseology. Fig. 26-1 delineates the differences.

Beckman (1975) describes two groups of alcoholic women, one with "primary" alcoholism and one with "secondary" alcoholism who manifest alcoholism in conjunction with (and probably as a secondary characteristic of) depression. In one study 27% of alcoholic women were classified as "secondary" alcoholics.

Incidence and prevalence

Conservative estimates of the number of adult women with alcohol-related problems range from 1.5 million to 2.25 million (Noble, 1978). The latter figure, based on data from national household surveys, may underestimate the extent of the problem because of the widespread use of male-oriented measures of problem drinking. Others believe that underestimation results from the greater social stigma associated with female alcoholics, which may prevent women from seeking treatment. Sandmaier (1977) estimates that from 3 to 5 million women suffer from problems with alcohol. Fewer women drink than men, (61% versus 76%) and among those women who do drink, the incidence of heavier and problem drinking is considerably lower (Noble, 1978). As a result, nearly all abuse and alcoholism research and treatment efforts have been directed toward the male population.

The drinking patterns are different for men and women. Practically all that is written about alcoholism—characteristics of clients, etiology, and treatment programs—is based on the male alcoholic (Blume, 1979). Often the research data on females are thrown out because their numbers are smaller and they present a different picture from the male subjects. The reader should view all re-

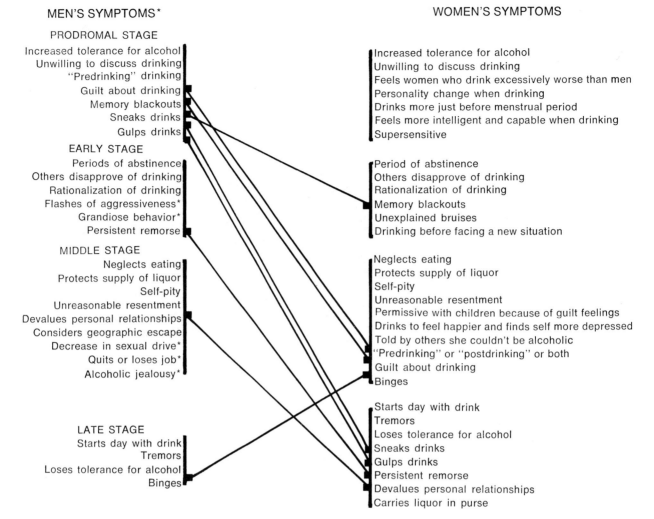

Fig. 26-1. Stages of alcoholism in men and women. * = reported by men only. (From Jones, J. E.: Symptoms of alcoholism in women: a preliminary report. Reprinted by permission from *Quarterly Journal of Studies on Alcohol*, vol. 36, pp. 1564-1569, 1975. Copyright by Journal of Studies on Alcohol, Inc., New Brunswick, N.J. 08903.)

search data on alcoholism as applicable only to men unless the researcher speaks specifically about women.

In the past few decades, the rate of increase in alcohol use among women has far surpassed that for men. Among college students, the proportion of male drinkers rose 3% between 1953 and 1974, while female drinkers increased by 12% (Sandmaier, 1977a). According to a 1974 Gallup Poll, women are "catching up."

Sandmaier notes that as more women drink, clearly more women risk developing alcohol problems. Some recent studies estimate that about one third of the 9 to 10 million alcoholic people in the United States are women. These estimates too may be conservative since they are primarily derived from public clinics, which many women avoid in favor of the privacy of the physician's offices. About 40% of physicians surveyed in a 1972 study reported seeing as many women alcoholic patients as men.

One third of AA's new members from 1975 to 1978 were women. Many believe that half of the nation's alcoholics are women, but they are simply less visible because of greater fear of exposure (Sandmaier, 1977a).

Blume (1979) cites case finding as male oriented since, traditionally, alcoholics have been identified from court records of drunken drivers or public inebriates and from industry. Women are found infrequently among those arrested or in programs sponsored by industry. In fact, in the recent past, a female would get arrested for drunk driving only if there was another cause, such as sassing the officer. When pamphlets about alcohol treatment intended only for male employees were accidentally put in *all* pay envelopes, a large number of women workers showed up for treatment (Blume, 1979).

Men get into treatment because of problems with the law and jobs, whereas women get into treatment because of problems with family relationships and health. One study found that 80% of the employed women alcoholics never missed a day of work because of drinking (Horn and Wanberg, 1973). Case finding for women would be more profitable if medical records were examined. Women problem drinkers go to their family physician, and twice as often as men they are put on psychoactive drugs. In one study, 86% of the women problem drinkers initially went to their physician with another complaint and casually mentioned alcohol intake. They were reassured that they could not possibly be alcoholic (Blume, 1979). Blume concludes that even when alcoholic women are recognized, they are not referred; if seen by a physician, often they are not diagnosed, and usually no mention is made of problems with alcohol. Even if a diagnosis of alcoholism is made, medical records show that either there is no referral for treatment or that the treatment programs are inadequate—designed primarily for men. Blume suggests that case finding for women would be much more effective if there were television messages telling women where to seek help.

Research data on the incidence of alcoholism among black Americans are scant. Harper (1976) indicates that black Americans differ from whites in that they tend either to drink heavily or not at all. A large proportion (51%) of black women are nondrinkers.

Lindbeck (1972) estimates that rates for alcoholism are nearly equal among males and females in the upper socioeconomic class. In Spain, alcoholism appears to be classless (Fernandez, 1976). The ratio of female to male alcoholism in Spain has altered dramatically over the past 20 years from 1:9 in 1954 to 1:4 currently. The rates of female to male alcoholism in the British Isles has increased from 1:4 or 5 in 1973 to 1:3 in 1976.

Beckman (1975) wonders if alcoholism is the ransom women pay for their emancipation. Even if true, Dr. Ernest Noble, Director of the National Institute on Alcohol Abuse and Alcoholism, has stated, "It is clear that the answer to female alcoholism is not to return women to their former status . . . attempts to limit the life choices of any human being—male or female—can only be detrimental to basic mental health."

Given these concerns, there is considerable interest in the social factors that contribute to alcoholism in women and their relationship to broader changes occurring in women's roles.

Social factors

Problem drinking rates are lower among ethnic groups whose drinking customs, values, and sanctions are well-established, known, and agreed upon by group members. Problem drinking rates have been found to be much higher among cultural groups with marked ambivalence toward alcohol (Beckman, 1973).

The proportion of women who drink drops considerably with increasing age, regardless of other social factors (Noble, 1978). However, there is a higher incidence of heavier and problem drinking in the 35 to 64 age group than in either the younger or older age groups. The sole exception to this pattern occurs for divorced and separated women under age 35 (Noble, 1978). Carver and associates (1976) found the majority of women alcoholics to be between 40 and 60 years of age. Much of the literature* shows women turning to excessive drinking later in life than men. Craddick (1976) speculates that the excessive drinking may be related to middle-age identity crisis after the children have left home.

The effect of marital status varies with the age group. Among women under age 35, there is little difference between single and married women, but divorced and separated women have the highest incidence of problem drinking of any age group. Older women who are divorced, separated, or widowed show lower problem rates than those who are married (Noble, 1978). This suggests that the crisis of divorce or separation, rather than the status of being divorced, is responsible for the elevated rates of heavy drinking among younger women.

Among married women under age 65, those who are working have higher rates of problem drinking than those who are not employed outside the home, regardless of socioeconomic status (Noble, 1978). This finding may stem from peer pressure in the work situation to drink more frequently, or from conflicts stemming from the dual demands of the roles of wife and employee.

Concerning education, one community in Canada evidenced a bimodal distribution of alcoholic women with a substantial number at the two extremes—primary school education or less, and postsecondary education (Carver et al., 1976). Women alcoholics have been shown to be in many ways a heterogeneous group, who frequently had an alcoholic parent (Noble, 1978; Bromet and Moos, 1976; Beckman, 1975).

Keil (1978) interviewed 876 women aged 21 to 65 in a household survey in Pennsylvania and analyzed the effects of a variety of predictors on abstinence and drinking. The drinkers were more likely to: (1) belong to religious groups that were without proscriptions against drinking or were ineffective in enforcing such proscriptions; (2) attend religious services less than once a week, (3) have mothers who drank, (4) have European, black, Puerto Rican, or Chinese background, (5) be 21 to 32 years old, (6) have 10 to 17 years of education, (7) associate with peers who drink, (8) work full-time, attend school or, if homemakers, be retired from work outside the home or attend school in addition to being a home-

---

*Kramer, 1976; Bromet and Moos, 1976; Carver et al., 1976; Schucket, 1972; Craddick, 1976; Beckman, 1975; Mulford, 1977.

maker. These findings differ from other studies, especially in regard to age and years of education. Even the profile of alcoholic women is incomplete at this time.

Psychologic factors

There is a widespread belief that female alcoholics show more psychopathology than male alcoholics. Female alcoholics are more likely to be admitted to hospitals as psychiatric patients (Schucket and Gundersen, 1975) and they are admitted more often and for longer periods of time (Beckman, 1975). Female alcoholics show more adult personality maladjustments than males, but that may be because women in general have higher rates of mental illness (Beckman, 1975). In almost every category of psychologic/psychiatric disturbance, Khantzian (1976) reports that alcoholic clients (both men and women) are more disturbed than typical clients on inpatient psychiatric units.

Alcoholic women report more emotional problems than do alcoholic men (Wechsler, 1978) and greater sexual dissatisfaction (Sclare, 1977). The incidence of suicide in women alcoholics has been found higher only in the group with secondary alcoholism. Females have a later age of onset of symptoms, a shorter duration of drinking before entering treatment, and a comparable age at hospitalization (Mulford, 1977; Schuckit, 1972).

Women alcoholics have fewer severe symptoms such as delirium tremens but more physical illness than men (Beckman, 1975). A study of the different ways that 100 female and male alcoholics sought treatment found that significantly more females were admitted as a result of an acute complication: unconsciousness, attempted suicide, mental confusion, neurologic disorders, etc., while the males generally sought treatment under less dramatic circumstances. Associated drug abuse was also more common among the female than the male alcoholics (Dahlgren and Myrhed, 1977b).

Beckman (1978a) speculates that what appears to be greater pathology in women could be a result of their alcoholism and the greater social disapproval and rejection associated with it, rather than an indication of more initial maladjustment and disturbance. The greater stigma placed upon female intoxication has contributed to the tendency for women as well as society to ignore the problem. The alcoholic woman is likely to share society's opinion of herself, and this stigma/guilt/shame factor is one of the main difficulties in treatment (Johnson and Garzon, 1977). Stafford and Petway (1977) studied a random sample of white, middle class people and found no difference between the stigma attached to male or female alcoholism; alcoholics and drunken persons of both sexes were greatly stigmatized. If greater stigma is associated with alcoholism in women, Stafford and Petway believe it originates in their self-perceptions rather than

in the perceptions of others; women have a greater need for social approval, which would make stigmatization more devastating for them than for male alcoholics. Research from the 1960s clearly indicates that society views female intoxication with disgust while viewing male intoxication with indifference or amusement (Gomberg, 1976). Perhaps the attitude toward women is not changing but society is merely getting less tolerant of male alcoholics.

The earlier rejection of female intoxication was related to women's roles in child care and sexual behavior (Gomberg, 1976). It was believed that drunken women would be unsafe as mothers and have "loose sexual morals." Though we do not know if there is a relationship between sexual behavior and alcohol, a 1974 college study reported that alcohol is the drug of choice for the male's sexual seduction of the female. The females perceive that alcohol increases their level of sexual arousal (Bowker, 1977). Wilson and Lawson (1976) report a negative relation between increasing levels of alcohol consumption and sexual arousal in women (as measured by vaginal pressure pulse readings). Interestingly, the majority of subjects reported enhanced sexual arousal with increasing levels of intoxication. Women's subjective estimates of the effect of alcohol were diametrically opposed to their vaginal pressure pulse readings. The effect of alcohol on women's sexuality remains an open question but there is no doubt that society greatly stigmatizes alcoholism in either sex.

Beckman (1975) advises not focusing on whether or not women are sicker or more stigmatized than men, but on the differences between the male and female alcoholic. We especially need to develop a body of knowledge about the drinking patterns of women. Women alcoholics are more likely than men to have depressive symptoms with both attempted and completed suicides. Men are more likely to be sociopathic with a much poorer treatment prognosis (Schuckit and Gundersen, 1975). Alcohol and heavy drinking in women are more likely to be linked to psychologic stress and a specific precipitating circumstance (Beckman, 1975), whereas men tend to drift into greater dependence on alcohol to cope with everyday problems (Mulford, 1977). Domestic stress or a specific life event crisis in the family setting are the reasons that women drink heavily whereas job stress accounts for the men's drinking (Sclare, 1977; Browne-Mayers et al., 1976; Carver et al., 1976). According to Sandmaier (1977):

The crises women cite most often as precipitating factors in alcohol abuse are divorce, death of a family member, a child leaving home, miscarriage, abortion, infertility, hysterectomy, menstrual difficulties, menopause, and post-partum depression. Significantly, all of these crises are relative to important functions defining the traditional female role, particularly the childbearing/mothering function. Since many women still identify themselves primarily through these functions, any occurrence which would undermine feelings of adequacy in these areas would be likely to be very threatening. But if a woman's identity and sense of self-worth derived from a broader base, these crises might well be less traumatic and therefore less likely to trigger alcohol abuse (p. 3).

Seventy-eight percent of alcoholic women who had ever been married reported obstetric or gynecologic problems as compared to 35% of the controls reporting such problems (Beckman, 1975). One fourth of the married alcoholics said they were unable to have children, as compared to 4% of married controls. Women who drink to deal with depression have a better long-term prognosis but a higher immediate suicide risk (Schuckit and Morrisey, 1976).

In one study more than 50% of the married alcoholic women had alcoholic spouses but only 10% of the married alcoholic men had alcoholic spouses (Dahlgren and Myrhed, 1977a). Alcoholic women are more likely to have spouses and parents who are heavy drinkers.

Health problems

There is a higher incidence of alcohol-related disorders among women than among men (Ashley, et al., 1977; Morgan and Sherlock, 1977) even though the length of time for drinking behavior is similar and the quantity consumed may be similar or less. Women were reported by Ashley and associates (1977) to have significantly more fatty liver, hypertension, obesity, anemia, malnutrition, gastrointestinal hemorrhage, and ulcers requiring surgery. The only significant increase for men was in obstructive lung disease. A study of liver function test results showed that the incidence of chronic advanced liver disease was higher among women (86%) than among men (65%) (Morgan and Sherlock, 1977). Women, however, were less likely to develop primary liver cell cancer. The commonest mode of presentation was a raised aspartate transaminase concentration with or without hepatomegaly.

Research findings indicate that women show higher mortality rate from alcohol-related disorders than do men (Hill, 1978; Dahlgren and Myrhed, 1977a; Metropolitan Life, 1977). Deaths among Swedish men and women from 1963 to 1969 were 3.0 and 5.6 times higher, respectively, than expected for men and women in the general population (Dahlgren and Myrhed, 1977a). Mortality among the alcoholic women was significantly higher than expected for diseases of the respiratory system and cirrhosis of the liver. The men had significantly higher than expected mortality from diseases of the circulatory system, neoplasms, and acute alcohol poisoning. The true impact of alcohol abuse is hard to measure because of considerable underreporting of alcoholism as cause of death in the United States. If mentioned as a contributory cause on the death certificate, it is not picked up (Metropolitan Life, 1977). Even so, from 1963–1964 to 1973–1974, the death rates from alcoholic disorders rose 71% in nonwhite women and 36% in white women. The figure for the nonwhite women is particularly striking since 50% of black women are abstainers.

Russell (1976) found that birth weights of 499 infants born to women with an alcohol-related psychiatric diagnosis were significantly lower than those of control infants (matched on sex, year and county of birth, maternal age, race, and education). Differences in birth weights between controls and babies of alcoholic women increased as the duration of maternal drinking and alcohol intake increased. Russell concludes that maternal drinking during pregnancy is associated with biologically significant adverse effects in intrauterine growth. The fetal alcohol syndrome is clearly a factor to be concerned about, especially with the recent increase in alcohol consumption among women of childbearing age.

Etiology

When women are asked why they drink, the following answers are given: they drink when they are tense or nervous, to relax and forget worries, to relieve feelings of loneliness and inferiority, to feel more acceptable socially, or because they cannot adequately fulfill a satisfying role within the family (Beckman, 1978a). A popular theory relates drinking to conflicts about dependency—heavy drinking gets these needs taken care of without the drinker ever having to ask (Beckman, 1978b). This theory, along with the notion that alcoholics drink to feel more powerful, has been tested with men only. Beckman suggests that women drink to feel more like women and that alcoholic women are more similar to other women than to alcoholic men.

A central feature of alcoholism in women is not dependency but preoccupation with inadequacy and a sense of futility about being able to make do for oneself (Beckman, 1978a). When self-esteem was measured in seventy-one drug-dependent subjects, females were found to have lower self-esteem than males. No such sex difference was found in a control group. In another study, Beckman (1978a) found also that the self-esteem of women alcoholics was lower than that of men alcoholics and of "normal" nonalcoholic women, but was similar to that of women in treatment for psychiatric disorders not related to misuse of alcohol or drugs.

Another theory explaining why some women become alcoholics derives from Rotter's internal-external locus of control (Obitz and Swanson, 1976). A group of fifty alcoholic women and a control group of forty women social drinkers completed Rotter's scale and a scale meas-

locus of control over drinking. The alcohol abusers perceived themselves as having less control on both the internal-external scale and drinking-control tests than did the social drinkers. The alcohol abusers were found to be significantly more externally oriented than either the controls, normal men and women, or alcoholic men.

In recent studies of the effect of sex hormone levels on drinking behavior, it was found that women taking oral contraceptives or hormone supplements metabolized alcohol more slowly than women not taking oral contraceptives (Jones and Jones, 1976a; Jones et al., 1976). Both the women taking oral contraceptives and those taking hormone supplements obtained significantly higher peak blood alcohol levels than the male group despite the administration of alcohol according to body weight. The authors conclude that estrogen may act to decrease the rate of ethanol metabolism in women. Belfer and Shader (1976) found that 67% of menstruating alcoholic women and 46% of nonmenstruating alcoholic women related drinking to their menstrual cycle, particularly to premenstruum. The relationship of drinking to premenstrual tension remains uncertain, however, since contradictory findings continue to be reported.

Sex-role conflicts have been cited as an important factor in the etiology of alcoholism in women. Wilsnack (1976) as well as Scott and Manaugh (1976) found that on a conscious level, alcoholic women valued traditionally feminine goals and life-styles as much as did normal women. However, Wilsnack found that unconscious measures of sex-role identity showed less "femininity" and more "masculinity" among the alcoholic women than among the control group. Wilsnack suggests that alcoholic women may drink to resolve the conflict between their unconscious, socially defined "masculine" strivings (assertiveness, independence) and society's narrow definition of "femininity," which does not allow for the expression of these strivings. Beckman (1978b) writes that sex-role conflict in the women alcoholic is a myth, pointing to the limited evidence of such conflict: fewer than one fourth of the alcoholic women studied show evidence of the "unconscious masculinity" and "conscious femininity" pattern. Among these conflicted women, lower self-esteem is a more important variable, says Beckman, adding that masculine identification (as in the successful career woman) is not maladaptive.

Sandmaier (1977b) summarizes the reasons why women drink as follows: dependence on men, depression, sex-role conflicts, and specific crises such as divorce or a child leaving home; low self-esteem, increased anxiety and guilt, and a host of "nuts-and-bolts" problems derived from her role in society; lack of job skills, few or no economic resources, and primary responsibility for children, which may prevent women from entering a treatment program. By the time a woman gets help, her alcohol problem is likely to be more serious than that of her male counterpart. She also is more likely to be cross-addicted, and to have a history of psychiatric care.

Treatment

Since most research on alcoholism has been done on male alcoholics, few of the results can be utilized in predicting the success of treatment programs for women. Some 39,000 women are treated annually through programs directly funded by the National Institute on Alcohol Abuse and Alcoholism (NIAAA). The total number of women receiving treatment during 1975 represented about 22% of the total treatment population. The great majority of the female treatment population is young in comparison to men (under age 18). Women generally have reported self-referral for treatment or were referred by family or friends (NIAAA, 1977). Browne-Mayers (1976) reports 11% self-referrals with a majority being pressured by spouse or family. Other referrals were for physical illness or from industry. The smallest number of referrals came from psychiatrists, social workers, physicians, or legal sources. Women showed greater improvement than men after 180 days of treatment. Overall, it is apparent that the NIAAA programs are having greater success with the women than with the men (NIAAA, 1977). No studies have attempted to assess effective treatment modalities for black women (Gaines, 1976).

Successfully treated alcoholic women have been found to be more likely than the unsuccessfully treated to change social groups to friends who drink little or none. They also report a lower attendance at drinking functions; have improved social relationships with family, friends, and people in general; are involved in AA; and had other successful experiences in general. The unsuccessfully treated women frequently have an alcoholic father, alcohol-related illnesses, and use other drugs. In one study favorable prognosis was associated with low socioeconomic status, low educational attainment, low occupational status, and a high degree of intelligence (Beckman, 1975).

Reducing rates of alcohol consumption is considered by Whitehead and Ferrence (1976) to be important in the prevention of alcoholism. Suggested methods include taxation and pricing mechanisms on alcoholic beverages, banning advertising, raising the legal drinking age, and enforcing strict laws about drinking and driving.

Gomberg (1976) suggests that treatment considerations must include recognition of the heavier social disapproval with which women often approach a treatment situation, and understanding of the fact that women will have fewer marketable skills and in greater need of vocational help than male clients.

Treatment programs for women should include all-women therapy groups, child care, and health services (Sandmaier, 1977b). Provision for child care and women therapists are frequently recommended (Johnson and Ganzon, 1977; Calobrisi, 1976; Artz, 1976). One program that takes the "whole woman" approach is Interim House in Philadelphia. It serves only women, is staffed almost entirely by women, and deals with alcohol problems in the context of a woman's total experience in society (Sandmaier, 1977b). The staff seek to find out what women need and what is preventing them from getting it. The needs are many: decent jobs, further education, parenting skills, medical care, emotional growth, healthy personal relationships. An all-female program can help women develop a sense of identity that they may have lacked by always being known as somebody's wife, girlfriend, sexual partner, or mother. These women have not succeeded as mothers and most have no work histories. The programs at Interim House include individual and group counseling, family therapy, psychodrama, sexuality sessions, yoga, Alcoholics Anonymous meetings, and job training and education at nearby schools. Since opening in 1973, approximately 125 women have completed the 6-month program. Sixty-five percent have remained sober at least 1 year after leaving the program.

Therapy issues emerging repeatedly include fear of expressing anger, guilt about children, hostility toward the mother, difficulties in relating to men, and fear of independence or of "making it" in the outside world. Many of these issues are dealt with by psychodrama. One of the most important services at Interim House is the adequate child care available through provision of a home for women and their children while the women recover from alcoholism. The women and children learn healthier ways of relating to each other as a part of carrying out daily living activities.

Theorists such as Sandmaier are committed to the notion that alcoholism in women is related to their restricted sex-role identity in society and their low self-esteem. If they do not succeed at traditional "feminine" roles and behaviors, they are overwhelmed with anxiety and inadequacy. Frequently, women have fewer job skills, minimal economic resources, and major responsibility for children; they drink to cope with life stresses and delay treatment because of stigma and because there is no one else to care for their children (Sandmaier, 1977b).

The interventions mentioned earlier to improve the status of women in this society should also help prevent alcoholism in women. Teaching the family physician and nurse practitioner to recognize and refer alcoholic women could reach a substantial number of women before extensive health-related problems occur. Television advertising could help educate the public and get women into treatment programs earlier.

Beckman (1975) points to the need to determine which aspects of the wife and mother role the alcoholic is not performing adequately, and then to provide resocialization or relearning for more adequate handling of these roles. Another approach is to suggest alternatives to the traditional feminine roles that might prove more gratifying.

Alcoholic women report that individual therapy is more helpful while men rank group therapy as more helpful (Beckman, 1975). Though many writers think that family therapy would be efficacious, research on its effects has been plagued by small samples, absence of controls, and disappointing results (Dinaburg et al., 1977). Ferrera reported on fourteen alcoholic women/nonalcoholic spouse dyads in therapy in which the couples insisted throughout that the excessive drinking by the wife was the only problem in an otherwise happy relationship. Since the mean length of marriage for the sample was 18 years, he considered these couples had stable (though pathologic) marriages and going for therapy was a sham (Dinaburg et al., 1977). Other studies have reported some success with family therapy for alcoholism; however, none were controlled and there were no posttreatment follow-ups. Dinaburg et al. suggest that family therapists should work in conjunction with self-help groups such as AA and use other adjuncts such as medication or sexual therapy. Family therapy with female alcoholics should be considered an "experimental" procedure on the basis of the data available (Dinaburg et al., 1977).

Studies on the effect of chemotherapy in treating women alcoholics show no difference between treated and untreated groups (Blume, 1979). There needs to be additional research on treating women with antianxiety agents premenstrually. Also, since lithium is effective with male alcoholics, its value should be assessed with female alcoholics. With lithium treatment there is some concern about teratogenic effects (Blume, 1979). Certainly, those women with secondary alcoholism will benefit from treatment of their depression.

It is widely believed that Alcoholics Anonymous (AA) offers the most successful treatment method, but scientific data supporting this are lacking, and most women have not felt comfortable in this primarily male subculture.

Antabuse is another treatment method whose real value has not been effectively determined. The drug works by causing the person to become very sick (nausea and vomiting) if she drinks alcohol after taking the drug. This is part of the behavioral treatment that views alcoholism as a learned response. The sickness induced by drinking causes an aversive rather than pleasant association with drinking. While the success of behavioral methods in the treatment of alcohol abuse has been limited, more research is indicated based on scattered reports of success.

Sandmaier (1977a) suggests a number of prevention strategies that promote an individual's self-development and general emotional health, thereby indirectly lessening the likelihood of alcohol abuse. These interventions place emphasis on improving interpersonal relationships, using one's talents and abilities to the fullest extent possible, and developing coping skills for survival in a complex, stress-filled society. Some examples include:

1. Consciousness-raising groups
2. Body awareness workshops
3. Natural highs (relaxation techniques such as yoga, TM)
4. Assertiveness training
5. Sexuality discussion groups
6. Sports and exercise
7. Parent effectiveness training
8. Women's support groups
9. Job counseling and training
10. Creative outlets

Drug abuse

In the United States drug abuse among women is rapidly increasing for both prescribed psychotropic drugs and drugs purchased illegally on the street. Of 8,516 Australian adults screened by Medicheck for drinking and drug-taking patterns, 25% of the women took either psychotropic drugs (mainly tranquilizers) or analgesics regularly (Reynolds et al., 1976). Those who drank everyday were among the highest drug users. Regular drug taking is predominantly a female characteristic (in Australia). Suffet and Brotman (1976) have summarized the major United States research findings on female drug use as follows: women are usually initiated into illicit drug use by men; rates of illicit drug use are lower among females than males, although the difference narrows among younger persons and among those who subscribe to more liberal values and life-styles; women are more likely than men to use psychotherapeutic drugs; and female opiate addicts are often involved in deviant activity such as prostitution. Suffet and Brotman (1976) predict that as women rebel against the old double standard, which denied them certain personal freedoms granted to men, we will begin to see a greater parity in rates of male and female drug use, especially among

teenagers and young adults. They also predict that the whole question of psychotherapeutic pill use will be examined closely.

It is assumed that use of psychotherapeutic drugs serves, intentionally or not, as a device for perpetuating women's unequal social status. It relieves the manifestations of the strains felt by women, but does nothing to remove the underlying causes. To the degree that the women's movement achieves social equality for women, thereby alleviating sexual strain, drug use will decrease. A countervailing force, however, is that as women gain equality in the work place, they will probably be subject to the same pressures now experienced by men in regard to career mobility, job responsibilities, dislocations and uncertainties in the employment market, and so on. Possibly working women will adopt the predominant pattern and turn to alcohol.

In regard to heroin addiction, Suffet and Brotman (1976) note that the proportion of women in the addict population is increasing but there is evidence that heroin is being replaced to some degree by illegal methadone, the use of which is growing among both sexes. Women who enter the addict world will continue to run the risk of prostitution or other illegal activity and the risk of giving birth to an addicted infant. Reduction of such risks depends mostly on significant changes in the social opportunity structure, say Suffet and Brotman. "As long as our society chooses to stigmatize and punish addicts, instead of providing more widespread help, and so long as our society restricts instead of opens opportunities for good housing, genuine education and satisfying work, especially for those groups most vulnerable to addiction, we have virtually guaranteed the continued existence of a large addict population—both male and female—in our midst." (Suffet and Brotman, 1976)

REFERENCES

Abernethy, V.: Cultural perspectives on the impact of women's changing roles on psychiatry, Am. J. Psychiatry 133:657-661, 1976.

Alberti, R., and Emmons, M.: Your perfect right, San Luis Obispo, Calif., 1974, Prometheus Books.

Alsbrook, L.: Marital communication and sexism, Social Casework 57:517-522, 1976.

Appleton, W. S., and Davis, J. M.: Practical clinical psychopharmacology, New York, 1973, Mediom Press.

Artz, J.: Can minorities be invisible: If not, why not? Am. J. Drug Alcohol Abuse 3:181-183, 1976.

Ashley, M. J., Olin, J. S., and Le Riche, W. M.: Morbidity in alcoholics: evidence for accelerated development of physical disease in women, Arch. Intern. Med. 137:883-887, 1977.

Aslin, A. L.: Feminist and community mental health center psychotherapists' mental health expectations for women, Dissert. Abstr. Int. 35(11-B):5630-5631, 1973.

Avery, D., and Winokeu, G.: Mortality in depressed patients treated with electrocommulsine therapy and antidepressives, Arch. Gen. Psychiatry 33:1029-1037, 1976.

Bardwick, J.: The sex hormones, the central nervous system and affect variability in humans. In Franks, V., and Burtle, V., editors: Women in therapy, New York, 1974, Brunner/Mazel, Inc.

Barrett, B.: Enterprising principles of counseling the low-income black family, Non-White Concerns in Personnel and Guidance 5:14-22, 1976.

Barrett, C.: The development and evaluation of three therapeutic group interventions for widows, Dissert. Abst. Int. 35:3569-3570, 1975.

Beck, A. T., and Greenberg, R.: Cognitive therapy with depressed women." In Franks, V., and Burtle, V., editors: Women in therapy, New York, 1974, Brunner/Mazel.

Beckman, L. J.: Women alcoholics: a review of social and psychological studies," J. Stud. Alcohol 36:797-824, 1975.

Beckman, L. J.: Self-esteem of women alcoholics," J. Stud. Alcohol 39:491-498, 1978a.

Beckman, L. J.: Sex-role conflict in alcoholic women: myth or reality, J. Abnorm. Psych. 87:408-417, 1978b.

Belfer, M. L., and Shader, R. I.: Premenstrual factors as determinants of alcoholism in women. In Greenblatt, ?., and Schuckit, M., editors: Alcoholism problems in women and children, New York, 1976, Grune & Stratton, Inc.

Bem, S. L.: Androgy vs the tight little lives of fluffy women and chesty men, Psych. Today 9:58-59, 1975.

Benedek, E. P.: Editorial practices of psychiatric and related journals: implications for women, Am. J. Psychiatry 139:89-92, 1976.

Benson, R.: The forgotten treatment modality in bipolar illness: psychotherapy, Dis. Nerv. Syst. 36:634-638, 1975.

Bernardez-Bonesatti, T.: Women and anger: conflicts with aggression in contemporary women, J. Am. Med. Women's Assoc. 33:215-219, 1978.

Birdbaum, J.: Life patterns and self-esteem in gifted family-oriented and career committed women. In Mednick, M., Langri, S., and Hoffman, L., editors: Women and achievement: social and motivational analysis, New York, 1975, Halsted Press.

Bloom, L. Z., Coburn, K., and Pearlman, J.: The new assertive woman, New York, 1975, Dell Publishing Co., Inc.

Blume, S. B.: Alcoholism: the search for sources. Presented at the North Carolina Alcoholism Research Authority, Raleigh, 1979.

Bowker, L. H.: Drug use among American women, old and young: sexual oppression and other themes, San Francisco, 1977, R and E Research Associates.

Brandon, S.: Psychiatric illness in women, Nurs. Mirror Midwives J. 134:17-18, 1976.

Bromet, E., and Moos, R.: Sex and marital status in relation to the characteristics of alcoholics, J. Stud. Alcohol 37:1302-1312, 1976.

Broverman, I. K., and others: Sex role stereotypes and clinical judgments of mental health, Consult. Clin. Psychol. 34:1-7, 1970.

Brown, G., Bhrolehain, M., and Harris, T.: Social class and psychiatric disturbance among women in urban populations, Sociology 9:225-254, 1975.

Brown, P., Perry, L., and Harburg, E.: Sex role attitudes and psychological outcomes for black and white women experiencing marital dissolution, J. Marriage Family 39:549-561, 1977.

Browne-Mayers, A. N., Seelye, E. E., and Sillman, L.: Psychosocial study of hospitalized middle-class alcoholic women, Ann. N.Y. Acad. Sci. 273:593-604, 1976.

Brown, T. R., and Sharon, T. J.: Suicide prediction: a review, Life-Threatening Behavior 2:67-97, 1972.

Bumbalo, J., and Young, D.: The self-help phenomenon, Am. J. Nurs. 73:1588-1591, 1973.

Butler, P.: Techniques of assertive training in groups, Int. J. Group Psychother. 26:361-371, 1976.

Caldwell, B.: What does research teach us about day care for children under 3, Child. Today 1:1-13, 1972.

Calobrisi, A.: Treatment programs for alcoholic women. In Greenblatt, M., and Schuckit, M. A., editors: Alcoholism problems in women and children, New York, 1976, Grune & Stratton, Inc.

Carter, C. A.: Advantages of being a woman therapist, Psychother. Theory Res. Pract. 8:297-300, 1971.

Carver, V., Huneault, N., and Pinder, L.: Characteristics, service patterns and needs of female alcoholics in Ottawa-Carleton. Presented at the 11th Annual Conference, Canadian Foundation on Alcohol and Drug Dependences, Toronto, Ontario, 1976.

Cassel, J. C.: Psychiatric epidemiology. In Caplan, G., editor: American handbook of psychiatry, vol. 2, New York, 1974, Basic Books, Inc.

Chesler, P.: Men drive women crazy, Psych. Today 5:18, 1971.

Chesler, P.: A word about mental health and women, Ment. Hygiene 57:5-7, 1973.

Cohen, E. S., Harbin, H. T., and Wright, M. J.: Some considerations in the formulation of psychiatric diagnoses, J. Nerv. Ment. Disorders 160:422-427, 1975.

Cohen, P. M., and Burdsal, C. A.: Factor analytic examination of role attitudes of married women, Psychol. Rep. 42:423-424, 1978.

Cole, J., and Davis, J.: Antidepressant drugs. In Freedman, A., Kaplan, H., and Sadock, B., editors: Comprehensive textbook of psychiatry, vol. II, ed. 2, Baltimore, The Williams & Wilkins Co.

Craddick, R. A., Leipold, V., and Leipold, W. D.: Effect of role empathy on human figures drawn by women alcoholics, J. Stud. Alcohol 37:90-97, 1976.

Crary, W., and Crary, G.: Depression, Am. J. Nurs. 73:472-475, 1973.

Dahlgren, L., and Myrhed, M.: Alcoholic females. II. Causes of death with reference to sex differences, Acta Psychiatr. Scand. 56:81-91, 1977a.

Dahlgren, L., and Myrhed, M.: Female alcoholics: ways of admission of the alcoholic patient, Acta Psychiatr. Scand. 56:39-47, 1977b.

Dalton, K.: The premenstrual syndrome, Springfield, Ill., 1964, Charles C Thomas, Publisher.

Darroch, D. B.: Media images and medical images, Soc. Sci. Med. 9:613-618, 1975.

Davis, J. M.: Which patients need ECT? Med. World News, Oct. 1975.

Dellas, M., and Gaier, E. L.: The self and adolescent identity in women: options and implications, Adolescence 10(39):399-407, 1975.

Densen-Gerber, J., Wathey, R., and Speller, M. L.: Women and addiction: the sociologic autopsy, Leg. Med. Ann. 1976:261-269, 1977.

Detre, T. P., and Jarecki, H. G.: Modern psychiatric treatment, Philadelphia, 1971, J. B. Lippincott Co.

DeRosis, H., and Pellegrino, V.: The book of hope: how women can overcome depression, New York, 1976, Bantam Books.

Dicken, C.: Sex roles, smoking and smoking cessation, J. Health Soc. Behav. 19:324-333, 1978.

Dimascio, A., Klerman, G. L., and Prusoff, B.: Relative study of amitriptyline in maintenance treatment of depression, J. Nerv. Ment. Dis. 160:34-41, 1975.

Dinaburg, D., Glick, I. D., and Feigenbaum, E.: Marital therapy of women alcoholics, J. Stud. Alcohol 38:1247-1258, 1977.

Doherty, E. G.: Are differential discharge criteria used for men and women psychiatric inpatients, J. Health Soc. Behav. 19:107-116, 1978.

Dohrenwend, B. S.: Stressful events and psychological symptoms, NIMH Grant MH-10328 and MH-13356, 1971.

Dohrenwend, B. S.: Social status and stressful life events, J. Personal. Soc. Psych. 28:225-235, 1973.

Dohrenwend, B. P., and Dohrenwend, B. S.: The problem of validity in field studies of psychological disorders, J. Abnorm. Psych. 70:52-69, 1965.

Dowsling, J. L.: Chemical trap: a physician's perspective. Presented at the Conference on the Clinically Dependent Woman, Toronto, Ontario, 1977.

Eisenberg, L.: Caring for children and working: dilemmas of contemporary womanhood, Pediatrics **56:**24-28, 1975.

Endicott, J., and Spitzu, R. L.: A diagnostic interview: the schedule for affective disorders and schizophrenia. Presented at the American Psychiatric Association Meeting, Toronto, Canada, May 1977.

Faulkner, A. C., Heisel, M. A., and Simms, P.: Life strengths and life stresses: explorations in the measurement of the mental health of the black aged, Am. J. Orthopsychiatry **45:**102-110, 1975.

Feed, S.: Feelings of adjustment. In Nye, I., and Hoffman, L., editors: The employed mother in America, Chicago, 1963, Rand McNally & Co.

Fernandez, F. A.: State of alcoholism in Spain covering its epidemiological and aetiological aspects, Br. J. Addict. **71:**235-242, 1976.

Fodor, I. G.: The phobic syndrome in women: implications for treatment. In Franks, V., and Burtle, V., editors: Women in therapy, New York, 1974, Brunner/Mazel, Inc.

Forbes, L. H.: Mental stress and the changing role of women, J. Am. Med. Women's Assoc. **32:**376-379, 1977.

Frank, J.: Bewildering world of psycho-therapy, J. Soc. Issues **28:**27-42, 1972.

Friedman, A. S.: Interaction of drug therapy and marital therapy in depressive patients, Arch. Gen. Psychiatry **32:**619-637, 1975.

Gaines, J. J.: Alcohol and the black woman. In Harper, F. D., editor: Alcohol abuse and black America, Alexandria, Va., 1976, Douglass Publishers.

Galassi, M. D., and Galassi, J. P.: Assertion: A critical review, Psychother. Theory Res. Pract. **15:**16-29, 1976.

Galassi, M. D., and Galassi, J. P.: Assert yourself: how to be your own person, New York, 1977, Human Sciences Press.

Garai, J. E.: Sex differences in breakdown of mental health, Genet. Psychol. Monogr. **81:**131-132, 1970a.

Garai, J. E.: Sex differences in identity intimacy, Genet. Psychol. Monogr. **81:**133-134, 1970b.

Garai, J. E.: Sex differences in motivation and life goals, Genet. Psychol. Monog. **81:**128-129, 1970c.

Gartner, A.: Self help and mental health, Soc. Policy **7:**28-40, 1976.

Gartner, A., and Riessman, F.: Self-help in the human services, San Francisco, 1977, Jossey-Bass, Inc., Publishers.

Gayford, J. J.: Alcoholic illness: who cares? Royal Soc. Health J. **96:**186-188, 1976.

Gershan, S.: Lithium. In Arieti, S., editor: American handbook of psychiatry, New York, 1975, Basic Books, Inc.

Golden, J. S., and Golden, M. A.: You know who and what's her name: the woman's role in sex therapy, J. Sex Marital Ther. **2:**6-16, 1976.

Goldstein, M. Z.: Preventive mental health efforts for women medical students, J. Med. Educ. **50:**289-291, 1975.

Gomberg, E. S.: Female alcoholic. In Tarter, R. E., and Sugarman, A. A., editors: Alcoholism, Reading, Mass., 1976, Addison-Wesley Publishing Co., Inc.

Gordon, R. E., and others: Psychiatric problems of the 1970's, Int. J. Soc. Psychiatry **22:**253-264, 1976-1977.

Gossop, M.: Drug dependence and self-esteem, Int. J. Addict. **11:**741-753, 1976.

Gove, W. R.: The relationship between sex roles, marital status, and mental illness, Social Forces **51:**34-44, 1972.

Gove, W. R., and Geerken, M. R.: The effect of children and employment on the mental health of married men and women, Social Forces **56:**66-76, 1977.

Gove, W. R., and Tudor, J.: Adult sex roles and mental illness, Am. J. Sociology **78:**812-835, 1973.

Goy, R. W.: Experimental control of psychosexuality. In Edwards, R. G., editor: A discussion of the determinants of sex, Philosophical Transactions of the Royal Society of London, Series B, vol. 259, London, 1970, The Society, pp. 149-162.

Gray, J.: Anxiety, Hum. Nature, July 1978, pp. 40-45.

Guttentag, M., Salasin, S., and Legge, W. W.: Women's utilization of mental health services studied, Evaluation **3:**30-31, 1976.

Guttman, D., and others: The impact of needs, knowledge, ability, and living arrangements on decision making of the elderly. Final Report, AOA Grant No. 90-A-522, Washington, D.C., 1977, Catholic University of America.

Halleck, S.: The treatment of emotional disorders, New York, 1978a, Jason Aronson.

Halleck, S.: Therapy is the handmaiden of the status quo. In Backer, B., Dubbert, P., and Eisenman, E., editors: Psychiatric/mental health nursing, New York, 1978b, D. Van Nostrand Co.

Hamblin, R. L., and Jacobsen, R. B.: Suicide and pseudocide: a reanalysis of Mariss data, J. Health Soc. Behav. **13:**99-104, 1972.

Hare, N., and Hare, J.: Black women 1970. In Bardwick, J., editor: Readings on the psychology of women, New York, 1972, Harper & Row, Publishers, Inc.

Harper, F. D.: Etiology: why do blacks drink? In Harper, F. D., editor: Alcohol abuse and black America, Alexandria, Va., 1976, Douglass Publishers.

Heiman, E. M., and Kahn, M. W.: Mental health patients in a barrio health center, Int. J. Soc. Psychiatry **21:**172-204, 1975.

Hilberman, E., and Munson, K.: Sixty battered women, Victimology **2:**460-471, Fall, 1977-1978.

Hill, S. Y.: Biological consequences of alcoholism in women. Presented at the NIAA Workshop on Alcoholism and Alcohol Abuse Among Women, Jekyll Island, Ga., 1978.

Hoff, L. A.: People in crises, Menlo Park, Ca., 1978, Addison-Wesley Publishing Co.

Hoffman, L. W., and Nye, F. I.: Working mothers: an evaluative review of the consequences for wife, husband, and child, San Francisco, 1974, Jossey-Bass, Inc., Publishers.

Hollister, L. E.: Clinical pharmacology of psychotherapeutic drugs, New York, 1978, Churchill Livingstone.

Horn, J. L., and Wanberg, K. W.: Females are different: on the diagnosis of alcoholism in women. Proceedings of the First Annual Alcoholism Conference, NIAAA, 1973, pp. 332-354.

Horner, M.: The motive to avoid success and changing aspirations of college women. In Bardwick, J. M., editor: Readings in the psychology of women, New York, 1972, Harper & Row, Publishers, Inc.

Horney, K.: Our inner conflicts, New York, 1945, W. W. Norton Co., Inc.

Horney, K.: Neurosis and human growth, New York, 1950, W. W. Norton Co., Inc.

Horwitz, A.: Some pathways into psychiatric treatment—some differences between men and women, J. Health Soc. Behav. **18:**169-178, 1977.

Ineichen, B.: Neurotic wives in a modern residential suburb: a sociological profile, Soc. Sci. Med. **9:**481-487, 1975.

Jacobson, S., Deykin, E., and Prusoff, B.: Process and outcome of therapy with depressed women, Am. J. Orthopsychiatry **47:**140-148, 1977.

Jacobson, S., Fasman, J., and Dimascio, A.: Deprivation in the childhood of depressed women, J. Nerv. Ment. Disorders **160:**5-14, 1975.

Jakubowski, P. A.: Assertive behavior and clinical problems of women. In Rawlings, E., and Carter, D., editors: Psychotherapy for women, Springfield, Ill., 1977, Charles C Thomas, Publisher.

Jakubowski, P. A.: Self-assertive training procedures for women. In Rawlings, E., and Carter, D., editors: Psychotherapy for women, Springfield, Ill., 1977, Charles C Thomas, Publisher.

James, J. E.: Symptoms of alcoholism in women: a preliminary survey of AA members, J. Stud. Alcohol **36:**1564-1569, 1975.

James, J. E.: Sex differences in equalitarianism and anxiety in ninth grade students, Adolescence **18:**59-61, 1975.

Joesting, L., and Joesting, P.: Sex differences in egalitarianism and anxiety in ninth grade students, Adolescence **10**:59-61, 1975.

Johnson, S., and Garzon, S.: Women and alcoholism: past imperfect and future indefinite. Presented at the Midwinter Research Conference of the Association for Women in Psychology, St. Louis, Feb. 1977.

Johnson, F., and Johnson, C. R.: Role strain in high-commitment career women, J. Am. Acad. Psychoanal. **4**:13-36, 1976.

Jones, B. M., and Jones, M. K.: Alcohol effects in women during the menstrual cycle, Ann. N.Y. Acad. Sci. **273**:576-587, 1976a.

Jones, B. M., and Jones, M. K.: Women and alcohol: intoxication, metabolism, and the menstrual cycle. In Greenblatt, M., and Schuckit, M. A., editors: Alcoholism problems in women and children, New York, 1976b, Grune & Stratton, Inc.

Jones, B., Jones, M. K., and Paredes, A.: Oral contraceptives and ethanol metabolism, Alcohol Techn. Rep. **5**:28-32, 1976.

Kaplan, B. H., Cassel, J. C., and Gore, S.: Social support and health, Med. Care **15**(Suppl):47-58, 1977.

Keil, T. J.: Sex role variations in women's drinking: results from a household survey in Pennsylvania, J. Stud. Alcohol **35**:859-868, 1978.

Khantzian, E. J.: Drug-alcohol problems in women: a clinical perspective. Presented to Senate Subcommittee on Alcoholism and Narcotics, Washington, D.C., Sept. 1976.

Kjervik, D. K., and Palta, M.: Sex-role stereotyping in assessments of mental health made by psychiatric-mental health nurses, Nurs. Res. **27**:166-171, 1978.

Kleiman, G. L.: Combining drugs and psychotherapy in the treatment of depression in drugs in combination with other therapies, New York, 1975, Grune and Stratton, Inc.

Klein, D. F., and Davis, J. M.: Diagnosis and treatment of psychiatric disorders, Baltimore, 1969, The Williams & Wilkins Co.

Konstam, V., and Gilbert, H.: Fear of success, sex-role orientation and performance in differing experimental conditions. In Bardwick, J. M., editor: Readings on the psychology of women, New York, 1972, Harper & Row, Publishers, Inc.

Kramer, R.: Why some women turn to drink. Parents Mag. **68**:116-119, Nov. 1976.

Larson, R.: Thirty years of research in the subjective well-being of older Americans, J. Gerontol. **33**:109-125, 1978.

Levine, S.: Sexism and psychiatry, Am. J. Orthopsychiatry **44**:327-336, 1974.

Levy, L.: Self-help groups: types and psychological processes, J. Appl. Behav. Sci. **12**:310-322, 1976.

Levy, R.: Psychosomatic symptoms and women's protest: two types of reaction to structural strain in the family, J. Health Soc. Behav. **17**:121-133, 1976.

Lieberman, M., and Bond, D.: The problem of being a woman: a survey of 1700 females in consciousness-raising groups, J. Appl. Behav. Sci. **12**:363-379, 1976.

Lieberman, M., and Borman, L.: Self-help and social research, J. Appl. Behav. Sci. **12**:397-403, 1976.

Liem, R., and Liem, J.: Class and mental illness reconsidered: the role of economic stress and social support, J. Health Soc. Behav. **19**:139-156, 1978.

Lindbeck, U. L.: The woman alcoholic, a review of the literature, Int. J. Addict. **7**:567-580, 1972.

Luda, F., Glezen, P., and Clyde, W.: Respiratory disease in group day care, Pediatrics **49**:428-437, 1972.

Maccoby, E., and Jacklin, C.: The psychology of sex differences, Palo Alto, Calif., 1974, Stanford University Press.

Mamalis, S. A.: Maurice Levine essay award paper, 1973. The psychoanalytic concept of feminine passivity: a comparative study of psychoanalytic and feminist views, Compr. Psychiatry **17**:241-247, 1976.

Maracek, J.: Psychological disorders in women: indices of role strain. In Frieze, I. N., and others, editors: Women and sex roles: a social psychological perspective, New York, 1977a, W. W. Norton Co., pp. 255-276.

Maracek, J., and Kravetz, D.: Women and mental health: a review of feminist change efforts, Psychiatry **40**:323-328, 1977b.

Marieskind, H.: Women's health movement, Int. J. Health Serv. **5**:217-223, 1975.

Marktush, P. E., and others: Epidemiologic study of migraine symptoms in young women, Neurology (MINNEAP) **85**:430-435, 1975.

Marram, G.: The group approach in nursing practice, St. Louis, 1978, The C. V. Mosby Co.

Martin, J.: Fetal alcohol syndrome: recent findings, Alcohol Health Res. World **1**:8-12, 1977.

Mason, K. A., Czajka, J. L., and Arber, S.: Change in U.S. women's sex-role attitudes, 1964-1974, Am. Sociolog. Rev. **11**:573-596, 1976.

McCranie, E. W., Horowitz, A. J., and Martin, R. M.: Alleged sex-role stereotyping in the assessment of women's physical complaints: a study of general practitioners, Soc. Sci. Med. **12**:111-116, 1978.

McCune, S. D.: Assertiveness training, NLN Publication, no. 52-1647, 1976, pp. 17-23.

McDowell, C.: Leisure counseling: selected lifestyle processes, University of Oregon, Center of Leisure Studies, 1976.

Mechanic, D.: Sex, illness, illness behavior, and the use of health services, J. Hum. Stress **2**:29-40, 1976.

Messer, S., and Lebrer, P.: Short-term groups with female welfare clients in a job-training program, Profess. Psychol., Aug. 1976, pp. 352-358.

Metropolitan Life: Mortality from alcoholism, Stat. Bull. **58**:3-5, 1977.

Metropolitan Life: Recent trends in suicide, Stat. Bull. **57**:5-7, 1976.

Miles, H., and Hays, D.: Widowhood, Am. J. Nurs. **75**:280-282, 1975.

Miller, J. H.: Differential treatment of women and men in comprehensive community mental health centers, Dissert. Abstr. Int. **37**(1-Bi):470, 1976.

Miller, J. B.: Psychoanalysis and women, New York, 1973, Penguin Books.

Moeller, M.: Praxis in Psychotherapies **29**:181-193, 1975.

Money, J., and Ehrhardt, A.: Man and woman, boy and girl, Baltimore, 1972, The Johns Hopkins University Press.

Morgan, H. G., Burns-Cox, C. J., Pocock, H., and Pottle, S.: Deliberate self-harm: clinical and socio-economic characteristics of 368 patients, Brit. J. Psychiatry **127**:564-574, 1975.

Morgan, M. V., and Sherlock, S.: Sex-related differences among 100 patients with alcoholic liver disease, Brit. Med. J. **1**:939-941, 1977.

Moscato, B.: Sex-role stereotyping: a crucial issue in psychiatric theory and practice. In Kneisl, C., and Wilson, H. S., editors: Current perspectives in psychiatric nursing: issues and trends, St. Louis, 1978, The C. V. Mosby Co.

Mostow, E., and Newberry, P.: Work role and depression in women: a comparison of workers and housewives in treatment, Am. J. Orthopsychiatry **45**:538-548, 1975.

Moulton, R.: Some effects of the new feminism, Am. J. Psychiatry **134**:1-6, 1977.

Mulford, H. A.: Women and men problem drinkers; sex differences in patients served by Iowa's community alcoholism centers, J. Stud. Alcohol **38**:1624-1639, 1977.

Nathanson, C. A.: Illness and the feminine role: a theoretical review, Soc. Sci. Med. **9**:57-62, 1975.

National Institute on Alcohol Abuse and Alcoholism: Women in treatment for alcoholism: a profile, Program Analysis and Evaluation Branch, Rockville, Md., 1977.

Noble, E.: Alcohol and health. Third Special Report to the U.S. Congress on Alcohol and Health from the Secretary of Health, Education and Welfare, U.S. Department of Health, Education, and Welfare, 1978.

NOW Task Force: (Women on words and images): Dick and Jane as victims: sex role stereotyping in children's readers, Princeton, N.J., 1972.

Oakley, A.: The sociology of housework, New York, 1975, Pantheon Books, Inc.

Obitz, F. W., and Swanson, M. K.: Control orientation in women alcoholics, J. Stud. Alcohol **37:**694-697, 1976.

O'Connell, A. N.: The relationship between life style and identity synthesis and resynthesis in traditional, neotraditional, and nontraditional women, J. Perspect. **44:**675-688, 1976.

Paige, K. E.: The effects of oral contraceptives on affective fluctuations associated with the menstrual cycle, Psychosom. Med. **33:**515-537, 1971.

Pearlin, K., and Schooler, C.: The structure of coping, J. Health Soc. Behav. **19:**2-21, 1978.

Percell, L., Bermick, P., and Beigel, A.: The effects of assertive training on self-concept and anxiety, Arch. Gen. Psychiatry **31:**502-504, 1974.

Pinder, L., and Boyle, B.: Double jeopardy employee: the woman alcoholic in the workplace. Presented at the second Canadian Conference on Occupational Alcoholism and Abuse, Ottawa, Ontario, May, 1977.

Pines, M.: A child's mind is shaped before age 2, Life **71:**63-68, Dec. 7, 1971.

Powell, B., and Reznikoff, M.: Role conflict and symptoms of psychological distress in college-educated women, J. Consult. Clin. Psychol. **44:**473-479, 1976.

Prange, A. J., Jr.: Antidepressants. In Arieti, S., editor: American handbook of psychiatry, vol. 5, New York, 1975, Basic Books, Inc.

President's Commission on Mental Health: Mental health—nature and scope of the problems; and Community support systems. Task Panel Reports, vol. II, Washington, D.C., 1977, U.S. Government Printing Office.

President's Commission on Mental Health: Mental health of women. Task Panel Reports, vol. III, Washington, D.C., 1978, U.S. Government Printing Office.

President's Commission on Mental Health: Research; and Public attitudes and use of media for promotion of mental health. Task Panel Reports, vol. IV, Washington, D.C., 1978, U.S. Government Printing Office.

Rawlings, E., and Carter, D.: Psychotherapy for women, Springfield, Ill., 1977, Charles C Thomas, Publisher.

Renne, K. S.: Health and marital experience in an urban population, J. Marriage Family **33:**338, 1971.

Reynolds, I., Harnas, J., and Gallagher, H.: Drinking and drug taking patterns in 8,516 adults in Sydney, Med. J. Australia **2:**782-785, 1976.

Rice, J. K., and Rice, D. G.: Implications of the women's liberation movement for psychotherapy, Am. J. Psychiatry **130:**191-196, 1973.

Riessman, F.: How does self-help work, Soc. Policy **7:**41-45, 1976.

Rimm, C.: Assertive training used in treatment of chronic crying spells, Behav. Res. Ther. **5:**372-374, 1967.

Rivkin, M. O.: Contextual effects of families on female responses to illness. Unpublished Ph.D. dissertation, Johns Hopkins University, Baltimore, 1972.

Roeske, N. A., and Lake, K.: Role models for women medical students, J. Med. Educ. **52:**459-466, 1977.

Russell, M.: Intrauterine growth in infants born to women with alcohol-related psychiatric diagnosis. Presented at the Seventh Annual NCA-AMSA Medical-Scientific Conference, Washington, D.C., May, 1976.

Sandmaier, M.: Alcohol programs for women: issues strategies and resources, Washington, D.C., 1977a, U.S. Government Printing Office, #241-186/1132.

Sandmaier, M.: Women helping women, Alcohol Health Res. World **2:**17-23, 1977b.

Schuckit, M.: The alcoholic woman: a literature review, Psychiatry in Medicine **3:**37-43, 1972.

Schuckit, M., and Gunderson, E. K.: Alcoholism in Navy and Marine Corps women: a first look, Military Med. **140:**268-271, 1975.

Schuckit, M. A., and Morrissey, E.: Alcoholism in women: some clinical and social perspectives with an emphasis on possible subtypes. In Greenblatt, M., and Schuckit, M. A., editors: Alcoholism problems in women and children, New York, 1976, Grune & Stratton, Inc.

Sclare, A. B.: Alcohol problems in women. In Madden, M., and others, editors: Alcoholism and dependence, New York, 1977, Plenum Press.

Scott, E. M., and Manaugh, T. S.: Femininity of alcoholic women's preferences on Edwards personal preference schedule, Psychol. Reports **38:**847-852, 1976.

Seiden, A. M.: Overview: research on the psychology of women. I. Gender differences and sexual and reproductive life, Am. J. Psychiatry **133:**995-1007, 1976a.

Seiden, A.: Overview: research on the psychology of women. II. Women in families, work, and psychotherapy, Am. J. Psychiatry **133:**1111-1123, 1976b.

Serbin, L. A., and O'Leary, L. D.: How nursery schools teach girls to shut up, Psychol. Today **9:**56-58, 1975.

Shepherd, M., and others: Minor mental illness in London: a general practice survey, Br. Med. J. **2:**1359, 1964.

Show, H. L.: The national drug abuse conference, Br. Med. J. **2:**934-943, 1977.

Silverman, J.: The women's liberation movement: its impact on marriage, Hosp. Community Psychiatry **26:**39-40, 1975.

Silverman, P.: The widow as a care-giver in a program of preventive intervention with other widows, Ment. Hygiene, pp. 540-547, 1970.

Snyder, B. J.: A note on the importance of cultural factors in suicide studies, Suicide Life Threat Behav. **7:**230-235, 1977.

Stafford, R., and Petway, J. M.: Stigmatization of men and women problem drinkers and their spouses. Differential perception and leveling of sex differences, J. Stud. Alcohol. **38:**2109-2121, 1977.

Stevens, S.: The mad housewife syndrome. In Kneisl, C., and Wilson, H. S., editors: Current perspectives in psychiatric nursing: issues and trends, St. Louis, 1978, The C. V. Mosby Co.

Stone, W. V., and Gilbert, R.: Peer confrontation groups: what, why, whether, Am. J. Psychiatry **74:**583-588, 1972.

Strangert, K.: Respiratory illness in preschool children with different forms of day care, Pediatrics **57:**191-195, 1976.

Stunkard, A. J.: The success of TOPS, a self-help group, Postgrad. Med. **18:**143-147, 1972.

Suffet, F., and Brotman, R.: Female drug use: some observations, Int. J. Addict. **11:**19-33, 1976.

Suter, B., and Domino, G.: Masculinity-femininity in creative college women, J. Pers. Assess. **39:**414-420, 1975.

Symond, A.: Phobias after marriage. In Smeller, J., editor: Psychoanalysis and women, New York, 1974a, Penguin Books.

Symonds, A.: The liberated woman: healthy and neurotic, Am. J. Psychoanal. **34:**177-185, 1974b.

Symonds, A.: Neurotic dependence in successful women, J. Am. Acad. Psychoanal. **4:**95-103, 1976.

Symonds, A.: The psychodynamics of expansiveness in the success-oriented woman, Am. J. Psychoanal. **38:**195-205, 1978.

Tavris, C., and Offin, C.: Longest war, New York, 1977, Harcourt Brace Jovanovich, Inc.

Teitelbaum, M., and Mantel, N.: Socioeconomic factors and the sex ratio at birth, J. Res. Sci. **3:**23-41, 1971.

Toffler, A.: Future shock, New York, 1971, Bantam Books.

Tracy, G., and Gussow, Z.: Self-help health groups: a grass roots response to a need for services, J. Appl. Behav. Sci. **12**:381-396, 1976.

Tregeman, S., and Kassinone, H.: Effects of assertive training and cognitive components of rational therapy on assertive behaviors and interpersonal anxiety, Psychol. Rep. **49**:535-542, 1977.

Udry, J. R., and Morris, N. H.: Distribution of coitus to the menstrual cycle, Nature **220**:593-595, 1968.

Verbrugge, L. M.: Females and illness: recent trends in sex differences in the United States, J. Health Soc. Behav. **17**:387-403, 1976.

Warren, R.: Stress, preliminary support systems and the blue collar woman. In McGurgan, D., editor: New research in women and sex roles, Ann Arbor, 1976, University of Michigan Center for Continuing Education of Women.

Wechsler, H.: Epidemiology and male/female drinking over the last half century. Presented at the NIAAA Workshop on Alcoholism and Alcohol Abuse Among Women, Jekyll Island, Ga., Apr. 1978.

Weissman, M. M.: Sex differences and the epidemiology of depression, Arch. Gen. Psychiatry **34**:98-111, 1977.

Weissman, M. M., and others: Assessing depressive symptoms in five psychiatric populations: a validation study. Unpublished. Jan. 1977b.

Weissman, M. M., Kasl, S. V., and Klerman, G. L.: Follow-up of depressed women after maintenance treatments, Am. J. Psychiatry **133**:757-760, 1976.

Weissman, M. M., Prusoff, B., and Pincus, C.: Symptom patterns in depressed patients and depressed normals, J. Nerv. Ment. Dis. **160**:15-23, 1975.

Weissman, M. M., and Kerman, G. L.: Psychotherapy with depressed women: an empirical study of content themes and reflection, Br. J. Psychiatry **123**:55-61, 1973.

Weissman, M. M., and others: The depressed woman as mother, Soc. Psychiatry **7**:98-108, 1972.

Weissman, S. H.: The incidence of primary psychiatric illness in women attending general medicine clinic, Dis. Nerv. Syst. **38**:150-153, 1977.

Whitehead, P. C., and Ferrence, R. G.: Women and children last: implications and trends in consumption for women and young people. In Greenblatt, M., and Schuckit, M. A., editors: Alcoholism problems in women and children, New York, 1976, Grune and Stratton, Inc.

Whittenburg, D., and Stoy, D.: Effects of TV stereotyping: a depression and hysteria in women. Unpublished paper, University of North Carolina–Chapel Hill School of Nursing, Chapel Hill, N.C., 1978.

Wiksnack, S. C.: Impact of sex roles and women's alcohol use and abuse. In Greenblatt, M., and Schuckit, M. A., editors: Alcoholism problems in women and children, New York, 1976, Grune & Stratton.

Wilson, G. T., and Lawson, D. M.: Effects of alcohol on sexual arousal in women, J. Abnorm. Psychol. **85**:489-497, 1976.

Wilson, H., Kneisl, C.: Psychiatric nursing, Palo Alto, 1979, Addison-Wesley, Publishing Co., Inc.

Wolpe, J.: Psychotherapy by reciprocal inhibition, Stanford, 1958, Stanford University Press.

Women and MH Project: Women to women services, Soc. Policy **7**: 21-27, 1976.

Women and work, Employment and Training Administration, U.S. Department of Labor, Monograph no. 46, 1977.

Yalom, I. D.: Theory and practice of group psychotherapy, New York, 1970, Basic Books.

Index

t indicates table, *n* indicates footnote.